Title of Video	Page # in Textbook

Rebhun's

DISEASES OF
DAIRY CATTLE

Second Edition

Rebhun's
DISEASES OF
DAIRY CATTLE

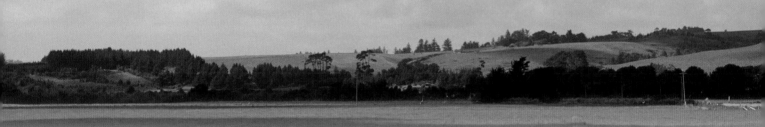

Thomas J. Divers, DVM, Dipl ACVIM, ACVECC

Professor, Large Animal Medicine
Department of Clinical Sciences
College of Veterinary Medicine
Cornell University
Ithaca, New York

Simon F. Peek, BVSc, MRCVS, PhD, Dipl ACVIM

Clinical Professor
Large Animal Internal Medicine, Theriogenology, and Infectious Diseases
School of Veterinary Medicine
University of Wisconsin
Madison, Wisconsin

With 625 illustrations

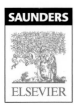

SAUNDERS

ELSEVIER

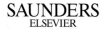

SAUNDERS
ELSEVIER

11830 Westline Industrial Drive
St. Louis, Missouri 63146

REBHUN'S DISEASES OF DAIRY CATTLE   ISBN-13: 978-1-4160-3137-6
Copyright © 2008, Elsevier Inc.

Notice

Knowledge and best practice in this field are constantly changing. As new research and experience broaden our knowledge, changes in practice, treatment and drug therapy may become necessary or appropriate. Readers are advised to check the most current information provided (i) on procedures featured or (ii) by the manufacturer of each product to be administered, to verify the recommended dose or formula, the method and duration of administration, and contraindications. It is the responsibility of the practitioner, relying on their own experience and knowledge of the patient, to make diagnoses, to determine dosages and the best treatment for each individual patient, and to take all appropriate safety precautions. To the fullest extent of the law, neither the Publisher nor the Editors/Authors assume any liability for any injury and/or damage to persons or property arising out of or related to any use of the material contained in this book.

The Publisher

Previous edition copyrighted 1995.

Library of Congress Control Number: 2007920423

Publishing Director: Linda Duncan
Publisher: Penny Rudolph
Managing Editor: Teri Merchant
Publishing Services Manager: Pat Joiner-Myers
Project Manager: David Stein
Design Direction: Maggie Reid
Cover Art: Agri-Graphics, Ltd.

About the cover: Lantland AJ Kat, pictured on the cover, was a 94 4E cow bred and owned by Lantland Farms of Horseheads, NY and a 274,891 pounds lifetime producer. She was successfully treated at Cornell in July 1998 for abdominal pain and cecal dilation. She was one of the last cows treated by Dr. Rebhun.

Printed in China.
Last digit is the print number: 9   8   7   6   5   4   3   2

Contributors

Alexander de Lahunta, DVM, PhD, Dipl ACVIM, ACVP
James Law Professor of Anatomy
Department of Biomedical Sciences
College of Veterinary Medicine
Cornell, University
Ithaca, New York

Thomas J. Divers, DVM, Dipl ACVIM, ACVECC
Professor, Large Animal Medicine
Department of Clinical Sciences
College of Veterinary Medicine
Cornell University
Ithaca, New York

Norm Ducharme, DMV, MSc, Dipl ACVS
Professor of Large Animal Surgery
College of Veterinary Medicine
Cornell University
Ithaca, New York

Francis H. Fox, DVM, Dipl ACVIM
Professor Emeritus
College of Veterinary Medicine
Cornell University
Ithaca, New York

Susan Fubini, DVM, Dipl ACVS
Professor of Large Animal Surgery
Department of Clinical Sciences
College of Veterinary Medicine
Cornell University
Ithaca, New York

Franklyn Garry, DVM, MS, Dipl ACVIM
Professor, Department of Clinical Sciences
Colorado State University
Fort Collins, Colorado

Lisle W. George, DVM, PhD, Dipl ACVIM
Professor, Dept of Medicine and Epidemiology
School of Veterinary Medicine
University of California
Davis, California

Robert O. Gilbert, BVSc, MMed Vet, MRCVS, Dipl ACT
Professor of Theriogenology
Senior Associate Dean
College of Veterinary Medicine
Cornell University
Ithaca, New York

Charles Guard, DVM, PhD
Associate Professor
Population Medicine and Diagnostic Science
College of Veterinary Medicine
Cornell University
Ithaca, New York

Robert Hillman, DVM, MS, Dipl ACT
College of Veterinary Medicine
Cornell University
Ithaca, New York

Sheila M. McGuirk, DVM, PhD, Dipl ACVIM
Professor, Department of Medical Sciences
School of Veterinary Medicine
University of Wisconsin
Madison, Wisconsin

Simon F. Peek, BVSc, MRCVS, PhD, Dipl ACVIM
Clinical Professor
Large Animal Internal Medicine, Theriogenology, and
    Infectious Diseases
School of Veterinary Medicine
University of Wisconsin
Madison, Wisconsin

Ronald Riis, DVM, MS, Dipl ACVO
Associate Professor of Ophthalmology
Department of Clinical Sciences
College of Veterinary Medicine
Cornell University
Ithaca, New York

Danny W. Scott, DVM, Dipl ACVD
Professor of Medicine and Dermatology
Department of Clinical Sciences
College of Veterinary Medicine
Cornell University
Ithaca, New York

Bud C. Tennant, DVM, Dipl ACVIM
James Law Professor of Comparative Medicine
Department of Clinical Sciences
College of Veterinary Medicine
Cornell University
Ithaca, New York

David C. Van Metre, DVM, Dipl ACVIM
Assistant Professor
Department of Clinical Sciences
College of Veterinary Medicine and Biomedical Sciences
Fort Collins, Colorado

Frank L. Welcome, DVM
College of Veterinary Medicine
Cornell University
Ithaca, New York

Robert H. Whitlock, DVM, PhD, Dipl ACVIM
Associate Professor of Medicine
Department of Clinical Studies
New Bolton Center
School of Veterinary Medicine
University of Pennsylvania
Kennett Square, Pennsylvania

Amy E. Yeager, DVM, Dipl ACVR
Staff Veterinarian
Imaging
Cornell University Hospital for Animals
Ithaca, New York

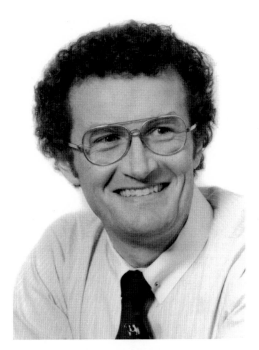

William C. Rebhun
July 24, 1947–March 24, 1999
Professor of Medicine
Cornell University

It gives me great pleasure to write the dedication of this book in honor of Dr. William C. Rebhun. Dr. Rebhun (Bill) was a student of mine from 1967 to 1971 and, after he spent 2 years in a large animal practice, I asked him to return to the College of Veterinary Medicine at Cornell University and teach in the large animal clinics. His return to Cornell was one of the highlights of my 60-year (and counting) career. Dr. Rebhun was the ultimate diagnostician, likely the best I have ever trained. His understanding of the diseases of dairy cattle was nearly impeccable, and his ability to define every detail during the physical examination was phenomenal. Following completion of the physical exam, he could quickly assimilate all the findings such that a practical, proper, and precise treatment plan could be presented to the owner. He was a veterinarian who mastered the three C's: completeness, confidence, and communication; these distinguish the most outstanding veterinarians.

Bill was a competitive individual who worked extremely hard and played hard. He was not a spectator but an active participant in numerous sports, particularly softball. A rugged individualist, he was also a true outdoorsman and an avid hunter. His presence in the clinical arena was commanding, comforting, candid, often passionate, and always appreciated. He had a remarkable gift for accurately recalling and relaying experiences. He had a prodigious and exact memory, and candid, uncompromising honesty. These qualities were evident in his relationships, both professional and personal. He was entertaining in a wide spectrum of situations. These traits were also evident in the classroom. Bill was quick to use past situations and cases, both good and bad, as teaching material. He was quick to use mistakes he had made or witnessed to emphasize a point. Bill respected the opinion of others and relished the academic exchanges with colleagues. He was opinionated and passionate when expressing his own ideas. He admired and respected the talented individuals around him and held his head high and his mind open, always striving to learn—even in his final months.

I am certain that Bill would be pleased with the outstanding contributors, all of whom worked with Bill during their careers and made this second edition possible.

Although the trend in dairy practice for at least the past two decades has been toward group (herd health) medicine, we should all remember that the foundation for all bovine practitioners should be "recognition of the sick animal, rapid identification of the disease process, and providing appropriate therapy." Building from Dr. Rebhun's first edition of the text, this group of outstanding collaborators/authors brings to the readers the state-of-the-art knowledge of diagnosis and treatment of the sick dairy animal. This is the text that everyone who has an interest in diagnosing and treating sick dairy animals should refer to. This book will further strengthen Dr. Rebhun's legacy.

Francis H. Fox, DVM, Dipl ACVIM
Cornell University
Class of '45
Professor Emeritus

Preface

Our goal in writing this book was twofold: first, to provide the most up-to-date and comprehensive book available on diseases of the individual dairy cow and, second, to honor Dr. William Rebhun. It was a privilege to have both worked with and learned from Bill, and we shall be forever indebted to him for knowledge gained. Dr. Francis Fox eruditely describes Bill in his dedication, and those who knew Bill, either student, colleague, or client, will warm to Dr. Fox's description of Bill's humor, pragmatism, and, above all, professionalism. It is in the spirit of his commitment to the art, as well as to the science, of bovine medicine that this book is dedicated.

When planning this book, we contacted international experts, all of whom had worked closely with Dr. Rebhun and are currently involved in treating dairy cows. As testimony to Dr. Rebhun's legacy, every potential author contacted readily agreed to help by contributing to this second edition of *Rebhun's Diseases of Dairy Cattle*. To all these contributors, we are grateful and say thank you. Appropriately for a book dedicated to Dr. Rebhun's memory, this group of contributors hails from North America, each one a recognized expert in his or her field; as a consequence, we sincerely hope that much of the information contained within the text will also be useful and relevant to the worldwide audience.

Many chapters have major changes from the first writing of the book due to newer diagnostics and treatments; yet we have purposefully retained many of Dr. Rebhun's thoughts and words, which remain state of the art and practical. As the trend of bovine practice has moved toward herd health and production medicine, we have tried to include some of this in each chapter; however, similar to Dr. Rebhun's first edition, the second edition primarily focuses on diseases of the individual dairy cow. We hope you find this book useful for diagnosing and treating dairy cattle diseases and that it will be useful as a reference in veterinary curricula.

This edition also features a DVD that includes 58 real-time videos of neurologic, ultrasound, and endoscopic case studies—cutting-edge technology and imaging techniques that make the text even more relevant to today's practitioners.

We also wish to thank Dr. Bridget Barry, Dr. Rebhun's wife, for her considerable time spent retrieving Bill's case photographs and her support of this project from its very inception. We would also like to thank Anne Littlejohn at Cornell for her help with the manuscript preparation and Teri Merchant and David Stein at Elsevier for seeing this project through start-to-finish. Thank you Bridgett, Anne, Teri, and David.

Finally, we would both like to thank our families, Nita, Shannon, Bob and Laurie, Emma, Michael, and Alexander, who are the real center of our lives. For T.J. Divers, he would like to thank his father for allowing him to spend 25 years with the family dairy and Drs. George Lawrence, Al Rice, Dilmous Blackmon, John McCormick, Robert Whitlock, and Lisle George for teaching him both the art and science of dairy medicine. For S.F. Peek, he would like to express his love and gratitude for the support of his parents, Bill and Lorna, and his heartfelt thanks for the good fortune and privilege to have had the opportunity to learn so much over the years from Drs. Tom Divers, Bill Rebhun, and Bud Tennant.

Thomas J. Divers
Simon F. Peek

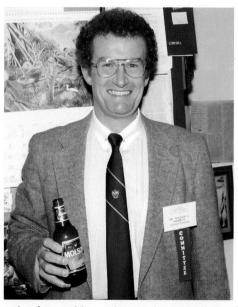

Photograph of Dr. Rebhun taken at the Cornell Conference, March 1996—an image his friends and colleagues will always remember.

Contents

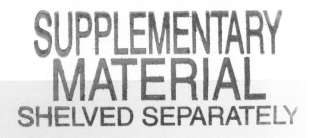
SUPPLEMENTARY MATERIAL SHELVED SEPARATELY

PART I

Examination
and Assessment

CHAPTER 1

The Clinical Examination

Thomas J. Divers and Simon F. Peek

The clinical examination consists of three parts: (1) obtaining a meaningful history, (2) performing a thorough physical examination including observations of the environment, and (3) selecting appropriate ancillary tests when necessary.

The goal of the clinical examination is to determine the organ systems involved, differential diagnoses, and, ideally, a diagnosis. In most cases, an accurate diagnosis will be reached by an experienced clinician. In difficult cases, the clinician, even when experienced, may formulate only a differential diagnosis that requires further information before an accurate diagnosis can be made.

The clinical examination is an art, not a science. The basic structure of the clinical examination can be taught, but the actual performance and interpretation involved require practice and experience. Clinicians who are lazy, who are poor observers, or who fail to interact well with clients will never develop good clinical skills.

The clinical examination is a search for clues in an attempt to solve the mystery of a patient's illness. These clues are found usually in the form of "signs" that are demonstrated to the examiner through inspection, palpation, percussion, and auscultation. Signs are the veterinary counterpart to the symptoms possessed by human patients. *Stedman's Medical Dictionary* defines a *symptom* as "any morbid phenomenon or departure from the normal in function, appearance, or sensation experienced by the patient and indicative of a disease." A sign is defined in the same source as "any abnormality indicative of disease, discoverable by the physician during the examination of the patient." Although somewhat pedantic, the veterinary interpretation of these terms has evolved to connote that animals cannot have symptoms, only signs. We cannot help but believe that sick cattle "experience" departures from normal and indicate that to experienced clinical examiners. However, we shall evade this pedantry and use the idiomatic "sign" throughout this text.

Signs are not the only clues that contribute to a diagnosis. Knowledge of the normal behavior of cattle, an accurate assessment of the patient's environment, the possible relationship of that environment to the patient's problems, and ancillary tests or data all may figure into the final diagnosis. A "tentative" diagnosis may be reached after the history is taken and physical examination is performed, but ancillary data are required to translate the "tentative" into the "final" diagnosis.

The major stumbling block for neophytic clinicians remains the *integration* of information and signs into a diagnosis or differential diagnosis. The inexperienced clinician often focuses so hard on a single sign or a piece of historical data that the clinician "loses the forest for the trees." These same "trainees" in medicine are frustrated when a cow has two or more concurrent diseases. In such situations, the signs fail to add up to a textbook description of either disease, and the examiner becomes frustrated. A cow with severe metritis and a left abomasal displacement (LDA), for example, may have fever and complete anorexia. Such signs are not typical for LDA, so the inexperienced clinician may want to rule out LDA. The clinician must recognize that concurrent disease may additively or exponentially affect the clinical signs present. The clinical signs may cancel each other out, as may be seen in a recumbent hypocalcemic (subnormal temperature) cow affected with coliform mastitis (fever) that has a normal body temperature at the time of clinical examination.

Much is made of "problems" possessed by sick animals and people. These problems constitute the basis of the Problem-Oriented Medical Record. We do not disagree with this thought process, but in fact it adds nothing to the skill or integration ability of a good diagnostician. It is longhand logic that allows other clinicians or students to follow the thought processes of the clinician writing the problem-oriented record. Therefore it may be valuable in communications among clinicians concerning a patient. The major "problem" with the problem-oriented approach is that it does not make a bad diagnostician a good one. The clinician who cannot integrate data or recognize signs cannot recognize problems and will not formulate accurate plans. Therefore the problem-oriented approach is not a panacea and in fact is merely an offshoot of the thought processes that a skilled diagnostician practices on a regular basis.

HISTORY

Obtaining an accurate and meaningful history or *anamnesis* is an essential aid to diagnosis. History may be accurate but not meaningful or may be misleading in some instances. The clinician must work to ask questions that do not verbally bias the owner's or caretaker's answers. When obtaining the history, the clinician also has the opportunity to display knowledge or ignorance regarding the specific patient's breed, age, use, and conformation. When the clinician appears knowledgeable concerning the patient, the owner is favorably impressed and often will volunteer more historical information. When the clinician appears ignorant of the patient and dairy husbandry in general, the owner often withdraws, answers questions tersely, and loses faith in the clinician's ability to diagnose the cause of the cow's illness. Therefore part of the art of history taking is to communicate as well as possible with each owner. Bear in mind that owners are proud of their cattle, care for them, and have large economic investments in them. The clinician enhances credibility with dairy farmers by displaying knowledge and concern regarding the sick cow, the herd, and the dairy economy.

Where should a history begin? Usually the owner has called the veterinarian to attend to a specific problem, and this problem may be easily definable or it may be vague. For example, a chief complaint of mastitis is specific as to location of the problem but not specific as to the cause, whereas a complaint of a cow "off feed" is very vague and requires a much more detailed history. For dairy cattle, several key questions usually need to be answered by an accurate history. In some instances, however, some of these questions may be omitted when the clinician can answer the question by observation. The following are examples of typical questions that should be asked while obtaining a history.

1. When did the cow freshen? Or, where in her lactation is she?
2. When did she first appear ill, and what has transpired since that time? Did you take her temperature?
3. What have you treated her with?
4. Has she had other illnesses this lactation or in past lactations?
5. What does she eat now?
6. How much milk was she producing before she became ill, and what is she producing now?
7. What has her manure been like?
8. What other unusual things have you noticed?
9. Have any other cows (calves) had similar problems? If so, what has been the end result?

Other information may be necessary. In most instances, the experienced clinician already will know breed, sex, approximate age, use, and other husbandry information. However, in some instances, specific age information may be necessary. The clinician can appear very observant by asking question three regarding treatments by the owner when it is obvious that the cow has had injections. Question eight is open-ended and may yield valuable information from an observant owner or totally useless information from an unobservant owner. The clinician should be as complete as necessary in obtaining information but should avoid asking meaningless questions because they may annoy or confuse the owner. Frequently when students are first gaining experience, they ask impertinent questions of owners; imagine the concerned owner, whose cow has an obvious dystocia, being asked what he feeds the cow. In such instances, the inexperienced clinician or student is trying to be thorough but has upset the owner, who usually will reply, "What difference does that make? She's trying to have a calf!"

Another important aspect of history is to determine the duration of the disease. The general terms used to distinguish duration include peracute, acute, subacute, and chronic, although various experts disagree on the exact length of illness to define each category. Rosenberger suggests the following:

Peracute = 0 to 2 days
Acute = 3 to 14 days
Subacute = 14 to 28 days
Chronic ≥ 28 days

These durations are somewhat longer than those commonly used in the United States, and in general we would suggest:

Peracute = 0 to 24 hours
Acute = 24 to 96 hours
Subacute = 4 to 14 days
Chronic ≥ 14 days

The interpersonal skills necessary for effective history taking and "bedside manner" in a veterinarian are similar to those used by physicians. The veterinary clinician, however, has to establish a doctor-client relationship, whereas the physician must foster a more direct doctor-patient relationship. A good relationship, together with the skills and interactions that create a good one, is the secret to acceptance by the human client just as for a human patient.

Experienced clinicians adjust to the owner's personality. Highly knowledgeable and educated clients require a much different use of language and grammar than do poorly educated clients who may be confused by or misunderstand scientific terms and excessive vocabulary.

The history also should clarify any questions regarding the signalment that the clinician cannot ascertain by inspection alone. Because we are concerned with the bovine species only, the use (dairy), sex, color, breed, size, and often age of the animal are apparent by inspection. It may be important to determine whether valuable cattle would be retained only for breeding use if production should decrease drastically. The various components of the signalment are important to recognize because certain diseases occur more commonly in some breeds, colors, ages, and sex than in others.

PHYSICAL EXAMINATION

The physical examination begins as soon as the bovine patient comes into the clinician's view.

General Examination

A general examination consisting of inspection and observation is performed. The experienced clinician often makes this general examination quickly and sometimes while simultaneously obtaining verbal history from the owner. The general examination may be as short as 30 seconds or as long as 5 minutes, should further observation be necessary. As part of the general examination, the clinician needs to establish the habitus—the attitude, condition, conformation, and temperament—of the sick animal.

Attitude

The attitude or posture may suggest a specific diagnosis or a specific system disorder. The clinician must have basic knowledge of the normal attitude of dairy cattle, calves, and bulls before interpreting abnormal attitudes. The arched stance and reluctance of the animal to move as observed in peritonitis may indicate hardware disease, perforating abomasal ulcers, or merely a musculoskeletal injury to the back. A cow observed to be constantly leaning into her stanchion may have either nervous ketosis or listeriosis. A cow standing with her head extended, eyes partially closed, and exhibiting marked depression could have encephalitis or frontal sinusitis. A bull lying down with a stargazing attitude may have a pituitary abscess. A periparturient recumbent cow with an "S" curve in her neck is probably hypocalcemic. All of the attitudes in the above examples are abnormal and indicative of disease. Many attitudes are not specific, however. A cow affected with hypocalcemia, for example, will often open her mouth and stick out her tongue when stimulated or approached, but some nervous cattle assume this attitude even when healthy. An arched stance with tenesmus may be observed in simple vaginitis, coccidiosis, or rectal irritation but may be observed occasionally with liver disease, bovine virus diarrhea, and rabies.

Cattle stand typically by elevating their rear quarters while resting on their carpal areas, then rising to their forelegs. It is unusual for cattle to get up on their front legs first as do horses, but some cattle, especially Brown Swiss cows, cows with front limb lameness, or late pregnant cattle, do this normally. Therefore once again, it is important to be familiar with normal variations. It is impossible to enumerate all the possible abnormal attitudes assumed by cattle, but Table 1-1 is a partial list.

Condition

The condition of the animal is another component of the habitus that is assessed during the general examination. Condition is judged both subjectively and experientially in most instances. The clinician may assess the condition of a calf or an adult cow in comparison with the animal's herdmates, as well as with the bovine population in general. Excessively fat cattle are predisposed to metabolic diseases during the periparturient period and, when suffering musculoskeletal injuries, may become recumbent more easily than leaner cattle.

Cattle may be thin yet perfectly healthy. When a cow loses weight and is thin because of illness, she generally appears much different than her herdmates. Healthy, thin cattle have normal hair coats and hydration status, appear bright, and possess normal appetites. Emaciated cattle that have lost weight because of chronic illness have coarse, dry hair coats, leathery dehydrated skin, and appear dull. The clinician must remember that severe acute disease may cause weight loss of 50 pounds or more per day. The condition of the animal correlates largely with the duration of the illness. Extreme emaciation is associated with chronic problems such as parasitism, chronic abscessation, chronic musculoskeletal pain, Johne's disease, advanced neoplasia, and malnutrition.

The body score of dairy cattle is a system designed to add some objectivity to the subjective determination of condition. Body score is used in herd management to assess the nutritional plane of the cattle and to correlate this to milk production, relative energy intake, and stage of lactation. Body score is arrived at subjectively by observation and palpation of the cow's loin, transverse processes of the lumbar vertebrae, and tail head area from the rear of the animal. Scores are recorded in half point gradations from 0 to 5 with 0 being very poor and 5 being grossly fat. Ideal scores have been suggested as 3.5 for calving cows, 2.0 to 2.5 for first service, and 3.0 for drying off (see Chapter 14).

Conformation

The conformation of the animal is the third component of the habitus to be assessed during the general examination. Familiarity with normal conformation is an obvious asset when observing conformational defects that may predispose to or indicate specific diseases. For example, udder conformation in the dairy cow is extremely important, and cattle with suspensory ligament laxity are prone to teat injuries and mastitis. Calves with kyphosis may have vertebral abnormalities such as hemivertebrae. Splayed toes may predispose to interdigital fibromas, and weak pasterns often lead to chronic foot problems. A crushed tail head allows chronic fecal contamination of the perineum and vulva, with the

TABLE 1-1   Some Examples of Abnormal Attitudes Assumed by Cattle

Arched back, anorexia, abducted elbows ("Painful stance")	Peritonitis, pleuritis
Arched back, anorexia, limbs placed further under body than normal, reluctance to stand	Polyarthritis
Arched back, normal appetite, legs placed further ahead (front) and behind (back) body than normal	Musculoskeletal back injury
Bloat, elevated tail head, weather vane head and neck, legs placed further ahead and behind body than normal, anxious expression, ears erect, nictitans protruding	Tetanus
Recumbent with forelegs extended	Musculoskeletal injuring to forelegs—usually carpus
Lateral recumbency but alert and responsive	Occasionally normal for brief time
	Usually indicative of musculoskeletal pain causing reluctance to flex one or more limbs
	Ventral abdominal pain caused by udder swelling, udder hematoma, ventral abdominal hernia, or cellulitis
Recumbency with "S" curve neck, depressed, or comatose	Hypocalcemia
Lateral recumbency, opisthotonos, depression	
Calves	Polioencephalomalacia or other central nervous system (CNS) diseases
Cows	Occasional hypomagnesemia or CNS disease or other CNS diseases
Recumbency, hyperexcitability	Hypomagnesemia, occasional hypocalcemia
Grinding teeth, blindness with intact pupillary responses, depression	Lead poisoning, polioencephalomalacia
Grinding teeth, pushing nose against objects	Chronic abdominal pain, sinusitis, musculoskeletal pain
Colic	Indigestion with small intestinal gas and fluid accumulation
	Small intestinal obstruction
	Pyelonephritis or other urinary tract abnormality
	Cecal distention or volvulus
"Praying position" with rear raised but resting on carpi	Laminitis
Tenesmus	Vaginitis, rectal irritation, coccidiosis, rabies, hepatic failure, BVD
Dog-sitting position	May be normal before raising rear quarters in some Brown Swiss and occasionally in other late pregnant cattle, some lamenesses
	If cow cannot raise rear quarters but can raise front end, it may indicate a thoracolumbar spinal cord lesion
Hind feet under body, forefeet in front of body, reluctance to stand or move	Acute laminitis or severe forelimb lameness
Hind feet standing on edge of platform with heels non–weight-bearing	Sore heels, overgrowth of claws, sole ulcers
Hind feet in gutter with rear legs extended behind body	Spastic syndrome, too short a platform for cow, heel pain
Hind feet in gutter with rear legs extended behind body and lordosis	Chronic renal pain, chronic pyelonephritis, other causes of colic
Forelimbs crossed, reluctance to move	Bilateral lameness of medial claws
Chewing on objects, biting water cup, licking pipes, licking and chewing skin, aggressive behavior, collapse	Nervous ketosis or organic CNS disease

potential for reproductive failure or ascending urinary tract infection. Chronic cystic ovaries may change the conformation appearance of many cows so that they display thickened necks, prominent tail head, relaxed sacrosciatic ligaments, and flaccid perineum.

Temperament

Temperament is the fourth component of habitus and should be evaluated from a distance in addition to when the animal is approached during general examination. From practical and medicolegal standpoints, it is imperative that the clinician anticipates unpredictable or aggressive patient behavior whenever possible, lest caretakers, the clinician, or the animal itself be injured. Dairy bulls should *never* be trusted, even when they appear docile. Dairy cattle with newborn calves should be approached cautiously because many people have been injured or killed by apparently quiet cows that suddenly became aggressive to protect a calf. Some dairy cattle are naturally wild and vicious. They should be approached with extreme care or restrained in a chute if possible. Fortunately, most dairy cattle are rather docile and, unless startled or approached without warning, may be examined thoroughly without excessive restraint.

As a general rule, free-stall cattle are wilder than cattle housed in conventional barns, but there are exceptions. The manners and nature of the owner (or herdsperson) are directly reflected in the contentment or lack thereof observed in the herd. Some herds consist of truly quiet and contented cows, whereas in other herds all cattle will act apprehensive, jumpy, and fear all human contact. These latter herds, without exception, are handled roughly and loudly and frequently are mistreated. The veterinarian will quickly learn to adjust to the variable husbandry of herds within the practice. The increase in size of herds coupled with the impersonal nature of free-stall housing has decreased the family farm husbandry that had allowed more human/cow contact.

> NOTICE TO THE HELP
> THE RULE to be observed in this stable at all times, toward the cattle, young and old, is that of patience and kindness. A man's usefulness in a herd ceases at once when he loses his temper and bestows rough usage. Men must be patient. Cattle are not reasoning beings. Remember that this is the Home of Mothers. Treat each cow as a Mother should be treated. The giving of milk is a function of Motherhood; rough treatment lessens the flow. That injures me as well as the cow. Always keep these ideas in mind in dealing with my cattle.
> W. D. Hoard, Founder of Hoard's Dairyman (Circa 1885)

Occasionally cows that are transported or moved from familiar to unfamiliar surroundings will go wild and become extremely apprehensive or aggressive. These cattle may act as if affected by nervous ketosis but frequently are not.

The clinician should question the owner as to perceived changes in the temperament of the patient. Docile animals that become aggressive warrant consideration of nervous ketosis, rabies, and other neurologic diseases. Vicious cows that become docile again should be thought of as either very ill or perhaps affected with organic or metabolic CNS disease.

People unfamiliar with dairy cattle anticipate kicking as the major risk in handling cattle. It is true that cattle can "cow kick" with a forward-lateral-backward kick, but some cows also kick straight back with amazing accuracy. Not discounting the dangers of being kicked, clinicians should be aware that a cow's head may be her most dangerous weapon. Anyone who has been maliciously butted or repeatedly smashed by a cow or a bull's head understands the inherent dangers.

Entire herds of cattle or large groups of cattle within a herd that suddenly become agitated, apprehensive, vocal, or refuse to let milk down signal to the clinician the possibility of stray electrical voltage. Occasional spontaneous demonstrations of anxiety or agitation in cattle at pasture may also be associated with ectoparasitism.

Hands-on Examination

Once the general examination and history are complete, the hands-on part of the physical examination should begin and proceed uninterrupted. It is important that the clinician is allowed to initiate and complete the hands-on examination in the absence of interference by others and during a period when other environmental interference (e.g., feeding, movement of cattle in the immediate vicinity) is kept to a minimum. A "group" approach to physical examination or one that is performed within a distracting environment only serves to minimize the reliability of physical diagnostics and will challenge even the best diagnostician.

Because dairy cattle are less apprehensive when approached from the rear, the physical examination starts at the rear of the animal. Adult dairy cattle are accustomed to people working around the udder, and their reproductive examinations or inseminations are frequent enough such that their overall anxiety is less when the examination starts at the hindquarters. Approaching the head or forequarters causes the cow to become more excitable, and this alters baseline parameters such as heart rate and respiratory rate.

The examination begins with insertion of a rectal thermometer—preferably a 6-inch large-animal thermometer—to obtain the rectal temperature. The thermometer should be left in place for 2 minutes (except for digital thermometers that provide rapid readings), during which time the animal's pulse rate is determined by palpation of the coccygeal artery (6 to 12 inches from the base of the tail) and a respiratory rate recorded by observation of thoracic excursions. The clinician should use this 2-minute period to further observe the patient and its environment and to determine the habitus. The rear udder should be palpated, as well as the supramammary lymph nodes, during the time temperature is taken. Enlargement of the supramammary lymph nodes necessitates consideration of mastitis, lymphosarcoma, and other diseases capable of causing local or general lymphadenopathy. The mucous membranes of the vulva may also be inspected to detect anemia, jaundice, or hyperemia, as well as observed to detect any vulvar discharges. The veterinarian's sense of smell is also used during this time. The distinct, fetid odor of septic metritis, necrotic vaginitis, or retained fetal membranes; the necrotic odor of udder dermatitis; the sweetish odor of melena; or the "septic tank" odor of salmonella diarrhea may be apparent to the trained clinician. If manure stains the tail, is passed during the examination, or has accumulated in the gutter behind the cow, the veterinarian should assess the consistency and volume of the manure visually as compared with herdmates on the same diet. Extreme pallor of the teats and udder may suggest anemia in cattle such as Holsteins that often have fully or partially nonpigmented teat skin. Inspection from the rear also may suggest a "sprung rib cage" on the left or right side, suggestive of an abomasal displacement.

Body Temperature

The normal body temperature range for a dairy cow is 100.4 to 102.5° F (38 to 39.17° C). Other authors allow the upper limit to reach 103.1° F, but this is above normal for the average dairy cow in temperate climate ranges. Calves, excitable cattle, or cattle exposed to high environmental heat or humidity may have temperatures of 103.1° F or higher, but this should not be considered normal for the average cow unless these qualifications exist. True hypothermia may occur as a result of hypocalcemia when ambient temperature is less than body temperature, exposure in extreme winter weather, and hypovolemic or septic shock. False hypothermia may occur when pneumorectum exists or the rectal thermometer has not been left in place long enough. Hyperthermia may be of endogenous origin (fever) or exogenous (heat exhaustion, sun stroke). Usually exogenous causes of hyperthermia can be explained readily based on the general examination and assessment of the environment. It should be noted that hypocalcemic cows or recumbent cows—especially if they are darker colored than white—can become hyperthermic when unable to move out of the sun or when ambient temperatures are greater than their body temperature. The fine distinction between 103.1 and 102.5° F as the upper limit of normal

temperature has resulted from our observation of scores of hospitalized cattle with confirmed chronic peritonitis but which maintain daily body temperatures between 102.5 and 103.1° F. Therefore unless exogenous hyperthermia is suspected, rectal temperatures above 102.5° F should alert the clinician to inflammatory diseases. A normal body temperature does not rule out all inflammatory infectious diseases! At least 50% of the confirmed traumatic reticuloperitonitis patients in our clinics, for example, register normal body temperatures. This phenomenon also has been observed by other authors.

Fever may be continuous, remittent, intermittent, or recurrent. Remittent fevers go up and down but never drop into the normal range. Intermittent fevers fall into the normal range of body temperature at some time during the day. Recurrent fever is characterized by several days of fever alternating with 1 or more days of normal body temperature.

It must be emphasized that fever is a protective physiologic response to sepsis, toxemia, or pyrogens. It is the body's means of destroying organisms and instigating protective defense mechanisms. Fever in cattle should not be masked by antiinflammatory or antipyretic medications. Cattle do not have the tendency for laminitis secondary to fever that is observed in horses. Therefore the primary disease—not the fever—should be treated. Fever provides an excellent means of assessing the clinical response of the cow or calf to appropriate therapy of the primary disease.

Pulse Rate
The normal pulse rate for adult cattle is 60 to 84 beats/min. Calves have a normal pulse rate of 72 to 100 beats/min. Various authors disagree on the normal pulse rates of cattle, but these figures constitute an average for a nonexcited animal. Interpretation of extraneous factors affecting the pulse rate must be left to the clinician who is performing the examination and taking environmental factors and habitus into consideration.

Tachycardia is an elevated heart rate (pulse rate) and is present when the patient is excited or has any of a number of organic diseases. Tachycardia, although abnormal, is not system specific and may exist in infectious, metabolic, cardiac, respiratory, neoplastic, or toxemic conditions. Tachycardia also is present in painful diseases, including musculoskeletal pain. With musculoskeletal pain, a large difference in pulse rate will be found between when the animal is recumbent (lower) and when it stands.

Bradycardia is a lower-than-normal heart rate (pulse rate) and is present in very few conditions in cattle. Pituitary abscesses, vagus indigestion, and botulism are the major diseases considered to result in bradycardia in cattle. Not all cattle with these conditions have bradycardia, however. It has been reported also that normal cattle deprived of feed and water for hours frequently develop bradycardia. We frequently find this in cattle that are not systemically ill but are held off feed in preparation for anesthesia and elective surgery. Except for an occasional cow with ketosis, we have not observed development of bradycardia in sick cattle that have been off feed for a prolonged time. It may be that veterinarians seldom see normal cattle off feed for long periods because we are only called to examine sick cattle. One exception is the "broken drinking cup" in confined cattle, in which the animal does not eat because she has had no water for 1 or more days. Hypoglycemic and/or hyperkalemic calves also may have bradycardia.

Pulse deficits or arrhythmias encountered when obtaining the pulse rate may dictate further consideration of both cardiac and metabolic disease.

Respiratory Rate

The normal respiratory rate for a dairy cow at rest ranges from 18 to 28 breaths/min according to Gibbons and 15 to 35 breaths/min according to Rosenberger. The frequency, depth, and character of respiration should be assessed. Depth is increased by excitement, exertion, dyspnea, and anoxia. Calves at rest breathe 20 to 40 times per minute. Some calves with pneumonia have normal respiratory rates when standing but elevated rates when lying down. Metabolic acidosis results in both increased depth and rate of respiration. High environmental temperatures and humidity also increase the rate and depth of respiration. Depth of respiration is decreased by painful conditions involving the chest, diaphragm, or cranial abdomen. The depth and rate of respiration are decreased in severe metabolic alkalosis as the cow compensates to preserve CO_2.

The character of respiration may be normal costoabdominal, thoracic, or abdominal. Thoracic breathing occurs in those with peritonitis and abdominal distention in which either pain or pressure on the diaphragm, respectively, interferes with the abdominal component of respiration. Abdominal breathing is noted when cattle are affected with painful pleuritis, fibrinous bronchopneumonia, or have severe dyspnea caused by pulmonary conditions such as bullous emphysema, pulmonary edema, acute bovine pulmonary emphysema, proliferative pneumonia, and other conditions that result in reduced tidal volume of the lower airway.

Dyspnea is synonymous with difficult or labored breathing but is used also to describe an increased rate of breathing (i.e., simple dyspnea). Polypnea and tachypnea are perhaps better words to describe an abnormal elevation of respiratory rate. Hyperpnea implies an increased depth of respiration. The examiner should note whether the maximal dyspnea occurs with inspiration (inspiratory dyspnea), expiration (expiratory dyspnea), or equally during inspiration and expiration (mixed dyspnea). Classically inspiratory dyspnea tends to originate from the upper airway, whereas expiratory dyspnea usually incriminates the lower airway. Mixed dyspnea occurs in many conditions such as anoxia, severe pneumonia, and narrowing of the lower tracheal lumen. Audible respiratory noise, mostly on inspiration, is characteristic of an upper respiratory obstruction. The head and neck are often abnormally extended in cattle with respiratory dysfunction, and when pneumonia is present the cattle often cough after rising.

Left Side

Once the initial portion of the hands-on physical examination is completed at the rear of the animal the examiner moves to the left side of the cow.

Auscultation of the Heart and Lungs

Auscultation of the heart should be completed at the three sites that correspond to the pulmonic valve, aortic valve, and mitral valve (see Chapter 3). If the animal is excited by the presence of the examiner near her forelimb, the heart rate may be higher than the pulse rate previously obtained. Heart rate, rhythm, and intensity of heart sounds should be assessed during auscultation of the heart. The heart rate or frequency of contraction should fall within the normal limits as described for pulse rate. The rhythm should be regular, and the intensity or amplitude of cardiac sounds should be even and commensurate with the depth of the thoracic wall. For example, the heart sounds are relatively louder in a calf than a fat dairy cow. The clinician must auscult many calves and adult cattle to learn the normal intensity or amplitude of the cardiac sounds. A "pounding" heart with increased amplitude of heart sounds is heard in extreme anemia, following exertion, and in some cases of endocarditis.

Relative increased amplitude is observed in extremely thin animals and cattle with consolidated ventral lung fields. Decreased intensity of heart sounds may be associated with shock, endotoxemia, severe dehydration, or an extremely thick chest wall, as in adult bulls or fat cattle. Extremely decreased or "muffled" heart sounds occur bilaterally in those with pericarditis, pneumomediastinum, and diffuse myocardial or pericardial infiltration caused by lymphosarcoma. Decreased or muffled heart sounds unilaterally may occur with unilateral thoracic abscesses, diaphragmatic hernias, thoracic neoplasia including lymphosarcoma, or tuberculosis.

The first heart sound, or systolic sound, occurs during the start of ventricular systole and usually is thought to be associated with closure of the atrioventricular valves and contraction of the ventricles. The second heart sound, or diastolic sound, occurs at the start of diastole and is thought to be caused by closure of the aortic and pulmonic valves. Many dairy cattle have a split first heart sound that results in a gallop rhythm (e.g., bah-bah-boop, bah-bah-boop). This split first heart sound is attributed to asynchronous closure of the atrioventricular valves or asynchronous onset of contracture of the ventricles and should be considered in most cases a normal variant.

Heart murmurs, or bruits, are abnormal and should be assessed as to valvular site of maximal intensity, relation to systole and diastole, and loudness or intensity. Grading systems such as those used in small animals may be applicable when describing bovine heart murmurs (e.g., a grade II/VI holosystolic murmur), but in cattle this is a very subjective evaluation because few practitioners will encounter enough cattle with heart murmurs to be objective about the intensity of the murmur. Heart murmurs occur in those with congenital cardiac anomalies, acquired valvular insufficiencies, endocarditis, anemia, and some cardiac neoplasms, and may occur as a result of dynamic or positional influences in cattle in lateral recumbency. Cattle receiving a rapid infusion of high volume intravenous fluid may have a transient murmur associated with fluid administration.

The heart sounds may radiate over a wider anatomic area than the normal cardiac location when conducted through fluid (pleural effusion) or solid (consolidated lung tissue) media. Such radiation of sound should be considered abnormal. In sick adult cattle, heart sounds also may radiate through an extremely dry rumen, becoming audible in the left paralumbar fossa. This has been classically described in cattle with primary ketosis, but the phenomenon is not limited to this disease.

Splashing sounds associated with the heart beat usually suggest a pericardial effusion, most commonly associated with traumatic or idiopathic pericarditis. Thoracic or lung abscesses located adjacent but external to the pericardium also occasionally may give rise to splashing sounds should liquid pus in the abscess have been set in motion by the beating heart. These splashing sounds would most likely be unilateral, as opposed to bilateral splashing sounds coupled with muffling of the heart sounds present in pericarditis patients.

Atrial fibrillation is the most common cardiac arrhythmia in dairy cattle and is associated with hypochloremic, hypokalemic metabolic alkalosis. Hypocalcemia also may be contributory, but hypokalemia seems to be the most consistent finding in cattle affected with atrial fibrillation. Some clinicians have found atrial fibrillation in a small percentage of cattle with endotoxemia secondary to gram-negative mastitis. A rapid (88 to 140 beats/min) erratic heart rate of varying intensity and a pulse deficit characterize the physical findings in atrial fibrillation. When atrial fibrillation is suspected, simultaneous auscultation of the heart and palpation of the facial artery or median artery are indicated to determine a pulse deficit. Cardiac arrhythmias other than atrial fibrillation are rare in adult dairy cattle. Calves affected with white muscle disease and calves that are hyperkalemic may have cardiac arrhythmias.

Following auscultation of the heart, auscultation of the left lung field should begin. The entire lung field should be ausculted and subsequently the trachea ausculted to rule out referred sounds from the upper airway. The caudal border of the lung field extends approximately from the sixth costochondral junction ventrally to the eleventh intercostal space dorsally. If auscultation detects any abnormalities, thoracic percussion and thoracic ultrasound should be performed to further aid diagnosis. The anterior ventral portion of the lung that lies under the shoulder should be carefully ausculted by forcing the stethoscope under the shoulder/triceps muscles. A comparison of sounds between both sides and different locations on the chest should be emphasized. Cattle with severe pneumonia often do not have crackles and wheezes, but auscultation of a tracheal or "sucking soup sound" in the thorax is indicative of lung consolidation. It is also helpful to have the owner hold the cow's mouth and nose shut for 15 to 45 seconds to force the cow to take a deep breath. Alternatively increased respiratory effort, thereby exaggerating abnormal lung sounds, can also be achieved by holding a plastic bag over the cow's muzzle, forcing her to inspire an ever increasing fraction of CO_2 and diminishing fraction of O_2 over a 1- to 2-minute period. In addition to enhancing adventitious lung sounds, other signs of lower airway disease may include a rapid intolerance of the procedure and development of dyspnea, or the initiation of spontaneous and frequent coughing during the rebreathing period. Calves can be backed into a corner, and the examiner can hold the nose and mouth shut to auscultate the lungs without additional help.

During auscultation of the heart and lungs in the left hemithorax, the examiner may also palpate the jugular and mammary (superficial abdominal) veins for relative degrees of tension, pulsation, or thrombosis. In addition, the superficial cervical lymph node, peripheral skin temperature (ear and lower limbs), and skin turgor may be evaluated at this time.

Assessment of the Rumen and Abdomen

The examination proceeds to the left abdomen and begins with assessment of the rumen. Palpation and auscultation of the rumen should be performed. Auscultation in the left paralumbar fossa for a minimum of 1 minute will quantitate and qualitate rumen contractions. Palpation of the left lower quadrant and paralumbar fossa may aid this evaluation and is a better means of determining the relative consistency of rumen contents. Healthy cattle have one or two primary rumen contractions per minute. Hypomotility suggests stasis caused by endotoxemia, peritonitis, hypocalcemia, or other causes. Hypermotility may suggest vagal indigestion. During auscultation of the rumen, the left superficial inguinal lymph node should be palpated, and the hair coat and skin may be further assessed.

The examination continues with simultaneous auscultation and percussion of the left abdomen to detect resonant areas (pings) indicative of gaseous or gas/fluid distention of viscera in the left abdomen. In descending order of frequency of occurrence, these would include left displacement of the abomasum, rumen gas cap, pneumoperitoneum, rumen collapse, and abdominal abscesses secondary to rumen trocharization (see Chapter 5). When pings are identified, simultaneous ballottement and auscultation should be performed to determine the relative amount of fluid present.

Right Side

The right thorax is evaluated next.

Auscultation of the Heart and Lungs

Auscultation of the right heart and lung fields is similar to that performed on the left side. In general, the heart sounds on the right side are slightly less audible than those on the left side because the majority of the heart lies in the left hemithorax. Auscultation of the right heart requires the examiner to force the head of the stethoscope as far as possible cranially under the right elbow of the cow. Murmurs originating from the right atrioventricular valve are best heard on the right side around the third intercostal space at the level of the elbow. Although the right lung is larger than the left, the clinical basal border of the lung remains clinically identical to that found on the left side. Once again, during auscultation of the right hemithorax, the examiner should assess the ipsilateral jugular vein, mammary vein, superficial cervical lymph node, skin turgor, peripheral skin temperature, hair, and skin. Suspicious areas discovered during auscultation of the right hemithorax may be evaluated further by percussion.

Assessment of the Abdomen

Evaluation of the right abdomen begins with simultaneous percussion and auscultation of the entire abdominal area. Many viscera and conditions in the right abdomen may give rise to pings (see Chapter 5). Simultaneous ballottement and auscultation will allow a relative assessment of the quantity of fluid present in a distended viscus when pings have been identified. The fingertips should be used for determination of localized abdominal pain in the right abdomen. Deep pressure is exerted in the intercostal regions, paralumbar fossa, and right lower quadrant. This same technique may be used to palpate an enlarged liver that protrudes caudal to the thirteenth rib.

Ventral Abdomen

The next step in the physical examination is the determination of localized abdominal pain in the ventral abdomen. Several means have been suggested for this determination. We prefer the examiner to be positioned in a kneeling position near the right fore udder attachment. A closed fist is rested on the examiner's left knee, and gentle but deep pressure is applied intermittently to specific areas to the left and right of midline as the examiner moves forward until the xiphoid area is reached. The cow should be allowed 2 to 5 seconds between compressions of each area to allow her to relax before pressure is applied to the next area. An average of 8 to 10 deep pressure applications is used while the examiner observes the patient's head and neck for signs indicative of pain. When a painful area is identified, the cow usually will lift her abdomen off the examiner's fist, then tighten her neck musculature and show an anxious expression. She may also close her eyelids, open her eyelids widely, groan audibly, guard her abdomen, or abduct the elbows excessively. The examiner does not need to watch the abdomen because one will feel the cow's abdomen lift away. Subtle or chronic peritonitis cases may demonstrate only tightening of the neck musculature or show facial expressions indicative of pain. Peracute cases may show more violent reactions, and the patient may either move away from the examiner or kick—especially if the patient is a nervous cow. Other examiners prefer the withers pinch technique, in which firm pressure is applied to the withers area with one or both hands by grasping the withers and pinching. The normal cow should lower the withers to avoid this contact. A cow with peritonitis may be reluctant to lower her withers and thereby "push" against the painful peritoneal surface. This technique requires more subjective analysis because many nervous cows are reluctant to respond to the withers pinch.

Mammary Gland

Evaluation of the mammary gland is then conducted by palpation and examination of mammary secretions in all quarters. The conformation and suspensory weaknesses may be evaluated but have been noted, usually during the general examination, by observation. Dry cows are assessed first by palpation, and secretion is examined only if palpation detects firmness or heat suggestive of mastitis in one or more quarters. Milking cows routinely require a strip plate evaluation of the secretion in each quarter. The strip plate should have a black plate to highlight abnormalities, and a normal secretion from one quarter is left as a pool on the strip plate so that potential abnormal secretions can be milked into it. Other tests such as the California mastitis test or pH strips may follow the use of the strip plate. Generalized edema and focal areas of induration, abscessation, edema, or fibrosis detected by palpation of the udder should be recorded. The teats should be examined individually for teat end abnormalities, condition of the skin, inflammatory or neoplastic conditions, frostbite, photosensitization, edema, or evidence of previous injury.

At the Head

Once the udder and teats have been examined, the cow's head is examined. Because examination of the head leads to the most patient apprehension, this part of the examination is left to next to last and followed by rectal examination. The head should be assessed for symmetry, nasal discharges, relative air flow from each nostril, cranial nerve deficits, and relative enophthalmos or exophthalmos. The eyes will be sunken as a result of dehydration or extreme emaciation. Specific examination may include ophthalmic examination and inspection of mucous membranes for hemorrhages, icterus, anemia, erosions, or ulcerations. The frontal and maxillary sinuses should be evaluated by percussion. Lymph nodes should be palpated. If previous physical findings suggest the possible diagnosis of rabies, then examination of the head should be performed with great caution, and examination of the oral cavity should be performed with gloved hands. The jaws and tongue should be manipulated to evaluate their strength and the teeth inspected for excessive or uneven wear, fractures, or loss. The age of the cow may be estimated by examination of the teeth.

The palate and oral mucous membranes should be examined with the aid of a focal light for erosions or ulceration. The odor of the breath and oral cavity should be noted. Those examiners who can smell ketones on the cow's breath may be able to evaluate this parameter. A manual oral examination is performed if foreign bodies, inflammatory lesions, or masses are suspected in the oral cavity or pharynx, larynx, or proximal esophagus. The muzzle should be examined for the degree and symmetry of moisture present because Horner's syndrome may result in ipsilateral dryness of the affected muzzle and nares as the most apparent clinical sign. Motor and sensory function of the facial musculature and skin should be assessed if cranial nerve lesions are suspected; this is especially important if listeriosis or otitis interna/media is a possible diagnosis. Although most dairy cattle have been dehorned, those with horns should have the horns palpated to detect horn fractures or fractures of the skull at the cornual base of the horn.

Rectal Examination

Before completing the physical examination, a rectal examination is mandatory in appropriate size cattle. Rectal examination allows evaluation of the reproductive tract, palpation of the dorsal and ventral sacs of the rumen, the left kidney, iliac and deep inguinal lymph nodes, urinary bladder, proximal colon, pelvic bones, and ventral aspect of the lumbar and sacral vertebrae. The rectal examination may confirm many causes of abdominal distention suspected by the external examination, including cecal distention/volvulus, small intestinal distention, ruminal enlargements, rumen collapse, pneumoperitoneum, some right-sided abomasal displacements with volvulus, some abdominal or pelvic abscesses, fat necrosis, and occasional neoplastic lesions. Caudal abdominal or pelvic adhesions and rectal tears also may be confirmed by palpation examination. When reproductive abnormalities such as metritis, dystocia, uterine torsion, or retained placenta are detected or suspected, a manual vaginal examination is indicated following cleansing and preparation of the vulva and perineum. Vaginal examination is indicated also if pyelonephritis is suspected because palpation of unilateral or bilateral ureteral enlargement is better performed via vaginal rather than rectal examination. Following the rectal or vaginal examination, cattle with pelvic pain should be observed for persistent tenesmus, and if present epidural administration may be required.

Obtaining Urine for Analysis

Urine should be obtained, ideally before rectal examination, by repeated stroking of the cow's escutcheon and vulva using the flat of one's hand, straw, or hay to stimulate urination. Urine obtained in this manner should be tested with multiple-reagent test strips or tablets for urinary ketones and other abnormal constituents that might suggest further evaluation via a catheterized urine sample.

Additional Evaluations

If lameness or musculoskeletal abnormalities are suspected, specific examination of the limbs, feet, or additional observation of the cow may be indicated. These procedures will be discussed in Chapter 11.

ANCILLARY TESTS

At the completion of the physical examination, the examiner may have arrived at a specific diagnosis or may have formulated a differential diagnosis requiring ancillary tests or special system evaluation to arrive at a final diagnosis. Some ancillary procedures are available immediately, whereas others require laboratory evaluation or special equipment that may require economic decisions before undertaking.

Ultrasound

If an ultrasound machine with a sector probe is available, then an ultrasound examination is often the most useful ancillary test that will provide immediate information in many sick cattle. Pneumonia, endocarditis, pleural and pericardial effusion, intestinal distention, thickened intestinal wall, abdominal abscessation, and many other abnormalities can be immediately determined by ultrasound examination. With time, on-site ultrasound examination of sick cattle will likely become a more common occurrence.

Abdominal Paracentesis

Abdominal paracentesis is indicated when peritonitis is suspected or exfoliative cytology may be helpful to diagnosis. The procedure is performed best in the ventral abdomen to the right of midline but medial to the right mammary vein. The left abdomen and midline are contraindicated because the rumen visceral peritoneum lies in direct apposition to the parietal peritoneum and usually results in a contaminated tap. If the right ventral abdomen fails to produce fluid, paracentesis may be attempted lateral to the right fore udder in an area devoid of obvious mammary vessels. In either event, the selected area should be clipped and surgically prepared before abdominal paracentesis. The tap is performed with a 3.75-cm, 18-gauge needle with the needle advanced carefully to avoid gut contamination. It is much more difficult to obtain abdominal fluid in cattle than it is in horses, but the procedure can be an extremely useful aid to confirm peritonitis in questionable cases. Normal values for bovine abdominal fluid vary, but in general total protein should be no greater than 3.0 g/dl, and total white blood cell (WBC) count should not exceed 5000 to 6000 cells/μl. One author also implies that neutrophils making up greater than 40% of the WBC and less than 10% eosinophils are more important indicators of peritonitis than are the aforementioned protein and total WBC values.

Thoracocentesis and Pericardiocentesis

Thoracocentesis and pericardiocentesis may be indicated for pleural fluid accumulation, suspected thoracic abscesses or neoplasms, and pericardial transudates or exudates. These procedures are performed following surgical preparation of the specific area (usually the lower third, fourth, or fifth intercostal space) and use an 8.75-cm, 18-gauge spinal needle advanced as far as necessary. Obviously the relative risk of this diagnostic step needs to be discussed with the owner before the procedure, but concurrent ultrasound examination can make this a much less risky procedure than was previously the case.

Arthrocentesis

Arthrocentesis is indicated for cytologic and culture study when septic arthritis or degenerative joint disease is suspected. This procedure requires surgical preparation and uses needles of various lengths, depending on the exact joint involved.

Aspiration

Aspiration may be required to diagnose fluid-filled masses occurring anywhere on the cow's body. In most instances, aspiration will differentiate abscesses, hematomas, and seromas. The procedure is contraindicated should physical examination make hematoma (proximity to a major vessel or anemia) the most likely diagnosis. Therefore on a practical basis, aspiration is used to differentiate seromas that do not require drainage from abscesses that subsequently require surgical drainage.

Aspiration of tracheal secretions (tracheal wash) for cytologic examination and culture can provide valuable information about cause and treatment of respiratory diseases. The procedure can be performed by clipping the mid-neck region directly over the trachea. After proper scrubbing and local infusion of lidocaine, a small cut is made through the skin on the midline and directly over the trachea. A 14-gauge needle is placed into the trachea, and a 16-gauge catheter is introduced. Once the catheter is in the trachea, 20 to 30 ml of sterile preservative-free saline is flushed into the trachea and aspirated back. The procedure is most easily performed if two halters (with one lead on the right side and one on the left side) are placed on the cow and just before making the tracheal puncture, the cow's head is elevated and tied on both sides. In calves the head can be elevated manually. After collection of the sputum it is important that the fluid be placed in appropriate transport vials for delivery to the laboratory.

Biopsy

Biopsy may be required for solid masses, such as neoplasms, granulomas, and fat necrosis, or for specific organ histopathology, such as the liver, kidneys, mammary glands, and lungs. Tru-Cut (Baxter Healthcare Corp., Valencia, CA) biopsy needles are the most versatile instrument for this purpose and are applicable to most lesions and organs listed above. Lesions in the upper or lower respiratory tract may require special biopsy devices, which are used through the channel of an endoscope. Once again, surgical preparation of the site and scalpel puncture of the prepared skin before percutaneous biopsy of organs or tissues are required.

Urinary Catheterization

Urinary catheterization may be required to obtain urine should exogenous contamination of voided urine be anticipated or should urine culture be required. A Chambers catheter works well for this procedure, and bovine practitioners need to become practiced in catheterization, lest the suburethral diverticulum confound proper catheterization.

Milk Sampling

Examination of the milk and the California mastitis test are part of the routine examination for all lactating dairy cattle, and this is further discussed under the section on mastitis (see Chapter 9).

Hematology and Serum Chemistry

Blood collection for laboratory analyses may be required for many different reasons. Routine complete blood count (CBC) and chemistry panels are most valuable in assessing the sick cow that has no obvious problem on physical examination. Specific laboratory data will be presented in each chapter for specific diseases. Normal values used at our clinics are listed in Tables 1-2 and 1-3.

TABLE 1-2	Normal Complete Blood Count Values	
Hematocrit (HCT)	%	23.1-31.7
Hemoglobin (HB)	g/dl	8.6-11.9
Red blood cell (RBC)	million/μl	5.0-7.2
Mean cell volume (MCV)	fl	41.2-52.3
Mean corpuscular hemoglobin (MCH)	pg	15.3-19.2
Mean corpuscular hemoglobin concentration (MCHC)	g/dl	35.7-38.1
Red cell distribution width (RDW)	%	16.7-23.0
White blood cell (WBC)*	thousands/μl	5.6-12.7
Segment N	thousands/μl	1.1-5.7
Band N	thousands/μl	0-0
Lymphocyte	thousands/μl	2.3-9.3
Monocytes	thousands/μl	0-0.6
Eosin	thousands/μl	0-2.0
Basophils	thousands/μl	0-0.2
S + IV Platlets	thousands/μl	210-710
Mean Platelet Volume	fl	5.5-7.2
Total Solids-Refractometer	g/dl	5.9-8.1

Calves < 6 weeks of age normally have more neutrophils than lymphocytes. Their PCV and blood glucose are also higher than normal adult values.

TABLE 1-3	Hitachi (917) Reference Ranges—Cornell University	
Na	mEq/L	134-145
K	mEq/L	3.9-5.3
Cl	mEq/L	94-105
Total CO_2 (venous)	mEq/L	25-35
Anion gap	mEq/L	17-24
Blood urea nitrogen	mg/dl	10-25
Creatinine	mg/dl	0.4-1.0
Glucose	mg/dl	31-77
Alkaline phosphatase	IU/L	23-78
Aspartate aminotransferase	IU/L	53-162
Iron	mg/dl	113-226
TIBC	mg/dl	362-533
γ-Glutamyltransferase	IU/L	11-39
Calcium	mg/dl or mmol/L	8.3-10.4 ionized ≥4 mg/dl or 1.0 mmol/L
Phosphorous	mg/dl	4.2-7.7
Total protein	g/dl	7.2-9.0
Albumin	g/dl	3.2-4.2
Globulin	g/dl	3.5-5.8
Total bilirubin	mg/dl	0-0.1
Direct bilirubin	mg/dl	0-0
Lipase	IU/L	1-35
Cholesterol	mg/dl	73-280
Creatine kinase	IU/L	77-265
Lactate dehydrogenase	IU/L	659-1231
Magnesium	mg/dl	1.7-2.2
Triglyceride	mg/dl	7-323
Bile acids	Umol/L	9-455 Too variable to be of use in dairy cattle
Glutathione Peroxidase Heparin blood	Eu/g of Hb (whole blood)	≥60
pH venous		7.35-7.50
PCO_2 (venous)	mm Hg	41-50
Bicarb	mEq/L	24-34
Total CO_2	mEq/L	25-35
Osmolality	mOs/kg	270-300
Osmol gap	mOsm/kg	0-15

Nonesterified free fatty acids (NEFFAs) . 0.4 mEq/L in a late pregnant cow (2 weeks to 2 days prior to freshening) suggest excessive negative energy balance.

Beta hydroxybutyrate > 1400 μmol/L or 14.4 mg/dl suggest threefold increased risk for ketosis (subclinical or clinical); clinical ketosis cows often have BHBA > 3000 μmol/L or 26 mEq/dl.

SUMMARY FOR CLINICAL EXAMINATION

As our clinical experiences increase, pattern recognition becomes an increasingly important armamentarium for arriving at an accurate diagnosis. Enhanced pattern recognition can both improve diagnostic accuracy and lower the number of diagnostic tests required. It has been our experience that if pattern recognition becomes the predominant means of reaching a diagnosis without completing a thorough clinical examination and/or seeking to understand a probable pathophysiologic explanation for the clinical signs, diagnostic clinical accuracy will actually decline (Figure 1-1). The experienced practitioner must guard against excessive reliance on pattern recognition.

SUGGESTED READINGS

Eddy RG, Pinsent PJN. In Andrews A, Blowey RH, Boyd H, et al, editors: *Bovine medicine,* ed 2, Oxford, UK, 2004, Blackwell, pp135-138.

Gibbons WJ: *Clinical diagnosis of diseases of large animals,* Philadelphia, 1966, Lea and Febiger.

Perkins GA: Examination of the surgical patient. In Fubini SL, Ducharme NG, editors: *Farm animal surgery,* St. Louis, 2004, WB Saunders, pp 3-14.

Radostits OM, Gay CC, Blood DC, et al: *Veterinary medicine,* ed 9 Philadelphia, 2000, WB Saunders, pp 3-40.

Rosenberger G: *Clinical examination of cattle.* Dirksen G, Gründer H-D, Grunert E, et al, collaborators, and Mack R, translator. Berlin, 1979, Verlag Paul Parey.

Terra RL. In Smith BP, editor: *Large animal internal medicine,* ed 3, St. Louis, 2002, Mosby, pp 1-14.

Wilson JH: The art of physical diagnosis, *Vet Clin North Am Food Anim Pract* 8(2):169-176, 1992.

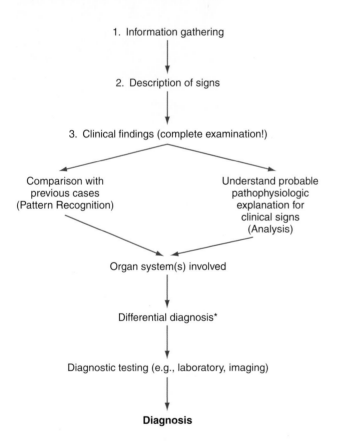

*A list of differential diagnoses for each clinical sign can be found at http://www.vet.cornell.edu/consultant/consult.asp

Figure 1-1

Summary of steps in establishing an accurate diagnosis.

CHAPTER 2

Therapeutics and Routine Procedures

Thomas J. Divers and Simon F. Peek

VENIPUNCTURE

The jugular vein is the major vein used to administer large volumes of intravenous (IV) fluids in dairy cattle. The middle caudal vein ("tail vein") is used for collection of blood samples and for administration of small volumes (less than 5.0 ml) of medications. If the tail vein is used for drug administration, only aqueous agents that will be nonirritating (should they leak perivascularly) should be used because it is harder to avoid some degree of leakage at this location than when a well-seated needle is used in the jugular vein. The mammary vein should not be used for either blood sampling or drug administration because complications of mammary venipuncture may have disastrous results, such as mammary vein thrombosis or phlebitis (see Figures 3-20 and 3-21), persistent unilateral mammary edema, and endocarditis. In general, it is contraindicated to use the mammary vein therapeutically unless the cow has a life-threatening illness and is in a compromised position, such that the jugular vein is inaccessible. Cattle with bilateral jugular vein thrombosis also may necessitate the risk of mammary vein venipuncture. In severely dehydrated calves, it is necessary occasionally to use a cephalic or dorsal metatarsal vein should the jugular veins become thrombosed during repeated fluid administration. Before any venipuncture, the overlying skin and hair should be moistened and smoothed down with alcohol. The vein should be "held off" by applying digital pressure proximal to the heart from the site of venipuncture (Figure 2-1). Neophytes seldom apply pressure of sufficient magnitude or duration before venipuncture and consequently have difficulty palpating or viewing the distended vein. Experienced clinicians are very patient and allow the vein adequate time to fill with blood, making venipuncture easier. Choke ropes or chains seldom are necessary in routine jugular venipuncture but may be helpful in extremely dehydrated patients. Utilizing gravity by allowing the head to hang over the side of a raised platform or table or even by hanging the calf over a stall divider or gate can distend the jugular vein significantly to facilitate venous access in very dehydrated calves. Commercial instruments such as Witte's neck chain and Schecker's vein clamp are available aids used in Europe.

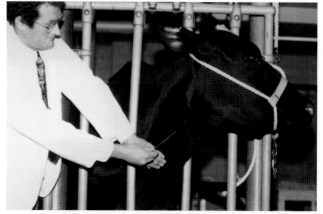

Figure 2-1

Jugular venipuncture. The cow is restrained forward in the stanchion and has her head tightly secured by a rope halter tied with a quick-release halter tie. The jugular region has been swabbed with alcohol, and the vein is held off by pressure on the heart side of the venipuncture site. A pointer indicates the distended vein.

Jugular venipuncture may be performed with a variety of needles, but the needle must be suited to the drug's viscosity, volume, and the duration of time anticipated for delivery. Stainless steel 14-gauge needles that are 5.0 to 7.5 cm in length are favored for most fluid infusions that do not exceed 2 to 4 L and that are to be administered promptly. Although many practitioners use disposable 14-gauge needles that are 3.75 cm in length, these needles are too short and so sharp that, with minimal patient struggling, such complications as laceration of the intima of the vein or perivascular administration of medications may occur. These shorter, disposable needles are acceptable for recumbent or extremely well-restrained cattle only. In general, venous complications such as thrombosis and perivascular injections are more common with the shorter needles. The longer 5.0- to 7.5-cm stainless steel needles are long enough to remain well positioned within the vein, are less sharp and therefore less likely to lacerate the intima of the vein and thus tend to cause less frustration to the practitioner faced with an unruly patient. The disadvantage of stainless steel 14-gauge needles is that they require cleaning, sterilization between uses, and periodic sharpening with an Arkansas stone. Cleaning and sterilization between uses are extremely important in preventing spread of bovine leukemia virus (BLV) and bacterial infections. Although most practitioners prefer 14-gauge needles, some practitioners successfully use 12-gauge, 5.0- to 7.5-cm stainless steel needles to allow an even more rapid administration of solutions such as dextrose and balanced electrolytes through the jugular vein. Careful pressure over the venipuncture site following removal of the needle is important in preventing hematoma formation, which may contribute to venous thrombosis.

When an indwelling IV catheter is to be placed in the jugular vein, a selected area in the cranial one third of the jugular furrow should be clipped and prepared surgically before inserting the catheter. Catheters may be secured by skin sutures, adhesive tape, cyanoacrylate to the skin, or by combinations of these techniques. Catheter placement is similar to placement of stainless steel needles, but a much greater length of catheter must be threaded into the vein. It is imperative that the vein distal to the site of placement remains compressed during the procedure. Because cattle, and especially dehydrated cattle, have an extremely thick hide, skin puncture with a no. 15 scalpel blade aids greatly the placement of IV catheters in dehydrated cattle or young calves.

Puncture of the middle caudal vein ("tail vein") is performed by inserting a needle on the ventral midline of the proximal tail. The exact distance from the anus may vary depending on the animal's size, but the site is usually 10.0 to 20.0 cm from the anus. The vein and artery are thought to run side by side as far as the fourth caudal vertebrae; the artery then usually runs ventral to the vein. However, this anatomy often varies. When performing tail vein venipuncture, the clinician must provide restraint by elevating the tail perpendicular to the top line. Forgetting to do this may result in a painful lesson in restraint. The tail is raised with the clinician's less adroit hand, and the venipuncture is performed with the preferred hand (Figure 2-2). Needles already should be connected to the syringe that holds the drug or with a Vacutainer (Becton Dickinson, Franklin Lakes, NJ) partially inserted so that the entire procedure can be done with one hand. Needles should be 18 or 20 gauge and 2.5 to 3.75 cm in length. The needle is inserted on the ventral midline perpendicular to the longitudinal axis of the tail and advanced until it gently strikes bone. Aspiration of blood is then attempted. If successful, the drug is administered or blood collected. If unsuccessful, the needle is gently backed off the bone 1 to 5 mm, and aspiration is attempted again. Use of the middle caudal vein for administration of small volumes (less than 5.0 ml) of medications and blood

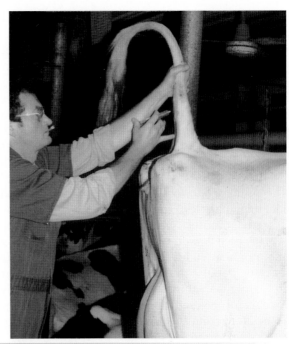

Figure 2-2

Middle caudal (tail) venipuncture.

collection has largely replaced jugular venipuncture for these procedures in dairy cattle. Tail bleeding is far less stressful to the patient, avoids bellowing and excessive restraint, and is quicker because one person performs both restraint and venipuncture. Although primarily valuable for blood collection in adult daily cattle, the tail vein may be used for blood collection in heifers of 300 kg or more. The procedure is more difficult in heifers of this size, however. Tail bleeding should not be attempted in young calves, lest permanent damage to caudal vessels occur.

Selection of appropriate needles for intramuscular (IM) injections in cattle requires consideration of density or viscosity of the drug to be administered, size of the patient, and desired depth of injection. Needles of too narrow bore prolong the time necessary for injection, often causing increased patient apprehension, struggling, or kicking. Needles too large of bore allow leakage of the administered drug from the site and cause more bleeding. Most aqueous-based drugs can be administered IM via an 18-gauge, 3.75-cm needle in adult cattle, whereas injection of oil-based or more viscous drugs (e.g., penicillin, oxytetracycline HCL) is facilitated by a 16-gauge, 3.75-cm needle. Most practitioners use disposable needles for IM injections to avoid the bothersome task of cleaning and sterilizing used needles. Increasing concerns regarding carcass spoilage as a result of the IM administration of therapeutic and biologic agents in grade dairy cattle have prompted a move toward subcutaneous administration of many products (antibiotics, hormones) that were previously given IM. Carcass trimming with subsequent lost revenue from meat is a relevant issue because the slaughter value of a culled dairy cow represents a significant revenue stream for many modern producers.

In dairy calves less than 2 months of age, a 20- or 18-gauge, 2.5-cm needle may be better for IM injections. In all instances, judgment is essential because the difference between a 1-week-old Jersey calf and an adult Holstein bull dictates selection of a needle based on the individual patient.

The primary site for IM injections in cattle is the caudal thigh muscles, especially the semimembranosus and semitendinosus. Occasionally the caudal biceps femoris is used as well (Figure 2-3). The gluteal region should not be used for IM injections in calves or adult dairy cattle because of the relative lack of musculature in a "dairy-type" animal. Injections in this area risk temporary or permanent injury to the sciatic nerve branches traversing the gluteal region when repeated IM injections or an IM injection of irritating drugs is necessary. Gluteal injections are especially contraindicated in dairy calves (Figure 2-4). Although many textbooks and publications advocate IM injections in the gluteal regions, this procedure should be avoided in dairy cattle.

Other available sites for IM injections include the triceps brachia (triceps) and the caudal cervical muscles (Figure 2-5). From a practical standpoint, dairy cattle generally are more excited by injections in their front end

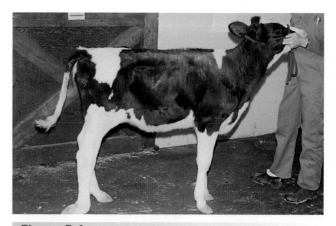

Figure 2-4

Sciatic nerve injury secondary to intramuscular injection in the gluteal region of a Holstein calf.

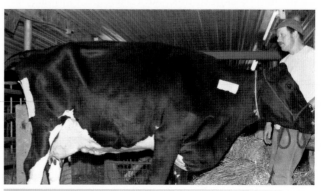

Figure 2-5

Site (white tape) for intramuscular injection of small volumes in the cervical musculature. Be sure to inject dorsal to the cervical vertebral region if this site is chosen.

than by injections in their hind end. If a cow is well restrained with a halter, IM injections can be made safely in the caudal cervical or triceps region. In poorly restrained cattle, those injection sites frequently cause wild and aggressive behavior. Most dairy cows tolerate IM injections in the caudal thigh muscles without kicking. However, unnecessary prolongation of the injection because of improper needles, multiple IM injections, or failure to prepare the patient for the "shot" all may lead to violent behavior. In addition, some dairy cattle are dangerous and require additional restraint before IM injections to avoid injury to themselves or their handlers.

The caudal cervical muscles in a calf provide an easily accessible site for IM injections of less than 5.0 ml of nonirritating solutions. The clinician can restrain the calf by straddling its neck and bending the calf's head to one side while the injection is made (Figure 2-6).

Selecting a clean site (free of manure and moisture) and swabbing it with 70% alcohol should precede IM injections. The needle is held by the hub between the

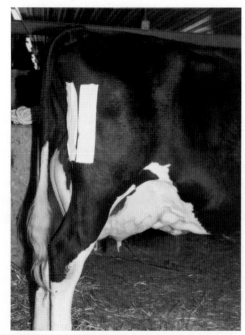

Figure 2-3

Caudal and caudolateral (white tape) thigh sites for intramuscular injections.

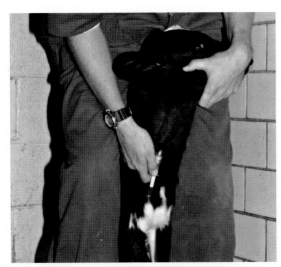

Figure 2-6

Restraint and positioning of a young calf for jugular venipuncture. An intramuscular injection in the caudal cervical musculature can be performed in a similar manner.

thumb and forefinger, and the cow is slapped repeatedly with the back of the clinician's hand near the site of the injection. Quickly rotating the hand, the clinician then slaps the needle into the selected IM site. The needle must be submerged all the way to its hub. A visual inspection for blood coming from the needle is made, and if none is seen, the syringe of medication is quickly attached to the needle. Aspiration on the syringe plunger will detect needles placed within vessels. If blood is aspirated, the injection is aborted, and the needle should be placed at a different site. If no blood is observed, the injection is made as quickly as possible. Up to 20 ml of drug may be deposited at an IM site in an adult cow, but probably no more than 5 ml should be placed at any one site in a young calf. Consideration of the drug's irritability to tissue may also influence specific volumes deposited at IM sites.

For cattle restrained in stanchions, usually little additional restraint is necessary. For cattle in free stalls or cows that appear apprehensive, haltering and tail restraint by an assistant may be necessary.

Subcutaneous injections are indicated for certain antibiotics and calcium preparations in adult cattle. In calves, balanced fluid solutions and certain antibiotics are administered. The recommended sites for subcutaneous injections in dairy cattle are (1) caudal to the forelimb at the level of the mid-thorax where loose skin can be grasped easily; and (2) cranial to the forelimb in the caudal cervical region where loose skin can be grasped easily. Care must be taken to avoid hitting the scapula with the needle!

It is important to avoid injury or irritation to the forelimbs when injections at these sites are made, and irritating drugs or excessive volumes should be avoided,

lest the animal experience pain associated with forelimb motion (Figure 2-7). To speed the administration, a large-gauge needle, such as a 14-gauge needle, should be used for adult cattle, and a 16-gauge needle should be used for calves. A disposable 3.75-cm needle is sufficiently long for this purpose. A 500-ml bottle of calcium borogluconate usually is divided into three or four sites (e.g., left and right side front of forelimbs, left and right side caudal to forelimb), whereas an antibiotic injection may be made at one site in the morning, another in the evening, and yet another site the following day. Calves requiring subcutaneous balanced fluid solutions may receive 250 to 1000 ml at a single site, depending on the size of the patient. During the injection, the bleb of fluids should be gently compressed and spread out by the clinician to distribute the fluids, improve absorption, and decrease leakage following withdrawal of the needle. Subcutaneous injections of irritating drugs or dextrose-containing solutions must be avoided.

Intraperitoneal injections seldom are performed in dairy cattle, with the exception of calcium solutions administered to hypocalcemic cows by laypeople untrained in venipuncture. Some over-the-counter calcium-dextrose solutions come complete with instructions recommending intraperitoneal injections through the right paralumbar fossa. Although this technique may be lifesaving for severely hypocalcemic cows, it also is dangerous for the following reasons:

1. Depending on the position of the cow and length of the needle used, the solution may enter subcutaneously, IM, intraperitoneally, or into a viscus such as the proximal colon.
2. Chemical peritonitis occurs if dextrose is present in the calcium solution.
3. Large intestinal adhesions are possible complications.

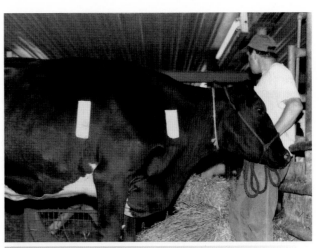

Figure 2-7

Sites cranial and caudal to the forelimb (white tape) for subcutaneous injections.

In adult dairy cattle, a needle at least 5.0 cm in length would be necessary for intraperitoneal injection, and risks of damage to viscera are minimized by rolling a recumbent cow to her left side before puncturing the right paralumbar fossa.

Complications of jugular IV injections include hematoma formation, thrombosis, thrombophlebitis, perivascular injections of irritating drugs, endocarditis, and Horner's syndrome (see Chapter 3, Figures 3-19 and 3-5). The most irritating and dangerous drugs commonly administered IV in cattle are 40 to 50% dextrose, 20% sodium iodide, and calcium. Avoiding perivascular deposition of these three drugs is extremely important. Good technique and adequate restraint are the keys to avoiding complications from IV injections.

Complications of caudal vein injections include hematoma formation, thrombosis, thrombophlebitis, and sloughing of the tail (Figure 2-8).

Complications of IM injections include tissue necrosis with subsequent lameness; peripheral nerve injury, especially sciatic nerve branches in the gluteal region or tibial branches in the caudal thigh muscles of calves; clostridial myositis; and procaine reactions. Peripheral nerve injury can be prevented best by avoiding the gluteal region when performing IM injections. In calves, palpation of the groove separating the biceps femoris and semitendinosus proximal to the stifle and injecting medial or lateral to this groove will help avoid sciatic nerve injury. Clostridial myositis is always a risk when injecting irritating drugs that may create a focal area of tissue necrosis and subsequent anaerobic environment in the IM site. Although *Clostridium chauvoei* (blackleg) spores may be in tissue locations already, most clostridial myositis secondary to IM injections is caused by *Clostridium perfringens* or *Clostridium septicum*. Currently prostaglandin solutions are the most commonly

incriminated solutions to result in clostridial myositis (see Chapter 15, Figures 15-1 and 15-2). Using sterile syringes, sterile needles, and avoiding contamination of multidose drug vials are important preventive measures. In addition, IM injections should not be made through skin covered by dirt or manure without first cleaning the site.

Procaine reactions occur when procaine penicillin preparations inadvertently enter a vein. Subsequent hyperexcitability, propulsive tendencies, shaking, collapse, or other neurologic signs may develop within 60 seconds of the injection. Clinicians or veterinary students who have made IM injections resulting in procaine reaction adamantly say that they "checked for blood by syringe aspiration before injection and definitely were not in a vessel!" Indeed these clinicians probably were not in a vessel at the start of the injection, but by pushing to force the thick procaine penicillin out of the syringe through an 18-gauge or smaller needle, they inadvertently forced the needle tip into a vessel. Entering a vessel can happen to anyone, but it can be best avoided by using needles that are big enough to both detect blood when aspirating before injection and to deliver the drug quickly IM without undue force on the syringe. When a procaine reaction does occur, leave the patient alone—do not try to restrain the animal and keep people away from the animal to avoid human injury. Procaine reactions seldom are fatal unless a large amount of drug enters the bloodstream. It is common for laypeople or inexperienced clinicians to mistake the classic procaine reaction for a penicillin "allergy" or hypersensitivity; the latter generally has more obvious signs of vasoactive amine release with systemic and/or cutaneous evidence of anaphylaxis. However, distinguishing the two is important because a procaine reaction does not necessitate cessation of penicillin therapy, merely more careful attention to injection technique.

Complications of subcutaneous injections include chemical and infectious inflammation. Chemical inflammation with eventual tissue necrosis and sterile abscessation is common should dextrose or calcium dextrose combinations be injected subcutaneously. Infectious inflammation, phlegmon, and eventual abscessation may result from poor skin-site preparation or technique. Common signs include painful, diffuse swellings that gravitate ventrally from the subcutaneous injection site, lameness and stiff gait caused by pain associated with forelimb movements, fever, and depression (Figure 2-9). Treatment consists of hydrotherapy, warm compresses, analgesics, and eventual drainage.

Various cannulas and commercial mastitis tubes are available for intramammary infusions. Individual sterile plastic cannulas (2-cm) with syringe adapters are used most commonly for infusion of noncommercial

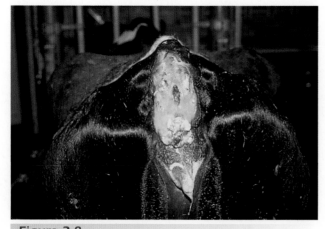

Figure 2-8

Complete sloughing of the tail in a Holstein cow following perivascular injection of phenylbutazone.

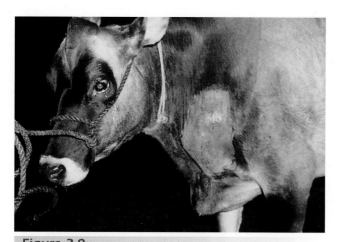

Figure 2-9

Painful cellulitis and abscessation of the caudal cervical region secondary to subcutaneous calcium-dextrose solution administration in a Jersey cow.

mastitis products, whereas stainless steel 14-gauge, 5.0-10-cm blunt-tip teat cannulas are sometimes used to facilitate milk-out from injured teats or for diagnostic probing of obstructed teats.

In all instances and regardless of the cannula used, the teat and teat end should be prepared aseptically before insertion of the cannula through the streak canal. After cleaning the teat thoroughly, the teat end should be swabbed repeatedly with alcohol before the cannula is inserted and again after the cannula is removed (see also Chapter 8). Large-volume infusions (greater than 100 ml) may be administered via gravity flow with the aid of simplex tubing and a sterile teat cannula.

Instruments used to deliver medications to the pharynx, esophagus, or rumen require passage through the oral cavity; the only exception is nasogastric intubation. Balling guns, oral specula and stomach tubes, a variety of dose syringes, and drenching devices are available for use in cattle. These instruments have tremendous potential to cause injury to cattle when used improperly or in a rough manner. Veterinarians should train laypeople in the proper use of instruments intended for oral delivery of medications to cattle because most injuries to the pharynx, soft palate, or esophagus of cattle are iatrogenic and caused by laypeople.

BALLING GUNS

Balling guns are available as single-bolus or multiple-bolus instruments. Single-bolus instruments require two people for administration, unless the person holding the cow's head releases the head each time a bolus is administered. Obviously the patient becomes harder to catch each time the head is released. Multiple bolus magazines have become popular because they avoid the need for "reloading."

Both types of balling guns are safe when used properly, and both are lethal weapons if used improperly. Before passing a balling gun into the patient's oral cavity, a quick assessment of the patient's size is mandatory. The administrator of the bolus using a balling gun should ask the following questions: Where is the pharynx in this patient? How much of the instrument should be advanced into the oral cavity? Balling guns passed too far caudally abut the soft palate or dorsal pharyngeal wall, thereby allowing pharyngeal injury when forceful expulsion of a bolus or multiple boluses occurs. In adult Holstein cattle, commercial balling guns are in correct position when the holding finger rings (not the plunger finger ring) are resting against the commissure of the patient's lips (Figure 2-10). However, this same position in a Jersey cow or a yearling Holstein places the bolus too far caudally in the oral cavity, thereby risking pharyngeal injury when the bolus is forcibly discharged.

Adult cattle balling guns should not be used in calves or young stock without extreme care. Smaller balling guns are available for calves and are preferable. Multiple-dose balling guns with sharp ends should be avoided. Gentle introduction and lubrication of balling guns, as with most instruments used in the oral cavity, will limit iatrogenic injuries. Balling guns should be of single-piece construction to avoid accidental loss of the magazine portion of the instrument into the rumen (which may occur with two-piece instruments!).

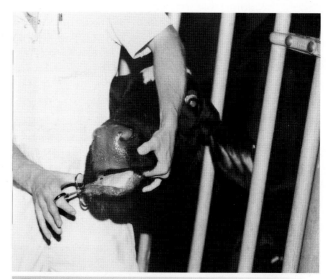

Figure 2-10

Proper position for delivery of medication using standard balling gun in an adult Holstein cow. Note that the operator's opposite hand is used to restrain the head and exert gentle fingertip pressure on the patient's hard palate such that the cow opens her mouth. In smaller cattle, the depth of insertion of the balling gun into the oral cavity needs to be adjusted to avoid pharyngeal injury.

STOMACH TUBES

Before passage of a stomach tube through the oral cavity of a cow, a speculum or gag must be used to guard the tube. Both the tube and some types of specula have the potential to cause iatrogenic injury. Stomach tubes should have smooth, tapered ends, appropriate flexibility, and measurement markers. A variety of gags are used to prevent cattle from chewing on or "eating" the stomach tube. Properly used gags present little potential for patient injury. However, a pipe and Fricke speculum are the oral specula used most commonly in dairy cattle and are potentially dangerous instruments. The length of a Fricke speculum exceeds the length of a cow's oral cavity so that the operator can safely hold a portion of the speculum external to the patient's mouth. Introducing a Fricke speculum too far caudally into the patient's oral cavity causes repeated gagging, coughing, and interferes with passage of the stomach tube because the tube repeatedly contacts the pharyngeal wall rather than the pharyngeal cavity when advanced. Overzealous forcing of the tube in this incorrect position results in injury to the patient. Before using a Fricke speculum, the patient should be "sized up" to determine how much of the speculum should be advanced into the oral cavity (Figure 2-11). The speculum should be continually grasped during the procedure or the cow may swallow the speculum.

A variety of stomach tubes are available. For cattle, a tube should have some flexibility, and the flexibility should be adjustable by temperature so that either warm or cold water can be used to add flexibility or add rigidity, respectively. Tubes that are too soft and flexible

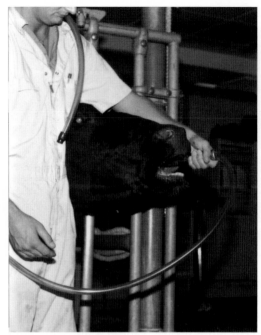

Figure 2-12

Passing a stomach tube with the aid of a Fricke's speculum. Note that the veterinarian uses his left arm to both restrain the head tightly to his body and to hold the speculum. The right hand is used to advance the tube. The patient's head should be held straight, not pulled to either side, as this makes passage of the tube difficult and potentially injurious to the patient's pharynx.

will double back during passage, whereas tubes that are completely inflexible risk iatrogenic injury to the pharynx, soft palate, or esophagus. Stomach tubes for adult cattle should have at least ¾-inch outside diameter (1.88 cm) to speed delivery of medications or evacuation of gas (Figure 2-12). Tubes of smaller diameter plug with rumen digesta too easily. Larger tubes, up to the "ultimate tube"—the Kingman—require excellent patient restraint, an appropriate gag or speculum, lubrication of the tube, and appropriate head position of the patient (Figure 2-13).

The Kingman tube is used to evacuate abnormal rumen contents or for rumen lavage. It may be used in cases of selected frothy bloats, lactic acidosis, and extreme fluid overload of the rumen. When passing a Kingman or other large-diameter stomach tube, the cow's head must be held straight forward and not pulled to the side because these tubes cannot be passed around a "corner." The cow's head should not be held higher than horizontal or normal position during passage of the tube should regurgitation around the tube (a frequent complication) occur. This technique will help to avoid inhalation of regurgitated rumen contents.

The increasingly common practice of routine or therapeutic drenching of periparturient and postparturient

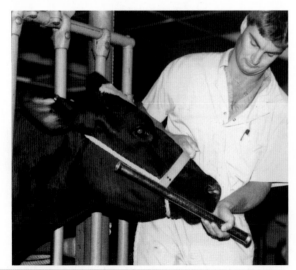

Figure 2-11

Determining the length of Fricke's speculum to be advanced into the oral cavity of patient before stomach tubing.

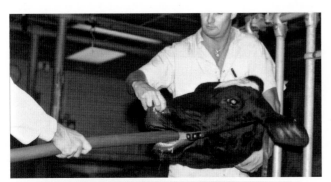

Figure 2-13

Passage of a Kingman tube with the aid of a cut-out wooden gag attached by a head strap. It is imperative that the patient's head and neck be held straight and that the head not be elevated. This position facilitates passage of the well-lubricated tube and minimizes the chances of inhalation should regurgitation occur.

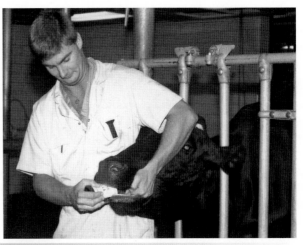

Figure 2-15

Drenching a cow. Fingertip pressure on the hard palate with the off hand facilitates introduction of the drench bottle. The cow's head is held horizontally, straight ahead, and close to the operator's ribs.

cattle has led to the widespread use of the McGrath pump (Figure 2-14) on modern dairies. This apparatus has the advantage of only requiring one person to position and then administer the fluids because it is maintained in place by a built-in set of nose tongs. Veterinarians should not hesitate to train laypeople in the proper restraint, positioning, and administration techniques when using this or any other stomach tube/oral drenching device because inadvertent aspiration and drowning are tragic but occasional consequences of their use by unqualified or poorly trained personnel.

Common sense, lots of lubrication, and gentle technique are minimal requirements for veterinarians using large-bore stomach tubes.

DOSE SYRINGE AND DRENCH BOTTLES

Oral medicaments such as rumenatorics and propylene glycol often are administered by oral drenching or dosing. These techniques are less likely to injure the oral cavity or pharynx physically but do risk inhalation pneumonia when performed inappropriately.

Once the cow's head is restrained, the drench bottle or syringe is introduced into the oral cavity at the commissure of the lips on the same side as the operator. Introduction is facilitated by finger pressure directed on the patient's hard palate by the operator's hand that is holding the patient's head (Figure 2-15). The cow's muzzle should be held so that the head from pole to muzzle is horizontal to the ground or slightly higher. Holding the head too high or twisting the head to the side interferes with swallowing and risks inhalation of irritating chemicals. Allowances for spillage should be made when calculating the drug volumes to be administered.

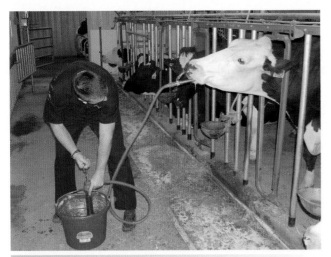

Figure 2-14

McGrath pump. The pump is passed into the esophagus and verified by palpation to be in the correct location before the nose tongs are used to secure the device in place. Fluids can then be administered by bilge pump by just one person.

ESOPHAGEAL FEEDERS

Popular for delivery of colostrum or electrolyte solutions to newborn or young calves, esophageal feeder devices are potentially dangerous when used by impatient or poorly trained laypeople. Pharyngeal and esophageal lacerations are all too common iatrogenic complications, and inhalation pneumonia is a less common complication. Laypeople should only be allowed to use these devices following training by a veterinarian. Proper disinfection of esophageal feeders that have been used to administer colostrum, milk replacer, or electrolyte solution is an important preventative measure in the control of infectious enteric disease in calves.

MAGNET RETRIEVERS AND OTHER INSTRUMENTS DESIGNED TO RETRIEVE HARDWARE FROM THE RETICULUM

All of these instruments are extremely dangerous to patients. Although some clinicians have had success with these instruments, they cannot be recommended because of an extremely high complication rate associated with their use. Iatrogenic pharyngeal lacerations are the most common complications encountered.

ORAL CALCIUM GELS OR PASTES

Tubes similar to those used to hold caulking compound have been marketed with various calcium and ketosis preparations for oral administration to dairy cattle. Although most of the nozzles have been shortened, some tubes may still have extremely pointed and sharp delivery tips that can result in soft palate or pharyngeal laceration when advanced roughly or in an overzealous manner into the oral cavity of patients. Products with sharp or elongated tips should have the tips cut off before introduction into the cow's mouth.

NASOGASTRIC INTUBATION

Nasogastric intubation with soft rubber tubing is the preferred method for tube feeding neonatal calves. A soft rubber stallion urinary catheter is passed through the ventral meatus into the esophagus (Figure 2-16). Verification of the tube's placement within the rumen is made by blowing through the end while ausculting the rumen through the left paralumbar fossa. This technique is easy to perform; easy on the patient; avoids injury to the oral cavity, pharynx, or esophagus by mechanical devices used in oral tubing; and can be done by one person.

The stallion urinary catheter should be flexible and made of either rubber or soft polyethylene. Once the catheter is in place, colostrum, milk, or fluids may be administered by attaching a funnel or dose syringe to the end of the tube. The tube may be taped in place should ongoing fluid needs be anticipated, but patients usually are more comfortable without indwelling nasogastric tubes. Larger nasogastric tubes may be used for larger young stock or adult cattle and are preferred by some practitioners to oral intubation. Nasogastric tubes may be used to force feed cows that persistently regurgitate during oral-pharyngeal tubing.

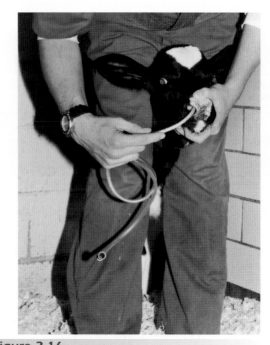

Figure 2-16

Introducing a soft rubber stomach tube into the ventral meatus of a calf.

GENERAL PRINCIPLES FOR ADMINISTRATION OF ORAL MEDICATIONS

Restraint is best provided by a stanchion or head gate that limits the patient's mobility and allows the operator to grasp the head without being thrown about or injured. When a cow is approached from the front, she tends to back away and lower her head. Cows that have received oral medications or have been subjected to nose lead restraint in the past will lower their muzzle to the ground to make it difficult to grasp. Cows that are in tie stalls are more difficult to restrain for oral medications and may require use of a halter to minimize bidirectional movement.

The cow's head is grasped with the operator's less adroit hand and the head held tightly to the operator's body (Figure 2-17). Holding the head tightly allows the operator to move with the cow and also prevents butting injuries that can break human ribs or cause other injuries. The operator is braced by standing with feet placed at least shoulder width apart and with the upper body holding the patient firmly. When a stanchion or head gate is available, the operator also may rest against these objects to further prevent movement.

Once securely positioned, the operator exerts pressure on the patient's hard palate using the hand that is holding the cow. This gentle pressure causes the patient's mouth to open and allows medications or devices to be

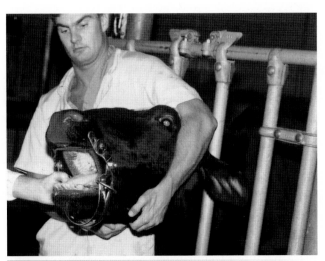

Figure 2-17

The cow's head is held tightly to the operator's body, and the head is restrained in a horizontal, straight ahead position while examination of the oral cavity is performed with the aid of a Weingart bovine mouth speculum.

positioned. Common errors to be avoided during oral medication procedures include:

1. Use of a halter: A cow cannot open her mouth if it is held tightly shut by a fastened halter. The halter must be removed or loosened or a nose lead used for restraint rather than a halter.
2. Keep the head straight forward: Excessive twisting or pulling the head to the side makes swallowing difficult for the patient and may increase the likelihood of pharyngeal injury when stomach tubes are used. Never attempt to pass a large-bore stomach tube with the patient's head twisted to the side.
3. Do not hold the head too high: Holding the head such that the muzzle is higher than the poll increases the likelihood of inhalation pneumonia, allows stomach tubes to enter the trachea more easily rather than the esophagus, and makes swallowing difficult.
4. Lack of lubrication: Always lubricate, even if just with water, any instruments being introduced in the oral cavity. This helps avoid iatrogenic injury

VAGINAL EXAMINATIONS

Vaginal examinations are performed to evaluate or medicate the postpartum reproductive tract, to monitor or assist parturition, to palpate the ureters in patients suspected of having pyelonephritis, to allow urinary catheterization, and for various other procedures. Before vaginal examination, the tail should be tied to the patient or held by an assistant. A thorough cleaning of the entire perineum should then be performed with mild soap and clean, warm water. Iodophor soaps, Ivory

soap, or tincture of green soap are acceptable soaps for this preparation. Sterile lubricant or mild soap should be used to minimize vulvar or vaginal trauma when the sleeved hand and arm of the examiner are introduced into the reproductive tract.

Following the vaginal examination, all soap and vaginal discharges should be washed away from the perineum, escutcheon, and rear udder, and the area dried. If discharges have reached the teat ends, these should be cleaned and dipped in teat dip. This latter step emphasizes regard for overall cleanliness and udder health specifically.

RECTAL EXAMINATIONS

Although the procedure of rectal examination is simple, the skills necessary for rectal palpation of the reproductive tract and viscera are complex and require thousands of repetitions. We believe that neophytes should be required to wear latex rubber gloves and sleeves when performing rectal examinations on cattle. These gloves not only allow more sensitive touch but help protect the patient from inevitable rectal irritation associated with neophytic palpators and plastic sleeves. Adequate lubrication of glove and sleeve, back-raking and removal of excessive manure in the rectum, patience, and gentle manipulations are critical to obtaining diagnostic information from the patient during a rectal examination.

URINARY CATHETERIZATION

Before urinary catheterization, the patient's tail is restrained, and the perineum is cleaned and scrubbed as described above for the vaginal examination. Sterile gloves and lubricant should be used. A sterile Chambers catheter is ideal for the urinary catheterization of cows. One gloved hand is introduced into the vestibule and used to identify the suburethral diverticulum. This is less than one hand's length from the lips of the vulva in most cattle and lies on the ventral floor of the vestibule. The urethra's external opening is a slit in the cranial edge of the vaginal origin of the diverticulum. The urethra is tightly compressed by smooth muscle tone and is much less obvious than the suburethral diverticulum. Therefore it is best to loosely fill the diverticulum with a single finger and introduce the sterile, lubricated catheter dorsal to that finger so as to avoid diversion of the catheter into the diverticulum. Gentle, patient manipulation will allow the catheter to enter the urethra along the cranial edge of the diverticulum's juncture with the vaginal wall. Once the urethra is entered, gentle pressure easily advances the catheter into the urinary bladder. Sterile technique is extremely important because urinary tract infections can be induced easily by dirty or traumatic catheterization, as frequently happened when dairy cows were catheterized routinely to obtain urine for ketone evaluations. *Corynebacterium renale* and other normal inhabitants of the caudal reproductive tract, as well as contaminants, can be introduced to the urinary tract by poor catheterization techniques.

CAUDAL EPIDURAL ANESTHESIA

Caudal epidural anesthesia is required in cattle for both medical and surgical reasons, such as:
1. Relieve straining and tenesmus during dystocia
2. Relieve straining and tenesmus when replacing a uterine or vaginal prolapse
3. Relieve tenesmus secondary to colitis, rectal irritation, or vaginal irritation
4. Provide anesthesia for surgical procedures involving the perineum (e.g., Caslick's surgery)

The site of caudal epidural anesthesia is the space between the first and second caudal (CA1-CA2) vertebrae. Usually this space is identifiable as the first movable joint caudal to the sacrum. Lifting the tail up and down allows palpation to identify this movement. Crushed tail heads or previous sacrocaudal trauma may make identification of the CA1-CA2 space difficult. Once the space is identified, the area should be surgically prepared and an 18-gauge, 3.75-cm sterile needle used to deliver the anesthetic. Very large (greater than 800 kg) cattle or adult bulls may require a longer 18-gauge needle. The cow's tail is moved up and down gently to allow the CA1-CA2 space to be palpated, and the needle is inserted on the dorsal midline over the space. The needle then is gently and carefully advanced in a ventral direction until the resistance to advancement suddenly stops and/or a negative pressure "sucking" sound is heard, indicating that the needle has entered the epidural space. The sensation as one advances the needle into the epidural space has been referred to as "popping into the space" and is identical to that experienced during cerebrospinal fluid (CSF) collection. Once the needle has been positioned, the selected anesthetic may be injected. Resistance to flow should be minimal to nonexistent should the tip of the needle be in fact positioned in the epidural space. Many clinicians attempt to confirm proper needle placement by dropping one or two drops of anesthetic from the syringe tip into the needle hub. If the needle is properly placed, then these drops quickly flow from the needle hub into the epidural space. If the needle is improperly positioned, then tissue resistance will prevent the drops from leaving the needle hub.

The volume of anesthetic (usually 2% lidocaine) injected during caudal epidural anesthesia should be as little as possible to avoid ascending anesthesia that could affect locomotion or hind limb function. In most instances, 3 to 6 ml of 2% lidocaine is sufficient to establish anesthesia, relieve tenesmus, and so on. The animal

should be standing or in sternal recumbency and should not have its front end lower than the hind, lest anesthetic too easily ascend the epidural space. Animals that develop any degree of limb paralysis or weakness following caudal epidural anesthesia should be confined to an area with good footing and hobbled loosely to prevent musculoskeletal injury until the anesthetic wears off. One of the major postoperative complications of true spinal (lumbar) anesthesia in cattle is musculoskeletal injury during the recovery period as the patient repeatedly attempts to rise despite its neurologic deficits. Lumbar anesthesia seldom is used in our hospital because of fear of this aforementioned complication.

Once the anesthetic is delivered to the epidural space, the needle should be removed. Needles left in place because of anticipated repeat dosing (e.g., prolonged dystocia) can lacerate the spinal nerves inadvertently, resulting in permanent neurologic deficits.

Longer-acting anesthetics than lidocaine should be considered only as a final option for a patient requiring repeated epidural anesthesia because these drugs may create irreversible complications and prolonged anesthesia. If repeated administration of anesthetics is expected, an epidural catheter (commercially prepared kits can be purchased or one can use sterile Silastic tubing that will fit through a 14-gauge needle) can be placed in the epidural space. A sterile gauze should be glued over the site following placement of the catheter in order to maintain sterility.

BLOOD TRANSFUSIONS

Blood transfusions may be life saving for patients that are suffering extreme anemia, acute blood loss, thrombocytopenia, and other coagulation defects that result in hemorrhage, as well as for neonatal calves that failed to receive adequate passive transfer of immunoglobulins. Despite these and other well-known indications, whole blood transfusions are performed with reluctance (and sometimes not at all) by many veterinarians, primarily because of concern over improper collection or administration techniques that result in inefficient or prolonged procedures. Therefore blood transfusion must be simple, rapid, and easy on donor, recipient, and veterinarian for the technique to be practiced. The following blood transfusion technique outlined is simple, rapid, and has evolved through many years as we have sought to minimize frustration and wasted time associated with earlier techniques.

The donor cow should be a large healthy cow, preferably known to be BLV negative and free of persistent bovine virus diarrhea virus (BVDV) infection. The stage of lactation or gestation is flexible, but an open cow destined for culling after her current lactation is ideal. Blood typing is seldom necessary because cattle have a large number of blood types. However, if major and minor cow matching is available (as for a hospital patient), blood typing procedures minimize the potential for incompatibility if the cow requires multiple transfusions. Four to 6 L of whole blood may be taken from large (≥700 kg) healthy cows without risk. The donor cow should be sedated with 15 to 25 mg of xylazine IV, a jugular site clipped and prepped, and the animal confined to a stanchion or head gate in which her head can be restrained tightly by a halter or nose lead. A choke rope is placed around the caudal one third of the cervical area, and a 15-cm, 8-gauge trochar is placed in the jugular vein. Blood is collected into wide-mouth 1- to 2-liter bottles that contain 35.0 ml of 20% sodium citrate/L as an anticoagulant (Figure 2-18). The blood is then caught in the collection bottles by free flow while the administrator gently swirls the bottles to ensure an adequate mixture of blood and anticoagulant (Figure 2-19). This technique allows collection of 4 to 6 L of whole blood in less than 10 minutes. Following collection of the desired quantity of blood, the choke rope is released, the trochar withdrawn, and external pressure applied to the jugular collection site for 2 minutes. Commercial transfusion needles, lines, and bags may also be used, but the collection process is slower.

The recipient is prepared for jugular catheterization, and a 14-gauge IV catheter is placed. The collected blood is administered at a slow-to-moderate rate through a blood administration set with in-line filter (Travenol Infuser, Travenol Laboratories Inc, Deerfield, IL). Although rapid administration may be necessary in selected emergency situations, too rapid administration may result in tachycardia, tachypnea, or collapse. Administration time varies from 30 to 120 minutes in most cases.

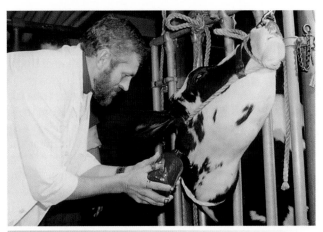

Figure 2-19

Collection of blood from a well-restrained donor cow.

Sedation and adequate restraint of the donor coupled with rapid collection via the large trochar and choke rope alleviate the donor and veterinarian frustration and apprehension that are often associated with alternative means of blood collection. Incompatibility, although uncommon, will be manifested in the recipient by signs of urticaria or anaphylaxis. Urticaria, edema of mucocutaneous junctions, tachycardia, and tachypnea observed in the recipient dictate that blood transfusion cease and appropriate treatment (most commonly antihistamines) of the allergic reaction be provided. Crossmatching or random selection of another donor must then follow.

CEREBROSPINAL FLUID COLLECTION

CSF may be collected from either the atlantooccipital (AO) or lumbosacral space (LSS) in cattle, and veterinarians should be familiar with both sites because a patient's status may dictate a preferential site. Recumbent or severely depressed patients may have CSF collected from either site. However, ambulatory patients usually are tapped at the LSS because an AO tap requires sedation or anesthesia. Suspected diagnoses also may influence the decision of site selection. When meningitis or encephalitis is suspected, an AO tap may be preferred, whereas with a suspected spinal abscess or lymphosarcoma, the LSS may be chosen. Although tapping "close to the lesion" is often a clinical preference, we have found little concrete evidence that this approach makes a significant difference in diagnostic yield for CSF. With the exception of rare spinal abscesses or lymphosarcoma masses that have been tapped into at the LSS, abnormalities of the CSF usually will be reflected in the fluid, regardless of collection site.

AO collection usually is easier than LSS collection, but AO collections require that the patient be recumbent, depressed, or sedated sufficiently to make the procedure

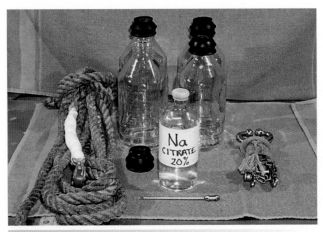

Figure 2-18

Equipment necessary for blood collection from a sedated donor cow includes a choke rope, four or more wide-mouth 1-L glass bottles, 20% sodium citrate solution (35 ml/L as an anticoagulant), halter or nose leads, and a 15-cm, 8-gauge trochar.

possible without risk of iatrogenic injury. The area from the poll cranially to the axis caudally is clipped and surgically prepared. The prepped area is usually 15 to 20 cm in length and 5 to 10 cm in width. The external occipital protuberance (cranial) and a line drawn transversely across the cranial aspects of the wings of the atlas (caudal) serve as landmarks. Approximately equidistant from these landmarks, on the dorsal midline, is the site for AO CSF collection. The patient's head is ventroflexed so that the muzzle is pushed toward the brisket. The patient's neck should be straight, not turned to the side. An 8.75-cm, 18-gauge needle with stylet is preferred for adult cattle or bulls, and a 3.75-cm, 20-gauge needle is used for neonatal calves. The needle is advanced ventrally, carefully but directly. The exact direction (slightly cranial/slightly caudal) will vary based on the selected site of the puncture. The most common displacement is to advance too far cranially such that the needle encounters the skull. This does not pose a major problem and allows the veterinarian to "walk" the needle off the skull to the AO space. The distinct decrease of resistance encountered when the needle perforates the dura mater and enters the subarachnoid space must be anticipated carefully and the stylet withdrawn to check for CSF whenever the administrator suspects that the space has been entered. Although the AO site is usually 5.0 to 7.5 cm ventral to the skin and on the median plane, distance estimates are not helpful because the cranial- or caudal-angle variations may add 2.5 cm versus a direct perpendicular approach. Practice on cadavers is the best way to become experienced with CSF collection techniques.

LSS puncture in cattle is not as difficult as in the horse because the needle travels much less distance from the skin to the LSS in cattle. The LSS usually is palpable as a depression caudal to the L6 vertebral dorsal spine and cranial to the dorsal spine of S2 (S1 not usually palpable). The site also is medial to the tuber sacral and intersects a transverse line drawn from the caudal aspects of the tuber coxae. This area and a surrounding 15 to 20 cm square area is surgically clipped and prepared before puncture. An 8.75-cm, 18-gauge spinal needle with stylet is sufficient for most cattle, but a longer needle may be necessary for cows greater than 750 kg and adult bulls.

A scalpel puncture of the skin over the selected site may greatly decrease skin resistance on the spinal needle, thus making adjustments in needle position easier. The needle is advanced ventrally and usually 10 to 15 degrees cranial or caudal on the median plane. The needle must remain perpendicular to the long axis. A less distinct "pop" accompanies puncture of the dura at the LSS than at the AO site, but a distinct decrease in resistance usually is felt as the subarachnoid space is entered. The patient frequently jumps, kicks, or otherwise reacts to the needle entering the subarachnoid, thereby signaling a successful tap. This response is

transient, and CSF may be aspirated from the needle once the patient relaxes. As opposed to AO puncture, LSS puncture usually requires that the CSF be aspirated rather than collected free flow because of gravitational differences in the techniques and any actual CSF pressure differences that may exist.

Aseptic technique during CSF collection is imperative to protect both the patient from iatrogenic infection and the veterinarian from zoonoses such as rabies. CSF is aspirated slowly into sterile syringes and then placed in ethylenediaminetetraacetic acid (EDTA) tubes (for cytology) and sterile tubes for culture. The stylet is replaced, and the needle withdrawn.

Specific abnormalities of the CSF are discussed in Chapter 12. Our laboratory considers normal CSF values for cattle to be:
Pressure (mm H_2O) < 200
Protein (mg/dl) < 40
Nucleated cells (per μl) < 5

ABDOMINAL PARACENTESIS

Abdominal paracentesis (AP) is used to collect peritoneal fluid as an ancillary aid toward diagnosing cattle with abdominal disorders. The most common indication for AP in cattle is to rule in or out the existence of peritonitis in a patient. Extraction of abdominal fluid (AF) also may be helpful for other purposes such as to provide exfoliative cytology when visceral lymphosarcoma or other tumors are suspected, confirm intraabdominal blood loss, detect rupture of the urinary bladder when suspected, and confirm ascites.

Because healthy cattle often have little AF, several sites of collection may have to be attempted before a successful AP is performed. The most common site for AP is the intersection of a longitudinal line between the ventral midline and right mammary vein and a transverse line drawn midway between the umbilicus and xiphoid. If this site is unsuccessful, then a site on the same longitudinal line but closer to the umbilicus or most pendulous portion of the abdomen may be attempted (Figure 2-20). As a last resort, the lower right abdomen just lateral to lateral support ligaments of the udder may be an attempted site for AP (Figure 2-21). The left abdomen should not be used because the rumen fills the entire left abdomen in most cows and may extend somewhat to the right of midline as well. Abdominal ultrasound examination is very helpful in evaluating location, amount, and ecogenicity of AF and can be used to determine proper location for the AP.

During clipping and surgical preparation of an AP site, large subcutaneous vessels should be noted and avoided during needle puncture of the abdomen. The patient should be restrained by a halter and tail restraint for AP.

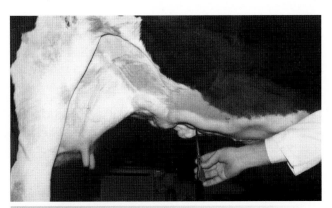

Figure 2-20

A pointer is directed to a potential abdominal paracentesis site on a longitudinal line between the ventral midline and the right mammary vein. Obvious subcutaneous blood vessels should be avoided when selecting a site.

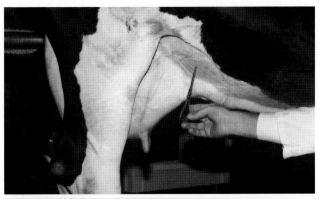

Figure 2-21

A pointer is directed to the alternative site for attempted abdominal paracentesis when sites between the midline and right mammary vein are unsuccessful.

In adult cattle, a 16- or 18-gauge, 3.7- to 5.0-cm sterile needle is popped through the skin and then advanced carefully until it pops through the parietal peritoneum. Alternatively, a blunt 14-gauge, 5.0-cm sterile stainless steel teat cannula can be used following a small scalpel puncture of the skin at the selected site. In addition to minute advancements of the needle, the needle hub should be twisted to vary the location of the needle opening. When successful, fluid dripping or flowing from the needle is collected in EDTA tubes and prepared for cytologic examination. Additional fluid can be collected for culture if indicated. In calves, a 2.5-cm, 20-gauge or 18-gauge, 3.75-cm needle is recommended, and great care should be practiced to avoid puncture of a viscus. Normal AF, light yellow in color, in cattle has <5000 nucleated cells/μl and total protein <2.6 g/dl.

The most common error occurring during AP in cattle is entering a viscus. This not only contaminates the needle but also the gut fluid may be confused with AF and subsequently sent for analysis. In addition, leakage

of ingesta from iatrogenic gut punctures may result in subclinical or clinical peritonitis—especially in calves. Normal periparturient cattle occasionally have increased amounts of AF that is a physiologic transudate. This fluid needs to be differentiated from fluid associated with peritonitis and from allantoic fluid.

In general, when peritonitis is suspected, a large volume of AF indicates a grave prognosis. For example, cattle having diffuse peritonitis from abomasal perforation tend to have large volumes of AF—so much so that nucleated cell counts of this fluid may fall within the normal range (≤5000/nucleated cells/μl) because of the dilutional effect of this massive inflammatory exudate on the relatively limited neutrophil pool of cattle. Although the protein value of this fluid will be elevated (greater than 3.5 g/dl), consistent with an inflammatory peritonitis, the low cell count creates confusion. Therefore the volume and protein levels of the fluid are the major parameters used to assess diffuse peritonitis—especially acute diffuse peritonitis. Localized peritonitis caused by traumatic reticuloperitonitis or smaller perforating abomasal ulcers may yield "textbook" values for AF. Localized peritonitis tends to cause a suppurative exudate confined by fibrin and therefore has elevated protein and nucleated cell counts. This fluid also may have a foul odor; be colored dark yellow, reddish, or orange; and have flecks of fibrin present. Frequently it is difficult to obtain AF from cattle with localized peritonitis because of "walling-off" or loculation of the fluid by fibrin. Therefore several sites may have to be tried before fluid is obtained. Similarly samples obtained from different sites may have greatly varying compositions (Figure 2-22) because of lessening degrees of peritonitis at greater distances from the site of origin. The use of ultrasound to

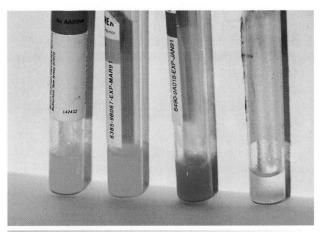

Figure 2-22

Abdominal fluid samples collected from different abdominal sites of a cow having localized peritonitis secondary to a perforating abomasal ulcer. Although all samples had elevated nucleated cell counts and total protein values, the samples closer to the site of peritonitis (tubes on left) had greater abnormalities.

identify pockets of AF may be useful when taking samples of fluid and is deemed very necessary ancillary data for a patient.

AF obtained by AP is an ancillary aid, not an absolute diagnostic tool. Frequently the values obtained from analyses of AF fall into the gray zone of normal versus abnormal. Various authors argue over the cellular contents of "normal" bovine AF. Cell count references may be found that range from less than 5000/μl to less than 10,000/μl. The reported ratio of neutrophils, mononuclear cells, and eosinophils found in normal bovine AF also varies. Despite these limitations, AP may yield diagnostic information that allows differentiation of surgical versus medical conditions of some patients. Abdominal paracentesis is specifically indicated in cattle whenever peritonitis is included in the differential diagnosis. In addition, those patients suspected of having abdominal neoplasia, hemoperitoneum, uroperitoneum, and ascites should have AP performed.

Contraindications for AP include extreme abdominal distention caused by distention of viscera that would necessitate surgical exploration regardless of AF values and extreme abdominal distention associated with a viscus that might be punctured during AP.

THORACOCENTESIS AND PERICARDIOCENTESIS

Thoracocentesis seldom is practiced on cattle simply because large volume accumulations in the pleural cavity are rare. Bacterial bronchopneumonia commonly causes fibrinous anteroventral bronchopneumonia with some exudative fluid, but the volume seldom is significant enough to warrant thoracocentesis for drainage. In addition, the tendency of cattle to develop fibrinous adhesions between the visceral and parietal pleurae makes pleural fluid difficult to collect when loculated within a labyrinth consisting of small pockets of exudate.

Occasional cases of pleural fluid accumulation have been observed; they occur secondary to lymphosarcoma or other neoplasms, thoracic trauma, lung abscessation, and acute perforation of the diaphragm by ingested hardware. Thoracic abscesses tend to be unilateral and may originate either from a primary thoracic site of infection or from a previous migration of hardware from the reticulum into the thorax. Thoracocentesis is an essential ancillary aid for diagnosis of these conditions.

Thoracocentesis is performed on the hemithorax, which is considered to harbor the most fluid, as determined on auscultation, percussion, and ultrasound examination if available. Usually auscultation and percussion are sufficient for diagnosis of pleural fluid accumulation in field situations because thoracic

ultrasound and radiography may not be available. In performing thoracocentesis in the absence of ultrasound guidance, the fifth intercostal space in the lower third of the thorax between the elbow and the shoulder is clipped and surgically prepared. The cow is restrained by halter and tail restraint. If the patient is not in respiratory distress, then mild sedation or local infiltration of the site with 2% lidocaine may be helpful. If the patient is suffering respiratory distress, then it is best to be direct and minimize sedation or additional needle punctures.

For diagnostic purposes, an 18-gauge, 8.75-cm spinal needle with stylet is an excellent choice for thoracocentesis. In small or average size cattle, a 14-gauge, 5.0-cm blunt-tip stainless steel teat cannula may be used following scalpel puncture of the skin. For drainage of fluid or evacuation of thick exudates such as those present in a thoracic abscess, a 20- or 28-French chest trochar with stylet may be required and previous scalpel puncture of the skin essential to allow thoracocentesis with these large trochars. Thoracocentesis of adult bulls and large, mature dairy cows often requires incision of the subcutis and outer intercostal musculature to pass an appropriately large diameter chest trochar for drainage.

Particular care to avoid cardiac puncture with needles and trochar is essential during thoracocentesis. The initial thrust or force necessary to direct the needle, cannula, or trochar through the chest wall must be immediately dampened as the pleural space is entered. This can be accomplished by holding the instrument with sterile, gloved hands and sterile gauze such that one hand provides the driving force while the opposite hand acts as a "brake" that allows only 4 to 5.0 cm of the instrument to make initial penetration beyond the skin. Further introduction under less forceful and careful advancement is then possible. Pericardiocentesis is simply an extension of thoracocentesis and is performed to confirm a diagnosis of pericarditis. Despite the tremendous enlargement of the pericardial sac, at least an 8.75-cm needle or trochar should be used to ensure penetration of the pericardium. Caution must be exercised to avoid cardiac puncture, and the procedure should only be performed following discussion with the owner. Rarely pericardiocentesis may cause rapid death in a patient with septic pericarditis—not as a result of cardiac puncture but rather because of a rapid alteration in the physiologic gas/fluid pressure gradient within the pericardial sac. Gas produced by bacteria in the pericardium acts to inflate the pericardium away from the heart, thereby lessening possible restrictive pressures. If pericardiocentesis results in a rapid loss of this gas because of needle puncture of the dorsal pericardial sac, then the pericardium and remaining septic fluid may exert a rapid pressure change on the heart in this heretofore "compensated" patient. Therefore even without cardiac puncture, pericardiocentesis does occasionally cause fatalities. Undoubtedly pericardiocentesis is best and most safely performed under ultrasound guidance.

Following thoracocentesis for diagnostic purposes, needles and cannulas are removed. Thoracic trochars or drains may be anchored in place should continuous or intermittent drainage be anticipated. A Heimlich's valve should be attached to the exposed external end of the drain to prevent pneumothorax when continuous drainage is selected. Most thoracic drain tubes tend to kink as they pass through the intercostal region; this kinking often increases to cause occlusion or necessitate replacement within several days.

ABSCESS DRAINAGE

Abscesses are an extremely common problem in dairy cattle. Subcutaneous abscesses and IM abscesses are the most common types observed, although mammary gland abscesses also are observed with some frequency.

Subcutaneous abscesses occur over pressure points, limbs, and facial regions. IM abscesses almost always evolve from dirty injections, but some cases lack a history of any injections and may evolve from skin puncture from a variety of objects in the environment. Subcutaneous and IM abscesses range from softball to beach ball size.

Abscesses eventually "soften" and drain spontaneously in most cases, but this may require weeks or even months. In addition, the lesions cause patient discomfort or pain, often interfere with locomotion or normal recumbency, and risk secondary problems such as endocarditis, glomerulonephritis, or amyloidosis. Therefore abscesses should be drained surgically whenever possible because this procedure allows a selection of drainage sites that improve chances of effective drainage and minimize subsequent recurrences.

Although abscesses are much more common than seromas or hematomas, the veterinarian should be careful to rule out these two types of lesions because drainage is contraindicated. Once the best site for potential ventral drainage of the suspect abscess is chosen, the skin at this site is clipped and surgically prepped. A 16-gauge, 3.75-cm disposable needle is used to aspirate some material from the lesion. If blood or serum jets from the needle hub, the needle is withdrawn, pressure is applied to the puncture site, and no further therapy is used. More commonly, however, when the needle is introduced, nothing flows from the hub. This dilemma is caused by the thick pus typical of that caused by *Arcanobacterium pyogenes*, which fills most abscesses. Pus can be aspirated by attachment of a syringe or by withdrawal of the needle and observing typically thick yellow-white pus clogging the needle and hub. Although use of a wider bore needle would encourage flow of pus, these

needles may be so large as to risk exogenous wicking of bacteria into sterile seromas or hematomas that are tapped. Therefore the 16-gauge needle seems the best for the initial aspirate in cattle.

Once needle confirmation has been obtained, a scalpel is used to drain the abscess, and a quick and rapid procedure is performed only with simple restraint if judgment dictates or with mild sedation (15 to 30 mg of xylazine) in most cattle. A liberal incision (≥5.0 cm) is essential for adequate and continued drainage. Large necrotic clumps of tissue and inflammatory debris should be removed manually from the core of the abscess. Following initial drainage, the patient's caretaker should be instructed in the following aftercare:

1. Each day the incision should be cleansed, and a gloved hand should be used to open the incision.
2. For large abscess cavities, flushing the cavity with dilute iodophor, hydrogen peroxide, or saline solutions is indicated to encourage removal of necrotic or inflammatory debris for 5 to 7 days.
3. Systemic antibiotics are not necessary in most abscess patients but would be indicated for severe or recurrent cases.

LIVER BIOPSY

Although not considered a routine procedure, liver biopsy may be necessary to confirm diffuse liver disease or focal liver lesions identified with the aid of ultrasound.

Liver biopsy in adult cattle is performed following sedation of the patient, surgical preparation of a site on the right eleventh intercostal space at the level of the mid-paralumbar fossa, local infiltrative anesthesia, scalpel puncture of the skin, and introduction of a Tru-Cut (Tru-Cut Biopsy Needle, Baxter Healthcare Corp., Valencia, CA) biopsy instrument or other liver biopsy needle. The instrument is usually advanced slightly cranial and ventral to the selected site.

The procedure can usually be performed blindly, but without question the use of ultrasound to identify the exact liver location is extremely helpful to successful biopsy.

DEHORNING

Dehorning of dairy cattle has long been accepted as a routine management necessity in most areas of the United States. Although veterinarians and owners agree that this task should be performed at as early an age as possible, it is inevitable that labor or time constraints develop on some farms with resultant dehorning remaining necessary for cattle 6 to 24 months of age.

Veterinarians must understand and be able to perform proper dehorning technique for various ages of calves and cattle. Laypeople who dehorn livestock almost never attend to details such as local anesthesia, cleanliness or antisepsis, and hemostasis. In addition, complications such as sinusitis and tetanus are much more common when cattle are dehorned by laypeople. Dehorning techniques will be discussed from their simplest to most complex.

Anesthesia and Restraint for Dehorning

Local anesthesia by cornual nerve blockade is performed before any dehorning technique. This minimizes operative pain to the patient and also allows the veterinarian to institute postoperative hemostasis without causing excessive stress or pain to the patient. The cornual nerve is a branch of the zygomatic temporal nerve and runs from the caudal orbit to the horn slightly below the temporal line. The nerve lies deeper near the orbit and more superficial along the caudal portion of the temporal line. Depending on the size of the animal being dehorned, 3 to 10 ml of 2% lidocaine is used to block the cornual nerve with an 18-gauge, 3.75-cm needle. Smaller needles may be acceptable for young calves.

In addition to local anesthesia, some practitioners use sedative analgesics such as xylazine to minimize the need for further restraint. Although this may be impractical when large numbers of calves have to be moved through chutes or stanchions, it may be helpful for fractious patients and is definitely indicated for bulls. Dosage depends on the size of the animal, degree of sedation desired, and facilities.

Restraint is imperative for effective and proper dehorning. Baby calves simply can be hand held or haltered. Larger calves (older than 4 months) should be tightly secured with a halter and stabilized by stanchion or held by an assistant whose hip provides a solid object against which the side opposite the dehorning site is positioned. Stanchions or chutes are ideal for calves >6 months of age. Such head gates allow the calf to be caught easily and will prevent excessive struggling. The calf may be restrained by a halter or nose lead, which allows the calf's head to be pulled to one side, then the other, to allow proper positioning for dehorning. A nose lead is preferable to halters in large calves and adults because it provides better restraint and does not interfere with effective hemostasis as a tight halter does, which may either accentuate or mask bleeding because of pressure caudal to the horn region. Adequate anesthesia and restraint for dehorning cannot be overemphasized because without it, the procedure will be prolonged. When the procedure is performed improperly, horn regrowth is possible, patient struggling and apprehension increase, the opportunity for patient injury increases, and handlers and the veterinarian become frustrated.

Electric or Heat Dehorning

This technique is the simplest form of dehorning because it can be done as soon as a horn bud can be palpated in baby calves, requires no hemostasis, can be performed by one person, and with it postdehorning complications are virtually eliminated.

The age for calves is usually 2 to 8 weeks; they are dehorned only if the emerging horn buds are distinctly palpable. Local anesthesia infiltration of the cornual nerve below the temporal line is provided by 5 ml of 2% lidocaine on each side. If a long hair coat is present, hair may be clipped over the horn buds. Electric or battery-heated dehorners that have been preheated before the onset of dehorning then are applied such that they surround the horn bud completely, thereby causing a thermal burn to skin circumferential to the horn and peripheral to the germinal epithelium. The dehorner is rotated slightly under gentle pressure to ensure uniformity of heat distribution. A "copper brown" ring in the burned tissue usually indicates sufficient cautery to prevent horn growth. During the procedure, the calf is held by an assistant or the veterinarian straddles the calf and holds its head to one side while dehorning the contralateral side, then switches hands while the head is pulled to the opposite side.

There are no disadvantages to electric or heat dehorning, but some owners fail to use the technique because of various factors: poor management that allows calves to get too large for effective electric dehorning; aesthetics (i.e., some people cannot stand the odor of burning hair and flesh); or cosmetics—some owners who show cattle believe that gouge dehorning performed at 4 to 12 months of age yields a more cosmetic head for show purposes.

Roberts or Tube Dehorners

This instrument, as with electric dehorners, is designed for dehorning young calves that remain in the horn bud stage. Following local anesthesia, restraint, or sedation, the tube with a sharpened circumferential edge is applied, twisted while pushed through the skin surrounding the horn bud, then rotated to flick off the horn bud and surrounding skin. Hemostasis is attained as necessary, and an antiseptic dressing is applied. The method is quick and effective.

Gouge or Barnes Dehorners

Once the horn has developed beyond the bud stage and develops an elliptical base, gouge dehorners usually are necessary to ensure complete dehorning and excision of enough skin peripheral to the horn origin to prevent regrowth. Gouge or Barnes dehorners are available in two sizes and can be used in most calves 3 to 10 months of age, depending on breed and size. Wooden or metal tubular handles are available, and an elliptical sharpened metal edge is formed when the handles are held together. Spreading the handles apart causes the sharpened edge to excise skin peripheral to the horn and the horn. The gouge must have a large enough circumference to remove skin circumferential to the horn itself effectively, thus preventing regrowth of the germinal epithelium. The long axis of the elliptical cutting surface is laid over the long axis of the elliptical horn base once the head has been restrained and anesthesia administered. A sharp, quick cut coupled with pushing the cutting edge toward the skull is important to proper dehorning: it will not only cause complete dehorning but also will allow effective hemostasis by exposing bleeding arteries subcutaneously, rather than in an interosseous location. Hemostasis is completed by pulling bleeding cornual arteries with artery forceps, followed by topical application of an antiseptic spray or solution.

Keystone Dehorners

Keystone dehorners are necessary for heifers or young bulls with large horn bases and for adult cattle. Large wooden handles operate the guillotine-type blades that remove the horn (Figure 2-23). Keystone dehorners are heavy, somewhat cumbersome and dangerous, but effective if used properly. To make a "good cut" that effectively removes the horn and a surrounding zone of skin

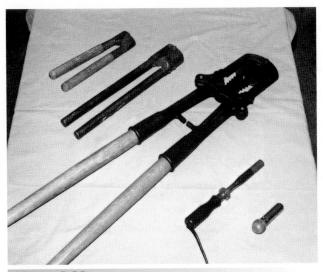

Figure 2-23

A variety of common dehorning instruments. From top to bottom: small Barnes gouge, large Barnes gouge, Keystone dehorner, an electric dehorner, and a Roberts or tube dehorner.

to prevent horn regrowth from the germinal epithelium, the patient has to be well restrained and positioned in a stanchion or head gate. The patient's head is pulled to one side and the "inside horn" (further from the veterinarian and closer to the stanchion) is removed. The patient's head then is pulled to the opposite side and the remaining horn removed. Positioning of the Keystone dehorner such that it properly cuts the ventral aspect of a large horn to allow subcutaneous exposure of the cornual artery branches requires that the cow's head be tipped toward the veterinarian and the distal portion of the dehorner be pushed closer to the skull. Anesthesia, restraint, hemostasis, and topical antiseptic care are performed as previously described.

In addition to complications associated with any open sinus dehorning (acute sinusitis, chronic sinusitis, or tetanus), Keystone dehorning has on rare occasions caused skull fractures in mature adult cattle.

Power Dehorners

Mechanical guillotine-type power-driven dehorners are available commercially. They are used when large numbers of heifers or adults require dehorning or when the veterinarian seeks to reduce the work required in using gouges or Keystone dehorners. The techniques are similar to those described for the Keystone dehorner, and once again adequate restraint is essential to proper technique. Extreme care must be exercised in the use of these devices because injuries to assistants or the veterinarian are potential hazards of using any power equipment.

Obstetric Wire

Obstetric wire is used to dehorn bulls and other large cattle that have horn bases too large for Keystone dehorners. Wire frequently is used to dehorn bulls, even yearling bulls, with wide horn bases and horns that protrude perpendicular to the longitudinal plane. Heifers especially have horns that curl upward as they project from the skull, whereas bulls often have horns that project outward, making it difficult to position dehorners properly to ensure a successful cut. Too often an improper cut with gouges or Keystone dehorners leaves a bull with a shelf of bone on the ventral horn base. This not only allows growth of horn ("skurl") but also precludes adequate hemostasis of the cornual artery because the artery is cut transversely and the cut end remains embedded in bone. Wire, on the other hand, can be positioned on skin below the shelf of bone and a proper cut completed as the horn is sawed off, using a sawing motion while holding the wire with obstetric wire handles. As with Keystone dehorners, the inside horn (closer to the stanchion) is removed as the head is tilted toward the veterinarian.

In addition to local anesthesia, it is preferable to sedate bulls or other animals being dehorned with obstetric wire because the procedure requires more time and much more effort for the veterinarian to complete horn removal. Proper removal technique allows hemostasis because the cornual artery is exposed in a subcutaneous location. Aftercare is standard.

Dehorning Saws

Box-type saws have been used to dehorn cattle, and the technique is similar to that used with obstetric wire. Saws, like wire, make dehorning more laborious than gouges or Keystone dehorners and are not widely used on dairy cattle.

Cosmetic Dehorning

Cosmetic dehorning is not as popular in dairy cows as in beef cows. Cosmetic dehorning requires careful aseptic technique, is more time consuming, and is more expensive than other techniques. The only advantages of cosmetic dehorning are to allow "shaping" of the head for aesthetic or show value and to attain rapid wound healing resulting from primary closure of the wounds.

The surgical procedure is done after sedation of the patient, local anesthesia, clipping of the entire poll region, surgical prep, and aseptic technique. Skin around the horn and peripheral to the germinal epithelium is incised, undermined, and loosened. Sterile obstetric wire is placed under the skin incision, and the horn is removed at a level below the skin. The skin incision may need to be elongated slightly toward the poll to allow adequate undermining of skin such that skin closure can be accomplished over the area formerly occupied by the horn. Closure with a continuous pattern of heavy suture material is then performed. Preoperative and postoperative antibiotics and tetanus prophylaxis should be considered for patients undergoing cosmetic dehorning.

Hemostasis for Dehorning

Although some veterinarians do not attempt to control bleeding caused by dehorning, fatal blood loss occurs on rare occasions as a complication of dehorning and justifies professional attention to hemostasis. Adequate hemostasis only requires that bleeding from the cornual artery be controlled. This can be accomplished only following a proper cut that exposes the cornual artery in a subcutaneous location. The cornual artery is a branch of the superficial temporal artery and runs caudally along the temporal line usually before branching just anterior to the horn into a dorsal and ventral branch. The dorsal branch is smaller and usually is exposed by dehorning

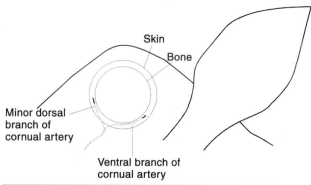

Figure 2-24

Schematic illustration of the cornual artery and typical subcutaneous locations of the ventral and dorsal branches after they are sectioned by a proper dehorning cut. The artery is represented by dotted lines where it remains buried, and the solid dark lines represent the cut ends that become apparent after dehorning. These cut ends then are pulled with artery forceps to establish hemostasis.

on the cranial edge of the cut. The ventral branch is larger and usually is obvious on the ventral aspect of the cut (Figure 2-24). Improper cuts that fail to remove all of the bone in the ventral aspect of the horn leave the cut ends of one or both of these arteries pulsing blood directly out of the remaining horn. When this occurs, the ends of the arteries cannot be grasped or ligated. Proper cuts expose both branches subcutaneously and allow the arteries to be grasped with artery forceps and "pulled." The ventral branch should be grasped, gently stretched, and pulled caudally until it breaks. If bleeding is still evident in the dorsal branch, this artery should be grasped, gently stretched, and pulled directly dorsal until it breaks. When the ventral branch is stretched sufficiently, it often is unnecessary to pull the dorsal branch because the artery breaks off proximal to the origin of the dorsal branch. Pulling these arteries until they break causes rapid hemostasis because bleeding is thereby confined within tissue or bone and clotting occurs more easily. Proper dehorning technique and adequate anesthesia allow rapid, practical hemostasis.

CASTRATION

Castration seldom is necessary for dairy animals because most male offspring are culled or used as sires. However, owners may request castration of male calves being raised for veal, baby beef, dairy beef, or oxen. Many castration techniques exist—it is beyond the scope of this textbook to delve into all of them. We use bloodless techniques with the Burdizzo's emasculatome for bull calves less than 6 months of age because of the lessened potential for complications and minimal stress on the patient. The Burdizzo's emasculator is applied to two sites on each spermatic cord for 60 seconds per application. The veterinarian should be sure to stretch each testicle when applying the emasculatome so that the penis and urethra are not damaged and to move the spermatic cord being clamped to a lateral location in the scrotum to avoid damaging the blood supply to the entire ventral half of the scrotum.

Other bloodless techniques such as elastrator bands may be used, but these suffer from seasonal concerns such as the presence of maggots in wounds during warm weather and also nonseasonal concerns regarding tetanus or improper application.

Many veterinarians prefer surgical castration to ensure complete removal of the testicles. Although bloodless techniques are highly successful when done with proper technique, concern about incomplete castration may influence some owners to prefer surgical castration. Surgical castration can be performed following bilateral scalpel incision on the lateral skin of the scrotum or following excision of the ventral quarter to one third portion of the scrotum. Individual preference dictates open versus closed castration techniques following scrotal incision. Regardless of technique, the use of an emasculator is recommended to minimize hemorrhage. Disadvantages of surgical castration include potential wound complication, maggots, tetanus, blood loss, and a greater stress to the patient. The major advantage is assurance of complete castration.

NOSE RING PLACEMENT

Proper placement of a nose ring helps prevent subsequent loss of the ring associated with ripping the ring through the muzzle during restraint. Rings are commonly placed in young bulls as they reach puberty and begin to show dominant or aggressive tendencies. It may be necessary to install a larger nose ring as the bull approaches maturity. Nose rings of several sizes are available commercially. The ring selected for an individual bull should be large enough to allow it to be grasped easily with fingers or bull leader and yet not so large as to become easily tangled on objects and torn out.

The nose ring is designed to facilitate restraint, leading, and management of bulls. Without a nose ring, it is impossible to manage individual bulls safely. Group-housed bulls, as observed in AI studs, do not have nose rings installed because their collective activity and aggressiveness risk trauma that could rip out the ring. Nose rings are inserted as bulls leave the group to be managed individually.

Particularly aggressive or difficult to catch bulls may require a short chain leader attached to the nose ring to allow the ring to be grasped more easily.

Nose rings occasionally are installed in heifers that are thought to be sucking teats in group housing situations. These nose rings have a "picket fence" aluminum plate attached that acts as a prod to the heifer being sucked so that such heifers no longer stand and allow the problem heifer to suck them. Nose rings are rarely applied to adult cows but have been used to make particularly aggressive show cows more manageable in the show ring.

Proper installation of a nose ring requires that a nose lead be used to extend the bull's head straight forward. The bull's head should not be turned. With the head fully extended and the nose lead tightly fixed, a no. 22 scalpel blade attached to a scalpel handle is quickly directed through the nasal septum. The back of the scalpel blade should abut the nose leads as the cut through the septum is completed. Dr. R.B. Hillman uses a 1.0- to 1.5-cm trochar rather than a scalpel blade. The trochar stylet acts as a guide for the ring as the trochar is withdrawn and the ring threaded through the nasal septum. Keeping pressure on the nose lead ensures that the ring will be placed as far forward in the nasal septum as possible. This avoids the septum cartilage and potential complications from cartilage injury. Special nose ring pliers that act as combined nose leads, scalpel, and insertion guide are available commercially.

Once the septum has been incised, insertion of the nose ring is easily accomplished by projecting the tapered end of the open ring through the incision, closing the ring tightly, and placing the small screw that holds the ring closed tightly in position. Dropping or losing this tiny screw is a common source of frustration and can be avoided by carefully holding the screw between one's teeth until it is needed.

Proper placement of nose rings minimizes the likelihood of nasal and muzzle lacerations caused by the ring being pulled out. Improper placement or excessive tension on a ring can cause this drastic injury and creates an injured bull without any practical means of being restrained or led. Repair of nose ring pullout lesions has been described and is indicated for valuable bulls. Sedation of the patient is coupled with local anesthesia provided by blocking sensory innervation through bilateral blocks at the infraorbital foramina; large mattress sutures of steel or other nonabsorbable material are used in the repair.

Dr. R.B. Hillman has extensive experience in repair of nose ring tears because of his supervision of bull health for the Cooperative bull stud in Ithaca, New York. He suggests primary closure with large mattress sutures that are preplaced before knotting (so that the entire wound can be seen), followed by simple interrupted sutures to oppose the skin edges. Dr. Hillman prefers heavy sutures. In addition to sedation with xylazine and local infiltration anesthesia, Dr. Hillman restrains the patient by tying it to a tilt table in the standing position so that the head can be restrained securely to the table.

REMOVAL OF DEWCLAW

Removal of the medial hind dewclaws is a routine practice for heifer calves on some dairy farms. Managers on these farms believe that this practice minimizes self-induced teat injuries. Although a controversial topic, no question exists that some mature cows or cows with pendulous udders do injure teats with medial dewclaws rather than medial claws of the digit. This can be proven by applying a dye to the medial dewclaw and then observing the cow's udder and teats several hours later to see where contact occurs.

Medial dewclaw removal is performed bilaterally in calves as a prophylactic measure and may be performed unilaterally or bilaterally in adult cows that repeatedly develop self-induced udder or teat injury.

The skin around the medial dewclaw is clipped and surgically prepared. An adult cow should be restrained in a head gate or stanchion and have the limb to be operated raised by a rope as in hoof trimming. Alternatively a tilt table may be used if available. Calves can be restrained by an assistant or sedated. Local anesthesia via local infiltration, ring block, dorsal metatarsal vein injection following tourniquet application, or specific nerve blocks should be performed. Sedation with xylazine may be helpful—especially in adult cattle—because of the drug's analgesic properties. In baby calves, heavy serrated scissors may be sufficient for removal of the medial dewclaw, whereas a sterile Barnes or gouge-type dehorner works very well in adult cattle. Care should be taken to avoid injury to deeper structures when amputating the medial dewclaws while being sure to remove a ring of skin peripheral to the dewclaw base so that regrowth cannot occur. Following removal, an antiseptic dressing and snug bandage are applied to protect the wound and speed hemostasis. The bandage is removed in 1 week, when it is either replaced or the wound left open and treated.

TAIL AMPUTATION

Many dairy farmers today are amputating the tails on all cows. This practice has gained popularity through the recommendation of animal scientists who maintain that tail docking improves cow cleanliness, improves udder hygiene, and lessens environmental soiling from tail switching. The practice also is popular with milkers because it prevents tail switching in the face. It remains to be seen if this practice will continue to be popular or if it will be a passing fad. Tail docking does not correct dirty management practices or lack of bedding. It does not improve sound premilking, milking, and postmilking hygiene or technique and there is no decrease difference in milk quality. Furthermore, although proponents

of tail amputation dispute this, cattle should have a defense against those insects that a tail can flick away.

Tails are docked at the level of the ventral vulva or just ventral to the lips of the vulva. This leaves enough tail to protect the perineum and perhaps allow tail restraint on the animal. An elastrator-type band is used to amputate the tail. The procedure may be performed on calves, heifers, or adult cows. Following placement of the bands, the tail distal to the band undergoes progressive dry gangrene and falls off in 2 to 8 weeks. The upper limit of the time range is met when bands are placed directly over a coccygeal vertebra rather than closer to an intervertebral location. Those wounds that expose bone obviously will take longer to heal.

Possible complications include chronic infections, osteomyelitis, ascending neuritis-myelitis, clostridial myositis, and tetanus.

Cattle should not have their tails docked unless the owners are willing to provide excellent insect control measures and practice excellent overall hygiene and cleanliness. Tail docking is not an excuse for dirty management. There have been a number of studies published in recent years examining the effect on fly control and insect avoidance behavior, as well as the animal welfare and pain issues associated with tail docking in cattle. At the current time tail docking is illegal in several European countries but still permitted in the United States. The available literature suggests that tail docking of calves may cause distress to the animal, and there is no conferred benefit in terms of udder cleanliness and the rate of intramammary infections in lactating cows with docked tails compared with those that have not had their tails amputated under conventional free-stall housing practices.

RESTRAINT

Restraint of any species is more art than science. Selection of the proper restraint for a given veterinary procedure requires common sense, judgment, and humane considerations. Experience plays a major role in selection of restraint techniques, and this experience is modified based on factors such as the patient's "personality," the owner's personality, the facilities available, the normal time required for completion of the necessary procedure, and the restraint skills of the assistants or handlers available.

There is an old adage that "the minimum restraint that allows the procedure to be performed quickly and effectively is the correct amount." It would be nice if we never had to restrain cattle, but this is not the case. However, erring on the side of too little restraint risks injury to the veterinarian, handlers, and patient. The potential for professional liability and malpractice suits must be considered with every patient that we, as veterinarians, treat. Too little restraint also may cause the patient to become increasingly apprehensive, wild, and progressively violent because a simple procedure has now become a prolonged adventure. Each time the procedure is restarted in a poorly restrained animal, the animal anticipates the procedure and becomes more violent. In addition, the handler and veterinarian become progressively frustrated, and so lose time and tempers. Too little restraint may result from lack of facilities or lack of knowledge.

Restraint is necessary to protect handlers, assistants, the veterinarian, and the patient itself. Kicking may be a vice or a defense mechanism for cattle. Cattle occasionally kick straight backward but usually "cow kick" by pulling the hind leg forward and then abducting the leg before kicking in a curved lateral and backward stroke. Vicious cows can kick straight back with one or both hind legs, causing severe injuries to handlers. Obviously if both hind legs kick simultaneously, the cow has to lower her head and put weight on the forelimbs. Such kicks may deliver a blow as high as a man's face to a person behind the cow and can be devastating. Cows that kick sideways often "crowd" a person that approaches them; most cows "crowd" people that approach from the side, but not all such cows kick. Being caught between a pipe partition or wall and a cow pushing all her weight against you is not a pleasant experience but is well known to people who handle cattle.

Very nervous cattle that bellow and jump about when they anticipate restraint, injections, or handling are dangerous simply because they are frightened. Thus they may become defensive and, in such a mood, can trap or trample a person.

Most people with even a rudimentary level of animal husbandry realize that cattle kick, but few realize the dangers presented by a cow's head when used in a defensive or aggressive way. A cow's head should never be approached without caution, and a person should stand beyond striking distance of the head unless the head is tightly restrained. Even loosely haltered or held heads can quickly break ribs or cause other damage to handlers. A cow's head only needs about 4 to 6 inches of freedom to generate sufficient force to hurt handlers or cause fractures. Therefore when restraining a cow's head with a halter or nose lead, the head must be tightly extended with no slack allowed. Similarly, when holding a cow's head for oral examination or to deliver oral medication, the head must be held tightly to the hip and upper body. Angry, demented, or protective (of a newborn calf) cows may attempt to charge, butt, or pin a person to the ground. The cow may charge straight ahead or swing the head back and forth, delivering blows with each change of direction. Not a year goes by when the lay press fails to report fatalities as a result of handlers' being mauled or killed by one of their own cattle protecting a newborn calf. Bulls obviously have an even greater potential to maim or kill humans. A dairy bull should never be trusted. Dairy bulls have a long legacy of unpredictability and have seriously injured many experienced dairy handlers who became overconfident or "in a hurry" when working in a bull pen.

Rarely, aggressive or frightened cattle will strike at a human with the forelegs. This usually happens when the cow's head is restrained for an IV injection or some other procedure involving the head or neck. Veterinarians and handlers should take care not to kneel too close to a cow because of this possibility.

Much variation in cattle behavior, handling, and husbandry exists on different farms. Small farms that have conventional housing and a great deal of contact time between the cattle and handlers are less likely to have vicious or wild cattle. However, rough handling, abusive handlers, constant yelling, or beating of cattle can occur in any environment. Free-stall or pastured cattle may be wild and only tractable when previous intense effort by experienced "cow people" has trained them not to fear approach by humans or haltering. The larger the herd, the less likely individual cattle will have been halter trained. Automatic lock-in head gates or stanchions and chutes are necessary to safely handle and treat wild cattle.

AN APPROACH TO DAIRY CATTLE RESTRAINT

Ownership of dairy cattle does not necessarily impart the knowledge, judgment, and techniques needed for proper restraint of these animals. Therefore the veterinarian must balance the need for proper restraint with a consideration of the owner's wishes or suggestions. It is best to allow the owner an opportunity to suggest restraint unless it becomes obvious that the owner's technique will not work. For example, when first visiting a farm it is courtesy for the veterinarian to say "please catch her head up while I prepare this bottle of ... to give her intravenously." The veterinarian can then observe routine restraint practice on the farm in question. Does the owner prefer a halter or nose lead? Many owners of registered and show cattle always use a halter and consider a nose lead offensive and unnecessary. Therefore a new veterinarian that immediately tries to put a nose lead in cows on this farm might not be called again.

Good dairy people also will warn the veterinarian about dangerous or nervous cows, and this should be an obligation of owners. Veterinarians may need to instruct dairy people in restraint for therapeutics or surgery to ensure safety to humans and beasts.

Cows should be approached slowly and made aware of the approach by verbal communication. Never touch a cow suddenly or move quickly toward her. It is preferable to approach tied cows on the same side that they are milked—given that this may be unknown in free-stall cows. Tied cows often are apprehensive when approached from the off-milking side, and this can be avoided by observing where the vacuum and pipeline stopcocks are located between cows. An assistant or handler should stay at the cow's rear end on the same side as the veterinarian if the veterinarian has to approach the animal's fore end. This prevents "crowding." Gentle cows can be reassured by the handler's scratching the tail head or rubbing the scapula and withers. An assistant should prevent the rear end of the cow from swinging across any posts positioned near the cow when the veterinarian is working near the rear of the cow. Loose cows can be made to stand briefly in a corner or moved into an open area by a person being positioned on each side of the animal. Moving slowly and deliberately without excessive noise is most effective and least likely to upset other cows in the barn. If one cow is roughly handled or mistreated, the entire herd may become apprehensive. Cows in tie stalls or free stalls that move sideways or back and forth should be restrained by a halter so that directional movement is limited.

Restraint of the Head

Rope halters are the most practical and gentle means of restraint. These suffice for most basic restraint and jugular injections, as well as for leading cows. Halters should be attached so that the free end tightens under the jaw and appears on the left side, which is the standard side from which to lead a cow. Positioning two halters on a wild cow to allow two people to lead her from opposite sides is generally worthless because the cow then pulls both people in a straight line. The principle of using one halter allows the leader to pull a wild cow's head to one side, forcing her to circle rather than escape. Nose leads are used when more restraint is necessary because of the cow's being wild or when very quick but painful procedures are necessary. Nose leads should not be used to lead a cow because the cow's normal response to nose leads is to pull back against them or to violently charge forward trying to either loosen them or reduce tension exerted by them. Neck straps are helpful to grasp the cow but provide poor restraint for large or wild cows. Bulls often are led by a long rope running from a neck strap or halter through the nose ring or by a snap on rope attached to the nose ring. Bulls also may be led by a bull leader attached to the nose ring. Whenever bulls are moved, a linear array of partition pipes placed close enough to allow a human to escape, but not the bull, is ideal.

Small to moderate sized cows that are calm can be restrained by having one person bend the cow's head around the handler's torso with the aid of a halter or fingers placed in the cow's nose (Figure 2-25).

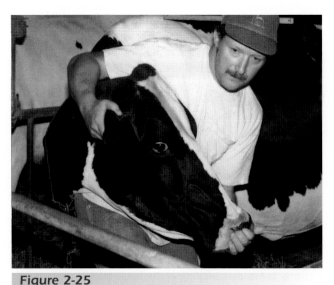

Figure 2-25

Manual restraint for intravenous injections or other minor procedures.

Whenever restraining a cow's head, the head should be pulled upward and to the side to gain more leverage. A cow allowed to hold her head too low has more mechanical advantage and thus compromises the restraint. Blindfolds are advocated as adjuncts to some restraint in Europe, but we have no experience with this technique. Calves may be restrained for injections, venipuncture, and examination by straddling the calf's neck and backing the calf into a corner.

Tail restraint is effective for minor, quick procedures such as IM or subcutaneous injections, collecting blood from the middle caudal vein, infusing a quarter, opening an obstructed teat, or draining an abscess. Effective tail restraint is provided with one hand while the opposite hand of the holder applies pressure to the cow's hip area on the same side as the veterinarian works (Figure 2-26). Tail restraint may be combined with sedative-analgesics or local anesthesia for teat surgery or other painful procedures. Proper tail restraint discourages kicking and keeps the cow steady. In tie stalls or loose housing, a halter should be applied before tail restraint to prevent excessive side-to-side or back-and-forth movement by the cow. Dry bedding or non-slip surfaces are important adjuncts to tail restraint, lest the cow slip backward or sideways while being restrained. Overzealous or sadistic tail restraint by extremely strong individuals can fracture caudal vertebrae, resulting in neurologic deficits to the perineum and tail. In contrast, failure to put some force into raising the tail to a vertical position results in lack of restraint. Therefore judicious pressure and experience are necessary to generate effective restraint by this method.

Antikicking devices seldom are used by veterinarians but are routinely used by milkers for specific cows that repeatedly kick at milking units or milkers. Antikicking

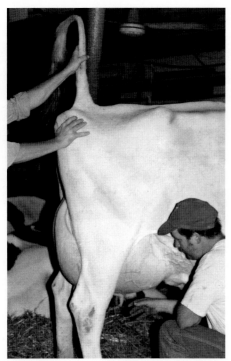

Figure 2-26

Tail restraint. Note that the holder also applies pressure to the cow's hip area on the side where the procedure is being performed. Thus if the cow reacts in a dangerous fashion, she can be pushed away from the person performing the procedure.

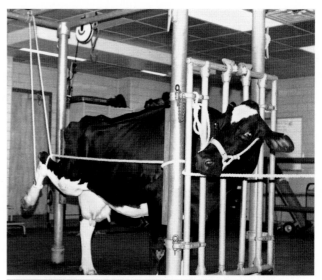

Figure 2-27

Raising a hind limb with the aid of a 30-foot soft nylon or cotton rope equipped with a quick-release honda and an overhead beam or beam hook. The cow is pulled forward in the stanchion, tied with a halter to reduce forward and backward movements, and tied toward the hind limb being lifted if there is a post or support available for her to lean against on the offside. The half-hitch loop in the rope must be maintained in the caudal gastrocnemius region for most efficient mechanical advantage.

hobbles and Achilles tendon (gastrocnemius) clamps are used by some farmers but have largely been replaced by flank clamps that are positioned more safely and easily than hobbles. One other disadvantage of hobbles is that cows that fight those devices tend to "double-barrel" kick by kicking out backward simultaneously with both legs.

Several methods exist to raise a hind limb for hoof trimming. A stanchion or trimming chute provides the ideal restraint for raising hind legs (Figure 2-27). However, veterinarians should be familiar with other methods because the structure of certain barns may not allow the use of beam hooks or pulleys.

Forelimbs are more difficult to lift and restrain than hind limbs. Regardless of technique, forelimb work contributes to "veterinary back pain" and sweat. A tilt table obviously is preferable for hoof trimming but is not always available. Typical techniques for lifting a forelimb are illustrated in Figures 2-28 and 2-29.

Ropes encircling the flank area or heart girth region that are tightened to effect may restrain some cattle effectively to prevent kicking and excessive movement. Whenever restraining a standing cow for foot care or other therapeutic and surgical procedures, her head should be tied via halter to prevent forward and backward movement. Preferably the cow's head should be pulled toward the side being worked on.

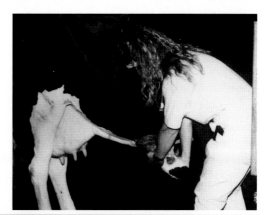

Figure 2-28

Manual lifting of the forelimb for examination of the foot. The patient's head is restrained by a halter and tied toward the opposite side in an effort to reduce weight bearing on the limb being examined. In some instances, a bale of straw or wooden block may be used to rest the limb and reduce back strain for the examiner.

Modifications of encircling flank and heart girth ropes also are used to cast cattle. Several methods have proven valuable, and most practitioners utilize modifications of Hertwig's method or Szabo's method to cast cattle for ventral abdominal surgery, correction of uterine torsion,

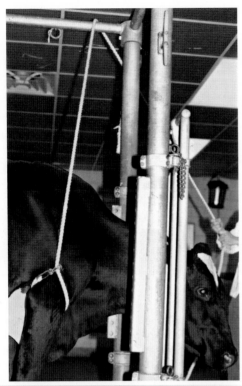

Figure 2-29

Another method to relieve weight bearing or "leaning on the examiner" is to lift the forelimb with the aid of a rope loop taken to the offside over a beam or beam hook and then tied so that the foot is easier to lift and hold. The cow also should be restrained with a halter and tied to the offside.

or teat surgery (Figure 2-30). These methods can be used in both sedated and nonsedated cattle.

*   *   *

"The cow is the foster mother of the human race. From the day of the ancient Hindoo to this time have the thoughts of men turned to this kindly and beneficent creature as one of the chief sustaining forces of human life."

W. D. Hoard, Founder of Hoard's Dairyman, Copyright 1925, by W. D. Hoard and Sons, Co.

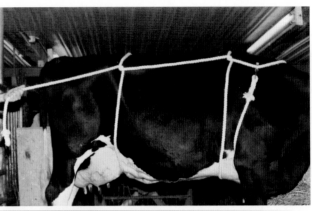

Figure 2-30

Commonly used modification of Hertwig's method to cast a cow. The forward loop is directed between the forelimbs to avoid choking the cow. The forward loop can be secured by either a bowline knot or, as illustrated here, a quick-release honda.

SUGGESTED READINGS

deLahunta A: *Veterinary neuroanatomy and clinical neurology*, ed 2, Philadelphia, 1983, WB Saunders.

deLahunta A, Habel RE: *Applied veterinary anatomy*, Philadelphia, 1986, WB Saunders.

Fox FH: Personal communication, Cornell University, Ithaca, New York, 1970.

Hillman RB: Personal communication, Cornell University, Ithaca, New York, 1984.

Leahy JR, Barrow P: *Restraint of animals*, ed 2, Ithaca, NY, 1953, Cornell Campus Store.

Perkins GA: Examination of the surgical patient. In Fubini SL, Ducharme NG, eds: *Farm animal surgery*, St. Louis, 2004, WB Saunders, pp 3-14.

Rosenberger G: *Clinical examination of cattle*, Berlin, 1979, Verlag Paul Parey, Dirksen G, Grunder H-D, Grunert E, et al, (collaborators) and Mack R (translator).

Stöber M: Surgery for the cattle practitioner: nose ring torn out—nasolabioplastic operation, *Bov Pract* 23:153-155, 1988.

Wheeler R: Facilities and restraining devices. In Fubini SL, Ducharme NG, eds: *Farm animal surgery*, St. Louis, 2004, WB Saunders, pp 51-57.

PART II

Diseases of Body Systems

CHAPTER 3

Cardiovascular Diseases

Simon F. Peek and Sheila M. McGuirk

EXAMINATION OF THE CARDIOVASCULAR SYSTEM

The cardiovascular system is assessed by observation of the animal's general state, mucous membrane appearance, and presence of venous distention or pulsation, as well as by examination of arterial pulse quality and rate and auscultation of the heart rate and rhythm.

Inspection of the patient may raise suspicion of cardiac disease if edema is observed in the submandibular space, brisket, ventral abdomen, udder, or lower limbs, or if abdominal contours suggest the presence of ascites. Obviously this requires differentiation from hypoproteinemic states, vasculitis, thrombophlebitis, lymphadenitis, or other less common diseases. Dyspnea, tachypnea, and grossly distended jugular or mammary veins are possible signs of cardiac disease that may be observed during general inspection of the patient. Weakness and exercise intolerance are other signs that require consideration of cardiac disease. In calves, overt abnormalities such as microphthalmos, wry tail, or absence of a tail signal the possibility of an accompanying ventricular septal defect, and ectopia cordis is grossly apparent by inspection of the thoracic inlet or caudal cervical area. However, many cases of congenital heart malformations occur in the absence of other defects.

During physical examination, mucous membranes should be evaluated for pallor, injection, or cyanosis. The visual appearance of the oral mucous membranes can vary with normal pigmentation patterns specific to the breed (e.g., Brown Swiss and Channel Islands cattle) and often appear pale to the inexperienced examiner in variably pigmented breeds such as Holsteins. In general, inspection of conjunctival and vulval mucous membrane appearance and refill time is preferable. Cyanosis is rare in dairy cattle with the exception of animals that are dying of severe pulmonary disease. However, cattle having advanced heart failure, right to left congenital shunts, and combined cardiopulmonary disease may have cyanotic mucous membranes. Capillary refill time often is prolonged in cattle with advanced cardiac disease.

Close inspection of the jugular and mammary veins for relative distention and presence of abnormal pulsation is a very important part of every physical examination. Proficiency and practice at palpation of major veins is essential before an examiner can differentiate an abnormal finding from the normal range of variation found in cattle of various ages and stages of lactation. Normally mammary veins are more sensitive indicators of increased venous pressure than jugular veins and therefore should be palpated routinely during the physical examination. Jugular veins should be observed during the general inspection and again during thoracic auscultation. Jugular veins should not be palpated until the end of the physical examination because many cattle become apprehensive when the neck region is palpated; this apprehension and subsequent excitement could affect baseline parameters or data being collected during the physical examination. This evaluation of the jugular veins, if deemed necessary, should be done at the end of the physical examination during examination of the head.

Mammary veins should be palpated by applying fingertip pressure. First the vein is palpated gently to detect pulsations suggestive of right heart failure; then the vein is compressed against the abdominal wall by gentle fingertip pressure. The amount of pressure necessary to compress the vein against the abdominal wall normally is minimal. When the vein is difficult to compress or, more commonly, seems to roll away from the fingertips, increased venous pressure from right heart failure may be suspected. These evaluations of the mammary veins obviously are subjective techniques but can be helpful adjuncts to other physical examination findings when practiced during every physical examination. Although pulsations in the mammary veins are considered abnormal findings suggestive of right heart failure, an occasional healthy older cow with a large udder and rich mammary vein branching may have slight mammary vein pulsation and distention.

Evaluation of the jugular veins for pulsation and distention requires differentiation of the "notorious" false-jugular pulsation commonly observed in thin-necked dairy cattle from pathologic true jugular pulsation and distention. False or normal jugular pulsation is a product of reverse blood flow from atrial contraction at the end of diastole and expansion of the right atrioventricular (AV) valve during systole. Passive jugular filling during systole also may contribute, as does a "kick," or referred carotid artery pulsation. False jugular pulsation arises as a wave that winds its way from the thoracic inlet to the mandible when the cow has her head and neck parallel to the ground. When the head and neck are raised, the false jugular pulse may only ascend a portion of the cervical area or may disappear. A true jugular pulse fills the whole jugular vein rapidly when the head and neck are parallel to the ground or slightly raised. This rapid filling is similar to filling a garden hose with the end held off when water to the hose is turned on full force. In addition, distention of the jugular veins is more obvious with true jugular distention as found in right heart failure (Figure 3-1). When confusion exists, the jugular vein may be held off near the ramus of the mandible, blood forced distally toward the thoracic inlet, and the vein observed. Emptying the vein in this fashion will eliminate a false jugular pulse, but a true jugular pulse will refill the emptied vein quickly and indicates right heart failure, increased central venous pressure, or right AV valve insufficiency. Some examiners suggest applying light pressure that partially occludes the jugular vein at the thoracic inlet, thereby mildly distending the jugular vein. This is thought to eliminate false (or normal) jugular venous pulsations from a referred carotid arterial impact. In general, the degree of gross distention of the jugular veins in cattle having right heart failure is more impressive than the degree of pulsation (see video clip 1).

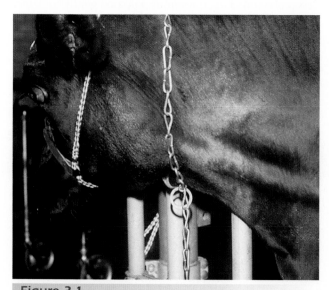

Figure 3-1

Obvious distention of the jugular vein in a cow having heart failure secondary to endocarditis.

Taking the arterial pulse may be helpful in the assessment of cardiac disease. The middle coccygeal artery is the first artery palpated for pulsation during the physical examination. The facial artery is utilized when treating recumbent (hypocalcemic) cattle, and the median artery is the most convenient to palpate when performing simultaneous cardiac auscultation and pulse monitoring. Pulse rate, rhythm, and quality should be assessed. Pulse quality implies considerations of the size, strength, and duration of the pulse wave and distention of the artery. Most cattle with heart failure have decreased pulse strength, unevenness of the pulse, increased pulse rate, or a pulse rate that is different than the heart rate. Abnormalities in pulse rate or rhythm should alert the examiner to the possibility of cardiac arrhythmias.

Proficiency at auscultation of the heart requires some basic knowledge, willingness to auscult both sides of the thorax carefully during every physical examination, and patience. Many cattle object to stethoscope placement over the sites on the chest wall necessary for cardiac auscultation and will adduct the forelimb tightly against the thorax. This is noticed especially on examining the right side, where cardiac auscultation in cattle requires the stethoscope to be placed very cranial in the axillary area around the third intercostal space. Dairy bulls and large or fat cows have thick chest walls that reduce the intensity of heart sounds. Heart sounds are easier to hear on the left side of normal cattle. The pulmonic valve region is best heard in the left third intercostal space at a level between the shoulder and elbow. The aortic valve region near the heart base is best heard in the left fourth intercostal space at approximately shoulder level. The mitral (left AV) valve region coincides with the cardiac apex and is best heard at the left fifth intercostal space just above the elbow. The right AV (tricuspid) valve is heard far forward in the right third intercostal space at a level halfway between elbow and shoulder.

Although clinicians generally discuss two heart sounds in normal cattle, it is possible to hear four heart sounds in some cattle as it is with horses. Although the potential for four heart sounds is somewhat confusing and may be impossible to differentiate in most clinical patients, examiners should be aware of these facts. The first heart sound (S1) heralds the beginning of systole, is associated with the final halting of AV valve motion after closing and is best heard at the apex regions coinciding with AV valves in the cow. A slight splitting of S1 into separate mitral and tricuspid valve components is possible but is rarely audible in normal cattle. S1 tends to be of lower frequency and longer duration than S2.

S2 usually is not as loud as S1 and coincides with aortic and pulmonic valve closure. Current theory suggests that valve closing sounds associated with the generation of S2 result from the sudden halt in valve motion when it closes. Asynchronous closure of the aortic and pulmonic valves results in audible splitting of S2 in many normal cattle, especially during the inspiratory phase of the respiratory cycle.

Although S1 and S2 comprise the major heart sounds for cattle, S3 and S4 have been described. Ventricular vibrations at the end of rapid filling in early diastole are thought to cause S3, a low frequency sound seldom heard in cattle. S4 sometimes is heard late in diastole and is related to atrial contraction. In cattle with tachycardia, it has been suggested that S4 may in fact closely precede S1 and be mistaken for a split S1. The tripling or quadrupling of heart sounds that resembles a horse's cantering gait is commonly referred to as a gallop rhythm and occurs in the higher range of normal heart rates or when tachycardia exists in some cows. Gallops are diastolic sounds related to atrial contraction (S4 gallop), to ventricular filling (S3), or to both (summation gallop). A prominent and persistent gallop rhythm in a cow with tachycardia may be the first indication of heart disease.

The heart rate of normal cattle is 60 to 84 beats/min. Neonatal calves may have normal heart rates as high as 110 to 120 beats/min, but frequently heart rates this high are brought about by the excitement of being handled or in anticipation of being fed. Not everyone agrees on the aforementioned range of normal heart rates for cattle, and several points should be addressed regarding this topic. Oxen and fat, persistently dry cows used only for embryo transfer may have a slower metabolism than lactating dairy cattle. Therefore somewhat like draft horses, these cattle may have heart rates at the low end of the normal range or even less than 60 beats/min. Conversely healthy but excited, nervous, or aggressive cattle may have heart and pulse rates more than 84 beats/min when approached by any examiner. Therefore the range of 60 to 84 beats/min really is an average and must be interpreted in light of the patient, its surroundings, and its intended use. Following the work of McGuirk et al with fasted cattle, a low normal range of 48 beats/min has been proposed. However, fasted healthy cattle seldom are encountered in the world outside of academic settings, and veterinarians are not frequently asked to examine healthy fasted cattle. An exception may be a cow off feed secondary to the classic broken water cup syndrome because she will become anorectic secondary to water deprivation. Sick cattle seldom have a heart rate less than 60 beats/min only because they are anorectic. Sick cattle that do have heart rates less than 60 beats/min usually have a vagal nerve-mediated bradycardia. Therefore 60 to 84 beats/min is still our preferred normal range for heart rate in adult dairy cattle.

Excited or nervous cattle may have an increased intensity or loudness of the heart sounds in addition to an increased heart rate. Other conditions that increase the intensity of heart sounds may be relative or pathologic. Relative factors include thin body condition, younger animals with thin chest walls, and excitement.

Pathologic factors include anemia, the "pounding" heart rate sometimes heard in cattle with endocarditis, and displacement of the heart to a position closer to the thoracic wall by a diaphragmatic hernia or an abscess or tumor in the contralateral hemithorax. "Muffling," or decreased intensity of heart sounds, may occur for relative reasons such as the increased thickness or fat on the chest wall of adult bulls or heavily conditioned cattle. Muffling also results from pathologic conditions such as pericarditis, pneumomediastinum, diaphragmatic hernia, and displacement of the heart toward the opposite hemithorax by an abscess or tumor in the hemithorax being ausculted. Cattle in shock may have either decreased or increased intensity of heart sounds, depending on the duration and severity of the condition. "Shocky" cows that are weak but still ambulatory tend to have increased intensity of heart sounds, whereas those that are recumbent or moribund have decreased intensity.

Auscultation combined with percussion provides the best subjective means to estimate the position and size of the heart. Heart sounds may radiate over a wider area than normal when transmitted by consolidated lung lobes or pleural fluid or when there is cardiac enlargement.

In calves and thin adult cattle, palpation of the apex beat is possible around the left fourth or fifth intercostal spaces at a level halfway between the elbow and shoulder. Palpation of an apex beat on the right side of adult cattle seldom is possible unless profound cardiac disease or displacement of the heart to the right by space-occupying masses has occurred. Deep palpation with the fingertips over the intercostal regions overlying the heart may elicit a painful response in conditions such as endocarditis, pleuritis, traumatic reticuloperitonitis, and rib fractures.

As in other species, bovine heart murmurs are classified based on intensity and timing. Intensity may be ranked subjectively on a 1 to 6 basis, with 1 of 6 being a faint, barely detectable murmur; 2 of 6 as soft but easily discernable; 3 of 6 as low to moderate intensity; 4 of 6 moderate but lacking a thrill; 5 of 6 loud with palpable thrill; and 6 of 6 so loud that it can be heard with the stethoscope off the chest and evincing a palpable thrill. Classification relative to timing of the cardiac cycle further defines murmurs as systolic, diastolic, or continuous. Further division is provided by terms such as "early systolic" or "holosystolic." In general, systolic murmurs in cattle reflect AV valve insufficiency or, much less commonly, aortic or pulmonic stenosis, whereas diastolic murmurs reflect aortic or pulmonic valve insufficiency or rarely AV valve abnormalities. Benign systolic murmurs occasionally are heard in excited, tachycardiac calves or cows with anemia, hypoproteinemia, or in those being given rapid intravenous (IV) infusions of balanced fluids. Pathologic systolic murmurs most commonly are found in calves with congenital heart abnormalities such as ventricular septal defect or tetralogy of Fallot and in adult cows with endocarditis. Continuous murmurs are rare but may be encountered in calves having a patent ductus arteriosus or in cows with pericarditis. The point of maximal intensity for each cardiac murmur may add subjective data as to the valve involved in the cardiac abnormality.

Arrhythmias may be benign, pathologic, or secondary to metabolic disturbances in cattle. Sinus bradycardia and arrhythmia have been confirmed in cattle held off feed, in hypercalcemic adult cattle, and in hypoglycemic or hyperkalemic young calves. Sinus tachycardia may result from excitement, pain, hypocalcemia, and various systemic states such as endotoxemia and shock. Cattle with severe musculoskeletal pain often have normal heart rates while recumbent but have tachycardia when forced to rise and stand. Persistent tachycardia should be considered abnormal and may reflect cardiac disease unless other systemic conditions coexist.

Hyperkalemia may cause a variety of arrhythmias and is most commonly observed in neonatal calves that develop acute metabolic acidosis associated with secretory diarrhea caused by *Escherichia coli* or acute diffuse white muscle disease. Atrial standstill and other arrhythmias have been documented in diarrheic calves having metabolic acidosis and hyperkalemia. Extreme hyperkalemia (>7.0 mEq/L) may lead to cardiac arrest and should be corrected immediately, especially in calves that may require general anesthesia. Because severe hyperkalemia may be associated with pathologic bradycardias, even without confirmatory blood work, the experienced clinician should be alert to the therapeutic need for fluids that will specifically address hyperkalemia in severely dehydrated, diarrheic calves with discordantly low heart rates for their systemic state. Calves with white muscle disease also may have direct damage to the myocardium, which may be manifested by arrhythmias, murmurs, or frank cardiac arrest. Hypokalemia and hypochloremia in cattle with metabolic alkalosis may predispose to the most common arrhythmia of adult cattle—atrial fibrillation.

Hypocalcemia may be present or contribute to cattle having abdominal disorders that lead to metabolic alkalosis. Metabolic alkalosis may be a factor that triggers atrial fibrillation in cattle with normal hearts. Atrial fibrillation causes an *irregularly* irregular rhythm, with a rate that may be normal or increased (88 to 140 beats/min), depending on the presence of heart disease or the underlying predisposing condition. Atrial fibrillation is associated with irregular intensity of heart sounds. A pulse deficit may be present in any cow with a rapid or irregular cardiac rhythm, especially when the rate exceeds 120 beats/min. Atrial premature complexes (APC) may also occur in cows with gastrointestinal disease and electrolyte abnormalities. APC may preceed or immediately follow atrial fibrillation in some cows. Variation in intensity of the first heart sound during auscultation is characteristic of APC.

Other causes of arrhythmia in adult cattle include sporadic cases of lymphosarcoma with significant myocardial infiltration often causing atrial fibrillation, and ventricular or atrial arrhythmias associated with septic or toxic myocarditis. IV administration of calcium solutions is the major drug-related cause of arrhythmias in cattle, but intravenous administration of antibiotics or potassium-rich fluids occasionally prompts transient arrhythmias.

Sounds ausculted in pericarditis patients are variable, often confused with murmurs, and tend to change on a daily basis if affected cattle are available for daily re-evaluation. Classic pericardial "friction" rubs occur at different stages of each cardiac cycle unlike murmurs, which tend to occur at a distinct phase of each cardiac cycle. Squeaky sounds, often similar to that made in compression of a wet sponge, may be heard as a result of pericardial disease. Rubs caused by contact between fibrin on the visceral and parietal pericardium also may be heard. The heart sounds tend to be muffled, and either free fluid or fluid-gas interfaces may lead to splashing or tinkling sounds or to complete muffling of all sounds. During the acute phase of traumatic reticulopericarditis, the character of the sounds tends to change each day. In those with subacute or chronic disease, muffling of the heart sounds or distinct tinkling or splashing tends to be consistently present.

Presence of an arrhythmia or murmur alerts the examiner that the heart may be abnormal. However, heart failure may or may not be present. In cattle, right heart failure is more common than left heart failure. The general signs of right heart failure include:
1. Ventral edema—the edema may be diffuse or limited to specific regions such as the submandibular area, brisket, ventral abdomen, udder or sheath, and the lower limbs (Figure 3-2)
2. Jugular and mammary vein distention with or without pulsations
3. Exercise intolerance with or without dyspnea
4. Persistent tachycardia
5. Ascites with or without pleural fluid

In addition to the general signs, specific cardiac signs such as a murmur, arrhythmia, or abnormal intensity of heart sounds usually are present and contribute to the diagnosis. Probably the most difficult set of differential diagnoses involves diseases that result in hypoproteinemia. Hypoproteinemia also causes ventral edema and may cause exercise intolerance and tachycardia. However, hypoproteinemia would not cause jugular and mammary vein distention and pulsation.

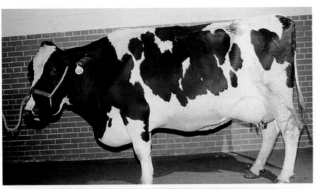

Figure 3-2

Submandibular, brisket, ventral, and udder edema in a cow in right heart failure caused by pericarditis.

Therefore venous distention and pulsation coupled with abnormal heart sounds or rhythm are the key signs when diagnosing heart failure in dairy cattle.

Left heart failure causes dyspnea, pulmonary edema, and exercise intolerance and may lead to cyanosis and collapse or syncope. Specific left heart failure seldom occurs in cattle, but left side failure combined with worsening, antecedent right heart failure may develop as the animal progresses into fulminant congestive heart failure.

Ancillary Procedures

Electrocardiography

The electrocardiogram (ECG) is essential for definitive categorization of arrhythmias in cattle. Vector analysis of ECG tracings to determine cardiac chamber enlargements and other pathology seldom is used in cattle because ventricular myocardial depolarization tends to be rapid and diffuse rather than organized, as in some other species. ECG is also indicated when cattle have variation in heart sound intensity, require monitoring for anesthesia or treatment of cardiac arrhythmias, or show signs of heart failure. Cardiac ultrasound, however, has superseded the ECG as a diagnostic tool in determining chamber enlargement and other cardiac pathology.

The base-apex lead system is most commonly used in cattle. The base-apex lead system results in an ECG with large wave amplitude and is sufficient for evaluating most arrhythmias. The positive electrode is placed on the skin over the left fifth intercostal space at the level of the elbow; the negative electrode is placed on the skin over the right jugular furrow roughly 30 cm from the thoracic inlet; and the ground electrode is attached to the neck or withers. The resultant ECG recorded through the base-apex lead system has a positive P wave with a single peak, a QRS complex with an initial positive deflection followed by a large negative

deflection, and a variable (positive or negative) T wave (Figure 3-3, *A* to *C*).

Echocardiography

Two-dimensional echocardiography and Doppler echocardiography have greatly enhanced our ability to assess cardiac function and visualize anatomic variations and pathologic lesions in cattle. Valvular, myocardial, pericardial, congenital, and acquired lesions can be visualized in real time, measured, and monitored. Qualitative and quantitative assessment of the impact of congenital anomalies and monitoring treatment response of endocarditis, pericarditis, or other myocardial lesions are possible with the appropriate equipment and people trained to conduct and interpret a systematic cardiac examination. In short, echocardiography is now an essential component of a cardiology workup. Sector scanners utilizing a 3.5-mHz (or lower) transducer are most useful for adult cattle. A 5.0-mHz transducer may be helpful when evaluating neonatal calves suspected of having congenital anomalies or other cardiac conditions. Although some clinicians may lack the equipment or expertise with echocardiography, current graduates are being trained in the technique, and continued competition among manufacturers may allow more

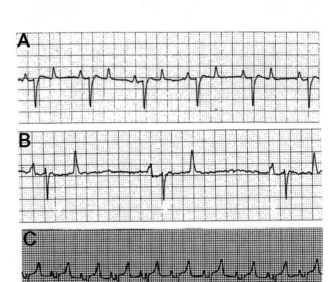

Figure 3-3

A, Normal sinus rhythm with a heart rate of 60 beats/min recorded from a 4-year-old Holstein cow. **B,** Sinus bradycardia with heart rate of 36 beats/min recorded from a 6-year-old Brown Swiss cow sick with abomasal ulcers. **C,** Sinus tachycardia with heart rate of 108 beats/min recorded from a 2-year-old Holstein with an acute leg injury.

veterinarians to own this equipment. In any event, referral for echocardiography is indicated for valuable cattle whenever cardiac disease is apparent but a specific diagnosis is lacking. In most cattle, a systematic examination can be conducted from the right parasternal window to provide a long axis four-chamber view of the heart, a long axis view of the left ventricular outflow tract, and a short axis view of the left ventricle just ventral to the mitral valve and at the papillary muscle level. From the same window, all four heart valves can be visualized, chamber sizes can be measured, myocardial functional measurements can be made, and abnormalities of the pericardium can be seen. Congenital lesions like ventricular septal defect (VSD) (Figure 3-4) and acquired pericarditis (Figure 3-5) are easily visualized by echocardiogram.

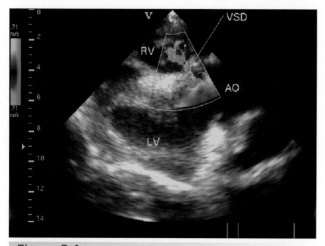

Figure 3-4

Echocardiogram of heifer calf with congenital ventricular septal defect.

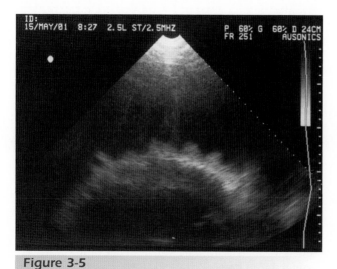

Figure 3-5

Echocardiogram of adult dairy cow with traumatic reticulopericarditis.

SPECIFIC CARDIAC DISEASES IN CALVES

White Muscle Disease

Myocardial damage from vitamin E and selenium deficiency may occur at any site in the heart and may be focal, multifocal, or diffuse (Figure 3-6). Signs may develop at any time from birth to 4 years of age but are more common in calves less than 3 months of age. Specific cardiac signs are variable and include arrhythmias, murmurs, exercise intolerance, cyanosis, dyspnea, congestive heart failure signs, and acute death. Signs may be subtle or dramatic, depending on the magnitude and locations of myocardial damage. Sudden death can occur spontaneously or following exercise or restraint. Other signs of white muscle disease such as stiffness, difficulty in prehension or swallowing, inhalation pneumonia, and myoglobinuria may or may not be present. Dyspnea may be directly related to the cardiac lesions or may be caused by Zenker's degeneration in the diaphragm or intercostal muscles. Tachycardia (>120 beats/min) and arrhythmias are the most common specific cardiac signs, but murmurs may be present as well.

Diagnosis can be confirmed by measuring blood selenium values, urine dipstick testing to look for positive "blood" (myoglobin) and protein, and serum biochemistry to evaluate creatine kinase (CK) and aspartate aminotransferase (AST) enzymes. If the heart is the only muscle involved, serum enzymes may not be greatly elevated; however, the heart seldom is the only area involved.

Treatment should be instituted immediately with vitamin E and selenium injected at the manufacturer's recommended dosage. Although some commercial preparations include label instructions that include IV use, it is suggested that vitamin E/selenium be given intramuscularly (IM) or subcutaneously to avoid the occasional

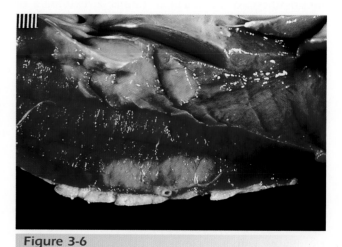

Figure 3-6

A pale focal area of Zenker's degeneration of myocardium from a calf that died of diffuse white muscle disease.

life-threatening anaphylactic-type reaction seen with these products. The calf should be kept in a small box stall, straw bale enclosure, or hutch, so it can move about but not run freely, lest further muscle damage be precipitated. If pulmonary edema is present, furosemide (0.5 to 1.0 mg/kg) may be given once or twice daily. Concurrent aspiration pneumonia would require intense antibiotic therapy. Vitamin E and selenium injections are repeated at 72-hour intervals for three or four total treatments. Herd selenium status and preventive measures to address the problem should be discussed. Calves that survive for 3 days following diagnosis have a good prognosis.

Hyperkalemia

Cardiac arrhythmias or bradycardia associated with hyperkalemia is primarily observed in neonates having severely *acute* diarrhea. Enterotoxigenic *E. coli* causing secretory diarrhea, metabolic acidosis, low plasma bicarbonate values, and hyperkalemia appears to be the most common causative organism. Rotavirus or coronavirus also may be involved in calf diarrhea, but they seldom produce as profound a metabolic acidosis as *E. coli*.

Less common causes of hyperkalemia include severe diffuse white muscle disease involving heavy musculature of the limbs, ruptured bladders, renal failure, urinary obstructions, and nonspecific shock.

Hyperkalemia reduces the resting membrane potential, which initially makes cells more excitable, but gradually (with further elevation in potassium and further reduction in resting membrane potential) the cells become less excitable. Atrial myocytes seem more sensitive to these effects than those within the ventricles. Cardiac conduction is affected, and several characteristic ECG findings evolve in a typical sequence that correlates well with increasing K^+ values: ECG changes include peaking of the T wave, shortening and widening of the P wave, prolongation of the PR interval, eventual disappearance of the P wave, widening of the QRS complex, and irregular R-R intervals (Figure 3-7). Atrial standstill characterized by bradycardia and absence of P waves may occur and has been documented in association with hyperkalemia in diarrheic calves. Further progression may lead to AV block, escape beats, ventricular fibrillation, asystole, and death.

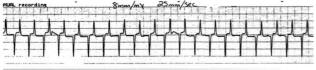

Figure 3-7

Base-apex lead ECG recording in a calf with a K of 8.6 mEq/L; despite the tachycardia of 130 beats/min, the peaked T waves and flattening of the P waves is very apparent.

In neonates, hypoglycemia is the major differential diagnosis when bradycardia is present. Septic myocarditis or white muscle disease also may be considered if an arrhythmia is present.

Calves less than 2 weeks of age that have developed acute diarrhea, are recumbent, dehydrated, and have bradycardia or arrhythmia should be suspected of being hyperkalemic. Obviously only an acid-base and electrolyte analysis of blood and an ECG can confirm this. However, these may not be available in the field. The consequences of underestimating the life-threatening importance of the heart and K^+ relationship in these patients are severe.

Calves suspected to be hyperkalemic based on history, physical signs, and arrhythmia or bradycardia should receive alkalinizing fluids and dextrose. Being neonates, hypoglycemia may contribute to bradycardia when this sign is present. One way to treat metabolic acidosis and hyperkalemia is by IV infusions of 5% dextrose solution containing 150 mEq $NaHCO_3$/L. Usually 1 to 3 L is necessary, depending on the magnitude of the metabolic acidosis and bicarbonate deficit. Glucose and bicarbonate help transport K^+ back into cells, and the glucose also treats or prevents potential hypoglycemia. Once the acute crisis has been resolved, the calf may be safely treated with balanced electrolyte solutions containing potassium. Calves with diarrhea, despite having plasma hyperkalemia, have total body potassium deficits and require potassium supplementation. This may be true even in the acute phase of disease, but when serum K^+ is 5.0 to 8.0 mEq/L there is no time to worry about a "total body potassium deficit." We have treated hundreds of calves as suggested above, and those with a venous blood pH of 7.0 or greater have a good to excellent prognosis unless they have had failure of passive transfer of immunoglobulins and subsequent septicemia. Specific insulin therapy as an adjunct to bicarbonate and glucose to correct hyperkalemia is not necessary in calves.

Congenital Heart Disease

Virtually all types of congenital cardiac anomalies occur in cattle. Most congenital anomalies appear to be sporadic, but inheritance may play a part in some of the most common anomalies. The most common congenital anomalies in cattle appear to be VSDs (Figure 3-8), tetralogy of Fallot, atrial septal defects, and transpositions of great vessels.

Most congenital cardiac defects cause distinct murmurs. Calves affected with the most common defects such as VSDs, atrial septal defects, tetralogy of Fallot, or aortic or pulmonic stenosis usually have systolic murmurs. Patent ductus arteriosus, which is rare as a single defect in calves, can cause a systolic or continuous murmur.

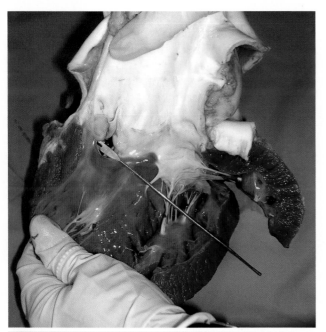

Figure 3-8

Image obtained at necropsy of a calf with VSD.

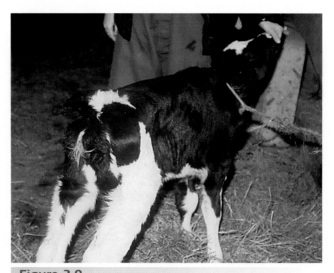

Figure 3-9

Congenital absence of the tail in a 1-day-old Holstein heifer that also had a VSD.

Most calves with congenital cardiac defects appear normal at birth but eventually are noticed to have dyspnea, poor growth, or both. Many calves with congenital heart defects are eventually examined by a veterinarian because of persistent or recurrent respiratory signs or generalized ill thrift. The respiratory signs may be real in the form of pulmonary edema associated with heart failure and shunts or be caused by opportunistic bacterial pneumonia secondary to pulmonary edema and compromise of lower airway defense mechanisms. The owners may already have treated the calf one or more times for coughing, dyspnea, and fever, only to have the signs recur. Usually only one calf is affected, thus making enzootic pneumonia an unlikely diagnosis. Regardless of whether pulmonary edema or pneumonia plus pulmonary edema are present, veterinary examination usually detects the cardiac murmur that allows diagnosis. Venous pulsation and distention of the jugular veins may be present, but calves seldom show ventral edema as distinctly as adult cattle with heart failure.

Calves with congenital heart defects that do not develop respiratory signs usually show stunting compared with herdmates of matched age. The degree of stunting varies directly with the severity of the congenital lesions in regard to blood oxygenation but usually becomes apparent by 6 months of age and is very dramatic in calves that survive to yearlings. Some cattle with small defects survive and thrive as adults, but this is rare.

VSDs are the most common defects in dairy calves and are found in all breeds. In Guernseys and Holsteins, VSD may be linked to ocular and tail anomalies. Microphthalmos and tail defects, including absence of

tail, wry tail, or short tail, frequently signal VSD (Figure 3-9). Sometimes ocular, tail, and cardiac defects all are present in the same calf, but it is more common to find tail or ocular pathology plus VSD. Depending on the size of the VSD, affected calves have a variable life span. Prognosis for most is hopeless because of eventual respiratory difficulty and stunting. However, calves do, in rare instances, survive to productive adult states. The genetics of these multiple defects (eye, tail, and heart) have not been investigated in Holsteins but have been assumed to be a simple recessive trait in Guernseys.

Tetralogy of Fallot and other multiple congenital defects that allow right to left shunting of blood provoke marked exercise intolerance, cyanosis, and dyspnea and may lead to polycythemia secondary to hypoxia. Prognosis for long-term survival is grave in these calves. Ectopia cordis in a calf creates a dramatic sight, with the heart beating under the skin in the neck, but is *extremely* rare.

SPECIFIC CARDIAC DISEASES IN ADULT CATTLE

Neoplasia

The heart is one of the common target sites of lymphosarcoma in adult dairy cattle. Many cattle with multicentric lymphosarcoma have cardiac infiltration based on gross or histologic pathology, but fewer of these cattle have clinically detectable cardiac disease. When the heart is a major target site, cardiac abnormalities are more obvious. The heart seldom is the only organ affected with lymphosarcoma. Therefore detection of cardiac abnormalities coupled with other suspicious lesions (e.g., enlarged peripheral lymph nodes, exophthalmos, melena, and paresis) simply helps to make a lymphosarcoma diagnosis more definite.

Depending on the anatomic location and magnitude of the tumors, cattle with cardiac lymphosarcoma may have arrhythmias, murmurs, jugular venous distention, jugular venous pulsations, or muffling caused by diffuse cardiac or pericardial involvement. Muffling and splashing sounds are possible if a pericardial transudate or exudate is present. The most common site of tumor involvement is the right atrium, but nodular or infiltrative tumors can be found anywhere in the myocardium or pericardium (Figure 3-10). The color and consistency of the tumors may vary. Mediastinal lymph nodes also are commonly involved. Cattle with signs of heart disease should be thoroughly examined for other lesions consistent with lymphosarcoma. When multiple lesions exist, the diagnosis is easy. However, cattle examined because of vague signs such as hypophagia and decreased milk production that are found to have tachycardia or other cardiac abnormalities can present diagnostic challenges. Although ECG and thoracic radiographs have seldom helped make a definitive diagnosis, ultrasound may be very helpful to image nodular or large masses of lymphosarcoma. Thoracocentesis and pericardiocentesis to obtain fluid for cytologic evaluation are the most helpful ancillary aids when cardiac lymphosarcoma is suspected. A complete blood count (CBC) and assessment of bovine leukemia virus (BLV) antibody status are indicated, but a positive BLV agar gel immunodiffusion (AGID) or radioimmunoassay (RIA) test does not ensure an absolute diagnosis because most positive cattle never develop tumors (see the section on Lymphosarcoma in Chapter 15). Therefore simply assuming a cow with a positive BLV test and heart abnormality detected on physical examination

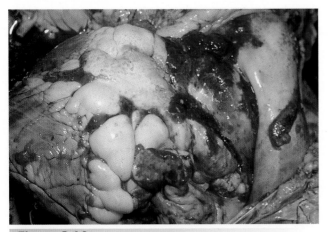

Figure 3-10

Lymphosarcoma in the heart of a cow that died as a result of multicentric lymphosarcoma. Multifocal areas of yellow-red friable tumor infiltrate are present scattered over the epicardium, great vessels, and right atrium.

has lymphosarcoma may be an incorrect assumption. A double line-positive BLV-AGID may add further weight to the suspected diagnosis, as would the finding of a persistent lymphocytosis in a set of CBC results. Clinical identification of masses in other locations or cytology from thoracocentesis or pericardiocentesis provides the best means of definitive diagnosis.

Fever usually is absent in cattle with cardiac lymphosarcoma. Occasional cattle with large tumor masses in the thorax or abdomen may have fever because of tumor necrosis or nonspecific pyrogens produced by neoplasms. Secondary bacterial infections of the lungs or other body systems also may lead to fever, which confuses the diagnosis.

Prognosis is hopeless for cattle with cardiac lymphosarcoma, and most cattle with the disease die from cardiac or multisystemic disease within a few weeks to a few months. Successful attempts at chemotherapy have not been reported to our knowledge. One author has successfully prolonged life up to 6 months in a few cattle with cardiac lymphosarcoma that had significant pericardial fluid accumulations by intermittent pericardial drainage. Occasionally valuable cattle may justify such treatment to allow a pregnancy to be completed or to be superovulated. However, as with many catabolic conditions, owners should be cautioned that maintaining the dam with advanced heart disease for more than a few weeks may produce a gestationally dysmature fetus even if the pregnancy is carried to term, or may seriously affect the cow's ability to superovulate or even produce viable oocytes for in vitro fertilization. There is also the risk of vertical transmission of BLV from dam to fetus in utero, which is greater should the dam have clinically apparent tumors. In one late pregnant cow with severe pericardial effusion caused by lymphosarcoma, we were able to maintain the cow for several weeks by surgically opening the pericardial sac into the pleural cavity, which significantly improved venous return to the heart and the overall condition of the cow. The cow was also treated with isoflupredone.

Neurofibroma, although uncommon, frequently causes arrhythmia and variable intensity of heart sound in affected cattle and bulls. Further the cardiac arrhythmia may coexist with paresis or paralysis caused by neurofibroma masses in the spinal canal. Because lymphosarcoma more commonly causes paresis coupled with cardiac disease, this combination of signs is most suggestive that lymphosarcoma is present. Although perhaps a moot point because both diseases are fatal, further medical workup of neurofibroma patients fails to provide confirmation of lymphosarcoma. To date, postmortem examination has been the only means of definitive diagnosis for cardiac neurofibroma. Examiners talented in ultrasound may be able to diagnose these lesions based on the typically gnarled, raised cords of tumor involving the cardiac nerves.

Myocardial Disease

Infections

Septic Myocarditis. Neonatal septicemia caused by gram-negative bacterial organisms, acute infection with *Histophilus somni,* and chronic infections in any age of cattle resulting from *Arcanobacterium pyogenes* are the most common cause of septic myocardial lesions in cattle. Septicemic calves, calves suspected of having *H. somni* infection, or calves with chronic infections should be suspected of having septic myocarditis if an arrhythmia or other signs of abnormal cardiac function develop during their illness. White muscle disease, hyperkalemia, and hypoglycemia should be considered. Septicemic calves have a guarded prognosis, and septic myocarditis worsens it. Septic myocarditis foci in adult cattle with chronic, active infection or abscesses associated with mastitis, localized peritonitis, foot lesions, or chronic pneumonia are more commonly identified by pathologists than clinicians. Although tachycardia is likely to be present, this finding often is assumed to result from the primary illness rather than from myocarditis. As with calves, adult cattle with septic myocarditis may have paroxysmal cardiac arrhythmias that alert the clinician to the diagnosis. Definitive diagnosis has been difficult in the living patient because test for cardiac muscle enzymes may lack specificity for cardiac muscles. Increased concentration of troponin I may be used to help diagnose myocardial disease. An ECG showing atrial or ventricular premature depolarizations in a calf or cow with evidence of sepsis or a walled-off infection can be used to lend credence to the diagnosis.

Treatment of the primary disease remains the most important part of managing septic myocarditis. If the primary problem and myocardial lesion can be sterilized, the heart may return to normal function.

Septic myocardial disease of adult cattle, as in calves, usually follows septicemia or chronic infections. Septicemic spread of infectious organisms, thrombi, or mediators of inflammation may be involved in the pathophysiology of myocardial injury that occurs in septic cattle. Although relatively uncommon, development of persistent tachycardia with or without an arrhythmia in a patient with infectious disease may suggest myocarditis. Tachycardia is so nonspecific that most examiners attribute the tachycardia to the primary disease rather than secondary myocarditis. Only when the myocardial damage causes signs of heart failure does a diagnosis of myocarditis become easier. Acute death is possible. Arrhythmia, if present, must be assessed using ECG and blood electrolytes and acid-base status to rule out atrial fibrillation associated with metabolic abnormalities. Dairy cattle are most at risk for myocarditis with acute septic diseases such as severe mastitis, metritis, pneumonia, and infection caused by *H. somni.* Occasional cases also occur secondary to chronic localized infections such as digital abscesses that predispose to bacteremia. Depending on the size and location of the myocardial lesion, clinical signs range from subclinical to overt heart failure. ECG evidence of ventricular arrhythmias would suggest myocardial damage, but supraventricular arrhythmias are possible as well. Unfortunately definitive premortem diagnosis is impossible without advanced echocardiographic or invasive cardiac technique. Treatment must be directed at the primary disease. Minor myocardial lesions away from nodal and conduction tissue may heal or fibrose asymptomatically, whereas large or multifocal lesions may lead to heart failure, persistent tachyarrhythmia, or sudden death.

Toxins

Ionophores such as monensin and lasolocid are capable of damaging myocardial and skeletal muscle when ingested in toxic amounts. Improper mixing of ionophores into rations is the most common error that may lead to toxicity, but accidental exposure to concentrated products also is possible. Obviously this is a potential concern for calves and heifers being fed milk replacer or feeds containing ionophores. Fortunately cattle are much more resistant to the toxic effects of ionophores than are horses, but there is a narrow margin of safety, especially in young calves.

Many poisonous plants are theoretically capable of myocardial injury, but in reality few are likely because of increased confinement of heifers and adult cattle. *Eupatorium rugosum* (white snakeroot), *Vicia villosa* (hairy vetch), *Cassia occidentalis* (coffee senna), *Phalaris* sp., and others are capable of toxic myocardial damage. Gossypol also is capable of causing myocardial damage when fed in toxic amounts. This fact is of special concern given the increased incidence of feeding cottonseed to dairy cattle. Copper deficiency, especially when chronic, occasionally has been linked to acute myocardial lesions, resulting in death ("Falling disease" in Australia). Many other organic and inorganic toxins have the potential for causing myocardial damage but create more obvious pathology in other body systems and thus will not be discussed here.

No specific treatment is available for toxic myocarditis. Common sense dictates identification and removal of the toxin from the environment, alongside immediate administration of laxatives, cathartics, and/or protectants to decrease absorption and accelerate intestinal transit. Vitamin E and selenium administration and specific supportive treatment for cardiac disease should be instituted, but the prognosis for animals already with congestive heart failure is grave.

Parasitic and Protozoan Infections

Cysticerca bovis may cause myocardial lesions, but these appear rarely in dairy cattle in the northeastern United States. This is the larval form of *Taenia saginata,* the common human tapeworm. Contamination by human sewage of feedstuffs, pastures, or fields puts cows at risk for this disease.

Although *Toxoplasma gondii* is capable of infecting cattle, the clinical disease appears rare because cattle rapidly eliminate parasites from tissue. Cattle are exposed to and infected by *T. gondii* via ingestion of feedstuffs contaminated by cat feces.

Sarcocystis sp. is a common cause of myocardial disease in cattle. Although most infestations are asymptomatic, clinical illness characterized by hemolysis, myopathy, myocarditis, weight loss, rattail, and other signs is possible. *Sarcocystis* sp. requires two hosts, and carnivores or humans usually are the hosts that shed sporocysts in fecal material that subsequently contaminates cattle feed (see Chapter 15). Cattle then become the intermediate host as intermediate stages of the parasite invade endothelial cells and later stages encyst in muscle—including the myocardium. Subsequent ingestion by carnivores of beef containing cysts continues the cycle.

Histopathologic identification of sarcocystis cysts in myocardium of cattle is very common but seldom deemed significant. Certainly, however, heavy exposure to the organism could provoke significant myocardial damage.

Parasitic or protozoan myocarditis usually requires histopathology or serology for diagnosis. Treatment would be best provided by preventive measures to avoid contamination of cattle feeds by carnivore or human feces.

Inherited Myocardial Disease

A dilated cardiomyopathy has been described in Canadian Holstein-Friesians. This condition appears in Canadian black and white Holsteins and expresses itself as heart disease between 19 and 78 months of age. Although most cattle develop clinical signs within 4 years of birth, some have lived for 6 to 7 years.

Most cases are presented because of signs referable to heart failure such as ventral edema, exercise intolerance, inappetence, dyspnea, tachycardia, muffled heart sounds, and jugular and mammary vein distention and pulsation. Although tachycardia is fairly consistent, other auscultation findings such as arrhythmias, murmurs, or varying intensity of the heart sounds vary in each case. Hepatomegaly consistent with chronic passive congestion of the liver secondary to right heart failure also was present in some patients.

Echocardiography and ECG recordings are required for diagnosis. Ultrasound is the best aid to confirm dilated cardiomyopathy.

Long-term prognosis is hopeless, but affected cattle may be helped in the short term by management with cardioglycosides, and furosemide is indicated if pulmonary edema exists. McGuirk suggests digoxin

at 0.86 μg/kg/hr as an IV infusion. This obviously requires diligence, IV catheterization, and hospitalization, or else a very attentive owner. Alternatively, 3.4 μg/kg IV every 4 hours may be utilized but creates greater variation in blood levels and increases the risk of digoxin toxicity. Furosemide is used at 0.5 to 1.0 mg/kg twice daily if pulmonary edema is present. Inappetent cattle may benefit from 50 to 100 g KCl orally each day to maintain potassium levels when being treated with digoxin. Ideally daily or every other day blood acid-base and electrolyte status should be assessed.

Endocarditis

Etiology

Bacterial endocarditis is the most common valvular disease or endocardial disease in adult dairy cattle. It also is one of the few treatable heart conditions of cattle. Therefore early suspicion, diagnosis, and appropriate treatment improve the prognosis.

Cattle with chronic infections such as septic musculoskeletal conditions, hardware disease, abscesses, lactic acid indigestion, chronic pneumonia, metritis or mastitis, and thrombophlebitis are at risk for bacterial endocarditis. In addition, cattle with long-term IV catheters have increased risk of endocardial infections. Bacteremia appears essential to the pathophysiology of bacterial endocarditis in cattle.

A. pyogenes is the most common organism isolated from the blood and endocardial lesions of cattle affected with endocarditis, but *Streptococcus* sp., *Staphylococcus* sp., and gram-negative organisms may also cause the disease. The right AV valve (tricuspid) is the most commonly infected valve with the left AV (mitral) being the second most common (Figure 3-11). Other valves or the endocardium adjacent to valves may also occasionally be the site of infection (Figure 3-12). Owner complaints regarding affected cattle include recurrent fever,

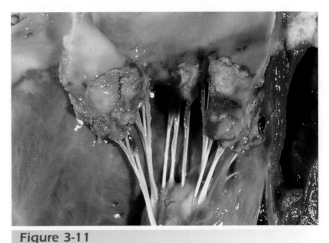

Figure 3-11

Bacterial valvular endocarditis with vegetative lesions in a cow. *(Photo courtesy Dr. John M. King.)*

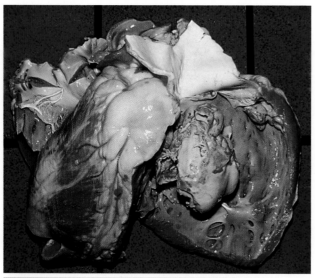

Figure 3-12

Large vegetative endocarditis lesion involving the valves and adjacent endocardium in the ventricle. *(Photo courtesy Dr. John M. King.)*

weight loss, anorexia, poor production, and sometimes lameness.

Signs

Persistent or intermittent fever, tachycardia, and a systolic heart murmur are the most common signs found in cattle having endocarditis. A "pounding" heart or increased intensity of heart sounds also is common, although the heart sounds may vary in intensity or even be reduced in some patients. Vegetative endocarditis may also occur in the absence of an auscultable murmur.

Some cattle with endocarditis appear painful when digital pressure is exerted on the chest wall over the heart region. Fever usually is present, has been present historically, or develops intermittently following initial examination. Some cattle with endocarditis never have fever recorded but do show other signs of illness and a systolic heart murmur or other cardiac signs.

Signs of heart failure may develop along with increased distention and pulsations of the jugular and mammary veins. Tachycardia is a consistent finding, and dyspnea may develop, especially after bacterial showering of the lungs. Arrhythmias are unusual and paroxysmal but may be observed in approximately 10% of patients.

Lameness, often shifting, and stiffness may be observed. Synovitis and joint tenderness sometimes are obvious, but in other patients exact localization of the lameness is difficult. Bacteremia to joints or epiphyses and immune-mediated synovitis have been suggested as origins of this lameness in endocarditis patients.

Laboratory Data

Nonregenerative anemia commonly results from chronicity of the primary infection, the endocardial infection, or both. Neutrophilia is common and was found in 24 of 31 cases in one report, whereas absolute leukocytosis was found in 14 of 31. In this same report, serum globulin values were greater than 5.0 g/dl in 19 of 23 endocarditis patients that had globulin measured. Elevated globulin was believed to be consistent with the chronicity of infection.

Blood cultures are an important diagnostic test, but echocardiography provides the definitive diagnosis. A patient suspected of having endocarditis should have a series of blood cultures submitted rather than a single time-point sample. Although blood cultures in adult cattle may be negative in as many as 50% of endocarditis patients tested, isolating the causative organism from the bloodstream provides the best opportunity for appropriate and successful treatment with a specific antibiotic. Venous blood cultures should be collected after the jugular vein has been clipped and prepared aseptically. The cow should have been held off systemic antibiotics for 24 to 48 hours before culture attempts, if possible. Although one blood culture attempt is better than none, it is preferable to obtain a series of three to four cultures when economics allow. The interval between collections of multiple samples has been debated by clinicians for decades. Some clinicians culture only during a fever spike, some at 3- to 30-minute intervals, some at 6- to 8-hour intervals, and some once daily. We prefer to obtain three cultures at 30-minute intervals in febrile patients and intervals of several hours in nonfebrile patients suspected of having endocarditis.

Diagnosis

Early signs of reduced appetite and production, fever, and tachycardia certainly are not specific for endocarditis. A pounding heart or systolic murmur should suggest the diagnosis and dictate further workup. Diagnosis may be overlooked because of more obvious primary problems such as abscesses, infected digit or other musculoskeletal infection, suspected hardware disease, or thrombophlebitis because these conditions may also cause fever and nonspecific signs of illness. Therefore heart murmurs, a pounding heart, or early signs of heart failure in addition to tachycardia merit consideration of a diagnosis of endocarditis. Lameness and stiffness may be difficult to differentiate from primary musculoskeletal disease or painful stance caused by peritonitis but can be important clinical signs that aid diagnosis. Because of fever, tachycardia, and sometimes polypnea, cattle having endocarditis often are misdiagnosed with pneumonia or traumatic reticuloperitonitis.

Diagnosis of endocarditis usually is based on the patient's history and clinical signs. However, a positive blood culture and echocardiography allow definitive

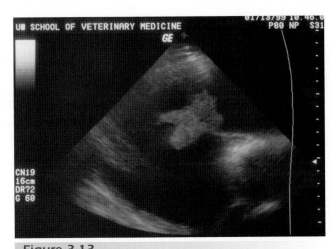

Figure 3-13

Echocardiographic image of endocarditis of the tricuspid valve of a cow.

diagnosis. Blood cultures, as mentioned previously, may or may not be successful; however, when positive, they allow appropriate selection of antibiotics. Definitive diagnosis based on two-dimensional echocardiography has proven to be one of the most impressive uses of ultrasound since its widespread use in diagnostics began 10 years ago. Veterinarians trained in echocardiography now have a tool to confirm bacterial endocarditis in most patients (Figure 3-13).

Treatment

Long-term antibiotic therapy is required to cure bacterial endocarditis in cattle. Thus cattle selected for treatment must be deemed valuable enough to justify the cost of antibiotics and discarded milk that will be incurred. A successful blood culture allows selection of an appropriate antibiotic based on sensitivity or mean inhibitory concentration (MIC) values. Because endocarditis in cattle usually is caused by *A. pyogenes* or *Streptococcus* sp., some clinicians assume penicillin will work and do not bother to do blood cultures. This assumption would be a worthwhile gamble if economics dictate that laboratory costs be minimized.

Therefore penicillin and ampicillin are the drugs of choice for bacterial endocarditis in cattle caused by *A. pyogenes* and most *Streptococcus* sp. Although ceftiofur currently has the advantage of "no withdrawal," it is more expensive and has been overused and abused by clinicians who hope the drug will cure all infections of dairy cattle. Penicillin (22,000 to 33,000 IU/kg twice daily) or ampicillin (10 to 20 mg/kg twice daily) is administered for a minimum of 3 weeks. If gram-negative organisms or penicillin-resistant gram-positive organisms are isolated from blood cultures, an appropriate bactericidal antibiotic should be selected based on MIC or antibiotic sensitivity testing.

Based on work by Dr. Ray Sweeney and others at the University of Pennsylvania, rifampin (rifamycin) has been shown to establish therapeutic blood levels after oral administration to ruminants. Unfortunately there is significant variability in blood levels between treated cattle, which may limit its treatment potential. Rifampin is a unique antibiotic that gains access to intracellular organisms or walled-off infections by concentrating in macrophages. Rifampin always should be used in conjunction with another antibiotic because bacterial resistance may develop quickly when the drug is used alone. The dosage is 5 mg/kg orally, twice daily for cattle. Although some maintain this dosage is too low, it has seemed effective clinically when used in conjunction with penicillin not only for chronic *A. pyogenes* endocarditis but also for pulmonary abscesses. Therefore if economics allow, oral rifampin has been reported to improve treatment success in cattle with bacterial endocarditis.

Occasionally cattle will become significantly anorectic while receiving rifampin (more so than was noted in association with the primary disease), but in many cases this apparent intolerance to the drug is overcome if administration is discontinued for several days and then reinstituted at the same or lesser dose.

In addition to antibiotic therapy, those cattle showing venous distention, ventral edema, or pulmonary edema require judicious dosages of furosemide. Because many endocarditis patients have reduced or poor appetites, overuse of furosemide may lead to electrolyte depletion (K^+, Ca^{++}) and dehydration. Therefore when furosemide is used, the drug should be administered on an "as-needed" basis, and 0.5 mg/kg once or twice daily usually is sufficient.

Because cattle with endocarditis often appear painful or stiff and may have either primary musculoskeletal disorders or secondary shifting lameness, aspirin is administered at 240 to 480 grains orally twice daily. Unfortunately aspirin does not appear to minimize platelet aggregation and is unlikely to prevent further enlargement of vegetative lesions. Free access to salt should be denied of cattle showing signs of congestive heart failure.

Treatment continues for a minimum of 3 weeks. Positive signs of improvement include increasing appetite and production, as well as absence of fever. The heart murmur persists and may vary as treatment progresses. Resolution of the heart murmur and tachycardia coupled with echocardiographic evidence of resolution of the endocarditis lesions are excellent prognostic signs. Many cows that survive are, however, left with persistent subtle or obvious heart murmurs caused by valvular damage. This should not be a concern as long as other signs indicate resolution of infection and heart failure is not present. Cattle with venous distention, ventral edema, or other signs of right heart failure have a worse prognosis than cattle diagnosed before signs of heart failure. However, mild to moderate signs of heart failure should not be interpreted to mean a hopeless prognosis because supportive treatment may alleviate these signs while antibiotic therapy treats the primary condition.

Prognosis for endocarditis patients is guarded. Sporadic case reports tend to highlight successfully managed individual cases, but further case series are necessary to suggest accurate recovery rates. Of 31 cattle affected with endocarditis that were admitted to our hospital between 1977 and 1982, 9 responded to long-term antibiotic (8 penicillin and 1 tetracycline) therapy. Based on these data and the experience of other clinicians, the prognosis is better when the diagnosis is made early in the course of the disease. Repeated echocardiographic examination allows for monitoring and reassessment of the valvular lesions during and after treatment. With experience and the correct software, ultrasound examination also allows for specific evaluation of cardiac function (e.g., atrial diameter, fractional shortening) that may more accurately assess the degree of cardiac dysfunction and provide valuable prognostic information.

Pericarditis

Etiology

The most common cause of pericarditis in dairy cattle is puncture of the pericardium by a metallic linear foreign body that originated in the reticulum. It is apparent during laparotomy and rumenotomy in cattle that the heart lays very close to the diaphragmatic region of the reticulum. Therefore traumatic reticuloperitonitis occasionally causes septic pericarditis. Hardware that penetrates the reticulum in a cranial direction may puncture the pericardium or impale the myocardium. It can also infect the mediastinum or puncture a lung lobe. Both the foreign body and the tract of its migration can "wick" bacterial contaminants into the pericardial fluid, resulting in fibrinopurulent pericarditis.

Fibrinous pericarditis can also occur in septicemic calves or cattle having severe bacterial bronchopneumonia. This form of pericarditis rarely causes clinically detectable fluid accumulation and seldom leads to overt signs of heart failure as are typical in traumatic pericarditis. Idiopathic hemorrhagic pericardial effusion may also occur in adult cows, causing signs of right heart failure.

Signs

Signs of traumatic pericarditis include venous distention and pulsation, ventral edema, tachycardia, and muffled heart sounds bilaterally (Figure 3-14). Fever is usually, but not always, present. Tachypnea and dyspnea may be present in pericarditis patients with advanced heart failure. Cattle having traumatic pericarditis are

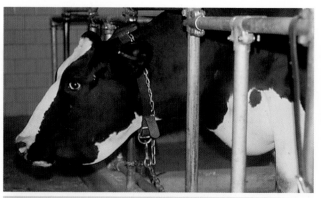

Figure 3-14

Anxious expression and severe ventral edema in a cow with traumatic pericarditis.

often reluctant to move, appear painful, and have abducted elbows.

Direct pressure or percussion in the ventral chest or xiphoid area elicits a painful response by the cow with traumatic pericarditis. Dyspnea is caused by a combination of lung compression by the enlarged pericardial mass, pulmonary edema, and reduced cardiac output. Auscultation of the heart reveals bilateral decreased intensity of the heart sounds. This muffling of heart sounds usually coexists with squeaky, rubbing sounds and splashing or tinkling sounds, but these sounds are not present in all cases. A fluid gas interface created by gas forming bacterial organisms in the pericardium creates the most obvious splashing sounds. Lung sounds may not be heard in the ventral third of either hemithorax because of the greatly enlarged pericardial sac's displacement of the lungs dorsally. In addition to these signs, there are two very important clinical facts associated with traumatic pericarditis in dairy cattle:

1. Most cows with traumatic pericarditis were observed by the owner to be ill 7 to 14 days earlier and may or may not have been diagnosed with traumatic reticuloperitonitis at that time. Frequently the signs of illness were vague and nonspecific, and veterinary attention may or may not have been requested. Typically these cattle improve or appear recovered from this previous illness only to become ill once again and have signs of cardiac disease. Certainly not all cattle have this two-phased clinical course, and some have peracute pericarditis or traumatic myocarditis and die within hours or days. When the history supports a two-phased clinical disease, it is assumed the cow transiently "felt better" after the foreign body left the reticulodiaphragmatic area and entered the chest, thereby alleviating the peritoneal pain and inflammation. Subsequent, worsening sepsis in the pericardial sac and eventual heart failure causes the second phase of disease that generally moves the owner to seek veterinary consultation.

2. During the acute and subacute phases of traumatic pericarditis, heart sounds may change on a daily basis. Muffling, tinkling, splashing, rubs, murmurs, and other sounds all may be present on one day, absent the next, and present again later. Pathology is dynamic as the relative amounts of fibrin, purulent fluid, and gas in the pericardium change. Chronic cases, on the other hand, tend to have bilateral muffling of heart sounds and a "far away" tinkling as fluid pus is jostled by heartbeats.

Laboratory Data

If the disease is subacute or chronic, neutrophilia is usually present. Cattle afflicted for greater than 10 to 14 days usually have decreased serum albumin and increased serum globulin; therefore total protein values are at least high normal and usually elevated. Hyperfibrinogenemia is typically present at all stages of the disease. Thoracic radiographs, although largely unavailable in the field, often dramatically demonstrate a greatly enlarged pericardium, fluid line, and gas cap above the fluid line. The causative metallic foreign body also may be apparent unless obscured by radiopaque pericardial fluid, fibrin and the cardiac shadow. Cows with idiopathic pericardial effusion generally have normal fibrinogen and globulin cencentrations. Serum liver enzymes may be elevated with serum pericardial effusion regardless of the cause.

Diagnosis

Although the clinical signs of traumatic pericarditis usually are sufficient for diagnosis, definitive diagnosis in the field can be accomplished by two-dimensional echocardiography, pericardiocentesis, or both procedures. Thoracic radiographs, if available, also may be definitive.

Fluid and fibrin in the pericardial sac are easily visualized with two-dimensional echocardiography. Heavy accumulation of fibrin coats the epicardium and visceral pericardium (Figure 3-15). This fibrin frequently has the appearance of "scrambled eggs" when seen on postmortem examination (Figure 3-16).

Pericardiocentesis can be performed with an 18-gauge, 8.75-cm spinal needle or chest trochar of similar length. Following clipping and standard prep of the left thorax, a skin puncture is performed with a scalpel in the fifth intercostal space just dorsal to the elbow. If continuous drainage is desired, a 20-French chest trochar and catheter may be introduced into the pericardium to effect further drainage. The fluid obtained is purulent and fetid. Fibrin clots frequently obstruct flow of the fluid through finer gauge needles or catheters. The purulent fluid greatly exceeds normal values for pericardial fluid (normal = protein <2.5 g/dl, white blood cell [WBC]≤5000/μl), and neutrophils are the major cellular component rather than the

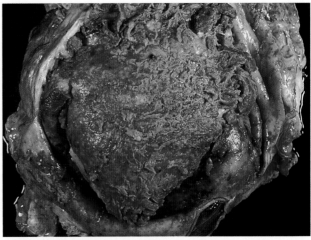

Figure 3-15

Traumatic pericarditis patient's heart and pericardium at necropsy. Purulent fluid has been rinsed away, but the severity of fibrin deposition is apparent as the epicardial surface of the heart is completely covered. The pericardium is greatly thickened and coated with fibrin. *(Photo courtesy Dr. John M. King.)*

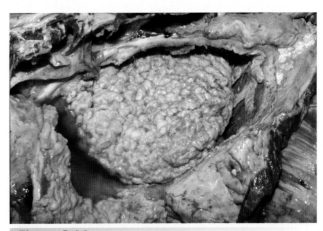

Figure 3-16

"Scrambled egg" appearance of epicardium and pericardial sac of an adult cow with pericarditis.

mononuclear cells normally found in pericardial fluid. Bacteria are easily detected in the gram-stained smears of this fluid.

The major reason for pericardiocentesis is diagnostic differentiation of traumatic pericarditis from diseases that may create similar signs. Lymphosarcoma with pericardial involvement and fluid accumulation is the major differential diagnosis. Occasional cases of idiopathic, nonseptic pericarditis have been documented, in which the clinical signs are very similar to those documented with septic pericarditis, but the fluid tends to be a sterile hemorrhagic transudate with low to moderate numbers of macrophages, neutrophils, and lymphocytes (see video clip 2). Cytology of pericardial fluid would clearly differentiate between these diseases. The prognosis for cattle with the idiopathic hemorrhagic form appears to be better following drainage and antiinflammatory therapy than for pericarditis associated with sepsis or neoplasia. The presence of flocculent, mixed echogenicity fluid with gas shadowing within the pericardium on ultrasound is also characteristic for septic pericarditis.

Pericardiocentesis is not without risk. Potential complications include pneumothorax, fatal arrhythmia, cardiac puncture leading to hemorrhage or death, and leakage of pericardial material into the thorax, resulting in pleuritis. Some, but not all, of these complications can be mitigated by performing the procedure using ultrasound guidance. Leakage into the pleural space is possible because most pericarditis patients do not have attachment of the fibrous pericardium to the parietal pleura. Pericardiocentesis performed on one of the author's patients yielded only gas from the needle and was associated with immediate anxiety, dyspnea, and death within 5 minutes. Postmortem examination confirmed that neither hemorrhage nor cardiac injury had occurred. The gas pocket and fluid distending the pericardium had been under positive pressure and may have become somewhat constrictive or altered compensatory mechanisms when suddenly relieved.

Given the hopeless prognosis usually associated with pericarditis, pericardiocentesis is a worthwhile risk to confirm the diagnosis before salvaging a cow suspected to have the disease.

Treatment

Treatment of traumatic pericarditis in dairy cattle usually is hopeless. Medical therapy with systemic antibiotics and drainage of the pericardial sac rarely, if ever, permanently cures affected cattle. Therefore most therapeutic efforts have been surgical. Thoracotomy and pericardiectomy or pericardiotomy have been performed in many fashions in an effort to provide drainage, search for the foreign body, and prevent fluid or later constrictive damage to the heart. Sporadic case reports and third-hand stories attest to the occasional success of pericardiectomy and fifth rib resections, but success is not common. Authors recommending rib-splitting thoracotomy and pericardiectomy reported that five of nine clinical patients recovered. Results from our clinic, as reported by Ducharme and co-workers, are much more pessimistic with only one of seven surviving thoracic surgery. Pericardiocentesis followed by fluid drainage may result in clinical improvement with prolongation of life to reach a short-term goal like calving. Despite a poor prognosis, surgery remains the treatment of choice for valuable cattle.

To improve a patient's chances of survival, surgery should be performed as early in the course of the disease as possible. Cattle with severe ventral edema and obvious heart failure are not good candidates for surgery. Removal of the causative wire during the thoracotomy

may be difficult but obviously is desirable. Usually the wire is mostly or completely in the thorax and would be difficult or impossible to remove through rumenotomy. However, we have observed patients with acute reticuloperitonitis *and* acute traumatic pericarditis from a single metallic foreign body that was still lodged in the reticulum and was removed through rumenotomy. These patients had clinically detectable pericardial effusions and radiographic evidence of foreign body penetration of the pericardium. Rumenotomy and intensive bactericidal systemic antibiotics are sometimes sufficient treatment of peracute or acute pericarditis in such cases. If pericarditis worsens despite systemic antibiotics and rumenotomy to retrieve the foreign body, thoracotomy may then be considered. Rumenotomy probably is most indicated in acute cases for which it is hoped that some portion of the metallic foreign object remains in the reticulum. Unfortunately it is difficult to know this without the benefit of radiographs, and although indicated in the field, an unsuccessful rumenotomy may further compromise the patient.

It is very disturbing that these "valuable cows" unfortunate enough to develop traumatic pericarditis were not administered a magnet prophylactically at some time in their lives by their owner. The routine administration of a magnet to heifers of breeding age and bulls before 2 years of age should be part of routine disease prophylaxis in dairy cattle.

Treatment of nonseptic pericarditis includes drainage of the pericardial fluid, systemic antimicrobial therapy, and administration of 5 mg of dexamethasone with or without 100,000 units of sodium penicillin into the pericardial space.

Cor Pulmonale

Etiology

Conditions of right heart dilatation, hypertrophy, and subsequent failure caused by pulmonary hypertension and increased pulmonary vascular resistance often is referred to collectively as cor pulmonale. This condition is uncommon and sporadic in dairy cattle. Most cases of cor pulmonale occur in cows known to have chronic pneumonia, bronchiectasis, and pulmonary abscesses secondary to bacterial bronchopneumonia, consolidated anteroventral lung lobes from previous pneumonia, or chronic lungworms. Severe chronic interstitial pulmonary disease, although rare, may also result in cor pulmonale in mature cattle with diffuse pulmonary fibrosis. In these instances, pulmonary hypertension initially may result from alveolar hypoxia and subsequent precapillary vasoconstriction. Chronic hypoxia and pulmonary hypertension in cattle may provoke hypertrophy of medial smooth musculature within pulmonary arteries and arterioles, causing further work for the right ventricle. We have treated one adult Holstein cow that had primary pulmonary hypertension.

The most common example of cor pulmonale is "brisket edema" or "mountain sickness" of beef cattle. This disease can occur in dairy cattle, and in fact Holsteins have been reported to be particularly sensitive. However, on a practical basis, to our knowledge, few dairy cattle in the United States are at risk because of a lack of exposure to high altitudes. Brisket disease may be seen at elevations of 1600 m (5249 ft) above sea level and tends to have increasing incidence at elevations above 1600 m. Definite genetic resistance or susceptibility is documented, and affected cattle must be returned to low altitudes early in the course of the disease to survive. Concurrent ingestion of certain plants such as *Astragalus* sp. and *Oxytropis* sp. (locoweed) is known to accentuate and accelerate brisket disease in animals at high elevations.

Pulmonary hypertension secondary to pulmonary and bronchial arteritis recently was observed as an endemic problem in a group of dairy calves. Periarteriolar sclerosis and vasculitis were identified pathologically and explained signs of right heart failure observed in the calves. Although unconfirmed, monocrotaline, a pyrrolizidine alkaloid, was suspected as the cause by the authors.

Signs

Dyspnea, tachycardia, ventral edema, and venous distention and pulsation characterize cor pulmonale. Therefore the signs are not unlike those found in other common heart diseases of cattle and require differentiation from cardiomyopathy, endocarditis, lymphosarcoma, pericarditis, and myocarditis.

Murmurs or a gallop rhythm may be ausculted, depending on valvular function, the degree of myocardial hypertrophy, or cardiac chamber dilation. Heart sounds have normal or increased intensity. Greatest attention should be directed toward the lungs to determine chronic abnormalities (e.g., consolidation) that may explain the right heart failure. Affected cattle appear more ill as the degree of dyspnea progresses.

Diagnosis

History of chronic pulmonary disease (or exposure to high altitude), ruling out other cardiac diseases, and finding signs consistent with right heart failure provide suggestive evidence of cor pulmonale. Two-dimensional echocardiography may add further evidence if right ventricular hypertrophy and dilatation is proven. Increased pulmonary arterial pressures, confirmed by cardiac catheterization, are diagnostic but limited to research facilities. Tracheal washes, thoracic ultrasound, or thoracic radiography may contribute to an understanding of the pulmonary problem in selected cases—especially cattle with chronic pneumonia, *A. pyogenes* pneumonia,

abscesses, or diffuse pulmonary fibrosis. Measurement of arterial blood gas concentrations may confirm the presence of underlying hypoxemia.

Treatment

In cattle affected with primary chronic pulmonary disease, treatment of the primary lung disease coupled with furosemide therapy may be beneficial. Cattle known to have had pneumonia in the past and mild but persistent chronic respiratory signs thereafter may benefit from a tracheal wash to establish cytologic and cultural aids to antibiotic treatment of the chronic lung problem. Baermann's technique should be performed if chronic lungworm infestation is suspected. Cattle at high altitude suspected to have brisket disease should receive oxygen and be moved to lower altitudes.

Furosemide is administered at 0.5 to 1.0 mg/kg twice daily as a diuretic. Although digoxin may be considered in these cases, those cattle that require digoxin require hospitalization and incur extreme expense. Therefore use of digoxin seldom is practiced. If digoxin is required for a select case, the recommended dosage is 0.86 μg/kg/hr IV.

Arrhythmias

Etiology

Arrhythmias in adult cattle can be caused by a variety of drugs, myocardial insults, and metabolic abnormalities. In calves, myocarditis, hyperkalemia, hypoglycemia, and white muscle disease have been discussed previously as factors involved in the pathogenesis of arrhythmias.

Myocarditis may be the most difficult of the adult cow causes to diagnose definitively and therefore is suspected when other known causes are eliminated. Toxic myocardial damage from ionophores and plant toxins, as well as septic or inflammatory mediators (myocardial depressant factor, tumor necrosis factor), must be considered when arrhythmias appear in cattle without gastrointestinal, electrolyte, or other typical predisposing factors.

Calcium solutions are well recognized as being capable of causing cardiac arrhythmias or death when administered IV to cattle. Both hypocalcemia and hypercalcemia have been associated with arrhythmias, and arrhythmias associated with hypercalcemia are thought to be mediated by vagal stimulation. In fact arrhythmias associated with hypercalcemia may be abolished by atropine. However, atropine seldom is used for this purpose because of its negative effects on the gastrointestinal tract of cattle. Atrial fibrillation has been associated with hypocalcemia and also has been reported following treatment of cattle with neostigmine that may have provoked increased vagal tone. Hypocalcemia and hypokalemia in cattle with primary gastrointestinal diseases seem to be major risk factors to the development of atrial fibrillation and atrial premature contractions in adult dairy cattle.

Oxytetracycline in propylene glycol vehicles may cause decreased cardiac output and stroke volume, as well as decreased heart rates and aortic pressures. Systemic hypotension and cardiac asystole also has been observed when these drugs are given IV to awake, healthy calves. It is common knowledge among bovine practitioners that oxytetracycline, especially when prepared in propylene glycol vehicles, should be administered slowly and as a solution diluted with saline or dextrose to avoid hypotension, collapse, or death in both calves and adult cattle.

Atrial fibrillation is the most common arrhythmia occurring in adult dairy cattle (Figure 3-17, *A* and *B*). A report suggests that atrial premature contractions in cattle with gastrointestinal disease may occur as commonly as atrial fibrillation. Atrial premature contractions often were associated with hypocalcemia and sometimes with hypokalemia in this study. Atrial premature contractions probably reflect vagotonia associated with abdominal distention or gastrointestinal diseases and are characterized using ECG by abnormal premature P waves (P′) from depolarization at an atrial site different from the sinus node. Atrial premature contractions usually result in a normal QRS-T on the ECG unless they enter the ventricle when it is partially refractory or if the AV node is refractory to excitement. In any event, it appears that atrial premature contractions may precede or predispose to atrial fibrillation. Sporadic irregularities rather than the irregularly irregular rhythm of atrial fibrillation are auscultated during atrial premature contractions in cattle.

Atrial fibrillation may occur with or without underlying heart disease and fortunately usually is a secondary event unrelated to primary heart disease. There may be a normal or fast heart rate, depending on the severity of the underlying condition, but the rhythm is always irregular with variation in the intensity of heart sounds and pulse deficits when the heart rate is rapid. There is an absence of P waves and presence of f (fibrillation) waves demonstrated by ECG recordings (see Figure 3-17).

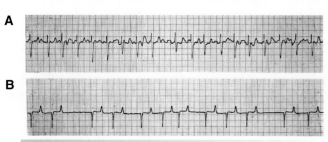

Figure 3-17

A and **B,** ECG recording from two different cows showing characteristic changes of atrial fibrillation. Both A and B demonstrate an irregular rhythm with normal QRS complexes but no P waves. In A, the f (fibrillation) waves are coarse and the heart rate is more rapid than in B, which demonstrates relatively fine f waves along with a normal heart rate.

Signs

Signs of atrial premature contractions and atrial fibrillation are nonspecific unless underlying primary heart disease is present, whereon general signs of heart failure also may be observed. Close observation of the jugular vein may reveal occasional abnormal pulsations in cows with atrial premature contractions. Signs of heart failure, such as venous distention or ventral edema, usually are not present in cattle with atrial fibrillation, except in advanced cases that have progressed to congestive heart failure. Because most cows with either atrial premature contractions or atrial fibrillation have a primary gastrointestinal or other medical disorder, the signs vary in each case. Without question, cattle with abomasal displacement and other diseases characterized by abdominal distention are most frequently affected by atrial fibrillation. Specific signs of atrial premature contractions or atrial fibrillation are associated with cardiac auscultation. Sporadic arrhythmias and variations in the intensity of S1 typify atrial premature contractions. Although the heart rate varies, perhaps dependent on the primary disease, it often is within the normal range. Atrial fibrillation, on the other hand, leads to more obvious abnormalities in cardiac auscultation. Marked irregularities in rhythm, tachycardia, and dramatic variations in the intensity of heart sounds are obvious. Pulse deficits may be present in cattle with rapid heart rates, and an absence of the S4 has been reported. Although exercise intolerance is possible with atrial fibrillation, cattle seldom show this sign because they are not "raced."

Atrial fibrillation also may occur as a result of primary heart disease (e.g., lymphosarcoma of the atrium and heart failure). This is a grave prognostic sign in such cases.

Diagnosis

Although cardiac auscultation is highly suggestive, ECG is necessary to make a definitive diagnosis of atrial premature contractions (Figure 3-18) or atrial fibrillation in cattle (see Figure 3-17). Key ECG findings in each condition are listed below and shown in the figures:

Atrial premature contractions = abnormal premature P waves (P′) = normal QRS-T unless occurring during refractory period of ventricle or AV node = sporadic

Atrial fibrillation = absence of P waves = F waves may be apparent = "irregularly irregular" rhythm = tachycardia (usually) = pulse deficit

Treatment

Treatment of atrial fibrillation in cattle seldom is necessary because resolution of the patient's primary medical or gastrointestinal problem generally results in return to normal sinus rhythm. Medical or surgical treatment of the primary problem coupled with correction of existing acid-base and electrolyte abnormalities is indicated for cattle whose problems include atrial fibrillation.

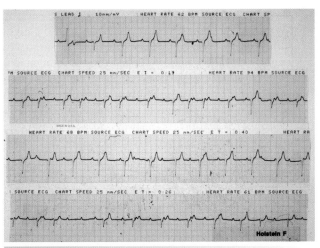

Figure 3-18

ECG recording from a cow with atrial premature contractions associated with concurrent gastrointestinal disease.

Routine administration of oral or subcutaneous calcium solutions as indicated and oral supplementation with 50 to 100 g of KCl orally, twice daily for 3 to 5 days are excellent empiric and supportive treatments for cattle with abomasal displacements or other causes of abdominal distention that also have atrial premature contractions or atrial fibrillation.

Occasionally atrial fibrillation persists several days to several weeks following resolution of the primary problem. Persistent atrial fibrillation raises concerns, lest the long-term condition lead to eventual heart failure. Heart failure has been suspected to result from prolonged (a course of years) atrial fibrillation in horses. Similar suspicions exist in cattle, but we know of no work that confirms this theory pathologically. In addition, cattle with atrial fibrillation that persists more than 1 month following resolution of a gastrointestinal or medical problem may in fact have myocardial disease causing atrial fibrillation or acquire heart disease because the noncontracting atria will develop progressive dilation that eventually results in tricuspid and mitral valve regurgitation, rather than one simply induced by electrolytes. It also is possible that some cows with persistent atrial fibrillation had it before the onset of their medical or gastrointestinal disease. Therefore discussions of appropriate criteria on which to base treatment are subjective. If medical or surgical therapy fails to resolve the primary illness in cattle also having atrial fibrillation, it is difficult to know how much the arrhythmia contributes to ongoing inappetence, depression, and decreased milk production.

If atrial fibrillation persists for 5 days beyond treatment or resolution of the primary problem, it is thought it should be treated with quinidine therapy. This may be premature in cattle that are clinically improved by resolution of their primary problem. Therapeutic intervention in cattle that are improving should be delayed at least 14 days because spontaneous resolution may occur during this time. Failure of cattle to resolve atrial fibrillation spontaneously may result from ongoing medical, gastrointestinal, acid-base, or electrolyte abnormalities. Treatment with quinidine or digoxin followed by quinidine may be expensive and requires careful clinical and ECG monitoring to avoid toxic side effects.

However, if atrial fibrillation persists beyond a reasonable time following resolution of a primary illness *or* is thought to be partially responsible for vague signs of illness in a patient *or* is thought to risk eventual heart failure, treatment may be considered. The following treatment protocols have been suggested:

1. Simple atrial fibrillation that has persisted despite resolution of primary disease:

   Quinidine 48.0 mg/kg in 4 L of saline or lactated Ringer's solution administered at a rate of 1 L/hr IV. Balanced fluids may be given concurrently via the opposite jugular vein.

2. Atrial fibrillation that is complicated by extreme tachycardia or that has not responded to previous quinidine therapy:

   Digoxin 0.86 μg/kg *per hour* or 11.0 μg/kg *thrice daily* IV for 4 to 5 days. Following this time, quinidine is administered as in (1) above.

   Digoxin—loading dose 22.0 μg/kg once *followed by* 0.86 μg/kg/hr for 2 to 4 days. Following this time, quinidine is administered as in (1) above.

In all treatment protocols, side effects of quinidine such as diarrhea, rumen hypermotility, and tachycardia must be anticipated. Signs of quinidine toxicity may include arrhythmias other than atrial fibrillation, prolonged QRS complexes, or collapse. If signs of toxicity appear, the rate of infusions should be slowed or stopped. IV sodium bicarbonate also may be administered. Some cattle are reported to show blepharospasm and ataxia just before conversion to normal rhythm.

Cattle having atrial fibrillation that persists despite therapy or cattle with ongoing primary illnesses may have myocardial disease or vagotonia that interferes with conversion to normal rhythm. Prognosis remains guarded for these patients and for untreated atrial fibrillation patients that remain in atrial fibrillation for more than 30 days following apparent successful resolution of their primary gastrointestinal or medical disease.

DISEASES OF VEINS

Thrombosis and Phlebitis

Etiology

Traumatic venipuncture and perivascular reactions to irritating drugs from attempted IV therapy are the major causes of venous thrombosis and thrombophlebitis. Dextrose solutions and calcium solutions that contain dextrose are the greatest offenders because of the tissue reaction that develops around hypertonic dextrose solutions. Tetracycline, phenylbutazone (not to be used in dairy cattle over 20 months of age), and IV sodium iodide also are capable of causing a severe thrombophlebitis when inadvertent perivascular leaking occurs.

Traumatic or repeated venipuncture may result in simple thrombosis, thrombophlebitis, or septic thrombophlebitis. Poor restraint, improper preparation of the vein for venipuncture, inexperience in venipuncture, and inappropriate selection of needles for IV therapy increase the risk of injury to veins. The common use of disposable 14-gauge needles for jugular venipuncture in cattle has increased the incidence of venous injury because these needles are only 3.75 cm (1.5 in) long—too short to be placed properly for adult cattle. Furthermore, these same needles are extremely sharp and can lacerate the intima of the vein if the cow moves at all. Prolonged use of indwelling IV catheters risks both thrombophlebitis and septic thrombophlebitis. Septic thrombophlebitis of any cause creates a major risk of endocarditis or pericarditis in cattle.

Dehydrated cattle and endotoxic cattle are especially prone to thrombosis during attempts at venipuncture. The normally thick bovine skin becomes even more difficult to penetrate when the animal is severely dehydrated. This is especially true in neonatal calves that are severely dehydrated by diarrhea. Repeated venipuncture efforts in those patients may injure the vein and cause thrombosis. Endotoxic patients and septicemic patients that are predisposed to coagulopathies may develop venous thrombosis very easily. Platelet activation and other coagulation factors may contribute to venous thrombosis in such cattle, even when an experienced clinician performed venipuncture. In some endotoxic or septic patients, gelatinous or "Jell-O-like" clots appear at the site of venipuncture within seconds of entering the intima of the vein. Further attempts at venipuncture often result in extension of the thrombus along the length of the vessel.

Although the jugular is the most commonly damaged vein in dairy cattle, mammary and tail veins may suffer damage occasionally. It is contraindicated to perform venipuncture in the mammary vein except in dire emergencies or when both jugular veins have been thrombosed. Injury to the mammary vein not only damages the vein but also causes persistent udder edema of both the forequarters and hindquarters on that side and will negatively impact future production.

Although most thromboses, thrombophlebitis, and septic thrombophlebitis are iatrogenic because of the aforementioned conditions, occasional cases develop spontaneously. Neonatal calves always are at risk for umbilical vein omphalophlebitis and consequential septicemic spread of bacteria to distant sites. In adult cattle, the mammary vein is the most common vein to suffer

spontaneous thrombosis, and this usually occurs during the dry period. Trauma by other cows butting the patient or simple pressure thrombosis caused by preparturient udder and ventral edema or excessive abdominal weight when lying on hard surfaces may contribute to this condition. Thrombosis and/or rupture of the perineal vein and caudal udder hematoma formation may occur in the region of the rear udder support and escutcheon (see the section on Udder Hematomas in Chapter 8).

Signs

Signs associated with simple thrombosis include palpable soft or firm clots within the vein. The vein may appear grossly distended by the thrombus or be of normal diameter. When the vein is held off below the thrombus, a fluid wave of blood cannot be balloted within the vessel. Acute thrombi tend to be soft or "Jell-O-like," whereas chronic or subacute thrombi may be firm to the touch. Edema may be apparent as a result of poor venous return in areas "downstream" from the thrombus. Therefore facial edema may appear with jugular thrombosis and ipsilateral udder edema with mammary vein thrombosis. Thrombosis may cause the patient mild pain, but it is not as painful as thrombophlebitis. "Needle tracks" or palpable swelling may be apparent in the skin overlying the site of thrombus formation.

Thrombophlebitis causes more obvious swelling in and around the affected vein. A perivascular component to the swelling and pain are more likely than with simple thrombosis (Figure 3-19). Palpable warmth to the swelling may be present, and subcutaneous edema usually appears downstream from the lesion. It may be difficult to differentiate a sterile thrombophlebitis from a septic thrombophlebitis. In general, fever and inappetence are

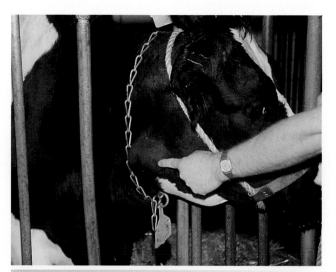

Figure 3-19

Thrombophlebitis of the right jugular vein in a cow that had repeatedly been administered dextrose by the owner.

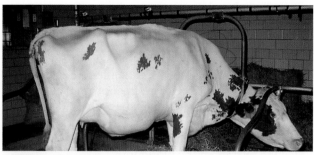

Figure 3-20

Thrombophlebitis of the right mammary vein in a Holstein secondary to owner-administered oxytetracycline and dextrose.

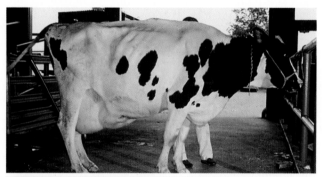

Figure 3-21

Septic thrombophlebitis of the right mammary vein that resulted in cellulitis cranial to the udder and septic endocarditis. Attempted blind-stitching of an abomasal displacement caused the original venous damage.

more common with septic thrombophlebitis. Both may be painful and warm, and when the jugular vein is involved, the patient may be reluctant to raise or lower its neck or eat. Ipsilateral Horner's syndrome develops in some cattle with jugular thrombophlebitis. Thrombophlebitis of the mammary vein causes marked ventral abdominal pain over the site and severe ipsilateral udder and ventral edema (Figure 3-20). Because septic thrombophlebitis predisposes to bacterial endocarditis in cattle, careful auscultation of the heart is indicated in all cases (Figure 3-21). Tissue necrosis associated with extremely irritating drugs (e.g., 50% dextrose, 20% sodium iodide, and phenylbutazone) placed perivascularly or resulting in thrombophlebitis eventually will cause sloughing, cellulitis, or sterile abscess formation. Bacterial contamination of such lesions ensures abscess formation and eventual drainage.

Severe thrombophlebitis involving the tail vein may result in sloughing of the entire tail (Figure 3-22).

Diagnosis

Clinical signs usually suffice for diagnosis. Two-dimensional ultrasound may be used to confirm the diagnosis, assess the extent of thrombosis, and detect fluid or pus

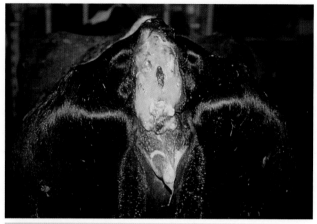

Figure 3-22

Tail slough secondary to perivascular injection of the tail vein.

accumulations that may be drained in septic thrombophlebitis.

Treatment

Simple sterile thrombosis requires no treatment other than avoidance of further injury to the vein. In acute cases, cool compresses may be applied to the site overlying the thrombus, but this only minimizes hematoma formation. If simple thrombosis is complicated by perivascular injection that risks thrombophlebitis, subcutaneous tissues around the swelling should be injected with normal saline in an effort to dilute the drug deposited in the perivascular region. In addition, warm compresses should be applied to the area several times daily.

Sterile thrombophlebitis is best managed by warm compresses and oral aspirin therapy (240 to 480 grains orally, twice daily for adult cows). Sterile thrombophlebitis may or may not eventually slough or abscess. Cases caused by irritating drugs are more likely to slough or abscess. Signs of improvement include stabilization or reduction in the degree of swelling, improved appetite and production, and less pain.

Septic thrombophlebitis requires intensive therapy lest further complications such as endocarditis occur. Warm compresses several times daily, systemic bactericidal antibiotics, and oral aspirin therapy are indicated. Unless culture results from a draining abscess or catheter tip indicate otherwise, procaine penicillin 20,000 to 30,000 IU/kg IM or subcutaneously twice daily should be chosen because of its activity against *A. pyogenes*. When septic thrombophlebitis associated with IV catheters occurs, the catheter tip should be cultured following its removal from the vein. An effort should be made to avoid further IV therapy in all patients having thromboses or phlebitis because injury to one vessel may predispose to multiple thromboses. When IV therapy is essential for patient management, extensive care is essential for future placement of IV catheters or injections. Therapy for septic thrombophlebitis usually is long term (several weeks), and relapses are common if therapy is halted prematurely. Occasional cattle with septic thrombophlebitis may have intermittent fever, depression, and inappetence, as well as swelling and pain at the site of venous injury. Such chronic thrombophlebitis is not as common as in horses but may require similar surgical removal of the affected area of vein. Positive signs for cattle being treated for septic thrombophlebitis include normal temperature; increased appetite and production; reduced pain, swelling, and heat at the site; and decreasing amounts of drainage in those cases suffering sloughing or abscess drainage.

The prognosis for simple thrombosis is fair. If further injury to the vessel is avoided, some veins recannulate with time. The prognosis for thrombophlebitis is guarded, and most affected veins do not recannulate. In addition, subcutaneous edema of the tissue "downstream" to the vein injury is more common and requires a longer time to resolve.

Prevention

Good restraint, proper technique and equipment, and clinician experience are the best ways to avoid iatrogenic vein injuries. Careful preparation of the selected vein and cutdowns through the skin with small scalpel blades are very important aids when injecting or catheterizing a vein in a known high-risk patient such as a severely dehydrated or endotoxic cow (see Chapter 2).

Lacerations

Etiology

Mammary vein lacerations are the most common life-threatening venous laceration in dairy cattle. Sharp objects or barbed wire is the usual cause of injury, and blood loss can be profound unless the animal is attended to quickly.

Signs

Small lacerations or penetrations lead to blood loss and hematoma formation, whereas complete lacerations lead to massive blood loss and exsanguination. Other than the obvious venous bleeding from the site, clinical signs are those associated with blood loss anemia. Weakness, polypnea, tachycardia, anxiety, and pallor of mucous membranes indicate a life-threatening degree of blood loss. Heart rates greater than 120 beats/min and respiratory rates greater than 60 breaths/min usually are associated with severe blood loss. These parameters, coupled with extreme pallor of the mucous membranes and weakness, dictate a need for whole blood transfusions.

Diagnosis

The diagnosis is self-evident. Because blood loss is peracute, the packed-cell volume (PCV) should not be used as a decisive parameter when assessing the need for a whole blood transfusion. Peracute blood loss does not allow time for physiologic vasodilation, and a cow with peracute severe blood loss may die with a normal PCV. Some clinicians rely on the respiratory rate, heart rate, mucous membrane color, and degree of weakness to judge the severity of the blood loss.

Treatment

Initial treatment includes temporary hemostasis by hemostats, ligatures, clothespins, or nylon ties followed by a complete physical examination to determine the severity of blood loss. If transfusion of whole blood is indicated (heart rate >120 beats/min, respiratory rate >60 breaths/min, and extreme pallor of membranes), at least 4 L of fresh whole blood should be administered. Following transfusion, surgical correction of the laceration with fine sutures or ligation of the vein should be performed. If the physical status of the patient tolerates it, the cow should be placed in dorsal recumbency to allow the wound to be explored, extended, and assessed before repair or ligature placement.

Because phlebitis and septic thrombophlebitis are potential complications, systemic bactericidal antibiotics such as penicillin or ceftiofur at standard dosages should be given and continued for 5 to 7 days. A belly wrap applied with self-adherent tape is useful as a pressure wrap following surgery.

Caudal Vena Caval Thrombosis

Caudal vena caval thrombosis secondary to rupture of abscesses near the hilus of the liver into the caudal vena cava is the most common clinical consequence of enteric origin liver abscesses in dairy cattle. Thrombi may form at the site of abscess rupture into the caudal vena cava or lodge between the heart and diaphragmatic region of the vessel. Thromboemboli traverse the right heart to lodge in the pulmonary arterial circulation leading to acute death, acute respiratory distress, or the more common caudal vena caval thrombosis syndrome with subsequent epistaxis, hemoptysis, anemia, and pneumonia. Endocarditis of the right heart valves is another common sequela. Further discussion of this syndrome is covered in Chapter 4.

Congenital Anomalies

Congenital portosystemic anastomoses have been identified in calves and usually result in poor growth and neurologic signs. They are further discussed in Chapter 12.

DISEASES OF THE ARTERIES

Rupture

Rupture of major arteries is rare in cattle. Occasional uterine artery tears occur in parturient cattle and are of unknown etiology. Trauma to the artery is suspected and may result from the vessel being trapped in the pelvis as extensive traction is placed on the calf during dystocia. The uterine artery also may experience extreme traction in some severe uterine torsions. Occasional cows having uterine prolapse suffer rupture of the uterine artery and exsanguinate (Figure 3-23). Copper deficiency has been suggested but seldom is confirmed as a cause of arterial rupture because it causes degeneration of the elastica within arteries. Deficiency of the enzyme lysyl oxidase, which contains copper, may prevent normal cross-linking of collagen and elastin. Although the aorta seems most at risk for rupture in copper deficiency, Drs. Charles Guard and John M. King have investigated several herds in New York that have had multiple cows die acutely from arterial rupture of the mesenteric arteries or aorta. Histopathology of arteries from affected cattle suggests copper deficiency, but copper levels have appeared normal. Therefore copper deficiency, although suspected, has not yet been proven. Major arterial rupture usually is fatal.

Aneurysms

One example of aneurysms in adult dairy cattle is presented by pulmonary artery aneurysms that develop proximal to septic thromboemboli in those with caudal vena caval thrombosis syndrome. These aneurysms later contribute to hemorrhage into the airways following dissection by septic thrombi that abscess.

We have observed several adult dairy cattle with persistent or intermittent colic that subsequently were

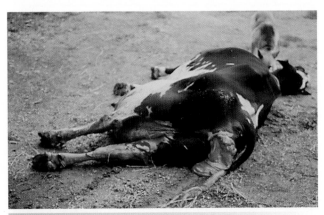

Figure 3-23

Fatal uterine artery rupture and uterine amputation in a cow that stumbled as a result of hypocalcemia and stepped on her prolapsed uterus.

shown to have mesenteric arterial aneurysms. Surgical removal of the aneurysms may be possible in some cases, but these cattle are likely to suffer arterial rupture and exsanguination eventually. If several cows are affected simultaneously, a toxin such as moldy clover or sweet vernal hay, which can prolong clotting times, should be suspected. For isolated cases the reason for the abdominal hemorrhage is generally unproven, although copper deficiency has been proposed as a causative factor.

Arterial Hypertrophy

Hypertrophy of the tunica media of pulmonary arteries and arterioles and subsequent pulmonary hypertension occurs as a response to prolonged hypoxia in "high altitude" disease or brisket edema of cattle. This situation leads to right heart failure and is further discussed under Cor Pulmonale earlier in this chapter.

Vasculitis

Although of nonspecific etiology, vasculitis may occur in conjunction with many infectious, parasitic, and immune-mediated diseases. In dairy cattle, malignant catarrhal fever is a cause of classic generalized vasculitis. Bovine virus diarrhea, bluetongue, *Salmonella* sp., *H. somni*, and *Erysipelothrix rhusiopathiae* are other potential causes of vasculitis in cattle.

Erythron

Evaluation of the erythron with CBC, stained blood smears, PCV, hemoglobin, and other parameters is primarily useful to clinicians monitoring anemia in cattle. It should be emphasized that the PCV for healthy lactating dairy cattle is lower than in many other species (see Table 1-2). Anemia usually is suspected based on physical examination findings and may be confirmed, quantified, and differentiated as to type based on evaluation of the erythron and leukon. Although a single CBC often allows classification of anemia into a regenerative or nonregenerative category, serial CBC analyses are required to follow trends in the erythron. Blood loss anemia and hemolytic anemia are "regenerative anemias," whereas anemias caused by chronic disease are termed "nonregenerative." Regenerative simply implies bone marrow response to anemia through increased erythropoiesis. Regenerative anemias in cattle frequently result in overt microscopic evidence of increased erythropoiesis such as increased anisocytosis, polychromasia, reticulocytosis, and occasionally even nucleated red blood cells (RBCs). In addition, an increase in mean corpuscular volume (MCV) and decreased mean corpuscular hemoglobin concentration (MCHC) are typical in regenerative anemias.

Physiologic hemoconcentration occurs with dehydration in calves and adult cattle. Because anemia may be counterbalanced by hemoconcentration, interpretations of PCV in sick cattle must always be made with consideration of the hydration status. True polycythemia (persistent elevation of PCV despite normal hydration) is rare but may occur as a result of familial, geographic, and pathologic conditions. Peracute severe blood loss as might occur in mammary vein lacerations or some abomasal bleeding ulcers does not immediately lower the PCV because physiologic vasodilation requires at least 12 to 24 hours. Therefore the degree of acute, obvious blood loss in a patient can be assessed best clinically by evaluating heart rate, respiratory rate, and mucous membrane pallor.

Definitions

1. Anisocytosis = variation in size of RBC. Normal to some degree in cattle = increases in regenerative anemias
2. Polychromasia = variable staining (toward blue) in Wright's type stains = indicates "young" RBC or reticulocytes still containing DNA
3. Basophilic stippling = blue granules, again indicative of DNA = also may be observed in chronic lead poisoning
4. Nucleated RBC = not unusual in cattle with severe but responsive anemia
5. Heinz bodies = precipitated hemoglobin deposits on the edge of RBC, observed in some hemolytic anemias. New methylene blue stain is helpful for detecting Heinz bodies and polychromasia in smears.
6. Poikilocytosis = uncommon in cattle RBC
7.

$$MCV = \frac{PCV \times 10}{RBC \text{ count in millions}/\mu l}$$

increase = usually regenerative anemia
false increase = blood not spun sufficiently for accurate PCV
8. Mean corpuscular hemoglobin

$$(MCH) = \frac{Hb \ (g/dl) \times 10}{RBC \text{ count in millions}/\mu l}$$

increase = increased number of reticulocytes = hemolysis
9.

$$MCHC = \frac{Hb \ (g/dl) \times 10}{PCV}$$

decrease = responding anemia with reticulocytosis = hemolysis
false decrease = blood not spun down sufficiently

Polycythemia

Relative polycythemia resulting from hemoconcentration is extremely common. Absolute polycythemia results from an absolute increase in PCV (usually ≥60%) that is repeatable, not associated with hemoconcentration, and does not lower in response to fluid therapy. Absolute polycythemia (absolute erythrocytosis) may be primary or secondary. Primary polycythemia also known as polycythemia vera is a rare myeloproliferative condition that usually causes excess production of WBCs and platelets, as well as RBCs. Plasma erythropoietin is decreased below normal levels in polycythemia vera.

Regardless of cause, progressive polycythemia eventually interferes with tissue oxygenation because of hyperviscosity and reduced cardiac output.

Secondary polycythemia is more common than primary polycythemia in cattle and implies a physiologic response to increased erythropoietin. Generally increased erythropoietin is a response to chronic tissue hypoxia. Therefore secondary polycythemia tends to occur in animals kept at high altitudes and in calves having congenital cardiac defects with right-to-left shunts. The chronic hypoxia associated with brisket disease or high altitude disease of cattle is capable of inducing polycythemia (see section on Cor Pulmonale). Tetralogy of Fallot and other severe congenital cardiac defects that create or progress to right-to-left shunting of blood also may cause secondary polycythemia.

Congenital polycythemia in Jersey cattle has been described as a recessive defect. These cattle are thought to have increased erythropoietin of unknown origin and have been grouped with secondary polycythemias.

Clinical signs associated with polycythemia are dyspnea, exercise intolerance, tachycardia, tachypnea, and very injected maroon or muddy-red membranes. Calves affected with polycythemia do not grow properly, regardless of whether the cause is cardiac or inherited. Funduscopic examination allows confirmation of hyperviscosity (Figure 3-24) in the retinal vessels. Retinal vessels are greatly increased in diameter, and the stars of Winslow (choriocapillaries on end) are very obvious. The hematocrit is consistently elevated over 55% and often greater than 60%.

Treatment is impractical in most polycythemia patients. This is especially true regarding congenital heart defects and inherited forms of the disease. Specific valuable cattle with high altitude hypoxia may benefit from phlebotomy and a return to lower altitudes. The practicality of the matter, however, dictates that extremely dyspneic cattle are most likely to benefit from phlebotomy, and these animals may die if restrained. If phlebotomy is accomplished, the PCV should be decreased below 50%, the animal moved to lower altitude, and symptomatic therapy given. Suspected hereditary polycythemia cases

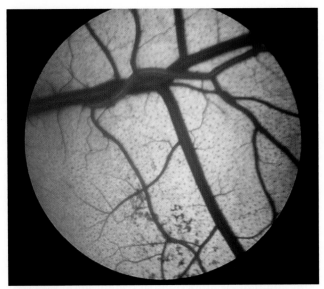

Figure 3-24

Dorsal view of the fundus of a calf that had polycythemia secondary to tetralogy of Fallot. The fundic vessels are greatly accentuated as is typical of hyperviscosity syndrome.

should be investigated genetically, and family members should be culled.

Anemia

Blood Loss Anemia

In addition to sporadic trauma and surgical procedures that result in severe blood loss, a long list of differential diagnoses exists for blood loss anemia in cattle. However, several common causes deserve comment.

Bleeding abomasal ulcers may cause acute or subacute blood loss in adult cattle. Melena is associated with most abomasal ulcers causing significant blood loss (Figure 3-25). Bleeding abomasal ulcers that result in anemia are rare, despite the fact that abomasal ulceration and perforation are common. Abomasal bleeding also may occur in association with chronic abomasal displacement in cattle. This combination of abomasal problems is most common in dry cows, bulls, and heifers that are not observed as closely as lactating cattle. Thus the abomasal displacement may have existed for days to weeks before diagnosis. The displaced abomasum distention, coupled with large volumes of hydrochloric acid, contributes to mucosal injury and subsequent ulceration with bleeding.

Lymphosarcoma of the abomasum may cause abomasal ulceration, hemorrhage, and blood loss anemia. The clinical signs may be difficult to differentiate from bleeding abomasal ulcers unless other signs of lymphosarcoma are detected during the physical examination.

Acute splenic rupture caused by infiltration of the spleen by lymphosarcoma may cause severe acute or

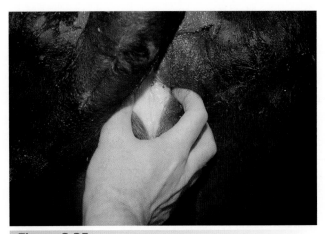

Figure 3-25

Extreme pallor of the vulvar mucous membranes in a cow that had severe blood loss associated with a bleeding abomasal ulcer.

peracute hemoperitoneum with resultant signs of blood loss anemia.

Caudal vena caval thrombosis syndrome may cause blood loss anemia after abscesses resulting from septic thromboemboli lodged in pulmonary arterioles erode into airways or lung parenchyma. Subsequent hemorrhage results in hemoptysis and epistaxis. Melena or fecal occult blood may be detected if the affected cow swallows sufficient quantities of blood. Epistaxis and blood loss also may occur as a result of granulomatous rhinitis and skull trauma.

Parasites are another cause of blood loss anemia. Lice are the most common ectoparasite to cause anemia in both calves and adult cattle in the eastern United States. In other geographic areas, fleas (*Ctenocephalides felis*) and ticks also may cause significant blood loss. Thanks to modern heifer management systems and routine deworming, endoparasites are uncommon but may result in blood loss, especially in pastured heifers. *Eimeria bovis* may cause life-threatening anemia as a result of intestinal blood loss. *Anaplasma marginale* infection may cause fever, jaundice, and severe extravascular hemolysis.

Pyelonephritis in cattle may result in anemia by either blood loss (acute and uncommon) or by nonregenerative mechanisms (chronic and common). Cattle having blood loss associated with acute pyelonephritis also may have colic as a result of blood clots obstructing ureters or urethra (see Chapter 10) and usually have fever. Anemia of chronic infection or perhaps that associated with decreased erythropoietin caused by chronic pyelonephritis may be involved in the anemia observed in chronic pyelonephritis patients. Blood loss anemia, sometimes severe, also occurs in association with thrombocytopenia caused by type 2 bovine virus diarrhea virus (BVDV) infection. Affected animals often have obvious petechial and ecchymotic hemorrhages on oral, vulval, and conjunctival membranes (see section on Thrombocytopenia).

Acquired or congenital defects in hemostasis may cause blood loss by a variety of mechanisms. Once hemostatic dysfunction exists, simple bruising, insect bites, injections, and other minor trauma may cause significant blood loss.

Rupture of the uterine artery during parturition or following uterine prolapse and sporadic rupture of other major arteries are other causes of acute blood loss. Self-induced trauma or laceration of a prolapsed uterus with subsequent hemorrhage has been observed in dairy cattle. Manual removal of a corpus luteum through rectal palpation to induce heat has fortunately fallen out of favor with bovine practitioners. This procedure occasionally resulted in severe blood loss or exsanguination.

Winter dysentery rarely causes severe blood loss from the colon in first calf heifers. Affected heifers have fresh clots of whole blood and severe dysentery and may require whole blood transfusions.

Nonregenerative Anemia (Anemia of Chronic Disease)

Chronic infections and neoplasms are most often associated with inadequate erythrocyte production or nonregenerative anemia. Chronic pneumonia with abscessation, chronic pyelonephritis, multiple abscesses secondary to musculoskeletal problems, endocarditis, and visceral abscesses may cause nonregenerative anemia. Chronic bovine virus diarrhea may rarely cause nonregenerative anemia, although BVDV-associated anemia is more commonly associated with acute disease, thrombocytopenia, and blood loss.

Cattle with chronic bilateral pyelonephritis may have depressed erythropoietin resulting from renal impairment to help explain their nonregenerative anemia. Chronic protein-losing nephropathies such as amyloidosis and glomerulonephritis also may cause nonregenerative anemia.

Lymphosarcoma may result in anemia through several mechanisms: nonregenerative anemia simply because of diffuse neoplasia, nonregenerative anemia caused by myelophthisis in sporadic adult cattle or calves with the juvenile form of lymphosarcoma, and blood loss anemia resulting from neoplastic ulceration of the abomasum or splenic rupture.

Bone marrow depression by chronic bracken fern intoxication may result in nonregenerative anemia plus blood loss anemia secondary to thrombocytopenia and subsequent hemorrhage. In regions where enzootic hematuria occurs in cattle pastured in bracken fern, blood loss anemia commonly accompanies the bladder lesions.

Iron deficiency anemia may rarely cause severe weakness in milk-fed calves. This usually occurs when the PCV is less than 15%. The anemia is characterized as a microcytic and hypochromic anemia. Serum iron will be extremely low, and iron binding capacity will be normal or high. Treatment with blood transfusion is usually curative.

Anemia through Hemolysis

Hemolytic anemias are associated with either intravascular or extravascular erythrocyte destruction. Although extravascular erythrocyte destruction is more common in most species, cattle have several forms of hemolytic anemia caused by intravascular destruction of erythrocytes. A very common cause of intravascular hemolysis in calves is water intoxication. Calves watered intermittently that are then given plentiful supplies of water may overdrink to the point that severe vasodilation occurs and RBC lysis follows. Hemoglobinuria and history are diagnostic. Low-grade fever also may be present resulting from RBC destruction, and neurologic signs develop in extreme cases. Similarly IV administration of hypotonic solutions is an occasional complication observed when electrolytes are not added or are added in insufficient quantities to large fluid containers (20 L of sterile water) before administration. Fever, trembling, hair standing on end, and hemoglobinuria are the clinical signs in the patient that identify the therapeutic error.

Intravascular destruction of RBC occurs in babesiosis (piroplasmosis) in cattle. Fever, anemia, depression, icterus, hemoglobinuria, and other signs associated with anemia occur in this disease. Leptospirosis in calves results in fever, intravascular hemolysis of RBC, and hemoglobinuria. Bacillary hemoglobinuria caused by *Clostridium novyi* type D (*Clostridium hemolyticum*) is another infectious disease causing intravascular hemolysis in cattle.

Heinz body hemolytic anemia results from a variety of oxidizing agents that denature hemoglobin. Complexes of globin, a protein, are then observed microscopically as Heinz body inclusions in RBC. Although rare in dairy cattle, Heinz body anemia has been observed in selenium deficiency and in cattle grazing on rye grass (*Secale cereale*), onions, and *Brassica* sp. Hemoglobinuria generally is observed in those with these diseases.

Postparturient hemoglobinuria may develop when lactating dairy cattle are fed a ration deficient in phosphorus. Intravascular hemolysis and hemoglobinuria associated with hypophosphatemia tend to appear during the first month of lactation. A depletion of adenosine 5′-triphosphate (ATP), secondary to phosphorus deficiency, may be involved in the RBC lysis in this condition.

Extravascular hemolysis occurs as a result of immune-mediated RBC destruction in anaplasmosis in cattle. Hemoglobinuria does not occur with this form of hemolysis. Autoimmune hemolytic anemia, as described in other species, is rare or has yet to be documented in cattle other than the RBC destruction that occurs with protozoan RBC parasites. Autoimmune RBC destruction has been suspected in some cattle with lymphosarcoma, but definitive documentation has not yet been provided. Neonatal iso-erythrolysis does not occur naturally in cattle, but the disorder has been observed when cattle were vaccinated against anaplasmosis and babesiosis with products of cattle origin. Subsequent passive transfer of maternal antibodies against specific blood types to calves from these cattle results in some calves showing isoerythrolysis.

The anemia sometimes present in cattle having the inherited disease erythropoietic porphyria ("pink tooth") (see also Chapter 7) is thought to be hemolytic in origin, although several other factors may be involved.

Determination of when an anemic patient requires whole blood transfusion must be made primarily based on the physical examination and secondarily based on PCV. In peracute blood loss, the PCV may be misleadingly high despite obvious pallor, tachycardia, polypnea, weakness, and other general signs that would indicate the need for a transfusion. When acute or subacute (24 to 72 hr) blood loss causes anemia, the usual PCV associated with the need for transfusion is in the range of 12% to 14%. Assuming normal hydration, a PCV greater than 14% seldom requires transfusion, and a PCV of less than 14% usually coincides with heart rates greater than 100 beats/min, respiratory rates of greater than 60 breaths/min, obvious mucous membrane pallor, and weakness. Heart rates that are greater than 120 beats/min and pounding, respiratory rates over 60 breaths/min, and obvious pallor all dictate a need for transfusion regardless of the PCV.

Chronic blood loss and nonregenerative anemias seldom require transfusions, and the slow, gradual development of anemia seems to allow physiologic compensation for the reduced numbers of RBCs. Cattle with chronic anemias may have PCV values of 9% to 10% without appearing in an anemic crisis.

Leukon

Cattle are unique in regard to the leukogram and its response to various diseases and stresses. Certain conditions, especially peracute inflammatory or endotoxic diseases, cause consistent changes in the leukogram, whereas other diseases, although infectious in origin, may be associated with normal or variable leukograms that shed little light on which disease the patient has. Despite having requested leukograms on thousands of bovine patients in an academic referral hospital, we find that the majority of these leukograms, regardless of the cause of illness, have been within normal limits. Despite this fact, the leukogram or, better yet, serial leukograms occasionally may aid greatly in the diagnosis and prognosis for a bovine patient.

WBC reference ranges used at the New York State College of Veterinary Medicine for adult cattle are listed in Chapter 1, page 14.

Stress and glucocorticoids reliably alter the leukogram to create neutrophilia, lymphopenia, and eosinopenia.

The numbers of monocytes appear variable. Concurrent inflammatory diseases may alter this typical "stress leukogram." For example, a cow with acute coliform mastitis that has been treated with dexamethasone may have a normal neutrophil count because of glucocorticoid-induced neutrophilia counterbalancing the expected neutropenia normally found in endotoxemia. This same cow could have a left shift with band (immature) neutrophils present and a lymphopenia in the absence of steroid administration. Cattle and their leukograms are exquisitely sensitive to exogenous corticosteroids. A single injection of 20 mg or more dexamethasone usually results in a stress leukogram characterized by neutrophilia, lymphopenia, and eosinopenia within 24 hours. Calves occasionally may have neutrophil counts of 20,000/μl or more following administration of dexamethasone. In addition to altering numbers of neutrophils, corticosteroids alter the function of neutrophils in a negative fashion. Whereas glucocorticoids are well known for their ability to be immunosuppressive, a single ketosis treatment dose of 0.02 mg/kg dexamethasone, however, is not associated with clinically significant immune function impairment. Neutrophil function may be impaired during the periparturient period and in cattle with retained fetal membranes.

A "degenerative left shift" wherein neutropenia coexists with the appearance of band neutrophils is typical of cattle with severe acute inflammation or endotoxemia. This helpful and, for the most part, consistent leukogram result is seen in dairy cattle affected with severe coliform mastitis, acute *Mannheimia hemolytica* pneumonia, severe Salmonellosis, severe postpartum gram-negative mastitis, and large perforating abomasal ulcers that cause diffuse peritonitis. Simplistic explanation of this phenomenon revolves around the fact that cattle have a limited bone marrow neutrophil pool to draw on in an acute emergency. Although the degenerative left shift remains a negative prognostic indicator and a positive indicator of severe infection or endotoxemia, it is so typical in cattle that it must be tempered by the patient's signs and response to treatment before using it as the sole basis of a prognosis. Cattle that have a degenerative left shift will often have a return to normal neutrophil numbers within 4 to 7 days following successful treatment of their acute infections. This time lapse may simply reflect the time necessary for resolution of a severe infection. If the infection requires more than 1 week for resolution, rebound neutrophilia usually will occur. Chronic infections may cause a neutrophilia, but many cattle with chronic infections such as visceral abscesses, musculoskeletal infections, chronic peritonitis, and other diseases frequently have normal neutrophil numbers despite having obvious infection. Neutrophilia seems more likely in resolving acute or subacute infections than in chronic infection. Certainly some cattle with chronic infections have neutrophilia, but the magnitude of the neutrophilia seldom is dramatic. It is rare to see an adult cow with more than 18,000 to 20,000 neutrophils unless exogenous corticosteroids have been administered to the animal.

Neutropenia also may be found during severe viral infections such as BVDV infection. Acute BVDV infection causes a leukopenia as a result of either a neutropenia, lymphopenia, or both. Because acute BVDV infection also adversely affects neutrophil function in addition to sometimes reducing absolute numbers, naive cattle acutely infected with BVDV have reduced ability to respond to concurrent or secondary infections until they form antibodies to resolve the BVDV infection. The immunosuppressive effect of acute BVDV infection and the potential for greater morbidity and mortality to be associated with concurrent infectious diseases such as Salmonellosis or Pasteurellosis should not be overlooked diagnostically during a herd outbreak of enteric or respiratory disease.

Absolute lymphopenia occurs in conjunction with stress, exogenous corticosteroid administration, some viral diseases such as BVDV, and some acute severe infections or endotoxemias. Frequently it is difficult to know whether the lymphopenia is associated directly with the disease or simply represents stress associated with a disease. Although eosinopenia should accompany lymphopenia when the cause is stress or corticosteroid administration, eosinophil counts have limited value in this regard. Absolute lymphocytosis that is transient is rare in dairy cattle and when present usually is associated with a neutrophilia in patients recovering from acute infection. Lymphocytosis that is persistent and repeatable usually indicates infection with BLV. Persistent lymphocytosis (PL) is a separately inherited condition that develops in association with BLV infection in certain lines of cattle. The Bendixen method of control of BLV was based on elimination of cattle with PL until a more modern understanding of the disease evolved. Cattle that are BLV positive and have PL may have a greater risk of developing lymphosarcoma than those cattle that are BLV positive without PL but this is controversial. In one study, PL was present in approximately one third of cattle infected with BLV. However, these percentages may vary in individual herds because genetic predispositions affect the trait of PL in response to BLV infection. The lymphocytosis in cattle with PL is generally refractory to stress or corticosteroid treatment. True lymphocytic leukemia does occur in a small percentage of cattle that develop lymphosarcoma following infection with BLV. Lymphocyte counts may range from 30,000 to 100,000 in such cases, and immature lymphocytes and lymphoblasts may be observed.

Eosinophils seldom are of diagnostic significance when interpreting the leukon of cattle. Geographic and management variations may alter the "normal numbers" expected as a result of parasite loads and other conditions. Eosinopenia concurrent with lymphopenia is consistent with stress or exogenous corticosteroid administration. Eosinophilia is rare in dairy cattle. Eosinophilia is thought to indicate heavy parasitism, histamine release, or some immune-mediated or allergic diseases. Unfortunately eosinophil numbers seldom convey useful clinical data. The same is true of basophils.

Monocytosis may be of some value in cattle because it generally is associated with chronicity. For example, a cow having chronic peritonitis may have a misleadingly normal neutrophil count with no left shift but also may have a monocytosis. Monocytosis, although not specific, should at least raise the clinician's index of suspicion for chronic infection. Although monocytosis is not a consistent finding in the peripheral blood of ruminants infected with *Listeria monocytogenes*, as in humans and rodents so infected, some cattle with listeriosis do have a classical monocytosis. (The name *L. monocytogenes* evolved from the tendency of monogastric animals to have a peripheral monocytosis in response to infection with the organism.)

Bovine Leukocyte Adhesion Deficiency (Bovine Granulocytopathy Syndrome)

Etiology

A fatal syndrome consisting of poor growth, chronic or recurrent infections, and persistent extreme neutrophilia has been observed in Holstein calves since the late 1970s. Affected calves had persistent neutrophil counts exceeding 30,000/μl, and some had counts exceeding 100,000/μl. Such calves were initially described subjectively as having a leukemoid blood response that required differentiation from myelogenous leukemia. Despite their neutrophilia, these calves seemed unable to mount normal defense against common pathogens and minor infections. Although the leukemoid calves sometimes survived for several months, most died before 1 year of age. True incidence of the disease was impossible to estimate because many "poor doing" calves eventually die in field situations without ever having a CBC or other diagnostics performed. A genetic immune-deficiency condition trait was suspected based on clinical observation of the condition in full siblings in a litter of embryo transfer offspring.

Reports from the United States and Japan on selected calves with the disorder suggested a granulocytopathy, and comparative studies of a canine granulocytopathy in Irish Setters and a leukocyte adhesion deficiency in humans brought about further suspicion of an inherited disorder in "leukemoid calves." Subsequently this was confirmed and termed bovine leukocyte adhesion deficiency (BLAD) by Kehrli et al as a genetic disease in Holsteins that represents a severe deficiency of neutrophil Mac-1 (CD11b/CD18). Recessive homozygotes are affected, and heterozygote carriers have intermediate amounts of the Mac-1 β subunit (CD18). Despite more than adequate circulating neutrophils, affected calves cannot effectively fight infections because their neutrophils have deficient β2 integrin expression, preventing adherence to vascular endothelium and subsequent migration into tissue sites of inflammation.

Signs

Affected calves have chronic or persistent infections and poor growth (Figure 3-26). Signs may appear early in life, although some calves live for several months. Relative exposure to a variety of routine pathogens may dictate somewhat the apparent age of onset reported by client histories. Diarrhea and pneumonia are typical signs, but persistent ringworm lesions, persistent keratoconjunctivitis, gingival ulcers, loose teeth, tooth abscesses, poorly healing dehorning wounds, and other lesions also are common. Infections thought to be clinically minor respond poorly or not at all to appropriate therapy. Recurrence of signs and multiple problems are typical.

Diagnosis

Persistent leukocytosis caused by neutrophilia without remarkable left shift is a hallmark of the disease. To date most affected calves studied have had greater than 30,000 neutrophils/μl in their peripheral blood. Although myelogenous leukemia is a consideration, neutrophil function tests differentiate these diseases because neutrophils in myelogenous leukemic patients have decreased neutrophil alkaline phosphatase activity. In addition, the leukemoid blood picture is characterized as a regenerative left shift, whereas BLAD calves have primarily a mature neutrophilia. Furthermore ex vivo tests of adhesion-dependent responses such as chemotaxis and phagocytosis can differentiate between BLAD animals and those with severe, chronic neutrophilia without β2 integrin deficits. Affected calves must be differentiated from calves with chronic abscessation of the thorax or abdomen and calves persistently infected with BVDV that show similar poor growth and apparent reduced resistance to routine pathogens.

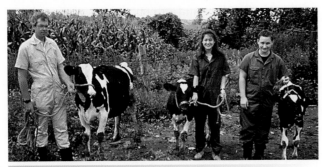

Figure 3-26

A normal heifer and two animals affected with BLAD. All three animals are 8 months of age and have been raised on the same farm. *(Photo courtesy Dr. Robert O. Gilbert.)*

Failure to confirm persistent infection with BVDV and ruling out visceral abscessation via radiographs, ultrasonography, and serum globulin values support the diagnosis. Definitive diagnosis alongside identification of carriers can be achieved by restriction analysis of polymerase chain reaction (PCR)-amplified DNA from a suspect individual to allow discrimination between normal, carrier (heterozygote), and affected (homozygote) animals.

Currently artificial insemination (AI) sires are being tested and identified as either carriers or noncarriers of BLAD. The routine genetic screening and identification of carriers by AI companies worldwide will eventually lead to the eradication of the disease. It is rare or nonexistent now.

Treatment

Treatment is only palliative, and most affected calves die before 1 year of age. Exact age of onset, progression, and true incidence are unknown because most sick calves never have a CBC performed. Theoretically it is possible that many BLAD calves die early in life and that only those that survive to develop chronic disease associated with poor growth are suspected to have the disease. Because variable expression of the glycoprotein deficiency is possible in homozygote recessives and in heterozygotes, it also is possible that mild forms of disease and prolonged survival occur.

DISORDERS OF COAGULATION

Inherited

A factor XI deficiency has been described in Holstein cattle and appears to be a recessive trait. Homozygote recessives bleed excessively or repeatedly following injuries or routine surgical procedures such as castration or dehorning. Hematomas commonly occur at venipuncture sites and may lead to venous thrombosis. Routine coagulation profiles may not show in vitro clotting abnormalities in heterozygote carrier cattle, even though such animals have less factor XI than normal.

Acquired

Thrombocytopenia

Etiology. Thrombocytopenia is the most common cause of abnormal coagulation in dairy cattle. Cattle normally have between 100,000 and 800,000 platelets/μl of blood. Platelet survival time is thought to be 7 to 10 days, and megakaryocytes in the bone marrow are the precursors of circulating platelets. Thrombocytopenia may result from decreased platelet production, increased platelet destruction, sequestration, or consumption.

Decreased platelet production generally implies a bone marrow insult. Therefore hemorrhage caused by

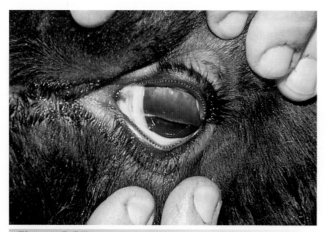

Figure 3-27

Subconjunctival hemorrhage and hyphema in a calf with thrombocytopenia secondary to BVDV infection.

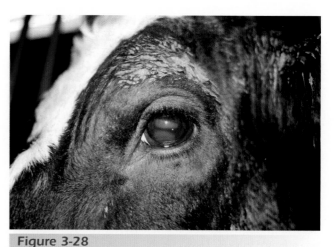

Figure 3-28

Hyphema associated with thrombocytopenia and DIC in an adult cow suffering from acute coliform mastitis.

thrombocytopenia may be the first clinically detectable sign of true pancytopenia. This is the situation with chronic bracken fern toxicity in cattle. Thrombocytopenia and leukopenia tend to be profound long before affected animals become anemic because of the longer normal life span of erythrocytes compared with granulocytes and platelets. Similar thrombocytopenia caused by decreased thrombopoiesis has been reported in association with intoxications resulting from ingestion of trichloroethylene-extracted soybean meal, furazolidone (in calves), and suspected mycotoxins in Australian cattle.

Decreased survival of platelets is probably the most common reason for clinical thrombocytopenia. Infectious diseases cause decreased platelet survival via several mechanisms. For example, an immune-mediated thrombocytopenia has been reported in cattle with East Coast fever, and although not specifically immune-mediated, the thrombocytopenia that occurs in association with certain strains of type 2 BVDV results from decreased platelet survival following viral infection. Thrombocytopenia in adult cattle and veal calves suffering natural acute BVDV infection has been observed, and studies confirm a thrombocytopenia beginning 3 to 4 days following experimental infection with type 2 strains of the virus. Platelet numbers in these cattle then decrease progressively over the next 10 to 14 days (Figure 3-27). Animals that survive this acute BVDV infection show a return to normal platelet numbers in conjunction with an increase in serum antibody titers against BVDV.

Infectious diseases also may initiate disseminated intravascular coagulation (DIC) with subsequent consumption of platelets. DIC has been suggested as the cause of thrombocytopenia in acute sarcocystosis and observed clinically in a variety of septicemic and endotoxic states in cattle. Septic metritis and septic mastitis are the most common endotoxic diseases to cause thrombocytopenia in adult cattle (Figure 3-28). Thrombocytopenia in these

cattle may either be caused by DIC or decreased survival for other reasons. In neonatal calves, thrombocytopenia is most commonly observed in association with neonatal calf septicemia.

Therefore infectious diseases may result in thrombocytopenia for a variety of reasons. However, those reasons usually affect platelet survival rather than production. Increased destruction, decreased life span resulting from platelet infection, consumption, vasculitis, and unknown factors contribute to thrombocytopenia in association with these infectious diseases. With the exception of BVDV infection and a few other diseases in which thrombocytopenia has been reproduced experimentally, most thrombocytopenia cases are sporadic and associated with a variety of disorders.

Trauma rarely has been associated with thrombocytopenia in cattle and may lower platelet numbers either by consumption or unknown mechanisms. We have confirmed occasional adult cattle with udder hematomas and cattle that are bleeding into a quarter as thrombocytopenic. It is not known whether the thrombocytopenia in these cattle represents cause or effect, but these patients showed no other evidence of systemic disease. Skull and orbital trauma apparently resulted in profound orbital hemorrhage secondary to thrombocytopenia in a calf (Figure 3-29, *A* and *B*) we treated. The calf completely recovered following a whole blood transfusion and replacement of the proptosed globe.

Immune-mediated thrombocytopenia—or thought to be immune mediated—rarely is observed in ruminants. Perhaps "idiopathic" thrombocytopenia is a better term because clinicopathologic confirmation of true immune-mediated thrombocytopenia seldom is possible in ruminants. Although perhaps more common in goats, idiopathic thrombocytopenia has developed in rare calves having no evidence of infectious disease, trauma, bone marrow depression, and so forth. Morris

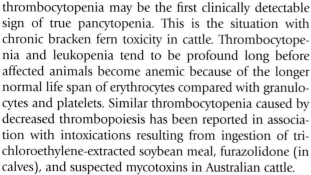

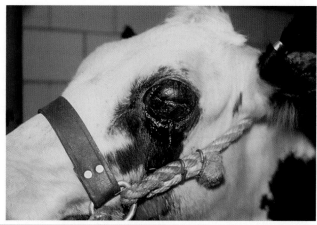
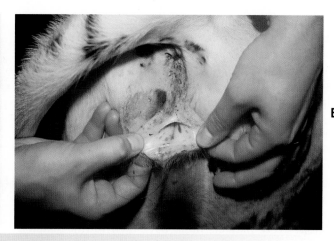

Figure 3-29

A, Proptosed globe secondary to orbital hemorrhage in a calf with thrombocytopenia following entrapment and struggling.
B, Petechial hemorrhages visible on the vulvar mucous membranes of the same calf as in Figure 3-29, *A.*

states, "The diagnosis of idiopathic thrombocytopenia must be based on small vessel hemorrhagic diathesis and severe thrombocytopenia in a horse with normal coagulation times and no other evidence of DIC." Although this statement refers to horses, obviously it also pertains to cattle because, in general, specific reagents to detect platelet-associated immunoglobulin (Ig) G, serum antiplatelet activity, and other confirmatory tests either have not been developed or are unavailable to most veterinarians.

Signs. Petechial hemorrhages on mucous membranes coupled with other signs of hemorrhage that may occur from small vessels anywhere in the body typify thrombocytopenic bleeding. Ecchymotic hemorrhages may accompany the petechial hemorrhages on mucous membranes such as the conjunctival, nasal, oral, or vulvar mucosa. Bleeding may occur from the skin at sites of injections or insect bites. Venipuncture causes bleeding, hematoma formation, and possible venous thrombosis. Epistaxis is common in cattle with thrombocytopenia and other signs of bleeding frequently accompanying inflammation or injury to specific sites. For example, cattle with thrombocytopenia associated with acute BVDV infection frequently have fresh blood or clots of blood in their feces because of the irritation of diarrhea. Hyphema, scleral hemorrhages, and hematomas may occur secondary to minor trauma, especially in stanchioned cattle. Melena and hematuria also are possible signs.

Clinical bleeding seldom appears until platelet counts drop below 50,000/µl and usually occurs when platelets are less than 20,000/µl. Obviously stress, trauma, and hydration factors may affect the incidence of bleeding at platelet values less than 50,000/µl. Many cattle with confirmed platelet numbers of less than 20,000 show no evidence of or tendency for bleeding. If stressed, however, or subjected to multiple injections, venipuncture,

bone marrow aspirates, rectal examinations, and so forth, these same cattle will begin to bleed.

Diagnosis. Absolute diagnosis of bleeding resulting from thrombocytopenia depends on:
1. Platelet count (usually less than 50,000/µl)
2. Ruling out DIC and other coagulopathies

Although this may be difficult in field situations, confirmation of thrombocytopenic purpura necessitates a coagulation panel to confirm normal values for prothrombin time, activated partial thromboplastin time, thrombin time, fibrinogen, and fibrinogen degradation products (FDPs). Bleeding time and clot retraction are abnormal. In essence, DIC is the major differential diagnosis, and the aforementioned tests differentiate primary thrombocytopenia from thrombocytopenia secondary to DIC.

Once the diagnosis of thrombocytopenia is confirmed by laboratory studies, clues to the cause of this disorder should be sought. Septicemia, endotoxemia, and recent trauma may be clinically obvious, whereas ingested toxins or parenteral drugs may require careful historical data and evaluation of the patient's environment. When no predisposing factor or cause can be determined, "idiopathic" or immune-mediated thrombocytopenia is the diagnosis. Fortunately, this latter category is *very* rare in cattle.

Bone marrow aspirates or biopsy is indicated whenever the etiology of thrombocytopenia remains obscure, granulocytopenia coexists with thrombocytopenia, or thrombocytopenia has been chronic or recurrent.

Treatment. Thrombocytopenia resulting in clinical bleeding requires therapy with a fresh whole blood transfusion and treatment of any primary condition. Ideally blood donors should be free of BLV and persistent BVDV infection. The volume of transfused blood will be somewhat dependent on the degree of patient blood loss that has occurred. The standard empiric quantities are a minimum of 1 L for a calf and 4 L for an adult cow, but greater volumes may be essential for severely anemic patients. Blood transfusions are "first aid" for thrombocytopenia, and the success of transfusion completely depends on whether platelet loss or lack of production will continue.

Specific and supportive therapy for primary causes such as endotoxemia, septicemia, trauma, and localized infections may allow a single whole blood transfusion to suffice for treatment of thrombocytopenia secondary to these disorders. Similarly calves or cattle with acute BVDV infection that are thrombocytopenic and bleeding usually require only one transfusion. These BVDV patients often have their lowest platelet counts approximately 14 days following infection. Therefore they are near recovery, and humoral antibodies are peaking at this same time. Whole blood transfusion and supportive care can save many of these patients.

Prognosis must be grave for patients having thrombocytopenia and granulocytopenia because pancytopenia should be suspected. Chronic bracken fern toxicity, furazolidone toxicity in calves, and other conditions that depress bone marrow are difficult to correct. Supportive therapy, whole blood tranfusions, and antibiotics to protect against opportunistic infections would be indicated in these patients. Bone marrow aspirates are essential to confirm the diagnosis.

If a primary cause cannot be found, and idiopathic thrombocytopenia is diagnosed, the clinical course is more difficult to predict. Idiosyncratic drug reactions should be ruled out by history, and drugs having the potential to cause thrombocytopenia should be discontinued. The patient must be monitored with daily platelet counts and physical examination to determine whether bleeding is continuing. Fecal occult blood, multistix evaluation of urine, and inspection of mucous membranes are important means of monitoring idiopathic thrombocytopenic patients. Further whole blood transfusions are not indicated unless signs of bleeding appear. Idiopathic thrombocytopenia patients that have persistent or recurrently low platelet counts of less than 25,000 and bleeding should have bone marrow aspirates evaluated. If the bone marrow is normal, low dose corticosteroids may be used in an effort to increase platelet numbers by increasing thrombocytopoiesis and counteracting a variety of immune mechanisms that may contribute to platelet destruction. Dexamethasone is preferable in our experience and may be therapeutic at doses as low as 0.05 mg/kg once daily. Most adult patients can be further reduced to 0.02 mg/kg once daily after 5 days. Most patients requiring corticosteroids for suspected immune-mediated thrombocytopenia can be weaned off medication within 30 days and do not tend to relapse.

Disseminated Intravascular Coagulation

Etiology. DIC is a complex coagulopathy characterized both by bleeding and excessive intravascular thrombosis. This apparent contradiction leads to a dramatic—and usually fatal—clinical appearance. Cattle suffering septicemia, endotoxemia, exotoxemia from clostridial infections, and other severe localized infections are at greatest risk for DIC. Septic mastitis and septic metritis are probably the two most common infections to cause DIC in dairy cattle. Fortunately DIC is uncommon in cattle.

Clinical signs of bleeding and thrombosis represent overstimulation of coagulation within vessels that eventually depletes coagulation factors to such a degree that bleeding evolves as a major sign. Fibrinolysis is excessive, and localized or regional tissue hypoxia occurs as a result of thrombosis. Subsequent major organ dysfunction (liver, kidney, brain, gut) may ensue. Because a serious primary disease already exists in patients that develop DIC, patients are further predisposed to organ failure and shock.

Products of inflammation (platelet activating factors) or infectious agents (endotoxin, clostridium α toxin) that encourage procoagulant activity or damage vascular endothelium may activate DIC. However, the exact mechanism by which DIC occurs is unknown, and it is impossible to predict patients that will have DIC complicate their already potentially life-threatening primary disease.

Clinical Signs. Rapid systemic deterioration in conjunction with vascular thrombosis and hemorrhage should cause suspicion of DIC in patients with serious primary inflammatory or gastrointestinal disease. Hemorrhages may be manifest as petechiae, ecchymoses, hematomas, or bleeding from body orifices. Melena or frank blood clots in the feces may appear—especially in cattle with enteritis. Microscopic or macroscopic hematuria may be present. Bleeding from injection sites and rapid venous thrombosis following venipuncture are typical signs. Epistaxis, hyphema, and visceral hematomas occasionally occur.

Major organ failure may be caused by reduced perfusion associated with thromboses. Lesser degrees of ischemia may cause renal (infarcts or tubular nephrosis), gastrointestinal (bleeding), neurologic (bleeding into central nervous system [CNS]), hemarthroses, or other signs.

As the patient's condition further deteriorates, venous thrombosis may frustrate attempts to improve the systemic state.

Diagnosis. Coagulation profiles and platelet counts are essential tests to confirm clinical suspicions of DIC in a patient. In all instances, a patient already seriously ill from a primary disease becomes "sicker" and has signs of thrombosis and bleeding. Because both may be caused by similar predisposing causes, DIC must be differentiated from simple thrombocytopenia. Other causes of bleeding such as hepatic failure, warfarin toxicosis, and inherited coagulopathies can only be ruled out by laboratory tests.

Textbook confirmation of DIC requires:

1. Decreased platelets
2. Prolonged prothrombin time, activated partial thromboplastin time, and thrombin time
3. Elevated FDPs
4. Prolonged bleeding time
5. Decreased antithrombin III (if available)

Realistically it is unusual to have all of these parameters fit the results suggested above in a patient suspected of having DIC. For example, the prothrombin time and activated partial thromboplastin time may or may not be outside the normal reference range for the laboratory and if abnormal may be only slightly prolonged. In addition, FDP results in large animals with DIC usually fall in the intermediate (10 to 40 µg/ml FDP) or suspicious range rather than being obviously elevated. Decreased fibrinogen levels are not typical of DIC in cattle and if identified may suggest liver disease. Therefore clinical cases of DIC may only fulfill two or three parameters for diagnosis. Those patients fitting the textbook parameters usually are in an advanced state and have a grave prognosis. Most DIC patients have thrombocytopenia, intermediate FDP (10 to 40) results, and may have slight prolongation of prothrombin time or activated partial thromboplastin time.

Treatment. Treatment of DIC is as poorly understood as the disease itself. Without question, intense treatment for the primary condition must continue. IV fluids are essential to counteract hypotension, tissue perfusion, and major organ failure. Nonsteroidal antiinflammatory drugs, especially flunixin meglumine (0.5 mg/kg body weight twice daily), may be helpful to patients having underlying gram-negative infections or enteric disorders. Severe thrombocytopenia or continued bleeding dictates replacement of clotting factors even though this may provide further substrate for ongoing coagulation. Therefore fresh whole plasma or, more likely in the field, fresh whole blood may be indicated.

Other therapy, such as heparin and corticosteroids, has been suggested, but there appears to be no scientific confirmation of their value in treating DIC, and in fact they may have deleterious effects in patients with DIC.

Prognosis for cattle with DIC is guarded to grave. Most patients with confirmed DIC die.

Coumarin Anticoagulants, Dicoumarol Toxicity, and Diffuse Hepatocellular Disease

Etiology. Rodenticides such as warfarin and brodifacoum that are coumarin derivatives, coumarin-containing sweet clover (*Melilotus* spp.) forages that have become moldy or sweet vernal grass, and diffuse hepatocellular disease may cause hemorrhage resulting from lack of liver origin clotting factors. Coumarin competes with vitamin Kl, a precursor of clotting factors II, VII, IX, and X. Excessive fungal growth during improper curing of sweet clover forages causes coumarin to be converted to dicoumarol and results in similar decrease in liver production of the aforementioned clotting factors. Diffuse hepatocellular disease also may prevent normal synthesis of these factors, but this is rare and generally seen only in advanced hepatic failure.

Because factor VII has a shorter plasma half-life than II, IX, and X, a prolonged prothrombin time tends to be the earliest laboratory coagulation abnormality found in patients with coumarin or dicoumarol toxicity. Subsequent prolongation of activated partial thromboplastin time and activated clotting time occurs as the disease progresses. Obvious external blood loss, hematomas, or occult internal hemorrhages causing profound anemia may appear in affected cattle.

Accidental ingestion of rodenticides containing coumarin derivatives or ingestion of sweet clover forages that are moldy tend to cause sporadic or endemic coagulopathies, respectively.

Toxicity of a given amount of ingested coumarin may be enhanced by hypoproteinemia, drugs that are highly protein bound (thus freeing more coumarin from protein binding), reduced hepatic function, and insufficient vitamin K in the diet.

Clinical signs tend to occur within 1 week of the ingestion of the toxic agent.

Clinical Signs. Ecchymotic hemorrhages, hemarthrosis, hematomas—especially over pressure points, epistaxis, melena, hematuria, and prolonged bleeding from injection sites or insect bites (Figure 3-30, *A* and *B*) all are possible signs. Although not common, petechial hemorrhages may be observed in some patients. In addition, moderate to severe anemia may be apparent resulting from internal or external blood loss and is apparent based on mucous membrane pallor, elevated heart rate, and elevated respiratory rate. Hypoproteinemia also is present when blood loss has been severe. Other less common clinical signs simply reflect bleeding into unusual locations as a result of incidental trauma. For example, seizures or neurologic signs may result from skull trauma. Prolonged bleeding may become obvious following minor surgical procedures such as dehorning in subclinical cattle.

Diagnosis. Clinical signs, history of exposure to sweet clover forages, or potential exposure to a coumarin-type rodenticide coupled with a prolonged prothrombin time and possibly prolonged activated partial thromboplastin time support the diagnosis when no other clotting abnormalities are identified. Platelet counts also should be normal. The absence of biochemical evidence of hepatic failure rules out liver diseases. Analysis of

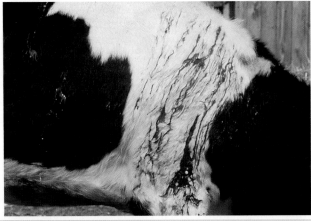
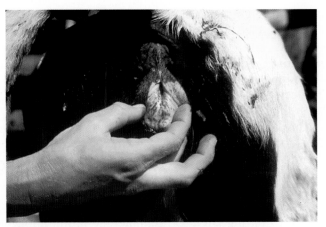

Figure 3-30

A, Streaks of blood originating from fly bites over the withers area in a calf that had eaten warfarin rodenticide. **B,** Petechial and ecchymotic hemorrhages of the vulvar mucous membranes of the same calf as in Figure 3-30, *A.*

blood, liver, or feedstuffs for dicoumarol may be available at some diagnostic or toxicology laboratories.

Treatment. All affected animals should receive vitamin Kl (1.0 mg/kg subcutaneously or IM). Treatment should be repeated twice daily and continue for at least 5 days. Affected animals that are severely anemic should receive 2 to 6 L of fresh whole blood in transfusions from healthy donor cattle (see also Chapter 2).

Vitamin K3 is *not* a substitute for Kl and in fact may be toxic. Most vitamin K3 products (menadione sodium bisulfite) have been taken off the market because of toxicity to domestic animals and humans.

Affected feed should be discarded and remaining feed inspected before allowing cattle access to it. Rodenticides should be managed carefully to avoid accidental ingestion.

CAUSES OF FATAL PERACUTE HEMORRHAGE IN CATTLE

Sudden death resulting from exsanguination may result in cattle from a variety of causes. When called to examine or necropsy a previously healthy animal that develops peracute anemia or dies from blood loss, the veterinarian should consider several diseases:
1. Obvious external blood:
   • Laceration of a major vessel such as occurs with mammary vein laceration
   • Caudal vena caval thrombosis with obvious bleeding from the mouth and nose
   • Bleeding from the abomasum with obvious melena
2. Occult or internal blood loss:
   • Manual removal of a corpus luteum during rectal palpation
   • Rupture of the spleen secondary to massive enlargement of the organ with lymphosarcoma
   • Rupture of a uterine or mesenteric vessel (consider both reproductive causes and copper deficiency)
   • Peracute abomasal hemorrhage without obvious melena

Thrombosis

Arterial and venous thrombosis are generally associated with septic causes, e.g., vena caval and related pulmonary thrombosis; jugular and vena caval thrombosis associated with septic phlebitis; uterine, mammary, or intestinal thrombosis associated with infectious/inflammatory diseases of those organs; and septic splenic thrombosis. Endocarditis may result in thrombosis of renal or pulmonary arteries. *Claviceps purpurea,* fescue foot, or ergotism may cause thrombosis of limb, ear, and tail arteries. Aortic and iliac artery thrombosis may occur in young calves (<6 months of age), resulting in an acute onset of posterior paralysis. Treatment of most of the above is generally unsuccessful.

SUGGESTED READINGS

Anderson DC, Schmalsteig FC, Finegold MJ, et al: The severe and moderate phenotypes of heritable Mac-1 LFA-1 deficiency: their quantitative definition and relation to leukocyte dysfunction and clinical features, *J Infect Dis* 152:668-689, 1985.
Anderson DC, Springer TA: Leukocyte adhesion deficiency: an inherited defect in the Mac-1 LFA-1 and p150, 95 glycoproteins, *Annu Rev Med* 38:175-194, 1987.
Araujo FR, Silva MP, Lopes AA, et al: Severe cat flea infestation of dairy calves in Brazil, *Vet Parasitol* 80:83-86, 1998.
Baird JD: Dilated cardiomyopathy in Holstein cattle: clinical and genetic aspects. In *Proceedings: 6th Annual Veterinary Medicine Forum* (American College Veterinary Internal Medicine), 175-177, 1988.
Bartol JM, Thompson LJ, Minnier SM, et al: Hemorrhagic diathesis, mesenteric hematoma, and colic associated with ingestion of sweet vernal grass in a cow, *J Am Vet Med Assoc* 216:1605-1608, 2000.
Buck WB: Toxic materials and neurologic disease in cattle, *J Am Vet Med Assoc* 166:222-230, 1975.

Buntain B: Disseminated intravascular coagulopathy (DIC) in a cow with left displaced abomasum, metritis and mastitis, *Vet Med Small Anim Clin* 75:1023-1026, 1980.

Callan RJ, McGuirk SM, Step DL: Assessment of the cardiovascular and lymphatic systems, *Vet Clin North Am Food Anim Pract* 8: 257-270, 1992.

Carlson GP: Diseases of the hematopoietic and hemolymphatic systems. In Smith BP, editor: *Large animal internal medicine,* ed 3, St. Louis, 2002, Mosby.

Carlson GP: Heinz body hemolytic anemia. In Smith BP, editor: *Large animal internal medicine,* ed 3, St. Louis, 2002, Mosby.

Carlson GP, Kaneko JJ: Influence of prednisolone on intravascular granulocyte kinetics of calves under nonsteady state conditions, *Am J Vet Res* 37:149-151, 1976.

Constable PD, Muir WW 3rd, Bonagura JD, et al: Clinical and electrocardiographic characterization of cattle with atrial premature complexes, *J Am Vet Med Assoc* 197:1163-1169, 1990.

Constable PD, Muir WW 3rd, Freeman L, et al: Atrial fibrillation associated with neostigmine administration in three cows, *J Am Vet Med Assoc* 196:329-332, 1990.

Corapi WV, Elliot RD, French TW, et al: Thrombocytopenia and hemorrhages in veal calves infected with bovine viral diarrhea virus, *J Am Vet Med Assoc* 196:590-596, 1990.

Corapi WC, French TW, Dubovi EJ: Severe thrombocytopenia in young calves experimentally infected with noncytopathic bovine viral diarrhea virus, *J Virol* 63:3934-3943, 1989.

Crispin SM, Douglas SW, Hall LW, et al: Letter: warfarin poisoning in domestic animals, *Br Med J* 2:500, 1975.

D'Angelo A, Bellino C, Alborali GL, et al: Aortic thrombosis in three calves with *Escherichia coli* sepsis, *J Vet Intern Med* 20:1261-1263, 2006.

Divers TJ: Blood component transfusions, *Vet Clin North Am Food Anim Pract* 21:615-622, 2005.

Ducharme NG, Fubini SL, Rebhun WC, et al: Thoracotomy in adult cattle: 14 cases (1979-1991), *J Am Vet Med Assoc* 2011:86-91, 1992.

Dyson DA, Reed JBH: Haemorrhagic syndrome of cattle of suspected mycotoxin origin, *Vet Rec* 100:400-402, 1977.

Evans ETR: Bacterial endocarditis of cattle, *Vet Rec* 69:1190-1206, 1957.

Evans IA, Howell RM: Bovine bracken poisoning, *Nature* 194: 584-585, 1962 [London].

Evans WC: Bracken fern poisoning of farm annuals, *Vet Rec* 76: 365-369, 1964.

Ferrer JF: Bovine leukosis: natural transmission and principles of control, *J Am Vet Med Assoc* 175:1281-1284, 1979.

Firshman AM, Sage AM, Valberg SJ, et al: Idiopathic hemorrhagic pericardial effusion in cows, *J Vet Intern Med* 20:1499-1503, 2006.

Fox FH: Personal observation, 1968, Ithaca, NY.

Fox FH, Rebhun WC: Warfarin poisoning with complications in a heifer, *Vet Med Small Anim Clin* 78:1611-1613, 1983.

Fregin GF: Arial fibrillation in the horse. In *Proceedings: 16th Annual Convention American Association Equine Practitioners,* 383-388, 1970.

Frelier PF, Lewis RM: Hematologic and coagulation abnormalities in acute bovine sarcocystosis, *Am J Vet Res* 45:40-48, 1984.

Gabor LJ, Downing GM: Monensin toxicity in preruminant dairy heifers, *Aust Vet J* 81:476-478, 2003.

Gentry PA: The relationship between factor XI coagulant and factor XI antigenic activity in cattle (factor XI deficiency), *Can J Comp Med* 48:58-62, 1984.

Gentry PA, Ross ML: Failure of routine coagulation screening tests to detect heterozygous state of bovine factor XI deficiency, *Vet Clin Pathol* 15:12-16, 1986.

Gentry PA, Tremblay RRM, Ross ML: Failure of aspirin to impair bovine platelet function, *Am J Vet Res* 50:919-922, 1989.

Giger U, Boxer LA, Simpson PJ, et al: Deficiency of leukocyte surface glycoproteins Mo1 LFA-1 and Leu M5 in a dog with recurrent bacterial infections: an animal model, *Blood* 69:1622-1630, 1987.

Gilbert RO, Grohn YT, Guard CL, et al: Impaired post partum neutrophil function in cows which retain fetal membranes, *Res Vet Sci* 5:15-19, 1993.

Goldman L, Ausiello D: The chronic leukemias. In Wyngaarden JB, Smith LH Jr, editors: *Cecil textbook of medicine,* ed 22, Philadelphia, 2004, WB Saunders.

Gross DR, Dodd KT, Williams JD, et al: Adverse cardiovascular effects of oxytetracycline preparations and vehicles in calves, *Am J Vet Res* 42:1371, 1981.

Hagemoser WA, Roth JA, Lofstedt J, et al: Granulocytopathy in a Holstein heifer, *J Am Vet Med Assoc* 183:1093-1094, 1983.

Harrison LR: A hemorrhagic disease syndrome of the vealer calf. In *Proceedings: 21st Annual Meeting American Association Veterinary Laboratory Diagnosticians,* 117-125, 1979.

Hayashi T, Yamane O, Sakai M: Hematological and pathological observations of chronic furazolidone poisoning in calves, *Jpn J Vet Sci* 38:225-233, 1976.

Howard JL: Monensin, lasalocid, salinomycin, narasin. In Howard J, Smith RA, editors: *Current veterinary therapy—food animal practice,* ed 4, Philadelphia, 1999, WB Saunders.

Hoyt PG, Gill MS, Angel KL, et al: Corticosteroid-responsive thrombocytopenia in two beef cows, *J Am Vet Med Assoc* 217:717-720, 674, 2000.

Jain NC: *Schalm's veterinary hematology,* ed 4, Philadelphia, 1986, Lea & Febiger.

James LF, Hartley WJ, Nielsen D, et al: Locoweed oxytropis-sericca poisoning and congestive heart failure in cattle, *J Am Vet Med Assoc* 189:1549-1556, 1986.

Jeffers M, Lenghaus C: Granulocytopaenia and thrombocytopaenia in dairy cattle—a suspected mycotoxicosis, *Aust Vet J* 63: 262-264, 1986.

Jensen R, Pierson RE, Braddy PM, et al: Brisket disease in yearling feedlot cattle, *J Am Vet Med Assoc* 169:513-520, 1976.

Jesty SA, Sweeney RW, Dolente BA, et al: Idiopathic pericarditis and cardiac tamponade in two cows, *J Am Vet Med Assoc* 226: 1555-1558, 1502, 2005.

Jubb KVF, Kennedy PC, Palmer N: *Pathology of domestic animals,* ed 3, vol 3, New York, 1985, Academic Press, Inc.

Kehrli ME Jr, Schmalstieg FC, Anderson DC, et al: Molecular definition of bovine granulocytopathy syndrome: identification of deficiency of the Mac-1 (CB11b/CD18) glycoprotein, *Am J Vet Res* 51:1826-1836, 1990.

Kimeto BA: Ultrastructure of blood platelets in cattle with East Coast fever, *Am J Vet Res* 37:443-447, 1976.

King JM: Personal communication, 1968, Ithaca, New York.

Krishnamurthy D, Nigam JM, Peshin PK, et al: Thoracopericardiotomy and pericardiectomy in cattle, *J Am Vet Med Assoc* 175:714-718, 1979.

Lacuata AQ, Yamada H, Nakamura Y, et al: Electrocardiographic and echocardiographic findings in four cases of bovine endocarditis, *J Am Vet Med Assoc* 176:1355-1365, 1980.

Littledike ET, Glazier D, Cook HM: Electrocardiographic changes after induced hypercalcemia and hypocalcemia in cattle: reversal of the induced arrhythmia with atropine, *Am J Vet Res* 37: 383-388, 1976.

Litwak KN, McMahan A, Lott KA, et al: Monensin toxicosis in the domestic bovine calf: a large animal model of cardiac dysfunction, *Contemp Top Lab Anim Sci* 44:45-49, 2005.

Mason TA: Suppurative pericarditis, treated by pericardiotomy in a cow, *Vet Rec* l05:350-351, 1979.

McGuirk SM: Treatment of cardiovascular disease in cattle, *Vet Clin North Am (Food Anim Pract)* 7:729-746, 1991.

McGuirk SM, Bednarski RM: Bradycardia associated with fasting in cattle. In *Proceedings: 4th Annual Veterinary Medicine Forum,* 2: 10–29-10–32, 1986.

McGuirk SM, Bednarski RM, Clayton MK: Bradycardia in cattle deprived of food, *J Am Vet Med Assoc* 196:894-896, 1990.

McGuirk SM, Muir WW, Sams RA, et al: Atrial fibrillation in cows: clinical findings and therapeutic considerations, *J Am Vet Med Assoc* 182:1380-1386, 1983.

McGuirk SM, Shaftoe S: Alterations in cardiovascular and hemolymphatic system. In Smith BP, editor: *Large animal internal medicine,* St. Louis, 1990, CV Mosby.

McGuirk SM, Shaftoe S, Lunn DP: Diseases of the cardiovascular system. In Smith BP, editor: *Large animal internal medicine*, St. Louis, 1990, CV Mosby.

Morley PS, Allen AL, Woolums AR: Aortic and iliac artery thrombosis in calves: nine cases (1974-1993), *J Am Vet Med Assoc* 209: 130-136, 1996.

Muller M, Platz S, Ehrlein J, et al: [Bacterially conditioned thromboembolism in dairy cows—a retrospective study of 31 necropsy cases with special consider of the causative complex] (German), *Berl Munch Tierarztl Wochenschr* 118:121-127, 2005.

Nagahata H, Noda H, Takahashi K, et al: Bovine granulocytopathy syndrome: neutrophil dysfunction in Holstein Friesian calves, *Zentralbl Veterinarmed A* 34:445-451, 1987.

Nicholls TJ, Shiel MJ, Westbury HA, et al: Granulocytopaenia and thrombocytopaenia in cattle, *Aust Vet J* 62:67-68, 1985.

Ogawa ERI, Kobayashi K, Yoshiura N, et al: Bovine postparturient hemoglobinemia: hypophosphatemia and metabolic disorder in red blood cells, *Am J Vet Res* 48:1300-1303, 1987.

Otter A, Twomey DF, Crawshaw TR, et al: Anaemia and mortality in calves infested with the long-nosed sucking louse (Linognathus vituli), *Vet Rec* 153:176-179, 2003.

Pipers FS, Rings DM, Hull BL, et al: Echocardiographic diagnosis of endocarditis in a bull, *J Am Vet Med Assoc* 172:1313-1316, 1978.

Power HT, Rebhun WC: Bacterial endocarditis in adult dairy cattle, *J Am Vet Med Assoc* 181:806-808, 1983.

Pringle JK, Bright JM, Duncan RB Jr, et al: Pulmonary hypertension in a group of dairy calves, *J Am Vet Med Assoc* 198:857-861, 1991.

Pritchard WR, Rehfeld CE, Mizuno NS, et al: Studies on trichlorethylene-extracted feeds. I. Experimental production of acute aplastic anemia in young heifers, *Am J Vet Res* 17:425-429, 1956.

Radostits OM, Gay C, Blood DC, et al: *Veterinary medicine. A textbook of the diseases of cattle, sheep, pigs, goats and horses*, ed 10, London, 2007, Saunders [with contributions by Arundel JH, Gay CC].

Rebhun WC, French TW, Perdrizet JA, et al: Thrombocytopenia associated with acute bovine virus diarrhea infection in cattle, *J Vet Intern Med* 3:42-46, 1989.

Reimer JM, Donawick WJ, Reef VB, et al: Diagnosis and surgical correction of patent ductus venosus in a calf, *J Am Vet Med Assoc* 193:1539-1541, 1988.

Renshaw HW, Davis WC: Canine granulocytopathy syndrome: an inherited disorder of leukocyte function, *Am J Pathol* 95: 731, 1979.

Rosenberger G: *Clinical examination of cattle*. Dirksen G, Grunder H-D, Grunert E, et al (collaborators) and Mack R (translator): Berlin, 1979, Verlag Paul Parey.

Roth JA, Kaeberle ML: Effect of glucocorticoids on the bovine immune system, *J Am Vet Med Assoc* 180:894-901, 1982.

Roth JA, Kaeberle ML: Effects of in vivo dexamethasone administration on in vitro bovine polymorphonuclear leukocyte function, *Infect Immun* 33:434-441, 1981.

Scott EA, Byars TD, Lamar AM: Warfarin anticoagulation in the horse, *J Am Vet Med Assoc* 177:1146-1151, 1980.

Step DL, McGuirk SM, Callan RJ: Ancillary tests of the cardiovascular and lymphatic systems, *Vet Clin North Am (Food Anim Pract)* 8: 271-284, 1992.

Stockdale CR, Moyes TE, Dyson R: Acute post-parturient haemoglobinuria in dairy cows and phosphorus status, *Aust Vet J* 83: 362-366, 2005.

Sweeney RW, Divers TJ, Benson C, et al: Pharmacokinetics of rifampin in calves and adult sheep, *J Vet Pharmacol Ther* 11:413-416, 1988.

Takahashi K, Miyagawa K, Abe S, et al: Bovine granulocytopathy syndrome of Holstein-Friesian calves and heifers, *Jpn J Vet Sci* 49: 733-736, 1987.

Tennant B, Asbury AC, Laben RC, et al: Familial polycythemia in cattle, *J Am Vet Med Assoc* 150:1493-1509, 1967.

Tennant B, Harrold D, Reina-Guerra M, et al: Arterial pH, PO_2, and PCO_2 of calves with familial bovine polycythemia, *Cornell Vet* 59:594-604, 1969.

Van Biervliet J, Krause M, Woodie B, et.al: Thoracoscopic pericardiotomy as a palliative treatment in a cow with pericardial lymphoma, *J Vet Cardiol* 8:69-75, 2006.

Vrins A, Carlson G, Feldman B: Warfarin: a review with emphasis on its use in the horse, *Can Vet J* 24:211-213, 1983.

Weldon AD, Moise NS, Rebhun WC: Hyperkalemic atrial standstill in neonatal calf diarrhea, *J Vet Intern Med* 6: 294-297, 1992.

Wessels J, Wessels ME: Histophilus somni myocarditis in a beef rearing calf in the United Kingdom, *Vet Rec* 157:420-421, 2005.

CHAPTER 4

Respiratory Diseases

Thomas J. Divers

DISEASES OF THE UPPER AIRWAY

These disorders are characterized by inspiratory dyspnea. The increased resistance to airflow caused by upper airway obstructions often creates audible inspiratory noise and results in referred airway sounds through the tracheobronchial apparatus. Sounds that have been "referred" to the lower airway from an upper airway obstruction may be misinterpreted as lower airway in origin unless the upper airway is examined and the trachea ausculted in such cases. If the respiratory sounds can be heard without a stethoscope, they are most likely originating from the upper respiratory tract. The upper airway examination should include detection of airflow from both nostrils, close examination of soft tissues of the head, and oral examination if necessary. Severe upper airway obstruction can cause open mouth breathing and head extension as the affected cow tries to decrease the resistance to airflow (Figure 4-1).

Mechanical or Obstructive Diseases

Congenital

Etiology and Signs. Congenital disorders including pharyngeal cysts of respiratory epithelial origin, nasal cysts, cystic nasal conchae, skull anomalies, laryngeal malformations, and branchial cysts have been observed in calves and adult cows. Inspiratory dyspnea with audible snoring sounds or stertorous breathing is a sign common to most of these problems. The condition may be present at birth or is most often observed within the first few months of life. The degree of dyspnea associated with these abnormalities tends to be progressive as a result of either enlargement of the lesion (cyst) or worsening upper airway edema and swelling from the mechanical overwork associated with respiratory efforts to move air through an airway narrowed by malformations.

Diagnosis. Specific diagnosis requires physical examination, including visual inspection of the nares and oral cavity, endoscopy, and skull radiographs (Figure 4-2). In addition, aspiration for cytology and cultures may be indicated for cystic lesions. Most cystic lesions will be secondarily infected.

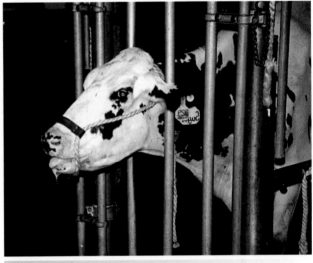

Figure 4-1

Open mouth breathing and neck extension in adult Holstein with retropharyngeal abscessation and pain associated with iatrogenic trauma.

Treatment. Method of treatment depends on the specific lesions found. Cystic conditions may be the most treatable because surgical removal offers some hope of being curative. Simple drainage or drainage with cautery of cystic lesions is not likely to be successful. Therefore referral of such cases to veterinary surgeons experienced in upper airway surgery is recommended so that complete excision of the secretory epithelium can be completed. Other conditions such as laryngeal malformations and skull anomalies have a poor prognosis.

Regardless of cause, symptomatic or supportive treatment may be necessary before diagnostic procedures are performed in calves with severe dyspnea, lest the stress of examination or endoscopy induce anoxia. A tracheostomy should be considered to allow safe diagnostic manipulation. Misinterpreting anoxic patient struggling as wildness requiring additional physical restraint is a frequent, and potentially fatal, error in judgment made by inexperienced clinicians. When a dyspneic animal struggles during examination, usually it is anoxic, frightened, and extremely anxious. All

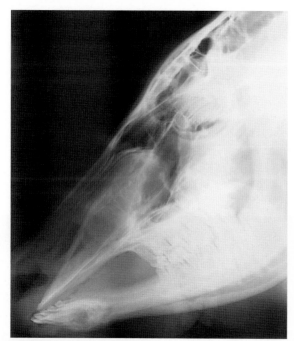

Figure 4-2

Radiograph of a conchal cyst in a 6-month-old heifer.

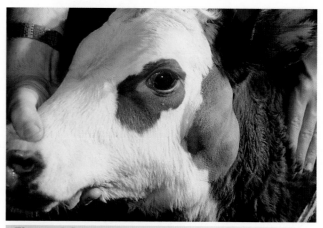

Figure 4-3

Juvenile lymphosarcoma in a 4-month-old Milking Short-horn calf presented because of inspiratory dyspnea.

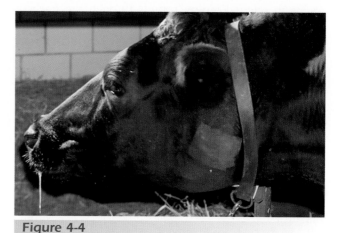

Figure 4-4

Adult Holstein with lymphosarcoma mass in the pharyngeal area that caused inspiratory dyspnea.

restraint of the head and neck should be relaxed, and the animal should be allowed to "get its breath." Continued restraint during these situations will result in asphyxiation of the animal.

Although the prognosis for congenital lesions varies with the specific diagnosis, generally it is guarded to poor.

Acquired

Etiology and Signs. Acquired mechanical or obstructive lesions of the upper airway may occur in calves or adult cattle. Most of the lesions represent enlargement or inflammation of tissues and structures external to the airway itself. Impingement into the upper airway by soft tissue masses such as pharyngeal abscesses, retropharyngeal cellulitis, necrotic laryngitis, pyogranulomatous swellings (e.g., wooden tongue), enlarged lymph nodes, neoplasms, foreign bodies, or enlarged maxillary sinuses compose the majority of lesions. Pharyngeal abscesses and necrotic laryngitis are probably the most common acquired causes of obstruction. Pharyngeal abscesses and retropharyngeal cellulitis may occur following traumatic injury to the mouth when an animal is treated with oral medication or may arise in calves with no history of pharyngeal trauma.

Regardless of cause, progressive inspiratory dyspnea is the primary sign observed in affected cattle. Fever may be present with pharyngeal abscesses or chronic maxillary sinusitis. Unilateral nasal discharge or reduced airflow from one nostril may be present with maxillary

sinusitis or unilateral neoplasms of the nasal pharynx or maxillary sinus. Lymphadenopathy may be present as a primary sign in neoplastic conditions, such as juvenile lymphosarcoma and adult lymphosarcoma (Figures 4-3 and 4-4), or as a secondary sign, in cases of soft tissue infections. Unilateral Horner's syndrome and progressive exophthalmos have been observed in slow-growing adenocarcinomas of respiratory epithelial origin in the nasal pharynx (Figure 4-5). Cattle with unilateral nasal obstruction often show more obvious respiratory signs during hot weather. One cow with Horner's syndrome would demonstrate open mouth breathing on hot days because of the nasal mucosal vasodilation and edema (Figure 4-6). A fetid odor may exist on the breath caused by chronic inflammation or tumor necrosis in some cattle. The owner may report a progressive course of stertorous breathing eventually leading to open mouth breathing. Inflammatory lesions often have a more acute course than neoplasms, but this is a generality rather than a rule. Obvious external swelling may be

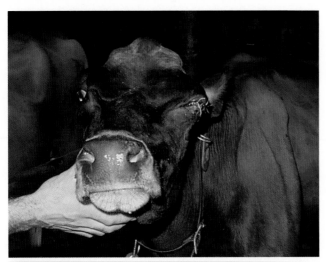

Figure 4-5

Aged Jersey cow with an adenocarcinoma of respiratory epithelial origin. The mass caused reduced airflow through the left nasal passage, left-sided Horner's syndrome, and exophthalmos. The eyelids have been sutured together to protect the eye.

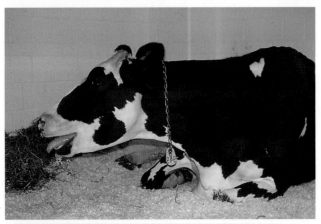

Figure 4-6

Open mouth breathing in a 5-year-old cow with unilateral Horner's disease (etiology unknown). The cow had no respiratory difficulties during the winter months.

present in certain conditions such as chronic maxillary sinusitis, pharyngeal or retropharyngeal abscesses, and lymphosarcoma.

Diagnosis. A complete physical examination followed by manual and visual inspection of the oral cavity is the first diagnostic procedure. Relative equality of airflow and the odor of the breath should be evaluated at the nostrils. If chronic maxillary sinusitis is suspected, the upper premolar and molar teeth should be examined closely for abnormalities.

Endoscopy should be performed in an effort to identify a specific lesion or the anatomic region of impingement of tissue into the airway. When performing endoscopy in a calf or cow with severe upper

airway dyspnea, most of the mucosal surfaces (e.g., soft palate, larynx, and respiratory pharynx) will be edematous from exertional or labored respiratory efforts. This edema should not be misinterpreted as the causative lesion (see video clips 3 to 5).

Skull radiographs may be necessary if physical examination and endoscopy fail to identify a lesion. Radiographs are helpful for definitive diagnosis of sinusitis, nasal or sinus cyst, and for identifying the location of soft tissue masses such as abscesses or tumors. In addition, radiographs would help to identify abscessed tooth roots in cases of chronic maxillary sinusitis and metallic foreign bodies.

Diagnostic ultrasonography, if available, may help in the assessment of soft tissue swellings. This technique also has been used to locate retropharyngeal abscesses and nonmetallic foreign bodies so that external drainage may be performed safely.

In the case of obvious or palpable swellings of the head or pharynx, aspirates for cytology and culture are indicated. Similarly, biopsies for histopathology are indicated for solid masses or enlarged lymph nodes.

Treatment and Prognosis. Treatment is most successful when external compression of the upper airway can be cured through treatment of an inflammatory lesion. Pharyngeal or retropharyngeal abscesses should be drained with liberal incisions that avoid vital structures. Internal drainage is preferred unless the abscess is close to the skin surface. External drainage is technically difficult in deep pharyngeal abscesses located more than a few centimeters below the skin surface. Vagus nerve damage, salivary duct laceration, and acute cellulitis are potential complications associated with opening the abscess. If drainage is not liberal, abscesses tend to recur. If recurrence is obvious, culture and sensitivity coupled with drainage through multiple sites are indicated. Daily flushing of the drainage sites is important. Systemic antibiotics should be administered for 1 to 2 weeks following drainage; *Arcanobacterium pyogenes* (*A. pyogenes*) and *Fusobacterium* spp. are the most common organisms cultured, so penicillin is the most commonly used antibiotic.

Chronic maxillary sinusitis should be treated by trephination of the sinus, removal of any teeth that have infected roots, daily flushing of the sinus with dilute disinfectants or sterile saline, and appropriate systemic antibiotics for 1 to 2 weeks.

In general, neoplasms have a hopeless prognosis, and the animal should not be treated. Juvenile lymphosarcoma often causes upper airway dyspnea via enlarged pharyngeal lymph nodes. Occasional adult-form lymphosarcoma cases have one or more very large (10 to 20 cm diameter) pharyngeal or mediastinal lymph nodes that will cause dyspnea. Lymphosarcoma usually results in death within 1 to 6 months of diagnosis. Adenocarcinomas originating in the respiratory pharynx in older cattle (i.e., more than 8 years of age) may have an insidious but progressive course over months to years. Therefore unlike cattle with lymphosarcoma, these animals may be allowed to survive for some time to deliver another calf or to undergo superovulation and embryo transfer. Only if the animal stops eating, develops severe respiratory distress, or is suffering from exposure damage from an exophthalmic eye will euthanasia be necessary. Cattle affected with primary squamous cell carcinoma, metastatic squamous cell carcinoma, or osteosarcoma originating in a sinus, bone, or periocular location occasionally may have enough tumor mass or lymph node metastases to develop inspiratory dyspnea. Cattle with squamous cell carcinomas frequently have a fetid breath odor from the primary tumor and should not be made to suffer unduly.

Inflammatory Diseases

Allergic Rhinitis

Also called summer snuffles, allergic rhinitis occurs primarily in cattle turned out on pasture in the spring and summer. Affected cows do not act ill but have a heavy bilateral nasal discharge and nasal pruritus. This condition also has been described as a familial problem in a group of Holstein-Angus cattle. Affected cattle may rub their nose so frequently that foreign bodies may be trapped in the nasal cavity, and significant self-induced trauma may ensue.

Granulomatous Rhinitis

Diffuse nasal granulomas are uncommon in dairy cattle in the northeastern United States. *Rhinosporidium* is the most common cause of granulomas that are observed. The granulomas develop on the nasal mucosa through the turbinate region, and as they enlarge, the nasal airway is progressively compromised. Therefore signs include a progressive inspiratory dyspnea, nasal discharge, and pruritus.

Frequently epistaxis is reported by the owner. Inspection at the nares with the aid of a focal light source allows observation of the tan or brown granulomatous masses in the nasal region. Endoscopy further defines the lesion. Biopsy for tissue culture and histopathology is indicated to determine the exact cause of the nasal granulomas.

Treatment consists of sodium iodide solution intravenously (IV; 30 g/450 kg once or twice at 24-hour intervals), followed by 30 g of organic iodide powder orally each day until signs of iodism occur.

Granulomas Caused by *Actinobacillus lignieresii* or *Actinomyces bovis*

Etiology and Signs. *Actinobacillus lignieresii* granulomas within the nasal cavity usually are unilateral masses within the external nares and appear as red, raised, fleshy masses that bleed easily and look very

similar to *Rhinosporidium* granulomas (Figure 4-7, *A* and *B*). Signs include a progressively enlarging mass in one nostril and inspiratory dyspnea as the lesion enlarges to occlude the nostril completely. The granulomas may originate at the site of nose-lead lesions of the mucosa near the nasal septum or at other mucosal sites of soft tissue injury from foreign bodies or fibrous feed. Progressive inspiratory dyspnea and nasal discharge are found in patients having granulomas deeper in the nasal cavity, larynx, pharynx, or trachea. *Actinomyces bovis* was responsible for multiple tracheal granulomas in a cow treated at our clinic.

Diagnosis. Granulomas can be confused with tumors on gross inspection. Therefore diagnosis requires biopsy for histopathology and tissue culture. Sulfur granules may be observed grossly on cut surfaces of these granulomas and suggest the diagnosis. Although usually found near the external nares, granulomas caused by

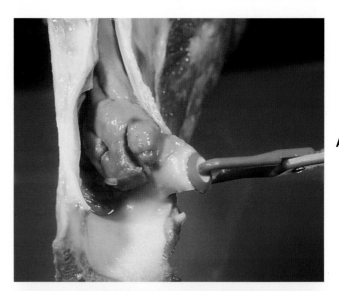

A

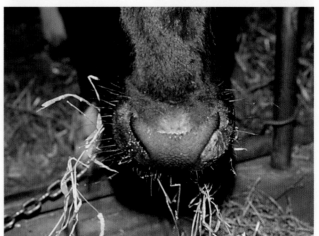

B

Figure 4-7

A, Necropsy specimen of nasal turbinate region showing *Rhinosporidium* granulomas. **B,** *Actinobacillus* nasal granuloma in a Holstein cow.

A. lignieresii or *A. bovis* could occur anywhere in the upper airway or trachea because these opportunists reside in the oral cavity and pharynx. When soft tissue infection occurs following injury to the mucosa, both organisms produce similar granulomas. Endoscopy and radiographs are necessary to identify granulomas at locations other than the external nares.

Treatment. Treatment for granulomas caused by *A. lignieresii* consists of excisional biopsy to debulk the mass to the level of nasal mucosa and sodium iodide therapy until iodism is observed. Usually this requires IV sodium iodide (30 g/450 kg) initially and at 2- to 3-day intervals for several treatments, or oral organic iodide (30 g/450 kg) daily following the initial IV dose. Cryosurgery has been used successfully on these granulomas following debulking. In severe or recurrent cases, antibiotic therapy may be necessary in addition to sodium iodide. Penicillin and ampicillin have been used to treat infection caused by *A. lignieresii*. Whenever possible, an antibiotic should be selected based on organism culture and sensitivity results. Usually the prognosis is good.

Granulomas caused by *A. bovis* are much more difficult to treat because this organism is poorly responsive to sodium iodide therapy. Treatment with penicillin (22,000 U/kg intramuscularly [IM], once a day), in conjunction with sodium iodide, may be effective. Surgical debulking of soft tissue granulomas also is indicated. The prognosis for those with lesions caused by *A. bovis* is guarded because of the limited clinical knowledge regarding treatment of this organism, and many owners may not treat for a sufficient time.

Frontal Sinusitis

Etiology and Signs. Frontal sinusitis in calves and adult cattle may be acute or chronic. Acute frontal sinusitis is more common and usually follows sharp dehorning techniques. Calves and cattle dehorned by laypeople are most at risk because of nonsterile equipment and techniques. Signs of acute sinusitis include fever (103.0 to 106.0° F/39.4 to 41.1° C), unilateral or bilateral mucopurulent nasal discharge, depression, and headache pain characterized by partially closed eyes, extended head and neck, head pressing or resting the muzzle on support structures (interestingly cattle with severe skeletal pain can often be found pressing their muscle against an object, which suggests this must be a pain relief point), and sensitivity to palpation on percussion of the sinus. When acute sinusitis follows recent dehorning, purulent drainage or heavy scabs may be observed at the wound in the cornual portion of the sinus. A multitude of bacteria such as *A. pyogenes, Pasteurella multocida, Escherichia coli,* and anaerobes may contribute to acute frontal sinus infection. Tetanus is another possible complication of acute frontal sinusitis if wound debris or scabs occlude the cornual opening to allow an anaerobic environment.

Chronic frontal sinusitis does not develop until months to years following dehorning and may be completely unassociated with dehorning because it occasionally occurs in animals dehorned by noninvasive techniques, polled animals, or animals with horns. Ascending respiratory tract infections, as in other species, are a cause of chronic frontal sinusitis and usually are caused by *P. multocida.* Chronic frontal sinusitis associated with old dehorning complications such as low-grade infection, bony skull fragments, or sequestra typically is associated with infection by *A. pyogenes* or mixed infections that may include *A. pyogenes, P. multocida,* anaerobes, or miscellaneous gram-negative organisms. Signs of chronic frontal sinusitis include gradual loss of condition and production that may be constant or intermittent; unilateral nasal discharge usually is observed, again as a persistent or intermittent complaint. Additional signs include head pressing, an extended head and neck, partially closed eyes, or resting of the muzzle on inanimate objects, all of which signal headache or pain. Intermittent or consistent fever is present. Bony expansions of the sinus may occur, causing asymmetric facial distortion—especially in cattle that do not have significant nasal discharge because of occlusion or obstruction of the ethmoidal meatus opening into the nasal cavity. In fact, some cattle will have intermittent bony swelling of the sinus that becomes less apparent during times of sinus drainage with subsequent nasal discharge. Palpation or percussion of the frontal bone overlying the affected sinus causes pain, and the patient is extremely apprehensive when the examiner approaches the head. Bony expansion of the sinus may result in ipsilateral exophthalmos and decreased air movement through the ipsilateral nasal passage (Figure 4-8). Neurologic

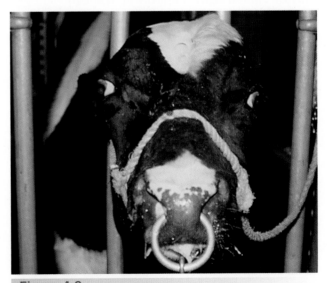

Figure 4-8

Chronic frontal sinusitis in a mature bull. The bull died from septic meningitis caused by the sinusitis.

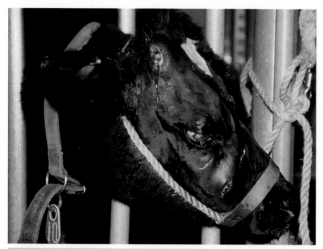

Figure 4-9

Orbital cellulitis, exophthalmos, and facial abscesses secondary to extension of chronic frontal sinusitis into the orbital soft tissue.

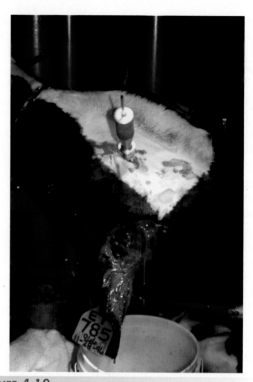

Figure 4-10

Sinus trephination with Steinmann pin to facilitate sample collection in a bull with chronic sinusitis. Note caudal trephination flap that has already been made in the dehorning site to facilitate sinus lavage.

complications, including septic meningitis, dural abscesses, and pituitary abscesses, are possible in neglected cases as a result of erosion of the bony sinus. Tetanus is another potential complication. Occasionally cattle with chronic frontal sinusitis have developed orbital cellulitis, pathologic exophthalmos, or facial abscesses from infectious destruction of the postorbital diverticula of the sinus, allowing soft tissue infection of the orbit (Figure 4-9).

Diagnosis. In acute cases, diagnosis is based on signs, history, and palpation and percussion of the sinus. Ancillary data are limited to bacterial culture and susceptibility testing to ensure proper antibiotic selection.

Diagnosis of chronic cases may be possible based only on clinical signs coupled with palpation and percussion of the sinus in selected cases. When mature animals are affected, however, it is important to rule out neoplasia and other differentials. Skull radiographs are helpful when available. Drilling into the sinus with a Steinmann's pin and collection of purulent material for cytology and bacterial cultures will confirm the diagnosis (Figure 4-10). Sedation and local anesthesia allow this procedure to be performed with minimal patient discomfort.

Treatment. In those with acute frontal sinusitis, treatment requires cleansing of cornual wounds, lavage of the sinus with saline or saline and mild disinfectant solutions, and appropriate systemic antibiotics for 7 to 14 days. Penicillin usually suffices, but selection of a systemic antibiotic is better based on culture and susceptibility testing. Tilting the patient's head to allow the sinus to fill and then twisting the head to empty the sinus facilitate lavage and drainage. Systemic analgesics such as aspirin or flunixin meglumine greatly aid patient comfort. The prognosis is good.

Treatment of chronic frontal sinusitis requires trephination of the sinus at two sites to allow lavage and drainage. One site is at the cornual portion of the sinus, and the second is located over the affected sinus approximately 4.0 cm from midline and on a transverse line connecting the caudal bony orbits (Figure 4-11, *A* and *B*). A third site caudodorsal to the rim of orbit and medial to the temporal ridge has been recommended, but we have found this site to be dangerous because it occasionally results in orbital soft tissue infection as compromised softened bone is penetrated. Further caution regarding trephination of the sinus should be practiced in animals less than 2 years of age because the rostral and medial rostral portions of the sinus may not be developed in younger animals. Attempts to establish rostral-medial drainage in these animals may risk invasion of the calvarium. Drains may be placed to communicate the two trephine sites and prevent premature closure of the wounds. Trephine holes should be at least 2.0 to 2.5 cm in diameter or they will close prematurely. Liquid pus is a positive prognostic sign, and pyogranulomatous or solid tissue in the sinus is a grave prognostic sign. Antibiotic selection must be based on culture and susceptibility testing and should be continued for 2 to 4 weeks. Analgesics such as oral aspirin are used to improve the patient's comfort.

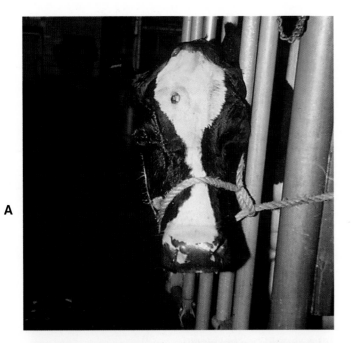

A

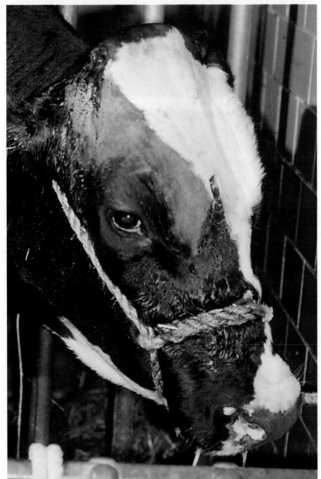

B

Prognosis is fair to good with appropriate therapy as described above unless neurologic signs have been observed. Neurologic signs and orbital cellulitis constitute severe and usually fatal complications of chronic frontal sinusitis. On several occasions, especially in animals less than 18 months of age, Dr. Rebhun performed enucleation successfully to allow orbital drainage necessitated by severe orbital cellulitis and ocular proptosis in addition to trephination of the affected sinus. Long-term wound care, antibiotics, and nursing are essential if treatment is elected for such complicated cases.

Laryngeal Edema

Laryngeal edema secondary to bracken fern intoxication has been described in calves. Termed the "laryngitic" form, this response leads to progressive dyspnea without obvious signs of hemorrhage as expected in older animals affected with bracken fern toxicity. Laryngeal edema has also occurred following vaccination of cattle, assumingly as part of an adverse immune response. Cattle with persistent upper airway obstruction and dyspnea caused by conditions associated with the soft tissues of the retropharynx and/or larynx may develop laryngeal edema as a secondary complication.

Necrotic Laryngitis (Calf Diphtheria)

Etiology and Signs. Necrotic laryngitis represents an atypical site of infection by the anaerobe *Fusobacterium necrophorum*, the organism responsible for calf diphtheria. Calf diphtheria is an infection of the soft tissue in the oral cavity following mucosal injury caused by sharp teeth in calves of 1 to 4 months of age. Calves affected with calf diphtheria usually have abscesses in the cheek region, have mild salivation, and may refuse solid feed (Figure 4-12). The infection spreads among calves fed from common utensils or those in such close contact that they may lick one another. When the larynx becomes infected in the atypical form of this disease, the affected calf develops a progressive inspiratory

Figure 4-11

A, Trephination sites surgically created to treat chronic frontal sinusitis in a 4-year-old Holstein cow. **B**, Trephination sites surgically created to treat chronic frontal sinusitis in a 3-year-old Holstein bull.

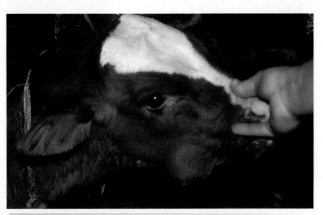

Figure 4-12

Typical cheek abscess observed in calf diphtheria.

dyspnea. Low-grade fever (103.0 to 104.5° F/39.44 to 40.28° C) may be present along with a painful short cough that is observed when the calf attempts to drink or eat. As the condition worsens over several days, both inspiratory and expiratory dyspnea may be apparent, but the inspiratory component always will be worse. A necrotic odor may be present on the breath.

Audible inspiratory efforts are heard. Harsh sounds of airway turbulence will be heard when a stethoscope is placed over the larynx; these sounds will be referred down the tracheobronchial tree to confuse auscultation of the lower airway.

Diagnosis. Endoscopy is helpful in confirming the diagnosis. In some calves, the lesions can be seen by using an oral speculum, but endoscopy is much easier and less stressful for the patient. If the calf is in extreme dyspnea or is anoxic or cyanotic, a tracheostomy should be performed before endoscopy. The larynx will be found to be uniformly swollen and may appear to have cartilaginous deformities in chronic cases (Figure 4-13). The laryngeal opening always is narrowed, and mucosal necrosis will be present in acute cases. Chronic cases may have laryngeal deformity and airway narrowing, but the necrotic, infected cartilage may be covered by normal mucosa (see video clips 6 to 8).

Treatment. Long-term therapy is required because infection of cartilaginous structures usually exists. Acute cases should be treated with penicillin (22,000 U/kg IM, twice daily). A tracheostomy is essential for treatment of calves that have severe dyspnea. This will provide a patent airway and rest the infected larynx from further exertional irritation while the infection is controlled. The prognosis for acute cases is fair.

Chronic cases have a poor prognosis because laryngeal deformity and cartilaginous necrosis or abscesses within the laryngeal cartilage already have developed. Treatment is similar to that described for acute cases but should be extended to 14 to 30 days in patients valuable enough to warrant treatment, or the necrotic cartilage should be surgically removed or debrided. A tracheostomy may be necessary for the reasons listed above, and some clinicians recommend concurrent treatment with sodium iodide in the hope of penetrating the deep-seated infection of cartilage. *A. pyogenes* frequently contributes to or replaces *F. necrophorum* as the causative organism in chronic infections because these two organisms are synergistic. For valuable cattle with the chronic form, referral to an expert surgeon familiar with the tracheolaryngostomy technique described by Gasthuys should be considered.

Tracheal Obstruction

Tracheal obstruction is not common but may occur from either intraluminal obstruction such as infectious bovine rhinotracheitis (IBR) infection or from extraluminal obstruction caused by abscess or lymphosarcoma or as a result of proliferative callus on the first ribs in calves (Figure 4-14). Congenital tracheal stenosis independent of rib injury has also been reported to occur within the cervical or thoracic portions of the trachea.

Diagnosis is generally easy if endoscopy and radiographs can be used to support the clinical examination. Most calves with tracheal obstruction resulting from proliferative rib callus are several weeks of age when

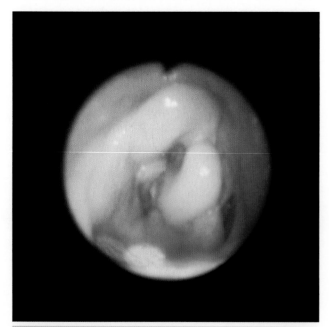

Figure 4-13

Endoscopic view of laryngeal deformity and profoundly narrow laryngeal airway in a 3-month-old Holstein calf that had necrotic laryngitis and chronic laryngeal cartilage infection caused by *F. necrophorum.*

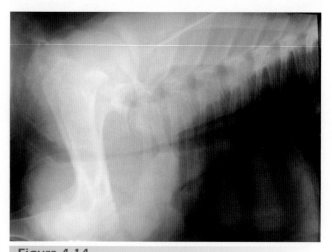

Figure 4-14

Radiograph of a 2-month-old calf with tracheal compression caused by callus formation on the first rib.

respiratory signs develop and have a history of dystocia at birth.

Treatment for intraluminal inflammatory obstruction would include nebulization with acetylcysteine, inhalational ceftiofur, and an appropriate bronchodilator (ipratropium inhaler and/or aminophylline or atropine systemically). Repair of the tracheal compression caused by proliferative callus formation has been described, but the procedure is technically difficult, and because of the young age of the animals, the prosthesis needs to be removed to permit normal growth of the trachea.

DISEASES OF THE LOWER AIRWAY

Bacterial Bronchopneumonia

This remains the most important cause of fatal respiratory disease in dairy calves and adult cattle. Virulent strains of *Mannheimia haemolytica* and *Histophilus somni* are primary pathogens capable of causing acute infections of the lower airway and lung parenchyma. These organisms do not always require the help of environmental and management stressors or other infectious agents to cause pneumonia. Chronic lower airway infections by *P. multocida* and *A. pyogenes* may cause pneumonia in calves either previously infected or coinfected with viral or *Mycoplasma* pathogens of the respiratory tract or in animals stressed by shipment, poor management, or ventilation insufficiencies. Chronic suppurative pneumonia in acute cattle may be the result of previous aspiration pneumonia; a combination of *P. multocida, A. pyogenes, Fusobacterium,* and *Mycoplasma* sp. are frequently cultured. Aspiration pneumonia associated with these same bacterial pathogens may also be observed in calves with white muscle disease, calves fed via an inappropriately large opening on the nipple of milk feeding bottles, premature calves with inadequately developed protective reflexes of the glottis, and calves with retropharyngeal diseases that interfere with normal upper airway reflexes. It is imperative for the bovine practitioner to understand the causes, predisposing factors, treatment, control, and prevention of these pathogens. In addition, it must be emphasized that the only way to diagnose and control contagious respiratory disease in cattle is to *know* the exact identity of the pathogens and predisposing causes. This can be accomplished only by careful history, thorough physical examination, collection of appropriate samples, and collaboration with a diagnostic laboratory capable of identifying all known bovine respiratory pathogens. The five major bacterial pathogens of the bovine lower airways currently are *M. haemolytica, P. multocida, Mycoplasma* spp., *H. somni,* and *A. pyogenes.* They will be discussed separately. Although other organisms may be involved, they seldom cause herd problems and will not be discussed.

Mannheimia haemolytica

Etiology and Signs. *M. haemolytica* is a gram-negative rod that may be a normal inhabitant of the upper airway but is not cultured from the upper airway of normal cattle as frequently as *P. multocida.* Several properties of *M. haemolytica* contribute to its pathogenicity. These include a capsule that provides defense against phagocytosis; production of an exotoxin (leukotoxin) lethal to alveolar macrophages, monocytes, and neutrophils; cell wall–derived endotoxin that helps to initiate complement and coagulation cascades; and the ability to reside in the upper airway among other nonpathogenic serotypes and then convert and/or overgrow under stressful stimuli to a pathogenic serotype, A1, that is more virulent. The cytotoxicity of the leukotoxin is associated with its ability to bind and interact with B2 integrin leukocyte function-associated antigen 1. Currently *M. haemolytica* is a leading cause of death as a result of respiratory infection in dairy cattle and calves in most areas of the United States. This organism is a primary pathogen not always needing assistance from other viral or *Mycoplasma* agents to establish lower airway infection, although it is well demonstrated that bovine herpesvirus 1 (BHV1) infection can activate genes that will increase leukotoxin binding, cytotoxicity to bovine mononuclear cells, and the severity of *M. haemolytica* infection. When a virus such as IBR, bovine respiratory syncytial virus (BRSV), or bovine virus diarrhea virus (BVDV) does infect a herd, mortality will be greatly increased if *M. haemolytica* bronchopneumonia is superimposed. In this situation, the bacteria may cause death because the viral infection compromises mechanical and cellular defense mechanisms. Mortality may approach 30% to 50% when a virulent *M. haemolytica* infection is superimposed on a preexisting viral infection (e.g., BHV1 or BVDV) in a herd. Cattle that are stressed are at great risk of *M. haemolytica* pneumonia because stress triggers both activation of the organism to a more virulent form, permits greater colonization of the virulent strain, and compromises the host defense mechanisms. Thus *M. haemolytica* is frequently isolated as the cause of "shipping fever pneumonia" associated with shipment of cattle, transport of cattle to shows, or recent purchase of replacement animals. Classic signs of pneumonia generally develop 1 to 2 weeks following any of these stresses. The morbidity and mortality percentages tend to be much greater for *M. haemolytica* pneumonia outbreaks than if *P. multocida* is found as the cause of shipping fever.

A great deal of variation in pathogenicity and antibiotic resistance exists for various isolates of *M. haemolytica.* Therefore the veterinarian must accept the fact that signs produced by these types will vary from mild to severe. Mild infections or less pathogenic *M. haemolytica* may mimic *P. multocida* with respect to clinical signs and response to therapy, whereas severe infections may be so drastic as to cause death within hours of the first clinical signs. In rare instances the death can be so peracute that toxicity is expected. A less pathogenic form has been seen causing high fever in recently fresh cows, all of which had a remarkably quick recovery following treatment with ceftiofur.

Signs of acute *M. haemolytica* pneumonia include fever, depression, anorexia, markedly decreased milk production, salivation, nasal discharge, moist painful cough, and rapid respirations (Figure 4-15). The fever may be as high as 108.0° F (42.22° C) but usually ranges between 104.0 and 107.0° F (40.0 to 41.67° C). Auscultation of the lungs reveals moist or dry rales in the anterior ventral lung fields bilaterally. Bronchial tones indicative of consolidation in the ventral lung fields are observed much more frequently than with acute *P. multocida* infections (Figure 4-16). Pleuritic friction sounds may be ausculted in some cases because of stretching or compression of fibrinous adhesions between the parietal and visceral pleura. The dorsal lung fields may sound normal on auscultation of animals with mild to moderate *M. haemolytica* pneumonia. In more severe cases, however, the dorsal lung may be forced to overwork because of the ventral lung consolidation. This overwork creates interstitial edema or bullous emphysema on occasion, and these pathologic changes cause the dorsal lung to be abnormally quiet on auscultation. Auscultation of the trachea will reveal coarse rattling or bubbling sounds caused by the inflammatory exudate free in the trachea. Palpation of the intercostal regions over the

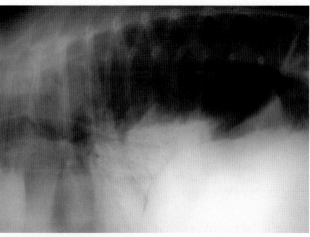

Figure 4-16

Thoracic radiograph of calf affected with severe *M. haemolytica* pneumonia. Cranioventral consolidation is highlighted by air bronchograms. Such lesions give rise to bronchial tones when the affected region of the lung is ausculted.

pneumonic lung causes the animal pain. Occasional cases will have an accumulation of transudative or exudative pleural fluid in the ventral thorax unilaterally or bilaterally that will cause a total absence of sounds when auscultation is performed.

More severe or neglected cases may show open mouth breathing (Figure 4-17), anxious expression, subcutaneous emphysema secondary to tracking of air from bullae rupture in the dorsal lung field, and have

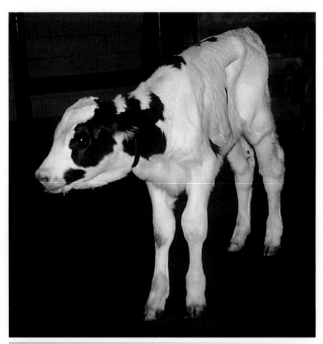

Figure 4-15

Calf affected with *M. haemolytica* pneumonia showing anxious expression, extended head and neck to minimize upper airway resistance, and ventral edema caused by both albumin loss into the severely infected lungs and gravitational edema.

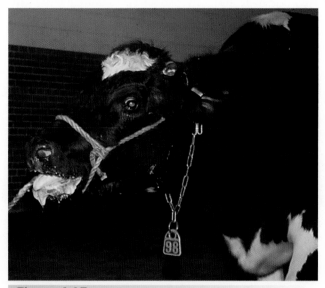

Figure 4-17

Cow affected with severe *M. haemolytica* pneumonia showing open mouth breathing, pulmonary edema froth at muzzle, anxious expression, dehydration, and extended head and neck to maintain a "straight line" upper airway.

harsh bronchial tones ventrally with inaudible lung sounds dorsally. Respiratory dyspnea is marked in such cases and affects both inspiratory and expiratory components, with the expiratory component being the most obvious. An audible grunt or groan may accompany each expiratory effort, and the animals are reluctant to move because of hypoxia and painful pleuritis.

A peracute rapidly consolidating form of *M. haemolytica* bronchopneumonia occasionally has been observed over the past 10 years in the northeastern United States and has resulted in high morbidity and mortality within affected herds. The causative *M. haemolytica* has proven extremely resistant to antibiotics. In some instances, it was resistant to all antibiotics approved for use in dairy cows. Signs in acutely affected cattle include high fever (106.0 to 108.0° F/41.11 to 42.22° C), marked depression, salivation, increased respiratory rate (60 to 120 breaths/min), complete anorexia and milk cessation, reluctance to move, absence of rales when the ventral lungs are ausculted, profound bronchial tones bilaterally that indicate consolidation of 25% to 75% of the ventral pulmonary parenchyma (Figure 4-18), and quiet or inaudible sounds in the dorsal lungs where the remaining pulmonary tissue has been subjected to extreme mechanical and physiologic stress to maintain gas exchange. Subcutaneous emphysema and pulmonary edema are common sequelae in these cattle. Ventral abdominal pain can be elicited in the cranial abdomen as a result of the fibrinous pleuritis present. This pain and absence of rumen activity coupled with the other signs have caused many veterinarians to confuse the initial case of rapidly consolidating pneumonia as peritonitis caused by hardware or perforating abomasal ulcer. The major reason for this error is the absence of rales with this form of *M. haemolytica*. Therefore we have had to "retrain" our

ears to auscult carefully for bronchial tones versus normal or harsh vesicular sounds. Careless auscultation of air sounds in the ventral lung field may not discriminate between bronchial tones and vesicular sounds. Acute infection with this form of *M. haemolytica* will result in progressive dyspnea and death in 12 to 48 hours unless the veterinarian is fortunate enough to choose as the first treatment an antibiotic to which the organism is susceptible.

Diagnosis. As with *P. multocida* pneumonia, accurate diagnosis of *M. haemolytica* bronchopneumonia requires culture of the organisms from tracheal wash specimens collected from *acute, untreated* cattle (Figure 4-19) or postmortem cultures of lung and lymph node specimens. Because mortality is greater for *M. haemolytica* than *P. multocida*, autopsy specimens often are the source of diagnostic material.

Once it is apparent that the disease is epidemic in the herd, the veterinarian should obtain appropriate cultures via tracheal washings or fresh lung tissue at necropsy from several animals so that the delay in accurate diagnosis and bacterial susceptibility to antibiotics is as short as possible.

Tracheal wash, nasopharyngeal swab, or autopsy specimens also should be cultured and/or antigen tested for viral pathogens, *H. somni*, and *Mycoplasma* sp. Serum for viral titers should be collected from several acute cases so that it may be compared with convalescent serum titers in the future, if the animals survive. In this way, some viral agents that are difficult to culture, such as BRSV, may be identified as primary or contributing causes of the respiratory outbreak. Having collected these samples for culture, antigen testing, and seroconversion, the veterinarian will now have a basis, albeit retrospective, to identify the pathogens involved and attribute the disease to *M. haemolytica* alone or combined with other pathogens. This will be of importance for future preventive measures.

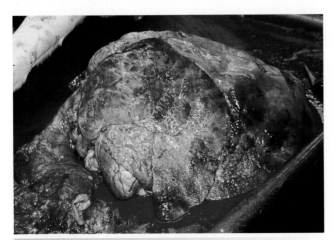

Figure 4-18

Necropsy view of lungs affected by peracute rapidly consolidating *M. haemolytica* pneumonia. Consolidation exists over 80% to 90% of the lung parenchyma, and fibrin is obvious on the visceral pleura. The clinical course of the disease was 36 hours.

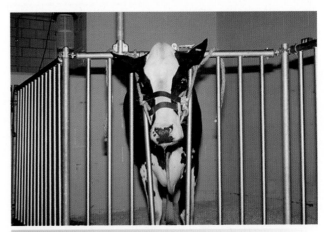

Figure 4-19

A cow being restrained with two halters in preparation of a transtracheal wash. This method of restraint helps keep the head and neck straight during the procedure.

Gross pathology specimens show a bilateral fibrinous bronchopneumonia with 25% to 75% or more of the lungs involved. The distribution is anterior ventral in all cases, and the affected lung is firm, meaty, friable, and discolored. Usually fibrin is present on both the visceral and parietal pleura. Increased amounts of yellow or yellow-red pleural fluid are found frequently. In acute cases with advanced pulmonary parenchymal consolidation or in chronic cases, the dorsal lung may have bullous emphysema or interstitial edema present.

A complete blood count (CBC) from acutely infected cattle usually will show leukopenia characterized by a neutropenia with a left shift as neutrophils move to the site of severe infection. Fibrinogen values are elevated.

Radiographs or ultrasonography is only of value for prognosing an individual valuable calf or cow. An estimation of degree of consolidation and subsequent abscess formation may be aided by these techniques and allow accurate prediction of outcome. However, these techniques seldom are necessary given the physical signs present.

Treatment. Broad-spectrum antibiotics constitute the major therapeutic defenses against *M. haemolytica* pneumonia. Once again, the veterinarian is forced to use "best guess" judgment when selecting an initial antibiotic in such cases. Following collection of appropriate diagnostic samples, antibiotic therapy should commence immediately. Because life-threatening signs usually appear in at least some of the affected cattle, the veterinarian is more likely to select broad-spectrum antibiotics immediately. The current popular antibiotics for cows and calves are shown in Table 4-1. Even when the causative bacterial organism is known, antibiotic therapy may be unable to cure the patient for a variety of reasons, such as the chosen antibiotic does not reach adequate tissue levels in the lung; the organism is resistant to the antibiotic; the organism is sensitive in vitro but in vitro inhibitory concentrations do not occur in the cow as a result of the dose, frequency of dosage, or other pharmacologic considerations; the drug may not be able to penetrate consolidated tissue or work in purulent tissue; and in vitro susceptibility tests may not reflect in vivo success of an antibiotic against a specific organism—thus the Kirby-Bauer disc assay has been criticized as too gross compared with mean inhibitory or bactericidal concentration tests that can give a concentration of drug that inhibits or kills an organism. This mean inhibitory concentration then can be compared with known achievable blood and tissue levels of the antibiotic in the cow to determine likelihood of successful treatment. The pathology may be irreversible or viral, and *Mycoplasma* or *A. pyogenes* pathogens may coexist to complicate the treatment plan. Textbook charts that quote percentages of isolates sensitive to various antibiotics are seldom helpful because both geographic differences in strains and temporal resistance patterns occur. Appropriate withdrawal times for any antibiotic selected for milk and slaughter residues must be known and observed and may shape decisions by the producer as to which antibiotic is chosen so that an immediate slaughter option is maintained.

The industry continues to seek the "silver bullet"—a magic antibiotic that will cure *all* cases of *Mannheimia*

TABLE 4-1   Dosages and Frequencies of Administration for Selected Antibiotics for Initial Therapy

Antibiotic	Dose	Frequency	Age
Ceftiofur	2.2 mg/kg *IM/IV +/or− aerosolution	Once or twice daily	Adult cattle and replacement heifers
Oxytetracycline HCI alone or in combination with sulfadimethoxine	11 mg/kg IV	Twice daily; use only in well-hydrated cattle	Adult cattle and replacement heifers
Florfenicol	20 mg/kg IM (neck only)	Every 48 hr	Replacement heifer
Erythromycin	5.5 mg/kg	Twice daily	Nonlactating cattle
Ampicillin	11.0-22.0 mg/kg	Twice daily	Adult cattle and replacement heifers
Enrofloxacin (Other fluoroquinolones available in some countries)	2.2-5.0 mg/kg*†	Once daily, Europe only	Adult cattle and replacement heifers
Tilmicosin	10 mg/kg SQ	Every 3 days	Replacement heifer
Tulathromycin	2.5 mg/kg SQ	Once or repeat in 5 days	Nonlactating dairy cattle

*Often used at higher dosages, but no objective data are available about efficacy of higher dosages.
†Prohibited in dairy cattle in the United States.

pneumonia. This silver bullet would take away the need for diagnostic work or preventive medicine, excuse management techniques that predispose to pneumonia, and of course would only be available through veterinarians. As a profession, we persist in overuse of every new antibiotic that becomes available. We ask these antibiotics to do things that cannot be done while ignoring older time-tested antibiotics. The silver bullet does not and will not exist.

Improvement in response to appropriate antibiotic therapy will appear as better attitude and appetite and a decreasing fever within 24 hours. A decrease of 2° F or more should be considered clinically indicative of improvement. The body temperature continues to decrease into the normal range over 48 to 72 hours in most cases that have been treated with appropriate antibiotics. Depending on which antibiotic is used, a minimum of 3 days of antibiotic treatment is often required, and more often 5 to 7 days of continuous therapy are necessary and less likely to result in recurrence.

Antiinflammatory medications are used by many veterinarians in conjunction with antibiotic therapy, as discussed under *P. multocida* pneumonia. If corticosteroids are used as part of initial therapy, we believe that 20 mg of dexamethasone or a comparable dose of prednisone for an adult cow is the maximum. This should not be used more than once, and it should not be used at all in pregnant cattle. Currently in our clinic, we do not use any corticosteroids in the treatment of *M. haemolytica* pneumonia. Flunixin meglumine or other nonsteroidal antiinflammatory drugs (NSAIDs) are sound therapeutic agents for use in those with *M. haemolytica* pneumonia for the first 1 to 3 days of therapy. Excessive dosage of NSAIDs or prolonged treatment with these agents should be avoided. Once again, aspirin is the safest drug for this purpose (at a dosage of 240 to 480 grains orally, twice daily for an adult cow or 25 grains/100 lb body weight twice daily for calves). Flunixin meglumine at 0.50 to 1.0 mg/kg is the most commonly recommended and only approved NSAID for treating bovine pneumonia and has been documented to improve clinical outcomes when combined with antibiotics compared with antibiotic treatment alone.

Antihistamines such as tripelennamine (1 mg/kg twice or thrice daily) are less commonly used these days but are still used by many experienced clinicians as supportive therapy. Atropine may be a useful adjunct in advanced cases showing marked dyspnea, open mouth breathing, or pulmonary edema. Atropine is used at 2.2 mg/45 kg body weight IM or subcutaneously (SQ), twice daily to decrease bronchial secretions and to act as a mild bronchodilator.

In severe cases, dehydration may be a complication because of toxemia and fever causing depression of appetite and water consumption. In addition, some cattle are so dyspneic that they are unable to take time to

drink, lest they become more hypoxic. Any IV fluid therapy that excessively expands the intravascular volume may cause or worsen existing pulmonary edema, and the fluid volume administered must be appropriate. Administrating fluids through a stomach tube is safer regarding pulmonary edema, but the procedure is very stressful to an already hypoxic animal. Clinical judgment is required for these decisions, and in most cases, it is best to hope that antibiotic therapy will improve the animal within 24 to 48 hours so that the cow or calf may hydrate itself through adequate water consumption. Adequate water, salt, and small amounts of fresh feeds should be used to promote appetite.

Any management or ventilation deficiencies should be remedied immediately, and fresh air is of the utmost importance. It is better that the animals be in the cold fresh air than in a poorly ventilated or drafty but warm enclosure. The worst environmental effects occur when cattle develop *M. haemolytica* pneumonia during hot, humid weather because the additional respiratory effort to encourage heat loss complicates existing hyperpnea. Intranasal oxygen is beneficial for affected cattle being treated in a hospital.

Prognosis always is guarded until signs of clinical improvement are obvious. Cattle improving within 24 to 72 hours have a good prognosis, whereas those that take more than 72 hours have a greater risk of chronic lung damage or abscessation.

Following endemic *Mannheimia* or *Pasteurella* infection in groups of calves, Drs. King and Rebhun observed occasional calves that developed peracute respiratory distress and dyspnea as a result of proliferative pneumonia 2 to 4 weeks after recovering from confirmed *Mannheimia/Pasteurella* pneumonia. At autopsy, resolving anterior ventral pneumonia from the previous *Mannheimia/Pasteurella* infection is observed in anterior ventral lung fields, and the remainder of the lung is diffusely firm, heavy, and wet. Histopathology confirms proliferative pneumonia. Viral cultures, fluorescent antibody (FA) procedures, and serology have been negative for other pathogens, including BRSV, which also may cause a delayed-effect hypersensitivity pneumonia but with different lesions. Following observation of a number of these secondary proliferative pneumonia cases in the necropsy room, they were able to recognize clinically and treat several calves with this problem. The calves had a history of being part of a pneumonia outbreak 2 to 4 weeks previously, then apparently recovering. A sudden onset of extreme dyspnea in one recovered calf typifies the clinical situation. Signs include mild fever, open mouth breathing, and diffusely quiet lungs. Treatment consists of atropine (2.2 mg/45 kg twice daily), furosemide (25 mg/45 kg once or twice daily), broad-spectrum antibiotics, and box stall rest in a well-ventilated area. Response to therapy is slow, but survivors gradually improve over 7 to 10 days.

Pasteurella multocida

Etiology and Signs. *P. multocida* is a gram-negative normal inhabitant of the upper airway of cattle and calves. The normal defense mechanisms of the lower airway prevent colonization of the lung by *P. multocida* via physical, cellular, and secretory defenses in the healthy state. *P. multocida* is, however, a likely opportunist any time lower airway defense mechanisms are compromised. Chemical damage to mucociliary clearance, such as is caused by ammonia fumes in poorly ventilated barns, may allow *P. multocida* the opportunity to colonize the lower airway. *P. multocida* also is found in mixed infections of the lung along with *H. somni*, *A. pyogenes*, *Mycoplasma* sp., and various respiratory viruses of cattle. *Fusobacterium* and other anaerobic organisms may also be present with chronic suppurative pneumonia in adult cattle.

The strains of *P. multocida* isolated from the lungs of cattle or calves frequently are sensitive to many antibiotics, including penicillin. This is in definite contrast to *M. haemolytica*, in which antibiotic resistance is much more probable. This difference will be important regarding treatment and prevention of *P. multocida* pneumonia.

The signs of acute *P. multocida* pneumonia include fever, depression, mild to severe anorexia, moist cough, increased rate and depth of respiration, and a decrease in milk production commensurate with the degree of anorexia. The fever ranges from 103.5 to 105.5° F (39.72 to 40.83° C) in most cases. Moist and dry rales will be ausculted in the anterior ventral lung field bilaterally and are classical findings in acute cases. Usually the dorsal lung fields are normal. Nasal discharge may be serous or mucopurulent in nature and is more apparent in calves than adult cows. The acute disease may occur in calves and cows of any age but tends to be more common in weaned calves and other grouped animals. When seen in younger animals, the acute disease usually is indicative of poor ventilation, excessive ammonia fumes, failure of passive transfer of immunoglobulins, and/or part of a diarrhea/pneumonia complex. All these predisposing factors are common in dairy calves placed in veal operations or other indoor group housing facilities. *P. multocida* has been found as the cause of neonatal septicemia in calves receiving inadequate colostrum. These septicemic calves may show signs of meningitis, septic uveitis, septic arthritis, and mucopurulent nasal and ocular discharge (Figure 4-20) in addition to the typical signs of acute *P. multocida* pneumonia.

Acute *P. multocida* pneumonia tends to occur as either an infectious epidemic or endemic disease in groups of housed calves or adult cattle and may affect 10% to 50% of the animals within a group. It is one of the causes of "enzootic pneumonia" in calves, but this is not the preferred term because it gives little information as to the exact cause of pneumonia. During an

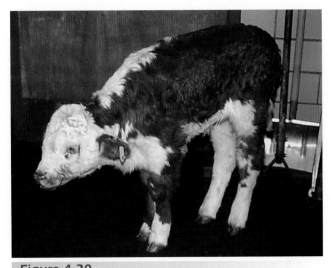

Figure 4-20

Neonatal calf with *P. multocida* septicemia. In addition to pneumonia, signs included fever, hypopyon, and mucopurulent nasal and ocular discharges.

acute outbreak, the degree of apparent illness and auscultable degree of pneumonia will vary greatly among affected cattle or calves. If only one animal in a group is infected, predisposing causes or stress unique to that animal should be sought when establishing a history (e.g., recent purchase, recent calving, possibility of BVDV-persistent infection [Figure 4-21], transport to a show, sale, or poor ventilatory management).

Chronic pneumonia resulting from *P. multocida* causes signs similar to the acute disease, but bronchial tones indicative of consolidation frequently are limited to the anterior ventral lung fields. The abnormal area may be missed unless the stethoscope is pushed under the shoulder and the calf or cow forced to take a deep

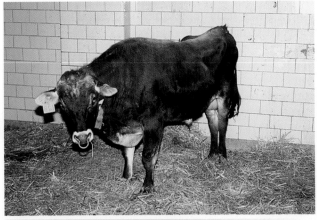

Figure 4-21

A 3-year-old Jersey bull at a stud facility developed *P. multocida* pneumonia without any environmental stress factors. The bull was later proven to be persistently infected with BVDV, which likely resulted in immunosuppression.

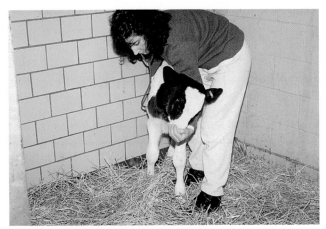

Figure 4-22

An easy method of properly auscultating the lungs in calves. To make the calf breathe deeply, the calf is backed into a corner and one hand is placed over the mouth and nose until the calf struggles, at which time the calf is allowed to breathe. Alternatively, in adult cows a plastic garbage bag can be used over the cow's nose and mouth to force deep breathing.

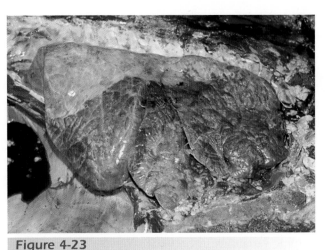

Figure 4-23

Necropsy findings in a calf that was affected with severe cranioventral pneumonia caused by *P. multocida*.

breath. In calves this can be accomplished most easily by holding the mouth and nose shut for a short period (Figure 4-22). Animals affected with chronic pneumonia may have marked exacerbation of dyspnea and an increased respiratory rate (≥60 breaths/min) if housed in poorly ventilated areas or where the environmental temperature exceeds 70.0° F (21.1° C). *A. pyogenes* is a common secondary invader in lungs chronically infected with *P. multocida*. Following acute epidemic *P. multocida* pneumonia, occasional affected animals may show signs of chronic pneumonia.

Diagnosis. *P. multocida* pneumonia may be suspected after obtaining the appropriate history from the cow's owner and finding typical signs complete with anterior ventral pneumonia and bilateral auscultable rales. However, confirmation requires culture of *P. multocida* from tracheal wash samples or autopsy specimens of *acute, untreated* affected animals. Neutrophils predominate the white blood cell components of the tracheal wash fluid, and gram-negative rods may be observed intracellularly in acute cases. The hemogram may show a degenerative left shift typical of acute infection in cattle or may be normal in mild cases. Chronic cases (≥2 weeks) may have neutrophilia, and adult cattle may show hyperglobulinemia in the serum.

Gross pathology of fatal acute cases includes bilateral anterior ventral pneumonia with the affected portion of lung being firm and discolored red or blue (Figure 4-23). Palpation of the firm affected lung is the key to gross pathologic diagnosis. Fibrin may coat the surface of the parietal or visceral pleura but tends to be less than that observed with *M. haemolytica*. Chronic cases will show

similar firm, pneumonic lung parenchyma but often have bronchiectasis and pulmonary abscesses.

Radiographs seldom are necessary but may be helpful for individual chronically infected calves or mature cattle to identify abscesses and degree of consolidation for prognostic purposes. Ultrasound examination will help define the severity of lung involvement.

Treatment. Antimicrobials and changes in husbandry or management constitute the integral components of effective therapy for *P. multocida* pneumonia. Many antibiotics have been used, including penicillin, ampicillin, erythromycin, and tetracycline. Sulfa drugs (trimethoprim-sulfa has been used in calves because it can be mixed with milk to bypass the forestomachs) also have been effective when administered either alone or in combination with antibiotics such as penicillin or tetracycline. Ceftiofur, a broad-spectrum cephalosporin, has been approved for use in *Pasteurella* pneumonia in cattle and has proven to be very effective. Tilmicosin (a macrolide) and florfenicol are also effective but currently not approved for use in adult dairy cattle. The practicing veterinarian must start antibiotic therapy without knowing results of cultures and antibiotic sensitivity tests. Therefore initial treatment is based on previous experience, geographic differences in antibiotic sensitivity, and economic factors. Animals that are febrile, anorectic, and dyspneic require treatment. Other animals that have mild fever and depression but continue to eat and do not act very ill may not require treatment. Individual or small groups of sick animals may be treated empirically if fatalities are not anticipated. However, if an epidemic situation is apparent, it always is best to do transtracheal washes from several animals before any treatment. Having done this, the veterinarian may start empiric therapy assured that definitive antibiotic sensitivity results will be forthcoming in 3 days. Thus if the animals fail to respond to the initial choice of antibiotic, a specific antibiotic may be selected based on the sensitivity results as soon as these are available.

Penicillin, tetracycline, florfenicol, ampicillin, or ceftiofur may be selected for initial therapy. Dosages and frequency of administration are listed in Table 4-1. Regardless of the antibiotic selected, all treated cattle should have temperature and attitudes recorded daily so that 24- and 48-hour evaluations can be assessed. A trend of decreasing temperature into the normal range should proceed at 1 to 2° F per day when an effective antibiotic is used; the attitude, appetite, and degree of dyspnea should improve along with the return to normal body temperature. Hjerpe has done extensive work in feedlot cattle to estimate probable efficacies of various antibiotics in pneumonia outbreaks. This material is an excellent reference, but the veterinarian must remember that geographic variations in bacterial serotypes and antibiotic susceptibility exist and that antibiotic resistance is likely to increase in years to come. Individual treatment generally is easier for dairy animals than beef animals. Antibiotics such as tetracycline, sulfa drugs, and tylosin have been added to feed and water to treat large groups of calves or heifers. This method may be utilized if the animals are not too sick to eat or drink. If affected cattle are completely off feed, this method is ineffective. When faced with an obvious epidemic, the veterinarian may choose to divide the animals requiring treatment into three groups—each group consisting of animals with mild, moderate, and severe signs. Each group then could be treated with a different antibiotic. Twenty-four hours after initial treatment, each group would be evaluated for relative degrees of improvement and all sick animals given the antibiotic that resulted in the most improved group.

Many practitioners use antiinflammatory agents in conjunction with antimicrobial therapy. The goals of antiinflammatory medications are to reduce fever, block specific parts or mediators of the inflammatory cycle, counteract endotoxins released by the cell wall of the causative gram-negative organisms, and result in symptomatic improvement through better appetite and attitude. The two general groups of drugs include corticosteroids and NSAIDs, such as aspirin and flunixin meglumine. Corticosteroids have a marked antiinflammatory and antipyretic activity that often leads to a "steroid euphoria" with resultant improved attitude and appetite within 24 hours. Although corticosteroids have these positive effects and also block several parts of the inflammatory cycle, they are dangerous if used repeatedly or in high dosages. Corticosteroids may reduce some of the chemotactic factors and lysosomal enzymes that cause a vicious cycle of increasing inflammation in the lung and tend to stabilize small vessels. However, they also partially or completely inhibit macrophage activation and antimicrobial peptide expression, which are serious detriments to the defense mechanisms of the lower airway. If the veterinarian elects to use corticosteroids, one treatment of low-dose

(10 to 20 mg/450 kg) dexamethasone may be given as part of the initial therapy and should not be used thereafter. This treatment cannot be used in pregnant cows because of the abortifacient qualities of dexamethasone. Corticosteroids have potent antipyretic properties, and this may lead to a false sense of security because the veterinarian may assume that the proper antibiotic has been used based on a decreasing fever 24 hours following treatment when in fact the antibiotic has not been effective and fever will return 24 to 48 hours later. I do not recommend the use of corticosteroids for bacterial pneumonia.

NSAIDs are safer than corticosteroids in the treatment of bacterial bronchopneumonia in cattle but are not without some disadvantages. Advantages include blockage of some prostaglandin-mediated inflammation within the lung, antiendotoxin effects, and antipyretic activity. Disadvantages include inability to gauge response to specific antibiotics based on body temperature alone as a result of the artificial decrease in fever caused by NSAIDs, and the possibility of toxicity manifested by abomasal ulceration or renal damage if treatment is excessive in frequency, dosage, or duration. Aspirin may be the safest of the NSAIDs and is given at 240 to 480 grains orally, twice daily for an adult animal, and flunixin meglumine at 0.50 to 1.0 mg/kg IV, once or twice daily may be the most effective. Occasionally aspirin and flunixin meglumine have caused abomasal ulceration when administered for a prolonged time to sick cattle. Renal toxicity also is a risk—especially in a dehydrated animal in which the cytoprotective and vascular effects of prostaglandins are essential during reduced renal perfusion. I prefer flunixin when NSAID therapy is selected, but similar to corticosteroids, these drugs are adjuncts, not essentials, for the treatment of bronchopneumonia caused by *P. multocida*.

Bronchodilators such as aminophylline have been used in cattle with pneumonia but do not appear to be beneficial clinically except when given by constant infusion to calves with respiratory distress. Atropine given parenterally or ipratropium by inhalation may be effective bronchodilators. If albuterol could be used in cattle, it might be beneficial because this drug has been shown in other species to act not only as a bronchodilator but also to improve mucociliary clearance. Parasympatholytic bronchodilators have been shown to be more effective in calves than sympathomimetic drugs.

Antihistamines are used as adjunctive therapy in bovine bronchopneumonia by many practitioners. Drugs such as tripelennamine hydrochloride (1 mg/kg IM or SQ, twice or thrice daily) are believed to improve the animal's attitude and appetite. These symptomatic observations may be valid, but because histamine has not been shown to be one of the major inflammatory mediators in *Pasteurella* pneumonia, no scientific evidence exists to justify the use of these drugs.

The recognition and correction of management problems or ventilation deficiencies may be as important, if not more so, than any of the previous pharmaceuticals when treating endemic *P. multocida* pneumonia. Because the organism primarily is an opportunist that gains access to the lower airway following insults to the physical, cellular, or secretory defense mechanisms, predisposing causes should be sought and corrected. In calves, poor ventilation, crowding, and poor husbandry relating to excessive ammonia fumes may be sufficient to allow *P. multocida* to descend from its normal habitat of the upper airway and colonize the lungs. Examples include changeable temperature and humidity when calves are grouped during the indoor housing season (especially fall, spring, and during winter thaws), broken fans, failure to clean large pens when calves have been in groups for weeks to months, lungworms, and drafts that the confined calves cannot escape. Fresh air is vital to recovery and should be provided even if it means allowing the animals access to outside air in inclement weather.

In adult cattle, all these factors above apply, but ventilation deficiencies predominate. In modern free stall facilities, transition cow management practices that add greater stress to an already changeable/stressful period appear to greatly impact the acquisition of acute pneumonia and progression to chronic disease. Frequent pen moves, overstocking, poor ventilation, and concurrent metabolic disease alongside some of the treatments and therapeutic practices used by producers all substantially increase the chances for postpartum respiratory disease to become a herd problem. Bronchopneumonia caused by *P. multocida* alone usually is a management problem. Although it certainly is recognized that previous viral infection or mixed infections (e.g., *Mycoplasma*) could and do predispose to *P. multocida* pneumonia in calves and cattle, it must be emphasized that management factors are very important. Secondary *P. multocida* pneumonia, such as that following viral respiratory infection, will be discussed in conjunction with viral diseases. Failure of cattle affected with *P. multocida* pneumonia to respond to appropriate antibiotic therapy based on culture and susceptibility results should alert the veterinarian to the fact that (1) *P. multocida* is not the only agent involved in the epidemic (i.e., a virus or *Mycoplasma* also may be present or was present—therefore viral isolation, paired serology, and so forth are indicated); (2) the predisposing management or ventilation problems have not been corrected; and (3) lungworms should be ruled out.

Vaccinations are included in the prevention section and are discussed on pages 107-109.

Histophilus somni

Etiology and Signs. With increasing frequency, *H. somni* has been identified as a pathogen of the lower airway in dairy cattle. It is occasionally identified as the cause of herd outbreaks of pneumonia in dairy cattle or calves in the northeastern United States. *H. somni* may be the only pathogen isolated or may be found in conjunction with *Mycoplasma* spp. or *Pasteurella* pneumonia in cattle. Although *H. somni* occasionally is isolated from the upper airway of normal cattle, this gram-negative organism is more commonly isolated in clinical pneumonia patients. A shift in the normal upper airway bacterial flora or stress activation of latent *H. somni* in the upper airway may contribute to lower airway infection.

The pathogenicity of *H. somni* and *Pasteurella* organisms is attributed to several characteristics: (1) an endotoxin derived from the cell wall lipopolysaccharides, (2) exotoxins that are lethal or damaging to alveolar macrophages, neutrophils, and vascular endothelium, and (3) chemotactic factors and possible hemolysins common to *H. somni* and other bacteria that act as inflammatory mediators. Vasculitis is a predominant feature of *H. somni* pathology. *H. somni*–stimulated platelets have also been shown to contribute to endothelial cell damage, which may play a role in pathogenesis of the vasculitis and thrombosis. In addition, *H. somni* has a propensity to cause disease in the heart muscle and sometimes the central nervous system.

The signs of *H. somni* bronchopneumonia in calves and adult cattle are indistinguishable from moderate to severe *P. multocida* pneumonia or mild to moderate *M. haemolytica* pneumonia. Affected animals have fever (103.5 to 106.6° F/39.72 to 41.44° C), an increased respiratory rate (40 to 80 breaths/min), depression, nasal discharge, occasional salivation, painful cough, and decreased milk production proportional to the degree of anorexia observed. Dyspnea may be marked in some cases, and these cattle will show anxiety and reluctance to move. Neurologic signs or septicemia caused by *H. somni* observed in feedlot animals is less common in dairy cattle and calves. If, however, any cattle develop neurologic signs during an outbreak of bronchopneumonia in a herd or group of calves, *H. somni* should be strongly suspected as the cause of the illness.

Auscultation of the lungs typically identifies bilateral anterior ventral pneumonia characterized by moist and dry rales with bronchial tones indicative of ventral consolidation identified in up to 50% of the cases. Tracheal rales may be ausculted as a result of the heavy mucopurulent exudate found in the trachea. Palpation of the intercostal spaces overlying the pneumonic regions may be painful to the animal.

Diagnosis. Because the signs usually are identical to those of *Pasteurella* pneumonia, the veterinarian should collect appropriate samples (tracheal washes for culture and bacterial sensitivities or autopsy cultures from lung and lymph nodes) and institute therapy. A failure of response to standard broad-spectrum antibacterial therapy typifies *H. somni* pneumonia. Usually an exact diagnosis as to etiology has to await culture and sensitivity results from diagnostic samples. CBCs are variable and nonspecific, with either a degenerative or regenerative left shift observed and elevated fibrinogen levels. Acute and convalescent serum may be helpful retrospectively if the diagnostic laboratory utilized for testing has the capability to establish *H. somni* titers.

Postmortem specimens will show anteroventral firm areas of pneumonia bilaterally. Fibrin may be apparent in the visceral and parietal pleura occupying the areas of pneumonia. In some cases, red blotches or hemorrhage is apparent. White microabscesses may be observed also.

Treatment. Although *H. somni* apparently is sensitive in vitro to many antibiotics including penicillin, clinical results in vivo are discouraging. Ampicillin is the drug of choice for *H. somni* pneumonia in calves and adult cattle. Ampicillin is used at 11 to 22 mg/kg twice daily by injection for 3 to 7 days in most cases. Cephalosporins also may be effective. Enrofloxacin reportedly has good efficacy against *Histophilus* sp. but currently is not approved for use in dairy cattle in the United States.

Response to ampicillin or other effective antibiotics will be manifested by a progressive decrease in body temperature to the normal range over 24 to 72 hours. For this reason, the treating veterinarian may find it best not to use NSAIDs or corticosteroids in *H. somni* pneumonia because these drugs decrease the temperature artificially through antipyretic effects and interfere with interpretation of appropriate antibiotic selection.

Just as in *Pasteurella* bronchopneumonia, ventilation or management factors that predispose to altered lower airway defense mechanisms should be corrected immediately. The prognosis is fair to good unless severe pneumonia and marked dyspnea are present.

Arcanobacterium pyogenes Chronic Suppurative Pneumonia

Etiology and Signs. *A. pyogenes* is a gram-positive coccobacillus that acts as a ubiquitous opportunist capable of establishing chronic pyogenic infections virtually anywhere in the cow's body. In the lung, it is a secondary invader that usually only establishes infection following suppression of host physical, cellular, or secretory defense mechanisms. Physical factors such as inhalation pneumonia also may allow *A. pyogenes* to infect the lung, and viral, bacterial, or *Mycoplasma* agents may precede infection with *A. pyogenes*. Immunosuppression caused by acute or persistent infection with BVDV has been followed by *A. pyogenes* pneumonia in calves and adult cows. Similarly, calves affected with bovine leukocyte adhesion deficiency (BLAD) frequently suffered *A. pyogenes* pneumonia. Pulmonary infection is aided by the proteases and hemolysins that the organism produces. These factors contribute to tissue necrosis and inflammatory events that perpetuate the organism's existence. *Fusobacterium* and other pathogenic anaerobic

organisms may be found concurrently with *A. pyogenes*, *P. multocida*, and *Mycoplasma* spp.

Signs are indicative of *chronic or recurrent infection*, the hallmark of *A. pyogenes* pneumonia. The history usually indicates illness of at least 1 week's duration or recurrent episodes of pneumonia over weeks to months. There may only be one (usually adult cattle) or a few animals (usually calves) affected out of a group or herd. In adult dairy cattle, it is common for clinical signs to develop following freshening (Figure 4-24). In some cases, there may be severe subcutaneous emphysema over the dorsum, suggesting a rupture of diseased alveoli associated with calving as a cause of the pneumomediastinum, subcutaneous emphysema, and sometimes pneumothorax. Although this should be considered in cattle with dorsal emphysema following calving, similar emphysema may be found sometimes in apparently healthy cattle following calving and of course in cattle with interstitial pneumonia. Affected animals may show low-grade fever (103.0 to 105.0° F/39.44 to 40.56° C), rapid respiratory rate (40 to 100 breaths/min), dyspnea characterized by exaggerated inspiratory and especially expiratory efforts (particularly when stressed), head and neck extension when lying down, cough, nasal discharge (Figure 4-25), rough hair coat, poor body condition, depression, inappetence, or decreased milk production. Some cattle maintain normal respiratory rates but exhibit the other signs. Chronic suppurative pneumonia should always be considered a differential for the "poor doing" cow. Auscultation of the lungs reveals moist and dry rales in the ventral 25% to 50% of both lungs in calves and one or both lungs in adult cattle, bronchial tones indicative of consolidation in the ventral lung fields, and coarse tracheal rales caused by a thick mucopurulent airway exudate. High environmental temperatures, high humidity, and poor ventilation exacerbate the clinical signs. A fetid smell may be

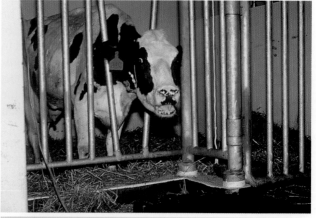

Figure 4-24

A 5-year-old cow with cough and respiratory distress following calving 5 days earlier. The cow had chronic suppurative pneumonia with acute onset of respiratory signs associated with stress of calving.

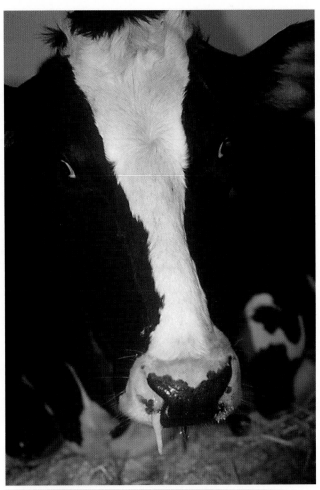

Figure 4-25

A mature Holstein cow presented to the hospital for poor production and weight loss. Although respiratory rate was within normal limits, the cow coughed after rising, had slight head and neck extension when lying down, and, as seen in this photo, had small and intermittent purulent nasal discharge. *P. multocida*, *A. pyogenes*, and *Mycoplasma* spp. were cultured from a tracheal wash. The cow improved dramatically following tetracycline therapy.

present following a cough if anaerobic bacteria are present. Auscultation during rebreathing, paying close attention to the cranioventral lung fields under the triceps musculature for the presence of bronchial tones indicative of consolidation, is important when investigating possible cases of mild to moderate chronic suppurative bronchopneumonia.

Diagnosis. History and physical signs are very suggestive of *A. pyogenes* pneumonia, but specific diagnosis requires culture of the organism from tracheal wash samples or lung tissue. There may only be one or a few animals affected with signs of chronic pneumonia following a preceding herd endemic of pneumonia caused by other organisms. Chronic or recurrent cases are referred to as "lungers" by some farmers.

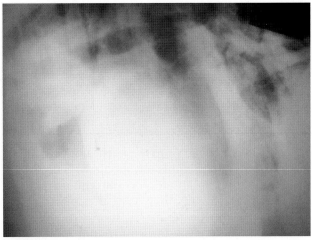

Figure 4-26

Radiograph of a cow with chronic suppurative pneumonia and a dramatic lobar consolidation.

Radiographs or ultrasonography of the thorax is helpful in establishing a prognosis because lung abscesses, bronchiectasis, and consolidation (sometimes remarkably severe in a single lobe) (Figure 4-26) are common in the affected lung (see video clip 9).

A CBC may show neutrophilia or be normal. Serum globulin often is in the high range of normal or elevated (≥5.0 g/dl), especially in adult cattle. The animal should be screened for persistent infection with BVDV via buffy coat viral isolation. Gross autopsy of fatal cases reveals anterior ventral consolidation with areas of purulent bronchiectasis and multiple pulmonary abscesses (Figure 4-27).

Treatment. Treatment is frustrating, and the prognosis is poor for pneumonia caused by *A. pyogenes*. Other causative organisms such as *P. multocida*,

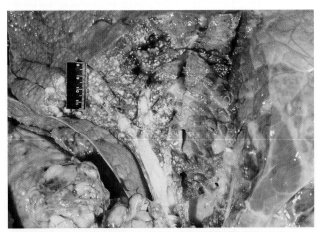

Figure 4-27

Necropsy view of cut section from the cranioventral lung region of a calf showing bronchiectasis and pulmonary abscesses typical of chronic *A. pyogenes* pneumonia.

M. haemolytica, Mycoplasma, and/or *Fusobacterium* also may be cultured from the tracheal wash sample. Penicillin is the drug of choice and should be given at 22,000 U/kg twice daily for 7 to 30 days. Although penicillin is effective against *A. pyogenes* in vitro, the pulmonary in vivo infection should be likened to an abscess because of the heavy accumulation of *A. pyogenes* pus in areas of bronchiectasis or encapsulated lung abscesses. If another pathogen, in addition to *A. pyogenes,* is isolated from the tracheal wash sample, appropriate antibiotic therapy should be selected for this organism as well. Ceftiofur, ampicillin, and tetracyclines are other commonly used therapies. Clinical treatment frequently results in short-term improvement followed by relapse when the animal is stressed or subjected to high environmental temperatures, humidity, or poor ventilation. Signs of improvement will be indicated by normal rectal temperature, improved respiratory function, and improvement in overall body condition and attitude. Many affected animals eventually succumb to the infection or are culled because of poor condition and production.

Mycoplasma Pneumonia

Etiology and Signs. Several types of *Mycoplasma* organisms, including *Mycoplasma dispar, M. bovis,* and *Mycoplasma bovirhinus,* have been isolated from the lungs of calves and cattle with pneumonia. In addition, *Ureaplasma* organisms and occasional isolates of *Mycoplasma bovigenitalium* have been found from lower airway infections in cattle. *M. dispar* and *M. bovis* probably are the two major types identified. The organisms may be normal inhabitants of the upper airway in some cattle. Experimentally, *Mycoplasma* spp. have caused pneumonia in calves when introduced into the lower airway. This pneumonia is characterized by peribronchiolar and peribronchial lymphoid hyperplasia and purulent bronchiolitis. Lesions usually are limited to the anterior ventral tips of the lung lobes, and the associated clinical signs are mild. Gross inspection at necropsy reveals ventral areas of lung lobes that are red-blue and firm, appear almost as atelectatic areas, and ooze purulent material from the airways on cut sections. *Mycoplasma* pneumonia has been described as a "cuffing pneumonia" because lymphoid hyperplasia appears around the airways and expands with time. *Mycoplasma* organisms have several properties that contribute to their pathogenicity, including inhibition of the mucociliary transport mechanism (at least in humans); they cause some degree of humoral and cell-mediated immunosuppression in calves; and they avoid phagocytosis by attaching to ciliated epithelium above the level of alveolar macrophages.

At our clinic, *Mycoplasma* frequently is isolated from acute and chronic calf pneumonia outbreaks and may be involved in up to 50% of chronic calf pneumonia

endemics that we investigate. However, *Mycoplasma* sp. seldom is the only pathogen isolated in these outbreaks, and *H. somni, P. multocida,* and *M. haemolytica* usually are isolated as well. Because *Mycoplasma* appears ubiquitous on many farms, we wonder whether the *Mycoplasma* infection has been present in the calves' lungs for a long time and contributes to impaired host defense against bacterial and viral pathogens or whether the *Mycoplasma* infection is acute along with the other pathogens. In herds with *Mycoplasma* pneumonia, *Mycoplasma* frequently can be isolated from almost all adult cows and calves—most of which appear healthy. Therefore the ubiquitous nature of the organism makes it nearly impossible for calves on these farms not to be infected. The subsequent low grade pneumonia and defense mechanism compromise caused by the *Mycoplasma* infection may precede the onset of clinical pneumonia caused by bacterial and viral pathogens. How significant *Mycoplasma* sp. is to the entire problem is difficult to determine, but we believe it increases the risk of calfhood pneumonia. In addition to pneumonia, *M. bovis* may also cause otitis media, mastitis, and arthritis once it becomes established in a herd. Some of the spread is likely from feeding infected milk. Effective control measures for *Mycoplasma* when it is ubiquitous on a premise are challenging and made more so because effective vaccines are not available. In endemic herds, the feeding of waste milk is a known risk factor for transmission of the organism to calves, and this practice should be actively discouraged. Pasteurization will remove the risk of *Mycoplasma* spread by this means but only makes economic sense on larger dairies or heifer-rearing operations.

Signs of pure *Mycoplasma* pneumonia may be very mild. In several calf and heifer outbreaks of pure *Mycoplasma* pneumonia, the only signs observed were coughing induced by stress or movement of the animals, a slight increase in the respiratory rate (40 to 60 breaths/min), and low grade fever (103.5° to 105.0° F/39.72° to 40.56° C). Most affected animals continued to eat and experienced only mild depression. Owners reported observing a slight mucopurulent nasal discharge in the animals in the mornings that disappeared after the animals became active, ate, and licked their noses clean. Tracheal washes grew pure cultures of *Mycoplasma,* and no other pathogens were identified by bacterial cultures, viral isolation, or retrospective paired serology. Pure *Mycoplasma* is the exception rather than the rule because, in our clinic, *Mycoplasma* usually is isolated in conjunction with other pathogens in the majority of pneumonia outbreaks in which it is involved. Signs of pneumonia in these instances are identical to those described for the specific bacterial or viral agents isolated. The *Mycoplasma* component does not have any unique clinical features except for its association with otitis media and arthritis, and perhaps that affected animals sometimes respond poorly to specific antibiotic therapy directed against the bacterial pathogen. When this occurs, a contributory viral or *Mycoplasma* infection should be suspected.

Diagnosis. This is totally dependent on culture of the organism from tracheal wash or necropsy samples. In pure *Mycoplasma* pneumonia, fatalities are rare, but typical *Mycoplasma* pneumonia gross lesions appear as red-blue firm areas in the anterior ventral lung. These areas resemble atelectatic areas but are firm, and pus may be expressed from the airways within these firm areas on a cut section. Histopathology demonstrates the "cuffing pneumonia" previously described.

In most instances in which *Mycoplasma* is merely one component of infection, gross necropsy lesions are typical of the other pathogens—usually anterior ventral consolidating bronchopneumonia typical of *Mannheimia*, *Pasteurella*, or *Histophilus* infection or abscessation caused by *A. pyogenes*. Occasionally *Mycoplasma* is isolated from lungs showing typical lesions of BRSV, BVDV, or other viral infections.

Treatment. Treatment for *Mycoplasma* pneumonia may be unnecessary in some pure *Mycoplasma* infections because the cattle do not appear extremely ill. In pure infections, oxytetracycline hydrochloride (11 mg/kg once or twice daily) is most frequently used. Erythromycin (5.5 mg/kg twice daily), tilmicosin (10 mg/kg SQ), tulathromycin (2.5 mg/kg SQ)or florfenicol (20 mg/kg IM in the neck) may provide effective therapy in some cases, but in vitro testing found widespread resistance to these antibiotics. Enrofloxacin or other fluoroquinolones are reported to be the most effective antibiotic against *Mycoplasma*, but these are not approved for use in dairy cattle in the United States. Because affected animals usually continue to eat, chlortetracycline or oxytetracycline (Terramycin, Pfizer) added to the feed in therapeutic levels may provide effective therapy for groups of weaned calves or heifers.

When *Mycoplasma* is isolated along with *P. multocida*, *M. haemolytica*, *A. pyogenes*, *Fusobacterium* sp., or *H. somni*, antibacterial therapy should primarily address the bacterial pathogen. If the *Pasteurella* or *Histophilus* isolate is sensitive to tetracycline or erythromycin, choosing one of these drugs may provide efficacy against both the bacteria and *Mycoplasma*. Fortunately, if treatment is directed against the bacterial pathogens and ventilation or management factors are corrected, the calves recover and the *Mycoplasma* may not require specific therapy.

At our clinic, we have investigated several chronic heifer and postweaning calf pneumonia problems in which *Mycoplasma* and *P. multocida* or *Mycoplasma* and *H. somni* have coexisted. These problems have been very difficult to solve. In these herds, the *Mycoplasma* seems to be ubiquitous and seems to infect calves very early in life. Calf hutches and individual rearing of calves may not be effective in preventing *Mycoplasma* infection in some of these herds, but calf hutches do seem to prevent bacterial infection in the calves. Therefore as soon as the calves are grouped following weaning, a pneumonia outbreak is caused by both bacterial and *Mycoplasma* components. Every new group seems to be affected, and attempts at prevention appear futile. Isolation of calves to a separate farm following immediate removal from their dams may be the only solution. Other recommendations for prevention of *Mycoplasma* infection in calves include avoiding feeding *Mycoplasma bovis*–infected milk, using separate feed buckets and bottles for every calf, and preventing calves from direct contact with other cattle.

Viral Diseases of the Respiratory Tract

Infectious Bovine Rhinotracheitis

Etiology and Signs. IBR (also known as BHV1, or "red nose") is an infection of the upper airway and trachea caused by BHV1. Infection may assume many forms in cattle, including respiratory, conjunctival, or infectious pustular vulvovaginitis affecting the caudal reproductive tract, infectious balanoposthitis of the male external genitalia, endemic abortions, and the neonatal septicemic form characterized by encephalitis and focal plaque necrosis of the tongue. Bovine herpesvirus 5 (BoHV5) may also cause outbreaks of encephalitis in young stock. The respiratory form of BHV1 is the most common and may occur alone or coupled with the conjunctival form. DNA variants of BHV1 initially described correlated to specific system disease, but recent genomic mapping has found no basis for these divisions. Abortions may occur in association with any of the forms of the disease, either during the acute disease or in the ensuing weeks following an endemic. Each infected herd seems to have one predominant clinical form of the disease, but occasional animals may also show signs of other forms during an endemic. Recent work suggests that genetic factors may play a role in the relative resistance of cattle to IBR virus and that this resistance may be mediated by type 1 interferon genotypes.

Like many other herpes viruses, IBR virus is capable of recrudescence when previously infected cattle harboring latent virus infection are stressed by infectious diseases, shipment, or corticosteroids. Immunity from natural infection or vaccination is short lived and probably does not exceed 6 to 12 months. Respiratory disease caused by IBR is associated with high morbidity but low mortality in susceptible animals. Fatalities seldom result from primary or recurrent IBR infections unless secondary bacterial bronchopneumonia, especially *M. haemolytica*, or concurrent viral infection with BVDV or BRSV occurs. (These viruses are discussed further in this section.) The IBR virus compromises the physical and cellular components of the lower airway defense mechanism by damaging mucociliary transport and the mucus layer and directly infecting alveolar macrophages. Therefore combination infections may result in high mortality because of multiple compromises of the lower airway host defense and possible immunosuppression—especially with concurrent BVDV infection. As stated previously, BHV1 infection up-regulates genes that activate receptors for the leukotoxin of *M. haemolytica* and contribute to the severity of that disease.

Because most dairy cattle and calves currently are vaccinated for IBR, owners and veterinarians sometimes overlook or fail to consider the possibility of IBR infection during acute respiratory outbreaks or herd abortions. However, the confusing array of bovine vaccines available to laypeople, outdated or mishandled vaccines, and inadvertent failure to vaccinate individual groups or herds of cattle still predispose to acute outbreaks of IBR.

The clinical signs of IBR-respiratory form include high fever of 105.0 to 108.0° F (40.56 to 42.22° C); depression; anorexia; rapid respiration (40 to 80 breaths/min); heavy serous nasal discharge that becomes a thick mucopurulent discharge during the first 72 hours of infection; a painful cough; a dried necrotic crusting of the muzzle; white plaques visible in the nasal mucosa, mucosa of the nasal septum (Figure 4-28), and sometimes on the external nares and muzzle (Figure 4-29); occasional mucosal ulceration of the muzzle and oral mucosa; coarse tracheal rales caused by mucopurulent exudate or diphtheritic membranes in the larynx and trachea; and referred sounds and rales from the upper airway heard over both lung fields (especially in the area of the major bronchi). Although bronchitis and bronchiolitis occasionally have been observed, most cases do not have pulmonary pathology unless secondary bacterial bronchopneumonia occurs. Bacterial bronchopneumonia usually occurs within 7 to 10 days following acute IBR infection in those instances in which bacteria complicate the viral infection. Devastating mortality may occur in stressed, recently transported or purchased animals that develop

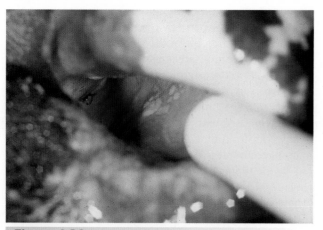

Figure 4-28

Classical IBR plaques on the mucosa overlying the nasal septum of a Holstein. The view is through the right nares, and a penlight is present in the right lower corner of the photo.

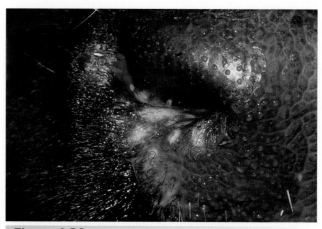

Figure 4-29

Plaques from IBR on the mucosa and mucocutaneous junction of the right nares region in a Holstein.

IBR infection concurrent with BVDV infection, BRSV infection, or virulent strains of *M. haemolytica* bronchopneumonia. In outbreaks in adult herds, the disease seems to cause the most severe signs in first-calf heifers and may severely affect their future milk production during the remainder of the first lactation.

Affected animals show signs for 7 to 14 days and recover after this time unless secondary infection occurs. Abortions may occur during the acute infection or in the subsequent 4 to 8 weeks. Although fetal mortality can occur at any stage of gestation, most abortions occur in cows in the second or third trimester of pregnancy. Direct fetal infection or stress and high fever may contribute to the abortions. The conjunctival form sometimes coexists with the respiratory form and is characterized by unilateral or bilateral severely inflamed conjunctiva and serous ocular discharge that becomes mucopurulent within 2 to 4 days. In addition, multifocal white plaques composed of lymphocytes and plasma cells appear grossly on the palpebral conjunctiva (Figure 4-30). Some cattle also have corneal edema in the peripheral cornea, but ulcerations do not occur (also see Chapter 13). BHV1 has a similar synergistic (increased pathogenicity) effect with *Moraxella bovis* in the eye as with *M. haemolytica* in the lung. Calves with the encephalitic form of IBR may demonstrate necrotic plaques on the ventral surface of the tongue or proximal gastrointestinal tract at autopsy (Figure 4-31).

Diagnosis. Usually the diagnosis of IBR is based on physical examination when characteristic signs and pathognomonic nasal mucosal plaques are present. Laboratory confirmation is possible by FA techniques during the acute stage (lesions less than 7 days are best). Scrapings of mucosal lesions and the white plaques in the nasal mucosa should be positive in almost all acute cases. In addition, viral isolation is possible during this time. Paired serum (acute and convalescent, 14 to 21 days later) samples provide another means of

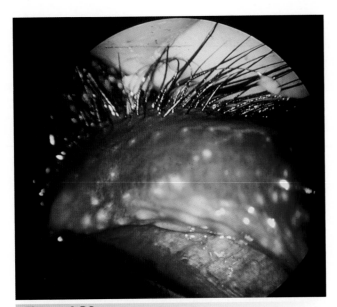

Figure 4-30

Multifocal white plaques on the palpebral conjunctiva of a Holstein affected with the conjunctival form of IBR.

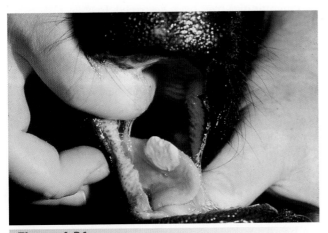

Figure 4-31

White plaque on the tongue of a neonatal calf infected with IBR.

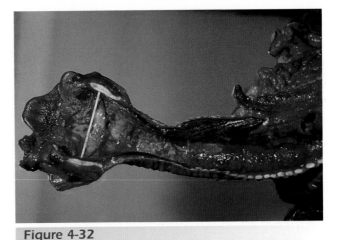

Figure 4-32

Severe mucosal necrosis involving larynx and trachea of a cow that died from IBR. Although fatal cases of pure IBR are rare, the pathology presented highlights the damage to the physical defense mechanisms of the lower airway that predisposes to secondary bacterial pneumonia. *(Photo courtesy Dr. John M. King.)*

positive diagnosis. One word of caution, however—individual sick cows with septic mastitis, septic metritis, bacterial pneumonia, and so forth may show typical IBR plaques as a result of recrudescence of latent virus of natural or live vaccine origin during their illness. A diagnosis of primary IBR should not be made in these cattle, although the plaque represents the only manifestation of BHV1 disease seen in such immunocompromised animals; importantly, they may be a contagious risk for in-contact and naive animals.

Necropsy of fatal IBR cases will show diffuse inflammation, necrosis, ulceration, and diphtheritic membranes throughout the nasal passages, larynx, and trachea (Figure 4-32). Characteristic white plaques will be visible in the inflamed nasal mucosa and sometimes in other areas of the nasopharynx or trachea. Oral mucosal ulceration sometimes occurs. Secondary bacterial bronchopneumonia or superimposed viral infections may mask some IBR lesions.

Bovine Respiratory Syncytial Virus

Etiology and Signs. BRSV has become one of the most important respiratory pathogens in dairy calves and adult cattle in the past 20 years. The virus certainly may have been present for much longer, but new diagnostic procedures, increased technology in virology, and recognition of the virus and its pathophysiology have heightened awareness of this disease. The virus is a pneumovirus within the paramyxovirus family and is distinctly different from the bovine syncytial virus (BSV), which is a spumavirus in the retrovirus family. There is no current evidence that the BSV is a pathogen in cattle. Respiratory disease caused by BRSV was first reported in Europe during the 1970s and has been recognized throughout the United States in the 1980s in endemic form in beef and dairy cattle. Experimental and natural diseases have been reported, and it is now accepted that BRSV is likely the cause of many poorly defined epidemics heretofore diagnosed as "atypical interstitial pneumonia" in calves and cattle. It also is likely that BRSV infection has proceeded, and predisposed cattle to, severe bacterial bronchopneumonia but gone undiagnosed because of overwhelming bacterial lesions.

The virus produces a humoral antibody response, which is helpful both for diagnosis and epidemiological surveys. Based on surveys completed in several regions of the United States, BRSV infection appears common in cattle because 50% or more of cattle surveyed have titers to BRSV. The virus has caused sporadic clinical disease in dairy cattle and calves and probably has gone undiagnosed frequently. Outbreaks of BRSV may be limited to calves, affect only adult cows, or can involve all animals in a herd. Morbidity is high, but mortality as a result of BRSV infection is much lower unless secondary bacterial bronchopneumonia ensues. The virus apparently does not infect alveolar macrophages but may damage physical defense mechanisms of the lower airway, such as mucociliary transport, and may lead to antigen-antibody complexes that subsequently engage complement and result in damage to the lower airway. Although experimental reproduction of the clinical disease has not been consistently successful in challenge studies, there have been recent studies that help explain the pathogenesis of the disease further. Two- to 6-month-old calves have been successfully infected and have marked production of inflammatory cytokines (tumor necrosis factor, interleukin 6, and interferon); these are thought to help promote viral clearance but may have a pathogenic role in causing airway obstruction. Previous work suggests that BRSV alters macrophage function sufficiently to short cycle and depress responsiveness of lymphocytes. In any event, interstitial pneumonia, secondary bacterial pneumonia, airway obstruction, and pneumothorax are very common following BRSV infection. Many unexplained facets of BRSV infection persist despite the proliferation of research on the virus. For example, BRSV infection often arises in herds that appear to have excellent management and have not purchased new cattle, shipped and returned existing cattle, or stressed animals in any apparent way. Where did the infection come from in these herds? Was it latent in a recovered animal, or was it introduced by regular visitors to the farm? Cattle are thought to be the reservoir, but it has not yet been shown how or why the virus activates, replicates, and spreads to cause all clinical epidemics.

Fortunately, because of increased awareness of BRSV in cattle, bovine practitioners are beginning to suspect the disease based on clinical signs and routinely seek virus identification, histopathologic confirmation of the virus, or serologic confirmation when acute epidemics of respiratory disease occur in cattle.

The signs of acute BRSV range from inapparent to fulminant. In most outbreaks, acute BRSV infection causes high morbidity in the affected group within several days to 1 week. Clinical signs include high fever (104.0 to 108.0° F/40.0 to 42.22° C); depression, anorexia, and decreased milk production; salivation and serous or mucoid nasal discharge; degree of dyspnea varies from simple increased respiratory rate (40 to 100 breaths/min) to open mouth breathing; and in all but the most mild outbreaks, a percentage of the affected cattle will have subcutaneous emphysema palpable under the skin of the dorsum, especially near the withers (Figure 4-33). Auscultation of the lungs in acute cases may reveal a wide range of sounds. Increased bronchovesicular sounds,

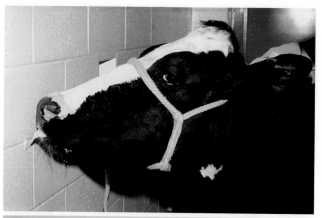

Figure 4-33

A mature cow representative of a herd outbreak with BRSV infection. This cow had respiratory distress and severe subcutaneous emphysema over the chest, back, and face (notice indentation of the halter on the face).

bronchial tones, fine crepitation caused by emphysema, and rales (usually as a result of secondary bacterial bronchopneumonia) have been described. In New York, practitioners have found the lungs may auscult as diffusely very quiet or almost inaudible in acutely affected cattle in some outbreaks. This has been a very important sign and initially appears in contrast to the outward signs of dyspnea displayed by these cattle. However, the relative deficit of airway sounds fits the existing pathology because pneumothorax and/or diffuse interstitial edema and emphysema compress the small airways and cause the lungs to be quieter than one would expect (Figures 4-34, A to C, and 4-35). This is the same phenomenon that occurs in proliferative pneumonia in which the alveoli and small airways are obliterated or reduced in size. If secondary bacterial pneumonia occurs, bronchial tones or rales are heard in the anterior ventral lung region, and the dorsal and caudal lungs become quieter because of mechanical overwork, increasing the degree of edema and emphysema. Dyspnea will be severe in such cases, and affected animals usually show open mouth breathing and an audible grunt or groan with each expiration. This dyspnea is more obvious if affected animals are stressed by handling or being made to move. Despite the high fevers and respiratory distress, affected cattle frequently do not look septic (e.g., severe depression, scleral injection) as with acute overwhelming bacterial pneumonia.

A biphasic disease may occur in some cattle with BRSV infection. The first stage or phase of the disease is characterized by mild or more serious signs as described above. The affected animals apparently improve over the next few days only to develop peracute severe respiratory distress several days to several weeks after their initial improvement. Because these animals initially appeared to have mild disease and responded to treatment, this secondary phase is entirely unexpected. Secondary acute

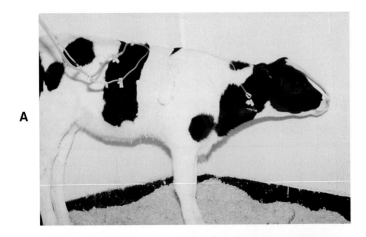

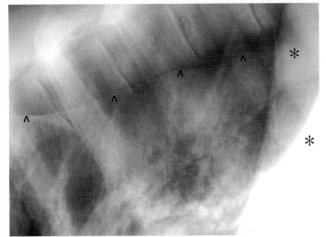

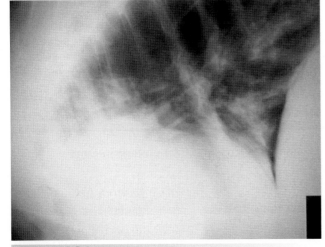

Figure 4-34

A, A 4-month-old calf with respiratory distress and pneumothorax caused by BRSV. **B,** Radiograph of the pneumothorax is shown. **C,** Radiograph of another calf on the farm infected with BRSV showing a large bullae in the lung. ^ , Top of lung; * , diaphragm.

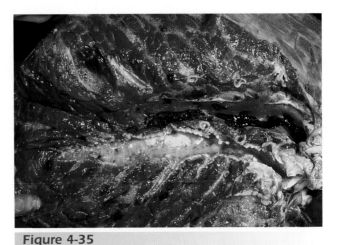

Figure 4-35

Cut section of lung at necropsy of a fatal case of BRSV pneumonia. Interstitial edema and emphysema are apparent. *(Photo courtesy Dr. John M. King.)*

dyspnea is thought to reflect an immune-mediated disease caused by hypersensitivity and/or a severe Th2 response in the lower airway and lung parenchyma and is frequently fatal.

Diagnosis. The signs of BRSV infection in calves or cattle may be suggestive of the diagnosis, especially when acute onset, high fever, and subcutaneous emphysema are found in several affected animals. These signs are rarely seen in calves younger than 6 weeks, but calves aged 2 to 6 months seem to be most commonly affected. Auscultation of the lungs in acute cases may be helpful if the lungs sound diffusely quiet despite obvious severe dyspnea. The veterinarian must be cautious in diagnosing BRSV based only on the finding of subcutaneous emphysema or pneumothorax in some animals. *Any* severe pneumonia (especially other interstitial pneumonias or severe consolidating bronchopneumonia) can also cause subcutaneous emphysema because the only remaining normal lung tissue (dorsal or caudal lung fields) is overworked to the point at which emphysema and interstitial edema are likely. Therefore subcutaneous emphysema may be *suggestive of but not pathognomonic* for BRSV. As with most of the diseases discussed thus far, laboratory confirmation is the only definitive means to confirm a diagnosis of BRSV. Viral cultures from tracheal wash fluid or necropsy specimens are indicated but often are not rewarding because BRSV is quickly cleared from the respiratory tract or a rapidly developing secretory antibody neutralizes the virus within the respiratory tract. The best results are from viral cultures or FA testing taken in the very early stages of the disease and quickly transported unfrozen to a diagnostic laboratory equipped with appropriate cell cultures. FA techniques may be used for tracheal wash samples, nasopharyngeal smears, and necropsy specimens of infected lung. Serology is helpful in establishing a diagnosis of BRSV because a marked humoral antibody titer occurs in response to the infection. Baker and Frey emphasize that antibody titers may increase early after acute infection and often peak before 2 weeks postinfection. Therefore collection of serum on day 1 and day 14 is very important when evaluating seroconversion. The same authors state that young calves may have titers derived from colostrum. These titers, indicative of passive immunity, are not protective against BRSV infection. Thus older calves, heifers, or adult animals are better populations to sample. Necropsy specimens may be very helpful in establishing a diagnosis. This is especially true if death has been acute and secondary bacterial pneumonia has not yet developed to somewhat mask the pulmonary lesions caused by BRSV. In pure BRSV infection, diffuse edema and emphysema may be present (see Figure 4-35). In addition, focal firm areas of pneumonia will be palpable throughout the entire lung. Lesions are not limited to any one area of lung tissue. If secondary bacterial bronchopneumonia coexists with BRSV, the anterior ventral lung fields usually are dark colored, firm, fibrin covered, and consolidated (Figure 4-36). In this instance, typical BRSV lesions of emphysema, edema, and scattered palpably firm areas will be found in the lung caudal and dorsal to the consolidated areas.

Several times at our clinic, we have obtained *Pasteurella* or *Mannheimia* isolates from tracheal wash specimens in BRSV outbreaks before BRSV was confirmed by the diagnostic laboratory. Cattle in these herd outbreaks failed to respond, or responded unusually slowly, when placed on antibiotics chosen for their specific *Pasteurella/Mannheimia* isolate. This poor clinical response is a signal that another pathogen is contributing to the herd problem. Subsequent laboratory procedures may identify the causative virus, but viral cultures often lag behind bacterial culture and sensitivities. Despite the clinical frustrations and economic consequences, the veterinarian must

show reasonable patience when requesting confirmation of viral diseases. It is best to make personal contact with the laboratory, explain the seriousness of the outbreak, provide appropriate samples, and ascertain the appropriate time required for viral isolation, FA techniques, or titers.

Treatment. Therapy for acute BRSV infection is symptomatic and supportive. Broad-spectrum antibiotics are indicated to counteract or discourage bacterial bronchopneumonia and should be initiated following collection of tracheal wash samples from acutely infected calves or cattle. Ceftiofur is initially used in most dairy animals until tracheal wash cultures have been completed. Once cultures are completed, specific antibacterial therapy may be instituted if bacterial pathogens are isolated.

NSAIDs may be helpful in acute BRSV infections. Aspirin or flunixin may be used in the same dosages mentioned previously. Corticosteroids have been recommended for treatment of BRSV infections in calves. Whereas calves or nonpregnant cattle with respiratory distress but minimal evidence of sepsis may receive some benefit from these drugs in diminishing the pulmonary pathology created by the BRSV, in a few cases a dramatic improvement in clinical signs can be observed. They certainly can predispose to secondary infections and abortions, and their use should be selective. Antihistamines also have been recommended for treatment of BRSV and may be used (tripelennamine hydrochloride at a dosage of 1 mg/kg IM, twice daily).

Any cattle that develop the second phase or second stage of BRSV infection, which appears as a hypersensitivity reaction, should receive antiinflammatory medication in addition to broad-spectrum antibiotics. The peracute onset and extreme dyspnea exhibited by these animals is usually fatal; therefore heroic therapeutic measures are indicated. Several drugs may be indicated, and clinical judgment will determine which drugs will be used. For an adult cow with this form of the disease, drugs that may be considered and their dosages follow:

1. Broad-spectrum antibiotics	Based on previous herd tracheal wash results
2. Dexamethasone	10 to 20 mg once daily (except in pregnant animals) IM or IV
3. Antihistamine	Tripelennamine hydrochloride 1 mg/kg IM twice daily
4. Atropine	0.048 mg/kg IM or SQ twice daily
5. NSAID	(e.g., flunixin 1 mg/kg IM or IV every 12 or 24 hours, aspirin 240 to 480 grains twice daily)
6. Furosemide	250 mg (if severe pulmonary edema is present) IV or IM once or twice daily

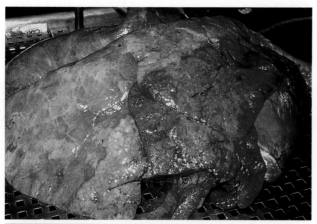

Figure 4-36

Necropsy view of lungs from a fatal case of BRSV combined with secondary *M. haemolytica*. This combination of pathogens killed 30 of the 55 heifers in the group within 10 days during inclement winter weather.

Intranasal oxygen (10 to 15 L/min) is usually used in our hospital and will often decrease the respiratory rate and effort. Nebulization with corticosteroids and antibiotics can be helpful, but a bronchodilator should be administered either before beginning the nebulization or at the same time. Systemic atropine and/or inhaled ipratropium and/or aminophylline (2 to 4 mg/kg every 12 hours) as a constant rate infusion can be used. In animals that develop pneumothorax, evacuation of free air from the pleural space can offer significant improvement. The complete mediastinum of cattle often confines pneumothorax to one hemithorax, but bilateral disease or severe unilateral lung collapse caused by pneumothorax may necessitate evacuation. Details regarding specific treatment of pneumothorax are given later in this chapter.

In summary, the veterinarian must allow for a wide range of severity in BRSV outbreaks. In some mild outbreaks, no animals will require treatment. On the other hand, severe outbreaks complicated by pneumothorax (Figure 4-37), emphysema, and/or bacterial pathogens may result in 10% to 30% mortality despite heroic treatment efforts. Vaccination will be discussed later, but the literature on BRSV vaccination is confusing, with some articles showing protection from inactivated or modified live vaccines, others demonstrating no protection from inactivated vaccines, and a few suggesting an adverse immune response on exposure to the virus. Most recently protection from challenge infection was good following the intranasal administration of a MLV vaccine marketed for parenteral administration.

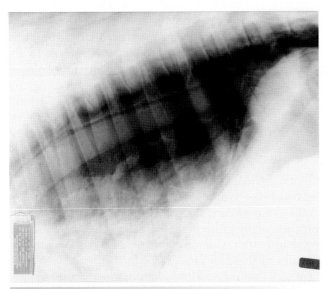

Figure 4-37

Radiograph of a yearling heifer with pneumothorax associated with BRSV infection. Note the unilateral lung collapse and "silhouetting" of great vessels, indicating concurrent pneumomediastinum.

Parainfluenza-3

Etiology and Signs. Parainfluenza-3 (PI$_3$) virus is capable of infecting the bovine respiratory tract and predisposing infected animals to more severe pneumonia when subsequently exposed to bacterial pathogens such as *M. haemolytica*. After experimental inoculation, the virus infects the upper and lower airways of calves with subsequent damage to ciliated epithelial cells, mucus layer, mucociliary transport, and infection of alveolar macrophages. As bronchitis and bronchiolitis ensue, purulent exudate fills some small airways. Despite this pathology, PI$_3$ infection is a mild disease unless complicated by secondary bacterial agents. Based on serologic surveys, most cattle probably have been exposed to PI$_3$ infection as calves. We seldom identify PI$_3$ in bovine respiratory outbreaks in dairy calves or cows in the northeastern United States. This may result from the fact that most dairy animals are vaccinated against this virus.

The signs of PI$_3$ infection include fever (104.0 to 107.0° F/40.00 to 41.67° C), depression, anorexia, nasal and ocular serous discharge, increased respiratory rate (40 to 80 breaths/min), tracheal rales, and occasional rales in the lower lung fields. Fatalities are uncommon, and recovery should occur over 7 days.

The signs of PI$_3$ complicated by bacterial pneumonia are simply those of a moderate to severe bacterial bronchopneumonia as previously described under the various bacterial pathogens. Response to specific treatment for the bacterial bronchopneumonia, however, would be less prompt and complete than anticipated for bacterial infection alone.

Diagnosis. The clinical signs of PI$_3$ infection in calves or cattle are not specific enough to allow definitive diagnosis. Therefore culture of the organism from acutely infected calves via tracheal wash, nasopharyngeal swabs, or necropsy specimens is necessary to identify this organism. Paired serum samples also are helpful because humoral antibody production is anticipated following infection. Isolation attempts may be fruitless if samples are not collected early in the course of the disease.

Fatal cases usually are complicated by secondary bacterial pneumonia—especially *M. haemolytica* or *P. multocida*. Therefore gross pathology lesions suggest bacterial bronchopneumonia, and a diagnosis of PI$_3$ is easily missed unless the veterinarian requests viral isolation and obtains paired serum samples from surviving animals.

Treatment. Treatment must address the frequent secondary bacterial pneumonia. There are no characteristic clinical signs to allow veterinarians to diagnose PI$_3$ specifically.

Bovine Virus Diarrhea Virus

BVDV is one of the major pathogens of dairy cattle and may cause a wide range of lesions or clinical syndromes. This pestivirus from the *Flaviviridae* family causes fever, mucosal erosions, diarrhea, abortions or reproductive failure, congenital anomalies, persistent infection of fetuses infected during 40 to 120 days of gestation, and many other signs. The disease will be discussed fully in Chapter 6. However, BVDV has been incriminated as a "respiratory virus" in cattle, and certain strains certainly can be isolated from the lower airway and alveolar macrophages of infected cattle. Some BVDV strains (genotypes 1a and 1b and biotype noncytopathogenic) are more commonly found in the lungs of cattle and are frequently associated with respiratory disease outbreaks. All strains of BVDV are immunosuppressive and predispose infected cattle to bacterial or other viral pneumonia. Naive cattle exposed to type 2 strain may develop severe interstitial pneumonia, thrombocytopenia, bone marrow necrosis, diarrhea, and acute death sometimes without having mucosal erosions. Additionally, a persistently infected calf or cow may suddenly develop bacterial pneumonia without other predisposing factors, and this scenario should always be considered as a possible reason for a single case of bacterial pneumonia in a herd.

During acute BVDV infection, high fevers occur in affected cattle early in the course of the disease. These cattle may show no other signs—no diarrhea, no mucosal lesions—and merely appear depressed and febrile at 106.0 to 108.0° F (41.11 to 42.22° C). Because the high fever necessitates increased physiologic heat loss, some cows have mild increases in their respiratory rate (40 to 60 breaths/min), but the lungs are normal on auscultation or may have slightly increased bronchovesicular sounds. These cattle are merely in the early stages of acute BVDV infection, and unless a superimposed bacterial infection develops, clinical pneumonia may not occur. If the animal seroconverts and responds to the BVDV in a normal fashion, no other signs may develop. Some cattle will progress from this early stage of fever with no other signs to blatant mucosal lesions and diarrhea 7 to 14 days following the original onset of fever. This situation has been observed in natural outbreaks and with experimental BVDV infection with certain strains of BVDV in naive cattle. Most cattle with BVDV have mild pulmonary lesions or normal lungs grossly and histologically unless an opportunistic bacterial pneumonia has developed. Naive cattle infected with the type 2 strain may die with severe interstitial pneumonia.

Acute BVDV infection causes profound immunosuppression in affected animals for 7 to 14 days or until they recover. Research documents the negative effects that BVDV infection has on neutrophil, macrophage, and lymphocyte function. Humoral and cell-mediated lymphocyte functions are depressed during acute BVDV infection. Leukopenia in the peripheral blood is a well-known feature of acute BVDV infection in cattle. Although naive or susceptible cattle fully recover immune function following the development of adequate

humoral antibody against BVDV, they are very susceptible to secondary infection *during* the acute BVDV infection and associated immunosuppression. Alveolar macrophages are frequently infected with BVDV, which would be expected to have a direct negative effect on lung protection against invading bacteria. Therefore the results are devastating if a cow or group of cows acutely infected with BVDV has the bad fortune to become infected with *P. multocida*, *M. haemolytica*, or *H. somni* pneumonia at the same time. Bacterial bronchopneumonia may progress rapidly because host defense mechanisms are negligible. In addition, cattle may die so quickly from severe pneumonia that necropsy identifies bacterial pneumonia as the cause of death. The existence of BVDV infection will only be confirmed if viral isolation or immunohistochemistry is performed, some affected cows develop signs of mucosal disease, or some fatalities demonstrate typical BVDV lesions as well as bacterial pneumonia at necropsy.

This situation most often develops in assembled groups of heifers or replacement heifers that are naive to BVDV and have lost maternal antibodies and subsequently encounter BVDV via a persistently infected animal. Other management-related stresses, transportation, pen reorganization, poor ventilation, and so on may also contribute to the development of bacterial pneumonia during concurrent BVDV infection.

In summary, BVDV by itself rarely causes major respiratory disease except for type 2 infections in naive cattle, which may cause interstitial pneumonia and acute death sometimes without the typical upper gastrointestinal tract lesions. Type 1 strains are commonly isolated from the lower airway and more recently pulmonary macrophages in BVDV outbreaks, and play a potentially important role in the bovine respiratory disease complex. Acute BVDV infection (any strain) may result in transient immunosuppression that predisposes to severe respiratory infections in cattle concurrently exposed to other respiratory pathogens. This immunosuppressive effect is not limited to the respiratory tract and certainly would contribute to drastic illness if a cow acutely infected with BVDV encountered septic mastitis, metritis, or salmonellosis.

Other Viruses

Several other viruses, including adenoviruses (types 3 and 7), rhinoviruses, and coronaviruses, have been shown experimentally to be potential pathogens of the bovine respiratory tract. Clinically there are no pathognomonic features of these viruses. Except for coronaviruses, diagnostic laboratories seldom identify these viruses in outbreaks of infectious respiratory disease in cattle or calves. The role coronavirus plays in the bovine respiratory disease complex is not clear. Coronavirus is commonly found in outbreaks, either acute or endemic, but can also be commonly found in healthy animals. It may be important if the farmer describes a "pneumonia-enteritis" complex in 1- to 8-week-old calves. The respiratory isolate is very similar to the enteric isolate.

Control and Prevention of Infectious Respiratory Diseases in Dairy Cattle*

The control of acute or chronic endemic respiratory disease within groups of calves or adult cattle consists of four components:

1. Definitive diagnosis of the causative agent(s)
2. Specific medical therapy
3. Correction of management, environmental, or ventilation deficiencies that contribute to or perpetuate the respiratory disease
4. Preventive medicine, including management techniques and vaccination

Most of these points have been addressed in the discussion of treatment for each of the infectious agents in this section. Field outbreaks of respiratory disease may be limited to individual groups such as weaned calves, breeding age heifers, milking cows, and dry cows, or may involve all animals on the premises. When only one group is affected, the veterinarian should try to determine what management, environmental, or ventilation conditions might have predisposed this group to infection. It also is necessary to elicit information from the owner such as vaccination history, previous outbreaks of respiratory disease, recent purchase of animals, recent movement of resident animals to shows, and other facts that may help to explain how the respiratory infection may have become established in a group of animals or the entire herd.

In the northeastern United States, calves housed indoors have a notoriously high incidence of pneumonia. This may be seen in calves of all ages or only in postweaning calves. The most common age for pneumonia in calves is 1 to 6 months. Infection may occur in every group of calves placed in a certain housing condition on the farm or only in calves kept in the main dairy barn. This type of high morbidity calf pneumonia has been termed "enzootic pneumonia," but this is a poor term because it does not help elucidate a specific etiology. The term has gained acceptance because it is often more indicative of management and ventilation deficiencies than a specific primary etiology. Respiratory viruses, bacteria, and *Mycoplasma* may be involved separately or in combination in these outbreaks. Although *P. multocida* and *M. haemolytica* are the most common bacteria found in such outbreaks, *H. somni* is also found in a small proportion of herd problems.

Chronic or recurrent pneumonia caused by bacterial pathogens other than *Mycoplasma* in milk-fed calves is best controlled by the use of calf hutches (Figure 4-38). Many farms have also had good success with plastic

*This section courtesy Dr. Chuck Guard, Cornell University, Ithaca, NY.

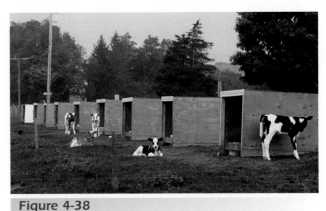

Figure 4-38
Plywood calf hutches with calves tethered.

hoop houses or curtain-sided barns with transparent roofs. Calves should be removed from the dam and calving pen as quickly as possible, aided in drying, and fed 4 quarts of colostrum before being moved to the hutch or calf barn. When the environment is managed in this way, most bacterial and viral pneumonias will be prevented, primarily by ensuring good ventilation that dilutes potential pathogens. *Mycoplasma* may be a herd problem even with good environmental management. Feeding of contaminated colostrum or waste milk is thought to be the primary means of transmitting *Mycoplasma* to young calves. Aerosol spread may subsequently occur to calves housed with or very near infected calves. Use of colostrum replacer, milk replacer, and pasteurization of waste milk are all alternatives to prevent exposure of young calves. Recent studies of heat-treating colostrum have shown that heating to less than pasteurization temperatures is very effective in killing important calf pathogens without damaging the immunoglobulins. Heating to 140° F (60° C) for 30 minutes eliminates *M. bovis* from colostrum. Standard pasteurization procedures have been used to successfully treat waste milk before feeding it to calves and are becoming common on larger dairies.

The major objection to the use of calf hutches by dairy farmers is the increased labor required to feed calves outdoors and the necessity to work outside in inclement winter weather. Both of these factors have probably contributed to the increased use of hoop houses and barns on larger dairies where employees care for calves. Regardless of the selected housing type, we recommend it be unheated and well ventilated. Calves have increased caloric requirements at low environmental temperatures and thus require additional milk or milk replacer. A rough estimate of the increase in energy needs is 50% at 20° F (−7° C) and 100% at −5° F (−21° C). Calves may be fed more volume twice a day or be fed an additional time at midday to meet these needs. The choice of bedding material influences the energy balance of the calf, with deep straw providing the greatest insulation benefit, wood shavings intermediate, and shredded paper the least. Despite the disadvantages to labor, calves reared in hutches appear to be at least risk of respiratory infection.

Cattle housed in tie stall barns are predisposed to infectious pneumonia where marked environmental temperature and humidity fluctuations occur during the indoor housing season. Late fall and early spring, as well as winter thaws, are the times most likely to vary widely in temperature and humidity. Increased humidity and ammonia accumulate in areas with inadequate ventilation. Ammonia dissolves in the suspended water vapor and is an irritant to the respiratory epithelium. Exhaled bacteria and viruses are included in microscopic droplets of moisture. Prevention of respiratory infections in these settings requires improvement in the ventilation to dilute the pathogens and remove the irritants. There is a wealth of information on techniques for designing or retrofitting appropriate ventilation systems available from agricultural engineers through the extension services of each state. If the walls or ceiling accumulate condensation or the odor of ammonia in the barn is noticeable, there is inadequate ventilation. Normally the inside temperature in these barns in winter should not exceed 50° F (10° C). All modern free stall barns in cold climates are now curtain-sided and can be adjusted according to weather conditions in the winter to allow adequate fresh air entry for removal of humidity and ammonia. A temperature gradient of only a few degrees between inside and outside temperatures is adequate to drive the necessary air exchanges for maintaining air quality inside the barn.

Whenever possible, prevention of infectious respiratory diseases in dairy cattle is more desirable than control measures. Prevention consists both of effective vaccination programs and management designed to reduce the probability of infectious respiratory disease. Currently, effective vaccines are available for IBR, PI₃, and BVDV. Vaccines against *H. somni* and *P. multocida*, although available, have not been proven to be of any benefit. Newer vaccines against *M. haemolytica* that are based on leukotoxins of this bacterium have been proven beneficial in reducing morbidity and mortality in feedlot cattle. No comparable data have been published for dairy cattle, but by extension a benefit is probable if mannheimiosis were to occur. Vaccination strategies for herds should be individually determined and include the assessment of risk for all age groups. Closed herds in isolated settings have a much lower risk of contagious pathogens than herds that continuously purchase animals or exhibit cattle. Regardless, primary immunization requires two doses of vaccine and is best done at an early age. Optimal response to vaccines occurs after the waning of colostrally derived antibodies. Thus current recommendations are to begin the primary series at about 3 months of age with the second dose administered 2 to 4 weeks later. Recent

research indicates the greatest response to immunization against IBR and BVDV occurs if the first two doses are a killed product and the subsequent booster is a modified live vaccine. All major vaccine producers offer combination products with options of killed virus or modified live virus that provide the four viral components in a single injection. The *M. haemolytica* leukotoxoids are usually a distinct product. Subsequent boosters are administered at frequencies that correspond to the perceived risk and usually at times or ages that offer some convenience to management. The duration of immunity following proper vaccination is mostly not known for each of the components of the routinely used products. Thus recommendations for low-risk herds may be annual revaccination of the entire herd, whereas high-risk herds may be given boosters two or three times per year. Alternatively, in many large herds adults are vaccinated in conjunction with the lactation cycle. For example, a modified live booster is given at 30 days in milk, and killed boosters are given at 120 and 240 days of gestation.

There have been recommendations in the face of endemic respiratory disease in calves to hyperimmunize young calves against viral and bacterial diseases by repeated vaccination at 2-week intervals. To date, there is no evidence this strategy has any merit. Rather, the environmental and management ideas discussed above are more likely to provide health and economic returns to the herd. Another widely used strategy for undifferentiated respiratory disease of recently weaned calves is metaphylaxis of the at-risk group. Current practice in many dairies is to wean a group of calves and move them within 1 week or so to group housing. This change, particularly when more than 10 calves in a group are moved at one time, seems to be a trigger for respiratory disease. Control has been achieved in many herds with mass medication at the time of a move with a single injection of a long-acting antibiotic such as oxytetracycline, tilmicosin, tulathromycin, or florfenicol or by feeding chlortetracycline and sulfamethazine pellets for 5 to 7 days. Herds that practice a more gradual assembly of large groups of calves or that simply have fewer calves seem to be at much lower risk for this problem.

As of this writing, there is a commercial vaccine available for *M. bovis* that has not yet been proven efficacious. Regulatory methods in the United States require that vaccines be safe and induce an immune response measured by the production of specific antibodies. Unfortunately, efficacy in preventing the target disease is not a requirement. Thus there are vaccines available for respiratory pathogens such as *P. multocida* and *H. somni* that appear to provide no benefit to the calf or cow. Efforts will no doubt continue to develop new immunization products with greater safety, efficacy, and efficiency. Veterinarians are encouraged to remain abreast of these new developments because new knowledge and technologies may make our current practices obsolete.

Parasitic Pneumonia

Dictyocaulus viviparus

Etiology and Signs. *Dictyocaulus viviparus* is the lungworm of cattle and causes parasitic pneumonia and bronchiolitis in calves and adult cattle. This parasite has a direct life cycle, so infection merely requires management factors that allow a buildup of the parasite in the environment and ingestion of the infective larvae by naive cattle.

Adult lungworms reside in the trachea and bronchi. Eggs produced by female adults hatch either in the trachea or before being passed in the feces. The progression to the infective third stage larvae requires only 5 days, and the larvae are then ingested during consumption of contaminated grass in a pasture or bedding in heavily contaminated box stalls. Ingested larvae traverse the intestinal wall to reside in mesenteric lymph nodes, moult to the fourth stage, and within 1 week migrate to the lungs through lymphatics or blood vessels. The final fifth stage is reached after the larvae arrive in the bronchioles. The prepatent period is approximately 4 weeks because this period is required for the larvae to mature to egg-laying adults.

Signs of primary infection include varying degrees of dyspnea, a characteristic deep and moist cough, and moist rales or crackles heard over the entire lung field. Coughing is more severe than with most other bovine pneumonias. Diffuse rales rather than rales limited to the anterior ventral lung fields are an important sign that differentiates lungworm from bacterial pneumonias. Severely affected calves or cows will show "heave"-like breathing with visible expiratory and inspiratory effort. In some cases, emphysema is present when heavy airway exudate results in extreme mechanical respiratory efforts. Fever (103.0 to 106.0° F/39.44 to 41.11° C) may be present in some cases, as opportunistic bacteria such as *P. multocida* invade the damaged lower airway and establish a secondary bacterial bronchopneumonia. Fever also may be present simply from exertion involved in breathing during warm weather or in poorly ventilated barns. Usually several animals in a group or the entire herd will show signs. Affected cattle will continue to eat unless severe dyspnea or coughing interferes with their ability to ingest feed. In those cases with severe dyspnea, frequent coughing, marked expiratory efforts, and open mouth breathing are noted.

In addition to the above signs of primary infection, veterinarians should be aware of the *reinfection or acute larval migration syndrome* that occurs in adult cattle with endemic *D. viviparus*. Although age-related immunity to *D. viviparus* exists in adult cattle in endemic areas, this immunity may be incomplete or may not be able to overcome heavy challenge. Although most ingested larvae are killed or fail to mature in previously infected cattle, heavy exposure apparently allows large numbers of larvae to reach the lungs and cause respiratory signs through either an immune-mediated means and/or from migration of large numbers of larvae into the lung. Signs usually develop 14 to 16 days following exposure to contaminated pastures. Coughing that is frequent and deep, as well as an increased respiratory rate, characterizes the syndrome. Milk production decreases acutely in affected cattle. Rales may not be present. Fecal examinations are usually negative for *Dictyocaulus* because the disease is a result of the L4 migration into the lung.

Diagnosis. In primary infections, the diagnosis is aided by history, physical examination findings, laboratory or postmortem confirmation, and knowledge of the life cycle of the parasite.

The characteristic deep moist cough and moist rales auscultated throughout the entire lung are the most significant clinical signs—especially if found in a majority of the cattle within a group. As with any parasitic disease, some affected animals ("weak sisters") will display more blatant signs than others, but most within the group will be affected. History may be very helpful if animals have been placed on pasture recently or confined by group housing (heifers) to pens having a base consisting of several months of manure accumulation.

Baermann's technique performed on fresh manure is indicated for specific diagnosis but is of limited value in prepatent *and* postpatent infections. Therefore Baermann's technique and tracheal washes should be performed on several animals. If larvae are found using Baermann's technique, the diagnosis is confirmed as a patent infection. In prepatent infections, tracheal wash samples may identify parasites, rule out other causes of pneumonia, and allow cytologic confirmation of eosinophilic inflammation typical of parasitic bronchitis/pneumonia. In postpatent infections, tracheal wash cytology indicates eosinophilic inflammation and may suggest chronic inflammation. Eosinophilic tracheal wash should be highly suggestive of parasitic pneumonia (Figure 4-39).

Necropsy findings in fatal infections vary with the stage of infection. In early prepatent infections, microscopic examination of bronchial exudate may be necessary to identify larvae, whereas in later prepatent infections, the larvae are obvious if the airways are properly opened and inspected. Eosinophilic bronchitis may be confirmed by histopathology. Patent infections are obvious because large numbers of mature parasites up to 8.0 cm in length are found in the airways (Figure 4-40). Secondary anterior ventral bacterial bronchopneumonia may be present, and interstitial emphysema is observed in occasional severe cases. In postpatent infections, chronic bronchitis, bronchiectasis, and secondary bronchiolitis obliterans may be observed.

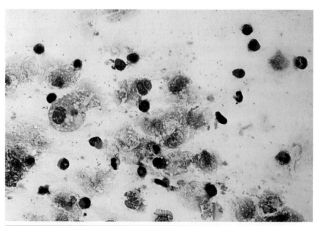

Figure 4-39

Wright-Giemsa stain of tracheal wash from a cow representative of a herd problem of chronic cough and decreased production. Lungworms *(D. viviparous)* were found to be the cause of the disease. The large number of eosinophils on this 40× slide is highly suggestive of lungworm infection.

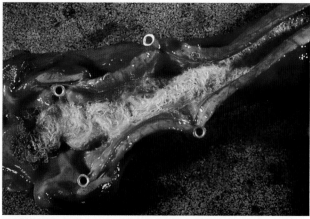

Figure 4-40

Necropsy specimen of trachea from fatal lungworm infection in a calf showing hundreds of *D. viviparous* lungworms. *(Photo courtesy Dr. John Perdrizet.)*

The reinfection syndrome is characterized by clinical signs of severe coughing in the majority of cattle following their introduction to infected pastures. Tracheal wash samples will reveal eosinophilic inflammation. Baermann's technique results will be negative. Necropsy lesions in the reinfection syndrome consist of small greenish-gray subpleural nodules, green exudate occluding small airways, and occasional green tinting of the interlobular septa. Histologically, eosinophils predominate, but lymphocytes, plasma cells, macrophages, and giant cells may be observed within the airways.

Treatment. Treatment of primary *D. viviparus* infection consists of an anthelmintic to destroy the parasite and, when necessary, antibiotic therapy to control secondary bacterial infection of the lower airway.

Levamisole phosphate (8 mg/kg body weight, SQ or orally), fenbendazole (5 mg/kg orally), albendazole (10 mg/kg orally), and ivermectin (0.2 mg/kg SQ) all have been recommended as treatments for primary *D. viviparus* infection. Levamisole has been very effective in our clinic but is no longer approved for use in dairy cattle, so fenbendazole would now be the first choice of treatment. Affected cattle should not be allowed back on infected pastures, and confined cattle should be removed from infected manure packs until the pens can be cleaned completely of manure and bedding.

Because the most common secondary bacterial invader is *P. multocida,* bacterial bronchopneumonia may be treated with tetracycline, ceftiofur, ampicillin, or penicillin. Secondary bacterial pneumonia may mask the presence of lungworms in calves or heifers. Such animals frequently appear to improve temporarily while on antibiotic therapy but then quickly relapse when antibiotics are withdrawn. Antibiotic therapy in these instances may cause resolution of fever and improved attitude but will not alleviate coughing or severe dyspnea. Only when further diagnostics are pursued in live patients or necropsies are performed in fatal cases will the true diagnosis be obtained and effective treatment instituted.

Although the reinfection syndrome appears to be an immune-mediated disorder, affected cattle appear to respond rapidly to levamisole injections according to Breeze. Without treatment, continued coughing and production losses persist in the affected animals for weeks.

Control. Control of *D. viviparus* infections requires management decisions regarding contaminated pastures. Because infective larvae have been shown to survive winter conditions, pastures should not be grazed in the early spring. Before being pastured, yearling heifers should be treated with anthelmintics effective against *D. viviparus,* and all animals should be treated routinely with anthelmintics at monthly intervals if the animals are to be placed on contaminated pastures. Moisture promotes survival and activity of infective larvae. Highlighting this fact, clinical lungworm infections in the northeastern United States are observed primarily during wet summers. Whenever possible, extreme care and additional anthelmintic treatment are indicated during wet summers and when animals are pastured in swampy, low-level endemic areas.

Ascaris lumbricoides

Etiology and Signs. Although reported rarely, *Ascaris lumbricoides,* the swine ascarid, has been identified as a natural and experimental cause of pneumonia in cattle. Exposure of susceptible cattle to large numbers of larvae occurs when the cattle are placed in bedded pens, corrals, or poor quality pastures previously used by pigs.

Clinical signs consisting of elevated temperature, elevated respiratory and heart rate, marked dyspnea, coughing, and an expiratory grunt develop 7 to 14 days after the cattle are exposed to ascarid ova. Auscultation of the lungs may reflect interstitial changes of pulmonary edema and emphysema. Therefore initial increased bronchovesicular sounds may be replaced by decreased sounds as further interstitial pathology and emphysema ensue. The clinical course lasts 10 to 14 days in most cases and occasionally may be fatal.

One experimental infection suggested that initial exposure to ascarid larvae resulted in very mild signs, whereas reexposure resulted in pronounced signs. This may imply an immune-mediated cause or component to the severe interstitial pneumonia.

Diagnosis. Diagnosis of this disease is difficult unless historical information leads to suspicion of exposure to *A. lumbricoides* ova. A tracheal wash sample may demonstrate an eosinophilic inflammatory pattern. Definitive diagnosis requires identification of the parasite or histopathology to study the larvae and associated interstitial pneumonia.

Treatment. Treatment is nonspecific and supportive in the hope that the normal life cycle of the parasite will eliminate the larvae. Prevention involves avoidance of environments used by swine.

Caudal Vena Caval Thrombosis

Etiology and Signs. Caudal vena caval thrombosis results in a variety of clinical respiratory syndromes in cattle. Septic thromboemboli originating from an abscess at the hilus of the liver shower the caudal vena cava, right heart, and pulmonary arterial circulation. Although most cattle do not show signs of illness when the shower occurs, some cattle experience acute death from massive pulmonary infarction or have an acute onset of profound respiratory distress at the time of a thromboembolic episode. Those cattle that have inapparent seeding of the pulmonary arteries or survive an acute respiratory distress episode caused by thromboemboli may eventually develop dyspnea, hemoptysis, and anemia. Epistaxis is the most common clinical sign observed in those cows with hemoptysis.

The pathogenesis of caudal vena caval thrombosis starts in the forestomach or abomasum and involves inflammatory or ulcerative mucosal lesions that allow bacterial seeding of the portal circulation with subsequent formation of liver abscesses. Therefore rumenitis, ruminal acidosis, abomasal ulcers, and similar disorders predispose to the condition. This same pathogenesis is responsible for "sawdust livers" in feedlot beef animals, but in dairy cattle, the abscesses usually are larger and fewer in number. Many dairy cattle have only one abscess. The location is much more important than the number of abscesses, however, because only those at the hilus of the liver or adjacent to the post cava represent significant risk (Figure 4-41). *F. necrophorum* or *A. pyogenes* are the most common organisms isolated from liver

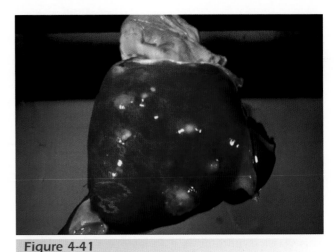

Figure 4-41

Multiple hepatic abscesses that were an incidental finding at postmortem in an adult dairy cow. Abscesses, although multiple, were small and located well away from the hilus. No evidence of embolic showering to other sites was evident at postmortem.

abscesses in dairy cattle. Most cattle with liver abscesses show no clinical signs of illness unless an abscess erodes into the vena cava or multiple large abscesses develop. This disease occurs sporadically in heifers and adult cattle but is rare in calves. This may be the result of calves being fed less intensive diets than heifers or lactating animals.

In caudal vena caval thrombosis, erosion of a liver abscess into the vena cava with formation of a septic venous thrombosis instigates the clinical disease, and the affected cow may show one of the following syndromes.

Sudden Death Syndrome

Acute rupture of a liver abscess into the caudal vena cava may result in massive thromboemboli to the right heart and pulmonary artery thrombosis, pulmonary infarction, exotoxemia or endotoxemia, and anoxia. Sudden death may result, and this syndrome represents one of the more common causes of acute death in adult dairy cattle. This sudden death may represent a hypersensitivity reaction following a previous clinically inapparent thromboembolic episode; however, sudden rupture of a large hilar abscess into the caudal vena cava or embolic movement of an existing large septic thrombus may cause enough direct pulmonary infarction to cause death without the need for a previous sensitizing episode. *F. necrophorum* toxins have also been shown to aggregate cattle platelets, and this may play some role in the development of thrombosis.

Acute Respiratory Distress Syndrome

This syndrome appears in one animal within a group or herd. The affected cow has peracute onset of respiratory distress, fever, labored breathing, and increased respiratory and heart rates. Pulmonary edema, subcutaneous emphysema, and open mouth breathing also may be observed. Auscultation of the thorax generally reveals reduced airway sounds resulting from pulmonary edema, pulmonary infarction, and bullous emphysema brought on by exertional respiratory efforts. Rales may be auscultated in some instances, but in general, the lungs are quieter than expected given the obviously labored respirations. The key to diagnosis is the fact that only one animal is affected with severe lower airway disease, and to the owner's knowledge, this cow has had no unique stress or previous problems.

Hemoptysis, Epistaxis, Chronic Pneumonia, Anemia Syndrome

This classic syndrome is associated with caudal vena caval thrombosis in cattle and results from singular or multiple episodes of thromboembolism from the hilar liver abscess and subsequent septic thrombosis residing in the caudal vena cava. Septic thromboemboli create pulmonary abscesses at their endpoint in pulmonary arteries, and aneurysms develop proximal to each of these abscesses within the affected pulmonary arteries. Because the pulmonary arterial branches in cattle course close to bronchi, eventual enlargement of the abscesses predisposes to their rupture into airways. Sudden discharge of purulent material into the airway creates septic bronchopneumonia followed immediately by minor or major hemorrhage from the arterial aneurysm now communicating directly into the airway. This hemorrhage may be sufficient to result in hemoptysis and subsequent epistaxis. Affected cattle are unthrifty and frequently have been treated for recurrent bronchopneumonia characterized by fever (103.0 to 106.0° F/ 39.44 to 41.11° C), increased respiratory rate, as well as rales, crackles, or wheezes within localized areas of the lung. Some affected cattle develop endocarditis caused by the septic thrombus in the caudal vena cava remaining as a source of chronic bacteremia through the right heart and pulmonary arteries.

Epistaxis or hemoptysis may be slight and intermittent or may be profound, acute, and result in sudden death (Figure 4-42). Epistaxis associated with coughing and chronic bronchopneumonia in dairy cattle indicates an extremely guarded prognosis because of the irreversible nature of the pathology in caudal vena caval thrombosis. Other signs such as ascites, generalized visceral edema, and diarrhea are possible if the thrombosis occludes the caudal vena cava and results in portal hypertension. Right heart failure and a chronic passive congestion of the liver may also develop in some chronic cases.

Diagnosis of Sudden Death Syndrome

The diagnosis of caudal vena caval thrombosis requires careful necropsy when sudden death results. Generally affected animals have appeared completely healthy before death. Only one animal is affected in the herd, and

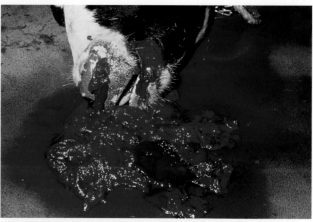

Figure 4-42

Massive pulmonary hemorrhage and acute death in a 3-year-old Holstein cow with hepatic-pulmonary abscesses. The cow was calving when the hemorrhage occurred.

the suddenness of death precludes physical examination or ancillary laboratory data. Necropsy will reveal a hilar liver abscess with rupture into the caudal vena cava (Figure 4-43). The lungs may show bullous emphysema, pulmonary edema, pulmonary infarction, and pulmonary arterial thrombosis.

Diagnosis of Acute Respiratory Distress Syndrome

Sudden onset of respiratory distress in a single cow within a herd raises an index of suspicion of acute caudal vena caval thrombosis. History and physical examination should exclude other causes of severe

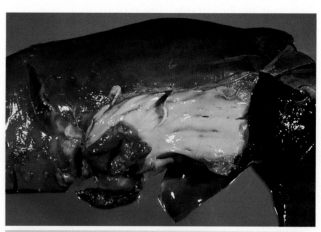

Figure 4-43

Necropsy specimen from a cow that died from rupture of a hilar liver abscess into the post cava. The site of rupture into the post cava is apparent as a rough-edged crater highlighted against the intima of the vein. The purulent remnants of the abscess appear to the left of the crater. *(Photo courtesy Dr. John King.)*

lower airway disease and acute respiratory distress. An elevated serum globulin (>5.0 g/dl) further raises the index of suspicion but cannot confirm the diagnosis. Chest radiographs, although not widely available in practice, are very helpful to the diagnosis because they usually demonstrate focal or multifocal pulmonary infarction and densities resulting from septic emboli, diffuse pulmonary edema, and bullous emphysema. In field situations, the affected cow is treated symptomatically and gradually may improve over 5 to 10 days. Subsequently, however, these animals usually develop hemoptysis, epistaxis, anemia, and chronic pneumonia typical of the classic signs associated with caudal vena caval thrombosis. The average lag phase between improvement from the acute syndrome and the onset of epistaxis is 3 to 6 weeks.

Diagnosis of Classical Caudal Vena Caval Thrombosis with Epistaxis, Hemoptysis, Anemia, and Chronic Bronchopneumonia

This form remains the most common clinical syndrome of caudal vena caval thrombosis. Elevated heart rate, increased respiratory rate, auscultable rales, persistent or recurrent fever, anemia, and hemoptysis are frequent signs. The owner may have observed epistaxis on several occasions or only once (Figures 4-44 and 4-45). Some affected cattle bleed out acutely with few premonitory signs. A heart murmur caused by anemia or endocarditis may be present. Generalized edema of the hind parts, ventrum, udder, and ascites may be present in some animals. If edema is generalized, diarrhea caused by gastrointestinal edema is observed. Frequently serum globulin is elevated (>5.0 g/dl), and a neutrophilic leukocytosis may be present in the hemogram. Thoracic radiographs or ultrasonography are helpful in identifying distinct

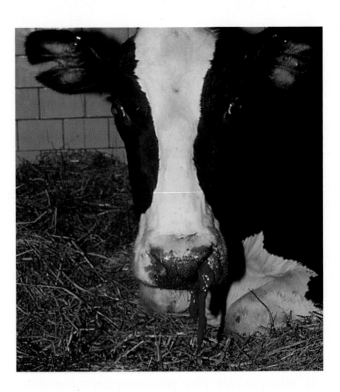

Figure 4-45

Severe epistasis and hemoptysis in a Holstein with caudal vena caval thrombosis (CVCT) that survived for 3 months after initial diagnosis of CVCT.

pulmonary abscesses, and occasionally the causative thrombus may be lodged in the caudal vena cava and identified on thoracic radiographs. Transabdominal ultrasound in the right eighth through eleventh intercostal spaces can also be useful to identify liver abscesses and allows visualization of the hilus and abdominal caudal vena cava close to the hilus. Endoscopy will help confirm the origin of hemorrhage in the lower airway and will allow collection of tracheal wash material for cytology and culture.

Treatment

Therapy for caudal vena caval thrombosis causing acute respiratory distress is symptomatic and includes:

Broad-spectrum antibiotics such as oxytetracycline, cephalosporins, or penicillin to control septic thromboemboli. *F. necrophorum* and *A. pyogenes* are the primary organisms found in these abscesses.

Furosemide (250 to 500 mg IM, twice daily per adult animal) if pulmonary edema is present.

Atropine (2.2 mg/45 kg body weight SQ, twice daily) as a supportive bronchodilator and to dry bronchial secretions.

Aspirin or another NSAID in standard dosages as an antiinflammatory drug. Initially flunixin meglumine may be used (250 to 500 mg/450 kg body weight) to counteract possible endotoxemia.

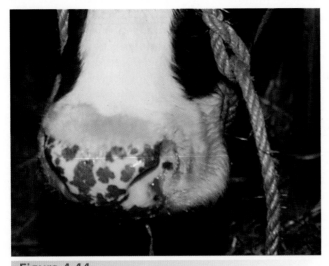

Figure 4-44

Slight epistaxis that was intermittently observed in a cow with caudal vena caval thrombosis (CVCT).

If improvement is observed, the animal should be maintained on long-term penicillin in the hope that the septic thromboemboli may be sterilized. Rifampin may be added to improve antibiotic penetration, but this represents extra-label drug use and is expensive. Prognosis is poor because a large thrombus tends to persist in the caudal vena cava, and constant or intermittent embolic showers are likely to continue. Few cattle have survived long term.

Treatment of caudal vena caval thrombosis with classic signs of pneumonia, epistaxis, hemoptysis, and anemia seldom is worthwhile because of the extensive pathology that exists. Valuable cattle may be treated with long-term penicillin (22,000 U/kg IM, twice daily) and aspirin (240 to 480 grains/450 kg body weight orally, twice daily). Penicillin is the antibiotic of choice, given the causative organisms, and aspirin may be safe for long-term use in an effort to discourage further platelet aggregation and thrombosis. Once epistaxis has been observed and confirmed to originate from the lower airway, prognosis is extremely guarded. Attempted therapy may be worthwhile in extremely valuable cattle in the hope that only a few pulmonary arterial abscesses have developed, giving the cow a chance to survive. However, it is rare for a cow with well-defined signs of caudal vena caval thrombosis to survive.

Control. Prevention or control of caudal vena caval thrombosis in cattle involves nutritional changes. Higly acidic diets that predispose to clinical or subclinical rumenitis and abomasal ulceration have to be tempered by buffers, prefeeding hay before high energy grains such as high moisture corn, or by feeding total mixed rations. Dairy rations should not be fed to yearling or bred heifers. High production herds are most at risk for rumenitis and abomasal ulceration secondary to intensive feeding of high-energy acid diets. Most cattle with liver abscesses are asymptomatic, and those having hilar abscesses probably suffered initiation of pathophysiology months to years before the onset of clinical signs. When more than an occasional case of caudal vena caval thrombosis appears in a herd, immediate evaluation of the herd's nutritional program is in order. One cow in a herd with caudal vena caval thrombosis is unfortunate but a common clinical problem. More than one cow in the same herd with caudal vena caval thrombosis, however, signals a potential serious economic loss and requires changes in the feeding program. Evaluation of the herd for subacute rumen acidosis is indicated under these circumstances and is described in Chapter 5.

Inhalation Pneumonia

Etiology and Signs. Inhalation pneumonia occurs when feed materials, milk, or medications enter the trachea and the animal fails to clear the airways of the material, and septic bronchopneumonia ensues. In calves, white muscle disease and iatrogenic inhalation pneumonia are the two most common causes. White muscle disease caused by selenium/vitamin E deficiency may affect the tongue, muscles of mastication, or muscles involved in swallowing and predispose to inhalation of milk or milk replacer as the affected calf tries to drink. Iatrogenic inhalation pneumonia in calves follows inadvertent intubation of the trachea with stomach tubes or esophageal feeders or, more commonly, from use of abnormally large holes on the end of nipple bottles. Nipple bottles used to feed calves should only drip milk when the bottle is turned upside down. Prematurity or dysmaturity may also predispose to inhalation pneumonia as a result of incompletely developed laryngeal protective reflexes. Inhalation pneumonia also may follow pharyngeal trauma by stomach tubes, esophageal feeders, or balling guns, resulting in dysphagia or neurogenic swallowing deficits. Crude or neophytic use of stomach tubes, feeders, and balling guns by laypeople causes most iatrogenic inhalation pneumonia.

In adult cattle, milk fever (parturient hypocalcemia) is the most common cause of inhalation pneumonia. The severely hypocalcemic cow not only is recumbent but also may lie in lateral recumbency and thus become bloated. Regurgitation of rumen ingesta may lead to inhalation because the cow's semicomatose state prevents her clearing the regurgitated ingesta from her pharynx and airway. Pharyngeal trauma caused by stomach tubes, magnet retrievers, and balling guns may injure vagal nerve branches traversing the pharynx. This neurogenic injury may lead to dysphagia and to defective eructation and regurgitation, and may predispose to inhalation pneumonia. Inadvertent intubation of the trachea during attempts at stomach tubing by an unskilled person creates a significant risk of inhalation in adult cattle as in calves. Choke, although rare in dairy cattle today, certainly represents a significant predisposing cause of inhalation pneumonia as well. Cattle that have choked on vegetables or feedstuff should be assessed carefully for early signs of inhalation pneumonia.

Neurologic disease constitutes another potential cause of inhalation pneumonia in cattle. Listeriosis and other diseases that affect the cranial nerves involved in deglutition, mastication, and swallowing food predispose to inhalation pneumonia, although our experience is that aspiration pneumonia associated with *Listeriosis* has rarely caused a clinical problem. Botulism represents an intoxication that may lead to inhalation pneumonia secondary to dysphagia.

Signs of inhalation vary with the relative volume and content of the inhaled material. For example, inadvertent administration of a large volume of fluid into the trachea results in immediate signs of dyspnea, respiratory distress, cyanosis, and repeated coughing. The affected calf or cow will expel some of the material from the nose or mouth as a frothy liquid before dying within minutes to hours. Smaller volumes of milk (calves with white muscle disease) or feed inhaled into the lower airway cause a septic or gangrenous pneumonia as the microorganisms contained in the causative material proliferate. In this instance, signs are progressive in nature and consist of a fever poorly responsive to antibiotics, dyspnea and rapid respirations, rales or bronchial tones in the anterior ventral lung fields (unless the animal was in lateral recumbency at the time of inhalation, in which case the major portion of the pathology may occur in one lung), and failure of response to antibiotic therapy. Rather than groups of animals being affected, as is typical with contagious pneumonia, only individual animals tend to be affected with inhalation pneumonia. However, when groups of calves are affected with white muscle disease, several calves may be affected with inhalation pneumonia at the same time.

Individual cattle with inhalation of rumen ingesta secondary to milk fever or other problems develop a progressive gangrenous pneumonia with fever, dyspnea, and toxemia. Rapid consolidation of affected lung tissue occurs, and bronchial tones and rales may be ausculted—usually in the cranioventral lung fields. Broad-spectrum antibiotic therapy is effective only if the amount of ingesta inhaled was relatively small. In most instances, the course is one of progressive deterioration over several days, ending in death. Sometimes inhalation of saliva or small amounts of water or feed as a result of dysphagia is treatable with broad-spectrum antibiotic therapy. We have had the best results with cattle that develop some degree of inhalation pneumonia secondary to dysphagia induced by pharyngeal trauma. Because the amount of inhaled material usually is unknown, treatment is indicated unless the animal shows profound dyspnea and cyanosis.

Treatment. Therapy for inhalation pneumonia incorporates broad-spectrum antibiotics directed against the microbes normally present in the material inhaled. Nonsteroidal antiinflammatory drugs also would be indicated for supportive therapy. Antibiotic therapy should be continued at least 2 weeks if symptomatic improvement occurs. Persistent fever, depression, dyspnea, and toxemia are negative signs and generally signal a fatal outcome.

Prevention. Inhalation of certain necrotizing or nonabsorbable chemicals (e.g., mineral oil) is uniformly fatal, and treatment is not indicated. Prevention of inhalation pneumonia can be practiced only when the problem is anticipated and is largely a matter of common sense. Therefore withdrawing feed from animals suffering from choke, dysphagia, and other known problems may be helpful. Prompt treatment of milk fever or other diseases that may prevent a cow from maintaining sternal recumbency is important in preventing aspiration pneumonia. Management practices such as routine or therapeutic drenching of postparturient cattle should only be performed by laypeople who

have been properly trained and provided with appropriate equipment. The feeding of milk to weak, premature, or dysmature calves should also be predicated on common sense and an awareness that normal protective airway reflexes may be overcome by impatient feeding practices (e.g., enlarging holes in nipples) or by allowing these calves to nurse with the head and neck hyperextended or dorsiflexed, as appears to be their instinctive habit. Feeding from buckets or a bottle with the head and neck in a neutral position parallel to the ground can lessen the risk of inhalation.

Thermal and Chemical Damage to the Lower Airway

Etiology and Signs. Barn fires and occasionally grass fires in pastures are responsible for thermal and smoke injury to the respiratory tract in cattle. Chemical damage may be mild, as a result of common gases such as ammonia, or severe, as in accidental exposure to anhydrous ammonia.

Thermal damage resulting from excessive heat and smoke inhalation has been well described for comparative species. The pathophysiology involves heat-induced edema and necrosis of the mucosal lining, pulmonary edema and congestion, destruction of the mucociliary apparatus, hyaline membrane formation, and filling of the small airways with proteinaceous fluid, sloughing tissue in the form of diphtheritic membranes, hyaline membranes, and inflammatory cell debris (Figure 4-46). Pathology tends to be progressive with increasing dyspnea as small airway occlusion develops hours to days following the original thermal and smoke insult. Therefore it is difficult to estimate the severity of the lesions immediately following the fire. Dyspnea characterized by an increased respiratory rate may be the only sign. Cattle with obvious facial burns, muzzle burns, or diphtheritic

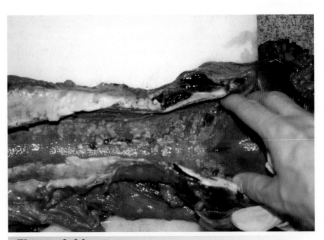

Figure 4-46

Postmortem specimen of trachea from cow that had died from smoke inhalation during a barn fire. Note the severe tracheal mucosal erosions and diphtheritic damage.

crusts in the nasal cavity should be suspected of having suffered significant smoke inhalation. Pulmonary edema is an early sign of severe thermal damage and suggests that subsequent pathology with hyaline membrane formation will follow. Other signs in severely affected animals include cough, tachypnea, wheezing, cyanosis, and stridor. In severe cases, respiratory distress will develop 1 to 24 hours following initial injury, and bacterial bronchopneumonia may develop within 1 to 4 days in cattle that survive the initial thermal injury. Carbon monoxide poisoning is a common cause of death for animals at the time of the fire or shortly thereafter.

Chemical damage resulting from high environmental concentrations of ammonia largely reflects poor management or inadequate ventilation within an enclosure. Excessive buildup of manure and urine without adequate ventilation will allow ammonia fumes to damage the physical defense mechanisms of the lower airway. Secondary bacterial pneumonias are the most common sequelae to this problem, and this topic has been discussed under bacterial pneumonias.

We have also observed a progressive increase in respiratory rate in some hospitalized cattle that have their bedding changed frequently and are kept in deeply bedded stalls for 2 weeks or more. This has occurred in all seasons of the year and does not seem to be simply temperature related. There is no coughing, and tracheal washes have not revealed a cause for the tachypnea. If the cows are put outside, the respiratory rates return to normal in 1 to 3 days.

Anhydrous ammonia is an extremely dangerous chemical that is widely used in agriculture today. It is used as a source of nonprotein nitrogen for forages and fertilization of various crops. The chemical seeks out water when it comes in contact with vegetable matter or tissue. Accidental exposure to anhydrous ammonia can be lethal to animals or humans who come in contact with the material. Because of the intense water affinity of the chemical, anhydrous ammonia seeks moist tissues such as the eye and respiratory tract. As a result of this contact, moist tissue rapidly desiccates followed by necrosis as the chemical dehydrates the tissue. Corneal edema, epithelial necrosis, and corneal stromal burns immediately develop in the eyes. The mucosa of the respiratory tract is burned, and following dehydration, sloughs and diphtheritic membranes fill the airways, leading to hypoxia or suffocation. Pulmonary edema develops rapidly, and death may occur peracutely or be delayed hours or days. Secondary bacterial pneumonias are possible if the animal survives the initial chemical injury.

Insecticides that are fogged into barns for fly control occasionally may induce chemical damage or sensitivity to the lower airway. The exact mechanism of action is not fully understood, but tachypnea, coughing, and mild dyspnea may be observed.

Diagnosis. The diagnosis of thermal or chemical injury is made by the history and physical examination findings. Ancillary information seldom is necessary. Endoscopy and thoracic radiographs may provide prognostic information for valuable animals but seldom are used in practice.

Treatment. Major treatment considerations for acute thermal injury of the airway include adequate oxygenation and establishment of an adequate airway. If laryngeal edema is so severe as to result in respiratory distress, a tracheostomy may be necessary. A tracheostomy should not be performed unless severe upper respiratory distress is present because the procedure further predisposes to secondary bacterial bronchopneumonia in burn patients. Oxygen administration is indicated if acute dyspnea suggests possible carbon monoxide poisoning.

Judicious dosages of furosemide (25 to 50 mg/45 kg body weight) may be necessary if pulmonary edema is present. Use of corticosteroids for acute pulmonary distress caused by thermal injury is controversial. Steroids have been proposed as initial therapy to "short cycle" parts of the vicious cycle of inflammation because they decrease mediators of inflammation, stabilize inflamed vasculature, and decrease edema of the upper and lower airway. If steroids are used, they should be given immediately rather than waiting for the subsequent pathology and respiratory distress that will follow thermal injury in the following 1 to 24 hours. Dosages vary but may be as high as 0.1 to 1.0 mg/lb dexamethasone as a one-time treatment. Abortifacient properties of the drug need to be considered before it is used on pregnant animals, and a significant risk associated with the use of steroids in the form of possible secondary bronchopneumonia also must be considered before dexamethasone's use. Dr. Rebhun commented that he had treated some barn fire victims with dexamethasone but that the results were hard to interpret. In one valuable yearling bull, a high dose of corticosteroids was used initially without respiratory consequences, but the bull developed a left displacement of the abomasum within 24 hours of treatment. The cause/effect relationship of the exogenous source of corticosteroids on the displacement never was confirmed but certainly was suspicious. NSAIDs may be used at regular dosages without the additional risks presented by corticosteroids. However, NSAIDs probably do not block the ongoing pathophysiology of lower airway disease corticosteroids. Prophylactic systemic antibiotics are reported not to influence the subsequent development of bacterial bronchopneumonia. Some literature regarding usage in humans discourages the use of prophylactic antibiotics for fear of allowing resistant strains of bacteria to emerge in the lower airway. In cattle, especially valuable ones, broad-spectrum antibiotics usually are used on a prophylactic basis, although no controlled data support their use. Tetracyclines may help decrease inflammation via their inhibitory effect on metalloproteinases. Disadvantages of tetracyclines would be that they are bacteriostatic and many commensal organisms may be resistant to the drug. If used, practitioners should be aware of their potential to cause nephrotoxicity, particularly in hemodynamically challenged patients. If tracheostomies or tracheal washes are performed, extreme care should be taken to minimize iatrogenic introduction of pathogens into the respiratory tract. As in thermal skin injury, *Pseudomonas* sp. and other opportunists are the major bacteria to invade damaged tissue.

Nebulization with antibiotics, bronchodilators, corticosteroids, acetylcysteine, and/or surfactant has also been used in affected cattle. Acetylcysteine has anticollagenase and antioxidant effects via its glutathione-promoting properties.

In chemical injury resulting from anhydrous ammonia, exposed animals and the entire environment should be sprayed with water to destroy residual fumes. Emergency personnel and fire companies should be summoned immediately so that gas masks and protective clothing are available for people spraying water in the area and repairing the leak. All humans in the area should move upwind and leave the area until the leak and fumes have been controlled. Cattle exposed but still alive should not be stressed and should be allowed access to as much fresh air as possible. No specific treatment is possible. Symptomatic treatment may include furosemide, prophylactic antibiotics, or oxygen therapy. Animals with chemically injured eyes should have topical antibiotic ointments and atropine ointments applied to the eyes several times daily.

Mycotic Pneumonia

Etiology and Signs. Mycotic or fungal pneumonia usually results from embolic dissemination of fungal organisms from other infected organs such as the rumen, abomasum, or mammary gland. Immunosuppression and immunosuppressive drugs (corticosteroids) predispose to fungal infection, as does intensive antibiotic therapy, which may deplete the bacterial flora and promote fungal growth. Lactic acid indigestion (toxic rumenitis) remains one of the leading causes of mycotic pneumonia. Pathophysiology evolves from chemical rumenitis to bacterial rumenitis and subsequent mycotic rumenitis—especially if the affected cow has been treated with antibiotics. Embolic infection of the lungs ensues as a result of seeding of the portal circulation and liver from the primary ruminal infection. Similarly fungal pneumonia has been observed as a sequela to severe septic mastitis in dairy cattle. Intensive antibiotic therapy and overzealous use of corticosteroids predisposed these animals to mycotic infections that became septicemic from the udder and then involved the lungs. Although *Aspergillus* spp. are the most common fungal organisms identified, theoretically any yeast or fungus could be causative.

Signs are nonspecific but consist of persistent fever unresponsive to antibiotics (104.0 to 108.0° F/40.0 to 42.2° C), increased respiratory rate, and variable abnormal lung sounds in one or both lungs. Rales and increased or decreased bronchovesicular sounds may be heard in individual cases. A primary site of severe infection such as the mammary gland, forestomach, or uterus usually is apparent, and the respiratory signs may be disregarded or difficult to identify. Multiple organ failure and neurologic signs frequently coexist or develop because of the fungal septicemia. Occasional cases of disseminated fungal disease with fungal pneumonia can be seen in septicemic calves or calves with severe enteritis that have received extensive antibiotic and/or corticosteroid treatment.

Diagnosis. Diagnosis is difficult and at best may only be suspected before the death of the individual. Tracheal washings may identify the organisms during cytology or culture procedures but also may be disregarded as evidence of upper airway contamination of the tracheal wash sample.

Gross and histologic pathology confirms the diagnosis. Discolored multifocal areas of pneumonia are present grossly (Figure 4-47), and hyphae are identified by histopathology.

Treatment. No successful treatment has been described for mycotic pneumonia in cattle, and the primary infection coupled with mycotic pneumonia or mycotic septicemia usually is fatal.

Prevention. Although intensive antibiotic therapy is necessary for certain infections in dairy cattle, practitioners should be aware that chronic localized infections in the udder, uterus, or gastrointestinal tract that are treated with long-term antibiotics may predispose to yeast or fungal overgrowth and potential embolic spread. Repeated IV therapy by practitioners or laypeople using drugs from multidose vials also may lead to

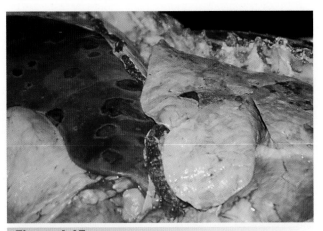

Figure 4-47

Necropsy specimen showing mycotic hepatitis (left) and pneumonia (right) secondary to lactic acid indigestion. Mycotic lesions appear similar to "targets" with red centers and pale peripheries.

direct mycotic septicemia, such as occurs occasionally in human abusers of IV drugs.

High or repeated dosages of exogenous corticosteroids are to be condemned in dairy cattle and may represent the most dangerous drugs currently predisposing to fungal infections. There are few, if any, dise/ases in dairy cattle that require high doses of corticosteroids for effective therapy. Corticosteroid use as initial therapy for severe infectious/inflammatory diseases should not be repeated. The low dosages of corticosteroids (10 to 20 mg of dexamethasone) utilized by many veterinarians as daily treatment for ketosis generally are safe if limited to 3 to 7 days and not used in cattle with severe infections such as septic mastitis, septic metritis, pneumonia, or toxic rumenitis.

Space-Occupying Masses in the Thorax, Lung Parenchyma, or Lower Airway

Etiology and Signs. Space-occupying thoracic masses involving the lung parenchyma, visceral or parietal pleura, or other structures in the thorax cause subtle or marked progressive dyspnea and may cause signs similar to congestive heart failure. Other clinical signs vary with specific lesions; for example, fever unresponsive to antibiotics would be present in cattle affected with thoracic abscesses or pleuritis, whereas fever may not be present in thoracic or mediastinal neoplasia.

Inflammatory lesions include thoracic abscesses and pleuritis (Figure 4-48). Thoracic abscesses usually are unilateral and result in detectable absence of lung sounds in the affected ventral hemithorax. Ipsilateral heart sounds may be absent or muffled, whereas contralateral heart sounds are louder than normal and accentuated by the displaced heart's proximity to the contralateral thoracic wall. Fever unresponsive to antibiotics, progressive dyspnea, venous distention and pulsation of the jugular and mammary veins, ventral edema, and

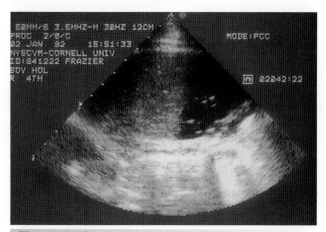

Figure 4-48

Sonogram of the thorax of a cow with septic pleuritis. The white echogenic spots in the black fluid suggest anaerobic infection and gas production.

a reluctance to move are other signs observed in cattle affected with thoracic abscesses. Etiology of thoracic abscesses sometimes is unknown, but penetration of the thorax by reticular foreign bodies and localized enlarging pulmonary abscesses from previous pneumonia have been confirmed at autopsy in several fatal cases. Previous history of pneumonia or hardware disease may suggest etiology in certain cases, but a specific etiology seldom is determined in surviving cattle. *A. pyogenes* is the organism isolated from most thoracic abscesses.

Pleuritis is rare in dairy cattle except when it accompanies severe consolidating bronchopneumonia of bacterial origin. As in other species, fever, progressive dyspnea, absence of lung sounds in the ventral thorax (unilateral or bilateral), and thoracic pain are typical. Although a fibrinous pleuritis is most common in cattle, when large amounts of pleural fluid are present, venous distention and apparent pulsations may be present in the jugular and mammary veins. Rare cases of pleuritis resulting from rupture of a parenchymal pulmonary abscess into the pleural space, penetrating thoracic wounds or foreign bodies associated with traumatic reticuloperitonitis, erosion of the diaphragm by an abscess associated with hardware or perforating abomasal ulcer, and rupture of the esophagus secondary to chronic choke or trauma also have been observed.

Pleural effusion may also occur as part of a nonseptic or septic pericarditis syndrome. We have had some cases of pericarditis/pleuritis in which the cause could not be determined. In one cow with fibrinous pericarditis (based on ultrasound appearance and a mixed cell type [neutrophils, lymphocytes, plasma cells] pericardial and pleural fluid cytology), there was a complete cure following pericardial injection of corticosteroids in addition to systemic antibiotics. Another cow had pleural effusion as a result of right heart failure caused by pulmonary hypertension. Although severe pleural effusion is not common in cattle with right heart failure, it may occur.

Seromas and hematomas may develop following trauma to the thoracic wall. These masses occasionally extend into the thorax itself. In these instances, apparent rupture or leakage of the seroma through the parietal pleura occurs. These seromas and hematomas may be associated with rib fractures or traumatic injuries at the costochondral junctions (Figure 4-49). Signs include progressive dyspnea, increased respiratory rate, venous distention and pulsation, normal temperature, absence of lung sounds ventrally in the affected hemithorax, absence or muffling of heart sounds in the affected hemithorax, and loud pounding heart sounds in the contralateral hemithorax caused by cardiac displacement.

Diaphragmatic hernias may cause dyspnea and absence of cardiopulmonary sounds in the affected thoracic area. Bloat is commonly observed in cattle having diaphragmatic hernia because the reticulum is usually the herniated organ.

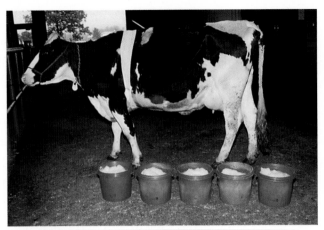

Figure 4-49

Mature Holstein with thoracic seroma or transudate secondary to traumatic injury at the costochondral region of the left thorax. Forty liters of transudative fluid have just been removed from the left hemithorax via thoracocentesis. The cow made a complete recovery.

Neoplastic masses may occur in the pulmonary parenchyma, pleura, lymph nodes, or thymus. Cardiac neoplasms will be discussed with other cardiac diseases. Thymic lymphosarcoma may be the most obvious neoplasm within this group. Thymic lymphosarcoma is recognized in cattle between 4 and 24 months of age and causes progressive dyspnea, bloat, or both. Swelling is obvious in the distal ventral cervical area and extends into the thoracic inlet. Some thymic lymphosarcoma masses are soft, fluid-like swellings on palpation (Figure 4-50), whereas others are firmer. Compression of the trachea and esophagus results in dyspnea and interference with eructation that varies with the size of the mass. Compression of the trachea, causing respiratory distress, may also occur in adult cattle with enzootic lymphosarcoma. Adult lymphosarcoma may cause tumor formation in the thorax as a result of lymph node, pleural, cardiac, and occasionally pulmonary involvement. Signs vary depending on the tumor numbers, size, and other organs affected. Occasionally lymphosarcoma patients will have fever caused by tumor necrosis, and this may be a misleading sign. Severe pleural effusion with many neoplastic lymphocytes may occur. The pleural effusion caused by lymphoma is often grossly discolored, having a bloody appearance.

Primary pulmonary tumors of epithelial origin described as papillary adenomas have been observed in young cattle at slaughter. These were reported as benign, multicentric tumors because metastases were not observed. Signs were not reported because these were incidental findings during slaughter inspection. Several case reports have documented malignant neoplasms such as bronchiolar adenocarcinoma in older cows showing signs of progressive dyspnea. Dr. Rebhun documented

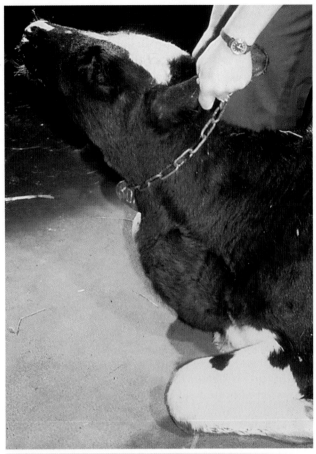

Figure 4-50

Thymic lymphosarcoma in a 6-month-old calf presented because of worsening dyspnea and intermittent bloat.

one older cow and one bull with massive pulmonary adenocarcinomas that resulted in progressive dyspnea, weight loss, and reduced lung sounds. Mesotheliomas originate from the pleura and tend to be multiple. They may enlarge collectively to create signs of progressive dyspnea, decreased lung sounds caused by massive pleural effusion, weight loss, and eventually lead to death.

Tuberculosis, although rare in dairy cattle because of regulatory control efforts, should be remembered as a potential cause of progressive dyspnea, coughing, weight loss, and signs of pneumonia. Enlarged thoracic lymph nodes associated with the infection may result in esophageal compression and bloat or obvious respiratory distress from tracheal compression.

Diagnosis. Diagnosis of space-occupying lesions in the thorax requires careful auscultation to detect differences in lung and heart sounds in each hemithorax.

Abscesses, seromas, or masses occupying one hemithorax will elevate the ipsilateral lung and push the heart toward the opposite hemithorax. Therefore in the affected hemithorax, lung sounds will be absent ventrally, and heart sounds will be muffled or absent. Auscultation of the opposite hemithorax will reveal uniformly increased bronchovesicular sounds and a loud "pounding" heart beat caused by the proximity of the heart to the thoracic wall on this side. Thoracic percussion also may be helpful in detecting the area of involvement. Because cattle affected with these problems often have increased central venous pressure as a result of impaired venous return, they may be confused with heart failure patients. An incomplete physical examination may lead to an erroneous diagnosis such as endocarditis or pericarditis if the examiner only auscults one hemithorax.

Once a lesion has been identified, further diagnostics are indicated. Thoracic radiographs and ultrasonography are indicated if a complete diagnostic workup is to be performed. Blood work may be helpful in the case of thoracic abscesses in that serum globulin usually is elevated ($\geq$5.0 g/dl) and neutrophilia may be present. The most direct diagnostic aid remains thoracocentesis with a suitable needle. Although a 5.0-cm needle will enter the pleural space of cattle, it is seldom long enough to invade the capsule of an encapsulated abscess or seroma. Therefore an 8.75-cm, 18-gauge needle is preferred for initial thoracocentesis through the lower fifth or sixth intercostal space on the affected hemithorax. If fluid or pus is obtained, the material is submitted for cytology and culture. If no fluid is obtained, biopsy of a mass lesion may be indicated.

Similarly, if thymic lymphosarcoma is suspected, aspirates for cytology or biopsies (True-Cut biopsy needle, Baxter Healthcare Corp., Valencia, CA) are indicated to allow definitive diagnosis. As previously mentioned, some thymic lymphosarcoma patients have a misleading fluctuant mass that appears fluid filled. Aspirate attempts yield no fluid, however, and biopsy will confirm the diagnosis. Juvenile cattle affected with thymic lymphosarcoma usually are negative for bovine leukemia virus when their serum is tested by agar gel immunodiffusion or radioimmunoassay.

Pleuritis or pleural effusion may be unilateral or bilateral. Careful auscultation and percussion should lead to suspicion of free pleural fluid because lung sounds usually are absent in the ventral aspect of the affected hemithorax. Dyspnea may be marked in cattle with large accumulations of pleural fluid. Pleural fluid does not displace the heart, as occurs in those with unilateral thoracic masses or abscesses. Therefore heart sounds are audible bilaterally and may appear to radiate caudodorsally by sound conduction through the pleural fluid. Pleural fluid must be differentiated from anterior ventral pulmonary consolidation. Bronchial tones usually are heard in consolidated regions of lungs, whereas *absence* of sounds is more typical of pleural fluid. Thoracocentesis is indicated to confirm pleural fluid accumulation; any sampled fluid should be analyzed using cytology and culture to differentiate infections from neoplastic or other causes. Ultrasonography and thoracic radiographs, if available, would help in the management of a valuable

cow affected with this problem. Ultrasonography is an extremely valuable tool for evaluating pleural disease in cattle. As more portable equipment becomes available, an ultrasound machine may be used with increased frequency as part of the evaluation for sick cows. Ultrasonography can quickly determine whether there is pleural effusion, abscessation, consolidation, or pleural surface masses. It can also be used as an aid for collection of samples via needle or biopsy. If available, thoracic radiographs are helpful to confirm or deny diaphragmatic hernia.

Thoracic tumors involving the lung parenchyma, pleura, or thoracic lymph nodes are difficult to diagnose unless thoracic radiographs and ultrasonography are available. Signs vary, and dyspnea and progressive weight loss occur despite symptomatic treatment. Thoracic lymphosarcoma may be suspected based on physical signs involving other sites or lymph nodes becoming obviously enlarged. A bovine leukemia virus agar gel immunodiffusion or enzyme-linked immunoabsorbent assay (ELISA) will be positive in most cows with clinical lymphosarcoma. This does not confirm a diagnosis but does add to the index of suspicion if lymphosarcoma is suspected. Bloat and tracheal compression may occur if mediastinal masses or lymphadenopathy become severe. Thoracocentesis may offer the best means of diagnosis in these unusual tumors because exfoliative cytology may help identify the tumor and allow proper prognosis.

Treatment. Therapy of unilateral thoracic abscesses and seromas involves drainage of the lesions through the thoracic wall. Because A. pyogenes is the usual causative organism of thoracic abscesses, a thick capsule often is present. Once the location of the abscess is confirmed by thoracocentesis, a large-bore (20 to 28 French) chest trochar is placed into the abscess cavity (Figure 4-51). The chest trochar is sutured in place, and the affected cow is started on penicillin (22,000 IU/kg, twice daily). Where ultrasonography is available, it may be used to confirm

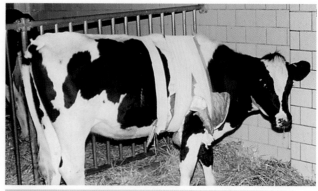

Figure 4-51

Yearling heifer with an encapsulated A. pyogenes abscess in the right hemithorax. A chest trochar has been placed to facilitate drainage.

pleural adhesions between parietal pleura and the abscess, allowing subsequent surgical thoracotomy coupled with rib resection to afford even more efficient drainage and exploration of the cause of the abscess. Complete drainage is the key to successful treatment. Lavage of saline or antibiotic and saline solutions through the indwelling trochar also has been used in some cases. Irritating solutions such as iodine products are contraindicated, however.

Cattle with seromas that are drained in this manner subsequently have a good prognosis. Abscesses require long-term antibiotic therapy and complete evacuation/drainage. Therefore the affected cow must be of substantial value to justify the medical expenses and associated loss of milk sales for several weeks. Cattle affected with thoracic abscesses may lose significant body condition during early treatment, but absence of fever, decreased venous distention, increased appetite, weight gain, and a return to normal thoracic sounds on auscultation are all signs of improvement.

Treatment for pleuritis and pleural fluid requires drainage of the fluid and appropriate antibiotic therapy to control associated pneumonia. If pleural fluid is caused by effusion from neoplastic conditions, treatment is rarely indicated. Hardware perforations of the diaphragm may result either in frank pleuritis with pleural fluid accumulation, thoracic abscess, or diaphragmatic hernia. When *A. pyogenes* predominates, a thick-walled thoracic abscess develops, resulting in chronic disease. If a mixed infection develops and a fluid pleuritis that is not encapsulated results, the affected cow has an acute disease with large amounts of septic pleural fluid free in the pleural space.

Surprisingly few cattle with bacterial bronchopneumonia develop clinically significant pleural fluid accumulation. Nonetheless, pneumonia remains the most common cause of pleural fluid accumulation. Diagnosis of pleural fluid accumulation unilaterally or bilaterally in a cow affected with severe pneumonia dictates drainage of this fluid. Pleural effusion associated with bronchopneumonia will result in fever unresponsive to antibiotics and marked dyspnea. Drainage is provided by daily thoracocentesis or continuous drainage until negligible quantities of pleural fluid are obtained. Appropriate systemic antibiotics should be selected based on culture and susceptibility results and maintained for at least 1 week beyond the last thoracocentesis.

Pneumothorax

Etiology and Signs. Dyspnea accompanied by increased respiratory rate and effort coupled with absence of bronchovesicular sounds in the dorsal lung fields unilaterally or bilaterally characterizes pneumothorax or bullous emphysema. Dyspnea may range from mild to severe. Some adult cattle appear very painful with pneumothorax. When severe dyspnea is present, open

mouth breathing and expiratory groan suggest a bilateral problem. Subcutaneous emphysema may be observed in some affected cattle. Pneumoretroperitoneum may be documented in some cattle with pneumothorax on rectal examination.

Auscultation of the affected hemithorax reveals increased bronchovesicular sounds in the ventral lung fields and absence of lung sounds dorsally. Body temperature is normal unless exertion, high environmental temperatures, or pulmonary inflammation leads to pyrexia. Severe exertion during parturition, exertion during restraint for treatment or surgery, penetrating thoracic wounds, or pharyngeal/laryngeal injury causing a pneumomediastinum that ruptures into the chest may cause pneumothorax. Primary pulmonary pathology associated with chronic bronchopneumonia and emphysematous bullae formation is the most common cause of pneumothorax in cattle. Fever may be present if primary pulmonary inflammation (BRSV, severe bacterial bronchopneumonia, acute bovine pulmonary emphysema [ABPE], among others) contributed to emphysema and resultant pneumothorax. BRSV is the most common infectious agent associated with pneumothorax in cattle. In these inflammatory diseases, auscultation of the ventral lung fields helps to define etiology. Ultrasonography may be helpful in diagnosing the pneumothorax (there is no normal sliding of the dorsal air line) and determining the cause (e.g., lung abscess).

Diagnosis. Auscultation and percussion suggest the diagnosis. Pneumothorax must be differentiated from bullous emphysema and pulmonary edema. Radiographs or ultrasonography will confirm the diagnosis but may not be available. If history, auscultation, and percussion suggest the diagnosis, thoracic puncture and vacuum evacuation of free air should be attempted through the dorsal ninth or tenth intercostal space. The presence of free air confirms the diagnosis, and airway sounds should return to the dorsal thorax following evacuation of free air. Tracheal wash samples for cytology and culture may be necessary to assess lower airway infection or inflammation.

Treatment. Therapy requires evacuation of air from the affected hemithorax and treatment of any primary problem such as pneumonia, puncture wounds, and so forth. Cattle with pneumothorax resulting from bacterial pneumonia have a guarded prognosis. Rapid improvement in the dyspnea should be anticipated when pneumothorax is the major problem. The clinician must remember that, except in exogenous puncture of the thorax, pneumothorax originates from damaged pulmonary tissue that has "leaked" air. Simple evacuation of the free air in the thorax will improve the affected animal temporarily but does not guarantee the problem will not recur. Owners need to be instructed to watch the patient carefully for recurrence of dyspnea if the damaged lung continues to leak. Most cattle, however, respond to one or two evacuations of the thorax. A technique for continuous drainage has been described by Dr. Peek in cattle that requires hospitalization and confinement.

Pneumomediastinum

Etiology and Signs. Pneumomediastinum most often accompanies severe pulmonary parenchymal diseases that result in emphysema and bullae formation. Subsequent leakage of air into the mediastinum occurs. Several of the causes of pneumothorax mentioned previously are also potential causes of pneumomediastinum. Pneumomediastinum is most common in postpartum cows. In some cases there is old pulmonary pathology predisposing to the pneumomediastinum, whereas other cases may simply result from the exertion of calving. Signs may be mild or impossible to separate from those caused by the primary pulmonary pathology. Mild dyspnea, subcutaneous emphysema, and bilateral muffled heart sounds are present in most instances. The muffled heart sounds are the only constant findings and are caused by air insulation of the cardiac sounds. The subcutaneous emphysema is mostly on the dorsum of the cow as the air migrates along the aorta and through the lumbar fascial planes. It can also be felt rectally along the aorta.

Diagnosis. Subcutaneous emphysema in a postpartum cow is highly suggestive of pneumomediastinum. The presence of bilateral heart sound muffling requires differentiation of this condition from pericarditis. This differentiation is aided by obvious pulmonary pathology coupled with an absence of signs of heart failure in most cases. If physical examination findings cannot definitely differentiate these problems, ultrasonography and radiographs are indicated. Pericardiocentesis is not indicated as an initial procedure because it may subject the patient to unnecessary risks. Thoracic radiographs demonstrate a very clear cardiac and aortic shadow because surrounding air highlights these tissues.

Treatment. Specific treatment for pneumomediastinum is not required unless the cow has labored breathing and a probable pneumothorax. Therefore therapy should be directed against any primary pulmonary pathology in addition to oxygen, bronchodilator, and antitussive therapy.

Noninfectious Causes of Acute Respiratory Distress in Cattle

Acute respiratory distress in cattle may occur with a variety of noninfectious pathologic changes. Some causes have well-documented pathophysiology, whereas others are more poorly defined and controversial. Terminology varies tremendously among pathologists and clinicians, resulting in much confusion regarding these disorders. Most acute diseases discussed here require gross or microscopic pathology to enable positive diagnosis. The clinician cannot differentiate most of these diseases based on physical examination alone. Textbook descriptions have confused the issue by using different synonyms and eponyms to characterize the problem.

Fortunately, as a collected group of respiratory problems, these diseases are uncommon and much less important than infectious causes of respiratory diseases in dairy cattle. Therefore they will be described individually as best as possible in this section. The reader should realize that the nomenclature of these diseases has changed in the past and is likely to change in the future. Specific therapy is addressed where indicated.

Acute Bovine Pulmonary Edema and Emphysema (Atypical Interstitial Pneumonia, Fog Fever)

Etiology and Signs. This acute disease of cattle develops within 2 weeks of the time cattle are moved to lush pasture. The exact composition of the pasture does not seem important because grasses, alfalfa, turnips, kale, and rape all have been incriminated. Similarly *Perilla* mint and moldy sweet potatoes may cause identical syndromes. Although not as well documented, we have seen similar clinical and pathological outbreaks associated with grass silages and ryegrass pastures. Affected cattle develop acute, severe respiratory distress characterized by reluctance to move, open mouth breathing, pulmonary edema, tachypnea, and hyperpnea. Temperatures are normal to slightly elevated unless environmental temperatures are very high.

The transformation of ingested L-tryptophan to indole acetic acid is followed by decarboxylation to 3-methylindole, which is the toxic metabolite of tryptophan. Following absorption of 3-methylindole into the systemic circulation from the rumen, the mixed function oxidase system metabolizes the chemical producing pneumotoxicity in Clara cells and type 1 pneumocytes. Experimental studies have confirmed that 3-methylindole is the toxic metabolite of tryptophan involved in ABPE. Calves seldom are affected, but adult animals over 2 years of age in good body condition appear most at risk.

Fortunately the disease is rare in dairy cattle in the United States because pasture management is more stringent and pasturing is practiced less commonly in confinement herds than in the beef industry. Dairy practitioners should be aware of ABPE but may never see a herd outbreak of this disease.

Signs. Profound dyspnea, reluctance to move, auscultable evidence of interstitial pneumonia (rhonchi and rales) in the ventral lung field, and quiet lungs dorsally secondary to emphysema and edema characterize the condition. Subcutaneous emphysema may be observed. Morbidity may approach 50%, and mortality quotes range from 25% to 50%.

Diagnosis and Treatment. Diagnosis is by history, clinical signs, and pathologic study of the lungs from fatal cases. Treatment is seldom helpful, although a variety of drugs have been used in an effort to save badly affected animals. Simple movement or mild restraint may be fatal to these anoxic animals. Therefore treatment is controversial and empiric. Furosemide (0.5 to 1.0 mg/kg) may lessen pulmonary edema. Atropine (0.048 mg/kg or 1/30 grain/100 lb body weight twice daily), antihistamines, NSAIDs, vitamins A and E, and cortisone all have been used with varying anecdotal results. Animals that are rested, removed from the pasture, and not severely affected usually recover in 1 to 2 weeks. Some cattle may fall into the category of "chronic lungers," this being caused by proliferation of type 2 pneumocytes and pulmonary fibrosis.

Prevention. Prevention is the best treatment and may be accomplished by feeding susceptible cattle monensin (200 mg/head/day) starting several days before they are introduced to lush pasture and for 7 to 10 days following being placed on that pasture. These drugs inhibit the metabolism of tryptophan to 3-methylindole.

Proliferative Pneumonia

Etiology and Signs. Proliferative pneumonia is another form of acute respiratory distress observed in dairy cattle. This condition occasionally has been observed to cause high morbidity within a herd but usually affects only one or a few cattle within a group. Acute onset of dyspnea characterized by hyperpnea, tachypnea, an occasional cough, open mouth breathing, and pulmonary edema is observed (Figure 4-52).

The term proliferative pneumonia derives from the characteristic gross pathology consisting of heavy, firm, wet lung that is diffusely affected. Histologic study of these lungs reveals obliteration of alveolar space by proliferating type 2 pneumocytes and interstitial edema.

The gross pathology and histopathology are characteristic. Unfortunately affected cattle show signs common to many diseases characterized by acute respiratory

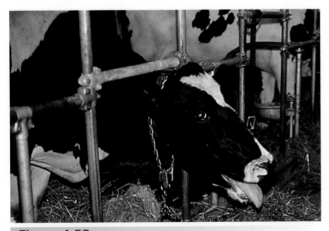

Figure 4-52

Holstein with acute severe dyspnea and open mouth breathing because of proliferative pneumonia.

distress. Clinical signs include low-grade fever (103.0 to 104.0° F/39.44 to 40.00° C), which may range higher (105.0 to 106.0° F/40.56 to 41.11° C) as a result of exertion and environmental factors. Auscultation of the lungs reveals diffuse reduction of airway sounds over the entire thorax. Proliferation of type 2 pneumocytes within the alveoli and interstitial edema contribute to the reduced lower airway sounds. Therefore although the affected cow has severe lower airway dyspnea, the lungs are very quiet on auscultation.

Other diseases, such as ABPE, diffuse pulmonary edema, acute dyspnea associated with embolic showering from a caudal vena caval thrombosis, nitrogen dioxide inhalation, and other causes of acute respiratory distress could lead to similar signs.

Not only is the disease difficult to diagnose accurately but also the exact cause or causes remain unknown. Nitrogen gases have been incriminated, and the disease has similarities to silo filler's disease caused by nitrogen dioxide (NO_2). However, calves and adult cattle that develop proliferative pneumonia frequently have not been exposed to silo gas or other environmental nitrogen gases. Other proposed etiologies include metabolites such as 3-methylindole (the cause of ABPE); Perilla ketone (*Perilla frutescens* or purple mint), which has been related to acute respiratory distress in cattle, sheep, rats, and mice and causes pneumotoxicity through preformed toxins absorbed from the rumen into the bloodstream; and moldy sweet potato toxicity, which is caused by 4-ipomeanol and related metabolites elaborated by the fungus *Fusarium solaria* from ipomeamarone and 4-hydroxymyoparone produced by the infected host potato. Once again, the 4-ipomeanol is pneumotoxic to Clara cells and alveolar epithelial cells after metabolic conversion by a cytochrome P450–dependent mixed function oxidase system.

The question remains—are all of these individual toxicities completely separate entities in cattle? It seems that the disease known as proliferative pneumonia may be a composite of these toxicities or may be caused by a yet-to-be-determined toxin common to the environment of dairy cattle.

Another form of pathologically confirmed proliferative pneumonia has been observed in dairy calves following previous infection with and recovery from *Pasteurella* or *Mannheimia* pneumonia. The disease occurs in a single animal among a group of calves affected by *Pasteurella* or *Mannheimia* pneumonia 2 to 4 weeks previously that had seemingly recovered. This single animal develops an acute severe respiratory distress syndrome with tachypnea, hyperpnea, elevated heart rate, open mouth breathing, fever (103.0 to 106.0° F/39.44 to 41.11° C), and pulmonary edema and may have an expiratory grunt. The animal is reluctant to move and may become cyanotic if stressed. The degree of respiratory effort makes it impossible to determine whether the pyrexia is caused by inflammation

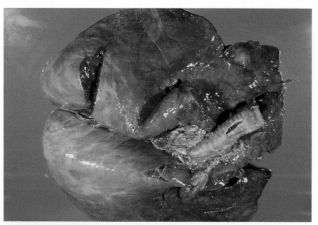

Figure 4-53

Necropsy specimen of lungs from a calf with acute proliferative pneumonia superimposed on resolving cranioventral bronchopneumonia. *(Photo courtesy Dr. John King.)*

or exertion. The lungs are very quiet on auscultation and have reduced sounds throughout all fields. If the previous pneumonia resulted in consolidation of anterior ventral lung lobes, bronchial tones may be heard ventrally and reduced sounds elsewhere. Usually both lungs are involved, but occasionally one lung has much more serious lesions. Unless treated quickly and intensively, the calf dies within 24 hours. Gross necropsy reveals diffusely heavy, wet, firm lungs with evidence of resolved or resolving anterior ventral pneumonia (Figure 4-53). Bacterial products resulting in a delayed hypersensitivity reaction are thought to be the cause of this problem. The 2- to 4-week interval between earlier signs of typical *Pasteurella/Mannheimia* pneumonia and subsequent acute proliferative pneumonia, as well as pathologic lesions, differentiate this syndrome from the "relapse" respiratory distress sometimes observed in BRSV infections. In addition, paired serum samples do not support BRSV as the cause.

Diagnosis and Treatment. Treatment of proliferative pneumonia is controversial because only lung biopsy or necropsy can confirm the clinical entity at hand. Lung biopsy via a Tru-Cut biopsy needle is a useful diagnostic step to aid diagnosis and treatment in valuable animals. Thoracic radiographs, if available, will demonstrate a diffuse pulmonary edema and mixed alveolar-interstitial pattern. Dr. King has recommended therapy with 1 g of atropine/1000 lb body weight daily IM or SQ. The mechanism of action is unknown, but in instances where endemic proliferative pneumonia has been confirmed by necropsy study, this therapy apparently has been beneficial to affected herdmates. When proliferative pneumonia is confirmed or strongly suspected, the following therapy is suggested:

Remove affected cattle from any source of toxic plants, nitrogen gases, or fumes; for example, if the only affected cows are confined near a silo chute or manure

pit, move them. Affected cattle should be moved only when their ventilation and environment need to be improved. Otherwise, any movement constitutes a severe stress.

Furosemide (0.5 to 1.0 mg/kg or 25 to 50 mg/100 lb body weight by injection once or twice daily) for the first 2 days of therapy if hydration status allows.

Atropine (0.048 mg/kg or 1/30 grain [2.2 mg] per 100 lb body weight twice daily).

Dexamethasone (10 to 20 mg once daily) for 3 days unless the affected cow is pregnant.

Broad-spectrum antibiotics for 5 to 7 days to protect against secondary bacterial pneumonia.

Respiratory Distress in Newborn Calves

Etiology, Pathophysiology, and Signs. This is a relatively common occurrence and may result from aspiration of meconium, congenital heart disease, white muscle disease, fetal lung pathology (e.g., herpes infection), or more commonly from dysmaturity/immaturity of the lung such as surfactant deficiency. It is especially common in premature, cloned, or in vitro fertilized calves (Figure 4-54). Some calves born as early as 6 weeks prematurely may have relatively normal pulmonary function, but this would be unusual. The abnormal compliance causes poor air exchange, hypoxia, pulmonary hypertension, and eventually right heart failure.

Diagnosis. Calves should develop a fairly normal respiratory pattern within the first hour after life, whereas newborn calves with respiratory distress syndrome (RDS) will have labored breathing that does not improve with time. There may be other signs of prematurity (e.g., small size, abnormally fine hair coat) in premature calves. Cloned calves may also have abnormally large umbilical vessels. Lung sounds are diffusely harsh and generally do not have rales. The heart rate will be high, but loud murmurs are usually absent unless the respiratory distress is caused by a congenital heart defect. An arterial sample

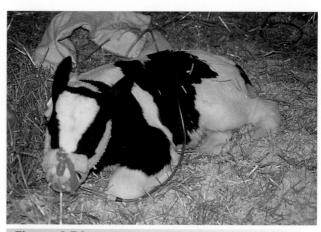

Figure 4-54

A newborn clone calf with hypoxemia being treated with intranasal oxygen.

can be collected from the brachial artery to confirm the severity of the hypoxemia. In some cases, the CO_2 will be elevated, and this can be confirmed by a venous sample (>45 mm Hg). If the CO_2 is elevated in a rapidly breathing calf, the PaO_2 will be extremely low. Pulse oximetry is useful in calves to confirm the hypoxemia and for monitoring therapy. A chest radiograph will reveal diffuse underinflation of the lung and parenchymal collapse. Some premature calves will have moderate to severe respiratory acidosis, hypercapnia, and hypoxemia but because of inappropriate/underdeveloped central responses will appear eupneic or only slightly tachypneic. Periodic assessment of preferably arterial blood gases, or at the very least venous blood pH and CO_2 tension, in the first day or two of life in premature calves is therefore recommended.

Treatment. Treatment must be early and vigorous if there is hope for survival. Vitamin E and selenium should be given IM. Intranasal oxygen must be administered and the calf given prophylactic antibiotics. One dose of corticosteroid (10 mg of dexamethasone) is often given and empirically does seem to help, especially following meconium aspiration. Although it is proven that corticosteroids given to cattle in the last 2 weeks of gestation improve lung function at birth in cesarean-derived calves, there is limited proof that postnatal-administered steroids will similarly accelerate lung maturation. It may be that postnatal-administered steroids, if they help at all, are inhibiting oxidative lung damage in the hypoxic calf. If surfactant is available, it should be given to the calf via intratracheal instillation via a tube, less commonly by direct injection, or it can be nebulized. Commercially prepared surfactant is preferred, but we have collected surfactant from healthy donor cows by bronchoalveolar lavage using 100 ml of sterile saline and then using the top (foamy) part of the collection for intratracheal administration or nebulization. We have also nebulized the affected calves with acetylcysteine while they were being administered an aminophylline drip. The aminophylline not only serves as a bronchodilator but also has antiinflammatory properties and helps maintain diaphragm strength. Fluids (crystalloids and colloids such as plasma) may be given IV as a continuous drip if needed. We have also administered thyrotropin releasing factor and/or thyroxin in hopes of increasing surfactant production. If pulmonary gas exchange cannot be sufficiently improved with the above and the owners request further treatment, the calf can be placed on a mechanical ventilator, but this is expensive. It is sometimes more difficult to keep calves quiet on a ventilator as compared with foals. Cloned calves with ascites and enlarged umbilical vessels seldom survive even when placed on the ventilator. Persistent pulmonary hypertension causes progression of right heart failure and sometimes reversion to fetal circulation patterns. Nitric oxide (ratio NO to oxygen = 1:9) can be administered through the oxygen line in hopes of decreasing the pulmonary hypertension (Figure 4-55). The

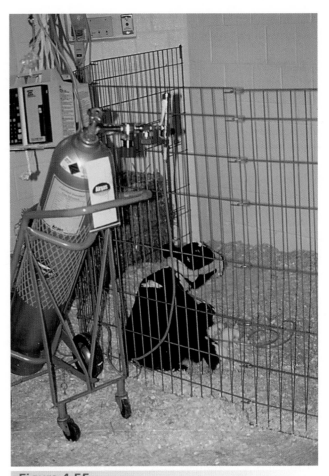

Figure 4-55

A 2-day-old calf with pulmonary hypertension receiving oxygen and nitric oxide.

chronic hypoxia results in acidosis and multiple organ failure.

Other Less Common Causes of Respiratory Distress

Silo Filler's Disease (Nitrogen Dioxide Poisoning)

Etiology and Signs. NO_2, a heavy yellow gas produced by anaerobic fermentation of fresh silage, may cause the same lower airway damage in cattle exposed to fumes as in humans. Because the gas is heavier than air, it lies on top of recently ensiled material—especially corn silage—and seeks out lower locations such as silo chutes. The major risk to farmers occurs when workers enter a silo chute or silo without first starting the blower in the silo loader to "wash out" NO_2. Cattle confined next to the silo chute are most at risk and may receive chronic low exposure toxicity or severe acute toxicity. Gaseous NO_2 seeks water that allows it to convert to nitric acid, which damages tissues. In the respiratory tract, nitric acid causes acute injury similar to anhydrous ammonia and subsequent obliterative bronchiolitis and interstitial fibrosis.

Affected cattle that have been chronically exposed to NO_2 have a chronic dry cough and increased respiratory rate greater than 40 breaths/min but few other symptoms. Cattle suffering acute severe exposure have a moist cough, more severe dyspnea (increased rate and effort), and pulmonary edema.

Diagnosis. Careful observation and history may be the key to diagnosis because the signs are nonspecific. Lung biopsy or necropsy is the only absolute means of diagnosis.

Treatment. Corticosteroids may be used judiciously in affected cattle. Cattle are very sensitive to dexamethasone, and 10 to 20 mg/day for several days would be appropriate therapy. Risk of secondary infection and abortifacient properties of dexamethasone need to be considered. Atropine and furosemide may also be indicated.

Farmer's Lung—Hypersensitivity Pneumonitis (Extrinsic Allergic Alveolitis)

Etiology and Signs. Hypersensitivity pneumonitis may occur in cattle and result in respiratory distress or chronic respiratory disease. In humans, many specific inhalant antigens may cause similar symptoms, but frequently *Micropolyspora faeni* and related organisms are incriminated. Wet hay that ferments excessively remains the biggest cause of this condition in farmers and cattle. The resultant dusty, moldy hay releases tremendous numbers of spores when bales are opened into the face of humans and animals. Large round bales also have been observed to cause the problem occasionally. A delayed hypersensitivity reaction is suspected.

Signs of acute experimental exposure include a sudden decrease in appetite and milk production, coughing, cranioventral pulmonary rales bilaterally, and transient fever. In natural cases, chronic cough without obvious illness remains the most common sign when this disease has been recognized in the northeastern United States. Usually more than 50% of the herd is affected, and herd production decreases 10% to 25% because affected cattle cough enough to interfere with normal consumption of feed. Auscultation of the lungs may reveal a few wheezes or may be normal. Signs lessen but do not stop entirely when animals are fed outdoors or go to pasture. Confinement and feeding the causative hay indoors accentuate the signs. Mortality is rare, but occasionally severe chronic cases have developed right heart failure. With the feeding of total mixed rations and the reduction in lifespan of dairy cattle in the United States, this disease has become less common. However, sporadic cases continue to be seen, not so much as a herd issue, but as an individual, older multiparous cow problem on traditional stanchion and tie stall farms.

Diagnosis. Diagnosis can be aided by history, observation, lack of profound illness in affected cattle, and high morbidity. Tracheal wash samples suggest lymphocytic inflammation with macrophages, lymphocytes, and some plasma cells. The serum of affected cattle may be analyzed for precipitins to *M. faeni* and other human antigens. When positive, this is suggestive but not definitive evidence because many normal cattle have positive antibodies.

Lung biopsy also may be a very helpful diagnostic aid if the value of the affected cow precludes necropsy. Necropsy inspection of the affected lungs reveals gray spots indicative of lymphocyte accumulations around small airways in the interstitium. Histopathology shows infiltration of lymphocytes and plasma cells in the interalveolar septa. Provocative testing utilizing the hay in question provides subjective causative evidence. Lungworms definitely should be ruled out by Baermann's technique, tracheal wash cytology, and necropsy, if necessary.

Treatment and Control. Because a large percentage of the herd may be affected, corticosteroids do not represent a wise treatment. Corticosteroids benefit acutely affected cattle or severe recurrent cases but cannot be used on a wide scale. Changes in management constitute both treatment and prevention. Feeding hay outside may give some relief, especially if the bales are opened several minutes or more before the cows being allowed access to the hay. Wetting the hay may be helpful. If economics allow, getting rid of the hay is the best policy and may solve the problem. Farmers who consistently make poor quality hay should be encouraged to consider haylage or at least including hay additives during harvesting that inhibit mold growth. Humans working with causative hay should consider the use of surgical masks or protective face masks to prevent symptoms of farmer's lung in themselves.

Bronchiolitis Obliterans

Etiology and Signs. This poorly described condition is observed occasionally in individual animals. A dry cough is the predominant sign in affected cattle, and Fox highlights the magnitude of the cough by quoting farmers who call only because the cow "coughs so hard she causes the milking machine to fall off." Auscultation of the lungs may reveal wheezes or abnormally quiet lung sounds. Although hyperpnea and tachypnea are present in addition to the dry cough, the affected cow does not otherwise appear ill.

The cause is unknown but probably involves chronic exposure to toxic gases, 3-methylindole, allergens, or other proposed causes of acute respiratory distress in cattle. The chronic damage that ensues may result in bronchiolitis obliterans—a pathologic diagnosis.

Diagnosis. Lung biopsy or histopathology following necropsy is required for definitive diagnosis.

Treatment. Dexamethasone often gives some relief to affected animals when administered judiciously at 10 to 20 mg/day. Appropriate contraindications should be considered.

Fibrosing Alveolitis

Etiology and Signs. This is a chronic debilitating respiratory disease of mature cattle. Affected cattle do not act ill but have an obvious increased respiratory rate and effort, as well as obvious coughing. Moist or dry rales may be ausculted over the entire lung field. Morbidity is low, but subsequent mortality is high because the disease is chronic and progressive.

The cause is unknown and may simply be the result of chronic exposure to some of the pneumotoxic materials previously discussed in this section. Chronic exposure to 3-methylindole, NO_2 or other gases, antigens known to cause hypersensitivity pneumonia, or unknown factors may result in diffuse fibrosis of the alveoli.

Diagnosis. Gross inspection of the lungs at necropsy reveals diffuse pale, heavy, firm lungs. The lobules are white and fleshy. Obliteration of alveolar air space by type 2 pneumocytes, macrophages, and other cells histopathologically explain the antemortem dyspnea. Lung biopsy is indicated if necropsy is not an option.

Treatment. No treatment is likely to be successful, but antiinflammatory drugs may be tried.

Anaphylaxis and Milk Allergy

Etiology and Signs. Respiratory distress often accompanies anaphylaxis induced by exogenous antigens such as vaccines, antibiotics, local anesthetics and feedstuffs, or endogenous antigens such as alpha-casein in milk.

In susceptible animals, signs usually develop within minutes following injection of biologics or antibiotics and consist of urticaria, edema of mucocutaneous junctions, and respiratory distress. Signs may be mild, with urticaria predominating, or severe, with collapse quickly following initial signs. Laryngeal edema may occur and be progressive over many hours. Certain biologics have been incriminated more than others in this regard. Antibiotic-induced anaphylaxis has been observed as a result of penicillin, tetracycline, sulfas, and other antibiotics. Penicillin may cause respiratory distress from a true anaphylaxis (usually hives accompany the respiratory distress) or as part of the procaine reaction. Biologics that cause an anaphylactic reaction in more than an occasional cow should be avoided unless suitable alternatives are not available. Many apparent anaphylactic crises may in fact be the result of endotoxins in certain biologics and cattle of certain genetic lines being more susceptible to such vaccine reactions.

Affected cattle appear apprehensive and restless, and their hair stands on end. The heart rate elevates, hives may develop, and frequent attempts to urinate and defecate may alternate with restless treading on the limbs. Dyspnea may be inapparent or obvious, with pulmonary edema, hyperpnea, and respiratory stertor. Cyanosis, cold clammy skin, and hypotensive collapse ensue in severe cases.

Milk allergy occurs most commonly in Channel Island breeds but may occur in any breed. The onset of signs may follow drying a cow off or a reduction in milking frequency to "bag" a cow for a show. Any delay in the normal milking interval may trigger this reaction in cattle sensitized to their own alpha-casein. The signs may be mild or severe as previously described. Hives, edema of mucocutaneous junctions, and respiratory signs develop to varying degrees.

A unique syndrome of collapse has been observed by many practitioners in cattle injected with concentrated vitamin E/selenium products. The reaction is observed within minutes of the IM injection, and collapse and dyspnea are the only signs. It is not known whether this represents anaphylaxis, accidental intravascular administration, or specific toxicity. Most cases recover, but fatal outcomes may appear in 10% to 20% of the cases.

Diagnosis. History and physical signs suffice for diagnosis.

Treatment. Treatment is commensurate with the severity of disease and consists of drugs such as epinephrine, antihistamines, corticosteroids, and furosemide. Recommended dosages for adult cattle include:

Epinephrine (1/1000 concentration), 2 to 10 ml IM or SQ; 2 to 4 ml can be given IV in severe cases

Tripelennamine HCl, 1 mg/kg IM or SQ

Furosemide, 0.5 to 1.0 mg/kg IM (if pulmonary edema is present)

Dexamethasone, 20 to 40 mg IV or IM if the cow is not pregnant

Flunixin meglumine, 1.1 mg/kg IM

For milk allergy, immediate milking out is indicated along with other symptomatic therapy (above) if the cow shows a serious allergic reaction.

In most cases, one treatment suffices, but in cattle with severe pulmonary edema or urticaria, several treatments at 8- to 12-hour intervals may be necessary for complete resolution.

SUGGESTED READINGS

Ahn BC, Walz PH, Kennedy GA, et al: Biotype, genotype, and clinical presentation associated with bovine viral diarrhea virus (BVDV) isolates from cattle, *Intern J Appl Res Vet Med* 3:319-325, 2005.

Antonis AF, Schrijver RS, Daus F, et al: Vaccine-induced immunopathology during bovine respiratory syncytial virus infection: exploring the parameters of pathogenesis, *J Virol* 77:12067-12073, 2003.

Aslan V, Maden M, Erganis O, et al: Clinical efficacy of florfenicol in the treatment of calf respiratory tract infections, *Vet Q* 24:35-39, 2002.

Autio T, Pohjanvirta T, Holopainen R, et al: Etiology of respiratory disease in non-vaccinated, non-medicated calves in rearing herds, *Vet Microbiol* 119:256-265, 2007.

Bednarek D, Kondracki M, Friton GM, et al: Effect of steroidal and non-steroidal anti-inflammatory drugs on inflammatory markers in calves with experimentally-induced bronchopneumonia, *Berl Munch Tierarztl Wochenschr* 118:305-308, 2005.

Bednarek D, Zdzisinska B, Kondracki M, et al: Effect of steroidal and non-steroidal anti-inflammatory drugs in combination with long-acting oxytetracycline on non-specific immunity of calves suffering from enzootic bronchopneumonia, *Vet Microbiol* 96:53-67, 2003.

Braun U, Pusterla N, Fluckiger M: Ultrasonographic findings in cattle with pleuropneumonia, *Vet Rec* 141:12-17, 1997.

Breeze R: Parasitic bronchitis and pneumonia, *Vet Clin North Am (Food Anim Pract)* 1:277-287, 1985.

Bryson DG, McNulty MS, McCracken RM, et al: Ultrastructural features of experimental parainfluenza type 3 virus pneumonia in calves, *J Comp Pathol* 93:397-414, 1983.

Carbonell PL: Bovine nasal granuloma—gross and microscopic lesions, *Vet Pathol* 16:60-73, 1979.

Confer AW, Fulton RW, Step DL, et al: Viral antigen distribution in the respiratory tract of cattle persistently infected with bovine viral diarrhea virus subtype 2a, *Vet Pathol* 42:192-199, 2005.

Cornish TE, van Olphen AL, Cavender JL, et al: Comparison of ear notch immunohistochemistry, ear notch antigen-capture ELISA, and buffy coat virus isolation for detection of calves persistently infected with bovine viral diarrhea virus, *J Vet Diagn Invest* 17:110-117, 2005.

Ducharme NG, Fubini SL, Rebhun WC, et al: Thoracotomy in adult cattle: 14 cases (1979–1991), *J Am Vet Med Assoc* 200:86-90, 1992.

Ellis J, Gow S, West K, et al: Response to calves to challenge exposure with virulent bovine respiratory syncytial virus following intranasal administration of vaccines formulated for parenteral administration, *J Am Vet Med Assoc* 230:233-243, 2007.

Ellis JA, West KH, Cortese VS, et al: Lesions and distribution of viral antigen following an experimental infection of young seronegative calves with virulent bovine virus diarrhea virus-type II, *Can J Vet Res* 62:161-169, 1998.

Ellis JA, West KH, Waldner C, et al: Efficacy of a saponin-adjuvanted inactivated respiratory syncytial virus vaccine in calves. *Can Vet J* 46:155-162, 2005.

Endsley JJ, Roth JA, Ridpath J, et al: Maternal antibody blocks humoral but not T cell responses to BVDV, *Biologicals* 31:123-125, 2003.

Ewers C, Lubke-Becker A, Wieler LH: Mannheimia haemolytica and the pathogenesis of enzootic bronchopneumonia [article in German], *Berl Munch Tierarztl Wochenschr* 117:97-115, 2004.

Fairbanks KK, Rinehart CL, Ohnesorge WC, et al: Evaluation of fetal protection against experimental infection with type 1 and type 2 bovine viral diarrhea virus after vaccination of the dam with a bivalent modified-live virus vaccine, *J Am Vet Med Assoc* 225:1898-1904, 2004.

Fingland RB, Rings DM, Vestweber JG: The etiology and surgical management of tracheal collapse in calves, *Vet Surg* 19:371-379, 1990.

Flock M: Diagnostic ultrasonography in cattle with thoracic disease, *Vet J* 167:272-280, 2004.

Francoz D, Fortin M, Fecteau G, et al: Determination of Mycoplasma bovis susceptibilities against six antimicrobial agents using the E test method, *Vet Microbiol* 105:57-64, 2005.

Fulton RW, Briggs RE, Ridpath JF, et al: Transmission of Bovine viral diarrhea virus 1b to susceptible and vaccinated calves by exposure to persistently infected calves, *Can J Vet Res* 69:161-169, 2005.

Fulton RW, Ridpath JF, Confer AW, et al: Bovine viral diarrhoea virus antigenic diversity: impact on disease and vaccination programmes, *Biologicals* 31:89-95, 2003.

Fulton RW, Ridpath JF, Saliki JT, et al: Bovine viral diarrhea virus (BVDV) 1b: predominant BVDV subtype in calves with respiratory disease, *Can J Vet Res* 66:181-190, 2002.

Fulton RW, Step DL, Ridpath JF, et al: Response of calves persistently infected with noncytopathic bovine viral diarrhea virus (BVDV) subtype 1b after vaccination with heterologous BVDV strains in modified live virus vaccines and Mannheimia haemolytica bacterin-toxoid, *Vaccine* 21:2980-2985, 2003.

Gevaert D: The importance of *Mycoplasma bovis* in bovine respiratory disease, *Tijdschr Diergeneeskd* 131:124-126, 2006.

Genicot B, Close R, Lindsey JK, et al: Pulmonary function changes induced by three regimens of bronchodilating agents in calves with acute respiratory distress syndrome, *Vet Rec* 137:183-186, 1995.

Grell SN, Ribert U, Tjornehoj K, et al: Age-dependent differences in cytokine and antibody responses after experimental RSV infection in a bovine model, *Vaccine* 23:3412-3423, 2005.

Guard CL, Rebhun WC, Perdrizet JA: Cranial tumors in aged cattle causing Horner's syndrome and exophthalmos, *Cornell Vet* 74:361-365, 1984.

Haines DM, Moline KM, Sargent RA, et al: Immunohistochemical study of Hemophilus somnus, Mycoplasma bovis, Mannheimia hemolytica, and bovine viral diarrhea virus in death losses due to myocarditis in feedlot cattle, *Can Vet J* 45:231-234, 2004.

Hasokusuz M, Lathrop SL, Gadfield KL, et al: Isolation of bovine respiratory coronaviruses from feedlot cattle and comparison of their biological and antigenic properties with bovine enteric coronaviruses, *Am J Vet Res* 60:1227-1233, 1999.

Hill JR, Roussel AJ, Cibelli JB, et al: Clinical and pathologic features of cloned transgenic calves and fetuses (13 case studies), *Theriogenology* 51:1451-1465, 1999.

Jolly S, Detilleux J, Desmecht D: Extensive mast cell degranulation in bovine respiratory syncytial virus-associated paroxystic respiratory distress syndrome, *Vet Immunol Immunopathol* 97:125-136, 2004.

Kadota K, Ito K, Kamikawa S: Ultrastructure and origin of adenocarcinomas detected in the lungs of three cows, *J Comp Pathol* 96:407-414, 1986.

Kelling CL: Evolution of bovine viral diarrhea virus vaccines, *Vet Clin North Am Food Anim Pract* 20:115-129, 2004.

Khodakaram-Tafti A, Lopez A: Immunohistopathological findings in the lungs of calves naturally infected with Mycoplasma bovis, *J Vet Med A Physiol Pathol Clin Med* 51:10-14, 2004.

Krahwinkel DJ Jr, Schmeitzel LP, Fadok VA, et al: Familial allergic rhinitis in cattle, *J Am Vet Med Assoc* 192:1593-1596, 1988.

Lathrop SL, Wittum TE, Brock KV, et al: Association between infection of the respiratory tract attributable to bovine coronavirus and health and growth performance of cattle in feedlots, *Am J Vet Res* 61:1062-1066, 2000.

Lathrop SL, Wittum TE, Loerch SC, et al: Antibody titers against bovine coronavirus and shedding of the virus via the respiratory tract in feedlot cattle, *Am J Vet Res* 61:1057-1061, 2000.

Lee WD, Flynn AN, LeBlanc JM, et al: Tilmicosin-induced bovine neutrophil apoptosis is cell-specific and downregulates spontaneous LTB4 synthesis without increasing Fas expression, *Vet Res* 35:213-224, 2004.

Leite F, Atapattu D, Kuckleburg C, et al: Incubation of bovine PMNs with conditioned medium from BHV-1 infected peripheral blood mononuclear cells increases their susceptibility to Mannheimia haemolytica leukotoxin, *Vet Immunol Immunopathol* 103:187-193, 2005.

Leite F, Kuckleburg C, Atapattu D, et al: BHV-1 infection and inflammatory cytokines amplify the interaction of Mannheimia haemolytica leukotoxin with bovine peripheral blood mononuclear cells in vitro, *Vet Immunol Immunopathol* 99:193-202, 2004.

Lockwood PW, Johnson JC, Katz TL: Clinical efficacy of flunixin, carprofen and ketoprofen as adjuncts to the antibacterial treatment of bovine respiratory disease, *Vet Rec* 152:392-394, 2003.

Loneragan GH, Gould DH, Mason GL, et al: Involvement of microbial respiratory pathogens in acute interstitial pneumonia in feedlot cattle, *Am J Vet Res* 62:1519-1524, 2001.

Mawhinney IC, Burrows MR: Protection against bovine respiratory syncytial virus challenge following a single dose of vaccine in young calves with maternal antibody, *Vet Rec* 156:139-143, 2005.

Mevius DJ, Hartman EG: In vitro activity of 12 antibiotics used in veterinary medicine against Mannheimia haemolytica and Pasteurella multocida isolated from calves in the Netherlands [in Dutch], *Tijdschr Diergeneeskd* 125:147-152, 2000.

Migaki G, Helmboldt CF, Robinson FR: Primary pulmonary tumors of epithelial origin in cattle, *Am J Vet Res* 35:1397-1400, 1974.

Morrow DA: Pneumonia in cattle due to migrating *Ascaris*, *Am Vet Med Assoc* 153:184-189, 1968.

Nicholas RA: Recent developments in the diagnosis and control of Mycoplasma infections in cattle. Proceedings of the 23rd World Buiatrics Congress, Quebec City, Canada, 2004.

Nowakowski MA, Inskeep PB, Risk JE, et al: Pharmacokinetics and lung tissue concentrations of tulathromycin, a new triamilide antibiotic, in cattle, *Vet Ther* 5:60-74, 2004.

Okada Y, Ochiai K, Osaki K, et al: Bronchiolar-alveolar carcinoma in a cow, *J Comp Pathol* 118:69-74, 1998.

Patel JR: Evaluation of a quadrivalent inactivated vaccine for the protection of cattle against diseases due to common viral infections, *J S Afr Vet Assoc* 75:137-146, 2004.

Patel JR, Didlick SA: Evaluation of efficacy of an inactivated vaccine against bovine respiratory syncytial virus in calves with maternal antibodies, *Am J Vet Res* 65:417-421, 2004.

Peek SE, Slack JA, McGuirk SM: Management of pneumothorax in cattle by continuous-flow evacuation, *J Vet Intern Med* 17:119-122, 2003.

Peters AR, Thevasagayam SJ, Wiseman A, et al: Duration of immunity of a quadrivalent vaccine against respiratory diseases caused by BHV-1, PI3V, BVDV, and BRSV in experimentally infected calves, *Prev Vet Med* 66:63-77, 2004.

Platt R, Burdett W, Roth JA: Induction of antigen-specific T-cell subset activation to bovine respiratory disease viruses by a modified-liver virus vaccine, *Am J Vet Res* 67(7):1179-1184, 2006.

Powers JG, Van Metre DC, Collins JK, et al: Evaluation of ovine herpesvirus type 2 infections, as detected by competitive inhibition ELISA and polymerase chain reaction assay, in dairy cattle without clinical signs of malignant catarrhal fever, *J Am Vet Med Assoc* 227:606-611, 2005.

Rebhun WC, King JM, Hillman RB: Atypical actinobacillosis granulomas in cattle, *Cornell Vet* 78:125-130, 1988.

Rebhun WC, Rendano VT, Dill SG, et al: Caudal vena caval thrombosis in four cattle with acute dyspnea, *J Am Vet Med Assoc* 176:1366-1369, 1980.

Rebhun WC, Smith JS, Post JE, et al: An outbreak of the conjunctival form of infectious bovine rhinotracheitis, *Cornell Vet* 68:297-307, 1978.

Rings DM: Tracheal collapse, *Vet Clin North Am Food Anim Pract* 11:171-175, 1995.

Ross MW, Richardson DW, Hackett RP, et al: Nasal obstruction caused by cystic nasal conchae in cattle, *J Am Vet Med Assoc* 188:857-860, 1986.

Roussel AJ, Hill JR, Hooper RN: Clone calves: medical challenges. Proceedings of the 23rd World Buiatrics Congress, Quebec City, Canada, 2004.

Shahriar FM, Clark EG, Janzen E, et al: Coinfection with bovine viral diarrhea virus and Mycoplasma bovis in feedlot cattle with chronic pneumonia, *Can Vet J* 43:863-868, 2002.

Shin SJ, Kang SG, Nabin R, et al: Evaluation of the antimicrobial activity of florfenicol against bacteria isolated from bovine and porcine respiratory disease, *Vet Microbiol* 106:73-77, 2005.

Slack JA, Thomas CB, Peek SF: Pneumothorax in dairy cattle: 30 cases (1990-2003), *J Am Vet Med Assoc* 225:732-735, 2004.

Smith DF: Branchial cyst in a heifer, *J Am Vet Med Assoc* 171:64-66, 1978.

Stipkovits L, Ripley P, Varga J, et al: Clinical study of the disease of calves associated with Mycoplasma bovis infection, *Acta Vet Hung* 48:387-395, 2000.

Stoffregen B, Bolin SR, Ridpath JF, et al: Morphologic lesions in type 2 BVDV infections experimentally induced by strain BVDV2-1373 recovered from a field case, *Vet Microbiol* 77:157-162, 2000.

Storz J, Purdy CW, Lin X, et al: Isolation of respiratory bovine coronavirus, other cytocidal viruses, and Pasteurella spp from cattle involved in two natural outbreaks of shipping fever, *J Am Vet Med Assoc* 216:1599-1604, 2000.

Sustronck B, Deprez P, Muylle E, et al: Evaluation of the nebulisation of sodium ceftiofur in the treatment of experimental Pasteurella haemolytica bronchopneumonia in calves, *Res Vet Sci* 59:267-271, 1995.

Taylor G, Bruce C, Barbet AF, et al: DNA vaccination against respiratory syncytial virus in young calves, *Vaccine* 23:1242-1250, 2005.

Thomas A, Nicolas C, Dizier I, et al: Antibiotic susceptibilities of recent isolates of Mycoplasma bovis in Belgium, *Vet Rec* 153:428-431, 2003.

Vangeel I, Antonis AF, Fluess M, et al: Efficacy of a modified live intranasal bovine respiratory syncytial virus vaccine in 3-week-old calves experimentally challenged with BRSV, *Vet J* 2006 (Epub ahead of print).

Vestweber JG: Respiratory problems of newborn calves, *Vet Clin North Am Food Anim Pract* 13:411-424, 1997.

Welsh RD, Dye LB, Payton ME, et al: Isolation and antimicrobial susceptibilities of bacterial pathogens from bovine pneumonia: 1994-2002, *J Vet Diagn Invest* 16:426-431, 2004.

Woolums AR, Anderson ML, Gunther RA, et al: Evaluation of severe disease induced by aerosol inoculation of calves with bovine respiratory syncytial virus, *Am J Vet Res* 60:473-480, 1999.

Woolums AR, Brown CC, Brown JC Jr, et al: Effects of a single intranasal dose of modified-live bovine respiratory syncytial virus vaccine on resistance to subsequent viral challenge in calves, *Am J Vet Res* 65:363-372, 2004.

Woolums AR, Gunther RA, McArthur-Vaughan K, et al: Cytotoxic T lymphocyte activity and cytokine expression in calves vaccinated with formalin-inactivated bovine respiratory syncytial virus prior to challenge, *Comp Immunol Microbiol Infect Dis* 27:57-74, 2004.

Zaremba W, Grunert E, Aurich JE: Prophylaxis of respiratory distress syndrome in premature calves by administration of dexamethasone or a prostaglandin F2 alpha analogue to their dams before parturition, *Am J Vet Res* 58:404-407, 1997.

Zecchinon L, Fett T, Desmecht D: How Mannheimia haemolytica defeats host defence through a kiss of death mechanism, *Vet Res* 36:133-156, 2005.

CHAPTER 5

Noninfectious Diseases of the Gastrointestinal Tract

Susan Fubini and Thomas J. Divers

DISEASES OF THE FORESTOMACH

Simple Acute Indigestion

Etiology

The term indigestion is used to describe a wide spectrum of clinical syndromes in cattle that range from simple intestinal inflammation to more severe disease forms and finally to lactic acidosis. The rumen is most commonly affected, followed by the small intestine. These two gastrointestinal site disturbances can occur together or independently. Cecal indigestion may be part of the cecal tympany syndrome; this is discussed later. Individual animals, or a few animals (if it is ruminal indigestion), can be affected at any one time. They may be at any stage of lactation, although indigestion seems to be more common in cows in the first weeks following parturition. The diagnosis of ruminal or small intestinal indigestion is made by using a combination of history, clinical signs, abdominal ultrasound (for small intestinal indigestion), rumen fluid analysis (activity and concentration of large and small protozoa are reduced, and new methylene blue reduction is increased), and ruling out other diseases through a complete physical examination.

Clinical Signs

Simple ruminal indigestion results in signs of anorexia, decreased milk production, cold extremities, and rumen dysfunction. Colic is common if there is small intestinal indigestion (Figure 5-1). Although rumen stasis or hypoactivity is typical, some cattle have increased rumen contraction rates but decreased strength of contractions. The cow's temperature, pulse rate, and respiratory rates are often normal with ruminal digestion, but tachycardia and tachypnea may develop in cows especially with small intestinal indigestion associated with colic. Abdominal distention may be present because of mild rumen distention, or gas and fluid distention may be present in the right lower quadrant, representing small intestinal distention. In small intestinal indigestion, enough fluid and

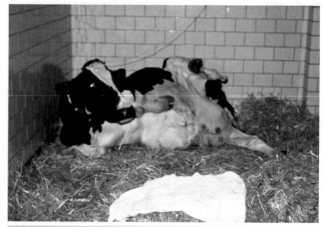

Figure 5-1

Severe abdominal pain in a Holstein cow caused by small intestinal indigestion and bowel distention. The cow developed diarrhea a couple of hours later and was normal the next day.

gas can accumulate in the small bowel to put severe tension on the mesentery, resulting in signs of colic such as kicking at the belly, bellowing, violent behavior, getting up and down repeatedly, and treading with the hind feet. In fact, this form of indigestion may be the most common cause of true colic in the dairy cow. Colic resulting from small intestinal indigestion can be difficult to differentiate from a mechanical small bowel obstruction. Extremely distended loops of small intestine, fibrin or crepitus on rectal examination, blood in the stool, or deterioration in cardiovascular signs all suggest a physical obstruction rather than simple indigestion. On abdominal ultrasound examination, fluid-filled and dilated loops of small intestine are typical of indigestion and obstruction, with hypomotility being most severe with prolonged physical obstruction and/or strangulation (Figure 5-2). The fluid responsible for small bowel distention results from stasis associated with indigestion and quickly appears as diarrhea as the cow responds to therapy or self-initiates gastrointestinal

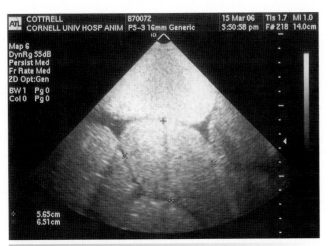

Figure 5-2
Ultrasound of the abdomen of the cow demonstrating small intestinal distention.

activity. Potential lameness sequelae including laminitis, sole ulcers, and toe abscesses may be observed in some cases 2 to 6 weeks after a rumen indigestion episode.

Ancillary Data

Laboratory data are seldom helpful in establishing an absolute diagnosis of simple indigestion. Hypocalcemia is the only biochemical abnormality anticipated with mild ruminal indigestion. Hypocalcemia and hypochloremia are common with small intestinal indigestion.

Treatment

Treatment for simple indigestion follows the two major principles suggested by Udall:
1. Reestablish normal gastrointestinal motility and establish normal flora
2. Evacuate the gastrointestinal tract with the intent of eliminating a causative agent

These two goals are accomplished by administration of oral laxative-ruminotoric mixtures and calcium solutions parenterally. Many laxative-antacid-ruminotoric mixtures are available, and each practitioner has a favorite. If the rumen has some activity, boluses of these mixtures may be acceptable, but the powdered form of these products should be mixed with warm water and administered through a stomach tube to ensure distribution of the product if rumen activity is severely depressed. In cases with ruminal tympany, a stomach tube should be passed routinely to relieve gas distention before administering treatment. Excessive treatment with alkalinizing products should be avoided because these can result in hypermagnesemia and metabolic alkalosis, which will further decrease ionized calcium. Calcium solutions are administered for all cases of simple indigestion because inappetence and gastrointestinal stasis coupled with calcium loss resulting from continued,

albeit reduced, milk production often leads to hypocalcemia. This hypocalcemia results in the clinical signs of cool peripheral parts and contributes to the already existing gastrointestinal stasis. For simple indigestion cases, 500 ml of calcium borogluconate intravenously (IV) or divided into four subcutaneous (SQ) locations is administered. Magnesium products (sulfate, oxide, or hydroxide) are commonly used as cathartics and/or alkalinizing products; in dehydrated cattle with low urine production, these may cause hypermagnesemia and clinical weakness when used excessively or repeatedly. Cows that demonstrate severe colic associated with small intestinal indigestion may require treatment with flunixin meglumine. Following treatment, a cow with small intestine indigestion should regain normal appetite and pass large amounts of loose manure within 12 to 24 hours. The patient's feces tend to remain watery or looser than normal for 2 to 3 days. Laxative therapy should be continued on a reducing dose basis for 2 to 3 days to ensure complete evacuation of causative feed material from the rumen. Although the diagnosis of simple indigestion often seems like an "excuse diagnosis" in a cow that is off feed and down on milk, the entity does exist, and the veterinarian should not hesitate to make this diagnosis if other diseases have been eliminated through careful examination. An important differential diagnosis is primary ketosis, and this should be ruled out by testing for urinary ketones. The two disorders also may coexist in some recently fresh cattle.

Moderate to Severe Acute Ruminal Indigestion

Etiology

More severe forms of ruminal indigestion may closely approximate lactic acidosis (lactic acid indigestion, toxic indigestion) and are difficult to categorize. There is a range of clinical signs possible, depending on the quantity and type of feed material ingested by the cow. A history of overingestion of grain or grain silage may exist. Although uncommon in modern dairy management feeding, bolus concentrate has historically been a common prelude to ruminal acidosis in cows (especially first calf heifers). A less common history would be that the cow had access to an apple orchard where large numbers of apples dropped from trees after a storm. Thus in cases of severe indigestion, the ingested material often is known as opposed to the usual case of simple indigestion, in which the causative feed material may not be known.

Clinical Signs

Signs of moderate to severe indigestion include a dramatic decrease in appetite and milk production, complete gastrointestinal stasis, cool peripheral parts, normal or subnormal rectal temperature, and normal or elevated heart and respiratory rates. Some affected cows are hypocalcemic enough to be recumbent and unable to rise. It should be emphasized that these cows have more severe signs than simple indigestion cases, including splashy rumen, dehydration, and tachycardia. As with any form of indigestion, clinical signs of lameness (laminitis) may occur 2 to 6 weeks later.

Ancillary Data
Hypocalcemia is a consistent finding, and acid-base-electrolyte values vary depending on the degree of lactic acidosis. Azotemia may be present.

Treatment
Treatment is similar to that described for simple indigestion, but slow IV or SQ administration of calcium solutions may be needed for recumbent cattle. Because rumen stasis is more severe, powdered ruminotoric-laxative-antacid products dissolved in water and 1 lb of activated charcoal administered through a stomach tube are recommended. If rumen fluid is readily regurgitated via the tube, rumen lavage would be indicated. If signs of severe indigestion occur within hours of known overingestion of rapidly fermentable feed material, a rumenotomy may be elected if, in the veterinarian's judgment, potential for lactic acidosis exists. This is a very difficult decision to make because medical therapy often will suffice and no clear-cut rules exist as to how much of any feed material constitutes a potentially lethal dose. Response to therapy should be gradual over 24 to 48 hours, and treatment may need to be repeated at 24-hour intervals. As gastrointestinal motility returns, loose manure usually is observed. Milk production may be slow to return to previous levels because of the precipitous decrease that occurs with this form of indigestion.

Fulminant Acute Lactic Rumen Acidosis

Etiology
Lactic acidosis (also called toxic indigestion, grain overload, rumen overload, and acute carbohydrate engorgement of ruminants) represents the most severe form of indigestion and is associated with overingestion of rapidly fermentable concentrate feed or the sudden change to a diet containing higher levels of finely ground rapidly fermentable feeds such as corn or wheat. Clinical examples of this may occur in feedlots where feeder steers are introduced to total concentrate diets rather than being gradually changed from high roughage to high concentrate feeds. Fortunately this is less often a herd problem in dairy cattle, but it has occurred when owners who have run out of one type of feed quickly change to another. For example, owners have switched cattle from pelleted grains containing some fiber to finely ground corn or wheat

grains and thus induced lactic acidosis. Sudden introduction of highly fermentable small grain silage into the herd can also result in lactic acidosis. Another problem that can lead to lactic acidosis in modern dairy management systems is improper mixing of total mixed rations (TMRs). In these cases, equipment failure or human error can lead to stratification of feedstuffs used in the TMR, and cows at one end of the feed line receive mostly roughage, whereas those at the other end receive mostly concentrate. Cattle that accidentally overeat grain by gaining access to the grain room or by getting loose and eating from a grain bin also may develop lactic acidosis. Both volume and type of concentrate are important, but even a few pounds of a finely ground concentrate such as barley may constitute a dangerous quantity if the cow's rumen flora is unfamiliar with the material. Because management factors often are involved, multiple animals in the herd tend to show signs. A basic understanding of the pathophysiology of lactic acidosis is essential for one to understand the signs that occur and be able to institute rational therapy. Within 6 hours of ingestion, the easily fermentable concentrate is broken down to lactic acid of both the D and L forms. Most of this occurs in the rumen, although substantial production of lactic acid may also occur in the lower gastrointestinal tract. The L isomer can be utilized rapidly, whereas the D isomer persists and results in D-lactic acidosis. *Streptococcus bovis* is the primary organism responsible for this conversion. As more and more lactic acid and volatile fatty acids are produced, the pH of the rumen contents decreases into the acid range. If sufficient substrate is available, the rumen pH may decrease to 4.5 to 5.0, at which time microbes other than *S. bovis* have been destroyed. Rumen stasis results. *S. bovis* continues to exist at this low pH and produces more lactic acid. Rapid accumulation of lactic acid in the rumen osmotically draws water into the rumen, causing the cow to dehydrate. In addition, the chemical or acid rumenitis damages the rumen mucosa, allowing plasma transudation into the rumen and endotoxin and escape of bacteria into the portal circulation.

Clinical Signs
Affected cattle are completely off feed, exhibit drastically decreased milk production, are dehydrated, and have elevated heart (90 to 120 beats/min) and respiratory rates (50 to 80 breaths/min). They typically have a splashy, totally static rumen, cool skin surface, subnormal temperature, and diarrhea or loose manure. Affected animals are weak and can be recumbent (Figure 5-3). Because of dehydration, titration of bicarbonate, hypotension, and high levels of lactic acid in the rumen and the blood, severely affected cattle have metabolic acidosis.

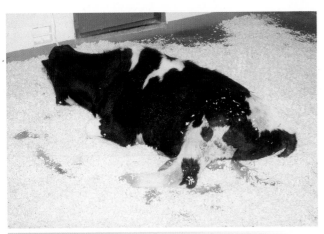

Figure 5-3

A Holstein steer with severe ruminal acidosis after eating recently ensiled oat silage. This steer, one of three affected, was unable to stand, severely dehydrated, obtunded, acidotic, and blind. This steer recovered after being treated with hypertonic saline and thiamine IV, draining rumen fluid via oral-rumen tube and administering 1 lb of activated charcoal intraruminally.

Ancillary Data and Diagnosis

Diagnosis of lactic acidosis is made by combining clinical signs with a detailed history of feeding in the herd. In acute cases, obtaining a rumen fluid sample through a stomach tube, percutaneous left flank puncture, or at necropsy examination of acute fatalities will reveal a rumen pH of 4.5 to 5.0. It must be emphasized that cattle with lactic acidosis that survive for 24 hours or more often have rumen pH values that increase to 6.5 to 7.0 because of the buffering effects of swallowed saliva and plasma dilution of the rumen contents. Other laboratory aids include acid-base and electrolyte values that tend to reflect a metabolic acidosis, a neutropenia with left shift in the hemogram, and marked azotemia. This is true even for fatal cases that survive 24 hours or more after ingestion of toxic quantities of grain. The systemic acidosis and acidemia are the result of increases in both D and L lactic acid. In some cases, the diarrhea or loose manure that is passed contains whole particles of the causative concentrate and may represent a clinical diagnostic clue.

Treatment

Treatment is difficult, and the veterinarian must decide whether medical therapy will suffice or a rumenotomy will be required. In addition, if signs have been present for 24 hours or more, the amount of rumen mucosal damage has already been determined and may not be affected by any treatment. When more than one cow is affected, the therapeutic difficulties multiply because the professional time commitment and expense of treatment are enormous.

Treatment must correct the rumen acidosis and attempt to discourage further lactic acid production. In an animal with a rumen pH of 5.0 or less, a heart rate greater than 100 beats/min, dehydration greater than 8%, and rumen distention and recumbency indicating a severe grain overload, a rumenotomy should be performed and the rumen contents evacuated. The rumen is then washed with water and emptied several times to remove as much lactic acid as possible. The cow is treated with laxatives, fresh hay in the rumen, rumen transfaunates if available, parenteral calcium, and IV fluid therapy. IV fluids should initially be hypertonic saline followed by balanced electrolyte solutions such as lactated Ringer's solution, and supplemental sodium bicarbonate is added if acidemia is severe (pH <7.15). Flunixin meglumine should be given (0.3 mg/kg every 8 hours) to combat excessive prostanoid production and shock. B vitamins should be administered for several reasons, one of which is that some cattle with ruminal acidosis develop polioencephalomalacia. The prognosis for severely affected cattle is poor. When such severe rumen acidosis affects a group of cattle or an individual animal of lesser economic value, the expense of treatment and the poor to grave prognosis that the condition carries for survival, let alone future production, should prompt at least consideration of salvage for slaughter.

Other treatments may be attempted for animals showing less severe signs and higher rumen pH values or when the number of animals affected precludes rumenotomies. One method involves passing a large-diameter stomach tube or Kingman tube and lavaging the rumen with warm water several times with the aid of a bilge pump. Several flushes with 10 to 20 gallons of water are necessary, and return flow of fluid must be effective for this treatment to be successful. Following lavage, antacid solutions such as 2 to 4 quarts of milk of magnesia, activated charcoal, and ruminotorics are administered, as well as supportive calcium solutions and IV fluids as indicated. Affected cattle should not be allowed to engorge on water because their atonic rumens will only distend again. Once rumen activity returns, free choice water may be made available. Another option that has been used successfully is to simply drain as much rumen fluid (Figure 5-4) as possible and administer 1 to 2 lb of activated charcoal into the rumen. This appears to be effective in binding rumen toxins (e.g., endotoxin). Additionally, affected cattle should receive SQ administered calcium solutions and IV administered isotonic fluids. Cows with moderate to severe rumenitis are generally treated with penicillin (10,000 to 20,000 IU/kg administered intramuscularly [IM] or SQ) in an effort to prevent bacteremia and liver abscess formation. Broad-spectrum antibiotics should not be used because these may predispose to fungal overgrowth.

Other treatments are empiric. They include antihistamines, penicillin solutions administered via a stomach

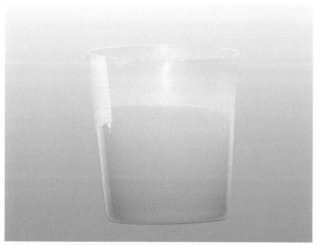

Figure 5-4

Sample of rumen fluid, pH 4.5, obtained from the steer in Figure 5-3.

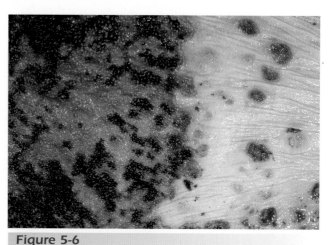

Figure 5-6

Mycotic rumenitis 7 days following acute lactic acidosis in a cow. The dark areas represent necrotic rumen mucosa that has sloughed in several focal areas to expose punched-out ulcerative lesions with red peripheries typical of mycotic rumenitis *(Courtesy John M. King, DVM.)*

tube in an effort to reduce the numbers of *S. bovis* organisms in the rumen, and roughage-only diets until the animals recover.

Cattle affected with lactic acidosis that survive the acute phase and have their rumen pH return to normal still are at risk for sequelae to the chemical rumenitis that has occurred. During the next several days, bacterial opportunists such as *Fusobacterium necrophorum* may invade the areas of chemical damage, attach to the rumen wall, and cause a bacterial rumenitis (Figure 5-5). If the animal lives 4 to 7 days or has been treated heavily with antibiotics or steroids, a mycotic rumenitis may occur in these previously damaged areas (Figure 5-6). Bacterial and mycotic opportunists invade the damaged rumen mucosa, ascend the portal circulation, and cause embolic infection of the liver, lungs, and other organs,

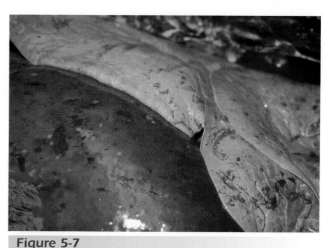

Figure 5-7

Embolic hepatitis and pneumonia secondary to lactic acidosis in a cow. The acute lactic acidosis occurred 7 days before these postmortem findings. The focal lesions in the liver and red areas in the lung represent bacterial and mycotic embolic lesions.

resulting in fever and, in severe cases, death (Figures 5-7 and 5-8). Fever resulting from mycotic infection generally is unresponsive to antibiotic therapy. Embolic infections of the brain may cause bizarre neurologic signs 7 to 14 days following the original clinical signs of lactic acidosis.

Subacute to Chronic Rumen Acidosis

This syndrome, also called subclinical ruminal acidosis (SARA), occurs more commonly in lactating cows than the previously discussed acute clinical syndromes of indigestion and/or ruminal acidosis and derives from modern feeding practices. In brief, feeding rapidly

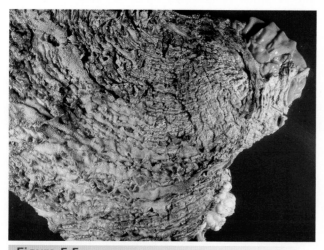

Figure 5-5

Chemical and bacterial destruction of the entire omasal mucosa as a result of lactic acidosis.

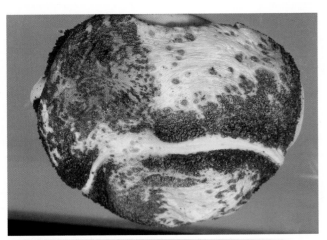

Figure 5-8

Widespread loss of rumen mucosa 2 weeks following acute grain overload. *(Courtesy John M. King, DVM.)*

fermentable concentrates and highly acid feeds allows a degree of rumen acidosis for a transient period after ingestion. During this period of acidosis, small areas of rumen mucosa are damaged by the same chemical mechanism that causes more widespread lesions in lactic acid indigestion. These small areas of rumenitis may act as entry points for opportunistic bacteria that subsequently ascend the portal circulation and result in liver abscesses. These may be single or multiple and, when located near the hilus of the liver, predispose the cow to caudal vena caval thrombosis syndrome. Dairy cattle seldom develop the "sawdust liver" or miliary liver abscesses of feeder beef animals despite the similar pathophysiology.

Subclinical rumen or relative acidosis also may be present on a continual rather than a transient basis in some feeding programs. In addition to liver abscesses and caudal vena caval thrombosis syndrome, these herds often have a high incidence of abomasal disease, indigestion, decreased or fluctuating dry matter intakes, diarrhea, decreased milk production, milk fat depression, and laminitis with subsequent lameness. Laminitis may result from release of various mediators, including endotoxins, from rumen microbes destroyed by pH decreases associated with subclinical rumen acidosis. Mediator absorption is enhanced by chemical damage to the rumen mucosa. When this syndrome is suspected, the veterinarian should collect rumen samples from several cows in the herd to analyze pH and rumen microflora. A pH less than 6.0 would be suspicious, although a normal pH does not rule out the disease because the pH will increase to normal following a period of anorexia! The other problem is in the collection of the sample because oral-ruminal collection is difficult and is often contaminated with saliva; rumenocentesis requires puncture of the rumen through the left flank. Additionally, commonly used pH paper is not accurate because the green

color of rumen fluid influences the interpretation. When sampling ruminal pH, practitioners should aim for the nadir in luminal pH; for component-fed herds, this is about 2 to 4 hours postfeeding, whereas in TMR-fed herds this point is reached about 6 to 8 hours postfeeding. In general, pH meters, appropriately maintained and calibrated before use, should be used whenever possible rather than pH paper for this purpose. Dr. Ken Nordlund at the University of Wisconsin has suggested that that a pH of less than 5.5 in 5 or more cows of a sample size of 12 should be used as an arbitrary cutoff point to define a herd problem with subacute rumen acidosis.

Correction or prevention requires natural or supplemental buffering of the diet, and a nutritional analysis should be performed to aid the dairy farmer, veterinarian, and any nutritional consultants in restructuring the diet to avoid relative acidosis. Sometimes this can be easily accomplished by feeding roughage before the concentrate to force natural buffering by saliva (i.e., that induced by roughage) that would precede the concentrate's entrance to the rumen. In other situations (e.g., where component feeding is still being practiced), a switch to a TMR may be indicated. However, the feeding of a TMR does not preclude the opportunity for subacute rumen acidosis. Each herd needs to be assessed and corrected on an individual basis, however, and generalities are not acceptable because feedstuffs, production levels, and management practices vary widely. Chronic indigestion of milk-fed calves is well described but will be discussed in the following section on bloat.

Ruminal Bloat

Bloat can be defined as obvious ruminal enlargement resulting in left-sided abdominal distention in both dorsal and ventral quadrants (Figure 5-9, *A* and *B*). When severe, bloat may cause generalized distention resulting from ventral sac enlargement into the right lower quadrant and crowding of the remaining abdominal viscera into the right dorsal quadrant. Causes of bloat may be divided into acute and chronic etiologies.

Acute Bloat

Etiology

Acute ruminal distention may be caused by either free gas or frothy ingesta. Acute free-gas bloats may occur in association with hypocalcemia and resulting ileus, esophageal obstructions or injuries, pharyngeal injuries that damage the vagal nerve roots controlling eructation, indigestion with tympany, and acute localized peritonitis with resultant ileus. Acute frothy bloat in dairy cattle almost always is associated with indigestion of unknown causes or sudden availability and over-ingestion of green forage such as succulent alfalfa.

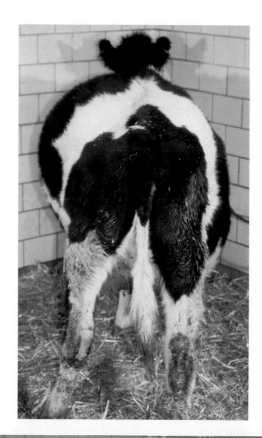

A

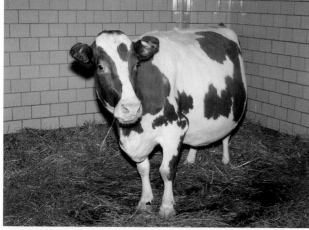

B

Figure 5-9

A, Ruminal tympany or bloat in a heifer. The left-sided distention is uniform and extends to the dorsal midline. **B,** Severe ruminal distention with ingesta in a cow with vagal indigestion caused by a perireticular abscess. A lack of respiratory distress, despite marked ruminal distention, is typical of ruminal distention caused by gas or nonfrothy ingesta.

Acute bloat can be classified into at least three categories determined by the physical properties causing the bloat:

1. Frothy bloat
   a. Frothy bloat results from stable froth of dietary origin that usually is higher in chloroplast membrane fragments and soluble protein. This type of bloat occurs with exposure to succulent legumes and clovers. Certain genetic strains of cattle may be more prone to frothy bloat than others. Show cows fed calf manna, a highly soluble protein feed, may also develop frothy bloat. Frothy bloat also occurs in some young calves with peritonitis or undetermined causes. This form of bloat is not relieved by a stomach tube.
2. Free-gas bloat
   a. Free-gas bloat occurs secondary to overingestion of grain, which promotes excessive volatile fatty acid production, lower pH, and then lactic acid buildup. This pathophysiology culminates in rumen stasis and free-gas bloat.
   b. Free-gas bloat results from mechanical, inflammatory, neurologic, or metabolic conditions that interfere with eructation or affect outflow (e.g., esophageal choke, vagal indigestion, hypocalcemia, listeriosis, or tetanus).
   c. Free-gas and sometimes fluid bloat occurs in calves following ruminal drinking of milk. This may occur within 30 minutes of milk feeding (usually by bucket), and the rumen fluid may have a putrid smell. Although the bloat is predominantly free gas, simultaneous ballottement and auscultation will produce a fluid "tinkling" in the left ventral quadrant associated with the inappropriately clotted milk. This is part of the clinical syndrome of chronic indigestion in milk-fed calves. In addition to ruminal bloat, calves may be depressed, have a poor appetite, be thin, weak, and have claylike feces.
3. Fluid and gas bloat
   a. Fluid and some gas bloat is seen acutely in calves with clostridial abomasitis-rumenitis and in cows with severe ruminal acidosis.

Clinical Signs

Clinical signs of acute bloat include a combination of acute onset, typical left-sided distention extending dorsally to the midline with a full paralumbar fossa, and rectal findings of ruminal distention extending into the right abdomen dorsally and ventrally. Dyspnea caused by increased abdominal pressure exerted on the diaphragm and thorax may be moderate to severe with acute frothy bloat.

Free-gas bloat causes a large gas ping on the left upper abdomen extending to the dorsal midline (Figure 5-10). In some cattle with free-gas bloat, an obvious ping may not be present. If a stomach tube can be passed easily and relieves the bloat, free-gas bloat is confirmed. Other physical signs and signalment data may allow a specific diagnosis of the cause of the bloat. For example, hypocalcemia may be considered if the cow is periparturient

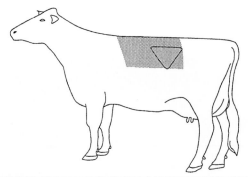

Figure 5-10

Left-sided pneumoperitoneum or rumen tympany.

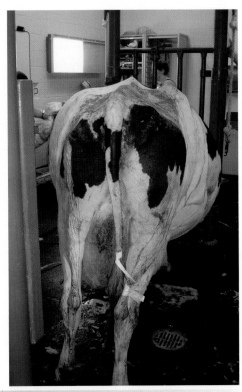

Figure 5-11

Severe abdominal distention and respiratory distress and hypovolemic shock caused by frothy bloat.

and shows signs of normal or subnormal temperature, cool peripheral parts, slow pupillary responses to direct light, recumbency, or weakness. Indigestion with tympany may cause few signs other than free-gas bloat, and signs other than free-gas bloat or signs referable to hypocalcemia mean other diseases must be ruled out. Animals with esophageal obstruction (choke), esophageal injury, or pharyngeal injury with perforation usually present with excessive salivation, an anxious expression, extended head and neck, bloat, and fever. Passage of a stomach tube would be impeded by a choke and be resisted by a cow with pharyngeal or esophageal injury. Frothy bloat is diagnosed based on the typical left-sided distention, less obvious pinging when simultaneous percussion and auscultation are performed, and failure to relieve the distention on passage of a stomach tube. The bloat may progress rapidly if it is frothy bloat, eventually distending both sides of the abdomen to its maximal limits (Figure 5-11) and causing respiratory distress, hypoxemia, poor venous return of blood to the heart, hypotension, and death.

Treatment

Treatment requires relief of the ruminal distention and correction of the primary cause. In instances of free-gas bloat caused by hypocalcemia, parenteral calcium therapy and passage of a stomach tube are required. Indigestion with tympany requires relief of the gas accumulation with a stomach tube and treatment with a parenteral calcium solution, as well as laxatives, antacids, and ruminotoric mixtures as necessary. In esophageal obstructions or choke, the obstruction must be relieved by gentle manual or mechanical manipulation. Localized peritonitis with secondary ruminal tympany must be treated with antibiotics, stall rest, and either a magnet, rumenotomy (for hardware), or dietary changes (perforating abomasal ulcers). If pharyngeal trauma is suspected, broad-spectrum antibiotics, gentle passage of a stomach tube, and analgesics may be indicated (see the section on Pharyngeal Trauma).

In cases of acute frothy bloat, passage of a stomach tube seldom produces dramatic relief of the rumen distention but does aid in diagnosis and allows treatment with surfactant agents such as Therabloat (poloxalene drench concentrate; SmithKline Beecham Animal Health, West Chester, PA) or vegetable oil to break down the froth. In some frothy bloats, a Kingman stomach tube may permit decompression, but this is not the rule, and in severe cases with thoracic compression, passage of the tube may, on rare occasion, cause acute death. Oral ruminotorics-laxative-antacid powders in warm water and parenteral calcium solutions also should be administered to encourage rumen emptying. Emergency rumenotomy (Figure 5-12) is the treatment of choice for progressive and severe frothy bloat. In a hospital environment, hypertonic saline administration, intranasal oxygen, and analgesics (flunixin) are helpful in stabilizing the cow during standing surgery.

Percutaneous rumen trocharization as a treatment for acute bloat of any cause is *contraindicated* in the dairy cow except in extreme cases when emergency decompression is necessary. Trocharization in the dairy cow ensures peritonitis, which may be fatal or may confuse the primary diagnosis by causing fever and signs referable to peritonitis—including bloat—over the following days.

Prevention of acute bloat is possible only when managerial changes have allowed ingestion of causative feedstuffs, including sudden availability to lush alfalfa pastures. Fortunately most dairy farmers are aware of

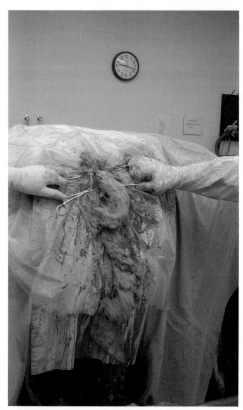

Figure 5-12

Frothy ingesta "exploding" from the rumenotomy site of the cow.

these dangers, and it seldom is necessary to educate owners concerning such hazards and appropriate preventative measures such as gradual introduction to succulent pasture, prefeeding with long-stem hay, pasture surfactant sprays, poloxalene salt blocks, or simple avoidance.

Chronic Bloat

Etiology

In calves, most cases of chronic bloat have a dietary or developmental etiology. Low fiber diets are the usual cause in calves fed only milk or milk replacers (Figure 5-13, *A* and *B*). Otherwise, these affected calves are healthy except for the free-gas bloat that develops shortly after eating. Calves that have been overtreated with oral antibiotics for systemic infections or diarrhea also may develop bloat associated with abnormal rumen flora. Calves affected with diarrhea and treated with methscopolamine or other parasympatholytic drugs may develop a paralytic ileus and subsequent bloat that persists for 24 to 72 hours after the administration of the drug. Although overdosage may have occurred, some calves develop bloat even after using the manufacturer's recommended dosages of methscopolamine.

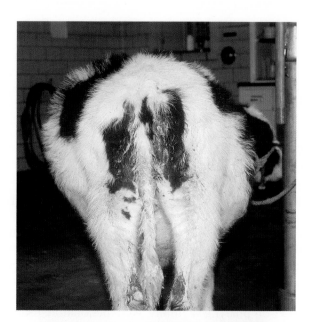

A

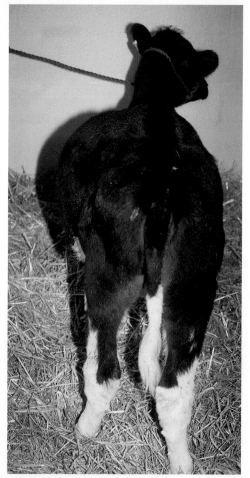

B

Figure 5-13

A, Chronic free-gas bloat in a calf on a low-fiber diet. **B,** Developmental free-gas bloat in an otherwise healthy calf.

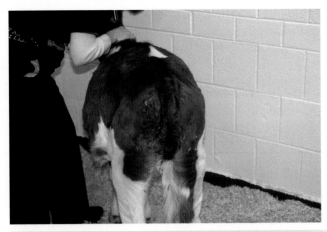

A

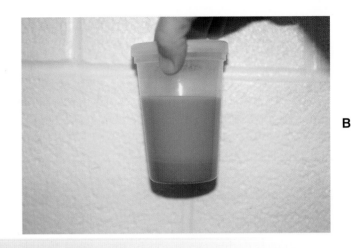

B

Figure 5-14

A, Acute ruminal bloat that occurred 1 hour after drinking milk replacer in a bucket. There had been several episodes of bloat in this calf, and its general condition and hair coat are adversely affected. **B,** Rumen ingesta collected from the calf.

Calves that have suffered severe bronchopneumonia occasionally develop free-gas bloat from damage to the thoracic portion of the vagal nerve or enlarged thoracic lymph nodes that cause failure of eructation. Left displacement of the abomasum (LDA) in calves may cause chronic or intermittent free-gas bloat, thereby confounding a diagnosis of LDA. Intermittent or chronic bloat associated with unthriftiness, inappetence, claylike feces, and abdominal distention occasionally occurs in 3- to 8-week-old dairy calves fed milk (mostly by bucket rather than bottle) (Figure 5-14, *A*). These calves are called "ruminal drinkers" because they have failure of the reticular groove reflex, thus causing milk to flow directly into the rumen rather than the abomasum. Ruminal parakeratosis and hyperkeratosis result in addition to metabolic and endocrine abnormalities. The calves may have excessive intestinal production of both D and L lactic acid and become severely acidotic from the D-lactic acid. The bloat may occur acutely within 1 hour after feeding but may also become chronic, and in some cases there may be enough milk putrefaction to cause the calf to become quite ill. Passage of a stomach tube may cause reflux of a gray fetid fluid (Figure 5-14, *B*).

Older calves that have been weaned off milk or milk replacers also may develop chronic free-gas bloat of dietary origin if fed a low fiber diet. Although this can occur on silage and grain diets, it is much more common in calves fed all-pelleted rations. Up to 10% or more of calves fed all-pelleted rations with no hay supplementation will develop chronic bloat that worsens shortly after they ingest pellets and then drink large quantities of water. Many other causes of chronic bloat also exist in postweaning calves but are more difficult to diagnose and treat. These include inherent tendencies of bloat as seen in dwarf animals and inherent defects in forestomach innervation or smooth muscle function. Other lesions such as abdominal abscess, umbilical or urachal adhesion, intestinal obstruction, LDA, focal peritonitis, and rarely abomasal impaction (Figure 5-15) may lead to chronic bloat as well.

Esophageal lesions also must be considered in the differential diagnosis of chronic bloat in the calf. These include pharyngeal and esophageal trauma induced by

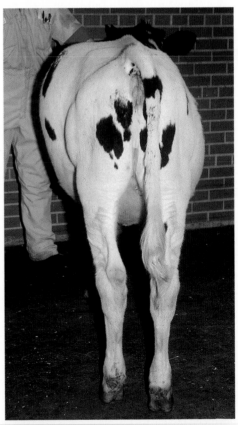

Figure 5-15

Abdominal distention characteristic of vagus indigestion in a calf with abomasal impaction.

balling guns, stomach tubes, or esophageal feeders. These lesions may damage the intricate vagal nerve branches responsible for eructation, swallowing, and forestomach motility. Esophageal motility disorders, although rare, should be considered as a cause of bloat in calves with a dilated esophagus. Thymic lymphosarcoma and enlarged mediastinal or pharyngeal lymph nodes resulting from the juvenile form of lymphosarcoma are the most common neoplastic causes of chronic bloat in calves. Diaphragmatic hernias are rare in dairy cattle but can result in acute or chronic rumen distention and bloat (Figure 5-16). Generally the reticulum is entrapped in the chest through the diaphragmatic rent. Signs include decreased cardiac and lung sounds and dullness during percussion in the ventral thorax (unilateral or bilateral), abdominal distention, bloat, vomiting, and dyspnea. Diaphragmatic hernias may be congenital or acquired as a result of trauma, parturition, or progressive weakening of the diaphragm adjacent to a hardware perforation and reticuloperitonitis.

Chronic bloat in adult cattle most often involves lesions of the vagal nerve. These lesions may occur anywhere from the brainstem to the pharynx to the abomasum. Causes similar to those described in calves may be involved, as can adult diseases such as listeriosis, hardware, reticular abscesses, liver abscesses, volvulus of the abomasum, abomasal impaction, advanced

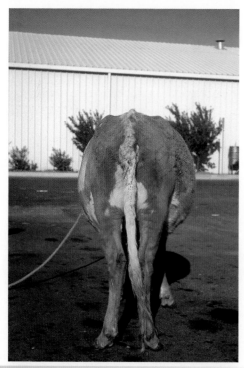

Figure 5-16

Chronic rumen bloat with ingesta and gas in a cow with a diaphragmatic hernia. The reticulum was believed to have been forced at calving through a congenital defect in the diaphragm.

pregnancy, and lymphosarcoma. These are discussed further in the section on Vagal Indigestion.

Forestomach neoplasms primarily include fibropapillomas of the distal esophagus or cardia and lymphosarcoma masses in the forestomach or abomasum. With fibropapillomas, a failure of eructation occurs because the tumor acts like a plug or one-way valve in the distal esophagus, thereby interfering with effective eructation. In lymphosarcoma and abomasal atony following correction of abomasal volvulus (AV), outflow disturbances with reflux of abomasal contents into the rumen, failure of eructation, or failure of motility all contribute to chronic rumen tympany. Rumen chloride content would be elevated (>51 mEq/dl) with abomasal reflux, and affected cows typically demonstrate moderate to severe hypochloremic, metabolic alkalosis on routine blood work.

Granulomatous lesions caused by *Actinobacillus lignieresii* and *Actinomyces bovis* may cause distal esophageal or reticular lesions that result in chronic bloat or indigestion. This is quite unusual, however.

Cattle with tetanus may have chronic (i.e., several days duration) bloat. In this instance, inability of the laryngeal, pharyngeal, and esophageal striated musculature to coordinate the intricate neuromuscular act of eructation because of tetany results in free-gas bloat. Bloat may also be observed in cows with listeriosis, botulism, or other neurological diseases.

In all cases of bloat, the veterinarian must confirm that the abdominal distention is caused by *ruminal* distention rather than pneumoperitoneum or LDA. In calves, simultaneous percussion and auscultation, ballottement, and abdominal palpation should differentiate abomasal, small intestinal, and cecal distention from that involving only the rumen. Observation, physical examination, and sometimes ultrasonography are extremely important in the calf because rectal examination is not possible. In adult cattle, rectal palpation coupled with other physical findings should easily confirm rumen distention.

The diagnosis of chronic bloat is confirmed by a combination of history and physical examination findings. Other causes of chronic abdominal distention such as ascites, displacement of the abomasum, cecal distention, and hydrops should be ruled out. In addition to abdominal auscultation and ballottement and rectal examination in cows, a stomach tube should be passed to determine whether the bloat is free gas or ingesta. Specific causes of chronic bloat should be sought through physical examination, ancillary data, and surgical exploration of the abdomen, if the value of the affected animal warrants this procedure.

Specific treatment depends on the specific cause of the chronic bloat. Because a portion of these cases involve lesions affecting the vagal nerve branches, treatment is discussed under Vagal Indigestion. Calves with unexplained chronic and/or intermittent free-gas bloat

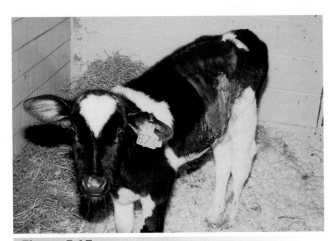

Figure 5-17

Surgically placed rumen fistula in a calf that had chronic free-gas bloat. The ingesta spilling down the side of the abdomen causes no problem.

are best treated by making a temporary rumen fistula (Figure 5-17). Calves with chronic or intermittent bloat and ill thrift because of ruminal drinking of milk can be weaned or fed via a bottle rather than a bucket. If they become acutely ill in association with feeding milk and bloat, an oral-rumen tube should be passed to drain as much fluid as possible from the rumen, and the calf should be treated with systemic antibiotics and fluids.

Chronic free-gas bloat in tetanus patients may be relieved by gentle passage of a stomach tube or preferably with a surgically prepared rumen fistula that provides continuous escape of gas and a portal through which to provide feed and water to the patient. The creation of a therapeutic fistula is an important aid to the successful treatment of tetanus cases because affected animals are typically unable to eructate or swallow, and repeated passage of a stomach tube significantly increases their anxiety and stress level.

Patients with free-gas bloat and ileus secondary to the administration of atropine or methscopolamine require passage of a stomach tube as frequently as necessary. These patients usually improve spontaneously 48 to 72 hours after the last administration of the offending drug.

Cows with ruminal bloat caused by abomasal outflow abnormalities causing reflux of abomasal content into the rumen generally have a poor prognosis.

Traumatic Reticuloperitonitis (Hardware Disease)

Etiology

Traumatic reticuloperitonitis after ingestion of metallic foreign bodies is one of the oldest diseases recognized in cattle but still occurs with alarming frequency under modern management. Unlike sheep and goats, cattle do not use their lips to discriminate between very fibrous feed and metallic objects in feedstuffs. Cattle also are given a great deal of chopped feed that may contain wire remnants, machinery parts, or other metallic debris.

Metallic foreign bodies, such as wire and nails, are the most common agents of hardware disease. In most cases, the wires range in length from 5.0 to 15.0 cm and tend to be slightly bent or have a crook at one end. Nails of all sizes also have been recovered from cattle with hardware disease as have, on occasion, hypodermic or blood collection needles. Many clinically normal cows will have metallic objects, sand, stones, fence staples, and some gravel in their reticulum. Such objects are ingested, drop into the rumen, and within 24 to 48 hours are propelled into the reticulum where they remain because of gravity or entanglement with the reticular mucosa. Nonperforating objects found frequently include nuts, bolts, washers, and short wire fragments (less than 2.5 cm). These objects may be found routinely on radiographic surveys or slaughterhouse specimens. Therefore exposure to metallic foreign bodies should be anticipated in dairy cattle. Although perforation may occur randomly at any time in a cow harboring a sharp metallic foreign body, physical factors may contribute to perforation and subsequent clinical signs. The prime example of such a physical factor contributing to perforation is advanced gestation and a heavily gravid uterus. During the last trimester, the combined weight and size of the gravid uterus may allow the organ to act like a pendulum as a cow gets up and down; this can apply physical pressure to the rumen and reticulum, contributing to perforation by an existing sharp metallic object. Clinical incidence of hardware disease in cattle in the last trimester of pregnancy is high enough to warrant inclusion of this disease in a differential diagnosis for any acute illness in heavily pregnant or dry cows. Diseases or conditions causing tenesmus or straining, such as parturition, also may cause increased abdominal pressure, possibly contributing to perforation.

Hardware disease usually occurs in heifers or cows older than 1 year of age. It is not known whether discrimination during prehension or absence of exposure to certain high-risk feedstuffs protects the animal during the first year of life.

In light of the likely exposure of most dairy cattle to metallic foreign bodies in feedstuffs, perhaps the greatest single factor in the causative development of hardware disease is failure to have administered a prophylactic magnet to the animal at 12 to 18 months of age. This should be considered a mandatory component of preventative herd health.

Signs

Once a metallic foreign body perforates the reticular wall, clinical signs develop. These signs are extremely variable and influenced by the anatomic region of perforation within the reticulum, depth of perforation, associated abdominal or thoracic viscera injury by the perforating object, physical features of the causative object, and the affected cow's stage of gestation or lactation.

Classic hardware disease causing acute localized reticuloperitonitis results in a sudden, dramatic, and often complete anorexia and cessation of milk production. Milk production may decrease to near zero within 12 hours and prompt the owner to seek veterinary attention for the cow. Affected cattle may have fever (103.0 to 105.0° F/39.44 to 40.56° C), normal to mildly elevated heart and respiratory rates, abducted elbows, an anxious expression, an arched stance (Figure 5-18), hypomotile rumen with or without mild tympany, scant dry feces, and abdominal pain localized in the cranial ventral abdomen near the xiphoid. When examined within 24 hours of onset, classic cases as described are relatively easy to diagnose. Many clinical cases show more variable signs (e.g., some cows stand up more than normal, whereas others lie down more than normal) and represent more difficult diagnostic challenges. In some cases, vague signs of partial anorexia, decreased milk production, and changing fecal consistency may be observed by the owner and may have been present for some time before veterinary attention is sought. Physical examination may reveal little beyond ruminal hypomotility or mild tympany suggestive of localized peritonitis, and cranial abdominal pain. In some mild cases, careful auscultation and observation may reveal treading with the hind feet because of the pain associated with localized peritonitis during ruminoreticular contraction. Affected cattle with less obvious signs may "grunt" or grind their teeth while being "poked" by a metallic foreign body embedded in the reticular mucosa or submucosa, or one that has penetrated full thickness and continues to cause pain intermittently. Occasionally cattle affected with hardware disease will "vomit" or regurgitate more material than

they can retain as a cud. This represents a neurogenic or pressure-related triggering of the regurgitation reflex from reticular irritation. In these less obvious cases, careful physical examination and attention to detail when assessing abdominal pain are important keys to the diagnosis.

An important point concerning patients with hardware disease is that the body temperature may be normal. This statement is in direct conflict with textbook descriptions of the disease and seems difficult to explain in light of the obvious peritonitis that exists in these patients. In a review of the case records from more than 200 cattle confirmed by surgery or necropsy to be affected with hardware disease, the body temperature was normal in more than half of these patients. This may relate to the subacute or chronic nature of the disease in these referral patients, or they may have had an initial fever spike after the acute perforation that was not recorded. The fact remains that the veterinarian may not be called to attend a hardware disease case during the acute phase, and hardware disease *should not* be ruled out by finding a normal rectal temperature.

Cattle affected with chronic localized peritonitis have signs of weight loss, poor hair coat, intermittent anorexia, decreased milk production, change in manure consistency, and rumen dysfunction with or without mild tympany. Such cows may have an arched stance and detectable abdominal pain as well.

Cattle affected with traumatic reticuloperitonitis that results in a diffuse peritonitis have much more severe signs than those affected with localized peritonitis. Cattle developing diffuse peritonitis resulting from hardware disease have fever, elevated heart rates (90 to 140 beats/min), elevated respiratory rates (40 to 80 breaths/min), total rumen and gastrointestinal stasis, a total cessation of milk flow and appetite, generalized skin coolness, reduced mucous membrane capillary refill time, scant loose manure, and often have an audible grunt or groan associated with expiration. The grunt or groan is most apparent when the animal arises, lies down, or is made to move about. Abdominal pain can be difficult to detect in these patients because the diffuse severe pain overwhelms any localized attempt to elicit pain by deep abdominal pressure. The animal will be reluctant to rise or move about and in most instances will progress to a shocklike state within 12 to 48 hours. As the animal's condition deteriorates, the body temperature also may plummet from the early fever to normal or subnormal. Risk of diffuse peritonitis is enhanced when a cow develops traumatic reticuloperitonitis in advanced gestation because the weight and movement of the gravid uterus tend to disseminate the peritonitis and make natural attempts at walling off the peritonitis difficult. Diffuse peritonitis caused by abomasal perforation is the principle differential diagnosis for cows with this presentation and signalment.

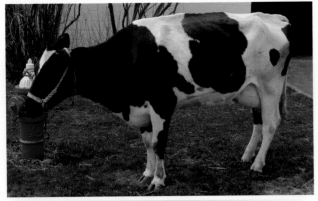

Figure 5-18

Classical appearance of a cow affected with traumatic reticuloperitonitis. The cow has an anxious expression, arched stance, and appears gaunt.

Ancillary Data and Procedures

Laboratory tests may be helpful in diagnosing confusing cases. Peritoneal fluid containing elevated total solids and white blood cell numbers supports a diagnosis of peritonitis. A complete blood count (CBC) may or may not be helpful because many patients with hardware disease have normal CBCs, although almost all have elevated plasma fibrinogen levels. Some patients with hardware disease with acute localized peritonitis and most patients with acute diffuse peritonitis will show a degenerative left shift in the leukogram. In chronic (longer than 10 days) hardware disease, serum globulin is often elevated (>5.7 mg/dl), and the leukogram may be normal or confirm mature neutrophilia. Cows with peracute, diffuse septic peritonitis caused by hardware disease may have hypoproteinemia as a result of fluid and protein loss into the peritoneal cavity, but this does not occur as commonly as with abomasal perforation. Because of forestomach and abomasal hypomotility or stasis, patients with hardware disease have a hypochloremic, hypokalemic, metabolic alkalosis that varies in severity in direct proportion to the degree of stasis. Cattle affected with subacute or chronic hardware disease that has caused complete rumen stasis may have a profound metabolic alkalosis with serum chloride values in the 40 to 50 mEq/L range. It is debatable whether alkalosis of this magnitude totally results from the disease present or is accentuated by oral administration of ruminotoric laxative medications before blood collection. Regardless of pathophysiology for alkalosis of this magnitude, the prognosis is not hopeless. The most helpful ancillary tests are abdominal ultrasonography and reticular radiography. Abdominal ultrasound should reveal an abnormal pocket of fluid and fibrin in the anterior abdomen (Figure 5-19). Radiography is the best test for confirming metallic penetration of the reticulum (or rarely rumen), the current location of the metal object, and the presence and size of perireticular abscesses (Figure 5-20, *A* to *D*). Unfortunately, this is the least available test for the practicing veterinarian because extremely powerful radiographic equipment is necessary to penetrate the reticular region in adult cattle.

Radiography of the reticulum has been a useful ancillary procedure in teaching hospitals and referral centers to aid in detecting reticular foreign bodies and abscesses of the reticulum or liver. The procedure is very helpful in confusing cases of abdominal disease or in confirmation of suspected hardware disease. Powerful radiographic units of 300 mA and 125 kVp using a 400 ISO speed film-screen combination are necessary for such studies. Experience with such radiographic studies and the subsequent surgical findings allow clinicians to diagnose, determine the need or approach for surgery, and prognosticate more specifically than possible without this ancillary aid. A portable unit has reportedly been used to take radiographs of the reticulum in cattle restrained in dorsal recumbency. However, it is difficult to keep cows in that position and the forced positioning of the cow could worsen the peritonitis.

Diagnosis

The diagnosis of traumatic reticuloperitonitis is based primarily on physical examination and is aided by laboratory work in less obvious cases. In cattle with obvious signs of peritonitis, perforating abomasal ulcers are the chief differential consideration. Perforating abomasal ulcers tend to cause pain in the midventral abdomen on the right side of midline, are usually associated with fever, and are most common 2 weeks before freshening and up to 100 days postpartum. Acute pyelonephritis or necrotic lesions of the cervix or vagina may present similar to hardware. With pyelonephritis, the urine may be discolored and rectal examination reveals an enlarged ureter. Cows with necrotic cervicitis or vaginitis are often febrile, depressed, stand either hunched up or stretched out, and have rumen atony, but unlike hardware cases, they strain and frequently aspirate air in the rectum. If an active magnet is already present in a cow having signs of peritonitis, abomasal ulceration is more likely than hardware disease. A compass can be used during physical examination to detect an active magnet in the reticulum. The compass is moved slowly into position behind the elbow on the left thoracic wall. A 60- to 90-degree deflection indicates the presence of a strong magnet in the reticulum. In cows with normal rectal temperatures, hardware disease must be differentiated from indigestion and ketosis. This can be done based on the absence of abdominal pain in patients with ketosis, while cows with hardware have evidence of abdominal pain in addition to ruminal hypomotility and negative to trace urinary ketones. A cow affected

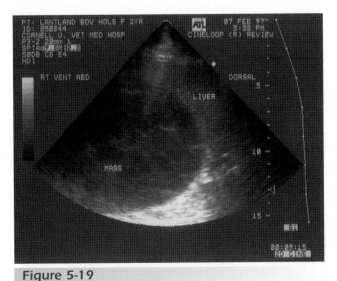

Figure 5-19

Sonogram of a large abscess in the anterior abdomen of a cow with hardware.

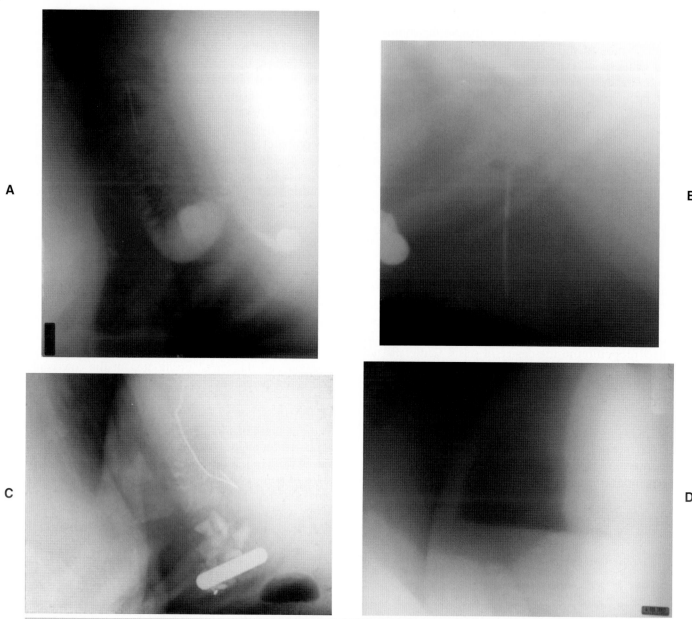

Figure 5-20

A, Radiograph of cow with traumatic reticuloperitonitis. Note fluid and gas interfaces around metallic foreign body suggestive of reticular abscess formation. **B,** Radiograph of cow with ventrally located draining fistula associated with traumatic reticuloperitonitis. The foreign body was a piece of bailing wire. **C,** Abdominal radiograph of a cow with hardware showing an abscess (gas) ventral to the reticulum floor. **D,** Radiograph of the anterior abdomen showing a fluid line of a large perireticular abscess.

with musculoskeletal diseases such as polyarthritis, laminitis, back pain, or trauma could be confused with one having hardware disease because of an arched stance, weight loss, anorexia, and decreased production. Physical examination should differentiate these diagnoses, however.

Treatment

Except for valuable cows, conservative treatment is indicated in most acute cases of traumatic reticuloperitonitis. This treatment consists of a magnet administered orally,

systemic antibiotics to control existing peritonitis, and stall rest to aid in the formation of adhesions; other symptomatic therapy such as oral fluids, ruminotorics, calcium solutions, and oral electrolytes also may be helpful. If dehydration is present and metabolic alkalosis is suspected or confirmed, fluid therapy and supplementation with potassium chloride orally (1 to 2 oz orally, twice daily) or IV are indicated. In severely alkalotic patients, alkalinizing ruminotorics should be avoided. Conservative therapy results should be evaluated within 48 to 72 hours. If the affected cow is beginning to eat and ruminate and production begins to increase, recovery can be anticipated. If the cow is not improving or if appetite and rumen activity wax and wane, rumenotomy may be indicated. Following oral administration of a magnet, the magnet first drops into the rumen. The magnet only moves to the desired location in the reticulum through effectual ruminoreticular contractions. Therefore if the rumen remains static, it is unlikely the magnet will move into the reticulum to grasp and hold the foreign body. It is revealing to note the number of cattle that are referred to teaching hospitals that possess a magnet or magnets within the rumen rather than the reticulum when the magnet has been administered as a therapeutic rather than prophylactic aid. If the affected cow already has a magnet at the time signs develop, exploratory laparotomy and rumenotomy may be indicated initially rather than conservative therapy. This situation may occur when the foreign body is extremely long (>15 cm) and extends off the magnet to a dangerous level or is not attached to a magnet, as in the case of an aluminum needle. Rumenotomy and object removal should be performed immediately in valuable cows to limit further movement of the object and worsening peritonitis. When laparotomy and rumenotomy are elected, it is best not to explore the serosal surface of the rumen and reticulum if adhesions are obvious. This will avoid dissemination of the peritonitis. During rumenotomy, a careful palpation of the entire reticulum is indicated to find the offending foreign body, which may remain only partially in the reticular wall. Left-sided laparotomy and rumenotomy allow for confirmation of the diagnosis, removal of the foreign body/bodies, and drainage of reticular abscesses into the lumen (Figure 5-21, *A* to *C*). Even with radiographic and/or ultrasonographic guidance, it can be challenging to identify and remove some foreign bodies that are embedded within mature, chronic, fibrous adhesions, and reaching a comfort level with abscess drainage by sharp scalpel incision into the reticular wall at the site of the adhesions takes some practice and experience. If there is a large reticular abscess, it could be drained via a ventral percutaneous approach, although cellulitis, reticular fistula, and dissemination of the peritonitis may occur.

Antibiotic therapy should be continued a minimum of 3 to 7 days to control existing localized peritonitis completely and to discourage secondary reticular abscesses at the perforation site. Penicillin, ceftiofur, ampicillin, and tetracycline all have been used successfully for this purpose.

In subacute or chronic cases in which chronic anorexia, dehydration, and severe alkalosis exist, IV therapy, antibiotics, and rumenotomy are indicated at the time of diagnosis. Conservative therapy is unlikely to be successful in these patients, and further supportive care with rumen transfaunates, calcium solutions, and long-term antibiotic treatment often are necessary.

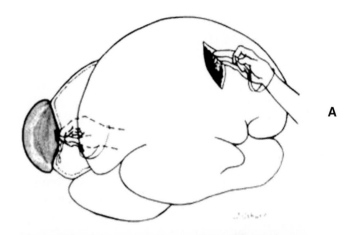

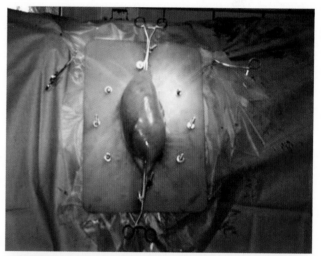

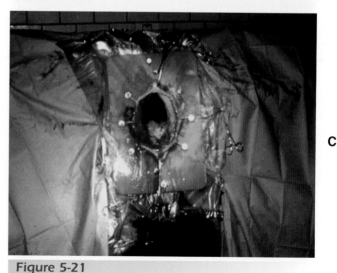

Figure 5-21

A, A drawing depicting rumenotomy and lancing a perireticular abscess into the reticulum. **B,** Left paralumbar fossa laparotomy with rumen wall attached to a "rumen board." **C,** Same cow as *B* with rumen open.

Sequelae

Cattle suffering from hardware disease may have myriad complications secondary to perforation and peritonitis. Septic pericarditis is perhaps the best-known complication and occurs when the metallic foreign body perforates in a cranial direction, perforating the diaphragm and pericardium (Figure 5-22, *A* and *B*). Reticular abscesses also are fairly common sequelae and often occur on the cranial or right wall of the reticulum where they directly, or indirectly, cause dysfunction of the ventral vagus nerve branches and result in signs of vagus indigestion. Signs of vagus indigestion vary from mild ruminoreticular disturbances to omasal transport difficulties or abomasal dysfunction/impaction. Septic pleuritis, pneumonia, thoracic abscesses, diaphragmatic hernias, and traumatic endocarditis are less frequent complications of a perforation of the diaphragm. Occasionally a

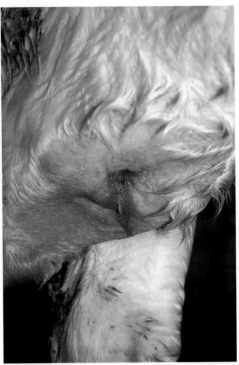

Figure 5-23

Reticular fistula through the sternum of a cow. Ingesta from the reticulum leaked from this fistula secondary to migration of a metallic foreign body.

metallic foreign body—usually a wire—associated with a ventral perforation migrates through the sternum or cranial ventral abdomen, resulting in a reticular fistula (Figure 5-23). Any perforation of the right wall of the reticulum may directly or indirectly, through associated inflammation and adhesions, injure, inflame, or irritate the ventral vagus nerve branches and result in signs of vagus indigestion. Therefore when hardware disease is suspected as the cause of vagus indigestion, a meticulous search of the right wall of the reticular mucosa is indicated during rumenotomy.

Prevention

All breeding age heifers or heifers 1 year of age, as well as young bulls, should receive strong prophylactic magnets. Not to recommend this for valuable cattle represents negligence, and the loss of a single valuable dairy cow because of traumatic reticuloperitonitis is inexcusable. Unfortunately hardware disease is still extremely common, and many cows die each year because the owner "forgot" to administer a magnet. Although occasional cows pass magnets through the gastrointestinal tract and some magnets do lose strength, the magnet remains the major means of preventing this disease. The effectiveness of magnets is apparent at slaughterhouses, where an impressive array of metallic foreign bodies are found trapped tightly to magnets. When purchasing magnets, the owner or veterinarian should assess the

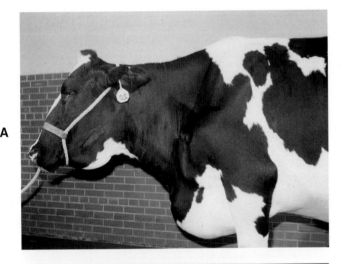

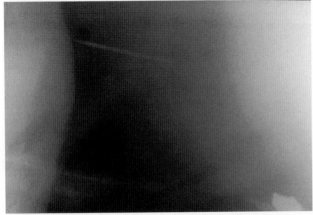

Figure 5-22

A, A cow with ventral edema, brisket edema, and intermandibular edema caused by pericarditis secondary to traumatic reticuloperitonitis. **B,** Radiograph of the anterior abdomen and ventral thorax of a 96-point cow with acute traumatic reticulitis. The wire has moved into the right thorax and was successfully removed via a standing thoracotomy.

strength of the magnet by testing it against metallic objects. Inferior magnets should not be purchased.

Large electromagnetic plates to trap metal can be incorporated into automatic feeding lines or silo unloaders and are available commercially; they are very helpful on large farms with automated feeding assemblies. Use of these plates should be encouraged because they tend to trap many pounds of dangerous sharp metallic objects each year.

Diseases Affecting the Vagus Innervation of the Forestomach and Abomasum—Vagus Indigestion

The vagus nerve may be damaged anywhere along its anatomic course to the forestomach and abomasum. Lesions capable of injuring, inflaming, or destroying the vagus nerve and its branches are discussed based on a regional basis, starting with the brainstem and progressing distally along the vagus nerve. All of these diseases lead to forestomach or abomasal dysfunction to some degree and have been included under the category Vagus Indigestion. Depending on the anatomic area involved and degree of damage to the vagus nerve or its branches, these diseases may cause a wide spectrum of forestomach or abomasal signs. In all cases, ruminal distention is present intermittently or constantly. This distention may be the result of functional or physical outflow obstruction from the forestomach, or failure of eructation causing free-gas distention. Physical or functional obstruction of the abomasum or pylorus may prevent outflow in more distal lesions.

The conditions discussed in this section are those that result in the syndrome called *vagus indigestion*. This syndrome must be thought of as a complex or set of signs secondary to a primary lesion along the course of the vagus nerve.

Signs

General signs suggesting vagus nerve damage include decreased appetite for several days or more, decreased milk production, abdominal distention that may be constant or intermittent but tends to be progressive, pasty manure that often varies in quantity in direct proportion to appetite and inversely with the degree of abdominal distention, and loss of body condition. Many cases develop bradycardia (heart rate 60 beats/min); however, not all cases develop this sign, and its absence should not rule out vagus indigestion. Bradycardia appears to be caused by reflex retrograde irritation of the vagus nerve, causing parasympathetic slowing of the heart rate. Bradycardia has also been associated with simple anorexia. Rumen contractions may be hypermotile, hypotonic, or atonic, and vagus indigestion has been categorized by some authors based on this sign. In some cases, rumen contractions occur more frequently than normal (3 to 6 contractions/min) but are ineffectual and fail to propel ruminoreticular ingesta into the omasum and abomasum, resulting in frothy ruminoreticular ingesta from constant churning activity.

The abdominal distention that develops is classical, with distention in the upper left, lower left, and lower right quadrants as the cow is viewed from the rear (Figure 5-24). In most cases, this distention results from progressive ruminal enlargement with the ventral sac enlarging toward the right. Therefore this typical distention results in an L-shaped rumen, as viewed from the rear or palpated per rectum. In severe cases, the rumen ventral sac not only fills the entire right lower quadrant of the abdomen but also may expand into the right upper quadrant so the rumen assumes a V shape. Extreme distention of the rumen into a V shape occasionally traps gas in the most dorsal region of the now expanded ventral sac, and this gas may result in an area of tympanitic resonance in the *right* upper quadrant. In very rare instances of true abomasal impaction or pyloric stenosis, the abomasum may be large enough to account for this right lower quadrant distention.

Depending on the primary lesions, signs of vagus nerve dysfunction may appear acutely or have a delayed onset. In most cases, onset of signs and typical abdominal distention occur several days to weeks after the affected cow initially developed signs of illness. Some primary lesions are relatively easy to diagnose, whereas others require extensive ancillary data or exploratory

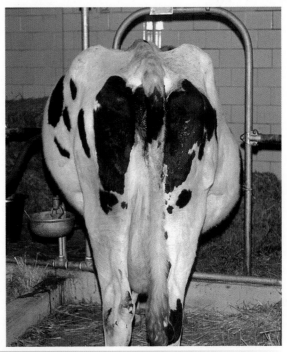

Figure 5-24

Classical appearance of abdominal distention in vagus indigestion with high left, lower left, and lower right quadrants affected.

surgery. In all cases, primary lesions resulting in the syndrome of vagus indigestion should be sought because prognosis directly depends on the primary cause. Having discussed the general signs of vagus indigestion, specific primary causes will next be discussed, and individual signs referable to each will be included when pertinent. Table 5-1 summarizes the clinical results of long-term follow-up evaluation for 112 cases of vagus indigestion and illustrates relative occurrence of the various primary lesions.

Vagus nerve nucleus lesions are rare, but occasionally cattle affected with listeriosis will show vomiting and

rumen inactivity as early signs, and this may reflect vagal nerve irritation. It also is possible that vomiting or normal regurgitation occurs but cannot be controlled when oral-pharyngeal neuromuscular function is impeded by specific cranial nerve deficits (V, VII, IX, X) at the brainstem level.

Pharyngeal trauma with typical signs of fever, dysphagia, salivation, extended head and neck, and soft tissue swelling in the pharyngeal area often results in vagal nerve dysfunction. This trauma invariably results from injudicious or unskilled use of balling guns, dose syringes, stomach tubes, specula, esophageal feeders, or magnet/foreign body retrieval apparatus when treating a cow. Vagal nerve dysfunction may be apparent as ruminal hypomotility, dysphagia, failure of eructation, and subsequent ruminal distention. Bradycardia is present in some cases. The complex neuromuscular act of eructation frequently is altered because vagus nerve branches controlling the pharynx, larynx, and cranial esophagus are subject to inflammatory or direct traumatic damage in these patients. Retropharyngeal abscess and pharyngeal foreign bodies may cause signs similar to those caused by pharyngeal trauma but are less common.

Esophageal lacerations from traumatic passage of stomach tubes, esophageal feeders, or magnet/foreign body retrieval apparatus may lead to severe cellulitis and associated vagus nerve dysfunction. Chemical or septic phlegmon with similar signs may follow perivascular injections of material intended for IV administration in the jugular vein. Fever, salivation, and severe inflammatory swelling in the cervical region usually accompany any signs of vagus nerve damage in these patients. Chronic choke may lead to esophageal necrosis and similar signs along with profuse salivation and reflux of ingested food or water.

Occasionally in calves and adult cattle, severe bronchopneumonia results in apparent inflammatory damage to the vagus nerve traversing the mediastinum. It is not known whether this syndrome involves direct inflammation of the nerve or indirect pressure from enlarged lymph nodes. In any event, the affected calf or cow develops signs of abdominal distention, ruminal tympany, and inappetence, despite apparent response of the pneumonia to broad-spectrum antibiotic therapy. Usually signs of ruminal tympany develop several days after the onset of the pneumonia. Passage of a stomach tube in these patients relieves and resolves a free-gas bloat, but the bloat recurs as a chronic problem and results in weight loss because the animal eats only during those times when the bloat is relieved. Failure of eructation seems to be the major cause of this recurrent free-gas bloat. Occasional cases of frothy-type bloat may occur in association with chronic bronchopneumonia in adult cattle, when pneumonic pathology involves thoracic branches of the vagus.

Neoplasms such as thymic, juvenile, or adult lymphosarcoma, neurofibromatosis, and pulmonary carcinomas

TABLE 5-1	Clinical Results of Long Term Evaluation for 112 Cattle Affected with Vagus Indigestion			
	Good	Moderate	Poor	Total
Pharyngeal trauma			1	1
Pneumonia			1	1
Fibropapilloma	1			1
Actinomyces granuloma		1		1
Lymphosarcoma			2	2
Toxic rumenitis			3	3
Traumatic reticuloperitonitis	13	3	16	32
Reticular abscess	10	1	4	15
Liver abscess	1	2		3
Abomasal ulcer (perforating)	3	3		6
Right displacement abomasum	4			4
Right torsion abomasum	3	3	20	26
RDA and perforating ulcer			1	1
Left displacement abomasum			1	1
Omasal impaction			1	1
Abomasal impaction			2	2
Abdominal abscess			1	1
Diffuse peritonitis	1		7	8
Advanced pregnancy			1	1
Idiopathic	1		1	2
	33	8	71	112

"Good" = remained in herd and returned to, or exceeded, previous production levels.

"Moderate" = remained in herd but was culled within one lactation.

"Poor" = died or was culled within 1 month of treatment.

sometimes may result in signs of vagus indigestion resulting from extraluminal compression of the esophagus or pressure on the vagus nerve and subsequent failure of eructation with chronic free-gas bloat.

Lesions at the cardia include fibropapillomas, other neoplastic processes, and granulomas caused by *Arcanobacterium* sp. or *A. lignieresii*. Generally lesions in this area mechanically occlude the distal esophagus during attempts at eructation or regurgitation and cause signs of vagal indigestion.

Most lesions involving the reticulum are located on the right or medial wall of the reticulum. These lesions damage the ventral vagal nerve branches with inflammation, pressure, or direct trauma. Traumatic reticuloperitonitis, reticular abscesses, liver abscesses, severe toxic rumenitis, and neoplasms such as lymphosarcoma would be included in this group. Some authors include adhesions of the cranial and medial reticulum in this category and imply that mechanical dysfunction results from these adhesions. Most authors, however, believe that neurogenic damage to the ventral vagal branches must occur even if adhesions are present. In this category, prognosis seems to vary depending on the cause. Traumatic reticuloperitonitis carries a variable prognosis based on the degree of peritonitis and involvement of the ventral vagal branches (13 of 32 cases had good outcomes), whereas reticular abscesses carry a more favorable prognosis (10 of 15 cases had good outcomes) (see Table 5-1) presumably because they tend to cause vagal nerve dysfunction by pressure on the nerve. This pressure dysfunction is alleviated by surgical drainage.

Lesions of the forestomach distal to the reticulum or involving the abomasum include a diverse group of problems such as lymphosarcoma (see video clip 10) and other neoplasms, diffuse peritonitis, peritonitis caused by perforating abomasal ulcers, abdominal abscesses, vagal nerve damage and possible vascular thrombosis secondary to right-sided AV, omasal impaction, and chronic or severe abomasal impaction. In general, prognosis is poor for cattle with signs of vagal indigestion secondary to these lesions (see Table 5-1) because of the extent of the pathology, the possibility of multiple sites being affected, and the likelihood of functional and mechanical outflow disturbances. In referral practice, a disproportionate number of cattle with right-sided AV are treated. Many of these cattle have been affected for 24 hours or more before referral, thereby being at high risk for subsequent signs of vagal nerve dysfunction. Usually these cattle appear to improve for 24 to 72 hours after surgical correction of their AV but then begin to show signs of an outflow disturbance. These cattle then develop bradycardia, typical ruminal distention, scant manure, poor appetite, and abdominal distention typical of an L-shaped rumen.

Most distention involves the forestomach compartments even though the abomasum was the primary problem. Recent work helps explain this syndrome. Because volvulus involves the abomasum, omasum, and reticulum, either neurogenic damage by stretching the ventral vagal branches or thrombosis of major vessels supplying the lesser curvature of the abomasum, omasum, and reticulum may result from prolonged volvulus. Most cattle that develop signs of vagal indigestion following right-sided DA and volvulus never recover despite attempts at therapy. Rumenotomy is seldom suggested for cows with vagus indigestion secondary to right-sided volvulus of the abomasum because the primary pathology is thought to be irreversible. Vagal nerve damage secondary to right-sided volvulus has an extremely poor prognosis with only 3 of 26 patients having a good outcome (see Table 5-1). Right-sided DAs and volvulus should be corrected on an emergency basis to minimize chances of vagal nerve damage or outflow disturbance. Valuable cattle that begin to develop symptoms of vagus indigestion following correction of right-sided volvulus of the abomasum by omentopexy may be considered for abomasopexy or abomasopexy following rumenotomy to ensure proper abomasal alignment that may improve outflow. The prognosis, however, remains guarded to poor.

Diagnosis of vagus indigestion is based on subacute to chronic history, typical abdominal distention, rectal findings of an L-shaped rumen (as viewed from the rear), and bradycardia (when present). The diagnosis is incomplete, however, until a primary cause of vagus nerve dysfunction is determined. The primary lesion is obvious in some instances, such as pharyngeal trauma, esophageal laceration, and vagus nerve dysfunction secondary to recent surgical correction of right-sided volvulus of the abomasum. In other instances, especially those with less common abdominal lesions or when associated with advanced pregnancy, the primary diagnosis may be difficult to determine unless exploratory laparotomy and rumenotomy are performed. Abomasal and sometimes ruminal impactions unrelated to any apparent vagal nerve injury sporadically occur. Abomasal impactions are a cause of decreased appetite and production in dairy cattle, and most have complete recovery following medical or surgical treatments and are likely unrelated to vagal dysfunction. Cows with abomasal impactions associated with vagal nerve dysfunction are much less amenable to treatment.

Clinical Pathology

In all cases, thorough physical examinations (including a rectal examination) should be performed. If a physical examination fails to reveal the primary lesion, ancillary tests may be helpful. CBC may indicate chronic or acute inflammation or suggest lymphosarcoma based on persistent lymphocytosis. Serum total protein, albumin, and globulin should be assessed. Elevated serum globulin may suggest reticular or liver abscess. Abdominal paracentesis is difficult to perform in cattle with vagal indigestion because the tremendous rumen distention leaves virtually no space for separation of the visceral and parietal peritoneum. Nevertheless, with ultrasound as an aid, abdominal fluid analysis may indicate peritonitis or lymphosarcoma. The right cranial paramedian location can be a rewarding location from which to obtain diagnostic fluid containing exfoliated neoplastic cells in cases of abomasal lymphosarcoma. Acid-base and electrolyte status is helpful in determining relative degrees of alkalosis. The clinician should not conclude, however, that severe alkalosis always indicates abomasal or pyloric disease because some cattle with subacute to chronic traumatic reticuloperitonitis have severe alkalosis. Somewhat surprisingly, most vagus indigestion patients have either normal acid-base and electrolyte values or mild hypochloremic hypokalemic alkalosis despite their apparent outflow disturbance. Gamma glutamyl transferase is elevated in approximately 50% of cows with liver abscess but overall has poor sensitivity and specificity for this disease.

Ancillary Tests

Abdominal ultrasound is very helpful in evaluating cattle affected with vagal indigestion. Ultrasound can help determine the nature of abdominal fluid and presence of fibrin or an intraabdominal abscess. Ultrasound can also be useful to image the abomasal wall to determine the size of the viscus and any evidence of neoplasia. Because of the poor sensitivity and specificity of biochemical markers of liver disease in cattle, transabdominal ultrasound is the most useful diagnostic aid in making a diagnosis of liver abscess. If facilities are available, radiographs of the reticulum are very helpful in detecting foreign body perforation of the reticulum, and radiographs of the pharynx or thorax can aid in the diagnosis of pharyngeal or thoracic lesions. If bovine lymphosarcoma is suspected, serum should be submitted for a bovine leukemia virus (BLV) agar-gel immunodiffusion test or enzyme-linked immunosorbent assay and a peritoneal centesis performed followed by cytologic examination for neoplastic lymphocytes.

Treatment

Some primary etiologies allow a sufficiently negative prognosis (neoplasms, vagus indigestion secondary to right-sided volvulus of the abomasum, and diffuse peritonitis) that exploratory surgery may not be necessary or indicated. Similarly, medical causes of vagus indigestion such as pharyngeal trauma, severe pneumonia, and other definable lesions that result in failure of eructation may only require symptomatic therapy for the primary problem. In cases of pharyngeal trauma or cellulitis, for example, broad-spectrum antibiotics, antiinflammatories, and analgesics would be indicated. If failure of eructation persists in these instances, however, use of a rumen fistula may alleviate chronic bloating and provide a means

of administering feed and water during the prolonged recovery. If the value of the affected cow warrants treatment and the suspected primary problem is abdominal in location, surgical intervention is necessary. Left-sided exploratory laparotomy and rumenotomy offer the best means of making a definitive diagnosis of the primary cause for the vagal nerve dysfunction. In addition to the diagnostic and prognostic advantages of these procedures, therapeutic advantages exist because the massively distended rumen may be emptied. This temporarily reduces the weight of the organ and also relieves pressure receptor dysfunction caused by massive distention of the rumen. Following rumenotomy, rumen and reticular pressure receptors may be better able to instigate effectual forestomach contracture if indeed the vagal nerve damage has not been extensive or permanent. In a few cows the passage of a Kingman tube may permit dramatic emptying of the rumen fluid, making the rumenotomy and exploratory exam easier for both the cow and the surgeon.

Adequate hydration and correction of acid-base or electrolyte deficits should be achieved by IV fluid therapy before surgery. If peritonitis is suspected, broad-spectrum antibiotics should be used as well. Usually oral medications or fluids are contraindicated because of existing functional outflow disturbance, although the administration of 1 lb of coffee by orogastric tube to adult cattle has had some dramatic effects on the passage of ingesta from the forestomach compartments and abomasum. Parenteral calcium solutions are indicated for those patients that are hypocalcemic secondary to reduced intestinal uptake coupled with continued calcium loss resulting from milk production.

Complete exploration of the abdomen should be attempted during left flank celiotomy. If extensive adhesions are found in the abdomen or around the reticulum, these adhesions should not be manipulated or broken down because this would be painful and may act to disseminate the existing peritonitis. Following exploration of the abdominal viscera, rumenotomy should be performed and the ruminal contents evacuated. Careful search of the forestomach compartments should be conducted with particular care devoted to the reticulum, cardia, and reticuloomasal orifice. The reticular mucosa should be lifted to detect adhesions between the visceral and parietal peritoneum. The abomasum and omasum should be palpated through the wall of the rumen. Abomasal impactions or extensive adhesions caused by perforating abomasal ulcers may be palpated at this time. Dislocation of the abomasum or pylorus associated with extensive adhesions also may be detected. In average size cattle, the surgeon may pass a hand into the omasal orifice to palpate the interior of the omasum and, occasionally by directing a hand ventrally, the interior of the abomasum. A methodical search of the reticular mucosa should be completed to rule out traumatic reticuloperitonitis and to detect any foreign bodies or tumors in the reticulum. Fibropapillomas should be removed. Palpation of the caudal esophagus will detect the occasional tumor or granuloma that may occur in this region. Reticular abscesses and liver abscesses resulting in vagal nerve dysfunction tend to be located along the right or medial wall of the reticulum, although the anterior-posterior orientation varies in each case. Usually reticular abscesses will be attached firmly to the reticular wall by adhesions, although liver abscesses generally are not. Large reticular or liver abscesses give the impression, based on palpation, that two omasums are present in affected cows. Usually the abscess is located anterior to the omasum. If a reticular abscess (Figure 5-25) is confirmed by firm adhesion of the mass to the reticulum and by an aspirate, the surgeon should proceed with drainage of the abscess into the reticulum by lancing the abscess as shown in Figure 5-21. When a liver abscess is confirmed (Figure 5-26, *A* to *C*), a second procedure through a ventral abdominal approach to establish drainage is indicated if the owner elects further attempts at therapy. Once exploratory survey of the forestomach compartments is completed, a transfaunate from a healthy cow's rumen should be administered and the rumen and body wall closed. If vagal nerve dysfunction characterized only by free-gas bloat exists, a rumen fistula may be placed surgically during closure of the abdomen; this will allow escape of rumen gas until healing of the primary condition occurs. Following the exploratory examination, if vagal indigestion signs are believed to be caused by advanced

pregnancy, the cow may need to be aborted at an appropriate time.

Postoperative care is dictated largely by the exploratory rumenotomy findings. The primary cause of the vagal nerve dysfunction should be treated specifically. If active peritonitis or abscess is present, broad-spectrum antibiotic therapy would be indicated. Fluid and electrolyte balance should continue to be assessed and treated. Daily rumen transfaunates, if available, should be administered. A laxative diet with adequate fiber (such as alfalfa hay) should be fed along with any other feedstuffs that may stimulate the cow's appetite. Parenteral calcium solutions are indicated if hypocalcemia is present. Recovery is slow but progressive; even in those cattle that respond to therapy, complete recovery usually requires weeks. Positive signs include improved appetite and milk production, lack of recurrent bloat, increased manure production, lack of rumen distention on rectal examination, and weight gain. Negative prognostic signs include a continued poor appetite, scant fecal production, recurrent bloat, and rumen and abdominal distention. Cattle that have had large amounts of ingesta removed from the forestomachs at surgery should not be allowed free access to feed, and particularly water, in the immediate postoperative period. Most cattle with substantial peritonitis will not want to eat or drink very much at this time anyway, and in many cases they look significantly worse for the first 24 to 48 hours after surgery. However, the occasional individual will gorge or drink excessively in the postoperative period and rapidly redistend the rumen if allowed ad libitum access.

Left Flank Abdominal Exploratory Laparotomy and Rumenotomy

This common surgical procedure (see Figure 5-21) provides direct access to the rumen of cattle, and indications for medical and research purposes have been reviewed by Fubini and Ducharme. In some instances, the rumen is so enlarged that it precludes any meaningful intraabdominal palpation. Following routine preparation and incision, the abdomen may be explored to some extent before rumenotomy. The surgeon should bear in mind that adhesions—especially those associated with the reticulum or abomasum—represent a potentially septic focus. Manipulation of such adhesions may lead to dissemination of infection and subsequent diffuse peritonitis. Depending on the size of the cow being explored, some of the abdominal viscera may be palpated by extending an arm over or caudal to the rumen. Usually, however, the right cranial abdomen is out of reach from this approach.

When performing a rumenotomy in cases of vagus indigestion or hardware disease, the interior of the rumen should be cleared of as much ingesta as possible. This will allow the surgeon to palpate the abdominal viscera through the wall of the rumen similar to the technique

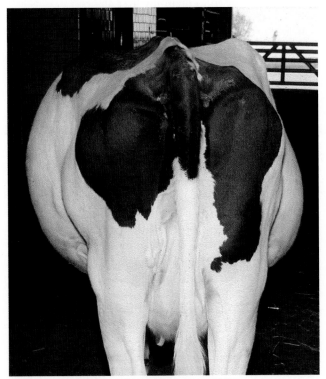

Figure 5-25

Vagus indigestion caused by a reticular abscess.

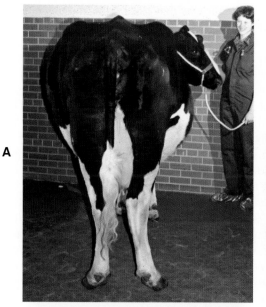

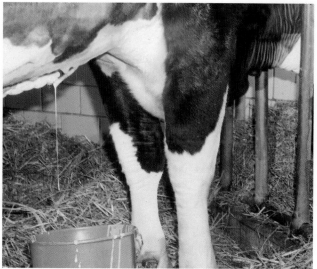

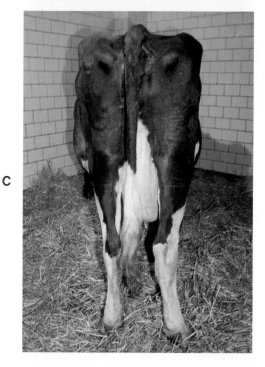

Figure 5-26

A, Presurgical vagus indigestion. This cow was found to have a large liver abscess at the time of rumenotomy. **B,** A chest trochar was used to drain the liver abscess following a second surgery performed in the right paramedian area to properly place the trochar. **C,** Postoperative appearance of the cow.

used in rectal palpation. The reticulum should be searched meticulously for foreign bodies. The wall of the reticulum should be grasped and inverted to detect adhesions. The distal esophagus should be entered to detect neoplastic or granulomatous masses. The reticuloomasal orifice should be entered with several fingers or the whole hand to palpate the interior of the omasum. In smaller cows, the surgeon may be able to advance through the omasum into the abomasum at this time. The omasum and abomasum should be palpated through the wall of the rumen. Abdominal abscesses associated with the reticulum, liver, or umbilical remnants likewise may be identified by palpation through the rumen wall.

If a reticular abscess is identified and is definitely adhered to the wall of the reticulum, aspiration to confirm abscess formation followed by incisional drainage of the abscess into the reticulum should be performed. If an abscess is identified but is found not to be adherent to the forestomach, it should be located carefully and approached by a second abdominal surgery for definitive drainage or marsupialization, assuming the cow's value dictates a second procedure.

In cattle suspected of having hardware disease, identification of the reticular adhesions helps confirm diagnosis and directs the surgeon's search for the causative foreign body. Methodical palpation of every "honeycomb" mucosal division in the reticulum should be performed. On many occasions in the teaching hospital, several surgeons have palpated for a foreign body and been unable to identify the object until aided by a more experienced surgeon. In these instances, the foreign body has been found lying flush to the reticular wall, having perforated several mucosal ridges, or has penetrated the wall to such a depth that only the very end of the wire or nail is palpable. Certainly many foreign bodies have been found to have fully penetrated and exited the reticulum to lie outside the organ. In these instances, efforts to retrieve tiny metallic objects are futile unless a ventral exploratory procedure is deemed possible. On rare occasions, it has been possible to retrieve foreign bodies from a ventral approach when previous rumenotomy or ultrasound has identified the object and its surrounding fibrous tissue. Several of these attempts have resulted in frustration, however, because of diffuse adhesions making removal of the foreign body impossible or the creation of diffuse peritonitis following radical procedures. Probably only those foreign bodies definitely palpated or visualized with radiographs or ultrasound ventral or caudal to the reticulum warrant a second abdominal exploratory procedure from a ventral approach.

Cows showing signs of vagus ingestion that are found to have primary reticuloperitonitis almost invariably have had perforation of the right or medial wall of the reticulum. The perforation, localized peritonitis, and associated inflammation in this location cause direct or indirect damage to the ventral vagal nerve branches on the medial wall of the reticulum. Therefore the methodical search for the foreign body should be directed to the right wall of the reticulum.

On rare occasions, placentae trapped in the reticulo-omasal orifice, plastic material, or other nonmetallic foreign objects are found. Rumenotomies have had to be performed to retrieve balling guns, parts of balling guns, Fricke specula, stomach tubes, and other pieces of equipment swallowed by cows during the administration of oral medications by laypeople and veterinarians alike. Before closure of the rumen, a good quality magnet should be placed in the reticulum. In some instances, it may be indicated to transfaunate the cow by giving rumen juices from a healthy cow into the rumen of the patient.

Listeriosis

Occasional cattle affected with meningoencephalitis caused by *Listeria monocytogenes* show rumen stasis and vomition as early signs. These signs may result from direct inflammation of the vagal nucleus in the brainstem that stimulates excess regurgitation or may be the result of an inability to retain regurgitated rumen ingesta because of inflammation involving cranial nerves such as V, IX, X, and XII. Those cattle with listeriosis that

have complete dysphagia will develop very firm rumen contents that may cause abdominal pain when deep abdominal pressure is exerted by the examiner. This pain has been confused with pain caused by peritonitis when the affected cow's cranial nerve deficits were not observed, leading to misdiagnosis of peritonitis.

Rumen Void Syndrome

This syndrome also has been called "rumen collapse" and is observed sporadically in cattle suffering from severe inflammatory diseases such as septic metritis, septic mastitis, or severe pneumonia causing complete anorexia of several days' duration. Physical examination usually identifies the primary inflammatory disease and a large area of tympanic resonance in the left upper quadrant of the abdomen. Simultaneous percussion and auscultation reveal a "ping" localized to the dorsal one half to one third of the left abdomen. This ping extends dorsally beyond the transverse processes of the lumbar vertebrae, includes the area of the paralumbar fossa, and an area cranial to the paralumbar fossa covering up to four to five rib spaces (Figures 5-27 and 5-28). The abdomen is *not* distended on the left side, but this ping creates great confusion because differential diagnosis of left displacement of the abomasum, ruminal tympany, and pneumoperitoneum must be considered. No fluid can be balloted in these patients, and this finding lessens the likelihood of an LDA. Rectal examination is necessary to confirm the problem and will reveal a collapsed dorsal sac of the rumen with no palpable rumen in the dorsal left quadrant and the left kidney pulled ventrally into the midabdomen. The dorsal sac of the rumen is not gas distended, ruling out ruminal tympany, and the rectum is not tightly compressed around the examiner's arm, ruling out pneumoperitoneum. Standing laparotomies were performed on several cattle with pings caused by rumen collapse before the syndrome was recognized. These laparotomies revealed a collapsed dorsal sac and left kidney pulled ventrally and medially into the midabdomen. Although

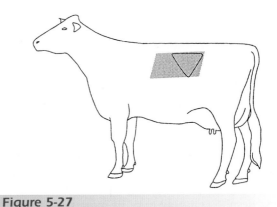

Figure 5-27

Tympanic resonance observed in rumen collapse.

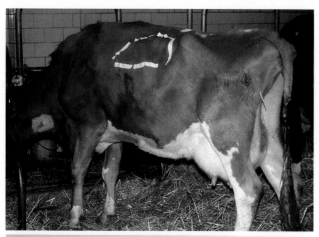

Figure 5-28

Area of tympanic resonance in a cow with rumen collapse secondary to septic metritis.

it is not understood why a ping occurs in these cattle, the characteristic clinical signs now allow diagnosis and avoid subjecting an already very ill cow to surgery.

Once a diagnosis of rumen collapse has been made and other causes of left-sided abdominal pings have been ruled out, treatment should be directed toward the primary disease. Systemic antibiotics are indicated for septic metritis, septic mastitis, or pneumonia. Further, local antibiotic therapy, along with evacuation of septic secretions, is indicated for mastitis and metritis patients. If endotoxemia is suspected, it should be treated with nonsteroidal antiinflammatory drugs (NSAIDs). Supportive therapy for hypocalcemia or ketosis should be used if indicated. Dehydration and acid-base electrolyte abnormalities should be corrected, and rumen stasis may be treated by ruminotorics, oral fluid and electrolyte therapy, or rumen transfaunates.

If therapy for the primary inflammatory disease is successful, the affected cow will begin to eat. The ventral extent of the ping will be located more dorsally each successive day during recovery as the rumen begins to fill and return to its normal position in the left upper quadrant. Prognosis is excellent if the primary disease is managed successfully because rumen collapse is merely a physiologic sign of prolonged anorexia rather than a pathologic gastrointestinal disorder.

Vomition

Vomition is observed sporadically in dairy cattle and may result from dietary or physical conditions. The most common cause of vomition is hyperacidity of the diet that usually affects only one cow in the herd. Why only one animal is affected is unknown. Such cows remain healthy, continue to eat, and do not show signs of distress despite vomiting once or more daily. It is important to determine when the vomiting has occurred

in relation to the time the animal ingested a given feed. Buffering by feeding roughage before the offending grain or silage or adding alkalinizing buffer to the feedstuff usually stops the problem. In rare instances, withdrawal of the causative feedstuff is necessary.

Vomiting also may be observed in those with traumatic reticuloperitonitis resulting from repetitive irritation of the reticulum, especially in the cranial reticulum near the cardia or when the foreign body is free in the ventral abdomen. Whether this irritation triggers receptors involved in regurgitation is unknown. In addition to vomiting, these cattle usually are ill with signs consistent with traumatic reticuloperitonitis. Treatment is as described in the section on Traumatic Reticuloperitonitis. Similar irritation that triggers the regurgitation reflex may be observed with distal esophageal or reticular warts and in diaphragmatic hernia. Rumen or reticular ulcers can also cause vomition, and the vomited ingesta were hemorrhagic in one case we have seen.

Some cattle affected with vagus indigestion will vomit. These cows usually have advanced signs of abdominal and rumen distention. Regurgitation may be associated with the release of a large amount of liquid rumen ingesta that cannot be retained in the oral cavity and therefore appears as vomition. It is also possible that attempts at regurgitation in the presence of greatly increased intraruminal pressure may predispose to vomiting.

As previously mentioned, dairy cattle affected with listeriosis may vomit in the early stages of the disease (Figure 5-29). This is thought to represent either irritation of the vagus nerve caused by inflammation of the vagal nucleus or inability to retain regurgitated ingesta as a result of cranial nerve deficits involving V, IX, X, and XII.

Vomiting has been observed in calves with white muscle disease. Although unusual, when it occurs, affected calves also may have dysphagia resulting from pharyngeal muscular dysfunction and may not be able to control regurgitated material. This may also be seen in calves with otitis media/interna. Inhalation pneumonia is a common sequela in calves so affected. Poisonous plants or toxins may cause vomiting in dairy cattle exposed to *Eupatorium rugosum, Hymenoxys* sp., *Andromeda* sp., *Oleander* sp., *Conium* sp., and other toxic plants. Because of modern management systems, however, dairy cattle are exposed to these plants only infrequently except in accidental exposure. Vomiting has been reported in cattle suffering from arsenic poisoning.

Dairy cattle with severe hypocalcemia resulting from parturient hypocalcemia may vomit as a result of increased intraruminal pressure and loss of smooth muscle tone. These animals are at greater risk of inhalation pneumonia because of their comatose condition than cattle that vomit because of other causes.

Passage of stomach tubes, especially large-diameter stomach tubes (4.0 to 5.0 cm diameter), may stimulate

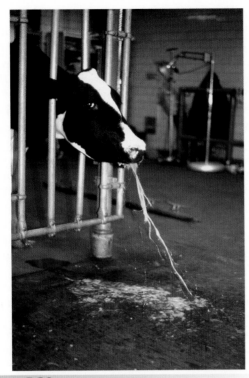

Figure 5-29

Vomiting and depression were the most noticeable clinical signs in this adult cow with listeriosis.

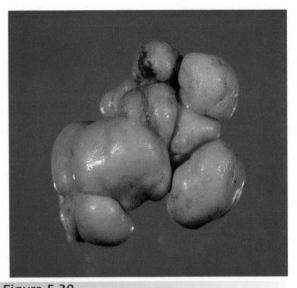

Figure 5-30

Fibropapilloma removed from the reticulum adjacent to the cardia. This mass acted as a valve to interfere with eructation and create signs of vagus indigestion in a cow.

vomiting in dairy cattle. This may be caused by pharyngeal or reticular irritation or be associated with the cow's primary disease (i.e., hardware disease) that has prompted the clinician to pass a stomach tube. If this repeatedly occurs and the cow needs to be tubed for feeding, a smaller tube passed through the nasal cavity will usually permit feeding without regurgitation.

Forestomach Neoplasia

Fibropapillomas are common in the distal esophagus, reticulum, or rumen of dairy cattle (Figure 5-30) but are seldom large enough or positioned so as to cause clinical problems. Large fibropapillomas located in the distal esophagus or cardia region may act as an impediment to eructation, thereby causing intermittent or chronic bloat. Bovine papilloma virus (DNA type 4) usually is the cause of alimentary tract warts in cattle. This virus causes fibropapillomata in the oral cavity, esophagus, and forestomach. In some parts of the world, ingestion of carcinogens such as bracken fern may encourage malignant transformation of fibropapillomas to carcinomas or squamous cell carcinomas. Cattle so affected are healthy otherwise and have normal appetites when not bloated. Rumenotomy offers the best means of diagnosis and surgical removal in such cases and has been performed successfully for fibropapillomas and fibromas. Seldom is the diagnosis suspected before rumenotomy, although

endoscopy may be used to examine the distal esophagus in suspected cases.

The other major neoplasm of the forestomach compartments is lymphosarcoma. Although more commonly found in the abomasum, lymphosarcoma may form singular or multiple lesions in the wall of the forestomach compartments and associated lymph nodes. In these instances, forestomach dysfunction characterized by bloat or signs of vagus indigestion may appear. Diagnosis may be suspected if other target organs, peripheral lymph nodes, or visceral masses palpated per rectum are identified by cytologic examination. Neoplastic cells are found in the peritoneal fluid of approximately 50% of cattle with abomasal lymphoma. In most cases, however, the lesions are identified on ultrasound examination or at the time of abdominal exploratory laparotomy. Treatment is rarely attempted. We have successfully used both isoflupredone and prednisone (alcohol base, 1 mg/kg IM daily) to improve clinical signs in late pregnant cattle such that the cow survives long enough to deliver a term calf. Although this has been successful in a few cases, the owners should be informed that the calf will likely be infected with BLV.

Rumen Fistulas as a Therapeutic Tool

Rumen fistulas have been used as a surgical means of treatment for chronic or recurrent free-gas bloat in dairy cattle and calves. For this procedure to be most effective, definitive diagnosis of the primary cause of free-gas bloat should be made. Therefore rumenotomy often precedes the rumen fistula procedure in cows. The cow or calf most likely to benefit from creation of a rumen fistula is one that is healthy and appetent whenever free-gas bloat is not present (failure of eructation). Thus if passage of a stomach tube easily relieves free-gas bloat in the patient and returns the animal to a normal appearance, rumen fistula may be considered a reasonable alternative to repeated passage of a stomach tube in cattle with chronic or recurrent free-gas bloat.

Failure of eructation because of previous reticuloperitonitis, pharyngeal trauma, or other causes of apparent vagus indigestion may benefit from this procedure if rumenotomy excludes other causes and definitely identifies the rumen distention as primarily a free-gas type. Similarly, calves that have had severe bronchopneumonia and that subsequently develop chronic free-gas bloat from possible vagal nerve irritation or inflammation in the thorax may benefit from this procedure if their pneumonia responds to antibiotic therapy. Rarely, no lesions are found by exploratory procedures and rumenotomy in such patients, and rumen fistulas are fashioned in the hopes of "buying time" for the animal and avoiding frequent passage of a stomach tube to relieve the free-gas distention.

Cattle with medical disorders also may benefit from the creation of a rumen fistula. The most common indications for this are pharyngeal trauma or lacerations and cattle with tetanus. In cases of pharyngeal trauma or lacerations, the animal usually has dysphagia, fever, and pharyngeal pain. The cow also may have forestomach dysfunction caused by vagal nerve branches being injured in the pharyngeal region. Therefore ruminal dysfunction or failure of eructation sometimes occurs. If the clinical recovery time is expected to be prolonged or if chronic free-gas bloat develops in such a patient, the rumen fistula will allow feeding, watering, and an escape route for rumen gas during recuperation. This also avoids frequent passage of a stomach tube in a cow that already has a very painful pharynx. In tetanus patients, free-gas bloat and inability to eat are common signs. Passage of a stomach tube to hydrate, feed, and debloat cows affected with tetanus is a painful and frightening experience for the animal. Therefore creation of a rumen fistula following sedation and local anesthesia early in the course of the disease allows a nonstressful means to feed and water the patient and to prevent bloat. A complete surgical description is available in a recent surgery text (Fubini and Ducharme).

DISEASES OF THE ABOMASUM

Abomasal Displacement

DAs (abomasal displacements) are the most commonly detected abdominal disorder and represent the most common reason for abdominal surgery in dairy cattle.

Etiology

Displacement may occur to the left (LDA) or to the right (RDA) side, but in the United States most displacements are to the left. Peak occurrence of DAs is during the first 6 weeks of lactation, but they may occur sporadically at any stage of lactation or gestation. Bulls and calves of any age may be affected with DA. DA in calves before weaning usually occurs as RDA, whereas after weaning, calves may displace to either side. RDA has been observed in calves as young as 3 days of age.

DAs in calves, bulls, heifers before calving, and dry cows may be chronic because of lack of suspicion of DA in these groups, as well as management factors that contribute to less careful observation when compared with milking cows. Although DA once was thought to occur mainly in pluriparous cows, the condition currently is common in first-calf heifers, and lactating cattle of any age may be affected. Some studies show an increased incidence in mature cattle over first-calf heifers. The exact cause of DA is unknown. Several factors may contribute to the development of DA, however:

1. Excessive production of volatile fatty acids caused by modern diets consisting of highly acid feed materials such as corn silage, haylage, and fermentable grains such as high-moisture corn.
2. Gastrointestinal stasis caused by metabolic or infectious diseases such as hypocalcemia, ketosis, retained placenta, metritis, mastitis, and indigestion. These factors are extremely important in the early postparturient period when gastrointestinal stasis with or without endotoxemia may allow abomasal stasis and gas production. These associated diseases also decrease the size of the rumen because of decreased appetite and may allow DA (especially LDA) to occur.
3. The deeper body capacity that has been selected in the modern dairy cow may allow more room in the abdomen for movement of the abomasum. Some lines of cattle and families of dairy cattle appear to have a higher incidence of DA than others. This has been especially apparent since embryo transfer was popularized.

A combination of these factors may be involved in any one case, but when a high incidence of DA occurs in a herd, investigation of the feeding regimen and management is in order. For example, buffers, prefeeding hay before fermentable feeds, or a TMR may help decrease frequency in herds with a high incidence of DA. Similarly herds with a high incidence of postparturient metritis may benefit from a cleaner calving environment, evaluation of selenium status, and dry cow nutritional analysis. Management procedures that create undue stress or diet changes during the periparturient period have been shown to contribute to DA.

Clinical Signs

Dairy cattle that develop simple LDA or RDA generally lose their appetite for high-energy feeds and decrease 30% to 50% in milk production. Therefore the initial chief complaint from the owner is "off feed and down on milk." Inspection of the cow may reveal an animal with a dull appearance and mild dehydration. Temperature, pulse rate, and respiratory rate are normal. Rumen contractions are present and moderate in strength. A sprung rib cage (Figure 5-31, *A* and *B*) may be present on the side of the displacement as the cow is inspected from the rear. This may be easier to appreciate with LDA because the rumen is no longer palpable in the left paralumbar fossa as the DA pushes the rumen to the right and balloons under the left rib cage. Simultaneous auscultation and percussion will reveal an area of high-pitched tympanic resonance ("ping") under the rib cage on the left or right side, corresponding to the location of the DA. Usually this ping lies on a line from the tuber coxae to the elbow but

may be of varying size. The ping should extend cranially at least to the ninth rib and often to the eighth rib (Figures 5-32, *A* and *B*, and 5-33). (This requirement is especially important for RDA in which proximal colon, displaced omasum, and cecal gaseous distention may be confused with RDA. Differentiation of right-sided pings will be discussed further in upcoming sections.) Ballottement coupled with auscultation will confirm the presence of a large fluid-filled viscus under the rib cage because a fluid

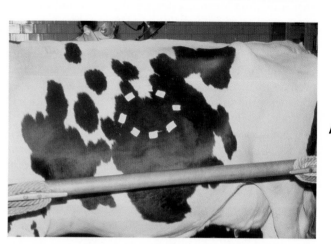

A

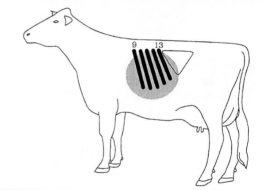

B

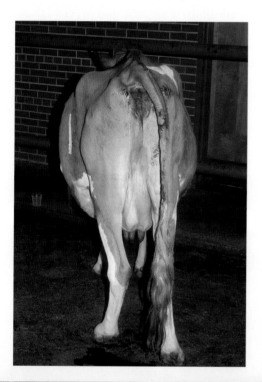

A

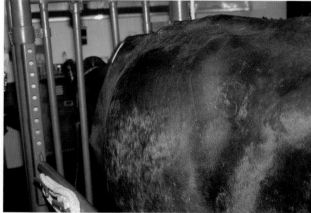

B

Figure 5-31

A, "Sprung" rib cage caused by left displacement of the abomasum (LDA) in a Guernsey cow. **B,** An even more dramatic "sprung" rib cage caused by an LDA. The abomasum of this cow could be palpated rectally.

Figure 5-32

A and **B,** Typical area of tympanic resonance indicative of a left displacement of the abomasum.

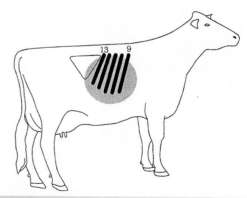

Figure 5-33

Typical area of tympanic resonance indicative of a right displacement of the abomasum.

wave creates a splashing sound with this technique (most dramatic with RDAs). Large DA will be visible as a quarter moon or half moon distended viscus appearing caudal to the thirteenth rib in the paralumbar fossa when viewed from the side (Figure 5-34). In most cases, rectal palpation of DA will not be possible. In extremely large LDA or RDA, it may be possible to just palpate the greater curvature of the abomasum, but this is not typical.

Although most DAs conform to the aforementioned anatomic ping location, variants do occur and deserve mention. The *typical* location of LDA in calves is caudal to the rib cage and extends dorsally to the paralumbar fossa (Figure 5-35). The chief complaint for calves with LDA is chronic or intermittent bloat. The ping and fluid present in the LDA are easily missed if the examiner confines pinging and ballottement to the area of the left rib cage. Rarely, LDAs in adult cattle are also identified in this location (Figure 5-36, *A*). Additionally, LDA and rumen pings may coexist, causing more rostral location of the LDA and adding some confusion in the diagnosis

(Figure 5-36, *B*). Rumen pings should not extend as ventral as LDA and may not have the fluid succussion or as high-pitched resonance sound as a LDA. Presence or absence of auscultable or palpable rumen contractions can be helpful in differentiating a confusing rumen/LDA ping; if rumen contractions are present, the ping is less likely to be a rumen ping. If the ping is relatively large and the rumen is against the body wall (based on rectal and external palpation), this would be more supportive of a ruminal ping rather than a LDA.

Other uncommon locations for LDA include (1) caudal to the left elbow in the area of the ruminoreticular junction, (2) dorsal to the rumen in cattle having an empty rumen or rumen collapse, (3) in the lower (ventral) left side of the abdomen, and (4) cranial and dorsal to the reticulum. This last position has been confirmed only once by Dr. N.G. Ducharme and myself following a radiographic finding of a gas-distended viscus in this area of a cow having intermittent anorexia. No ping was present on either side of the abdomen in this animal. Because of this variety in location, examiners should keep an open mind to clinical variations and ping over the entire left abdomen before ruling out LDA.

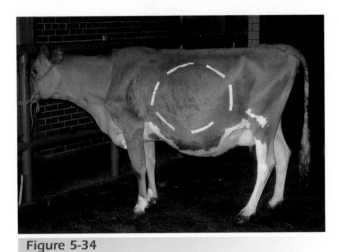

Figure 5-34

Large left displacement of the abomasum extending into the paralumbar fossa caudal to the thirteenth rib.

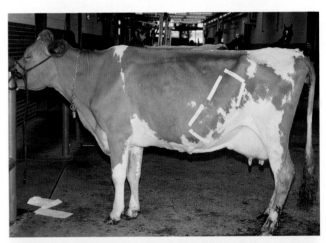

A

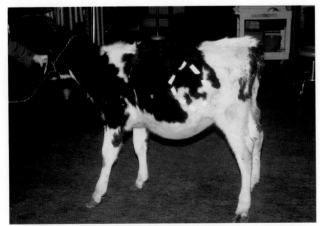

Figure 5-35

Typical location of a ping in a calf with a left abomasal displacement.

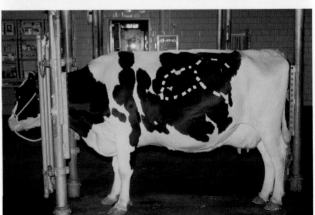

B

Figure 5-36

A, Guernsey cow with left displacement of the abomasum in caudal location. **B,** Coexisting left displaced abomasum and ruminal gas (ping) in a cow.

Signs of fever and pneumoperitoneum in a cow with LDA should alert the clinician to the possibility of abomasal perforation in addition to the displacement. Such cattle are found to have the abomasum adherent to the parietal peritoneum adjacent to the ulceration. A guarded prognosis must be offered, and surgical repair is best attempted from the ventral right paramedian approach.

Urinary ketones frequently are positive in cattle with DA. This ketosis may be the primary cause of a depressed appetite and rumen motility predisposing to DA, or secondary in a patient with DA that refuses high-energy feeds while continuing to produce milk. The strength of the urine ketone reaction may have some weak relationship between primary and secondary ketosis in cows with DAs, with strong reactions more likely an indication of primary ketosis.

Concurrent diseases such as metritis, mastitis, pneumonia, pyelonephritis, hypocalcemia, or musculoskeletal problems should be identified by completion of a thorough physical examination and treated appropriately.

Once a DA has been diagnosed, the value of the cow should be determined in light of past and present productivity, associated diseases, and genetic potential. If the cow's value dictates therapy, medical and surgical treatment should be planned to correct the DA.

Clinical Pathology

Cattle affected with DA without concurrent diseases have a characteristic hypochloremic, hypokalemic, metabolic alkalosis. With simple DA, metabolic alkalosis is mild to moderate and seldom requires intensive electrolyte correction. In chronic DA or in cattle with DA and associated diseases contributing to more drastic anorexia, acid-base and electrolyte disorders may require more vigorous therapeutic efforts. Table 5-2 shows normal values and approximate ranges of acid-base and electrolyte abnormalities in DA patients. Abdominal paracentesis is indicated if concurrent ulceration and displacement are suspected.

When laboratory tests are available and indicated, acid-base and electrolyte values constitute the most meaningful data for affected cattle that appear to be excessively dehydrated, weak, or have chronic histories. Cattle that are severely ketotic and therefore ketoacidotic may inconsistently have a blood pH in the acid range, a high anion gap, and a lower bicarbonate value than expected in cattle with simple DA. Assessment of urinary ketones always is indicated for cattle with DA and may help explain unexpected variations from the anticipated metabolic alkalosis found in most cattle with simple DA.

Paradoxic aciduria has been described as a consequence to prolonged or severe metabolic alkalosis associated with DA. This probably relates to hypochloremia (causing decreased passive sodium reabsorption in the proximal tubule), dehydration with increased sodium and water reabsorption in the distal nephron, and more importantly potassium depletion to such a degree that hydrogen ions must be excreted in the urine (to offset the increased sodium resorption) instead of potassium. Although interesting as a physiologic event, it does not change fluid and electrolyte therapy in our hospital because we always assume cows with DA have body potassium deficits except in rare cases of oliguric renal failure.

TABLE 5-2   Approximate Acid-Base and Electrolyte Status of Displaced Abomasum (DA) and Abomasal Volvulus (AV) Cattle

	pH	Cl⁻ mEq/L	K⁺ mEq/L	HCO₃⁻ mEq/L	Base Excess
Normal venous blood	7.35-7.50	97-111	3.7-4.9	20-30	−2.5-+2.5
Typical left DA	7.45-7.55	85-95	3.5-4.5	25-35	0-10
Typical right DA	7.45-7.60	85-95	3.0-4.0	30-40	5-15
Large right DA	7.45-7.60	80-90	3.0-3.5	35-45	5-20
Typical AV	7.45-7.60	75-90	2.5-3.5	35-50	10-25
Advanced AV	7.45-7.65	60-80	2.0-3.5	35-55	10-35
Very advanced AV with abomasal necrosis*	7.30-7.45	85-95	3.0-1.5	15-25	−10-0
Typical LDA with severe ketosis†	7.15-7.30	85-95	3.5-4.5	15-30	−10-0

*These cattle have very large AV and clinically severe dehydration, high heart rate, weakness, and may appear to be in shock. Therefore the acid-base and electrolyte status seem inconsistent. In fact, tissue necrosis and shock have superimposed metabolic acidosis on the preexisting metabolic alkalosis typical of AV.

†These cows do not appear to have serious abomasal problems and are not greatly dehydrated or weak. The acid-base status seems to contradict the anticipated metabolic alkalosis typical of LDA but can be explained by the severe ketoacidosis that affected the venous pH, anion gap, and so forth. The cows may be so ketoacidotic that nervous ketosis should be anticipated.

Treatment

Medical Therapy. In simple DA, economic factors, concurrent diseases, or veterinary and management time constraints may temporarily or permanently rule against surgical correction and dictate medical therapy. Although not as successful as surgery, medical therapy may be attempted in simple DA. Medical therapy usually includes oral laxatives, ruminotorics, antacids, or cholinergic medications designed to stimulate gastrointestinal motility and encourage evacuation of the gastrointestinal tract. Calcium solutions should be administered SQ or IV (slowly) if the patient is judged to be hypocalcemic. Potassium chloride (1 to 4 oz twice daily) may be administered orally in gelatin capsules, added to drinking water, or added to water administered by stomach tube. Some practitioners recommend the use of 0.5 to 1 lb of coffee mixed with warm water and administered via stomach tube. In addition to drugs, physical therapy consisting of "rolling" is a frequent component of the medical treatment for simple LDA. The cow may be cast onto either side and then is rolled into dorsal recumbency with the help of two or three people. The cow is rocked gently from side to side while in dorsal recumbency and maintained in this position for 2 to 5 minutes. During this time, the LDA should float or "balloon" to the ventral midline and return to a normal position. The longer the cow remains on her back, the more gas and sequestered fluid will escape the distended organ. The cow is then rolled down on the *left* side so that the rumen is always in contact with the left parietal peritoneum; this prevents rapid recurrence of the LDA. The cow is then forced to stand immediately. This procedure should never be performed on cattle with simple RDA because this may predispose to AV.

Following medical therapy alone or medical therapy including rolling, the cow should be encouraged to eat as much hay as possible to fill the rumen with roughage. This may act as a physical deterrent to recurrence of LDA, as well as encourage ruminal and subsequent gastrointestinal motility in the case of either LDA or RDA. Highly acidic feed components should be added to the diet gradually until full intake resumes. If concurrent diseases exist (e.g., metritis, mastitis, or ketosis), they must be treated at the same time, or medical treatment is severely compromised.

In one study performed in our practice, 30 of 100 cattle with simple LDA remained corrected for an entire lactation following one or two medical treatments that involved rolling and symptomatic medications. Although this study is not highly significant or highly successful, it illustrates the fact that medical therapy may hold some value when surgery is not deemed possible or practical.

Acupuncture therapy also has been proposed as a medical therapy for DA, but we have no experience with this technique.

The clinician must remember that once a diagnosis is made and correction of DA has occurred, the gastrointestinal tract has mechanically and functionally returned to normal. Therefore oral fluids and electrolytes usually suffice for correction of acid-base, electrolyte, and hydration abnormalities in those with simple DA. Potassium chloride may be administered in drinking water, through a stomach tube, or in gelatin capsules to help correct existing or suspected electrolyte abnormalities. It is common practice to administer 1 to 4 oz of potassium chloride orally, twice daily, to cattle with DA following correction. Cattle that are weak should be suspected of having hypokalemia (<3.0 mEq/L) and may require more intensive IV fluid therapy and potassium supplementation, although increased urine production from the IV administered fluids may enhance K losses. When supplementing potassium chloride, 1.0 g yields approximately 14 mEq.

To illustrate, assume a cow has severe metritis, LDA, inappetence, and weakness to such a degree that manual assistance by tail lifting is required to help her to rise. Hypokalemia should be suspected to be part of the reason for her weakness. Subsequent plasma electrolyte analysis determines $Cl^- = 85$ mEq/L and $K^+ = 2.5$ mEq/L. The cow weighs 600 kg (1320 lb). Consider that potassium ideally should be increased to 4.5 mEq/L. Therefore the cow needs a minimum of 2.0 mEq/L extracellular fluid (ECF) to be corrected.

$$\begin{array}{cc}
600 \text{ kg} & 180 \text{ L ECF} \\
\underline{\times\ 0.3 \text{ ECF}} & \underline{\times\ 2 \text{ mEq}}\ \text{KCl} \\
180 \text{ kg or } 180 \text{ L ECF} & 360 \text{ mEq KCl}
\end{array}$$

The cow would need 360 mEq of KCl to return extracellular K^+ levels to 4.5 mEq/L.

$$1 \text{ g KCl} \approx 14 \text{ mEq}$$
$$25.7 \text{ g KCl} = 360 \text{ mEq}$$

If IV administration (30 g KCl or 1 oz = 420 mEq) is chosen, the potassium chloride should be delivered at the rate of 40 mEq/L. If oral supplementation is chosen, the potassium chloride may be given in gelatin capsules or added to drinking water buckets. Using the oral route, 2 to 4 oz of potassium chloride is administered, once or twice daily, following repair of the LDA and treatment of metritis until the cow regains strength and appetite.

Occasional cows with hypokalemia fail to respond to potassium supplementation or saline-based fluids and develop progressively worsening hypokalemia despite intensive attempts to provide potassium. These cattle become weaker, often recumbent, and may show neurologic signs when serum potassium is less than 2.0 mEq. Affected cattle that do not respond to potassium supplementation and have low serum potassium values despite resolution of hypochloremia and alkalosis are frequently cows that have been treated aggressively for ketosis with glucose and corticosteroids, particularly extralabel doses of isoflupredone. Cattle that have potassium values less than 2.5 mg/L should be considered critical patients, and intensive potassium supplementation should be provided orally (sometimes up to 1 lb), 80 mEq/L slowly IV, or both. A specific predisposing factor to the development of severe hypokalemia and recumbency has been the repeated use of the drug isoflupredone acetate; however, not all cases appear to be associated with the administration of this combined mineralocorticoid/glucocorticoid drug. Some cases are associated with repeated treatments of dexamethasone. A more detailed discussion on severe hypokalemia is found in Chapter 14.

Surgical Correction. This discussion addresses available surgical options for simple DA. Individual training and experience of the veterinarian will dictate which surgical procedure will be chosen. Other factors, including concurrent disease, stage of gestation, and economic value of the animal, may further alter the decision as to the surgical procedure pursued. Advantages and disadvantages of each procedure will be discussed.

Right Paramedian Abomasopexy. This approach allows the best access to the abomasum and allows it to be inspected completely and relocated to the correct anatomic position. If performed properly, abomasopexy should result in a permanent adhesion of abomasum to parietal peritoneum. Nonabsorbable sutures are recommended for the abomasopexy procedure to ensure permanent adhesion formation.

Disadvantages of abomasopexy include the additional labor necessary to roll and restrain the affected cow in dorsal recumbency, the risk of incisional hernia or fistula formation, incisional infection resulting from contamination of the incision site, regurgitation during recumbency, and concern about ventral parturient edema and superficial abdominal vessels associated with the mammary circulation in cattle with large udders. The procedure also would be contraindicated in cattle concurrently affected with acute or chronic bronchopneumonia, certain musculoskeletal injuries, and late gestation cows. Despite the list of disadvantages, this procedure has been used successfully in thousands of cattle and is the procedure of choice for valuable cattle because it minimizes the risk of future DA and ensures correct anatomic relocation of the organ. Attention to surgical detail minimizes the chance of incisional problems following abomasopexy.

Right Flank Omentopexy. This standing procedure is favored by many clinicians for surgical correction of simple LDA or RDA. It can be performed with minimal assistance, allows manual reposition of the abomasum, and has few incisional risks. As in any procedure done with the animal standing, minimal risk of regurgitation exists so that there is no fear of operating on a DA cow with concurrent problems such as pneumonia or musculoskeletal disorders that may be worsened during dorsal recumbency. Among the disadvantages are that the entire abomasum frequently is not available for

inspection, the repositioning is relative rather than absolute, the integrity of the omentopexy may be affected by tears in the omentum or excessively fat cows, and future RDA is possible despite an intact omentopexy.

Left Flank Abomasopexy. This procedure is used by some surgeons to correct LDA. It has the advantages of a standing procedure as listed above and incorporates an abomasopexy through a continuous suture placed in the greater curvature of the LDA. The suture is placed such that each end of the nonabsorbable suture is left long and attached to a large needle. These two needles then are directed through the right paramedian ventral abdominal wall in the desired location. The abomasum is repositioned by the surgeon, and the long suture ends are tied by the assistant to the outside of the body wall.

Disadvantages include the possibility of exogenous infection following the sutures into the peritoneal cavity, malposition of the organ or sutures based on limited accessibility of the abomasum in the left flank in some LDA cattle, and failure of abomasopexy if the abomasum is not tightly opposed to the parietal peritoneum or if the sutures break.

A mirror-image procedure through the right flank has been recommended by some practitioners for correction of RDA in cattle.

Blind Tack Abomasopexy and Toggle-Pin Abomasopexy. These procedures have been applied by practitioners when economics dictate an inexpensive and quick alternative to more definitive surgical procedures in cattle affected with LDA. The cow is cast and rolled into dorsal recumbency and the gas-distended abomasum located by simultaneous auscultation and percussion in the right paramedian area. In the blind tack procedure, following minimal preparation of the surgical site, a large half circle upholstery needle attached to nonabsorbable suture is driven through the abdominal wall into the abomasal lumen and back out the abdominal wall. The suture is then tied. One or more sutures are placed in this fashion.

The toggle-pin procedure is similar in that two separate toggle pins attached to sutures are placed through a sharp cannula driven into the abomasal lumen. The ends of the sutures then are tied together. Proponents of this technique cite the advantage of being able to obtain abomasal contents through the cannula to confirm the low pH fluid as abomasal rather than ruminal in origin. This is rarely done; however, it is possible to smell the characteristic odor of abomasal gas through the cannula. Advantages are speed and low cost. Disadvantages are innumerable but include missing the abomasum, obstructing the abomasal body or pyloric region with an encircling suture (Figure 5-37), suturing the abomasum in a malposition, allowing leakage from the abomasal lumen into the peritoneal cavity, puncturing the wrong organ, phlebitis from injury to the mammary vein (Figure 5-38), and risking peritonitis via endogenous

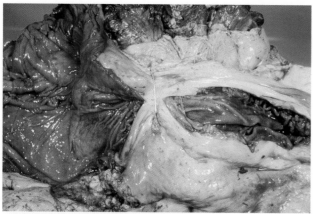

Figure 5-37

Blind stitch complication—the suture has completely obstructed the abomasal at the pylorus, resulting in the cow's death.

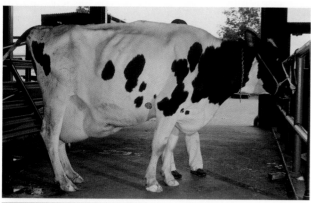

Figure 5-38

Phlebitis of the right mammary vein following blind stitch abomasopexy. This cow died because of endocarditis secondary to this phlebitis.

(abomasal contents) or exogenous (skin, hair, environment) means of contamination of the peritoneal cavity.

Severe complications have been documented subsequent to blind tack and toggle-pin procedures. We continue to see cattle referred because of complications such as toggle pins placed in the cecum, proximal colon, and rumen. Many of these complications have fatal outcomes even following referral and exploratory laparotomy in an often futile attempt to correct the problem. Therefore these procedures cannot be recommended for valuable dairy cows.

In defense of these procedures, in the hands of an experienced practitioner they can be a very cost-effective and labor-saving option in grade cattle. Complications of the toggle-pin procedure can be lessened by prompt identification of a problem in the immediate days following the abomasopexy, promptly removing the suture/toggle if a problem is noticed on the day following the procedure, and making sure that the toggle sutures are not left in place too long (>10 to 14 days).

Cows with simple LDA will show a marked increase in appetite and production in the 48 to 72 hours following the procedure; however, cattle with iatrogenic malpositioning of the abomasum, penetration of another viscus, or significant peritonitis will usually appear worse over this time period. At the very least, releasing the sutures and, at best, exploring the cow at this time may be indicated, but economics frequently dictate that conservative medical treatment is the chosen approach. Cattle that require an exploratory for toggle complications generally have a guarded to poor outcome.

Abomasal Volvulus Following RDA

AV or right-sided volvulus of the abomasum is a serious, life-threatening condition in dairy cattle and is characterized by moderate to severe dehydration, hypochloremic, hypokalemic alkalosis, and mechanical obstruction of abomasal outflow.

Etiology

Although it develops following RDA, incidence of AV following RDA is not known. Certainly it does not follow in all cases of RDA because many cattle can be affected with RDA for many days or even weeks without the complication of AV. Although the gas and fluid distention present in neglected RDA probably predispose to volvulus of the organ, it remains that many cattle with AV have acute (24 to 48 hours) histories of illness and most likely have not had long-standing RDA before AV.

AV may occur in cattle of any age or sex. Most cattle with AV develop the disorder during the 6 weeks following calving, similar to the peak occurrence of DA. Young calves (preweaning) that are affected with RDA frequently develop AV and unfortunately sometimes are erroneously diagnosed with ruminal bloat. The exact mechanism and direction of AV have been debated, but anatomic dissection studies confirm rotation around the lesser curvature that involves the abomasum, omasum, and reticulum. The resultant malposition places the omasum medial to the abomasum and the reticulum caudal to the omasum and medial to the abomasum.

Clinical Signs

Cattle affected with AV usually appear much more depressed, dehydrated, and anxious than cattle with simple DA. Appetite and milk production decrease acutely and dramatically following development of AV. Physical examination reveals normal temperature, a heart rate that varies from bradycardia (less than 60 beats/min) to 110 beats/min, normal or reduced (due to severe alkalosis) respiratory rate, cool peripheral parts, anxious expression (Figure 5-39), and dehydration (Figure 5-40). Frequently the distended abomasum appears as right-sided abdominal

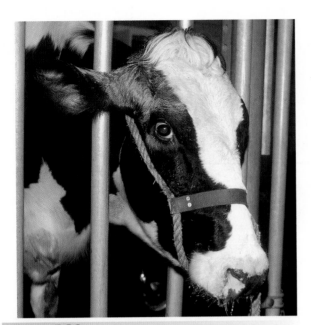

Figure 5-39

Anxious expression in a cow with abomasal volvulus.

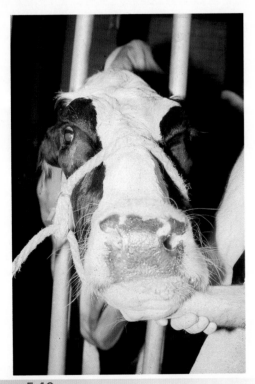

Figure 5-40

Severe dehydration (sunken eyes) in a Holstein cow with abomasal volvulus.

distention or "sprung rib cage" as viewed from the rear of the cow (Figure 5-41). The AV may be so large as to extend caudally behind the thirteenth rib, causing an obvious quarter moon or half moon distention that is visible and palpable in the right paralumbar fossa. Simultaneous auscultation and percussion will produce a large area of

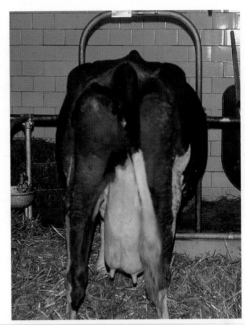

Figure 5-41

"Sprung" rib cage in a cow with abomasal volvulus.

tympanic resonance under the right rib cage. The area of "ping" usually extends cranially to the ninth or eighth rib and caudally to the thirteenth rib or into the paralumbar fossa as discussed previously (Figures 5-42 to 5-44) and may be larger than the ping associated with simple RDA (Figure 5-45). Combined ballottement and auscultation will confirm a large fluid wave within the AV on the right side. Rarely, the ping includes the entire paralumbar fossa or an extreme cranial location (Figure 5-46) and may indicate omental tearing with loosening of the abomasum from its attachments. Cecal dilatation, distention of the spiral colon, and/or pneumorectum or pneumoperitoneum may occur simultaneously with RDA, causing some confusion in the interpretation of the "pings" (Figures 5-45 and 5-47).

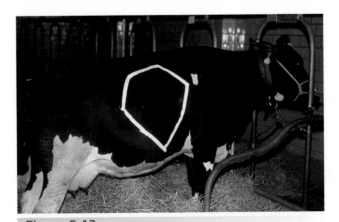

Figure 5-42

Tympanic area resulting from abomasal volvulus in a Holstein cow.

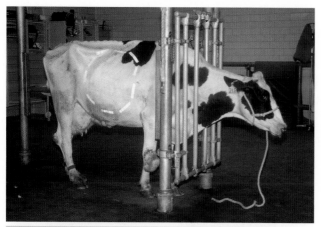

Figure 5-43

Large tympanic area of gas and succussible fluid in a cow with an abomasal volvulus.

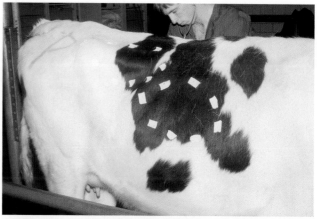

Figure 5-45

Typical area of ping in a cow with both a right abomasal displacement and pneumorectum.

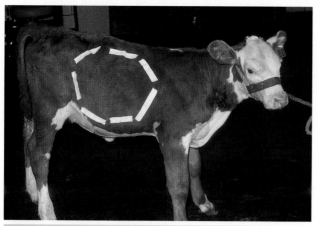

Figure 5-44

Tympanic area resulting from abomasal volvulus in a 4-week-old Hereford calf.

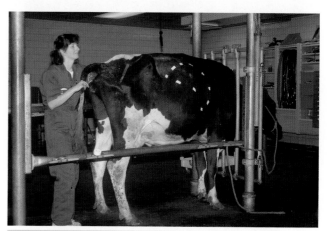

Figure 5-46

Marked cranial location of ping from a right displaced abomasum and omental tear.

In some cattle, it is difficult to differentiate RDA from early AV based on the physical examination. In general, cattle with AV will be moderately to severely dehydrated, have cool extremities, and appear more anxious than cattle with simple RDA. In addition, the examiner is more likely to palpate the distended abomasum per rectum in AV than in RDA. If the abomasum can be palpated per rectum in AV, one feels the distended greater curvature lying against the right flank area at arm's length. The greater omentum is palpable covering the organ in most instances and seems to help differentiate it from a distended cecum or proximal colon. Furthermore, it is difficult on rectal examination to get one's hand and arm between the abomasum and lateral body wall with an RDA or AV. With cecal distention, the examiner can usually palpate both the medial and lateral surface of the distended viscus.

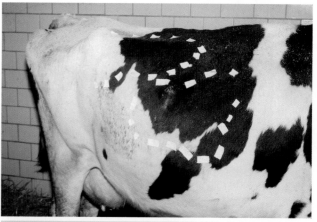

Figure 5-47

Holstein cow with abomasal volvulus and cecal dilation. Only by rectal examination could the more caudal-dorsal ping be determined to be cecal dilation instead of pneumorectum, pneumoperitoneum, or gas in the descending colon.

Slow, extremely shallow respirations occasionally are observed in cattle affected with AV. This physical sign often signals severe metabolic alkalosis with respiratory compensation as the animal attempts to retain carbon dioxide through decreased respiratory effort. Bloat also is observed in some cattle affected with AV and is probably secondary to the true mechanical outflow disturbance created from the abomasum and pylorus by AV or caused by secondary ileus preceded by hypocalcemia in some AV patients.

Clinical Pathology

Cattle affected with AV typically have hemoconcentration and moderate to severe hypochloremic, hypokalemic, metabolic alkalosis. Serum chloride concentrations range from 80 to 90 in early cases to 65 to 80 in neglected or severe cases. Plasma chloride values and base excess show a roughly direct correlation with the clinical prognosis in most cases. In extremely advanced AV, however, devitalization of the affected organs, shock, and lactic acidosis produce metabolic acidosis that overwhelms the previous metabolic alkalosis, while masking the laboratory severity of the metabolic disorder! Therefore a cow with a large AV, severe dehydration, cool peripheral parts, AV palpable per rectum, and weakness, but having measured acid-base and electrolyte values in the normal or metabolic acidosis range, probably has a grave prognosis. Marked elevation in plasma L-lactate could indicate poor systemic and/or abomasal perfusion. If metabolic acidosis is present, but hypochloremia and hypokalemia also are present, the possibility of severe ketoacidosis should be investigated and the prognosis adjusted accordingly. Respiratory acidosis is often present due to respiratory compensation for metabolic alkalosis or severe abdominal distention, which may compromise depth of respiration. Examples of anticipated or approximate acid-base and electrolyte values are provided in Table 5-2. Although many publications have detailed statistical correlations of prognosis for cattle with AV based on acid-base and electrolyte or anion gap or lactate values, clinicians must not fail to look at the patient when offering a prognosis. A cow should never be denied surgical repair based *only* on laboratory values if her physical parameters are fair to good. In general, the prognosis varies directly with chloride levels and hydration status, whereas it varies inversely with heart rate preoperatively, duration of AV, plasma lactate, and anion gap. If the cow is acidotic and recumbent, the prognosis is extremely grave.

Although ketosis and hypocalcemia may be present and require treatment in those with AV, they usually are overshadowed by acid-base and electrolyte abnormalities. Serum sorbitol dehydrogenase or ornithine carbamoyl elevations in cows with LDA suggest hepatic lipidosis, but with AV their elevations may be the result of systemic hypotension and/or inflammatory response. CBC and peritoneal fluid analysis are rarely helpful in cattle affected with AV unless the condition is advanced to a point where tissue necrosis, transudation, or exudation create a left shift in the hemogram and elevated white blood cells and protein in the peritoneal fluid.

Treatment

The most important treatment for AV is early recognition and correction. AV, as opposed to simple LDA or possibly RDA, is a progressive disorder, and the eventual outcome is dictated largely by the duration and nature of volvulus. Early suspicion by the owner with subsequent early diagnosis and surgical correction (<12 hours' duration) by the veterinarian offers a good prognosis in most instances. Those cattle affected with AV for longer than 24 hours probably have a less than 50% prognosis following surgical correction, and cattle affected longer than 48 hours generally have an extremely poor prognosis. These guidelines must be coupled with the physical examination findings because it is possible that a cow could have had RDA for 24 to 36 hours and have developed AV in the 12 hours before diagnosis, thus making the prognosis less grave.

Treatment consists of surgical correction of the volvulus and medical correction of dehydration and electrolyte and acid-base disturbances. Surgical treatment consists of either right flank omentopexy or right paramedian abomasopexy, depending on the preference and judgment of the surgeon. Other surgical approaches are contraindicated because they offer no direct means of access to the affected abomasum, omasum, and reticulum. The surgeon will encounter the omasum lying medial to the abomasum and the reticulum caudal to its normal location because of volvulus involving the lesser curvature of the abomasum, omasum, and reticulum. The right flank approach is less stressful, less likely to cause regurgitation, allows direct access to the volvulus for abomasotomy to drain fluid and gas, allows easier anatomic realignment of omasum and abomasum, and can be done with less help. The major advantage of right paramedian abomasopexy is exact relocation of the abomasum once correction of the volvulus is completed. This helps ensure that the greatly distended abomasum and pylorus will remain well positioned postoperatively as opposed to the right flank omentopexy, after which a greatly distended abomasum may tend to remain slightly displaced to the right following correction. Abomasopexy is arguably more difficult for the inexperienced surgeon in AV cases because of the anatomic difficulties and because it may allow regurgitation in patients with severe ruminal and abomasal distention. In either approach, manipulation of the omasum can be helpful when correcting the volvulus. The omasum is lifted or pushed dorsally and laterally in an attempt to reposition both omasum and abomasum.

Replacement of the abomasum is facilitated by removal of the gaseous distention via suction. In those with severe AV and more than 10 L of fluid present, abomasotomy (purse string a stomach tube into the viscus) to relieve fluid distention may be necessary and is more easily accomplished through a right flank surgical approach. Rehydration and correction of acid-base/electrolyte deficits may be performed postoperatively in early cases, but it may be necessary to address some of these needs preoperatively in severe cases, lest hypokalemia progress to diffuse muscular weakness. In early cases or cattle with AV that have mild dehydration, postoperative oral fluids (20 to 40 L water) and potassium chloride supplementation (30 to 120 g orally, twice daily) suffice for medical needs postoperatively because the gastrointestinal tract has been realigned and should have normal absorptive capacity. With moderate to severe dehydration and metabolic alkalosis, 1 to 2 L of IV hypertonic saline or 20 to 60 L IV physiologic saline with 40 mEq/L potassium chloride may be necessary to correct existing deficits. From a practical standpoint, oral administration should be used once the AV is surgically corrected except in extremely severe cases in which forestomach ileus persists postoperatively. Oral fluids probably are contraindicated preoperatively because they may worsen abdominal distention before surgery. Associated hypocalcemia or ketosis and any concurrent diseases should be treated as indicated. In our hospital it is routine practice to administer 500 mg of flunixin meglumine and 1 to 2 L of hypertonic saline IV and 500 ml of calcium SQ before surgery to correct an AV and to monitor ionized calcium following surgery.

Prognosis and Sequelae

Two major complications of AV—direct damage to vagal nerve branches and vascular thrombosis along the lesser curvature location of the volvulus—are responsible for most poor results or deaths following surgical correction and medical fluid therapy. Most cattle that survive surgery for AV and receive fluid therapy appear dramatically improved in appetite and attitude following this treatment for 24 to 72 hours. Clinical experience, however, indicates that a good prognosis cannot be offered until 96 hours postoperatively. Vagal nerve damage or vascular thrombosis (Figure 5-48, A and B), if present, usually results in failure of abomasal outflow by this time. If AV patients are diagnosed and properly treated within 1 to 4 hours after onset of clinical signs, these complications are much less common than in AV patients that are not surgically corrected for 24 hours. Either complication results in progressive abdominal distention, dehydration, bradycardia, decreased appetite, decreased fecal production, ineffectual rumen contractions, and weight loss that mimics the signs of vagus indigestion (Figure 5-49). The aforementioned signs

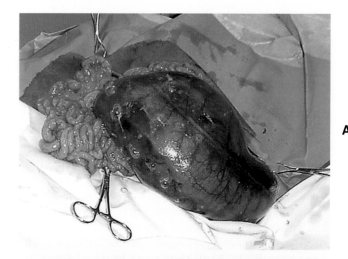

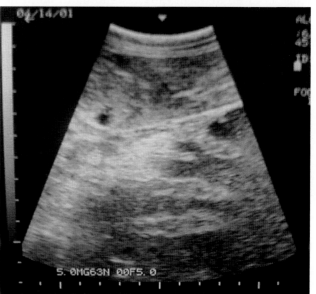

Figure 5-48

A, Purple discoloration of an abomasum with severe vascular compromise as a result of abomasal volvulus. **B,** Ultrasound of the right abdomen of the cow showing the distended abomasum and abomasal folds.

respond poorly to symptomatic therapy, but the cattle may survive for weeks before death occurs (see the section on Vagus Indigestion).

Occasional cattle with severe AV and subsequent abomasal devitalization die of abomasal perforation and diffuse peritonitis within 72 hours postoperatively, but this complication is rare in contrast to the two previously described complications that cause slow deterioration.

Without question, early recognition of illness by an experienced owner, coupled with early diagnosis and surgical intervention by an experienced veterinarian, improves the prognosis for cattle affected with AV. Cows with AV that are recumbent and cannot rise, even after correcting hypocalcemia, are often acidotic and have an extremely poor prognosis.

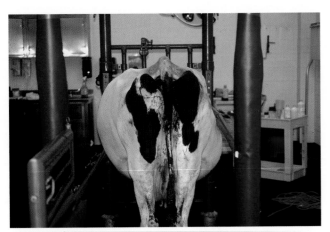

Figure 5-49

Vagal signs in a cow following correction of an abomasal volvulus. This is generally a poor prognosis, but this cow luckily lived.

Abomasal Ulcers

Etiology

Abomasal ulcers in dairy cattle and calves are common clinical problems. Intensive management and highly acidic diets consisting of concentrates and silage probably contribute to the pathogenesis of abomasal ulcers. Abomasal ulcers occur frequently in herds that feed high-moisture corn and corn silage as a major portion of the diet. Stress, although a poorly defined entity, also contributes in the recently fresh cow. Additionally, higher producing cattle seem predisposed to abomasal ulcers, and it is possible that the greater increase in cardiac output going to the udder may cause a relative underperfusion of the abdominal viscera, which could predispose to abomasal ulceration. Most clinically detectable abomasal ulcers in dairy cattle occur within the first 4 to 6 weeks of lactation. The second most common time in adult dairy cattle seems to be just before freshening and may be related to increased plasma cortisol and decreased abomasal perfusion caused by shunting of a higher percentage of cardiac output to the fetus. Young, rapidly growing calves also frequently are affected with abomasal ulceration and perforation. In many cases, predisposing factors may be difficult to determine, although feeding of large volumes of milk in only two daily feedings may be involved in the pathogenesis. Calves and adult cows treated with NSAIDs may also develop abomasal ulcers; we have commonly seen this in young calves receiving flunixin and in bulls being treated with NSAIDs for prolonged periods for musculoskeletal disorders. Lymphosarcoma may also cause bleeding abomasal ulcers in adult cattle.

Clinical Signs

Perforating abomasal ulcers may be seen in calves, bulls, older heifers, and milking cows at any stage of lactation or gestation. They are most common in cows during the first 6 weeks of lactation. Because the clinical syndrome can vary tremendously depending on the size and number of perforations, this discussion will be divided into a section on perforations that cause localized peritonitis and another on those that cause diffuse peritonitis. Perforating ulcers that cause localized peritonitis in cattle produce a syndrome similar to traumatic reticuloperitonitis. An acute leakage of abomasal contents occurs but is walled off by the omentum and fibrinous adhesions (Figure 5-50), and the abomasum becomes adherent to the parietal peritoneum and/or to the omentum. The septic reaction from the perforation may also be trapped and localized between the abomasum and diaphragm. Cows with localized peritonitis caused by a perforated abomasal ulcer are anorectic to a variable degree, usually febrile with a fever of 103.0 to 105.0° F (39.44 to 40.56° C), have rumen hypomotility or stasis, and have a painful abdomen. The cow will be reluctant to move, and deep palpation of the ventral abdomen usually will localize a painful area of the midventral abdomen to the right of the midline. In calves, the same signs are present, but ruminal tympany is more common secondary to ileus because of the localized peritonitis; calves with perforating abomasal ulcers seem to be more likely to develop diffuse peritonitis than adult cows. Occasionally some affected cattle will grind their teeth. Anatomic localization of pain is done more easily in acute cases. In subacute or chronic abdominal cases, pain may be difficult to localize, thereby making the differentiation of this syndrome from traumatic reticulitis difficult. Ultrasound examination may be helpful in determining the extent of the peritonitis. If the cow is known to have a magnet in her reticulum (either by history or by confirmation with a compass), abomasal ulceration is much more likely than hardware; conversely, if the cow is in the mid or late lactation stage, abomasal ulceration is less likely than hardware. Symptoms can vary widely depending on the size of the

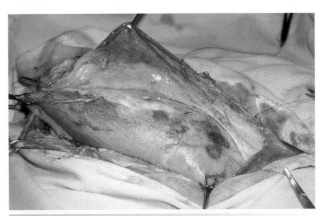

Figure 5-50

Fibrinous localized peritonitis on the abomasal serosa from a small perforating ulcer discovered during abomasopexy.

perforation and the resulting amount of localized peritonitis present. Cattle and calves affected with ulcers that cause diffuse peritonitis are much different on initial presentation than those with localized peritonitis. Massive leakage of abomasal contents (Figures 5-51 to 5-53) prevents localization of the infection. Signs include acute complete anorexia, complete stasis of the forestomach and distal gastrointestinal tract, fever (typically 104.0 to 106.5° F/40.0 to 41.39° C) that may be present for only a few hours, cold skin and peripheral parts, dehydration, a reluctance to move, an audible grunt or groan with each expiration if the animal is forced to move or rise, generalized abdominal pain, pulse rate elevated to 100 to 140 beats/min, severe depression, and progression to recumbency. Basically the animal is in a state of septic shock similar to that seen with severe coliform mastitis. Calves with perforated abomasal ulcers are often either found dead or, if alive,

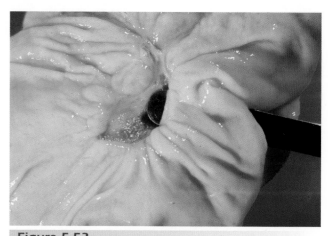

Figure 5-53

Large (3.0 cm) perforating ulcer in a cow that died with diffuse peritonitis. *(Courtesy John M. King, DVM.)*

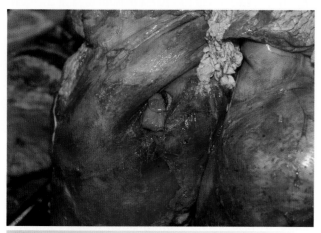

Figure 5-51

Large perforating abomasal ulcer that caused diffuse peritonitis and death in a cow. Abomasal mucosa protrudes through the full-thickness ulcer.

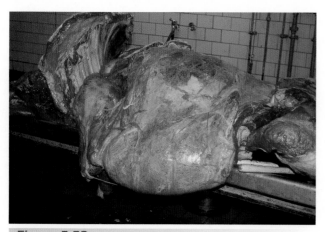

Figure 5-52

Diffuse peritonitis with large sheets of fibrin coating all the viscera following abomasal perforation.

are recumbent (Figure 5-54) and have abdominal distention and respiratory distress. The entire course of the disease can be peracute, with death occurring within 6 hours, or can be extended to 36 to 72 hours or longer if medical support is provided. The prognosis is grave, and if the body temperature begins to decrease or is subnormal when the animal is first attended, the animal usually dies within 12 to 36 hours.

Bleeding abomasal ulcers are uncommon in calves compared with perforating ulcers. In adult cows, they can be seen at any stage of lactation but are most common during the first 6 weeks of lactation. Bleeding abomasal ulcers can be categorized by the extent of abomasal hemorrhage.

Abomasal ulcers with slight bleeding are the most difficult to diagnose because signs are not profound. Asymptomatic cattle that have mild bleeding may pass small, tarry, partially digested blood clots intermittently in the manure, whereas symptomatic cattle show mild

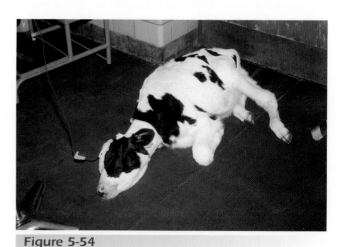

Figure 5-54

A 3-week-old calf with an acute onset of septic shock caused by a perforated ulcer.

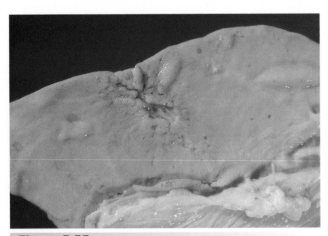

Figure 5-55

Abomasal mucosal ulceration. Such a lesion may result in mild hemorrhage from the abomasum. *(Courtesy John M. King, DVM.)*

chronic abdominal pain, periodic grinding of the teeth, capricious appetite, and intermittent occult blood present in the manure (Figure 5-55). Such symptomatic cattle appear interested in feed but stop eating after a few mouthfuls, as if aware of abdominal discomfort. Positive diagnosis is difficult and is made by elimination of other diseases, coupled with a normal abdominal paracentesis and positive fecal occult blood. A fecal occult blood test should be performed on a sample obtained before an extensive rectal examination to avoid false-positive results.

Cattle with bleeding abomasal ulcers causing major hemorrhage have normal temperatures but show obvious melena (Figure 5-56) and partial to complete anorexia. When complete anorexia and severe depression are apparent, the cow usually shows all the cardinal signs of massive blood loss. These signs include: pale to chalk white mucous membranes (Figure 5-57), a pulse rate elevated to 100 to 140 beats/min, weak pulse, rapid and shallow respirations, weakness, and cool extremities. A typical sweetish odor of digested blood can be detected around the melena-stained perineum or tail. Diagnosis usually only requires physical examination if melena is obvious (Figure 5-58, *A* and *B*). Manure may be normal consistency or more commonly loose. A packed-cell volume, total serum protein, evaluation of hydration status, and fecal occult blood test can be used for ancillary and confirmatory purposes.

Although most abomasal ulcers are *either* bleeding or perforating, occasionally an animal demonstrates signs consistent with both perforation and bleeding. Long-standing displacement of the abomasum predisposes to both perforation and bleeding. Therefore this syndrome tends to occur in animals not observed closely or not thought to be likely candidates for DA (heifers, bulls,

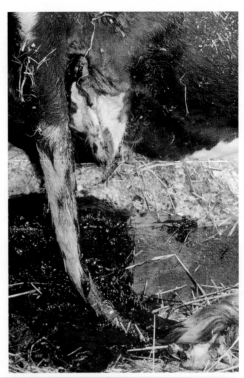

Figure 5-56

Black tarry feces (melena) caused by a bleeding abomasal ulcer.

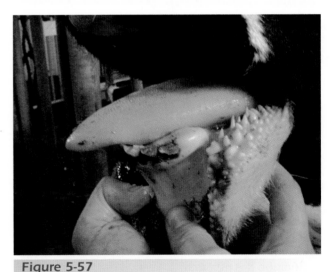

Figure 5-57

White mucous membranes of the mouth in a Holstein cow with bleeding abomasal ulcer and PCV of 14%.

and dry cows). These animals are often kept in group housing and are not observed carefully; partial anorexia in a single animal sometimes could go unnoticed for days or weeks.

Chronic distention of the displaced abomasum contributes to physical stretching or tearing of the abomasal mucosa and diminished perfusion. Furthermore, constant exposure of the compromised mucosa to large

A

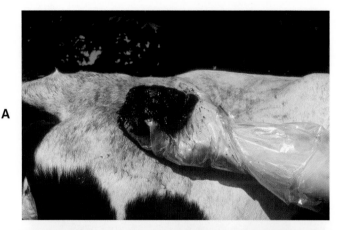

B

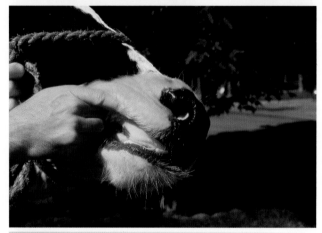

Figure 5-58

Melena **(A)** and pale membranes **(B)** of a cow with bleeding abomasal ulcer and PCV of 11%.

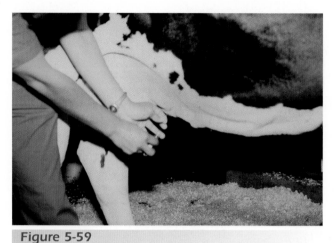

Figure 5-59

Most common location for performing a peritoneal centesis in a cow.

amounts of retained hydrochloric acid propagates ulceration. Hemorrhage results from multiple mucosal erosions and ulcerations that can deepen to cause major submucosal hemorrhage or frank perforation. Symptoms include anorexia, partial to complete ileus, melena, fever, elevated pulse rate, and abdominal pain. Displacement of the abomasum may be present, and abdominal pain will be most intense when pressure is exerted in the region of the displacement. Signs of pneumoperitoneum and fever also may be present if perforation has occurred.

Laboratory Data

The best ancillary aid to diagnosis of perforating ulcers causing localized peritonitis is abdominal paracentesis, which typically demonstrates increased numbers of white blood cells (>5000 to 6000/μl) and protein (>3.0 g/dl). Although it would be helpful to see bacteria either free or in macrophages as well in this fluid, these seldom are present because the cow has such an inherent ability to "wall off" localized peritonitis with fibrin. The peritoneal tap can most easily be performed just in front of the udder on the

right side and on either side of the mammary vein (Figure 5-59); an 18-gauge, 1.5-inch needle should be directed perpendicular into and through the abdominal wall until fluid is obtained. If there is a fetid smell to the fluid and the plasma protein is low, this suggests more diffuse peritonitis and a poor prognosis. Ultrasound examination can be of value in detecting pockets of fluid and fibrin. CBCs and serum biochemistry seldom are helpful in making a diagnosis, although an inflammatory leukogram in combination with an abnormally low chloride may be seen in some cases.

Similarly, in cattle affected with perforating ulcers that cause diffuse peritonitis, abdominal paracentesis confirms the diagnosis. A large amount of inflammatory exudate is obtained easily. The total solids and total protein always are elevated (>3.0 g/dl protein), but the white blood cell count may be surprisingly low (<10,000) in some acute cases. This low count, despite obvious massive peritonitis, is simply dilutional because the affected cow usually has gallons of exudate in the abdomen. A neutropenia with left shift frequently is present in the leukogram, and serum albumin, as well as total protein values, is low because of loss of protein into the peritoneal cavity. A similar dilutional effect on protein and cell levels in abdominal fluid may be observed in calves with diffuse peritonitis caused by abomasal perforation.

For cattle suspected of having bleeding abomasal ulcers, fecal occult blood tests, packed cell volume, and total protein constitute the major laboratory aids. Rarely the bleeding may be so acute that PCV and plasma protein do not accurately predict the severity of the blood loss; mucous membrane color, heart rate, and degree of weakness, in addition to measuring blood lactate, will provide an accurate measurement of the severity of blood loss.

Diagnosis

Diagnosis of perforating abomasal ulceration is based on physical signs, ruling out other causes of peritonitis, and the abdominal paracentesis. Obviously without exploratory surgery or necropsy, the diagnosis of abomasal ulceration is not truly confirmed. The correlation, however, between clinical signs observed in past nonsurvivors or in survivors that had surgery allows a high index of clinical suspicion for abomasal perforation. Diagnosis of bleeding abomasal ulcers is based on clinical signs of pale mucous membranes, high pounding heart rate, melena, and low packed-cell volume (PCV) and protein. In calves, primary perforating abomasal ulcers can be distinguished from abomasitis-ulcer syndrome by the abomasal fluid and gas distention with the abomasitis syndrome. Transabdominal ultrasound can be helpful in adult cattle (see video clip 11) but is particularly useful in calves with diffuse peritonitis, in which a large volume of anechoic abdominal effusion with fibrin can be visualized. Ultrasound examination can also help direct the abdominocentesis to areas of fluid accumulation in cases with low-grade peritonitis and adhesions.

Treatment

The management of perforating abomasal ulcers causing localized peritonitis requires dietary changes and medical therapy. The cow should be held off silage, high-moisture corn, and finely ground concentrates for 5 to 14 days or until clinical evidence of improvement exists. A more fibrous diet including high quality hay should be substituted. If ketosis becomes a complicating factor as high-energy feeds are withdrawn, a coarse calf grain or whole oats can be fed judiciously. Medical therapy includes stall or box stall rest and broad-spectrum antibiotics for 7 to 14 days (or until a normal temperature has been present for at least 48 hours) to control the peritonitis present. In valuable cattle or calves, IV histamine type 2 blockers can be administered (e.g., 1.5 mg/kg ranitidine every 8 hours). Calves that are still nursing may be given small amounts of milk frequently mixed with antacids. If other complications such as hypocalcemia or ketosis are found during the course of the disease, cows should be treated symptomatically. Corticosteroids and NSAIDs are *contraindicated* and should *not* be used because they may contribute to further ulceration; we have observed this to be the case, especially with the use of phenylbutazone or flunixin meglumine in cattle. Most patients require 5 to 14 days for recovery; dietary management should continue until the cow is fully recovered and totally appetent. For calves or on farms with a herd problem of perforating ulcers in calves, more frequent feeding is recommended.

Management of abomasal ulceration with diffuse peritonitis is difficult and highly unsuccessful because of the massive septic peritonitis present. Most commonly, therapy includes high levels of broad-spectrum antibiotics, continuous IV fluids specifically addressing the animal's current acid-base and electrolyte status, and other supportive drugs as necessary. Because of the shocklike state of these animals, most affected calves and cattle are acidotic rather than alkalotic; this fact is important when the clinician considers appropriate IV fluids. Peritoneal lavage should be considered. Few cattle and calves survive this problem, and massive abdominal adhesions are an expected sequela. Also, if lactating, these cows usually dry off for the remainder of the lactation.

Not all cows with diffuse peritonitis following ulcer perforation die on the day of the perforation. Some cows will survive for a few days, but if progressive abdominal distention, complete anorexia, and a decrease in plasma protein are noted, they seldom survive beyond 7 days despite the most intensive therapy.

It is the consensus of most experienced clinicians that perforating abomasal ulcers are best handled medically rather than surgically unless concurrent DA is present. Many reasons exist for this opinion. One is that fibrinous adhesions form quickly in the cow's abdomen; therefore even through a right paramedian abdominal incision, it may be difficult to expose or explore the abomasum sufficiently to surgically oversew or resect the affected area. Another reason is that the ulcerations can be multiple, and resection of all affected abomasum may be impossible. In diffuse peritonitis, the shocklike state of the cow generally results in it dying during surgery. The only cases that are considered for surgery are those with peracute histories (seldom seen in a referral hospital) or cows that do not appear to be responding to medical therapy but have not developed abdominal distention or a precipitous decrease in plasma protein. These latter cows typically stabilize for 24 to 72 hours but then again develop fever, rumen stasis, acute abdominal pain, and symptoms of further abomasal leakage as if fibrinous adhesions have not adequately walled off the perforation. Calves with peracute signs of diffuse peritonitis caused by large perforating ulcers have undergone surgery in an effort to find and oversew the causative ulcer. Medical therapy for shock, coupled with such surgery, has resulted in few survivors.

Usually abomasal ulcers with only slight bleeding can be managed easily by changing the diet as described under treatment of perforating ulcers and administering oral antacid protectants or astringents. Concurrent inflammatory or metabolic diseases, if present, also should be treated.

Abomasal ulcers with major hemorrhage are life threatening and must be treated by medical and dietary means. Dietary management and oral antacid protectants should be used as described under treatment of perforating ulcers. The major medical therapeutic decision is whether a whole-blood transfusion is necessary. If the mucous membranes are chalk white, the pulse rate is greater than 100 beats/min, and the respiratory rate is elevated, a blood transfusion usually will be necessary to allow time for the cow to compensate and respond to its blood loss anemia as the ulcer heals. As in any massive blood loss situation, whole blood transfusion is the only treatment that will stabilize the cow if the blood loss is severe, although isotonic crystalloids are indicated in addition to the whole blood. Whole blood is used to improve both oxygen-carrying capacity and perfusion pressure, whereas crystalloids help improve perfusion. Hypertonic IV fluids should be used only with life-threatening hypotension because they may disrupt clot formation as a result of rapid increases in blood pressure. In Dr. Rebhun's experience, a cow with normal hydration and subacute blood loss (24 to 72 hours) has a transfusion "trigger point" for PCV of 14%. With peracute hemorrhage, which rarely occurs in cattle with bleeding ulcers, PCV and plasma protein concentrations are not good indicators of blood loss in the first 12 to 18 hours of hemorrhage. Clinicians must always base the need for transfusion on clinical signs of pallor, increased heart rate, and increased respiratory rate along with PCV. Cows with PCV less than 14% usually have high respiratory rates, a pulse rate more than 100 beats/min, extremely pale mucous membranes, and will need a transfusion. Hydration status can greatly affect these parameters, and a dehydrated cow with a PCV of 16% to 17%, for example, still may require a transfusion. These guidelines apply to cattle that have experienced fairly rapid blood loss over 24 to 72 hours—not cattle that have chronic anemia with physiologic compensation that may be able to survive with a PCV of 8% to 9% if the blood loss has stopped.

Routine transfusion at this clinic totals 4 to 6 L of whole blood from a healthy cow to the affected animal. Larger volumes may be given provided the donor can tolerate, or is treated for, the volume depletion. Because the multiple blood types present in cattle make a transfusion reaction unlikely, cross-matching is not done. The ideal blood donor would be BLV-negative and not a persistently BVDV-infected animal. Usually one transfusion is sufficient to stabilize the cow until dietary and medical treatment aid healing of the abomasal ulceration. Also, the cow generally has a bone marrow very responsive to blood loss; it tends to self-correct and stabilize quickly once a transfusion has eased the critical situation. Although uncommon, some cattle require two or more transfusions over the first few days of treatment; one cow required seven transfusions during 8 days of continued blood loss from her abomasum. Although transfusions require professional time, they are lifesaving in most cases (even the cow transfused seven times) and thus are worthwhile, especially in a valuable dairy cow. Also, they need not be overly time consuming if the practitioner has the basic equipment

necessary and is well practiced in collecting and administering blood.

Abomasal bleeding can occur secondary to DAs, especially chronic displacements. If melena, anemia, and DA are all present in a cow, the cow should be stabilized, and the severity of its anemia should be assessed. If the PCV is greater than 14% and a transfusion is deemed unnecessary, the DA should be corrected surgically as soon as possible. If the PCV is less than 14% and the cow shows other physical signs of severe anemia (high heart rate, weakness, elevated blood lactate), a blood transfusion should be performed before surgical correction of the DA. Surgical correction of the DA relieves abomasal distention and acid pooling in the abomasum, and hemorrhage usually stops within 24 to 48 hours. Thus the DA appears to contribute to hemorrhage in these cases and warrants prompt surgical correction.

In cases of ulcers that are bleeding *and* perforating, physical examination should confirm the presence or absence of concurrent DA. If left or right displacement is present, the cow should be explored surgically from the right paramedian approach. If the abomasum is locked in an abnormal position by adhesions resulting from perforating ulcers, it will be necessary to decide whether the adhesions can be broken down manually without rupture of the abomasum. Then an attempt to dislodge the abomasum from adhesions to the parietal peritoneum is made, and if successful, abomasopexy and ulcer resection (or oversewing) can be completed (Figure 5-60). Surgical replacement of the organ to its

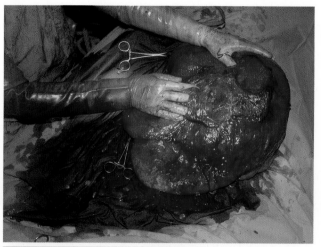

Figure 5-60

Massive adhesions on the surface of an abomasum that had a perforating ulcer subsequent to chronic LDA. The surgeon has successfully separated the adherent abomasum from the parietal peritoneum and delivered the organ through a ventral midline incision. The organ will now be examined for any leakage of ingesta, and an abomasopexy will be performed.

normal location generally will result in marked improvement in the abomasal ulcer symptomatology within 24 to 48 hours.

Dietary changes and broad-spectrum antibiotics should be used for 7 to 14 days following surgery in these difficult cases. Antihistamine H_2 blockers are not commonly used in the therapy of abomasal ulceration in adult cattle. Although primarily because of prohibitive costs, a lack of data exists to support efficacy of these products in the adult ruminant abomasum. Initial work showed little effect on abomasal pH of cattle following administration of cimetidine. However, recent work in sheep suggests that ranitidine may elevate abomasal pH significantly. Unfortunately, the dosage of ranitidine was so high as to be impractical and unaffordable. In calves, ranitidine could be used IV (1.5 mg/kg every 8 hours) or orally (10 mg/kg every 8 hours) mixed in milk. Oral omeprazole (4 mg/kg q 24hr) could also be used in milk-fed calves. Frequent feeding of milk via bottle will itself help increase abomasal pH. The pH can be further increased by adding commercially available antacids to the milk. Sucralfate may also have an additional protective effect and should be mixed in milk feeding four times daily.

Prognosis and Discussion

Prognosis for cattle and calves with perforating abomasal ulcers that cause localized peritonitis is good with dietary and medical management. It is important to continue broad-spectrum antibiotics until the peritonitis is well under control. Once fully recovered for 7 to 14 days, there does not appear to be a tendency for recurrent ulceration, and the animal may return to the herd as a productive individual. The most difficult cases are dry cows with large gravid uteri. These cows seem to have difficulty forming effective adhesions around the perforation. In addition, the gravid uterus may force the abomasum more cranially in the abdomen to lie against the diaphragm. Therefore if a perforating ulcer occurs in a dry cow, the abomasum may remain in this position, which would be considered abnormal in a lactating cow. Such cows may show variable appetites when placed on intensive rations after calving. In addition, we have observed two such dry cows that suffered perforating ulcers with localized peritonitis and adhesions to the diaphragm that subsequently developed septic pleuritis as the diaphragm suffered septic erosion (Figure 5-61). For these reasons, cows in an advanced state of pregnancy may have a more chronic course, may be more prone to multiple episodes of ulceration, and may subsequently develop diffuse peritonitis or omental abscesses. Consequently they have only a poor to fair prognosis.

Prognosis for cattle with perforating abomasal ulcers that cause diffuse peritonitis is grave. Most of these cases in cattle and calves result in death. Some animals can be normal at night and dead "suddenly" by the next

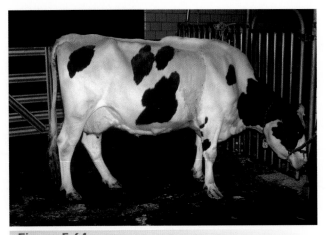

Figure 5-61

A 6-year-old Holstein with septic pleuritis caused by a perforated abomasal ulcer during late pregnancy with adhesions to the diaphragm and eventually necrosis of the diaphragm following calving.

morning. Others live long enough to be diagnosed but die within 24 to 48 hours despite supportive therapy. Infrequent survivors may be left with massive abdominal adhesions despite several weeks of broad-spectrum antibiotics before stabilizing. The current lactation, if the cow is milking, is ruined. Thus only extremely valuable dairy cattle warrant intensive treatment.

The prognosis for cattle with bleeding abomasal ulcers is good if the condition is diagnosed before severe anemia develops. Dietary and medical therapy as discussed above usually will result in a cure within 7 to 14 days. Even in those animals that require blood transfusions, prognosis is good if the clinician and owner are willing to spend the time necessary for effective treatment.

Occasionally lymphosarcoma can cause severe abomasal hemorrhage as the tumor infiltrates the abomasum. Although other lesions of lymphosarcoma usually are obvious on physical examination of these cattle, rare cases have no other lesions detectable at the time that anemia and melena are present. These animals do not respond to blood transfusions and die despite treatment. Neoplastic cells (Figure 5-62) may be observed on peritoneal fluid in approximately 50% of cattle with abomasal lymphoma of which bleeding and evidence of pyloric obstruction are the predominant clinical findings. At autopsy, typical lesions of lymphosarcoma are found (Figure 5-63, *A* and *B*). On very rare occasion abomasal perforation may occur. A thorough physical examination to rule out other lesions of lymphosarcoma always is indicated for cattle having melena. Serologic testing for BLV status may be indicated, but results must be interpreted carefully (see the section on BLV). Right paramedian abdominocentesis may reveal lymphoblasts and is a valuable procedure to perform in cattle over 2 years of age with signs consistent with

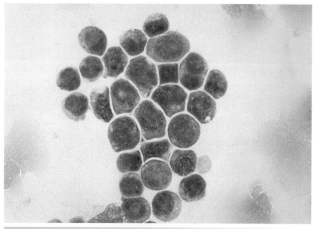

Figure 5-62

Neoplastic lymphocytes in the peritoneal fluid from a 2-year-old Holstein bull with a non-BLV lymphoma of the abomasum.

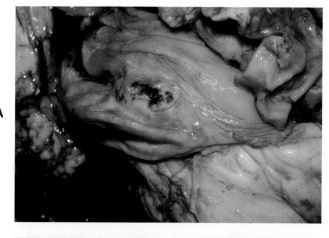

A

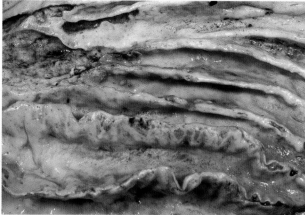

B

Figure 5-63

A and B, Necropsy views of the mucosal surface of an abomasum infiltrated with lymphosarcoma. A deep ulcer that had caused melena in this cow is apparent.

gastrointestinal bleeding caused by abomasal ulceration that are outside of the usual signalment range for early lactational ulcers.

Bleeding abomasal ulcers in calves are rare and sporadic, whereas perforating abomasal ulcers are quite common. The reason for this discrepancy between the calf and the adult cow is not known. Calves experiencing sepsis and concurrent enteritis or receiving parenteral nutrition appear to be at greatest risk for spontaneous abomasal ulcers that perforate.

Prognosis for cattle affected with ulcers that bleed and perforate is poor. Because these cases tend to be chronic or neglected or involve concurrent DA, the lesions can be severe. If displacement of the abomasum is present and can be corrected surgically, the prognosis for the ulcers improves. However, if the perforating ulcers have locked the abomasum in a displaced position or caused a great deal of peritonitis, the prognosis must be guarded to poor. Each of these cases must be assessed and prognosed individually.

Abomasal Fistulas

Abomasal fistulas infrequently develop following surgical abomasopexies or blind abomasopexy procedures such as the blind stitch and toggle-pin techniques. Intimate adhesion of the abomasal visceral peritoneum to the parietal peritoneum, coupled with intraluminal suture placement (unintentional during abomasopexy or intentional during blind tack procedures), can cause abomasal contents to seek an outlet through the body wall following the path of the incisional line (abomasopexy) or through-and-through sutures (blind stitch, toggle pin). In either event, the abomasopexy sutures have penetrated the abomasal lumen to allow egress of ingesta. Eventually the incisional line weakens or breaks down in surgical abomasopexy patients, allowing abomasal contents and mucosa to protrude to the exterior. In through-and-through techniques, the same phenomenon may occur as abomasal ingesta follows the nonabsorbable sutures through the body wall and abomasal mucosa migrates along the suture to the exterior body wall. In some cases, the mucosa eventually prolapses to the exterior and presents as a hemorrhagic, edematous mucosal surface (Figure 5-64). Blood loss may be severe at this time.

Diagnosis is made by observation and learning of a history of abomasopexy. If blood loss appears severe, laboratory data may be necessary for assessment of PCV and plasma protein in anticipation of whole blood transfusion. If the fistula has been chronic, acid-base and electrolyte status should be assessed because chronic chloride loss may have occurred, leading to advanced metabolic alkalosis. The prognosis somewhat depends on the size of the area that must be resected to correct the fistula but should be guarded in all cases.

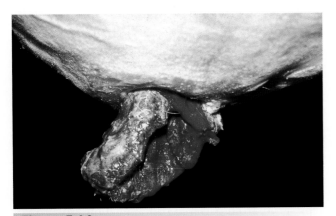

Figure 5-64

Abomasal fistula secondary to an abomasopexy.

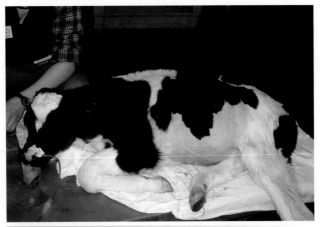

Figure 5-65

Abomasal distention and shock in a 6-week-old calf with acute abomasitis, tympany, and abomasal ulceration. Following surgical drainage of the abomasum, suturing two abomasal ulcers, and intensive medical therapy, the calf recovered.

Treatment consists first of medical therapy with systemic antibiotics, whole blood (if necessary), or replacement balanced-electrolyte solutions, as dictated by physical examination and laboratory data. Second, the abomasal fistula requires surgical resection using an en bloc abdominal wall resection that includes the abomasal adhesion to the parietal peritoneum. Hemostasis and closure of en bloc abdominal wall resection present time-consuming problems for the surgeon. Fistulas through abomasopexy incisions are often complicated by incisional hernias that also require resection, thereby creating a larger abdominal wall defect. Successful primary closure of the site following en bloc resection has been reported. In severe cases with huge body wall defects and infection, closure can be accomplished by through-and-through tension mattress sutures using heavy surgical steel sutures and quill sutures. Postoperatively, the wound is bandaged and the cow maintained on systemic antibiotics until the incisional area heals "from the inside out" completely in approximately 2 to 4 weeks. General anesthesia is highly desireable for these procedures.

Abomasitis, Abdominal Tympany, and Abomasal Ulceration Syndrome in Calves

Etiology

This is a clinical syndrome with characteristic clinical signs and pathological findings in nursing calves of which the exact etiology(s) remains unproven. *Clostridium perfringens* type A, *Sarcinia* sp. and *Salmonella typhimurium* DT104 have all been incriminated. Although outbreaks of the syndrome have been described in nursing beef calves and lambs, in dairy calves it is mostly sporadic and/or endemic on a farm.

Clinical Signs

Affected calves are milk-fed calves, often 2 to 4 weeks of age, which develop acute bloat, anorexia, rapidly progressive depression leading to recumbency, and

frequently shock. Affected calves may have diarrhea or colicky signs, although these are inconsistent findings. On clinical examination, the calves are noticeably distended (Figure 5-65) and have variable location and size, sometimes large, abdominal pings with easily succussible fluid in the ventral abdomen. Affected calves have tachycardia, cold extremities, and other signs of shock/poor perfusion. The progression of clinical signs can be rapid.

Laboratory Findings

Severely affected calves frequently have a metabolic (high lactate, high anion gap) acidosis. Other abnormalities include low serum chloride, azotemia, elevated PCV, and immature and toxic-appearing neutrophils. With severe abdominal distention and/or depression, respiratory acidosis (hypoventilation) may accompany the metabolic acidosis and cause acidemia less than 7.0.

Diagnosis

The diagnosis is based on the age of the calf, the characteristic clinical findings, and laboratory evidence of acidosis, dehydration, and sepsis. Differentials would include displaced abomasum, acute peritonitis caused by perforated abomasal ulcer or ruminal bloat, either idiopathic or resulting from ruminal milk accumulation. Calves with ruminal bloat would generally not be as sick as calves with abomasitis and would not have the amount of succussible fluid characteristically found with the abomasitis syndrome. Evidence of ruminal drinking and abomasitis may be concurrent in some calves, but this is not characteristic. Ultrasound examination often demonstrates an edematous and thickened wall of the abomasum (Figure 5-66). Significant abdominal effusion is rarely noted in calves

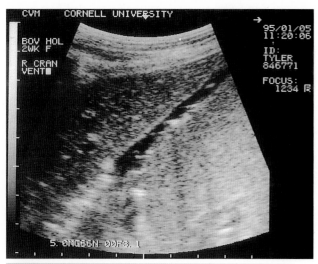

Figure 5-66

Ultrasound of the abdomen of a calf with abomasitis showing marked edema (black) of the abomasal wall. The liver is seen between the body wall and the abomasum.

with nonperforated abomasitis, but its presence should raise suspicion of full-thickness perforation and carry a grave prognosis.

Treatment

Calves with progressive signs associated with abomasitis should be treated intensively with colloids, crystalloids and systemic antibiotics. Colloids (plasma or hetastarch) may have particular benefit in severely affected calves because there is evidence of systemic inflammatory shock, leaky capillaries, and a predisposition for intestinal wall edema and pulmonary edema. Systemic antibiotics are indicated because there is high potential for translocation of *Clostridial* spp. or other intestinal bacterial from the gut to other organs. An oral-gastric/rumen tube should be passed because in some cases a large amount of fetid fluid is refluxed, which improves the clinical condition of the calf. It is unclear whether this reflux is part of the abomasal fluid or if rumen putrefaction plays a role in the disease in some calves. In many cases, there is no reflux. Regardless, penicillin is often administered orally in an attempt to decrease intestinal clostridial overgrowth. There is a technique of abomasal puncture described for lambs that have severe abomasal tympany, but this is untested in calves. *C. perfringens* C and D antitoxin is frequently given SQ or orally, but efficacy is unproven.

If the calves do not respond promptly to fluid therapy and passage of the oral-rumen tube and/or abdominal distention and signs of shock do not rapidly improve, a laparotomy to empty the abomasum and oversew any apparent abomasal ulceration sites should be performed. If there are no abomasal perforations and hypotension

can be reversed, the calves may have a fair to good prognosis. Affected calves may die quickly from acute peritonitis and/or severe hypotension, or some may linger following surgery and die several days later from peritonitis and adhesions.

Preventative recommendations are unknown, although it seems as if "greedy" nursers are most often affected, which suggests that either ruminal drinking or abomasal stasis may allow overgrowth of the causative organism. Because the problem can be endemic on some farms, a concentrated effort at routine disinfection of equipment, proper handling of the milk or milk replacer to avoid bacterial contamination, isolation of affected calves, and disinfection of their stalls all seem pertinent. One farm that had several cases of abomasitis in calves prevented further cases by administering oral penicillin mixed in the milk. Dividing the milk into increased number of feedings may also be helpful. Vaccination of adult cattle or calves with *C. perfringens* type C and D vaccines should not be expected to provide significant protection against any of the incriminated organisms. Anecdotal field observations have suggested that the condition may be more common in calves fed according to accelerated milk replacer programs, particularly when ad libitum access to water is denied. On rare occasion we have seen a similar condition in adult cows appearing similar to braxy (*Clostridium septicum*).

Abomasal Impaction

Etiology

Primary abomasal impaction in adults may be caused by extremely fibrous feed or pica with subsequent heavy ingestion of sand, nut shells, or rocks, or it may be idiopathic. Primary abomasal impaction resulting from extremely fibrous feeds and lack of water as seen in wintered beef cattle is rare in dairy cattle. Secondary causes, which are more common, include pyloric outflow disturbances secondary to ventral vagus nerve injuries, vascular or neurogenic damage secondary to AV, abdominal adhesions, pyloric masses or adhesions, and lymphosarcoma. Traumatic reticuloperitonitis and peritonitis associated with perforating abomasal ulcers are the most common causes of abomasal impaction at our clinic. These conditions may create either neurogenic or mechanical abomasal outflow disturbances. Other hospitals have diagnosed this condition more commonly, often without a known etiology.

In calves, idiopathic abomasal impaction may be observed in any breed but is most common in Guernseys. Calves having peritonitis for any reason also may develop abomasal impaction secondary to abdominal adhesions. Neurogenic damage to the vagus nerve in calves having AV or chronic DA also provides a risk of subsequent abomasal impaction.

Clinical Signs

Signs are not specific and are similar to those observed in all vagus indigestion patients. Progressive abdominal distention may occur over days to weeks, and the patient has an intermittent appetite, reduced manure production that is frequently loose or watery, weight loss, and decreased milk production. Diarrhea is common because primarily fluid ingesta escapes the abomasum and bypasses the impaction. Abdominal distention, if present, is like that of vagus indigestion with high left, low left, and low right distention. In other cases, the signs are not pronounced, and decreased appetite is the only clinical finding. Rumen contractions may be normal to absent to increased in frequency. In calves, the firm, enlarged abomasum sometimes can be palpated or visualized with ultrasound, but this is seldom possible in adult cattle. Rectal examination of adult cattle usually finds enlargement of the rumen dorsal and ventral sacs. Rarely the enlarged abomasum may be palpated in the right lower quadrant, but usually the enlarged ventral sac of the rumen occupies this position.

Cattle with abomasal impaction sometimes grind their teeth and may show evidence of pain in response to deep pressure in the midabdomen. Temperature, pulse rate, and respiratory rate usually are normal unless bradycardia secondary to vagal nerve irritation is present.

Ancillary Data

Varying degrees of metabolic alkalosis occur depending on the degree of HCl retention or reflux into the forestomach. Surprisingly, some patients with abomasal impactions have only moderate or no metabolic alkalosis, perhaps resulting from the insidious chronic progression of the disease, location of the impaction, and less than complete obstruction to outflow.

Diagnosis

The diagnosis of abomasal impaction is made during right-side exploratory laparotomy or left-side laparotomy and rumenotomy. For cattle showing signs of vagus nerve injury, diagnosis usually is made by palpation of the abomasum through the also distended rumen during rumenotomy. The majority of cattle with abomasal impaction have impactions of the pyloric antrum alone, whereas more severe cases have impaction of the abomasal body and pyloric antrum.

Treatment

Passage of a stomach tube through the reticuloomasal orifice into the abomasum during rumenotomy allows mineral oil or dioctyl sodium succinate to be delivered to the impaction. However, a one-time medical treatment such as this is rarely expected to work if there is vagus nerve injury. Laxatives, ruminotorics, and laxative feeds seldom are successful in those cases, although coffee (1 lb given in the rumen) has helped some cases. Definitive treatment for vagal indigestion/abomasal impactions may require abomasotomy performed on a recumbent patient, usually through a low right paracostal or ventral right paramedian approach. Prognosis is guarded for all nerve injury abomasal impactions, but some may be helped if specific causative lesions such as adhesions or malposition of the organ can be corrected. Abomasal impactions secondary to peritonitis of any type carry a poor prognosis. Idiopathic abomasal impactions may carry a good prognosis with massage via right flank laparotomy and administration of mineral oil, coffee (1 lb), or magnesium products for 2 to 5 days. Those with antrum impactions alone have a better prognosis than cows with abomasal body impactions.

Abomasal Neoplasia

The most important tumor involving the abomasum is lymphosarcoma. The abomasum is one of the favorite "target" regions for multicentric lymphosarcoma in cattle. The tumor may invade the wall of the abomasum diffusely or in multifocal fashion (Figure 5-67). The pyloric region may be obstructed, resulting in an outflow disturbance from the abomasum and forestomach compartments. On rare occasion biliary outflow may be obstructed, causing icterus and marked elevation in gamma glutamyl transferase. Serum chloride is almost always low (sometimes <70 mEq/L) and rumen chloride is high (>60 mEq/L) if the lymphoma is obstructing the pylorus. Affected cows may have progressive abdominal distention (Figure 5-68) and eventually become so weak they cannot rise. We have treated a small number of pregnant cows with lymphoma with Predef 2X (Pfizer, New York, NY) and on rare occasion had enough improvement that the cow remained alive until the calf was born. Owners were made aware of the fact

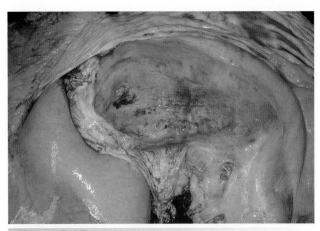

Figure 5-67

Necropsy view of an abomasum infiltrated with lymphosarcoma. The corrugations and raised areas are neoplastic lesions.

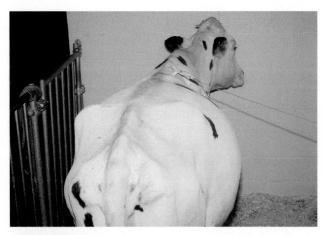

Figure 5-68

Slowly progressive and now severe abdominal distention caused by pyloric obstruction from pyloric lymphosarcoma, resulting in abomasal and forestomach compartment distention.

the calf was at high risk of being infected with BLV and would be predisposed to developing the neoplasia. In other cases, melena is the only sign observed as the neoplasia progresses to cause abomasal ulceration and hemorrhage. The diagnosis can usually be made by knowledge of the age of the cow (usually 4 years or older), clinical signs, evidence of tumorous disease elsewhere in the cow, BLV status of the cow, ultrasound examination of the abomasum (can usually be seen with diffuse involvement), and cytological examination of peritoneal fluid and blood. A low percentage of cows with lymphoma have blast cells in the peripheral blood, but approximately 50% of cows with abomasal lymphoma have tumor cells in the peritoneal fluid. Definitive diagnosis in some cases may require a right-side laparotomy and biopsy. Adenocarcinomas of the abomasum also have been described.

Obstructive Diseases of the Small Intestine

Mechanical obstructive diseases of the small intestine are not as common as forestomach and abomasal disorders, but they occur regularly enough to warrant concern in the differential diagnosis of abdominal distention in the cow and calf. The various obstructions will be discussed as a group with notations where appropriate concerning specific obstructive disorders.

Etiology

The cause of small intestinal obstructions such as volvulus, torsion, and intussusception is seldom apparent, although predisposing factors may be identified retrospectively during exploratory laparotomy or necropsy of affected cattle. For example, it is relatively common to

find a potential nidus of aberrant intestinal motility such as an *Oesophagostomum* sp. nodule or small polyp at the site of an intussusception in a cow. Intussusceptions are more common in calves than in cows and may occur in association with infectious diarrhea. Complete torsions on the mesenteric root have been observed following the casting and restraint of cattle for surgical procedures. Similarly, fibrous bands traversing the abdomen may predispose to intestinal entrapment and subsequent obstruction, especially in calves. Growing calves, especially those irritated by lice, may become obstructed by tichobezoars. In some herds, intraluminal obstructions are more common because of hemorrhagic bowel syndrome. Although uncommon, fecal impactions of the small intestine (most commonly ileum) do occur in cattle.

Signs

The general signs of small intestinal obstruction in the cow are distinct and include:

1. Acute onset of anorexia and gastrointestinal stasis
2. Abdominal distention especially of the right ventral quadrant
3. Colic
4. Absence of manure production
5. Fluid-distended bowel identified by ballottement and auscultation in the right lower quadrant of the abdomen (Figure 5-69)
6. Rectal and/or ultrasound findings of distended loops of small bowel
7. Progressive deterioration in the general physical status as regards hydration, attitude, and heart rate

These signs allow the diagnosis of small intestinal obstruction to be made with assurance in most cases, so that surgical treatment or slaughter may be discussed. Obviously variations exist in the signs depending on the duration of obstruction, age of the patient, and the type of obstruction present. Dehydration begins early in small intestinal obstruction and progresses rapidly. Metabolic alkalosis may be mild in distal small intestinal obstruction or severe in duodenal obstruction. The

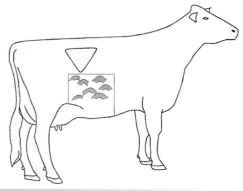

Figure 5-69

Typical area for small intestinal fluid distention.

heart rate tends to increase progressively because of pain and deteriorating hydration status but may be misleadingly normal in some small intestinal obstructions for which the cattle have received analgesics or in cases of long-standing (>24 hours) intussusception where the patient is no longer showing signs of colic. Hypocalcemia may occur secondary to absence of appetite, gastrointestinal stasis, and any milk production.

Severe colic is observed in patients with torsion of the root of the mesentery, volvulus of various sorts, and torsion of the distal flange. Severe colic in the cow is characterized by kicking at the abdomen (Figure 5-70), bellowing, lordosis (Figure 5-71), reluctance to stand for even a few seconds (Figure 5-72), and by the animal throwing itself down. Less severe colic may be noticed in intussusception with kicking at the abdomen, treading

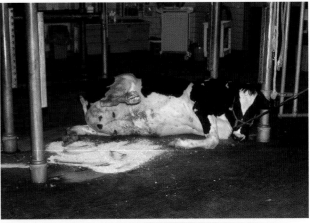

Figure 5-72

Marked abdominal pain in a cow with mesenteric volvulus.

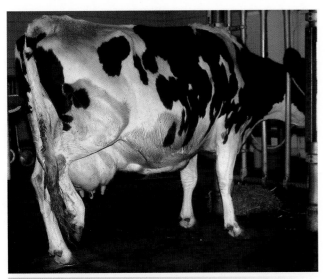

Figure 5-70

Colic characterized by kicking at the abdomen in a cow affected with intussusception. The wet hair in the right lower flank has been caused by the cow's right hind foot contacting the abdomen at this site.

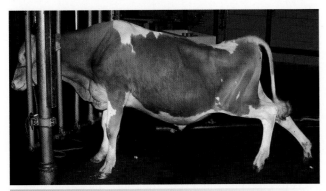

Figure 5-71

Severe colic characterized by lordosis in a Guernsey bull affected with small intestinal volvulus.

the hind feet, swishing the tail, and a preference for recumbency. We need to remember that the most common cause of colic in the adult dairy cow is small intestinal indigestion. Except for *C. perfringens* enteritis, calves rarely demonstrate marked colic with infectious bacterial, parasitic, or viral diarrheas. Cattle affected with intussusception may show colic during the first 12 to 24 hours of obstruction and thereafter have minimal signs of colic with anorexia, absence of manure, dehydration, and abdominal distention as the only outward signs of obstruction. This makes rectal and/or ultrasound examination imperative for diagnosis because cattle with intussusception may survive several days or up to 1 week with complete obstruction.

Confusion also may exist if a cow affected with small intestinal obstruction passes any manure. Certainly manure distal to the obstruction may be passed early in the course of intestinal obstruction, but in general cattle with small intestinal obstructions pass no manure. Occasionally red or raspberry-colored bloody mucus or blood clots descend the intestinal tract from the site of intussusception (Figures 5-73 and 5-74) and appear at the rectum. This is an especially helpful sign in the calf with suspected obstruction because rectal examination is impossible. Not all cases of intussusception show this blood-stained mucus nor is the finding always limited to intussusception. Abdominal distention worsens progressively in small intestinal obstructions and consists of two major components:

1. The small intestine proximal to the obstructions fills with fluid and gas, resulting in distention of the right lower abdominal quadrant and is detectable by simultaneous ballottement and auscultation.
2. The forestomach and abomasum distend secondary to the intestinal obstruction because of failure of normal outflow and reflux of small intestinal secretions. This results in left-sided abdominal distention that is proportional to the duration of obstruction.

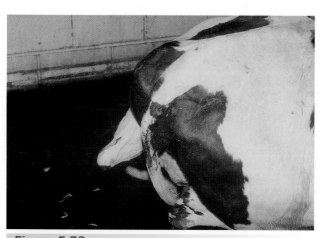

Figure 5-73

"Raspberry-colored" manure typical of that passed from devitalized small intestine.

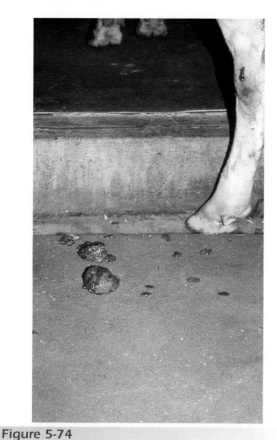

Figure 5-74

Scant manure with flecks of blood passed from a cow with intussusception.

Rectal examination findings of distended loops of small bowel provide the key to diagnosis in cattle affected with small intestinal obstruction. In addition, tight mesenteric bands, volvulus, or intussusception (Figure 5-75, A) may be palpated in some patients. Unfortunately rectal examination is not possible in calves and may be very difficult to perform in large cows

in advanced gestation because the gravid uterus occupies so great an area. In these cases, the cow or calf may need to undergo exploratory laparotomy to confirm the diagnosis. In young calves, entrapment of a segment of the bowel by an umbilical structure or another band is not unusual (Figure 5-75, B). Ultrasound is an important tool for evaluating cattle (cows and calves) with suspected small intestinal obstruction. Distended small intestines are usually readily visible in the right flank. The intestinal wall may be thickened, and with strangulating lesions there is no motility to the distended loops. With intraluminal obstruction such as a blood clot caused by the hemorrhagic bowel syndrome, motility may be increased or normal early in the obstructive disorder, but eventually hypomotility will result.

Hemorrhagic bowel syndrome has been the most common cause of small intestinal obstruction in our hospital

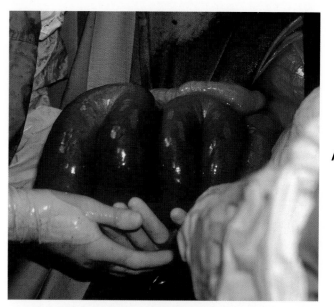

A

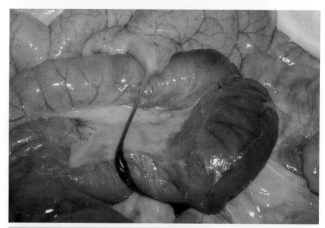

B

Figure 5-75

A, Intussusception in a cow. The coiled appearance of the affected bowel is typical. **B,** A segment of small intestine trapped by a band of undetermined origin in a 3-week-old "colicky" calf.

during the past 10 years. The cause of the syndrome is not known, but it is most common in third lactation cows, and the median time between parturition and onset is 104 days. Some farms have a relatively high incidence of the disease, whereas other farms have no cases. Farms that feed the highest energy diets seem to be at greatest risk for having cows with the syndrome. The disease appears to be disproportionately common in the Brown Swiss breed, but it has been seen in all of the conventional North American dairy breeds and even in bulls. *C. perfringens* A with a beta 2 toxin is found more commonly in the bowel of affected cattle compared with herdmates. Although a few cows have survived with medical therapy (Figure 5-76) and/or flank laparotomy (Figure 5-77, *A* and *B*) and drainage of the clot without resection, the prognosis, with or without surgery, is poor.

Differential Diagnosis

The differential diagnosis includes those diseases that may result in colic:

1. Simple indigestion with gas and fluid distention of the small intestine is the major differential diagnosis for small bowel obstruction. Occasionally cattle with indigestion have fluid and gas distention of the small intestine and subsequent tension on the mesentery preceding passage of this fluid ingesta as diarrhea. These cattle may show extreme colic and be misdiagnosed with intestinal obstructions. They tend to have gastrointestinal stasis, abdominal distention, increased heart rate, slight dehydration, hypocalcemia, hypochloremia, and either absent or scant manure production. Usually they *do not* have tightly distended loops of bowel per rectum. On ultrasound examination, the small intestine is dilated, but some motility is often present, especially after hypocalcemia is corrected. These cows may begin to pass

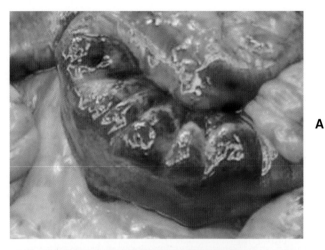

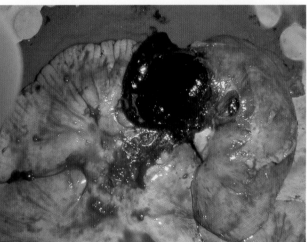

Figure 5-77

A, Small intestine at the time of surgery in a "colicky" cow with hemorrhagic bowel syndrome. **B,** Blood clot in the lumen of the intestine of the cow in *A*.

liquid manure on their own with resultant remission of signs or do so after symptomatic therapy with laxatives, ruminotorics, and calcium solutions. It is extremely important to recognize that a cow passing substantial quantities of manure *does not have a small bowel obstruction. Most cows with small bowel obstruction will not eat.* Although many cows with colic do not require surgery because of the high incidence of small intestinal indigestion, colic caused by enteritis in calves is not common, and a higher percentage of calves showing obvious colic signs have structural obstruction and would require surgery.

2. Acute pyelonephritis and other painful urinary tract problems such as renal calculi or ureteral calculi could cause signs of colic and thus may be confused with small intestinal obstructions. However, no abdominal distention is evident externally, no distended small bowel is palpated per rectum, and the cow usually is passing manure. Examination of the urinary system and urinalysis lead to proper diagnosis.

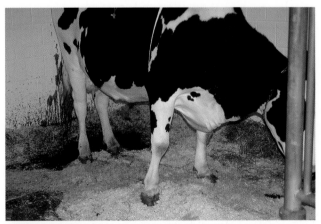

Figure 5-76

"Bloody" manure passed from a "colicky" cow believed to have hemorrhagic bowel syndrome. The cow passed blood in the manure for less than 12 hours and then recovered following fluid therapy and flunixin.

3. Cecal distention or volvulus may lead to signs of mild to moderate colic. This colic seldom is as violent as observed in small intestinal obstruction and usually consists of treading of the hind feet and occasional kicking at the abdomen. Abdominal distention involves the upper and lower right quadrants, and rectal examination is diagnostic of cecal distention or volvulus. Small intestinal distention proximal to a cecal volvulus may contribute to the observed colic.
4. Uterine torsion during the middle or final trimester of pregnancy causes mild colic with treading on the hind limbs. Rectal and vaginal examination will confirm this diagnosis.
5. Hematomas of the mesentery may also present as acute colic.

Treatment

The only treatment for small bowel obstruction is right-sided exploratory laparotomy, identification of the anatomic malposition, and correction thereof. Because prognosis varies tremendously depending on the exact obstruction identified, economics may dictate slaughter as an option for affected cattle deemed of marginal value, advanced cases, or those rapidly approaching a shocklike state. If the value of the animal dictates surgical exploration, a decision regarding on-farm surgery versus referral must be reached. Small bowel surgery in the cow is difficult under the best of circumstances and often requires trained assistants or more than one surgeon when complications occur or bowel resection is required.

Before surgery or during preparation, IV fluids should be administered as well as analgesics such as flunixin meglumine (1.0 mg/kg) to help stabilize the patient. Calves should be positioned in left lateral recumbency. If laboratory facilities exist, acid-base and electrolyte status, PCV, and plasma proteins should be assessed preoperatively to assist fluid therapy recommendations. In complicated cases in which resection of bowel is anticipated, most surgeons prefer left lateral recumbency and general anesthesia for adult patients.

The small bowel should be examined or "run" from the duodenum to the ileum or vice versa to identify the exact anatomic lesion. Difficulties revolve around the large amount of dilated small bowel that often needs to be exteriorized, manipulated, and replaced or resected (Figure 5-78). Excessive manipulation will lead to further intestinal injury and ileus. Some conditions such as abdominal fibrous bands, slight torsions of the mesentery, and volvulus of the distal flange require only anatomic repositioning or resection of the causative band. Other problems, such as complete torsion of the mesentery (Figure 5-79), mesenteric tears with entrapped bowel, volvulus of the intestine, and intussusception are more difficult and may require resection and anastomosis. Postoperatively, continued IV fluids, broad-spectrum antibiotics, calcium solutions, and judicious use of analgesics

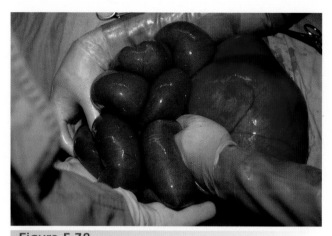

Figure 5-78

Distended loops of a small intestine proximal to an intussusception in a cow.

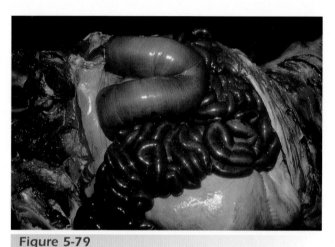

Figure 5-79

Complete 360-degree torsion of the mesentery in a cow.

may be required. If resection and anastomosis have been necessary, bactericidal antibiotics such as a penicillin derivative coupled with the extralabel use of an aminoglycoside or extralabel dose of ceftiofur are indicated for 3 to 7 days. Peritoneal lavage of warm balanced electrolyte solutions and bactericidal antibiotics also are used before final closure by some surgeons following resection and anastomosis.

The patient should begin to pass loose feces within 4 to 24 hours postoperatively. Intensive aftercare may be required, including colloid and crystalloid therapy and even partial parenteral nutrition in some cases. The major complications include further deterioration in blood flow and oxygenation of part of the small intestine, peritonitis, anastomosis breakdown, and adhesions that result in obstruction or abscess formation. The patient that maintains a normal temperature, has returning appetite, and continues to pass manure during the first 5 to 7 days postoperatively has a favorable prognosis.

Drugs Used to Alter Intestinal Motility

Various drugs affecting intestinal motility have been used to stimulate motility and manure production when postoperative ileus persists. In the past, metoclopramide (0.1 to 0.25 mg/kg SQ, once or twice daily) has been used primarily in postoperative calves having had intestinal surgery for small intestinal or cecal disorders. Postoperative prolonged ileus in such calves results in abdominal distention, mainly from failure of abomasal outflow and subsequent abomasal and forestomach fluid retention. Although experiments have not shown metoclopramide to affect abomasal motility, there is anecdotal evidence that it promotes abomasal and intestinal emptying in postoperative calves unless extensive intestinal adhesions exist. There is a report suggesting that bethanechol (0.07 mg/kg) coupled with metoclopramide (0.1 mg/kg) or bethanechol alone may be more effective than metoclopramide alone. Other work suggests that erythromycin (8.8 mg/kg) has a greater effect on abomasal motility than metoclopramide or neostigmine. Currently IV lidocaine has been the first-line treatment for postoperative ileus in calves more than 2 weeks of age; 1.3 mg/kg is given as a slow bolus over 10 to 15 minutes, and this is followed with a constant rate infusion of 0.05 mg/kg/min mixed in crystalloid fluids. Although unproven, younger calves may have delayed metabolism of the lidocaine, which could result in neurological or cardiac abnormalities.

Neostigmine is seldom now used to stimulate intestinal motility, although some clinicians do use this drug to treat vagus indigestion patients. Ranitidine and IV potassium penicillin may also have some prokinetic properties and are often administered to calves following intestinal surgery.

Atropine and methscopolamine reduce intestinal motility and should be avoided in cattle with gastrointestinal dysfunction. Ileus and bloat caused by those drugs persist for 24 to 96 hours and can only be reversed by time. Atropine sulfate (0.04 to 0.08 mg/kg) can be used safely if needed for respiratory or other medical problems. However, overdosage or chronic administration of these drugs is contraindicated in calves and cows with gastrointestinal disease (including diarrhea). Coffee, 0.5 kg P.O. to an adult cow, is effective in increasing motility.

MISCELLANEOUS CAUSES OF SMALL INTESTINAL OBSTRUCTION

Fat Necrosis

Fat necrosis may be observed in any breed of cattle and is characterized by hard masses in the mesentery and omentum that gradually cause partial or full extraluminal intestinal obstruction. More commonly, rectal constriction occurs, establishing a risk for iatrogenic rectal injury during palpation. Affected cattle usually are overconditioned middle-aged to old animals. Before complete obstruction, affected cattle frequently have diarrhea because the intestinal lumen is constricted from external pressure. Partial anorexia, loose manure followed by little or no manure, and occasional abdominal distention or mild colic characterize this vague illness. Hard masses associated with the omentum, mesentery, and around the small intestine, rectum, or colon can sometimes be palpated per rectum to confirm a diagnosis of fat necrosis. Differential diagnosis includes lymphosarcoma, intestinal adenocarcinoma, and abdominal abscesses. It is worth emphasizing that lesions of fat necrosis feel exceptionally hard, even compared with neoplasia, on rectal palpation. In valuable cattle, ultrasound-guided biopsy or exploratory laparotomy and biopsy to confirm the disease may be warranted. Prognosis for cattle affected with fat necrosis usually is hopeless, but rare cases have had localized masses that have been amenable to resection and anastomosis of affected bowel.

Neoplasia

Partial to complete intestinal obstruction has been observed in cattle affected with intestinal adenocarcinomas, lymphosarcoma, and, rarely, other tumors. Signs, as in fat necrosis, are vague. If obstruction becomes complete, abdominal distention and colic may be observed. Metabolic alkalosis can be marked in proximal small intestinal obstructions secondary to neoplasia. Physical examination may allow an index of suspicion for lymphosarcoma, but intestinal adenocarcinoma seldom is diagnosed short of exploratory laparotomy. If palpable per rectum, adenocarcinomas tend to be hard, whereas lymphosarcoma is firm and may have associated visceral lymphadenopathy. The prognosis is hopeless for lymphosarcoma and poor for adenocarcinoma unless all of the involved intestine can be resected.

Lesions Associated with Reproductive Tract Pathology

Adhesions of the small intestine secondary to puncture of the dorsal cranial vagina by infusion pipettes most commonly occur when laypeople attempt to infuse the uterus of a recently postparturient cow that has a uterus too heavy to retract. The ensuing chemical or bacterial peritonitis can involve the omental sling or small intestine through adhesions. Partial or full intestinal obstruction can result if extensive adhesions develop. Treatment consists of systemic broad-spectrum antibiotics and time. Prognosis varies with the degree of adhesion present. The affected cow should have complete reproductive rest and only be palpated once monthly to prognose her condition.

Traumatic rupture of the small intestine during calving has been observed by Dr. John King, Professor of Pathology at the New York State College of Veterinary Medicine. Most of these cattle die within 24 hours after calving. Lesions consist of rupture of the small intestine with subsequent massive fibrinous peritonitis. Apparently during labor and straining, a loop of bowel is trapped in the pelvic region by fetal pressure, and further pressure during fetal extraction leads to rupture.

At our hospital, we observed a multiparous cow that became anorectic and mildly colicky immediately following calving. The cow would tread with her hind feet, occasionally kicked at her abdomen, and preferred to lie down. She temporarily regained appetite and continued to pass manure for 1 week in response to symptomatic therapy but then relapsed with reduced manure production, inappetence, colic, and fever. Small bowel distention was found on rectal palpation. Surgical exploration confirmed a localized perforation of the small intestine that the mesentery had walled off as an abscess. Resection of the affected bowel resulted in full recovery. It was theorized that, during calving, this cow had severely bruised and compromised a loop of small bowel but not caused complete laceration.

Prolapse of the intestine through uterine rupture can follow dystocia or prolapse of the uterus. In general, the prognosis is hopeless, and the affected animal should be slaughtered. Heroic efforts may be indicated for valuable cattle, but the complicated surgery required, coupled with obvious peritonitis, makes survival unlikely.

OBSTRUCTIVE DISEASES OF THE CECUM AND COLON

Cecal Dilatation and Volvulus

Etiology
Although much less common than abomasal disorders, cecal disorders constitute a common cause of gastrointestinal dysfunction in dairy cattle.

Many of the same theories proposed to explain DA could be used to explain cecal dilatation or subsequent volvulus. Volatile fatty acid production occurs in the cecum just as in the abomasum. Modern diets consisting of high concentrate and silage levels provide a large amount of substrate for volatile fatty acid production throughout the cow's gastrointestinal tract. Additional factors such as hypocalcemia, endotoxemia secondary to metritis or mastitis, or indigestion that result in gastrointestinal ileus further predispose to cecal dilatation. In simple cecal dilatation, the cecum distends with gas and fluid to varying degrees, and the apex begins to rise in the abdomen from its normal location toward the pelvic inlet. Further distention of the organ leads to rotation of the cecum that tends to occur in a clockwise direction, as viewed from the right side. Although cecal

dilatation-volvulus may occur at any stage of lactation or gestation, the majority of cases occur early in lactation at the same time as the peak of metabolic disorders and DAs. Cecal dilatation-volvulus also may occur in calves and bulls, especially those fed highly fermentable concentrate such as high moisture corn. Many experienced practitioners will note that there are a surprising number of normal, healthy, dairy cattle in whom a mild to moderate degree of cecal dilation can be palpated during routine reproductive examination, suggesting that the condition can be subclinical in some individuals.

Signs
Inappetence, reduced manure production, and abdominal distention are the usual complaints and initial observations in cattle affected with cecal dilatations. Milk production decreases commensurate with the appetite reduction. Affected cattle have a normal body temperature, respiratory rate, and a normal to slightly elevated heart rate. As cecal dilatation progresses, mild to moderate colic manifested by treading on the hind limbs or kicking at the abdomen may be observed. Rumen contractions weaken and become less frequent, and intestinal motility is decreased. A right-sided ping will be detected by simultaneous percussion and auscultation. This ping will develop in the right paralumbar fossa and may extend one to three rib spaces cranial to the fossa (Figures 5-80, A and B, and 5-81). In advanced cases, the ping may extend into the mid or ventral right caudal abdomen. Fluid may be ballotted within a distended viscus in the right upper quadrant. Right-sided abdominal distention is apparent when the cow is viewed from the rear or from the right side. In early cases, this distention causes the right paralumbar fossa to appear "full." In advanced cases, both the upper and lower right abdominal quadrants appear distended, and an outline of a portion of the body of the cecum and sometimes the ascending colon may be seen outlined in the right paralumbar fossa. In cattle affected for more than 24 hours or in severe cases, dehydration may be mild to moderate, and cool peripheral parts, suggesting hypocalcemia, may be apparent. Rectal examination provides the key to diagnosis because the dilated cecum is easily palpable in the right caudal abdomen, and frequently the apex of the cecum is directed into the pelvic inlet such that the veterinarian palpates the organ and/or the ascending colon as soon as the wrist enters the rectum. If rotation of the body of the cecum has already occurred, more than one loop of cecum and spiral colon may be palpable in the right and central caudal abdomen. A serum chloride concentration can also be useful. Cattle with right-sided abomasal disorders typically are hypochloremic. Cattle with cecal disease do not usually have dramatic changes in serum chloride.

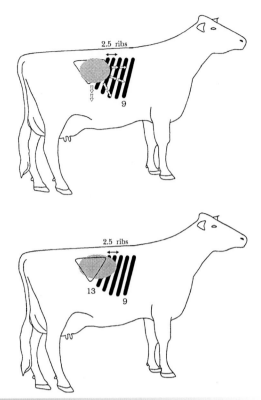

A

B

Figure 5-80

A, Area of ping resulting from mild cecal distention. The size of the ping (arrows) may increase if cecal distention worsens or cecal volvulus is present. **B,** Ping associated with distention of the proximal or coiled colon.

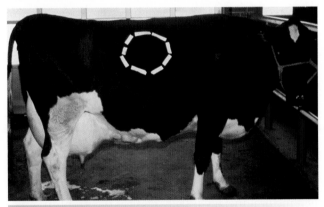

Figure 5-81

Area of tympanic resonance in a cow with cecal dilatation. This ping includes the last three ribs and the cranial portion of the right paralumbar fossa. Rectal examination would be essential to differentiate cecal dilatation from benign colonic distention and RDA or AV.

In those with cecal volvulus, signs are more remarkable and obvious. Milk production, appetite, and manure production decrease dramatically. Affected cattle are moderately to severely dehydrated, have obvious right abdominal distention, ruminal distention, and stasis,

have an elevated heart rate (80 to 100 beats/min), and have a large ping in the right caudal abdomen expanding from the paralumbar fossa cranially at least three rib spaces and often ventral to the paralumbar fossa; additionally, fluid is easily detected by ballottement combined with auscultation. In some cases, the ping is so expansive that differentiation from AV is necessary (Figure 5-82). Rectal examination reveals dilatation of the cecum with rotation or volvulus and dilatation of the proximal colon, and may reveal a distended ileum because the cecal volvulus kinks the ileocecal region. Rectal examination also rules out the major differential diagnosis—AV. Ultrasound examination can also help differentiate cases when it is not clear whether the problem is cecal volvulus or AV. Small intestinal distention will be present with cecal volvulus. Additionally, cows with cecal volvulus can be very colicky, which is rarely the case in those with AV (Figure 5-83).

In calves, right-sided abdominal distention, anorexia, greatly decreased manure production, dehydration, and an elevated heart rate (84 to 120 beats/min)

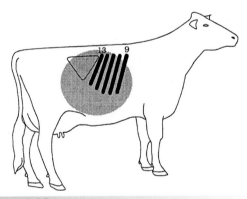

Figure 5-82

Ping typical of very large cecal volvulus or abomasal volvulus.

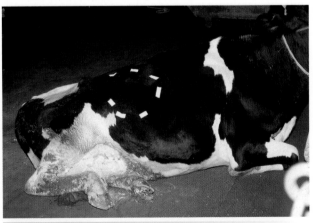

Figure 5-83

Area of tympanic resonance (ping) in a "colicky" cow with cecal volvulus. Succussible fluid was easily detected in the right flank.

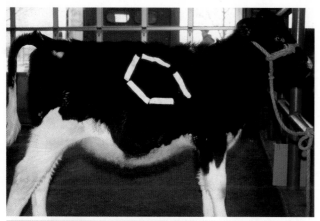

Figure 5-84

Area of tympanic resonance in a calf with cecal dilatation. Because the calf was too small for rectal examination, it would be difficult to differentiate cecal dilatation from right displacement of the abomasum because this area extends from the cranial paralumbar fossa forward to rib nine.

characterize cecal dilatation/volvulus. A large ping may be detected over the right caudal (and sometimes simultaneously over the left) abdomen, including the right paralumbar fossa and several rib spaces cranial to the fossa (Figure 5-84). Fluid may be heard to splash in a large viscus when the right abdomen is ballotted. Mild colic with treading, lying down, and kicking at the abdomen are common. Rectal examination is not possible because of the size of the patient, and the condition may be difficult to differentiate from AV in animals of this age. Ultrasound examination is helpful in distinguishing between the two disorders. As in adult cattle, however, the uniform distention of the paralumbar fossa and the outline of a distended tubular viscus in the flank area suggest cecal distention. In contrast, AV usually causes a half-moon viscus distention projecting into the paralumbar fossa caudal to the right thirteenth rib. Of particular importance in calves is the fact that cecal dilatation or volvulus may progress to necrosis and peritonitis within a relatively short time (24 to 72 hours) because of the fragile nature of the calf's intestinal tract. In such cases, fever and abdominal pain will be detected in addition to the other clinical signs.

Laboratory Data

Laboratory data seldom are diagnostic in cecal distention or volvulus. Mild to moderate metabolic alkalosis is the rule because a physical obstruction of the gastrointestinal tract has occurred. This obstruction may be partial in cecal distention, with mild alkalosis anticipated, or complete in cecal volvulus, with more dramatic metabolic alkalosis. Metabolic acidosis only occurs in advanced cases with bowel necrosis. Abdominal fluid is normal except in advanced cases in which protein levels exceed normal limits

because of vascular compromise and edema in the mesentery and cecum. In addition, those rare calves that have cecal perforation or leakage would have abdominal fluid values consistent with peritonitis.

Differential Diagnosis

The major differential diagnosis is RDA or volvulus. In general, abomasal problems cause a more cranial ping and abdominal distention under the right rib cage rather than the caudal abdomen. Adhesions and dilation of the spiral colon and a rare case of omasal dilation may be confused with a cecal volvulus. Small intestinal obstruction should be considered in cattle passing no feces and showing signs of colic. Rectal examination should allow differentiation of these problems.

Treatment

For cecal distention patients, the clinician must decide whether medical treatment will suffice or surgical exploratory procedure is necessary. The best candidates for medical therapy meet the following conditions:
1. Normal heart rate
2. Some manure production and appetite (usually for roughage)
3. Mild to nonexistent dehydration
4. Mild to moderate abdominal distention with the cecal apex palpable in the pelvic inlet per rectum
5. Probable hypocalcemia, which may be easily treated

For these patients, medical treatment consists of daily laxative ruminotorics, calcium solutions as needed, and treatment of any concurrent problems such as ketosis, metritis, or mastitis. Daily laxatives seem more effective (clinical impression) when administered mixed with warm water using a stomach tube rather than merely as oral boluses. Increasing appetite, manure production, and milk production are positive signs following treatment. Highly fermentable feeds should be offered only in limited quantities. Treatment must continue for 3 to 7 days and should not be stopped following initial signs of improvement, lest relapse occur. The cecal distention is monitored by rectal palpation or ultrasound of the organ and seldom returns to normal size and position in less than 5 days. If the animal continues to improve, continued medical therapy usually resolves the problem. Analgesics are not used, lest signs of abdominal pain be masked.

The following parameters are present in patients with cecal distention or volvulus that require surgical intervention:
1. Elevated heart rate
2. Little or no manure production and appetite
3. Detectable dehydration
4. Moderate to marked abdominal distention with the cecum and proximal colon very distended when palpated per rectum
5. Colic

IV fluid therapy and IV flunixin meglumine (0.5 to 1.0 mg/kg twice daily) are administered preoperatively. Perioperative antibiotics are appropriate. Surgical treatment consists of right flank laparotomy followed by typhlotomy. A long flank incision is indicated, as the cecal diameter may approach 18 to 30 cm in severe cases, and delivery of this greatly distended organ into the incision is difficult if the incision is too small. On entry into the abdomen, the cecum is gas decompressed "in situ" by a needle attached to tubing and a suction apparatus. This alleviates some of the distention. Once the cecum is externalized (Figure 5-85, *A* and *B*), a typhlotomy at the apex should be performed (Figure 5-86), the cecum emptied, the proximal colon and ileum "milked" of ingesta (Figure. 5-87), and a double-layer closure used for the typhlotomy.

In advanced cases with cecal necrosis or in recurrent cecal dilatation-volvulus patients, a partial typhlectomy may be necessary. Complete typhlectomy in cattle is a difficult procedure because of the intimate apposition of ileum to the cecal base, which is continuous with the proximal colon. Therefore in most instances, a partial typhlectomy removing the apex of the cecum and leaving the ileocecal region intact is performed to minimize the "balloon effect" and lessen the chances of future recurrences. In advanced cecal or cecocolic necrosis (Figure 5-88), complete typhlectomy and ileocolic anastomosis is the only alternative. This is an extremely difficult procedure for all but the most experienced surgeon.

However, typhlotomy, rather than the more complicated typhlectomy, usually is indicated for first-time surgical patients because recurrence rates for cecal dilation-volvulus are only reported to be approximately 10%.

Postoperatively, supportive therapy with laxative ruminotoric mixtures can be given on a daily basis for several days, and rectal palpation should be performed at 24- to 48-hour intervals to assess the degree of cecal distention. Loose manure for 48 hours is typical and desirable postoperatively. Antibiotic therapy is indicated for 3 to 7 days for typhlotomy patients, and broad-spectrum bactericidal antibiotic therapy for 5 to 14 days is indicated for typhlectomy patients. Highly fermentable feeds should be reintroduced gradually.

Prognosis is good for cecal distention-volvulus patients. Complications include recurrence in approximately 10% of the patients and the possibility of peritonitis or adhesions in those with complicated surgical procedures.

Colonic Obstructions

Colonic obstructions are sporadic in dairy cattle. In general, they are caused by regional inflammation resulting in adhesions or by space-occupying masses. Intraperitoneal injections through the right paralumbar fossa are

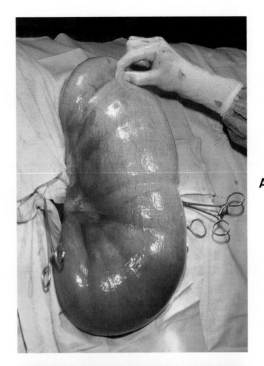

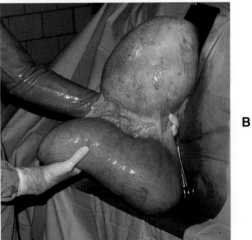

Figure 5-85

A, Cecal dilatation as the organ is exteriorized through a right flank laparotomy incision. **B,** Cecum (ventral) and proximal colon being exteriorized in a cow with cecal dilatation.

one cause of nonseptic or septic peritonitis that can result in partial or complete colonic obstruction. Concentrated dextrose solutions injected in this fashion are capable of inducing significant chemical peritonitis and subsequent adhesions and intestinal obstruction. Any intraperitoneal injection that penetrates the duodenum or proximal colon can allow leakage of ingesta with localized septic peritonitis and similar signs of obstruction. Fever usually is present in those patients with septic peritonitis. Similar inflammation or abscessation occasionally results from previous surgical procedures performed through the right flank.

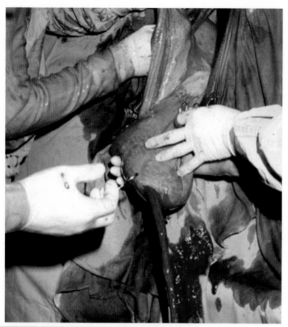

Figure 5-86

Typhlotomy and cecal content drainage in a cow with cecal volvulus.

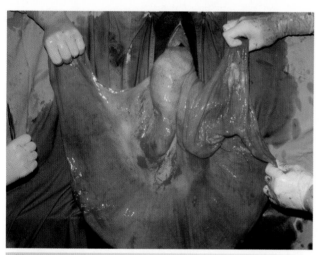

Figure 5-87

A large flaccid cecum following typhlotomy for cecal volvulus in a cow. The apex of the cecum appears at the left, and the proximal colon appears in the right upper area.

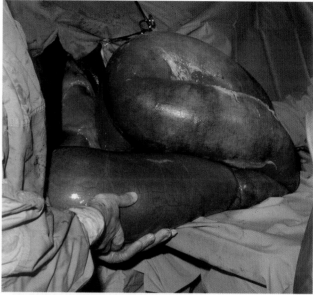

Figure 5-88

Infarcted cecum and fibrin on the visceral peritoneum of the cecum in a cow affected with severe cecal volvulus. These lesions necessitated typhlectomy.

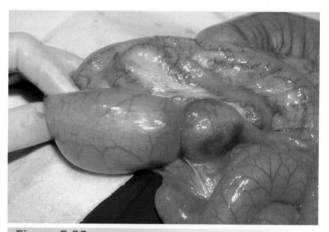

Figure 5-89

Intussusception of the descending colon in a 2-week-old Holstein calf. The calf had diarrhea for 3 days and then acute onset of colic and sudden absence of feces. On ultrasound examination, the cecum was distended with fluid. Surgery with intestinal resection and anastomosis were successful.

Spiral colon intussusception can also occur in calves and should be considered in those with diarrhea that suddenly pass no manure and become progressively distended (Figure 5-89). Calves with small colon obstruction will have fluid distention of the cecum that can be easily visualized by ultrasound examination. Space-occupying masses such as fat necrosis also may result in colonic obstruction.

Signs

Cattle affected with colonic obstructions have vague signs of anorexia, low volume production of loose manure, and decreased milk production. If the obstruction is complete, abdominal distention may be present. A ping is present in the right paralumbar fossa consistent with colonic or cecal distention. In cattle that have had intraperitoneal injections, the history may be helpful, and "needle tracks" with dried blood matting the hair below the injection site may be observed in the right paralumbar fossa. Rectal examination determines whether distended proximal colon, cecum, or fibrinous adhesions are present. Fever often is present in those cattle with localized septic peritonitis. Rectal examination and/or ultrasound also are beneficial in the diagnosis of fat necrosis because hard masses may be palpated or imaged in the right upper abdominal quadrant. In calves with spiral colon intussusception, a large homogeneous fluid-filled cecum can be visualized on ultrasound examination.

Treatment

In cattle with injection reaction obstructions, immediate therapy is symptomatic and consists of antibiotics and analgesics. If this is not successful after several days of treatment, a right paralumbar fossa exploratory celiotomy is indicated. Adhesions of the visceral colonic peritoneum and parietal peritoneum should be anticipated and a decision reached as to the practicality or potential for surgical bypass of the lesion. A similar determination is required for cattle affected with fat necrosis.

Prognosis

Unless medical therapy alleviates the signs of obstruction, prognosis is poor. Colonic bypass surgery is technically difficult, and only extremely valuable animals are candidates. The prognosis for cattle affected with fat necrosis that causes rectal or colonic obstruction is extremely poor.

Atresia Coli

This sporadic congenital defect results in complete obstruction of the gastrointestinal tract, and signs usually appear by 1 to 3 days of age. Etiology is unknown, but hereditary causes and damage subsequent to early pregnancy palpation of the embryo have been suggested as possibilities. Comparative literature suggests compromised vasculature during early embryogenesis as a likely cause. Holsteins constitute the majority of calves reported with this problem.

Signs

Abdominal distention (Figure 5-90) and absence of manure production signal this diagnosis. The anal sphincter and rectum appear normal, which distinguishes the condition from atresia ani. The owner may report some early passage of mucus after birth, followed by no manure after that time. Affected calves appear normal at birth and usually are willing to drink colostrum. Within 24 to 72 hours, however, they go off feed, become distended and depressed, and begin to dehydrate. Rarely, a calf will remain apparently healthy for 5 to 7 days. Calves with atresia coli usually have a normal temperature, elevated heart rate, and detectable fluid on ballottement of the right lower quadrant. Colic may be observed.

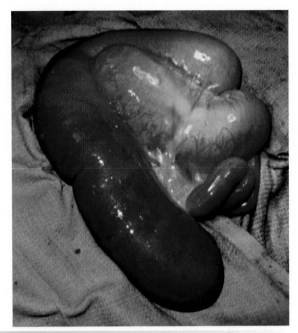

Figure 5-90

Severely distended proximal colon in a calf with atresia coli.

Laboratory Data

Blood work to evaluate PCV and plasma proteins is indicated, as are acid-base and electrolyte analyses. Some assessment of passive transfer of immunoglobulins also should be made before treatment because many atresia coli calves have inadequate immunoglobulin levels despite proper administration of colostrum. This fact suggests compromised absorption directly or indirectly associated with the atresia. If fever is present, an abdominal paracentesis may be indicated.

Treatment

The only treatment is to bypass the defect surgically by anastomosing proximal spiral colon to the descending colon distal to the atresia. Excessive attempts to determine colonic patency by means of passage of tubes or probes into the rectum are contraindicated. Before surgery, the calf may need to be stabilized with fluid and electrolyte supplementation, glucose, plasma or whole blood (if failure of passive transfer has occurred), and antibiotic therapy. The surgical procedure has been described in a number of surgical texts. Technical difficulties include possible anatomic confusion and the anastomosis of a relatively large-diameter section of proximal colon to the small-diameter descending colon. The major surgical complication is peritonitis, but medical complications such as neonatal enteritis, pneumonia, or septicemia also are possible. Electrolyte imbalances may also occur associated with the reintroduction of milk.

Prognosis

The prognosis is probably is no better than 50%—even in the hands of an experienced surgeon. Therefore only extremely valuable calves should be treated. The potential for genetic transmission has not been entirely ruled out and is being studied. The results of these studies may dictate future prognosis for this problem. If owners elect treatment, referral to surgeons experienced in this repair is recommended. Growth rates may be compromised, at least initially, in some animals that do survive the surgery.

Benign Distention of the Proximal Colon

Etiology

This syndrome results in gas and fluid accumulation in the proximal colon with a subsequent ping detected in the right paralumbar fossa region. Extent of this ping varies (Figure 5-91) but includes the right paralumbar fossa and may extend two to three rib spaces cranial to the paralumbar fossa. Location of this ping leads to confusion in differential diagnosis, and many cattle with benign colonic distention are diagnosed erroneously as RDA or cecal dilatation patients. In fact, benign distention of the proximal colon simply reflects gastrointestinal stasis, which may occur in septic or endotoxic conditions, or as a result of a primary gastrointestinal obstruction. Because the region of this ping overlaps that of a cecal dilatation, a rectal examination should be performed to rule out cecal dilatation. In cattle with benign proximal colonic distention, rectal palpation reveals mild to undetectable colonic distention. If palpable at all, the loops of colon are fluctuant and soft

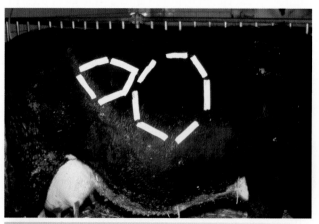

Figure 5-91

Two distinct areas of tympanic resonance in a cow affected with right displacement of the abomasum but also having benign colonic distention (caudal area). Ileus or passage of some gas and fluid from the displaced abomasum into the lower gastrointestinal tract during transportation may have resulted in the benign colonic distention in this case.

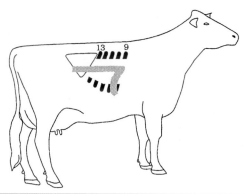

Figure 5-92

Ping resulting from distention of the proximal and descending duodenum.

rather than pathologically distended. In addition, there is no right-sided abdominal distention.

This syndrome merely represents a sign of gastrointestinal stasis and is not a primary diagnosis. Once rectal examination confirms this finding, the animal must be reassessed and a diagnosis sought.

Despite the caudal location of the ping associated with benign distention of the proximal colon, this ping is commonly misdiagnosed as a RDA. It must be emphasized that the RDA ping extends cranial to the ninth or even eighth ribs, unlike a benign proximal colon ping, which never extends more than three rib spaces cranial to the right paralumbar fossa.

Occasionally pings associated with the proximal and descending duodenum occur when small intestinal obstruction or recent DA has been present. This distention causes a ping along the course of the duodenum as illustrated (Figure 5-92). This ping is most obvious in cattle that have been rolled or recently transported to correct a preexisting LDA.

DISEASES OF THE DESCENDING COLON AND RECTUM

Extraluminal Compression of the Rectum

Etiology

Extraluminal compression of the rectum occasionally may accompany pelvic inflammatory or mass lesions. Signs are disparate because of variable etiologies, but straining to defecate and narrow liquid streams of feces are observed in most cases, regardless of specific signs. The most common diseases that cause extraluminal rectal compression are listed in Table 5-3 with diagnostic aids, treatment, and prognosis.

Diagnosis

Rectal examination confirms the diagnosis in most cases. It may be difficult to differentiate lymphosarcoma from fat necrosis unless other signs of lymphosarcoma

TABLE 5-3 Causes of Extraluminal Compression of the Rectum

Disease	Diagnosis	Treatment	Prognosis
Fat necrosis	Diffuse hard masses surrounding rectum on rectal examination Normal TPR	None	Hopeless
Lymphosarcoma	Firm masses in pelvis—often associated with pelvic lymph nodes or the reproductive tract	None	Hopeless
Perimetritis	Firm uniform pelvic soft tissue swelling—most prominent ventral to the rectum associated with reproductive tract but also surrounding the rectum and restricting movement Fever Occurs within a few days following parturition (usual history of dystocia)	Intensive systemic antibiotics analgesics	Poor
Abscesses	Rectal findings of large fluctuant or firm masses attached to reproductive tract or pelvic lymph nodes	Drainage Antibiotics Iodides	Fair to good with drainage; poor for multiple abscesses
Hematomas	Firm, often multiple masses within the pelvis Dystocia in history Very common in heifers	Rest	Good—most resolve in 30-60 days

are found during the physical examination. History of recent calving, presence of fever, and rectal and vaginal examinations confirm perimetritis. Pelvic abscesses may result from dystocia, uterine perforation during infusion with a pipette, or *Arcanobacterium pyogenes* abscesses that have ascended the lymphatics from deep musculoskeletal abscesses in the hind limb.

Vaginal examination should be performed to ascertain whether adhesions exist between the pelvic masses and the vagina. If adhesions are present, diagnostic aspirates, biopsies, and subsequent surgical drainage of abscesses may be performed through the vaginal wall. If adhesions between the mass lesions and vagina are absent, abdominal exploratory surgery would be necessary to confirm the diagnosis and attempt drainage of the abscess.

Postparturient pelvic hematomas are extremely common in primiparous cattle and possible in multiparous cattle. Dystocia is the usual cause. Hematomas can be singular or multiple and may be found at any location of the pelvic region, although most occur in the ventral or lateral pelvic areas. Treatment is not necessary. Rarely a massive hematoma may develop secondary to dystocia and cause severe anemia and rectal compression.

Laboratory Aids

In confusing cases, ancillary aids such as cytology from aspirates or biopsies may be indicated. Serum globulin levels usually are elevated in cattle affected with pelvic abscesses. Although laboratory aids seldom are necessary

in perimetritis patients, in severe cases the acute overwhelming infection usually results in a degenerative left shift in the hemogram, elevated fibrinogen, and a decrease in serum albumin secondary to protein loss into the massive cellulitis.

Treatment

Pelvic abscesses causing extraluminal rectal compression have a fair to good prognosis depending on location. In singular large abscesses, drainage may be attempted per vagina assuming solid adhesions to the vagina exist, or via laparotomy. Appropriate systemic antibiotics should be administered after drainage. Penicillin at 22,000 U/kg once or twice daily is suitable when *A. pyogenes* is isolated from the abscesses. Organic iodide powder may be fed at 1 oz/day for 2 to 3 weeks for its nonspecific activity against thick-walled abscesses. If drainage is not possible without contamination of the peritoneal cavity, prognosis is poor, but long-term penicillin therapy (3 to 6 weeks) and oral iodide powder for a similar length of time may be tried. The addition of rifampin to the antibiotic regimen may also be considered to improve abscess penetration, although this represents extralabel drug use; absorption is variable; and the drug is quite expensive.

Treatment of perimetritis is not highly successful but includes broad-spectrum intensive antibiotic therapy to control the mixed bacterial flora likely found in such cases. Analgesics such as flunixin meglumine also are indicated.

The prognosis for lymphosarcoma and fat necrosis is hopeless. Pelvic hematomas require no treatment other than rest and once-monthly rectal palpation to assess resolution. Most resolve within 30 to 60 days after freshening. Rarely, massive hematomas that cause anemia may require whole blood transfusions and carry a poor prognosis.

Rectal Lacerations

Etiology

Rectal lacerations result from ignorant roughness by neophyte examiners, frustrated or angry attempts at palpation on poorly restrained animals, and sadism. Occasional rectal lacerations have been blamed on inadvertent penile damage to the rectum during natural breeding. Inexperienced examiners cause most rectal lacerations. Although rectal lacerations are much less common in cattle than horses, they occur frequently enough to emphasize the need for gentle, well-lubricated rectal palpation. Plastic sleeves are to blame for some of the rectal lacerations that occur in dairy cattle. Neophyte examiners should be trained with rubber gloves and sleeves; it is not possible to palpate as carefully or gently with a plastic sleeve as it is with a rubber glove. Even experienced examiners using plastic sleeves often inadvertently cause rectal mucosal lacerations and bleeding.

Rectal lacerations in the cow generally are not graded, as are equine rectal tears, but a simple classification system would include mucosal injuries, submucosal and muscular layer injuries, and full-thickness injuries.

Signs

If rectal laceration occurs during rectal examination, signs are immediate in the form of fresh blood on the sleeve as it is withdrawn from the rectum and subsequent tenesmus. If the veterinarian has not been present for the causative rectal examination, signs will depend on the depth of the rectal injury and the time elapsed since injury. In injuries of less than full thickness, tenesmus, inappetence, and blood-stained fecal material may be present. Attempts at rectal examination will be greatly resisted with tenesmus and often bellowing.

In full-thickness injuries, the cow will become febrile with gastrointestinal ileus, elevated heart rate, and an arched stance. Septic peritonitis has occurred, and if the rectal tear communicates fully with the peritoneal cavity, the cow will usually be dead in less than 24 hours. In heifers that are examined and sent back to pasture, where they are not closely observed, sudden death may be suspected, and the exact cause will escape detection unless an autopsy is performed. If a full-thickness rectal tear remains retroperitoneal, the cow will still typically be febrile, have tenesmus, stand with an arched stance,

and have gastrointestinal ileus. Once again, rectal palpation will be greatly resisted. These animals will survive longer (2 to 7 days) than cattle with full-thickness lacerations directly entering the peritoneal cavity but still usually have a fatal outcome.

Diagnosis

Unless present for the causative injury, the veterinarian may not be confident of a diagnosis until a rectal examination is done. As soon as the rectal injury is palpated or suspected by the rapid appearance of blood on the examiner's sleeve and severe tenesmus, the rectal examination should be terminated. The veterinarian should administer epidural anesthesia immediately and perform a gentle rectal examination using either a rubber sleeve or a bare arm with plenty of lubrication. The extent of the injury then can be palpated gently and a diagnosis/prognosis reached. If no history of previous rectal examination exists, the veterinarian must keep in mind the possibly of sadism and decide judiciously if and when to discuss the possibility with the owner and authorities.

Treatment

If only mucosal injury has occurred, rest from rectal examinations for a minimum of 1 week along with laxative feeds (silage or green chop) are indicated. Epidural anesthesia may be required for 24 to 48 hours in some cases with extreme tenesmus. The prognosis is favorable.

If the injury extends to submucosal or muscular layers, rest from rectal examinations for a minimum of 1 month and prescription of a laxative diet are imperative. Once again, epidural anesthesia may be required for 1 to 4 days to minimize tenesmus in individual cattle that strain excessively such that they refuse feed and water because of the vicious cycle of straining—more pain—straining. Following 1 month of rest, an experienced examiner should perform a rectal examination and assess the rectal integrity. The prognosis is favorable, but only an experienced veterinarian should palpate such cows in the future.

If full-thickness rectal lacerations communicate with the peritoneal cavity, the cow should be slaughtered because fecal material will be in the abdomen and a hopeless prognosis must be offered. If full-thickness rectal lacerations communicate with the retroperitoneal space in the pelvic region, the prognosis is usually poor. However, some cattle with small full-thickness rectal lacerations in this area have healed following systemic broad-spectrum antibiotics, a very laxative diet, and rest from rectal examinations. The laxative diet and species difference in fecal consistency preclude the necessity for flushing the injured area free of impacted fecal material as might be necessary in a horse with a similar injury.

Rectovaginal Constriction in Jersey Cattle

This simple, autosomal, recessive defect results in constriction at the anorectal region and vulva-vestibule region. Fibrous tissue at these areas prevents rectal examinations and leads to dystocia. Jersey cattle with this defect also appear especially prone to severe parturient udder edema.

Atresia Ani

This condition is seldom encountered in dairy cattle. Affected calves show signs shortly after birth because they are unable to pass manure. Abdominal distention, depression, colic, tenesmus, and weakness will be observed if the condition is undiagnosed until 24 hours or more after birth. The rectal lumen usually bulges subcutaneously in the normal region of the anus when the abdomen is compressed. Although simple cutaneous puncture often allows fecal passage, these incisions often fibrose and lead to anal stricture, tenesmus, and abdominal distention. A rectal pull-through procedure has been advocated for best long-term results. Although heritability has not been documented, the ethics of performing this procedure in an animal with breeding potential are questionable.

Constipation

This condition is uncommon in cattle and, when observed, generally points to neurologic deficits or painful conditions that interfere with defecation. Neurologic conditions often are associated with trauma to the sacral area or severe spinal cord damage that results in atony and hypoalgesia of the anus. Possible causes of nontraumatic caudal spinal cord injury include lymphosarcoma, neurofibroma, and ascending cauda equine myelitis associated with tail head cellulitis caused by perivascular leakage of irritant drugs intended for coccygeal administration. Poor aseptic technique during repeated epidural administration is another possible cause of ascending myelitis.

Fractures of the base of the tail involving the sacrococcygeal junctional area may cause so much pain and can also cause neurologic defects that the cow shows signs of constipation. The most common cause of tail fractures in cattle is being ridden by other cows or bulls during standing estrus. Sadistic tail restraint that fractures the tail may also cause severe pain, constipation, tail head swelling, and flaccidity of the tail.

Treatment for tail fractures is symptomatic in most cases and includes analgesics, antiinflammatories, and laxative diets. Aspirin (240 to 480 grains orally, twice daily) or flunixin meglumine (200 to 500 mg IM, twice daily) may be used as an analgesic for 3 to 5 days.

Systemic dexamethasone (10 to 30 mg IM, once daily) may be helpful in acute cases (if the animal *is not pregnant*) to help reduce inflammation in the spinal nerves. Permanent tail paralysis may persist and result in a soiled perineum and tail, as well as possible vulvovaginal fecal contamination, which interfere with fertility. Surgical repair may be possible for show animals or very valuable breeding animals in which a fractured tail would be cosmetically unacceptable or potentially interfere with breeding.

Pneumorectum

Pneumorectum may be caused by conformational defects in the perineum, rectovaginal lacerations following dystocia, dyspnea, tenesmus for any reason, and rectal examination allowing air to enter the rectum. Pneumorectum usually does not require treatment because it does not cause illness unless it persists and becomes severe, in which case one or more epidurals may be needed as treatment. Cows can get into a vicious cycle of "sucking" air and straining such that they will become anorexic, Dr. Whitlock calls this malignant tenesmus. When a rectal examination is essential for diagnostic purposes (e.g., pregnancy) in a cow affected with pneumorectum, however, the examiner must know how to gently evacuate the air from the rectum. This may be accomplished by a gentle sweeping of the rectum until a contraction band can be grasped and pulled caudally to express the air from the rectum. The procedure may need to be repeated several times to complete evacuation and is quite successful except in instances of severe rectal irritation and tenesmus.

Pneumorectum also results in a right-sided abdominal ping that may be confused with other causes of right-sided abdominal distention (Figure 5-93). Because the rectum traverses the right upper abdominal quadrant, the ping occurs from the tuber coxae through the right paralumbar fossa and a variable distance cranially. The ping may extend to the dorsal midline. Although this finding creates a broad differential diagnosis (cecal

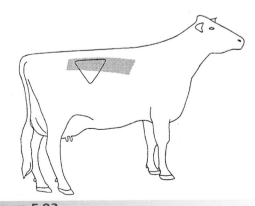

Figure 5-93

Typical pneumorectum ping.

distention, benign colonic distention, pneumoperito-neum) based on external percussion and auscultation, rectal examination should quickly identify pneumorec-tum and rule out other causes of tympanitic resonance.

MISCELLANEOUS ABDOMINAL DISORDERS

Pneumoperitoneum

Etiology

Pneumoperitoneum is defined as air or gas free in the peritoneal cavity. Whereas the most common cause of this disorder is exploratory laparotomy, other causes such as perforation/rupture of distended abdominal organs may result in pneumoperitoneum. Clinically appreciable pneumoperitoneum appears to be more commonly as-sociated with abomasal perforation rather than traumatic perforation of the reticulum. Pneumothorax or pneumo-mediastinum also occasionally progresses to involve the abdomen, thereby creating pneumoperitoneum.

Signs

Pneumoperitoneum causes mild to marked bilateral ab-dominal distention and a ping bilaterally in the upper third of the abdomen extending to the dorsal midline (Figure 5-94). Although more easily heard on the right side because of the rumen mass filling the left abdomen, this ping generally is detectable to some degree on both sides. Fluid is not present when the abdomen is ballotted over the area of the ping. When rectal examination is performed, the examiner will find the rectum uniformly compressed against the hand and arm by the pressure of air free in the peritoneal cavity. It is difficult or impossible to grasp structures through the wall of the rectum such that the examiner must just "touch" various organs with the fingertips. The rumen is difficult to palpate or auscult through the left paralumbar fossa because free air lies between the parietal peritoneum and visceral peritoneum of the rumen.

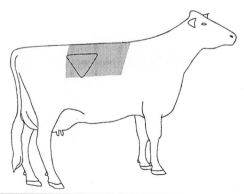

Figure 5-94

Right-sided pneumoperitoneum ping.

Although the above signs are present in all cases of pneumoperitoneum, other signs will be specific for distinct causes of pneumoperitoneum. For example, fever and abdominal pain also will exist in cattle with pneumoperitoneum secondary to a displaced aboma-sum that has developed a perforating ulcer. Cattle with pneumoperitoneum of thoracic origin would be dys-pneic in addition to the aforementioned signs. Uterine perforation during dystocia and penetrating abdom-inal wounds are other causes of pneumoperitoneum that would have additional distinct signs or historical features.

Diagnosis

The diagnosis is made by physical examination and rectal findings. This disorder must be differentiated from other causes of abdominal distention by careful auscultation/percussion and rectal evaluation (Table 5-4). When the ping is present bilaterally, there seldom should be confu-sion. If a cow has had laparotomy surgery recently, the cause should be obvious. A cow with LDA or RDA that suddenly develops signs of pneumoperitoneum and fe-ver should be suspected of having a perforating abomasal ulcer.

Treatment

In mild cases of pneumoperitoneum following explor-atory surgery, no treatment is necessary. In moderate to severe cases, affected cattle are so distended that dis-comfort and lack of appetite may result. Therefore the free air in the abdomen should be evacuated by suction through needle puncture in the right paralumbar fossa.

If pneumoperitoneum and fever are present in cattle with a recent history or physical signs of LDA or RDA, surgery through the ventral right paramedian approach should be performed in an effort to secure the aboma-sum and oversew the perforating ulcer (Figure 5-95). Some cattle will remain displaced to the left or right fol-lowing perforation, allowing adhesions of the displaced abomasum to the parietal peritoneum. In these cattle, the typical ping and fluid content of a displaced abomasum will be present along with the signs of pneumoperito-neum and fever. The pneumoperitoneum may mask or confuse the diagnosis of DA in such instances until the air is evacuated through aspiration (Figure 5-96). Local-ized abdominal pain also may be present in the area of the displacement when perforation coexists. Right para-median laparotomy to best gain access to the abomasum is recommended, but the prognosis is guarded because the abomasum may be affixed to the body wall by fibrin-ous adhesions and is prone to rupture or leak contents through the perforating ulcer when surgical manipula-tions detach the organ from the body wall. Systemic and peritoneal lavage antibiotics are indicated as supportive therapy.

TABLE 5-4 How to Differentiate Pneumoperitoneum from Other Pings

Side	Key Aid
Left	
Ruminal tympany	Rectal examination or stomach tube
Rumen collapse	Rectal examination
	No abdominal distention in rumen collapse
Right	
Cecal dilatation	Rectal examination—not bilateral
Benign colonic distention	Rectal examination—not bilateral—no abdominal distention in benign colonic distention
Pneumorectum	Rectal examination
Right abomasal displacement	Fluid present in RDA (ballottement) and RDA located midabdomen and cranial, rather than dorsal third, as in pneumoperitoneum

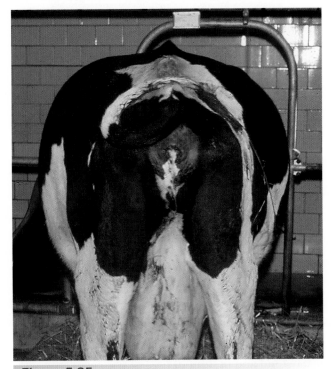

Figure 5-95

Pneumoperitoneum in a cow that historically had simple left displacement of the abomasum before shipment to our hospital. The cow had fever present at admission as well. Immediate surgical exploration from the right paramedian approach confirmed a small perforating abomasal ulcer, which was oversewn and an abomasopexy performed.

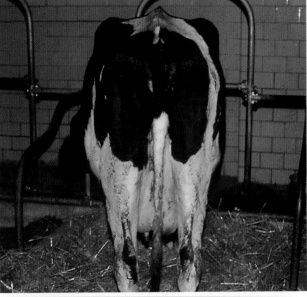

Figure 5-96

Postoperative view of the cow shown in Figure 5-95; this animal made a full recovery following the surgery and supportive antibiotic therapy.

Prevention

Prevention of severe pneumoperitoneum is only possible for those animals at risk because of exploratory laparotomy and is accomplished by an attendant pushing on the opposite side of the cow's abdomen to evacuate the air before final closure of the peritoneal sutures by the surgeon.

Peritonitis

Well-known causes of peritonitis in the dairy cow include traumatic reticuloperitonitis, perforating abomasal ulcers, improperly performed blind tack and toggle-pin procedures, and uterine rupture following dystocia. Less frequent causes of peritonitis exist, but because of both their rare occurrence and high mortality, discussion of these will be limited.

Small Intestinal Rupture

This condition results in rapid deterioration and often appears as sudden death. It may be observed in neonatal calves that apparently have been stepped on by their dam or other adult cows. It also occurs in adult cattle during parturition when a loop of small intestine is entrapped and subsequently squeezed between the maternal pelvis and the fetus within the birth canal.

Uterine Perforation by Pipette Injury

This lesion results in peritonitis or abscessation involving the uterus and is caused by neophytic or overaggressive attempts at uterine infusion—especially when attempting to infuse a cow with septic metritis less than 2 weeks postpartum when the cervix and uterus cannot possibly be elevated into the pelvis for routine infusion. This lesion is typically non–life-threatening but can limit the individual's future reproductive use and value.

Vaginal Perforation

Perforation of the vagina has been observed following natural mating, pipette injuries, dystocia, or sadism. Prognosis varies with the degree of contamination of the offending object.

Abdominal Abscesses

Although reticular and liver abscesses are well recognized and have been discussed as potential causes of vagus indigestion, other abdominal locations may harbor abscesses. These include the umbilical remnants or region and the omental bursa. Perforating abomasal ulcers are the most common cause of omental bursitis, bursal abscesses, or walled-off omental abscesses. Perforations of the visceral surface of the abomasum may allow ingesta to enter the omental bursa, the potential space between the superficial and deep sheaths of the greater omentum. Abscesses also may develop subsequent to rumen trocharization. Signs are not specific but include progressive inappetence, decreased milk production, abdominal distention, and usually fever unresponsive to antibiotic therapy. Ruminal abscesses can also be seen secondary to toxic rumenitis, but these tend to be confined to the wall of the organ. Occasional full-thickness ruminal perforations with associated peritonitis will occur because of penetrating foreign bodies, but this is not as common as traumatic reticuloperitonitis. Laboratory data may be helpful to the diagnosis because serum globulin often is elevated, serum albumin is decreased, and the abdominal fluid usually reflects inflammation with elevated total solids (>3.5 g/dl) and an elevated white blood cell count. Ultrasonography may help localize the lesion such that surgical drainage may be attempted. Appropriate antibiotic therapy is based on culture and sensitivity results from the abscess. The prognosis is poor.

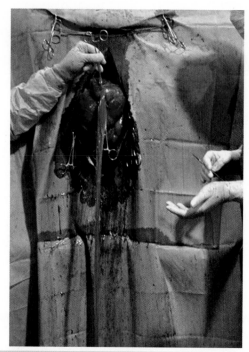

Figure 5-97

Drainage of omental bursitis in a cow that had a perforated abomasal ulcer.

Omental bursa abscesses (Figure 5-97) may be so large as to create a detectable fluid wave on ballottement of the right abdomen and a dull right-sided midabdominal ping resulting from gas accumulation dorsal to the large purulent fluid accumulation (see video clip 12).

Neoplasias of the abdomen other than lymphosarcoma are rare. Tumors such as mesothelioma (Figure 5-98, *A* and *B*) are occasionally seen and may cause massive peritoneal effusion.

Displacement of the Omasum

In the past few years we have seen several cows with displaced omasum into the upper right abdomen, both just behind and in front of the last rib. These cases were first brought to our attention by Dr. Chuck Guard and have been confirmed on exploratory laparotomy and at necropsy. Cows often have a several-day history of decreased appetite and production. A small ping can be heard over the area of the displacement, often high on the 13th rib. The omasum has been palpated rectally on a couple of the cows. An appropriate surgical repair method has not been determined at this time.

Idiopathic Eosinophilic Enteritis

This is a rare but well-documented cause of chronic diarrhea and weight loss in adult cattle. The clinical signs and age are nearly identical to Johne's disease. Plasma

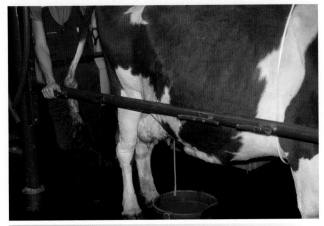

Figure 5-98

A, Ultrasound revealing massive peritoneal effusion in a 8-year-old red Holstein with mesothelioma. **B,** Drainage of the neoplastic peritoneal fluid seen in *A.*

albumin, although consistently low in clinical cases of Johne's disease, often remains within normal range in cattle with eosinophilic enteritis. Confirmation of the diagnosis is by biopsy of the small intestine and finding eosinophilic inflammation and edema within the intestine. Blood eosinophil count is normal. One-month treatment with systemically administered corticosteroids has been attempted in a very few cases and a favorable response was observed.

SUGGESTED READINGS

Abutarbush SM, Naylor JM: Obstruction of the small intestine by a trichobezoar in cattle: 15 cases (1992-2002), *J Am Vet Med Assoc* 229: 1627-1630, 2006.

Ahmed AF, Constable PD, Misk NA: Effect of orally administered cimetidine and ranitidine on abomasal luminal pH in clinically normal milk-fed calves, *Am J Vet Res* 62:1531-1538, 2001.

Ahmed AF, Constable PD, Misk NA.: Effect of orally administered Omeprazole on abomasal luminal pH in dairy calves fed milk replacer, *J Vet Med A Physiol Pathol Clin Med* 52:238-243, 2005.

Ames NK: Left displaced abomasum in dairy cows, *Agri-Practice* March:11-16, 1987.

Bertone A, Roth L, O'Krepky J: Forestomach neoplasia in cattle: a report of eight cases, *Compend Contin Educ Pract Vet* 7:585-591, 1985.

Bertone AL: Neoplasms of the bovine gastrointestinal tract, *Vet Clin North Am (Food Anim Pract)* 6:515-524, 1990.

Blood DC, Radostits OM, Henderson JA: *Veterinary medicine,* ed 6, London, 1983, Bailliére Tindall.

Bosshart JK: Telescoped intestines in cattle, *Cornell Vet* 20:55, 1930.

Braun U.: Ultrasound as a decision-making tool in abdominal surgery in cows. *Vet Clin North Am Food Anim Pract* 21:33-53, 2005.

Braun U, Gansohr B, Fluckiger M: Radiographic findings before and after oral administration of a magnet in cows with traumatic reticuloperitonitis, *Am J Vet Res* 64:115-120, 2003.

Braun U, Iselin U, Lischer C, Fluri E: Ultrasonographic findings in five cows before and after treatment of reticular abscesses, *Vet Rec* 142:184-189, 1998.

Brenner J, Orgad U: Epidemiological investigations of an outbreak of intestinal atresia in two Israeli dairy herds, *J Vet Med Sci* 65: 141-143, 2003.

Breukink HJ: Abomasal displacement, etiology, pathogenesis, treatment and prevention, *Bov Pract* 26:148-153, 1991.

Breukink HJ: Clinical consequences of ruminal drinking in veal calves. In *Proceedings: 14th World Congress on Diseases of Cattle 1986,* pp. 1157-1162.

Bristol DG, Fubini SL: Surgery of the neonatal bovine digestive tract, *Vet Clin North Am (Food Anim Pract)* 6:473-493, 1990.

Carlson SA, Stoffregen WC, Bolin SR: Abomasitis associated with multiple antibiotic resistant Salmonella enterica serotype Typhimurium phagetype DT104, *Vet Microbiol* 85:233-240, 2002.

Cebra ML, Cebra CK, Garry FB, et al: Idiopathic eosinophilic enteritis in four cattle, *J Am Vet Med Assoc* 212:258-261, 1998.

Chapman WL, Smith JA: Abomasal adenocarcinoma in a cow, *J Am Vet Med Assoc* 181:493-494, 1982.

Constable PD, Miller GY, Hoffsis GF, et al: Risk factors for abomasal volvulus and left abomasal displacement in cattle, *Am J Vet Res* 53:1184-1192, 1992.

Constable PD, St Jean G, Hull BL, et al: Intussusception in cattle: 336 cases (1964-1993), *J Am Vet Med Assoc* 210:531-536, 1997.

Constable PD, St. Jean G, Ring DM, et al: Preoperative prognostic indicators in cattle with abomasal volvulus, *J Am Vet Med Assoc* 198:2077-2085, 1991.

Cramers T, Mikkelsen KB, Andersen P, et al: New types of foreign bodies and the effect of magnets in traumatic reticulitis in cows, *Vet Rec* 157:287-289, 2005.

Davidson HP, Rebhun WC, Habel RE: Pharyngeal trauma in cattle, *Cornell Vet* 71:15-25, 1981.

Dennison AC, Van Metre DC, Morley PS, et al: Comparison of the odds of isolation, genotypes, and in vivo production of major toxins by *Clostridium perfringens* obtained from the gastrointestinal tract of dairy cows with hemorrhagic bowel syndrome or left-displaced abomasum, *J Am Vet Med Assoc* 227:132-138, 2005.

Depez P, Hoogewijs M, Vlaminck L, et al: Incarceration of the small intestine in the epiploic foramen of three calves, *Vet Rec* 158: 869-879, 2006.

deVisser NAPC, Breukink HJ: Pensdrinkers en kleischijters, *Tijdschr Diergeneeskd* 109:800-804, 1984.

Dirksen G: Digestive system. In Rosenberger G, editor: *Clinical examination of cattle,* Berlin, 1979, Verlag Paul Parey.

Dirksen G, Doll K, Einhellig J, et al: Abomasal ulcers in calves: clinical investigations and experiences [article in German], *Tierarztl Prax* 25:318-328, 1997.

Dirksen G, Stöber M: Contribution to the functional disorders of the bovine stomach caused by the lesions of the nervus vagus-Hoflund's syndrome summary, *DTW Dtsch Tierarztl Wochenschr* 69:213-217, 1962.

Doll K, Klee W, Dirksen G: Cecal intussusception in calves [article in German], *Tierarztl Prax Ausg G Grosstiere Nutztiere* 26:247-253, 1998.

Ducharme NG: Surgery of the bovine forestomach compartments, *Vet Clin North Am (Food Anim Pract)* 6:371-397, 1990.

Ducharme NG: Surgical considerations in the treatment of traumatic reticuloperitonitis, *Compend Contin Educ Pract Vet* 5:S213-S224, 1983.

Ducharme NG, Dill SG, Rendano V: Reticulography of the cow in dorsal recumbency: an aid in the diagnosis and treatment of traumatic reticuloperitonitis, *J Am Vet Med Assoc* 182:585-588, 1983.

Ducharme NG, Smith DF, Koch DB: Small intestinal obstruction caused by a persistent round ligament of the liver in a cow, *J Am Vet Med Assoc* 180:1234-1236, 1982.

Ducharme NG, Arighti M, Horney FD, et al: Colonic atresia in cattle: a prospective of 43 cases, *Can Vet J* 29:818-824, 1988.

Dunlop RH, Hammond PB: D-Lactic acidosis of ruminants, *Ann N Y Acad Sci* 119:1109, 1965.

Duran SH: pH changes in abomasal fluid of sheep treated with intravenous and oral ranitidine. In *Proceedings: 11th Annual American College Veterinary Internal Medicine Forum 1992*, p. 960 [Abstract].

Edgson FA: Bovine lipomatosis, *Vet Rec* 64:449, 1952.

Figueiredo MD, Nydam DV, Perkins GA, et al: Prognostic value of plasma L-lactate concentration measured cow-side with a portable clinical analyzer in Holstein dairy cattle with abomasal disorders, *J Vet Intern Med* 20:1463-1470, 2006.

Fox FH: The esophagus, stomach, intestines, and peritoneum. In Amstutz HE, editor: *Bovine medicine and surgery*, ed 2, Santa Barbara, 1980, American Veterinary Publications.

Fubini SL, Ducharme, NG, editors: *Farm animal surgery*, St. Louis, 2004, Harcourt Health Sciences.

Fubini SL, Ducharme NG, Erb HN, et al: Failure of omasal transport attributable to perireticular abscess formation in cattle: 29 cases (1980–1986), *J Am Vet Med Assoc* 194:811-814, 1989.

Fubini SL, Smith DF, Tithof PK, et al: Volvulus of the distal jejunoileum in four cows, *Vet Surg* 15:410-413, 1986.

Fubini SL, Ducharme NG, Murphy JP, et al: Vagus indigestion syndrome resulting from liver abscess in dairy cows, *J Am Vet Med Assoc* 186:1297-1300, 1985.

Fubini SL, Erb HN, Rebhun WC, et al: Cecal dilatation and volvulus in dairy cows: 84 cases (1977–1983), *J Am Vet Med Assoc* 189:96-99, 1986.

Fubini SL, Gröhn YT, Smith DF: Right displacement of the abomasum and abomasal volvulus in dairy cows: 458 cases (1980–1987), *J Am Vet Med Assoc* 198:461-464, 1991.

Fubini SL, Smith DF: Failure of omasal transport due to traumatic reticuloperitonitis and intraabdominal abscess, *Compend Contin Educ Pract Vet* 4:S492-S494, 1982.

Fubini SL, Yeager AE, Mohammed HO, et al: Accuracy of radiography of the reticulum for predicting surgical findings in adult dairy cattle with traumatic reticuloperitonitis: 123 cases (1981–1987), *J Am Vet Med Assoc* 197:1060-1064, 1990.

Garry FB, Hull BL, Rings DM, et al: Prognostic value of anion gap calculation in cattle with abomasal volvulus: 58 cases (1980–1985), *J Am Vet Med Assoc* 192:1107-1112, 1988.

Gold JR, Divers TJ, deLahunta A: Postanesthetic poliomyelopathy in a 7-day-old calf, *J Vet Intern Med* 19:775-778, 2005.

Gröhn YT, Fubini SL, Smith DF: Use of a multiple logistic regression model to determine prognosis of dairy cows with right displacement of the abomasum or abomasal volvulus, *Am J Vet Res* 51:1895-1899, 1990.

Grymer J, Ames NK: Bovine abdominal pings: clinical examination and differential diagnosis, *Compend Contin Educ Pract Vet* 32:S311-S318, 1981.

Grymer J, Johnson R: Two cases of bovine omental bursitis, *J Am Vet Med Assoc* 181:714-715, 1982.

Guard C: Bloat or ruminal tympany. In Smith BP, editor: *Large animal internal medicine*, ed 3, St. Louis, 2002, Mosby.

Habel RE: A study of the innervation of the ruminant stomach, *Cornell Vet* 46:555-633, 1956.

Habel RE, Smith DF: Volvulus of the bovine abomasum and omasum, *J Am Vet Med Assoc* 179:447-455, 1981.

Hagan HA: Fat necrosis in cattle, *J Am Vet Med Assoc* 59:682, 1921.

Herrli-Gygi M, Hammon HM, Zbinden Y, et al: Ruminal drinkers: endocrine and metabolic status and effects of suckling from a nipple instead of drinking from a bucket, *J Vet Med A Physiol Pathol Clin Med* 53:215-224, 2006.

Horney FD, Cote J: Congenital diaphragmatic hernia in a calf, *Can Vet J* 2:422-424, 1961.

Hutchins DR, Blood DC, Hyne R: Residual defects in stomach motility after traumatic reticuloperitonitis of cattle. Pyloric obstruction, diaphragmatic hernia and indigestion due to reticular adhesions, *Aust Vet J* 33:77-82, 1957.

Jafarzadeh SR, Nowrouzian I, Khaki Z, et al: The sensitivities and specificities of total plasma protein and plasma fibrinogen for the diagnosis of traumatic reticuloperitonitis in cattle, *Prev Vet Med* 65:1-7, 2004.

Jarrett WFH, Campo MS, Blaxter ML, et al: Alimentary fibropapilloma in cattle. A spontaneous tumor, nonpermissive for papillomavirus replication, *J Natl Cancer Inst* 73:499-504, 1984.

Kalaitzakis E, Roubies N, Panousis N, et al: Evaluation of ornithine carbamoyl transferase and other serum and liver-derived analytes in diagnosis of fatty liver and postsurgical outcome of left-displaced abomasus in dairy cows, *J Am Vet Med Assoc* 229:1463-1471, 2006.

King JM: Personal communication, 1980, Cornell University, Ithaca, NY.

King JM: Personal communication, 1987, Ithaca, NY.

Kleen JL, Hooijer GA, Rehage J, et al: Rumenocentesis (rumen puncture): a viable instrument in herd health diagnosis, *Dtsch Tierarztl Wochenschr* 111:458-462, 2004.

Koch DB, Robertson JT, Donawick WJ: Small intestinal obstruction due to persistent vitelloumbilical band in a cow, *J Am Vet Med Assoc* 173:197-199, 1978.

Leipold HW, Watt B, Vestweber JGE, et al: Clinical observations in rectovaginal constriction in jersey cattle, *Bov Pract* 16:76-79, 1981.

McDuffee LA, Ducharme NG, Ward JL: Repair of sacral fracture in two dairy cattle, *J Am Vet Med Assoc* 202:1126-1128, 1993.

McGuirk SM, Butler DG: Metabolic alkalosis with paradoxic aciduria in cattle, *J Am Vet Med Assoc* 177:551-554, 1980.

Neal PA, Edwards GB: "Vagus indigestion" in cattle, *Vet Rec* 82:396-402, 1968.

Ness H, Leopold G, Mullet W: Zur Genese des angeborenen Darmverschlusses (Atresia coil et jejuni) des Kalbes, *Monats Veterinarmed* 37:89-92, 1982 [Genesis of congenital ileum in calf (atresia coli et jejuni)].

Newton-Clarke M, Rebhun WC: Diaphragmatic herniation causing respiratory signs in a heifer, *Cornell Vet* 83:205-209, 1993.

Palmer JE, Whitlock RH: Perforated abomasal ulcers in adult dairy cows, *J Am Vet Med Assoc* 184:171-173, 1984.

Parker JL, Fubini SL: Abomasal fistulas in 8 dairy cows, *Cornell Vet* 77:303-309, 1987.

Pearson H: Dilatation and torsion of the bovine caecum and colon, *Vet Rec* 75:961-964, 1963.

Pearson H: Intestinal obstruction in cattle, *Vet Rec* 101:162-166, 1977.

Pearson H: Intussusception in cattle, *Vet Rec* 89:426-437, 1971.

Pehrson BG, Shaver RD: Displaced abomasum: clinical data and effects of periparital feeding and management on incidence. In *Proceedings: XVII World Buiatrics Congress, 1990*, vol I, pp. 116-121.

Rager KD, George LW, House JK, et al: Evaluation of rumen transfaunation after surgical correction of left-sided displacement of the abomasum in cows, *J Am Vet Med Assoc* 225:915-920, 2004.

Rebhun WC: Differentiating the causes of left abdominal tympanitic resonance in dairy cattle, *Vet Med* 86:1126-1134, 1991.

Rebhun WC: Right abdominal tympanitic resonance in dairy cattle: identifying the causes, *Vet Med* 86:1135-1142, 1991.

Rebhun WC: Rumen collapse in cattle, *Cornell Vet* 77:244-250, 1987.

Rebhun WC: The medical treatment of abomasal ulcers in dairy cattle, *Compend Contin Educ Pract Vet* 4:S91-S98, 1982.

Rebhun WC: Vagus indigestion in cattle, *J Am Vet Med Assoc* 176:506-510, 1980.

Richardson DW: Parovarian-omental bands as a cause of small intestinal obstruction in cows, *J Am Vet Med Assoc* 185:517-519, 1984.

Roberts SJ: Diaphragmatic hernia in a bovine, *Cornell Vet* 36:92-96, 1946.

Robertson JT: Differential diagnosis and surgical management of intestinal obstruction in cattle, *Vet Clin North Am (Large Anim Pract)* 1:377-394, 1979.

Roussel AJ, Brumbaugh GW, Waldron RC, et al: Abomasal and duodenal motility of cattle after administration of prokinetic drugs. In *Proceedings: 11th Annual American College Veterinary Internal Medicine Forum 1992*, p. 960 [Abstract].

Rutgers LJE, Van der Velden MA: Complications following use of the closed suturing technique for correction of left abomasal displacement in cows, *Vet Rec* 113:255-257, 1983.

Sattler N, Fecteau G, Helie P, et al: Etiology, forms, and prognosis of gastrointestinal dysfunction resembling vagal indigestion occurring after surgical correction of right abomasal displacement, *Can Vet J* 41:777-785, 2000.

Simpson DF, Erb HN, Smith DF: Base excess as a prognostic and diagnostic indicator in cows with abomasal volvulus in right displacement of the abomasum, *Am J Vet Res* 46:796-797, 1985.

Smith DF: Right-side torsion of the abomasum in dairy cows: classification of severity and evaluation of outcome, *J Am Vet Med Assoc* 173:108-111, 1978.

Smith DF: Surgical repair of atresia coli in a calf, *Compend Contin Educ Pract Vet* 4:S441-S445, 1982.

Smith DF: Treatment of left displacement of the abomasum. Part I, *Compend Contin Educ Pract Vet* 3:S415-S423, 1981.

Smith DF, Donawick WJ: Obstruction of the ascending colon in cattle. I. Clinical presentation and surgical management, *Vet Surg* 8: 93-97, 1979.

Smith DF, Erb HN, Kalaher KM, et al: The identification of structures and conditions responsible for right side tympanitic resonance (ping) in adult cattle, *Cornell Vet* 72:180-199, 1982.

Steen A: Field study of dairy cows with reduced appetite in early lactation: clinical examinations, blood and rumen fluid analyses, *Acta Vet Scand* 42:219-228, 2001.

Steenhaut M, DeMoor A, Verschooten F: Intestinal malformations in calves and their surgical correction, *Vet Rec* 98:131, 1976.

Sterner KE, Grymer J: Closed suturing techniques using a bar-suture for correction of left displaced abomasum—a review of 100 cases, *Bov Pract* 17:80-84, 1982.

Stöber M, Dirksen G: The differential diagnosis of abdominal findings (adspection, rectal examination and exploratory laparotomy) in cattle, *Bov Pract* 12:35-38, 1977 [This paper was originally published in German in *Berl Munch Tierzaztl Wochenschr* 89:129-133, 1976].

Stocker H, Lutz H, Kaufmann C, et al: Acid-base disorders in milk-fed calves with chronic indigestion, *Vet Rec* 145:340-346, 1999.

Stocker H, Lutz H, Rusch P: Clinical, haematological and biochemical findings in milk-fed calves with chronic indigestion, *Vet Rec* 145:307-311, 1999.

Stocker H, Rusch P: Chronic indigestion in milk-fed calves [article in German], *Schweiz Arch Tierheilkd* 141:407-411, 1999.

Svendsen P: Etiology and pathogenesis of abomasal displacement in cattle, Master's thesis, Cornell University, Ithaca, NY, 1969.

Tithof PK, Rebhun WC: Complications of blind-stitch abomasopexy—20 cases (1980–1985), *J Am Vet Med Assoc* 189:1489-1492, 1986.

Trent AM: Surgery of the bovine abomasum, *Vet Clin North Am (Food Anim Pract)* 6:399-448, 1990.

Troutt HF, Fessler JF, Page EH, et al: Diaphragmatic defects in cattle, *J Am Vet Med Assoc* 151:1421-1429, 1967.

Tulleners EP: Avulsion of the jejunum, with vaginal evisceration in a cow, *J Am Vet Med Assoc* 184:195-196, 1984.

Tulleners EP, Hamilton GF: Surgical resection of perforated abomasal ulcers in calves, *Can Vet J* 21:262-264, 1980.

Udall DH: *The practice of veterinary medicine*, Ithaca, NY, 1954, published by the author.

van Bruinessen-Kapsenberg EG, Wensing T, Breukink HJ: Indigestionen der Mastkalber infolge fehlenden Schlundrinnen-reflexes, *Tierärzt Umsch* 7:515-517, 1982.

Whitlock RH: Abomasal ulcers. In Anderson NV, editor: *Veterinary gastroenterology*, Philadelphia, 1980, Lea & Febiger.

Whitlock RH, Becht JL: Probantheline bromide and cimetidine in the control of abomasal acid secretion. In *Proceedings: 16th Annual Convention American Association Bovine Practice 1983*, p. 140 [abstract].

Whitlock RH: Cecal volvulus in dairy cattle. In *Proceedings: International Congress on Diseases of Cattle* 1:60-63, 1976.

Wittek T, Constable PD: Assessment of the effects of erythromycin, neostigmine, and metoclopramide on abomasal motility and emptying rate in calves, *Am J Vet Res* 66:545-552, 2005.

Wittek T, Constable PD, Morin DE: Abomasal impaction in Holstein-Friesian cows: 80 cases (1980-2003), *J Am Vet Med Assoc* 227: 287-291, 2005.

Wittek T, Furll M, Constable PD: Prevalence of endotoxemia in healthy postparturient dairy cows and cows with abomasal volvulus or left displaced abomasum, *J Vet Intern Med* 18:574-580, 2004.

Zust J, Pestevsek U, Vengust A: Impact of lactic acid fermentation in the large intestine on acute lactic acidosis in cattle [article in German], *Dtsch Tierarztl Wochenschr* 107:359-363, 2000.

Infectious Diseases of the Gastrointestinal Tract

David C. Van Metre, Bud C. Tennant, and Robert H. Whitlock

CALVES

Escherichia coli

Escherichia coli is a normal inhabitant of the gastrointestinal tract of warm-blooded animals and ubiquitous in the farm environment. Disease caused by *E. coli* in calves may present as enteric or septicemic illness and is an important cause of neonatal mortality in dairy calves. Failure of passive transfer and management practices that allow exposure of the neonatal calf to large numbers of *E. coli* are of central importance in the pathogenesis of disease. A plethora of *E. coli* serotypes exist on dairy farms. These gram-negative organisms are classified based on various serologic and antigenic parameters, including cell wall or somatic (O) antigens, capsular (K) antigens, pilar or fimbrial (F) antigens, and flagellar (H) antigens. Heretofore, pilus antigens were sometimes classified as K antigens, but recent reference to pilus antigens as F antigens reduces confusion in this area.

Septicemia (Septicemic Colibacillosis, Colisepticemia)

Etiology. Colisepticemia in neonatal calves can be considered a disease of poor management. Failure of passive transfer is the primary risk factor for this disease. Colostral transfer of immunoglobulins may be compromised by short dry periods, preparturient leaking of colostrum, assumption that a calf has nursed colostrum just because it is left with the dam for 24 hours, primiparous heifers that have poor-quality colostrum, and many other factors. In addition, poor maternity area and poor calf pen hygiene promote exposure of the calf to the multitude of strains of *E. coli* capable of causing septicemia. Filthy conditions, calving areas that are dirty, wet, overcrowded, or overused, and failure to dip navels are additional factors that predispose to this problem. Sanitation and hygiene with respect to collecting, storing, and administering colostrum are also emerging as important factors in the provision of adequate passive transfer and the prevention of colibacillosis.

Invasive *E. coli* of many subgroups are capable of opportunistic, septicemic infection of neonatal calves. Various reviews suggest an involvement of a multitude of possible *E. coli* types. Variations may be explained by geographic or environmental differences.

Calves with less than 500 mg IgG/dl are very prone to septicemic *E. coli,* and those with 500 to 1000 mg IgG/dl are defined as having partial failure of passive transfer and are also at increased risk. Adequate passive immunoglobulin that ensures at least 1000 IgG mg/dl serum (10 mg/ml serum) or preferably 1600 mg/dl serum is likely to prevent the disease.

Septicemia caused by *E. coli* most commonly occurs from 1 to 14 days of age. The onset of disease tends to occur earlier in this time frame when calves are exposed to high numbers of *E. coli* soon after birth (i.e., in the maternity pen). Poor or nonexistent transfer of passive immunoglobulins to the calf also hastens the onset of disease. Invasive *E. coli* may gain entrance through the navel, intestine, or nasal and oropharyngeal mucous membranes. Once invasion and septicemia occur, clinical signs develop rapidly and usually are apparent within 24 hours. Calves with partial failure of passive transfer or those exposed to less virulent *E. coli* strains may develop more chronic signs of disease over several days.

Septicemic calves shed the causative *E. coli* in urine, oral secretions, nasal secretions, and later in the feces, provided they survive long enough to develop diarrhea. Thus transmission may occur among communally housed calves, crowded calves, or uncleaned maternity stalls because of the heavily infected secretions of sick and septicemic calves. Because septicemic calves can shed large numbers of the organism before clinical signs are evident, contamination of communal pens and common-use feeding devices (e.g., esophageal feeding tubes) and direct contact with the infected calf or its feces or urine may promote spread of infection. Infected calves allowed to remain in the maternity area will amplify the level of environmental contamination, thereby placing other neonates born in that area at risk. Similar amplification may occur in calf housing areas and reinforces the biosecurity need for spatial and temporal separation between occupants, as well as the appropriate and routine disinfection of calf housing.

Clinical Signs. Peracute signs of depression, weakness, tachycardia, and dehydration predominate when

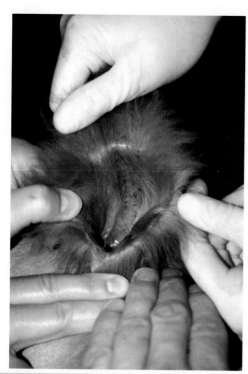

Figure 6-1

Ear of 5-day-old Jersey calf demonstrating petechial hemorrhage associated with *E. coli* septicemia.

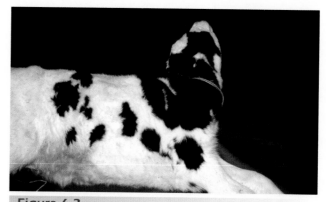

Figure 6-2

Seven-day-old Holstein calf with opisthotonus associated with *E. coli* meningitis and septicemia as a result of failure of passive transfer.

highly virulent strains of *E. coli* cause septicemia. Affected calves usually are less than 7 days of age and may be less than 24 hours old. Although often present early on, fever is usually absent by the time obvious clinical signs of disease occur, when endotoxemia and the resultant poor peripheral perfusion often render the animal normothermic or hypothermic. Exceptions to this rule are calves with peracute disease that collapse when exposed to direct sunlight on hot days—such calves can be markedly hyperthermic. Signs of dehydration are mild to moderate in most cases. The suckle reflex is greatly reduced or absent, and the vasculature of the sclerae is markedly injected. Petechial hemorrhages may be visible on mucous membranes and extremities, particularly the pinnae of the ears (Figure 6-1). The limbs, mouth, and ears are cool to the touch. Affected calves show progressive weakness and lethargy, often becoming comatose before death. Diarrhea is often seen but may not be apparent in peracute cases.

Evidence of localization of infection in certain tissues may become apparent in cases that survive the acute disease. Hypopyon may be present, as may uveitis, which is evidenced by miotic pupils with increased opacity to the aqueous fluid ("aqueous flare"). Hyperesthesia, paddling, and opisthotonus (Figure 6-2) are signs suggestive of septic meningitis. Lameness may result from bacterial seeding of joints and/or growth plates. Signs of omphalophlebitis may be present. Weakness, poor body condition, and recumbency secondary

to weakness or joint or bone pain may be present in chronic cases.

Clinical signs of acute septicemia may be difficult to differentiate from those of acute enterotoxigenic *E. coli* (ETEC) infection because dehydration, weakness, and collapse may be common to both. However, septicemic calves tend to be less dehydrated and have less watery diarrhea than calves with ETEC diarrhea; further, diarrhea tends to develop in the terminal stages of septicemia. Historical data may indicate other neonatal calves have recently shown similar signs or died at less than 2 weeks of age. Other differential diagnoses for acute colisepticemia include asphyxia or trauma during birth, simple hypothermia and/or hypoglycemia, septicemia caused by *Salmonella* spp., and congenital defects of the central nervous or cardiovascular systems. Polyarthritis caused by *Mycoplasma* spp. is an important differential diagnosis for septic arthritis secondary to colisepticemia but tends to be seen in older calves, and feeding unpasteurized milk is a significant risk factor for *Mycoplasma* disease. Salt poisoning, hypoglycemia, congenital neurologic disorders, traumatic injuries, and intoxications (e.g., lead) should be considered as differential diagnoses for meningitis secondary to colisepticemia. We have also seen several herds in recent years with young calves presenting with neurologic signs indistinguishable from meningitis for which the ultimate diagnosis was ionophore toxicity caused by overdosing before feeding milk replacer. Failure of passive transfer and meningitis were *not* involved.

Ancillary Data. Calves suffering from peracute *E. coli* septicemia often have elevated packed cell volumes resulting from dehydration and endotoxic shock. The total white blood cell (WBC) count is variable but is frequently low or within normal ranges. Generally a left shift is observed, and toxic changes (e.g., azurophilic cytoplasm, nuclear hypersegmentation, and Dohle bodies) are often apparent on cytologic examination of blood neutrophils. Plasma fibrinogen concentration is variable.

Hypoglycemia is a common finding, and metabolic acidosis, although common, usually is less severe than in calves recumbent as a result of ETEC. In fact, an acid-base and electrolyte determination that does not demonstrate a severe metabolic acidosis in a recumbent, diarrheic, dehydrated calf less than 14 days of age is a grave sign and usually portends septicemia. Severe hypoglycemia would be the only other laboratory finding that might indicate an easily treatable condition. Blood cultures provide the greatest specific diagnostic aid, but results may not be forthcoming in time to help the patient.

Acute, subacute, and chronic septicemic calves may have detectable clinical signs of localization of infection that allow a more definitive diagnostic test (e.g., cerebrospinal fluid [CSF] tap for patients showing signs of meningitis or joint tap to confirm septic arthritis) (Figure 6-3). In chronic cases, the serum immunoglobulin concentration (and serum total globulin concentration) may be normal or increased as a result of de novo synthesis of antibodies in response to the well-established bacterial infection.

Diagnosis. Whenever clinical signs suggest the diagnosis, the calf's serum immunoglobulin levels should be analyzed. Although adequate levels of IgG do not rule out the disease, calves with IgG ≥1600 mg/dl serum based on a single radial immunodiffusion test are unlikely to suffer septicemic *E. coli* infections. Specific laboratory evaluation of immunoglobulin levels is preferable to field techniques when confirmation of failure of passive transfer (FPT) is essential but may not provide rapid results in the field. Therefore even though dehydration may falsely elevate blood protein levels, these may be useful field tests. Adequate immunoglobulin levels are suggested by serum total protein ≥5.5 g/dl in clinically ill calves. Serum gamma glutamyl transferase (GGT) activity >50 IU/L is a reliable indicator of adequate passive transfer in ill calves, as is development of visible turbidity in the 18% solution of sodium sulfite turbidity test. Several commercial "quick tests" (e.g., Midlands Bio-Products, Boone, IA) are now available for determining IgG concentration in calves.

Blood cultures provide definitive diagnosis but usually provide this information too late to be of practical value. When multiple calves are affected, however, blood cultures can help to differentiate *E. coli* septicemia from septicemia caused by other pathogens (e.g., *Salmonella* spp.); this differentiation is relevant for determining the source of infection and initiation of preventive measures. Further, antimicrobial sensitivity testing of blood culture isolates may aid in directing therapy for subsequent cases. Clinicians and producers should be aware of the differences between specific antigenic strains of *E. coli* (e.g., ETEC) capable of producing severe disease in calves with adequate passive transfer and the everyday, commensal, and environmental *E. coli* often associated with sepsis caused by FPT. This is an important distinction, lest clients concentrate preventive efforts and management on specific vaccination programs rather than colostrum and neonatal calf management.

Treatment. Treatment of peracute *E. coli* septicemia usually is unsuccessful because of overwhelming bacteremia and endotoxemia in the patient. Signs progress so quickly that most septicemic calves are recumbent and comatose by the time of initial examination. Shock, lactic acidosis, hypoglycemia, and multiple organ failure are common in peracute cases.

If treatment is attempted, correction of endotoxic shock and acid-base and electrolyte abnormalities, effective antimicrobial therapy, and nutritional support are the primary goals. Intravenous (IV) balanced electrolyte solutions should contain dextrose (2.5% to 10%) and sodium bicarbonate (20 to 50 mEq/L if the plasma bicarbonate concentration is <10 mEq/L) to address hypoglycemia and metabolic acidosis. Adjustments of the concentration of dextrose and sodium bicarbonate in polyionic fluids can be guided by subsequent serum chemistry results. Maintaining normoglycemia in some peracute and acute septicemic calves can be extremely challenging due to consumption of administered glucose by bacteria. Antimicrobials used to treat neonatal septicemia should be bactericidal and possess a good gram-negative spectrum, such as ceftiofur, trimethoprim-sulfa, or ampicillin. Parenteral administration is necessary to achieve effective blood concentrations. Aminoglycosides such as gentamicin or amikacin can be used alone or in conjunction with the synergistically acting beta-lactam antibiotics (e.g., ceftiofur, penicillin, or ampicillin). The use of potentially nephrotoxic aminoglycosides in a dehydrated patient with prerenal azotemia must be weighed against the

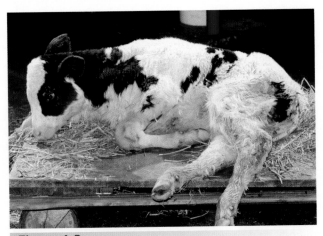

Figure 6-3

A 1-week-old calf affected with subacute *E. coli* septicemia. The calf has fever, diarrhea, dehydration, and a septic carpal joint. The calf had inadequate immunoglobulin levels.

potential bactericidal activity of the drugs. Given the present concerns regarding aminoglycoside use in food animals, use should be limited to situations in which other antibiotics have proven ineffective. Further, a minimum 18-month slaughter withdrawal must be enforced for calves that receive aminoglycosides. Use of fluoroquinolones (e.g., enrofloxacin, danofloxacin) in dairy calves is currently not permitted under federal law in the United States.

If the previous therapy stabilizes the patient, a transfusion of 2 L of whole blood from (preferably) a bovine leukemia virus (BLV) and bovine virus diarrhea virus persistently infected (BVDV-PI) free cow should be performed because failure of passive transfer is assumed or confirmed. This translates to a dosage of 40 ml of whole blood/kg for the calf. Bovine plasma, which is commercially available, may also be used at the same dosage rate as whole blood. Nutritional support ideally entails frequent feedings of small volumes of whole milk or good-quality milk replacer. Partial or total parenteral nutrition (TPN) may be considered for valuable calves, particularly those with concurrent and significant enteritis. Deep, dry bedding, good ventilation, and good nursing care are essential adjuncts to medical treatment.

Specific sites of localized infection also may require specific therapy. As an example, patients manifesting seizures because of meningitis may require diazepam to control seizures. Calves with septic joints often require joint lavage. In many cases, arthrotomy is necessary to remove fibrin clots from infected joints.

Chronic cases usually are cachectic, have polyarthritis and diarrhea, and have an extremely poor prognosis. Although recumbent, weak, dehydrated, and emaciated, these patients tend to have relatively normal acid-base and electrolyte values, so fluid therapy is of limited value.

Prevention: Colostrum and Management. Sporadic cases of *E. coli* septicemia are unfortunate events, but endemic neonatal calf losses resulting from this disease demand a thorough evaluation of management regarding dry cows, periparturient cows, and newborn calves. There are two basic questions that require answers: (1) are newborn calves being fed *sufficient volumes of high-quality colostrum soon enough* after birth? And, (2) is the environment likely to harbor large numbers of *E. coli* during the periparturient and neonatal period? In other words, two facets of the dairy operation must be carefully critiqued: colostrum management and the hygiene of the maternity area and neonatal calf pens. A few very basic concepts regarding colostrum should be understood:

1. Maternal immunoglobulin is concentrated in the mammary gland of the dry cow via an active transport mechanism during the last few weeks of gestation. Although IgG$_1$ is the major immunoglobulin transferred, IgG$_2$, IgM, and IgA are found as well. Resultant colostrum contains IgG at much higher concentrations than maternal serum and transfer of maternal antibody into colostrum temporarily decreases maternal IgG$_1$ levels.

2. A minimum of 40 dry days and a maximum of 90 dry days result in the best quality colostrum.

3. Assume dry cows that leak milk before parturition or collection of colostrum have lost the "best" colostrum.

4. Holstein calves must ingest at least 100 g of IgG$_1$ in the first 12 hours of life for adequate passive transfer of immunoglobulins. The immunoglobulin concentration in colostrum deemed "acceptable" ranges from 30 to 50 g IgG/L; obviously if larger volumes of more dilute colostrum are fed, adequate immunoglobulin mass would then be provided. However, most dairy calves simply allowed to nurse dairy breed dams to satiety will not voluntarily ingest an adequate volume of colostrum to meet their required immunoglobulin intake.

5. Certain genetic lines of cattle may be prone to low immunoglobulin levels in colostrum. For example, beef cattle tend to have higher levels than Holsteins. These may reflect genetic selection or merely reflect the dilutional effects of the greater milk volume in dairy cattle.

6. A colostrometer (a hydrometer that measures specific gravity of fluid indirectly measures solids and, it is hoped, immunoglobulin concentration) is a common on-farm tool used to assess colostrum quality. Colostrometer readings may be affected by the colostrum temperature; higher temperatures underestimate quality, whereas lower temperatures overestimate quality. Therefore readings should be made when the colostrum is at room temperature (20 to 25° C). That aside, there is considerable overlap in specific gravity readings among colostrums with low and high immunoglobulin concentration. Previous recommendations state the hydrometer should have a colostrum specific gravity reading of ≥1.050 at room temperature for adequate immunoglobulin levels. However, given the large number of variables that affect colostrum specific gravity (e.g., protein concentration, lactation number, cow breed, and temperature), use of the 1.050 cutoff value will misclassify many (two thirds) poor-quality colostrums as acceptable.

7. Recently a cow-side immunoassay kit (Colostrum bovine IgG quick test kit, Midlands Bio-Products, Boone, IA) has been demonstrated to identify poor-quality colostrums (those with IgG concentrations <50 g/L) with 93% specificity; in other words, this test appears to be superior to the hydrometer in accurately identifying poor-quality colostrum. Weighing the colostrum is another means of selecting high-quality colostrums. In a large study of

Holstein cows, the total volume of first-milking colostrum weighing <8.5 kg (18.7 lb) was shown to have significantly higher colostral IgG$_1$ concentration than colostrums weighing >8.5 kg. By discarding (or feeding to older calves) Holstein colostrums weighing >8.5 kg, a producer would likely increase the percentage of high-quality colostrums being fed to calves.

8. Pooled colostrum from each cow's first milking may not ensure adequate immunoglobulin content because the poor-quality (dilute) colostrums tend to lower the immunoglobulin concentration of the entire pool and may increase *Mycobacterium avium* subspecies *paratuberculosis* and leukemia virus infections.

9. Springing heifers' colostrum has traditionally been considered lower quality than older cows. However, based on immunoglobulin concentration, colostrum from heifers is comparable with cows beginning the second lactation. In theory, the younger heifers have less immunological "experience" than cows, so it is possible the antibody "spectrum" (the number of different antigens to which antibodies are produced) is less in heifers than cows. However, the impact of this theoretical issue on calf health remains unproven. Until contrary data are made available, heifer colostrum should be evaluated on the same basis as cow colostrum.

Given this current summation of colostral quality research, the following recommendations are made for newborn dairy calves:

1. High-quality colostrum cleanly collected from Johne's disease-negative and BLV-negative cows may be stored for use. If not fed within 2 hours of milking, colostrum should be refrigerated in sanitized 1- or 2-L containers until fed; use of larger containers may limit prompt cooling, thereby promoting bacterial overgrowth in colostrum. Fresh colostrum may be refrigerated for 1 week and frozen for 1 year. If frozen, thawing should be performed slowly in warm water. Microwave thawing, if done carefully, can be used to thaw colostrums without overheating and denaturation of colostral antibodies. However, if microwave thawing is used, thawing for short time periods, periodically pouring off the thawed liquid and using a rotating tray may help to limit overheating. Immunoglobulin content of colostrum can be determined by using a validated hydrometer. Colostrum should contain at least 60 g of IgG/L.

2. Calves should receive 4 L of high-quality first milking colostrum during the first 12 hours of life (3 L is often sufficient for Jerseys and Guernseys). The first 2 L should be fed within 1 to 2 hours after birth, and the second 2 L should be fed before 12 hours of life. Many operations have chosen to feed all 4 L by esophageal feeder in a single feeding to larger calves.

3. The exact means of feeding (nipple versus tube) is less important than the timing of colostrum feeding, the volume fed, and the total immunoglobulin mass contained in that volume of colostrum.

4. Passive transfer status can be tested directly by radial immunodiffusion (RID) or indirectly by measurement of serum total protein levels. In healthy, well-hydrated calves 2 to 7 days of age, adequate passive transfer is indicated by a serum IgG concentration >1000 mg/dl and a serum total protein >5.2 g/dl. If the serum sodium sulfite turbidity test is used, use of the 1+ endpoint (turbidity in 18% solution) as an indicator of adequate passive transfer status will maximize the percentage of calves correctly classified by this assay.

5. Regular evaluation of passive transfer status of all newborn calves in a herd allows the veterinarian to objectively monitor colostrum management over time. An on-farm testing method that has been scientifically validated (e.g., serum total protein, immunoassay kit, and sodium sulfite turbidity test) should be used.

6. Calves born prematurely or from difficult births may have a variety of physical problems (e.g., swollen tongue) and metabolic disturbances (e.g., hypoxia) that may impact their ability to suckle colostrum and/or absorb immunoglobulins from the gut. Special attention should be paid to these calves to ensure adequate colostrum ingestion, and subsequent testing of serum is recommended to allow early detection and correction of FPT. Calves fed colostrum of questionable quality, those not receiving their first colostrum feeding until after 12 hours of life, and calves of exceptional value also warrant testing for FPT. Calves found to have FPT should receive a 40-ml/kg dose of whole bovine blood or plasma from their dam or from a BLV- and BVDV-PI-negative cow.

7. Colostrum can become heavily contaminated with bacteria if good milking hygiene is not practiced at the first milking. Clean teats and udders, clean milking equipment, sanitized storage containers, and sanitized feeding equipment are necessary to limit the possibility of colostrum becoming a culture medium for pathogenic bacteria, including *Salmonella* spp. and virulent strains of *E. coli*. McGuirk and Collins have provided goals for bacterial contamination of colostrum:

   • Total bacteria: <100,000 colony forming units (CFU)/ml
   • Fecal coliforms: <10,000 CFU/ml
   • Other gram-negative bacteria: <50,000 CFU/ml
   • Streptococci (non-*Streptococcus agalactiae*): <50,000 CFU/ml
   • Coagulase-negative Staphylococcus: <50,000 CFU/ml

8. Esophageal feeders and bottles used to feed colostrum must not be used for older or ill calves and must be disinfected and dried between uses.

9. Colostral supplements are frequently used in place of colostrums. Some of these products may provide IgG concentrations that are reportedly adequate but do not supply IgA, vitamins, growth factors, and so on that are normally present in colostrum and often do not result in serum protein or immunoglobulin levels equal to that of colostrum-fed calves. Some of these products contain very low immunoglobulin mass. Although colostrum replacers containing immunoglobulins derived from serum, milk, colostrum, or eggs provide IgG for the newborn calf, none appear to be equal or superior to natural colostrum when used as a replacement. Use of such products has recently been implemented in certain herds as a tool to limit transfer of infectious agents to the calf via colostrum, such as *Mycobacterium avium* subspecies *paratuberculosis*, the causative agent of Johne's disease or bovine leukosis virus.

In addition to colostrum, maternity (calving) pen management practices that predispose to *E. coli* septicemia must be corrected. The importance of maternity pen hygiene cannot be overstated because no level of passive immunoglobulin transfer can protect completely against gross filth in the environment, and conversely even calves with partial or complete FPT may survive when cleanliness is exceptional. Dry cows should not be kept in filthy environments that allow heavy fecal contamination of the coat and udder. Maternity stalls or calving areas should be cleaned, disinfected, and adequately bedded between uses by different cows.

Newborn calves should be removed from the calving area as soon as possible after birth because they will inevitably incur fecal-oral inoculation as they attempt to nurse. Ideally calves should be moved from the maternity area into individual hutches, without being allowed to contact one another. This may not be feasible on larger dairies with limited manpower. In such situations, a small "safe pen" for calves can be constructed adjacent to the maternity pens. A safe area is a sheltered, fenced-in, well-drained, concrete-floor pen located in or near the maternity area. These typically measure approximately 20 × 20 ft. Walls should be constructed to prevent contact with cows or bedding from the maternity area. This small area can be cleaned and disinfected daily with relative ease, and fresh bedding can be added easily. A large gate to facilitate cleaning with a bucket loader should be installed at one end of the safe pen to facilitate efficient (and therefore regular) removal of all bedding before cleaning and disinfection, which should be rigorous and regularly scheduled. This pen becomes the holding area for all newborn calves in the maternity area. Personnel on the dairy are made responsible for moving newborn calves into the safe pen as soon as

possible after birth; use of gloves and footbaths will aid in preventing contaminating newborns with pathogens carried on boots or clothing. The calves are less likely to become rapidly inoculated with maternity area pathogens. The calves are kept here until the calf attendant can provide colostrum and move the calves to hutches. It is critical the safe pen be disinfected regularly and not be used as a long-term housing area for calves, or accumulation of pathogens is inevitable. On large dairies, particularly those experiencing high calf morbidity and mortality problems in the first 2 weeks of life, it may be cost-effective to dedicate one employee to the maternity pen whose sole responsibility is the prompt removal of newborn calves and colostrum administration. Only larger dairies will be able to implement this because 24-hour coverage will be necessary to monitor and care for all calvings.

Enterotoxigenic *Escherichia coli*

Etiology

ETEC produces enterotoxins that cause secretory diarrhea in the host intestine. Several types of enterotoxins have been identified, and a single ETEC may be capable of producing one or more enterotoxins. Both heat-labile (LT I, LT II) and heat-stable (STa, STb) enterotoxins have been identified in ETEC. In calves, ETEC producing the low molecular weight STa cause the majority of neonatal diarrhea problems.

Pathogenic ETEC must be able to attach to the host enterocytes to create disease. Once adhered, the organism releases enterotoxin, which induces the intestinal epithelial cell to secrete a fluid rich in chloride ions. Water and sodium, potassium, and bicarbonate ions follow chloride, creating a massive efflux of electrolyte-rich fluid into the intestinal lumen. Although some of this fluid is reabsorbed in the colon, the efflux of secreted fluid exceeds the colonic capacity for fluid absorption, and watery diarrhea results.

Because enterotoxins are nonimmunogenic, efforts to control ETEC in calves have centered on inducing antibody against fimbrial proteins. The type I fimbriae that allow pathogenic ETEC to attach to enterocytes are proteins that initially were categorized with capsular (K) antigens. Currently fimbriae are classified as F antigens. Unfortunately even the current literature still refers to K-99, K-88, and so forth, rather than the current designation, F-5 and F-4, respectively. In calves, F-5 (K-99) is the most commonly identified antigenic type and has received the most attention regarding diagnostics and vaccines for calves. However, ETEC possessing other fimbrial antigens or multiple fimbrial antigens including F-41, F-6, and some types still not widely identified are capable of causing diarrhea in calves. Some ETEC possess more than one type of fimbriae, and both F-41 and F-5 types may be isolated from an ill calf. Colostrum

TABLE 6-1 Fimbriae Antigens

Designations		
New	Old	Toxin
F 4	K 88	LT I
F 5	K 99	STa
F 6	987 P	STa
F 41		SIa

possessing passive antibodies against a specific ETEC fimbriae type will protect the newborn calf against that specific F type but will not cross-protect it against others (Table 6-1).

As for *E. coli* septicemia, ensuring prompt feeding of adequate levels of colostrum is extremely important to protect calves against ETEC. However, because of lack of cross-protection against various fimbrial antigens, even calves with excellent passive transfer are at risk to ETEC with F types other than those against which the dam has provided colostral antibodies. Colostrum containing antibodies against specific F types will prevent attachment of homologous ETEC to calf enterocytes by coating the fimbriae binding sites. Therefore colostral protection is a local effect of IgG in the gut. To be effective, colostrum containing antibodies against ETEC F antigens must be fed as early in life as possible, lest ETEC colonize the gut before colostrum has been consumed. Although one experimental design showed colostral F-5 antibodies to be effective up to 3 hours after experimental oral challenge with ETEC F-5, it is more practical to assume colostrum should "beat" the ETEC to the gut. Other management factors in addition to colostral feeding are also important in the pathogenesis of ETEC diarrhea. Conditions that allow or encourage buildup of ETEC in the dry cows, in the maternity or neonatal calf facilities, and/or in stored colostrum increase the risk of ETEC diarrhea, as is true with *E. coli* septicemia. Marrow products may also decrease the risk of ETEC by binding to toxin receptors and/or preventing proliferation of pathogenic bacteria.

Affected calves are usually 1 to 7 days of age, with most cases seen in calves less than 4 to 5 days of age. Calves are most susceptible to F-5 ETEC during the first 48 hours of life and thereafter begin to build resistance to those organisms. Concurrent infection with rotavirus may extend the age of susceptibility to ETEC diarrhea to approximately 10 days of age. In older calves, continued exposure to heavy inocula of pathogenic ETEC may result in intestinal colonization and shedding of the organism in normal or diarrheic stools, thereby facilitating new infections in neonates.

Clinical Signs

These signs vary from mild diarrhea with resultant spontaneous recovery to peracute syndromes characterized by diarrhea and dehydration that progress to shock and death within 4 to 12 hours.

Because of the multitude of ETEC types and variability in their pathogenicity, as well as the influence of passive transfer, individual farms may have sporadic or endemic problems resulting from ETEC. Mild disease is common on many farms and seldom is brought to a veterinarian's attention. These calves have loose or watery feces but continue to nurse (Figure 6-4). Spontaneous recovery or apparent response to the farmer's favorite "calf-scour" treatment (usually an oral antibiotic) is the rule. Owners usually call for veterinary assistance only when peracute cases develop, a high morbidity is apparent, calves fail to respond to over-the-counter medications, or mortality in neonatal calves is experienced.

Peracute cases may produce dehydrated, weak, and comatose calves within hours of the onset of the disease. Historically these calves usually have nursed normally and appeared healthy until signs develop. Dehydration and weakness are the predominant signs (Figure 6-5). Mucous membranes are dry, cool, and sticky. The suckle reflex is weak or absent.

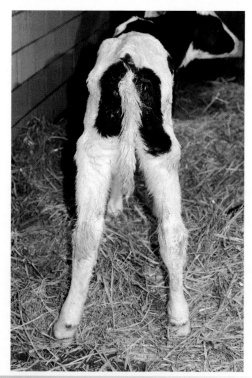

Figure 6-4

A 5-day-old calf with mild "calf scours" caused by ETEC. The perineum, tail, and hocks are stained by watery or soupy diarrhea. This type of diarrhea could be caused by enteric pathogens other than ETEC, and clinical signs are not specific for diagnosis.

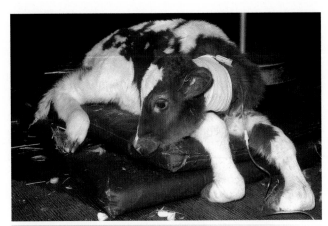

Figure 6-5

Peracute ETEC diarrhea patient that is recumbent, extremely dehydrated, and has severe metabolic acidosis.

Most peracute cases show evidence of voluminous diarrhea (Figure 6-6), with watery feces coating the tail, perineum, and hind legs. Some calves with peracute disease may not have diarrhea; however, the pooling of fluid in the intestinal lumen creates abdominal distention, and fluid splashing sounds can be detected by simultaneous auscultation and ballottement of the right lower abdominal quadrant. Mild, transient colic may be noted early in the disease course. Bradycardia and cardiac arrhythmia accompany the systemic signs in some peracute cases and result from hypoglycemia or hyperkalemia. Atrial standstill has been documented in some bradycardiac calves with hyperkalemia. Rectal temperatures usually are normal or subnormal if the calf is recumbent.

Because of the profound and peracute signs, differentiation of *E. coli* septicemia from peracute ETEC infection often is difficult in the field setting. In prodromal, peracute ETEC cases, the presence of massive fluid in the intestine, as evidenced by abdominal contour, simultaneous auscultation and ballottement, and/or abdominal ultrasonography, are key indicators that the characteristic voluminous diarrhea is impending. Further, on resuscitation with IV fluids, ETEC cases typically break with voluminous diarrhea, and provided the concurrent abnormalities in hydration, electrolyte, acid-base, and glucose status are addressed properly with IV fluids, calves with ETEC typically show rapid clinical improvement. In contrast, calves with *E. coli* septicemia show less voluminous diarrhea, and diarrhea typically develops late in the disease course. Also, unlike ETEC cases, calves with *E. coli* septicemia typically fail to demonstrate a dramatic clinical response to fluid resuscitation.

Acute cases show obvious watery diarrhea, progressive dehydration, and weakness over 12 to 48 hours. The character and color of the feces vary as well, but feces usually are voluminous, watery, and yellow, white, or green. Such calves may have low-grade fever or normal temperatures and deterioration in the systemic state and suckle response. Continued secretory diarrhea gradually worsens the hydration and electrolyte deficiencies; weight loss is apparent—especially if fluid intake is decreased by reduced suckling.

Translocation of bacteria from the gut into the systemic circulation is an uncommon event when ETEC is the sole agent involved because these organisms do not invade the deeper layers of the gut wall and incite minimal intestinal inflammation. Therefore evidence of localized infection (e.g., hypopyon, arthritis) is uncharacteristic of ETEC infection and more indicative of colisepticemia and/or septicemia secondary to other enteric diseases.

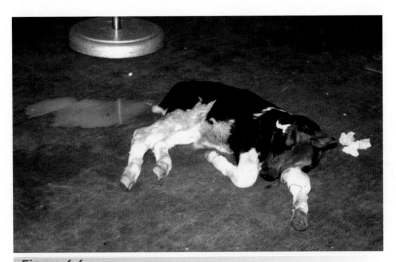

Figure 6-6

Peracute ETEC diarrhea with voluminous diarrhea. The calf had a plasma bicarbonate of 6, pH = 6.98, and K = 8.4 mEq/L. Following sodium bicarbonate therapy, the calf made a quick recovery.

Clinical Pathology

Peracute infections resulting from ETEC cause severe secretory diarrhea that result in a classical metabolic acidosis with low plasma bicarbonate and low venous pH. Hyperkalemia and hypoglycemia also are characteristic. Hyperkalemia results from efflux of K^+ from the intracellular fluid in exchange for excessive H^+ in the extracellular fluid (ECF). Reduced renal perfusion contributes to retention of K^+ in the ECF. Mild hyponatremia and hypochloremia are inconsistently present. Dehydration is generally greater than 8%, and corresponding elevations in packed-cell volume (PCV) and total protein are typical. The WBC count usually is normal, although elevated numbers of WBC may be present because of extreme hemoconcentration, and stress leukograms occasionally are discovered. Leukopenia, left shifts, and toxic cytologic changes in neutrophils are uncommon in ETEC infections, and those findings more likely support septicemia and/or salmonellosis.

Hypoglycemia is more likely to be present if the interval between feedings is prolonged; this finding is not present in all peracute cases. Blood values for a typical case are shown in Table 6-2. Mild azotemia resulting from prerenal causes (reduced renal perfusion) is common and should be kept in mind when use of potentially nephrotoxic drugs is considered in these patients.

Diagnosis

The diagnosis is suggested by the calf's age, physical signs, and laboratory data. Peracute ETEC may be difficult to differentiate from *E. coli* septicemia and salmonellosis in neonatal calves based on clinical signs alone. Response to appropriate fluid therapy strongly supports ETEC infection, as does confirmation of adequate patient serum immunoglobulins.

Definitive diagnosis requires isolation of an *E. coli* possessing pathogenic F antigens that allow intestinal attachment in calves having typical clinical signs. When submitting samples for culture, the clinician should indicate that ETEC infection is a possibility and should request typing of *E. coli* isolates for F antigens (by

immunofluorescence, slide agglutination, or polymerase chain reaction [PCR]) and, if available, for enterotoxin (by PCR or, rarely, by ligated gut loop assays). In fatal cases, ETEC can be cultured from the ileum; a section of ileum should be tied off, placed in a sterile container, and transported on ice packs to the laboratory. Isolation of ETEC from diarrheic feces of older calves is generally considered to reflect the presence of the pathogen in the calf population. In such cases, fresh specimens of jejunum and ileum should be examined carefully for histologic evidence of attachment of ETEC to enterocytes. These findings suggest participation in enteric disease by ETEC, rather than simple intestinal colonization by the organism. Obtaining samples for culture before antibiotic therapy, particularly when oral antibiotics are being given, is an important factor in the diagnostic workup of a potential ETEC outbreak.

Histologic examination of fresh samples of ileum and jejunum of affected calves greatly aids in confirming the diagnosis of ETEC infection. Sections of ileum should be cut into 2- to 3-cm lengths, then split longitudinally and swirled in 10% neutral buffered formalin solution to aid in rapid fixation of the mucosa. Samples for histology should not be tied off because this delays fixation of the mucosa. In classic ETEC infection, a dense population of gram-negative rods are found adherent to the mucosa of the ileum.

Because mixed infections with combinations of ETEC, rotavirus, coronavirus, and *Cryptosporidium* are common, feces and/or intestinal contents should also be analyzed for viral and protozoan pathogens. Salmonellosis also must be included in the differential diagnosis because many types of *Salmonella* sp. can cause severe diarrhea, dehydration, shock, and acid-base disturbances similar to ETEC. Fever, neutropenia, and a left shift are more commonly observed in *Salmonella* patients. In addition, enterotoxemia resulting from *Clostridium perfringens* must be considered, especially in peracute cases with abdominal distention but no diarrhea. Calves with clostridial enterotoxemia may be weak, dehydrated, or "shocky" but seldom have as dramatic a metabolic acidosis as that found in ETEC infections.

Treatment

Appropriate replacement and maintenance fluids constitute the primary therapy of ETEC infection in neonatal calves. Correction of metabolic acidosis and hypoglycemia and reestablishment of normal hydration status are imperative. Calves with peracute signs or those that are recumbent require IV therapy. Calves that can stand but show obvious dehydration, cool and dry mucous membranes, and have a reduced or absent suckle reflex also should initially be given IV therapy. Calves that are ambulatory and have a good suckle response usually can be treated with oral fluids.

Concentrations of required electrolytes based on subjective clinical parameters rather than objective laboratory

TABLE 6-2	Laboratory Data From a Typical Peracute ETEC Infection in a 7-Day-Old Holstein Calf	
Item Tested	Electrolyte (mEq/L)	Normal Range
Na =	127	132-150
K^+ =	8.1	3.9-5.5
Cl^- =	104	97-106
HCO_3^- =	12	20-30
Tot CO_2 =	10	26-38
Ven pH =	7.09	7.35-7.50

tests are empiric at best, but sometimes are necessary in field situations. Therefore rules of thumb include:

Recumbent calves 12% to 15% dehydrated—base deficit 15 to 20 mEq/L

Weak calves 8% to 12% dehydrated—base deficit 10 to 15 mEq/L

Ambulatory calves 5% to 8% dehydrated—base deficit 5 to 10 mEq/L

These rules of thumb are not absolute, and chronic low-grade bicarbonate loss and/or increased D-lactate production in the gut may create profound acidosis over a period of days in a calf having only minimal signs of dehydration. A 40-kg calf that is judged 10% dehydrated will need 4 L of fluid simply to address current needs. For all calculations of replacement electrolytes, a 50% ECF will be assumed for neonates. Therefore a 40-kg calf will be assumed to have $40 \times 0.5 = 20$ L ECF compartment. If this 40-kg calf has a venous plasma bicarbonate concentration of 10 mEq/L, and 25 to 30 mEq/L is the desired normal level, then 15 to 20 mEq of bicarbonate must be replaced in each liter of ECF. Therefore 20 L $\times$ 15 mEq = 300 mEq (20 L $\times$ 20 mEq = 400 mEq) would be necessary to correct the bicarbonate deficit associated with the metabolic acidosis.

Total CO_2 of venous blood also may be used to calculate base deficits in lieu of HCO_3 values.

Much research data and individual clinical opinions exist as to the most appropriate content of initial fluid therapy for ETEC infections in calves. An effective solution, first proposed by Dr. R. H. Whitlock, is formulated by adding 150 mEq of $NaHCO_3$ to 1 L of 5% glucose. This combination is used for the initial 1 to 3 L of IV therapy, depending on severity of measured or suspected metabolic acidosis. Glucose corrects hypoglycemia if present, and both bicarbonate and glucose facilitate potassium transport back into cells, thereby lessening the potential cardiotoxicity associated with hyperkalemia. Some reports minimize the importance of hyperkalemia and suggest using IV potassium in the initial fluid. These workers and others emphasize that dehydrated calves having severe ETEC-induced secretory diarrhea have a total body K^+ deficit despite having an elevated ECF [K^+]. Although this latter medical fact may be true, it seems risky to tempt fate by administering K^+-containing solutions as the initial therapy for a patient known to be hyperkalemic. This is especially true for a patient with bradycardia or arrhythmias because deaths occasionally have occurred when potassium-containing fluids have been given as initial therapy. Once plasma K^+ and HCO_3^- levels are quickly improved by the initial 1 to 3 L of 5% dextrose with 150 mEq $NaHCO_3$/L, potassium-containing fluids can be safely used. Balanced electrolyte solutions such as lactated Ringer's solution suffice for maintenance fluid needs, but supplemental $NaHCO_3$ and dextrose may be required to address continued secretory losses and anorexia. Response to treatment usually is dramatic in calves

with ETEC secretory diarrhea. Calves initially recumbent usually appear much improved following 2 to 4 L of appropriate IV fluids and usually can stand within 6 hours and begin to nurse within 6 to 24 hours of initial therapy. This type of prompt response strongly suggests a correct diagnosis and tends to rule out septicemia because septicemic calves seldom respond promptly, if at all. Depending on the setting (field versus clinic), maintenance or intermittent IV fluid therapy may be continued or replaced by oral fluids in those calves that quickly regain a suckle response and are eager to eat.

Antibiotic therapy for peracute ETEC infections remains controversial, with current concerns focused on antimicrobial residues in edible tissues and indiscriminate and unnecessary use of antimicrobials leading to resistance. However, in peracute cases, the overlap of many clinical signs with colisepticemia often prompts the clinician to include antimicrobial treatment in the therapeutic regimen. In a Canadian study, diarrheic calves ≤5 days of age were found to be at significantly greater risk of bacteremia than older calves; this age range obviously includes calves at risk for ETEC infection. Further, in cases with fever and severe debilitation, the veterinarian is often prompted to consider the possibility of complicating conditions such as bacterial pneumonia. Oral antimicrobial treatment offers the potential benefit of reducing the number of ETEC in the gut, and by reducing the source of enterotoxin, one might reduce the drive for hypersecretion. In his thorough review of the subject, Constable found published evidence supporting the logic and clinical efficacy of amoxicillin trihydrate (10 mg/kg orally every 12 hours) or amoxicillin trihydrate–clavulanate potassium (12.5 mg combined drug/kg orally every 12 hours) for at least 3 days for treatment of undifferentiated calf diarrhea. Repeated use of these products over the long term is likely to induce resistance; therefore long-term efforts must focus on prevention rather than treatment.

Recommended treatments for diarrheic calves with signs of severe systemic illness (e.g., fever, weakness that persists after fluid resuscitation) include ceftiofur (2.2 mg/kg intramuscularly [IM] or subcutaneously [SQ] every 12 hours), amoxicillin, or ampicillin (10 mg/kg IM every 12 hours). Extra-label drug use regulations apply to all of these regimens. Systemic antibiotics usually are continued for 3 to 5 days based on the calf's clinical response, temperature, and character of the feces. Most ETEC that result in high calf mortality have limited antibiotic susceptibility, and sensitivity testing or MIC levels should be determined when the herd history or clinical data suggest high morbidity and mortality from ETEC.

Feces usually remain more watery than normal for 2 to 4 days. If diarrhea persists beyond this time, concurrent infection with other organisms is likely. Other treatments for peracute cases may include flunixin meglumine (1.1 mg/kg IV or SQ every 24 hours) directed against potential endotoxemia, resolution of fever, and reduction of pain associated with fluid-filled bowel. Repeated dosages of this product carry the risk of renal and gastrointestinal injury because continued use of flunixin meglumine interferes with vasodilatory prostaglandin synthesis in the gut and kidney.

Milk or milk replacer should be withheld for no more than 24 to 36 hours, during which time a high-quality oral electrolyte energy source may be fed several times (four to six times) daily. Holding ETEC-infected calves off milk or replacer for prolonged times creates weight loss from inadequate energy intake and places calves at risk of starvation. Even though many oral electrolytes are supplemented with dextrose as an energy source, no commercial oral electrolyte solution provides enough energy for maintenance needs, especially for dairy calves in hutches during winter weather. Weight will be lost, and starvation may occur if these electrolyte solutions are fed as the only ration for more than 1 or 2 days. In highly valuable calves undergoing hospitalization, treatment with parenteral nutrition offers an excellent option to at least approximate maintenance calorific needs while the calf is nil per os (NPO). Calves with ETEC are so significantly catabolic that they will still lose weight despite calorific supplementation with IV lipid and amino acids. Careful monitoring of blood glucose for hyperglycemia and strict attention to aseptic technique, as well as catheter and fluid line maintenance, are important when administering parenteral nutrition. Consequently it is rarely practical outside of a referral hospital.

The alkalinizing potential of oral electrolyte solutions is of great importance, especially when those solutions are utilized as ongoing therapy for peracute cases following initial IV fluids, or when those solutions are used as sole therapy of less severely affected calves having ETEC. Continued HCO_3^- loss accompanying ETEC secretory diarrhea must be anticipated and treated. Therefore oral electrolyte solutions containing bicarbonate are most helpful. The optimal oral electrolyte solutions typically possess 70 to 80 mEq of alkalinizing potential per liter (as bicarbonate or acetate), dextrose, and electrolytes; these should be fed at 4 to 6 L/day. Oral electrolyte solutions that when mixed with water are nearly isotonic are preferred over those that are markedly hypertonic.

Concerns regarding adding oral electrolyte solutions to milk or milk replacers revolve around the alkalinizing solutions' tendency to interfere with abomasal clot formation. Therefore oral electrolytes are fed during separate feedings at least 30 minutes before or after a milk feeding. Calves do not digest sucrose effectively, and addition of table sugar to "home remedy" electrolyte mixtures will reliably worsen fluid and electrolyte losses in diarrheic stools. After 24 to 36 hours of oral electrolyte treatment, calves may be fed small volumes

of milk or milk replacer. Calves that respond rapidly to initial fluid resuscitation can be started back on small volumes of milk or milk replacer at an earlier time. During recuperation, calves should be deeply bedded in dry straw or similar bedding material and provided shelter from rain and snow. When milk feedings are resumed, feedings are best performed in small volumes frequently. If this is not possible, total milk or replacer should be divided into two to three daily feedings. Supplemental oral electrolyte solutions can be continued if ongoing fluid and electrolyte losses are assumed to result from continued diarrhea, and these solutions should be fed at intervals between milk or replacer feedings. Unless the calf is hypoglycemic or acidotic, isotonic electrolyte solutions are preferred because they allow a more normal abomasal transit than do hypertonic solutions.

Treatment of acute ETEC infections in calves that are ambulatory and still able to suckle may not require IV therapy. Cessation of milk or replacer feeding coupled with substitution of oral electrolyte-glucose solutions for 24 to 36 hours may be sufficient. Bicarbonate loss and resulting metabolic acidosis should not be underestimated, however. It is imperative to use highly alkalinizing electrolyte glucose solutions to provide 4 to 6 L of fluids per day. Parenteral antibiotics are indicated if the affected calf is febrile, and oral antibiotics may be administered when the herd medical history indicates involvement of a highly pathogenic ETEC. Milk or replacer should be restored after 24 to 36 hours, and electrolyte feedings should be used as fluid supplements in the intervals between milk feedings.

Mild ETEC infections seldom require veterinary care. Spontaneous recovery is the rule, and supportive care with oral electrolyte solutions frequently is used by owners in such cases. Use of over-the-counter remedies is widespread among dairy farmers treating mild ETEC infections or nonspecific "calf scours." Although little scientific evidence is found to justify these products, anecdotal testimonials from farmers exist for oral neomycin, tetracyclines, sulfas, and other antibiotics, oligosaccharides, or protectants. Over-the-counter calf diarrhea products that contain methscopolamine, atropine, or products that reduce intestinal motility are contraindicated and may cause bloat and ileus if overdosed. Bismuth subsalicylate is palatable and can be used safely in calves.

Prevention

This assumes prime importance when a high morbidity, significant mortality, or both occur on a dairy farm. It is not unusual to encounter 70% to 100% morbidity and mortality when virulent strains of ETEC are present. These strains also tend to be resistant to many antibiotics. The usual situation is that the owner tries multiple over-the-counter products on the first few affected calves and then calls for veterinary assistance to select a "better" antibiotic. One or more calves may die or require intensive therapy before a thorough investigation of the problem ensues.

The veterinarian must avoid the temptation to simply provide or suggest a "newer" or better antibiotic if the problem is to be solved. Feces must be submitted from *more than one* acutely affected calf. If necessary, bull calves should be raised in the identical manner as heifers just to allow them to develop disease and allow early sampling. A qualified diagnostic lab must identify the *E. coli* as an ETEC stain with attachment antigens and determine antibiotic susceptibility.

Management must be meticulously assessed as to cleanliness of dry cows, colostrum, feeding instruments, maternity areas, and newborn calf facilities. Evidence of successful passive transfer of immunoglobulins must be evaluated in several consecutive calves to rule out *E. coli* septicemia or poor colostral feeding as the major cause of ETEC infection. Culturing of colostrum at milking and from the bucket or bottle immediately before its feeding can be used to assess the cleanliness of colostrum milking procedures, colostrum storage, and feeding instrument hygiene. Readers are directed to the previous section on colisepticemia for more details on assessment of colostrum management.

If an ETEC with attachment antigens such as F-5 is cultured from the feces of more than one affected calf, preventive measures can be instituted. Management factors including colostral feeding must be emphasized, lest preventive vaccines are looked on by the farmer as a "silver bullet" that obviates any need for management changes. When specific F antigen ETEC are involved, a commercial bacterin containing these F types can be administered to the dry cows 6 weeks and 3 weeks before freshening or at manufacturer's recommended times. Autogenous bacterin manufacturers should be required to show data on endotoxin levels in bacterins because administration of endotoxin-rich vaccines to adult cattle can cause dramatic production losses and/or abortion. Calves born to dry cows in the next few weeks that are unlikely to form sufficient colostral antibodies in response to bacterins may be given commercially available oral monoclonal antibodies (Genecol 99 (*E. coli* antibodies), Schering-Plough Animal Health Corp., Union, NJ) against F-5 if this is confirmed as the attachment factor for the ETEC in question. Monoclonal antibody products must be given immediately after birth before colostrum is fed. Valuable calves at risk born to these same dry cows also may receive systemic antibiotics for the first 3 to 5 days of life in an effort to prevent infection with the ETEC identified, and selection of appropriate antibiotics should be based on antibiotic susceptibility testing of the causative organism.

Rarely a particular serotype of *E. coli* other than the F-5 pilus type is isolated from the small intestine of scouring neonatal calves. If the organism subsequently

is consistently confirmed as the pathogen (based on samples from multiple affected calves) and commercial dry cow vaccines have not altered the incidence of disease, an autogenous bacterin should be considered. However, the use of autogenous bacterins can only be justified when an absolute diagnosis of a highly pathogenic ETEC has been confirmed by isolates from several affected calves and commercial bacterins fail to stop the disease. Because free endotoxin content may be high in some autogenous vaccines made from gram-negative organisms, the manufacturer should "wash" the preparation to reduce endotoxin content, and data on endotoxin content in the final product should be requested. It is important to resist the temptation to initiate autogenous bacterin production using a nonspecific *E. coli* isolate obtained from one or more calves that merely had colibacillosis as a result of FPT.

Other *Escherichia coli* Diarrhea

Etiology

Although less common than ETEC, other forms of *E. coli* have been identified as causes of clinical calf diarrhea. Enteropathogenic are defined as those capable of attachment and effacement of intestinal cell microvilli. Attaching and effacing (AEEC) are EPEC that do not produce enterotoxins but may produce cytotoxins of various types. They do not possess *Shigella*-like invasiveness. These organisms have been isolated from calves with diarrhea that have histologic evidence of effacement of microvilli in the cecum, colon, and distal small intestine. Cellular degeneration may ensue if the organisms produce cytotoxins. These histologic changes enable differentiation of AEEC from ETEC that attach to enterocytes but do not cause histologic damage. Because the lesions typically involve the large intestine, dysentery and diarrhea may be observed. Malabsorption, maldigestion, and protein loss are characteristic of disease with AEEC or EPEC. Calves from 2 days of age up to 4 months of age may be infected, and other enteric pathogens often are present concurrently.

Shiga-like toxin-producing *E. coli* (SLTEC) are another type of *E. coli* that produce hemorrhagic colitis and the hemolytic uremic syndrome in humans. These organisms also have been called EHEC and occasionally have been found in calves. Some of these strains invade the mucosa to reside in the lamina propria of the large intestine and produce a severe hemorrhagic colitis. Ulcerative colitis with hemorrhage may be present grossly and microscopically in necropsy specimens. Those producing Shiga-like toxin (verotoxin) create enterotoxemia, inhibition of protein synthesis, and vascular damage in the involved intestine. Other less common strains of *E. coli* produce cytotoxic necrotizing factor (CNF), a potent cytotoxin that may be linked genetically to a plasmid that encodes fimbriae and toxins. This plasmid may be found in the same strains of *E. coli* responsible for calf diarrhea and septicemia in neonatal farm animals.

Clinical Signs

As observed with ETEC diarrhea, dehydration, depression, and weakness are common signs associated with EPEC, AEEC, and SLTEC (EHEC) infections in calves. Dysentery or fresh blood in the feces, when present, suggests severe colitis and distinguishes the disease from ETEC secretory diarrhea. Fever tends to be more common with AEEC and SLTEC because of mucosal damage and erosive or ulcerative damage to the intestine. Diarrhea is profuse in some calves and intermittent but blood and mucus tinged in others. Tenesmus may be observed as a result of colonic inflammation. Blood loss in the feces may be negligible with some AEEC or severe enough to cause anemia and hypovolemic shock in some with SLTEC (EHEC). Dysentery or frank blood in the feces always dictates that *Salmonella* sp. be ruled out as a cause of the diarrhea because clinical signs of AEEC and SLTEC (EHEC) can resemble closely those found in *Salmonella* patients. Affected calves usually are 4 to 28 days of age, and morbidity and mortality vary greatly.

Laboratory Data

Calves affected with EPEC, AEEC, and SLTEC have maldigestion and malabsorption and may have protein loss from erosive or ulcerative colonic lesions. Therefore total protein and the albumin fraction of serum may be low. Anemia may be present because of gastrointestinal blood loss. Total WBC counts may be normal or low with a left shift. Although shock and lactic acidosis may create a metabolic acidosis in recumbent patients, calves still standing tend not to have a remarkable base deficit because the pathophysiology of diarrhea is different than the secretory diarrhea of ETEC.

Diagnosis

Fecal cultures that confirm an *E. coli*-possessing cytotoxin, usually without enterotoxin or typical ETEC fimbrial antigens, are necessary to confirm the diagnosis. Categorization and typing of these organisms can only be performed by specialized diagnostic laboratories (Gastroenteric Disease Center, Pennsylvania State University, University Park, PA). Because coexisting enteric, bacterial, viral, or protozoan infection is present in most calves with AEEC or SLTEC, feces should be analyzed for rotavirus, coronavirus, ETEC, *Salmonella*, *C. perfringens* type C, and *Cryptosporidium parvum*. If the incidence of diseased calves with diarrhea is found to be high, fecal samples from several acute cases should be evaluated to ensure that the suspected AEEC or SLTEC is in fact the cause of calf diarrhea on this farm.

Treatment

Therapy is similar to that for ETEC infection except that whole blood transfusions of 2 L of blood may be necessary in calves with severe dysentery and fecal blood loss. Ceftiofur is the most frequently used parenterally administered antimicrobial for this disease. Broad-spectrum antibiotics such as gentamicin (6.6 mg/kg SQ or IV every 24 hours), amikacin (15 mg/kg SQ or IV every 24 hours), or trimethoprim-sulfa combinations (22 mg/kg IV or orally every 12 hours) are also used because of the microvillus or mucosal damage to the intestine, but these represent extra-label drug use in the United States. Prognosis is guarded for calves with AEEC or SLTEC infections unless intensive care is provided. Colonic, cecal, or distal ileal pathology may be so severe as to cause ulceration or perforation of the intestine in some cases. Because of the gross and histologic intestinal pathology, corticosteroids and prostaglandin inhibitors are contraindicated except when used once, in conjunction with initial shock therapy, because these drugs reduced cytoprotective mechanisms of the bowel.

Because of the maldigestion and malabsorption created by these organisms, oral electrolyte-energy sources may be less useful than in ETEC. These products, however, usually are recommended for at least the first 36 to 48 hours of therapy. Calves continuing to have diarrhea after 48 hours can be returned to milk or replacer feeding but may be candidates for TPN if they are valuable enough to warrant the expense.

Prevention

Because AEEC and SLTEC do not possess typical F-5 fimbriae, commercial dry cow bacterins and monoclonal antibodies against F-5 are unlikely to prevent future outbreaks. Therefore management procedures should be examined carefully and corrected when found deficient. If multiple isolates confirm a single AEEC or SLTEC strain, autogenous bacterins administered twice during the dry period may be considered. Colostral management (hygiene and feeding) and passive transfer of immunoglobulins must be assessed.

If rotavirus, coronavirus, *C. parvum*, or other enteric pathogens are found to be concurrent problems, these should be addressed from a management and preventative standpoint. The frequent association of these pathogens with AEEC and SLTEC raise concern that these pathogens may be the primary cause of intestinal injury, and AEEC or SLTEC in fact may be secondary.

The veterinarian responsible for herd health must consider the public health concerns associated with some AEEC or SLTEC. Currently the 0157:H7 strain has caused a great deal of bad publicity for cattle because cattle have been blamed as carriers of this organism that may infect people, causing severe colitis and occasionally hemolytic uremic syndrome. Therefore sanitation, disinfection, and careful handling of feces to avoid human exposure are indicated.

Rotavirus

Etiology

Rotaviruses are members of the *Reoviridae* family and are classified further via complicated division into groups (serogroups), serotypes, and subgroups. The rotaviruses cause diarrhea in multiple species, including humans. Although the rotaviruses share certain antigens and cross-infection of species occurs with some strains, in general resistance is specific, and cross-protection against heterologous strains is poor.

Calves usually are infected by group A serotypes and less commonly by group B serotypes. Initially identified by Mebus and co-workers, the Nebraska rotavirus isolate was used extensively for study and vaccine production. Other group A serotypes have been identified in the United States and abroad. Exposure to rotaviruses apparently is widespread in the cattle population based on serologic surveys. Older calves and adult cattle serve as carriers of the virus, shedding the virus intermittently in feces. In addition, up to 20% of healthy calves may shed rotavirus. As a rule, rotaviruses coexist with other neonatal enteric pathogens such as ETEC and *C. parvum* in herd calfhood diarrhea outbreaks. Experimental mixed infections of rotavirus with bovine virus diarrhea virus (BVDV) have been shown to result in more severe diarrhea than infection with either of these agents alone, suggesting some synergistic effect in pathogenicity.

Neonatal calves (<14 days of age) are at greatest risk for infection by enteric rotavirus, and most infections occur during the first week of life. Prevalence of infection in neonatal calves born on dairy farms harboring the virus is high, morbidity is high (50% to 100%), and mortality varies greatly. Clinical manifestations of disease and mortality in calves are influenced by several factors, including level of immunity to the virus, magnitude of viral inoculum, viral serotype, concurrent infection of the gastrointestinal tract or other systems, stress, and crowding. Germ-free calves infected by rotavirus have self-limiting diarrhea and rapid recovery. Infected calves in field situations may have inapparent, mild, moderate, or fatal disease. As is true with most enteric pathogens, the younger the patient, the higher the likelihood of severe disease because of losses of water, electrolytes, and body nutrient reserves secondary to diarrhea.

Rotavirus infection is limited to the small intestine and characterized by destruction of villous enterocytes and subsequent replacement of these columnar cells by immature and more cuboidal cells derived from the intestinal crypts. Although these new immature cells are resistant to further viral infection, they are unable to carry out the normal digestive and absorptive tasks necessary for villous enterocytes because of deficient disaccharidase and sodium-potassium ATPase activities. Therefore rotavirus diarrhea is characterized by maldigestion and malabsorption. To further complicate matters, the intestinal crypt cells continue their normal secretory function, which is no longer balanced by absorptive villous function. Thus net secretion outweighs absorption and contributes further to diarrhea. Increasing intraluminal osmotic pressure also may draw further water into the bowel as lactose and other undigested nutrients pass through the gut and are fermented in the colon to volatile fatty acids. Bacterial fermentation of undigested lactose creates both D- and L-isomers of lactic acid; in diarrheic calves, absorption of the slowly metabolized D-isomer may result in accumulation of this acid in the systemic circulation, thereby contributing to the development of metabolic acidosis. Water and electrolyte losses of variable severity occur in affected calves.

The level of local passive immunity conferred to calves by colostral intake somewhat determines the risk and relative severity of infection. Colostrum with a high virus-neutralizing antibody titer ($\geq$1:1024) against rotavirus is protective against experimental infection. However, unless colostrum or colostrum/milk combinations with titers this high continue to be fed, this local protection "wears off" within a few days, and the calf becomes susceptible to infection. Colostrum or colostrum milk/ combinations with lower virus neutralizing titers may impart partial protection. Feeding of colostrum having very high levels of IgG$_1$ antibodies against rotavirus soon after birth may establish high circulating humoral antibodies against rotavirus. Although this humoral protection will not, by itself, protect a calf from infection, a portion of these IgG$_1$ antibodies are secreted back into the intestine over time and are thought to confer additional local protection against infection.

Clinical Signs

No pathognomonic signs of rotavirus exist in dairy calves that allow differentiation of the disease from ETEC or other enteropathogens. In addition, infections may be subclinical, mild, moderate, or severe based on factors such as inoculum and serotype virulence of virus, immunity of the calf, concurrent enteric or other system infections in the calf, and other stressors.

Depression, reduced suckle response, diarrhea, and dehydration comprise the major clinical signs. Fever, salivation, and recumbency may be observed in some patients. Feces usually are watery and yellow in pure rotavirus enteritis. Because mixed infections are common, however, the color, consistency, and composition of the feces vary greatly.

Signs of depression, dehydration, and shock are more likely to occur in the youngest calves (<5 days of age) and seldom occur in calves more than 2 weeks of age. Recumbent calves usually have profuse watery diarrhea and abdominal distention of the right lower quadrant with fluid-filled small intestine.

Ancillary Data

Laboratory data are not specific enough to aid in the diagnosis of rotavirus enteritis in calves. Severely affected calves will develop a metabolic acidosis with low plasma bicarbonate. Other electrolytes and glucose values tend to be low but vary with severity and duration of disease.

Diagnosis

Diagnosis requires identification of rotavirus particles in the feces of acutely infected calves. Feces should be collected within the first 24 hours of illness and diarrhea. Feces submitted to qualified diagnostic laboratories are examined by electron microscopy to observe viral particles or subjected to testing using a latex agglutination or an enzyme-linked immunosorbent assay (ELISA) test to detect viral antigen. Fluorescent antibody (FA) stains also are available for tissue analysis from fatal cases. Because of the frequency of mixed infections, feces submitted from acute neonatal diarrhea cases should be analyzed for viruses, bacteria, and *C. parvum*. Feces from more than one acute case in the herd must be tested before staking an entire prevention program on one isolate. Affected calves should be assessed for adequacy of passive transfer of immunoglobulins to rule out FPT.

Treatment

Treatment is nonspecific and generally follows therapy described for ETEC regarding indications and types. Several differences are noted, however:

1. Because of villous enterocyte pathology, the efficiency of absorption of oral electrolyte/energy sources is likely reduced relative to ETEC infections. Obviously this comment is relative, not absolute, because generally less than 100% of the small intestinal villi are damaged. Therefore absorption of some proportion of the glucose, electrolytes, and water that comprise the oral fluids will occur, and aggressive oral fluid therapy (4 to 6 L/day) is still indicated in this disease. Isotonic electrolyte replacements may be preferable unless the calf is hypoglycemic. Electrolyte solutions containing glutamate mixed with yogurt may speed intestinal recovery, although this is not proven in the calf.

2. Maldigestion, as well as malabsorption, will influence the duration of diarrhea and digestibility of milk or milk replacers in viral enteritis patients. Once diarrhea from rotavirus becomes evident, the damage to the intestinal lining has already occurred, and only time and supportive care can allow the intestine to heal. Nutritional support is a critical component of that supportive care—particularly because rotaviral scours may persist for 3 to 7 days. Producers should be counseled that provision of milk or milk replacer is necessary in viral enteritis, even though the maldigestion of the milk nutrients may contribute in part to the pathologic process. Denial (for >24 hours) of milk feeding to a calf with viral diarrhea places the calf at significant risk for cachexia and may lower its resistance to opportunistic disease. Death from starvation may occur in such cases, particularly during times of inclement weather (Figure 6-7). To quote Dr. Chuck Guard, "If a calf scours for a week, and all that the calf is fed is oral electrolyte replacer, then that calf will be well hydrated and will have absolutely perfect blood electrolyte concentrations and acid-base balance on the day it starves to death." Producers should learn to live with the "more-in, more out" rule: The more milk goes in the front end, the more diarrhea comes out the back end. However, this process is not necessarily harmful because digestion and absorption of some fraction of milk nutrients is likely to occur, and these nutrients are necessary to support the tissue synthesis required to return the intestine to normal. Any exacerbation of fluid losses and acidosis that may result from maldigestion of milk nutrients can be offset by aggressive fluid and electrolyte replacement. Ideally the affected calf should be fed small amounts frequently with the addition of lactaid tablets!

3. Maturation of immature villous replacement cells of crypt origin will allow the intestinal tract to return

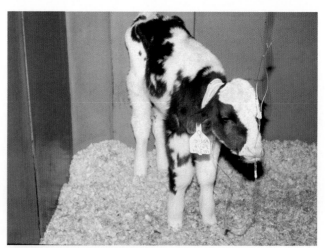

Figure 6-7

A 3-week-old red and white Holstein calf with chronic diarrhea and emaciation caused by rotavirus and *Cryptosporidium* infection. The calf was normally hydrated and had normal electrolytes but was deteriorating because of malabsorption/maldigestion and cachexia. This is one of the first calves we successfully treated using parenteral nutrition (1982).

to normal within several days to 1 week in most cases that recover.

IV fluid therapy is necessary for recumbent, extremely dehydrated, or "shocky" patients, and patients that have lost their suckle reflex. IV fluid therapy is best guided by acid-base and electrolyte determinations. If this is not practical or available, however, the most severely affected calves with acute diarrhea should be assumed to have metabolic acidosis, low bicarbonate, high potassium, and low glucose values. Guidelines for fluid therapy are available in the section on treatment of ETEC. Parenteral nutrition may be "life saving" in calves with cachexia.

Although there is no need for antibiotic therapy in pure rotaviral enteritis, the likelihood of mixed infections and the pathologic damage to enterocytes that fosters attachment of bacterial pathogens may be reason enough to treat severely affected calves with systemic antibiotics.

Control

Rotavirus is ubiquitous in cattle populations; therefore management procedures that decrease the magnitude of exposure of neonatal calves to rotavirus must be the focus of preventive efforts. Cleaning maternity pens between deliveries of different cows, immediately removing the calf from the dam (and thus exposure to feces), placing the calf in an individual hutch that has been cleaned and put on a new spot since removal of the last occupant, and feeding the calf from its own nipple bottle or pail rather than a common feeding device all help reduce spread of viral pathogens. Feces from a clinically diseased calf may contain hundreds of millions of viral particles per gram and can contaminate inanimate objects and workers' feet, clothing, and hands to be passed to a naive calf. The use of a safe pen can also be considered (see discussion in section on colisepticemia).

Vaccination of newborn calves or dry cows is somewhat controversial because passive humoral immunoglobulins derived from colostrum probably are not as effective as passive local immunoglobulins derived by continued feeding of colostrum or colostrum/milk combinations that contain high antibody levels against rotavirus. Oral modified-live vaccine (MLV) vaccination of newborn calves before feeding them colostrum has been practiced, but it is somewhat cumbersome for most management teams and risks bacterial infection because colostrum is withheld until several hours after the MLV oral vaccination to prevent inactivation of the vaccine by colostral antibodies. Although this vaccine protocol can induce cell-mediated immunity and secretory IgA and IgM against rotavirus of vaccine serotype, efficacy in field studies has been questioned.

Because colostrum, colostrum/milk combinations, or milk containing virus-neutralizing antibodies $\geq$1:1024 will protect the gut from infection by local means, feeding such material to calves for the first 30 days of life usually will prevent rotavirus infection. This also requires that the serotype of rotavirus to which the calves are exposed be the same as that from which the colostral antibodies have been derived. It also requires that management prevent overwhelming exposure of neonatal calves to challenge with this or other combined infections.

Boosting the level of rotavirus antibody in colostrum is a potential means to prevent enteric rotavirus infection if calves are fed adequate to large amounts of colostrum to achieve local protection. If colostrum is only fed for 1 or a few days, the local protective effect will "wear off," and the calf will become susceptible to rotavirus enteritis. Continued feeding of colostrum is ideal but often not practical. Initial postnatal ingestion of very high antibody-containing colostrum may in fact create high enough humoral antibody levels to create secretory IgG_1 antibodies into the gut. Boosting the level of colostral antibodies against rotavirus usually is done by vaccinating the dry cow with MLV or killed vaccines containing rotavirus and coronavirus. Currently the killed products generally are recommended, and the dry cow should be vaccinated 6 and 3 weeks before freshening (or according to manufacturer's recommendations) and subsequently given booster shots each year 4 weeks before freshening. No vaccine or antibody can overcome massive viral challenge, and conversely less concern for passive protection is necessary when management excels at reducing risk for the newborn calf. Given the practical limitations and expense of continued colostrum (or colostrum supplement) feeding of calves, the producer should focus on initial colostrum administration to newborns, maternity pen and hutch hygiene, dry cow vaccination, and controlling spread by fomites and personnel. Incidence of rotavirus diarrhea has been decreased on some farms by mixing some colostrum (10%) with milk or replacer for 30 days.

Being a nonenveloped virus, rotavirus is stable in the environment (6 months in fecal matter) and relatively resistant to the effects of some disinfectants. Decontamination of hutches and maternity pens requires thorough physical effort to remove fecal matter and other organic debris because most disinfectants show reduced, even negligible, activity in their presence. Application of appropriately diluted bleach, a phenolic, or a peroxysulfate disinfectant to a thoroughly cleaned solid surface, with provision of long (>10 minutes) contact time and subsequent sunlight exposure and drying, will effectively reduce the number of infectious rotavirus particles. Heavily soiled areas, such as the ground beneath calf hutches, may need to be stripped down to the packed surface and exposed to sunlight and dry conditions for several days to weeks (depending on weather conditions) before being considered habitable for the next calf.

Coronavirus

Etiology

Based on seroprevalence studies, the bovine coronavirus (BCV) responsible for calf diarrhea apparently is quite prevalent in U.S. cattle herds, as is rotavirus. A closely related strain of BCV has been isolated from feed lot cattle with respiratory and enteric disease. Winter dysentery in adult cattle has been associated with BCV, and the same strain that causes diarrhea in calves has been used to experimentally create winter dysentery in adult cattle. Therefore the upper age limit of susceptibility to infection by this agent is apparently longer than traditionally thought.

Although not as common as rotavirus as a cause of viral enteritis in dairy calves, coronavirus has been identified in neonatal calf diarrhea outbreaks—especially with mixed infections. Affected calves tend to be slightly older than calves infected with pure ETEC or pure rotavirus. They average 7 to 10 days of age at onset, with some observed as late as 3 weeks of age. The virus causes a severe enterocolitis characterized by villous enterocyte destruction in the small intestine and destruction of both ridges and crypts in the large intestine. Maldigestion, malabsorption, and inflammation all contribute to the pathophysiology of coronavirus diarrhea in calves. The virus is cytolytic, and affected villous enterocytes in the small intestine are replaced by cuboidal cells from the crypts, whereas the colonic lesions leave denuded mucosa in affected areas of the colon. The severity of this damage helps explain why coronavirus enteritis, unlike rotavirus, can kill calves even in a germ-free isolation facility. Thus in the natural setting, coronavirus enteritis creates a severe clinical diarrhea and can be associated with mortality >50% when combined with other viral, bacterial, or *C. parvum* infections.

Clinical Signs

Acute, severe diarrhea, as well as dehydration, reduced appetite or suckle reflex, and progressive depression and weakness are typical, albeit nonspecific, signs of coronavirus infection in calves. Because of the colonic pathology, mucus may be more apparent in feces. Coronavirus is also commonly found in the respiratory tract of young calves, and a pneumonia/enteritis complex may occur in those calves.

Ancillary Data

Coronavirus enterocolitis creates varying degrees of abnormalities in acid-base and electrolyte status also common to *E. coli* and rotavirus. In severe coronavirus infections or mixed infections that include coronavirus, metabolic acidosis and low plasma bicarbonate are the rule. Potassium values vary with the severity and duration of the diarrhea and acidosis. Hemoconcentration secondary to the diarrhea elevates PCV and total protein values. Leukograms are variable. Although of nonspecific etiology, the acid-base and electrolyte assessment is of greatest value for individual patient management.

Diagnosis

Submission of feces from calves with acute or peracute diarrhea provides the best diagnostic sample from live patients. Feces collected during the first 24 hours of diarrhea are best. Electron microscopy, ELISA, or PCR may be used to detect virus. FA testing of tissue samples obtained from both the small and large intestines is best for necropsy specimens. Because of the cytolytic nature of coronavirus, the virus can disappear rapidly from tissue. Therefore chronically affected calves are not good candidates for sampling.

Treatment

Treatment principles are the same as those previously listed under ETEC and rotavirus treatment. As with rotavirus, oral electrolyte/energy sources may be less efficiently absorbed in coronavirus infections because of enterocyte loss. However, even given these limitations, oral electrolyte-energy sources may contribute to the patient's well-being during the time of intestinal repair. Diarrhea is likely to persist to some degree for 1 week with coronavirus because of the severe enterocolitis. Systemic antibiotics are often indicated to help affected calves cope with secondary bacterial infection of the lung, gut, and other systems.

Control

Every effort should be made to control management factors that predispose calves to infection. These are described in the control of rotavirus. Because coronavirus is an enveloped virus, its persistence in the environment and resistance to disinfectants are considerably lower than those of rotavirus. Dry cows should be vaccinated at 6 and 3 weeks before calving with a killed rota-corona vaccine and boosted each year thereafter at 4 weeks prepartum. Because it is assumed that local antibody is more important than humoral antibody, the feeding of colostrum containing high antibody levels against coronavirus is advantageous, and when possible, such colostrum should be fed for the first 30 days of life. Recently specific antibody products have become available and can be administered to newborn calves at birth. One such product contains K-99 antibodies and coronavirus antibodies (First Defense, Bovine coronavirus–*Escherichia coli* antibody, bovine origin. ImmuCell Corporation, Portland, ME) derived from hyperimmune bovine colostrum. In an experimental challenge study with BCV, dairy calves fed a commercial product containing spray-dried bovine serum showed increased feed intake and higher scores for certain clinical parameters as compared with control calves. The expense of such products is considerable, and analysis of the cost and therapeutic benefit is often warranted before use.

Cryptosporidium **Infection**

Etiology

C. parvum causes diarrhea in neonatal calves that occurs most commonly from 5 to 28 days of age. *Cryptosporidiidae* are a family of coccidian protozoans grouped with the *Sarcocystidae* and *Eimeriidae* families in the suborder *Eimeriina*. Similar to other coccidia, members of the *Cryptosporidiidae* family have both sexual and asexual components to their life cycle but differ from other coccidia in having less host specificity. *Cryptosporidium* spp. are much smaller than *Eimeria* spp. and are therefore difficult to detect in fecal flotation. Laboratory techniques that use acid-fast stains or immunological techniques greatly aid detection. The true prevalence and pathogenicity of *C. parvum* in calves have only recently been appreciated.

Following the original description of the parasite in a calf, cryptosporidiosis was thought to be a novel or sporadic infection that most likely affected immunocompromised calves. During the 1980s, it became apparent that the organism was much more prevalent, epidemic to endemic on many farms, and a primary or component cause of neonatal calf diarrhea.

C. parvum can infect calves, lambs, young pigs, people, and other species such as suckling rodents. Public health concerns regarding spread of *C. parvum* from animals to people are real and require diligence in the diagnosis and management of this parasite. Genetic analysis of human and bovine isolates has revealed two distinct genotypes of *C. parvum*: genotype 1, which is transmitted solely among humans, and genotype 2, which has a larger host range, including cattle. This distinction is important for investigation of potential zoonotic cases of cryptosporidiosis: if the isolate from the affected person is genotype 2, a bovine or other animal source is possible, whereas an isolate of genotype 1 implicates human-to-human spread. A novel species of *Cryptosporidium* has recently been isolated from cattle in the northeast United States; the proposed species name is *Cryptosporidium bovis*. As genomic analysis continues to define the genus *Cryptosporidium*, further refinements in taxonomy are likely. Its role in diarrheal diseases of calves is not proven.

In cattle, neonates are at greatest risk of infection and disease because age-related resistance seems to be strong; this trend is less evident in humans. Veterinarians, students, technicians, and other individuals involved in handling affected calves, feeding equipment, bedding, or even clothing from in-contact individuals may develop clinical disease if strict hygienic measures are not followed. Immunocompetent hosts usually develop self-limiting diarrhea. However, the organism causes a particularly devastating disease in immunocompromised hosts, wherein persistent infections can occur.

The organism usually infects via the fecal-oral route, but contaminated ground water and contaminated feedstuffs can induce infection. The infective dose of cryptosporidium likely varies among individual animals and people, but the infective dose in a susceptible individual may be less than 100 oocysts. Given that infected calves may shed millions of infective oocysts in each gram of diarrheic stool, there is strong potential on many farms for accumulation of massive infectious challenge.

Sporulated oocysts are readily infective to neonatal calves and release sporozoites that infect primarily the small intestinal (but some colonic) enterocytes by infecting the microvillus brush border. A parasitophorous vacuole that resides adherent to the cell but outside the cytoplasm is formed. The life cycle phases of *C. parvum* then result in destruction of cells as the parasitophorous vacuoles break to release merozoites that infect other host cells. The subsequent sexual life cycle phase results in formation of oocytes infective to susceptible hosts. Villous atrophy, villous fusion, and inflammation of intestinal crypts ensue. Autoinfection within the intestine occurs, wherein specialized oocysts are released to infect other enterocytes without exiting the host. Clinical signs of diarrhea reflect a mixed pathophysiology of maldigestion, malabsorption, and osmotic effects with or without secretory and inflammatory factors. The autoinfection process has been hypothesized to account for occasional protracted or relapsing cases that can result in cachexia. Damage to the microvilli appears to predispose the calf to combined infections with *E. coli*, viruses, or *Salmonella* sp. Therefore it is unusual in dairy calves to find only *C. parvum* when investigating endemic calf diarrhea. However, because oocyst shedding typically begins with the onset of clinical signs and persists until several days after diarrhea resolves, fecal testing may tend to reveal this pathogen more consistently than rotavirus or coronavirus, which are shed early in the disease course and for a shorter period of time than *C. parvum*. This reiterates the importance of testing affected calves early in the disease course when investigating the etiology of calf diarrhea. Combinations of enteric pathogens in neonatal calves complicate treatment, worsen the clinical signs and prognosis, tend to result in higher mortality, and predispose to malnutrition. *C. parvum* may by itself produce severe diarrhea in immunocompromised calves and those exposed to inclement weather and/or poor nutrition.

Clinical Signs

Diarrhea, dehydration, and reduced appetite are the major clinical signs and thus do not differentiate *C. parvum* infection from bacterial and viral enteropathogens in neonatal calves. Morbidity tends to be greater than 50% in calves less than 3 weeks of age, and mortality is low unless mixed infections occur or supportive treatment is less than adequate. When *C. parvum* is the only pathogen, diarrhea usually persists for up to 7 days, but most calves do not lose their ability to nurse or their interest in nursing during this time. When mixed infections occur, dehydration, acid-base and electrolyte abnormalities, and dysentery are possible. Malnutrition is a possible sequela to *C. parvum* infections when poor supportive therapy and poor nutritional quality coexist with the rather chronic diarrhea. Malnutrition is quite common in *C. parvum*-infected calves raised outside in hutches during winter weather extremes in northern climates. Because these calves normally have greatly increased caloric needs over calves raised at moderate temperatures, maldigestion, malabsorption, and fluid losses greatly compromise their well-being.

Diagnosis

Microscopic identification of *C. parvum* oocytes is required for positive diagnosis but may require a trained microscopist! In most instances, standard flotation on feces from acutely affected calves is performed, but very fresh necropsy tissue samples of ileum and colon also may be examined following tissue preparation and staining. Acid-fast stains are commonly used to assist in the identification of *C. parvum*. Immunofluorescence, ELISA, and PCR are all believed to be more sensitive and specific than microscopy. Genetic analysis of bovine or human isolates may be performed to aid in epidemiologic investigations, particularly when zoonotic cases are suspected. Even when *C. parvum* is suspected and confirmed, mixed infections should be considered and feces submitted for bacteriologic and virologic evaluation.

Treatment

Treatment is supportive and consists of fluids by whatever route indicated by the severity of clinical dehydration. In addition, a high-quality source of nutrients such as whole milk or a quality milk replacer must be fed. If oral electrolyte energy sources are fed during the acute phase of diarrhea, they should not remain the only source of nutrients for more than 24 hours. Thereafter, milk or replacer should be fed at least twice daily and oral electrolyte/energy sources fed between milk feedings to compensate for the fluid losses caused by *C. parvum* diarrhea. During cold or extreme winter weather, hutch-sheltered or neonatal calves left outside should receive milk or high-quality replacer at least three times daily if twice-daily feeding fails to maintain body condition or *C. parvum* diarrhea, maldigestion, and malabsorption interfere with efficient utilization of nutrients.

Antibiotics are not necessary, although they may be indicated in mixed infections that include bacterial pathogens. Many drugs have been tested for efficacy against *Cryptosporidia*, but none have been found to be completely effective or economically justifiable. Standard coccidiostats are ineffective with the exception of lasalocid at doses so high as to be toxic to calves. Recent work in Europe and Canada has demonstrated that treatment with halofuginone lactate will reduce oocyst shedding and delay the onset of diarrhea in calves, but like many other investigated therapies, it does not significantly impact the incidence or severity of diarrhea in treated calves compared with controls. Paromomycin, nitazoxanide, azithromycin, and a few other drugs have shown some activity against *C. parvum*, and ongoing research to benefit AIDS patients will continue to drive discoveries in this area. These drugs could potentially be used in valuable calves with cryptosporidiosis. Halofuginone (100 µg/kg) for 7 days is approved in several countries for the preventative treatment of cryptosporidiosis in calves. In the near future, immunization of cows with subunit vaccines may increase the effectiveness of passive transfer of antibodies in limiting the severity of this disease in calves.

Control

Because treatment is not possible, prevention assumes supreme importance. Unfortunately many dairy farms fail to effectively control *C. parvum* once environmental contamination becomes extreme. Although diseased calves serve as the primary source of environmental contamination, oocysts are also spread by movement of laborers, equipment, and animals. Given the low dose of oocysts necessary to cause disease, the morbidity rate can become unacceptably high. Therefore control requires a careful, open-minded reexamination of all management practices related to calf rearing, including maternity pen hygiene, colostrum management, cleaning of feeding equipment, hutches, and the ground surrounding hutches, labor allocation, and the order by which laborers feed and handle calves.

First, calf facilities should include individual calf arrangements rather than grouping. Ideally newborn calves should be separated from the dam at birth and moved to a cleaned and disinfected calf hutch on new dry ground or concrete. Placing a calf in a hutch on the same ground as that used for the previous occupant will not work because *C. parvum* oocysts can persist for months in such areas, and the ground beneath used calf hutches is often heavily contaminated. Bedding from within and around hutches should be completely removed and disposed of, the ground stripped bare, and the bare ground allowed several days to weeks of sunlight exposure under dry conditions before being considered habitable for another calf. Moving cleaned hutches to new ground or placing them on concrete slabs that can be cleaned, disinfected, and allowed to dry between calves is the best technique. Because cryptosporidium oocysts are highly resistant to the effects of almost all disinfectants, hutches and feeding equipment must be vigorously and thoroughly scrubbed with soap and water and rinsed well with hot water to physically dislodge oocysts. Drying and ultraviolet light are relatively effective against the oocysts; therefore more hutches should be made available than would be occupied at any given time; a 20% vacancy rate for newly scrubbed hutches will often allow ample time for sun exposure and drying of recently emptied hutches. A peroxygen-based disinfectant (Virkon-S, Antec International, Sudbury, Suffolk, United Kingdom) has been shown to reduce the infectivity of *Cryptosporidium* oocysts under experimental conditions and is currently used in some veterinary hospitals to disinfect thoroughly cleaned surfaces. Newer generation, peroxygen-based compounds have also shown promise for reduction of oocyst viability.

Calves should have individual feeding implements, and removal of manure from the hutch should be done in such a way that calves are not exposed to manure from neighboring calves or hutches. When doing chores, laborers should move from young calves to older calves and from healthy to sick calves to limit spread of oocysts.

Salmonellosis (Calves)

Etiology

Salmonellosis as a sporadic cause of diarrhea has been long recognized in cattle, but intensive management systems have contributed to endemic disease in dairy calves, veal calves, and adult dairy cattle. Currently salmonellosis ranks as one of the two most important bacterial causes of diarrhea in adult dairy cattle (*M. avium* subspecies *paratuberculosis* being the other) and has surpassed *E. coli* in this respect in calves on many operations. *Salmonella* spp. are gram-negative, aerobic and facultative, anaerobic and facultative intracellular pathogens that cause a wide spectrum of clinical disease, ranging from peracute septicemias to inapparent carrier infections. Recent taxonomic and nomenclature descriptions have become confusing, but the pathogenic serotypes encountered in cattle are all classified within one subspecies of *Salmonella*, namely, *Salmonella enterica* subspecies *enterica*. For example, *Salmonella typhimurium*, as most veterinarians know it, is now precisely defined as *Salmonella enterica* subspecies *enterica* serotype Typhimurium. However, for simplicity and to avoid confusion, only the generic name followed by the serotype will be used throughout this text. Antigenic identification has been based on O (somatic or cell wall), H (flagellar), and Vi (virulence) antigens. Most current serogroups are divided by O antigens and listed by capital letters (e.g., A, B, C, D, and E). *Salmonella* type B—usually Typhimurium—has historically been the most common cause of enteric salmonellosis in calves and cattle in the northeastern United States, but types C (e.g., *S.* Newport, *S.* Infantis , and *S.* Montivideo) and E (e.g., *S.* Anatum, *S.* Muenster) are now commonly diagnosed. Most cattle isolates are *Salmonella* of types B, C, and E, which are not host-specific, or *Salmonella* Dublin (type D), which is host-adapted to cattle.

Other recent developments in bovine *Salmonella* research include a herd survey by Dr. Loren Warnick et al indicating that approximately 4% of cows and calves on New York dairy farms are shedding *Salmonella*. Multiple risk factors include free stall housing, access to surface water, eating forage from fields where manure has been applied, herd size in the study, presence of diarrhea, and recent antimicrobial treatment in cows. A small but concerning percentage of *Salmonella* isolates from other studies have been multidrug-resistant (MDR) isolates. These MDR isolates have included several serotypes such as Typhimurium DT104 and Newport. These MDR strains are resistant to tetracyclines, sulfas, and most beta-lactams (via the CMY-2 gene).

Some broad characterization of the clinical syndromes associated with certain serotypes can be made. With group B infections such as *S.* Typhimurium, as well as with many group E infections, a herd outbreak of diarrhea and septicemia may occur in adults and calves. Abortion or early embryonic death may occur as a result of acute endotoxemia and shock. However, few cattle appear to develop a chronic carrier state, and as the population develops immunity to the agent, clinical signs often dissipate within 1 to 2 months. Infections with group C *Salmonella* are more difficult to characterize because infection and clinical disease may persist in the herd for variable periods of time, suggesting the potential role of carriers in maintaining the organism over the long term. Infection may also be perpetuated over the long term by environmental contamination or by group C *Salmonella* continuously cycling through rodents, birds, or insects. Infection with the host-adapted *S.* Dublin (the most common group D isolate from cattle) is characterized by establishment of a higher percentage of carrier animals in the population. Once *S.* Dublin is established in the population, most adults experience asymptomatic infection and may serve as shedders (even in milk), and pneumonia, septicemia, and acute death become the primary manifestations of disease in calves. Some calves that develop infection and survive will become long-term carriers. *S.* Dublin is not common in northeastern dairies. Sporadic abortions may occur with *S.* Dublin.

Calves with acute, chronic, or carrier intestinal infections shed varying levels of organisms in their feces; this serves as the major source of infection to naive herdmates via fecal-oral transmission. Calves with peracute or acute disease often are septicemic and may shed organisms from other secretions such as saliva and urine. Fecal-oral transmission is the norm for types B, C, and E *Salmonella*; infection of the distal small intestine, cecum, and colon ensues. Mucosal injury causes maldigestion, malabsorption, and loss of protein and fluid. A secretory component to the diarrhea also is thought to contribute to further electrolyte and fluid depletion. *S.* Dublin is unique in that respiratory signs may predominate, and transmission may occur by various secretions and feces. Adult dairy cattle may be carriers and harbor *S.* Dublin in the intestine or mammary gland. Milk, colostrum, or feces from infected or carrier *S.* Dublin cows can be infective to calves. Clinical epidemics of many *Salmonella* types including *S.* Dublin are common in calves in the northeastern United States and other parts of the country. Geographic differences in serogroup prevalence do occur, but widespread transport of calves or adult cows and herds assembled from distant locations has tended to negate geographic limits for various *Salmonella* serogroups.

Factors that adversely affect the normal enteric flora tend to favor growth of *Salmonella*, which are common, albeit low, components of the gastrointestinal flora of carrier or "normal" cattle. Parturition, transport, concurrent disease, anesthesia, and withholding of feed and water are just a few of the stresses that cause intestinal ileus, reduced host immunity, and/or shifts in enteric bacterial populations that induce proliferation of *Salmonella*. In calves, antibiotics that alter the intestinal flora may also favor the growth of *Salmonella*. Once shedding of large numbers of organisms occurs in a carrier animal, naive calves are at increased risk if crowding, poor sanitation, use of common feeding implements or housing location, concurrent diseases, or stress are present. Both humoral and cellular immune mechanisms are involved in resistance to *Salmonella*. Calves persistently infected with BVDV are at high risk for developing acute salmonellosis with exposure to the organism.

Clinical Signs

Fever and diarrhea are the hallmark signs of *Salmonella* types B, C, and E in dairy calves. Fever may precede clinical signs of diarrhea but seldom is detected before calves begin to show diarrhea and appear ill. Fresh blood and mucus in the feces (some calves may have blood in feces before diarrhea) also are common with *Salmonella* enteritis (Figure 6-8). Blood-stained mucus or whole blood clots may be apparent based on the severity of infection and *Salmonella* type. Clinical signs associated with septic physitis, arthritis, meningitis, and pneumonia may be seen in some calves. Sporadic or endemic disease may occur, and although calves from 2 weeks to 2 months are most commonly affected, those of any age may develop the disease. Newborn calves deprived of colostrum that were purchased from different farms may have clinical signs within the first 3 days. Tremendous variation in clinical severity of disease exists based on the virulence and infecting dose of the *Salmonella*, and the age, immune status, and

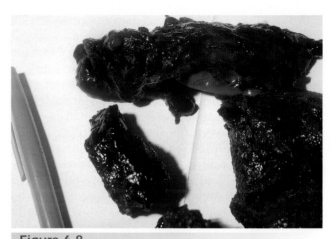

Figure 6-8

Blood in the stool from a calf with salmonellosis.

existence of concurrent disease in the calf. Type E *Salmonella*, such as *S.* Anatum, tends to cause mild signs of diarrhea and fever with variable morbidity and low mortality, whereas types B and C are more likely to cause high morbidity and variable mortality based on strain and exposure dosage of organisms. Neonatal calves have a greater risk of death caused by *Salmonella* because of septicemia and fluid losses leading to severe dehydration and electrolyte imbalances (Figure 6-9).

Peracute septicemia resulting from *Salmonella* types B, C, and D may cause death before diarrhea becomes obvious. These calves rapidly dehydrate into their intestinal tract, have abdominal distention as a result of filling of the small and large intestine and sometimes forestomach, and die secondary to bacteremia and endotoxemia induced by release of cell wall products of the gram-negative infective agent. Bacteremic calves shed large numbers of *Salmonella* in other bodily secretions and feces and quickly contaminate premises.

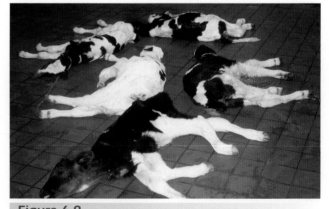

Figure 6-9

One day's death toll of neonatal calves from a dairy farm suffering high mortality in cattle of all ages during an epidemic caused by a highly virulent *S. typhimurium* strain.

Acute cases caused by types B, C, and E show classical acute diarrhea—often with fresh blood and mucus in the feces, as well as fever and dehydration. Feces are foul smelling (septic tank odor) and vary in color and consistency, with the most virulent strains causing profuse watery diarrhea with whole blood clots present. The infected calves are frequently bacteremic, and pneumonia, arthritis, physitis, and meningitis may occur.

Acute disease in calves usually is associated with high morbidity and variable mortality that depends on the strain of *Salmonella*. Fecal contamination of the environment is especially problematic when calves are housed in group housing, raised slatted stalls or crowded areas, or when born in a stall used both as a maternity pen and sick cow stall. Milk from adult cows shedding *Salmonella* in their feces or mammary gland and contaminated feeds or feeding devices are common sources. Chronic infection leads to chronic or intermittent diarrhea, weight loss, hypoproteinemia, and failure to thrive. Some chronically infected calves typically evolve from epidemics of acute salmonellosis in dairy calves and thus enhance the risk of exposure for naive herdmates.

Acute infection associated with *S.* Dublin may be much harder to diagnose because diarrhea may not be the principal sign. Fever, depression, and respiratory signs may be most obvious in acute *S.* Dublin infections in calves. Although diarrhea may be present, it is seldom the predominant clinical sign, which may lead to erroneous assumption of calf pneumonia. Fever and depression unresponsive to antibiotics may be observed. Abortions may also occur on the premises. Calves infected with *S.* Dublin are typically 4 to 8 weeks of age.

Laboratory Data

Peracute or acute infection with *Salmonella* types B, C, and E has variable effects on the patient's leukogram. A degenerative left shift with neutropenia and band neutrophilia is considered classical for severely affected animals, but it is not consistent, and many patients have neutrophilia or normal leukograms. Although blood may be present in the feces, hemoconcentration tends to mask mild anemia resulting from blood loss. PCV is normal or elevated because of dehydration. Total protein and albumin concentrations are usually normal or low because of protein loss into the gut and malabsorption. Renal function may be compromised by dehydration, reduced renal perfusion, endotoxemia, or nephritis secondary to bacteremia with renal infection. Peracute and acute infections cause inflammatory, secretory, and malabsorption-maldigestion types of diarrhea and result in metabolic acidosis and hyponatremia and hypochloremia. These electrolyte changes are particularly common in instances when the calf loses salts and water in the diarrheic stool but is only allowed access to water for rehydration. Potassium may range from high (peracute) to low (subacute, chronic) depending on severity and duration of diarrhea, subsequent fluid losses, and acid-base status.

Acute *S.* Dublin infection seldom results in profound acid-base abnormalities but may lead to mild electrolyte loss (Na, Cl, and K) and hypoproteinemia. The leukogram in *S.* Dublin-infected calves is extremely variable and reflects duration of infection. Acute cases may be neutropenic with a left shift, severely neutropenic, or have normal WBC counts. Subacute or chronic *S.* Dublin infections have a mild to moderate neutrophilia or stress leukogram.

Diagnosis

Regardless of the type or strain of *Salmonella*, isolation of the organism, coupled with history and clinical signs, confirms the diagnosis. Fecal cultures are the standard test necessary to identify types B, C, and E, whereas fecal, blood, transtracheal wash, or lung tissue samples may be necessary to identify *S.* Dublin. Fecal samples submitted from suspect calves should be sent to qualified diagnostic laboratories equipped to culture enteric pathogens. When neonatal calves are involved, the laboratory should be forewarned that *Salmonella* and *E. coli* are suspected. When affected calves vary from neonatal to several months of age, *Salmonella* is more likely than *E. coli* because the latter tends to more commonly affect only neonates. Sample handling is pivotal in reaching a definitive diagnosis, and practitioners should familiarize themselves with their local diagnostic laboratory requirements and recommendations for maximizing the chances of a positive culture from feces, environmental samples, or postmortem tissues. *Salmonella* are quickly overgrown by many other fecal organisms, and preenrichment or the use of specific selective transport media may be indicated for samples obtained in the field.

Calves that die peracutely should be necropsied and cultures obtained from the ileum, cecum, or colon. In addition, the mesenteric lymph nodes, gallbladder, and heart blood should be cultured. Calves that die following respiratory and enteric signs should have lungs and gut cultured for *S.* Dublin.

Although pathologists associate salmonellosis with gross enteric lesions such as diphtheritic membranes in the distal small intestine or large intestine, it must be emphasized that peracute *Salmonella* types B or C and acute *S.* Dublin infections often cause minimal demonstrable gross lesions. This fact has been borne out by observing necropsy specimens from many calf mortality epidemics and dictates routine bacteriologic assessment rather than empiric gross determination of etiology.

Subacute or chronic cases may have fibrinonecrotic or diphtheritic membranes scattered throughout the large and distal small intestine (Figure 6-10). Petechial hemorrhages and edematous mesenteric lymph nodes are other gross pathologic findings in some cases.

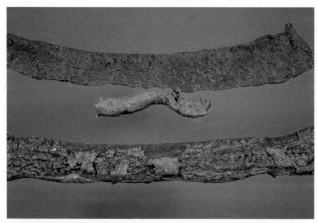

Figure 6-10

Classical fibrinonecrotic or diphtheritic membrane lining the intestine of a calf that died from subacute *S.* Typhimurium enterocolitis.

Treatment

Fluid and antibiotic therapy is the cornerstone of treatment for calves with salmonellosis. Decisions as to route of fluid administration are based on physical signs, severity of the diarrhea, and economic considerations. As with *E. coli* infections, calves that are "shocky," unable to rise, severely dehydrated, and those that have no suckle response should be given IV fluids. Calves that are ambulatory, able to suckle, and are only moderately dehydrated usually can be managed with oral and possibly SQ fluids. Peracute and acute salmonellosis caused by types B, C, or E may result in a metabolic acidosis similar to that found in ETEC infections. However, losses of Na^+ and Cl^- tend to be more severe in salmonellosis than those found in ETEC-infected calves. Bicarbonate-rich solutions are indicated in peracute *Salmonella* infections and should be considered when profound depression or shocklike signs accompany peracute diarrhea. Following correction of metabolic acidosis, balanced electrolytes may be used IV or oral fluids substituted (see section discussing treatment of ETEC). Oral electrolyte-energy solutions are helpful but limited by the maldigestion, malabsorption, and inflammatory lesions in the patient's intestinal tract. Diarrhea tends to persist longer in *Salmonella* than ETEC infections and may become chronic if the intestine is permanently damaged.

Whole blood transfusion occasionally is necessary because of fecal blood losses and more commonly necessary as a result of severe hypoproteinemia associated with albumin loss from the inflamed intestine. Whole blood (free of BLV and BVDV) is sometimes more economical than plasma for calves having severe hypoproteinemia.

Severe peracute infections that result in shock may necessitate one-time administration of corticosteroids or flunixin meglumine in conjunction with IV fluids. Continued or repeated use of full dosages of either of

these products warrants caution because their side effects on the gastric mucosa and renal vasculature appear to be augmented by volume depletion.

Antibiotic therapy for calves having salmonellosis is somewhat controversial and deserves comment.

Reasons not to use antibiotics:

1. Fear of creating antibiotic-resistant strains that may present a risk to humans and animals in the future.
2. Although antibiotic therapy may aid clinical recovery, it does not stop fecal shedding or positively affect the duration of fecal shedding!
3. Salmonellae are facultative intracellular organisms, and antimicrobial penetration into the infected host cell is often limited even for the antimicrobials that show in vitro efficacy against the organism.

Reasons to use antibiotics:

1. Bacteremia is common with salmonellosis of any type in neonates and is very common with *S.* Dublin.
2. Veterinarians cannot always predict which calves are septicemic and which are only endotoxemic when faced with signs of shock and severe diarrhea.
3. Although intracellular penetration of infected host cells by antibiotics may be limited, adequate blood concentrations of an effective antibiotic may limit spread of infection from the gut to other tissues by acting on the organisms that are free in the blood and ECF.
4. Clinical impressions suggest a shorter course of disease and higher recovery rate when antibiotics are used.
5. Secondary infections (e.g., joints) are possible in severely ill calves with salmonellosis.

Antibiotic therapy is justified for calves with peracute or acute signs that suggest overwhelming infection. Calves having mild signs, calves that are asymptomatic, and those with chronic disease do not appear to benefit from antibiotic therapy. Given the characteristically unpredictable nature of antibiotic susceptibility of *Salmonella*, selection should be based on culture and sensitivity. Currently many strains are resistant to beta-lactam antibiotics, macrolides, and tetracyclines but are frequently sensitive to aminoglycosides and trimethoprim-sulfas. Antibiotic therapy should be maintained at least 5 to 7 days for peracute and acute salmonellosis and is more likely to be necessary in type B and C infections than in type E. A decision not to use antibiotics for calves with salmonellosis is easier to enforce when mortality is low or nonexistent. This same decision is impossible to enforce when high mortality occurs because owners will not tolerate such losses and will demand antibiotics or change veterinarians in the hope of saving sick calves. Ultimately decisions on antibiotic use must be based on humane considerations weighed against the public health concerns related to induction of resistance in an organism with demonstrated zoonotic potential. Wholesale treatment of calves at risk and the use of oral antibiotics such as tetracycline for all calves in a group are contraindicated because these techniques are more likely to be ineffective or lead to antibiotic resistance. Antibiotics should be considered as potential components of the treatment regimen, with aggressive fluid and electrolyte replacement, good nursing care, and maintenance of adequate nutrition as primary considerations. Experience suggests that resolution of a salmonellosis problem on a dairy requires far more critical and influential decisions than antibiotic selection for individual cases.

Control

Although an individual calf sporadically becomes infected with *Salmonella* sp. as a result of stress or FPT, endemic infection is more the rule in dairy and veal operations. Infected calves shed large numbers of organisms into the environment, and contamination is worsened by the fluid characteristic of feces in diarrheic calves. Infection spreads quickly when calves are grouped in confinement or crowded into pens. Fecal contamination of feed, water, or feeding devices is common, and septicemic calves may shed organisms in body secretions and feces. *S.* Dublin–infected calves may shed organisms from body secretions, feces, or the respiratory tract. Inapparent or subclinical infections are common and represent a constant source of environmental contamination.

Cleanliness and disinfection of housing units are extremely important to the control of salmonellosis because a primary determinant of the severity of infection appears to be the magnitude of challenge or infective dose. Many severe outbreaks have resulted from contamination of feed, and this area deserves particular scrutiny in the herd investigation because this route serves as a very efficient means of oral inoculation of new hosts.

Detection of the carrier state by serologic or milk antibody testing has historically been possible for *S.* Dublin but at the time of writing is no longer available. Detection of carrier animals is difficult because of inapparent infections, variable patterns of shedding, and the failure of negative cultures to completely rule out a carrier state. Recovered animals continue to shed type B, C, and E organisms for 3 to 6 months, or more in some instances, and *S.* Dublin-infected animals may shed forever. Therefore control measures based on detection and elimination of carriers are more easily instituted when small groups are infected.

Vaccination against *Salmonella* sp. is controversial. Because cell-mediated immunity is a major factor in host resistance, killed bacterins that stimulate only humoral immunity give questionable protection. Vaccination of dry cows with specific *Salmonella* sp. bacterins may protect neonatal calves somewhat for the first 2 to 3 weeks of life but probably not thereafter. Autogenous bacterins

developed from the specific *Salmonella* sp. involved in an epidemic may be more helpful in this regard. Killed vaccines administered to neonatal calves have not performed well in research trials, primarily because calves appear to respond poorly to the oligosaccharide side chain antigens that comprise the protective antigens. Both commercial and autogenous bacterins must be used with caution because anaphylactic or endotoxic reactions are possible and are thought to represent an inherited hypersensitivity to endotoxin or other mediators. Aromatic-dependent *S.* Typhimurium and *S.* Dublin strains have been used as MLVs in calves and appear promising because they stimulate both cellular and humoral immune responses. In addition, subunit vaccines utilizing siderophore receptors and porins as antigens have shown promise in reduction of salmonella shedding in poultry and are now available for use in adult cattle.

Immunization of calves with commercial J-5 vaccines has been shown to reduce mortality from salmonellosis in an experimental challenge study; however, in a large field trial, J-5 immunization of calves did not affect survival to 100 days.

Control of epidemic salmonellosis in dairy calves entails the basic principles of infectious disease control. Isolation of active cases, hygiene, disinfection, education of handlers, and perhaps culling or depopulation may be required. Whole herd epidemics are frightening experiences that lead to tremendous public health concern. It is critical that the producer understands that once an outbreak is well established, control measures may mitigate the severity of the outbreak but often fail to immediately bring resolution. Patience, persistence, and communication are important.

Methods of *Salmonella* control in calves include:
- *Establish diagnosis* via culture and sensitivity; conduct investigation of the premises
  A. Several affected animals should be cultured in epidemics to confirm a common pathogen, although most clinically ill animals will be culture-positive on a single sample.
  B. Cultures of feces must always be performed.
  C. Colonic contents and mesenteric lymph nodes may be cultured from necropsy submissions.
  D. If *S.* Dublin is suspected, blood, tracheal wash, and/or lung tissue samples may be cultured in addition to feces.
  E. Carefully examine herd medical records, and conduct an inspection of the premises to characterize the spatial and temporal characteristics of the problem. Is there a common sick cow pen/maternity stall?
  F. Critique flush water flow patterns and traffic patterns of personnel and vehicles.
  G. Trace feedstuffs (including colostrum, milk, milk replacer, and water, as well as solid feeds) from their storage, preparation, transport to the

animals, and delivery to the animal. Consider the possibility of contaminated feed, feed storage areas and transport equipment, feeding utensils, or feed bunks/buckets as potential sources of oral inoculation of healthy animals. Culture, then disinfect, accordingly.

H. It is often useful to culture milk or milk replacer, water, and dry feeds for *Salmonella* spp. on their preparation or initial storage, during transport in containers, and after they are placed in the final container and presented to the calf (i.e., in a bucket or nipple feeder). This helps to identify potential sites of contamination and amplification of the organism. Producers often forget that milk and milk replacer are excellent culture media for *Salmonellae*, and small inocula can become tremendous pathogen loads as the organisms replicate in feeds.

• *Isolate* infected animals

A. This measure is relative and imperfect because some infected animals may *not* appear ill. However, calves with fluid feces, fever, dehydration, and the like should be isolated because they are shedding billions of organisms into the environment.

B. Salmonella control is often a numbers game, and reduction in pathogen load requires inspection of all facets of calf handling and colostrum/milk feeding. Carefully scrutinize each and every step of the process of calf handling from parturition (maternity area hygiene) through placement in the hutch or pen. Often the first material ingested by the newborn calf is directly from the maternity environment, immediately after birth, and before consuming colostrum. In a recent outbreak on a Colorado dairy, a colleague of the author, Dr. Rob Callan, isolated *Salmonella* Infantis from the nose and mouth of a newborn calf less than 5 minutes after being born. This calf had been pulled several yards across the ground of the maternity pen to a separate area where calves are then fed colostrum. In this situation, *Salmonella* was likely ingested well before consuming colostrum, greatly increasing the risk of infection. While maternity pen hygiene is essential for minimizing exposure to calves, prompt removal of calves to individual calf hutches can also aid in minimizing exposure. Washable industrial wheelbarrows and wheeled bins make for excellent transfer vehicles for moving calves from the maternity area to designated calf housing. Alternatively, a calf "safe pen" can be considered (see previous section on colisepticemia).

C. All feeding and cleaning implements should be scrubbed with soap and hot water, then disinfected between uses, and never used on healthy calves.

D. Distance can be an effective buffer for reducing pathogen load to calves. When possible, calves can be moved to new, well-protected ground that is well removed and upwind from adult cows and protected from water flow from the main operation.

E. If labor is spread thin, it may be easiest for the producer to hire additional labor or reallocate personnel such that certain person(s) is/are solely dedicated to the husbandry of calves. Disinfection and good hygiene take time, and personnel with multiple time demands often fail to fully and persistently implement good sanitation practices when handling calves.

F. Identify and remove all animals persistently infected with BVDV from the herd.

• *Therapy* for infected animals

A. Fluids to maintain hydration, acid-base balance, and serum electrolyte concentrations.

B. Additional protection from weather stress.

C. Maintain adequate nutrition.

D. Treat with appropriate antibiotics when indicated.

• *Physically clean environment*, improve hygiene, and disinfect premises

A. Separate calves from adult cattle (particularly critique flush water flow patterns and maternity pen hygiene because these are common sites of spread of infection from adults to calves).

B. Clear maternity stalls and disinfect between calvings. Consider use of a "safe pen" for calves (see previous section on colisepticemia) and cleanable, plastic wheeled bins or wheelbarrows for transfer of calves out of the maternity area.

C. Do not house young calves in a group.

D. Disinfect with a disinfectant approved to kill *Salmonella* sp. after physically cleaning organic debris from surfaces.

E. Being an opportunist, *Salmonella* spp. often flourish to cause disease in cattle populations under conditions of suboptimal nutrition or reduced immune function. Poor transition cow management, a high prevalence of animals persistently infected with BVDV, and alterations in feed intake brought about by temperature extremes or poor bunk management are examples of the "intangibles" that often determine whether *Salmonella* infection becomes problematic on a given operation.

• *Educate* the farm owner and workers regarding public health concerns

A. Farm workers, calf handlers, and their families *frequently* become infected by *Salmonella* sp. during calf epidemics, and workers must be educated on how to minimize this risk.

B. Insist on handlers wearing separate footwear and coveralls when handling infected calves. Allocate labor to prevent cross-infection from diseased calves to healthy calves. If certain personnel are responsible for all calves, have those individuals handle healthy calves first. Disinfect boots, hands, and implements. Be very careful about hygiene.

C. Do not drink raw milk from adult cows if any signs of enteric disease or abortion have been observed in the herd.

- Recognize that recovered animals will shed intermittently or constantly for some time and thus represent significant risk to uninfected animals and people. Therefore ongoing hygiene, disinfection, and surveillance are necessary.
- Immunization with modified live (preferred) or killed vaccines (commercially available orautogenous) should be considered as an adjunct measure to be used only when the aforementioned management changes do not result in satisfactory abatement of the problem. Producers should be reminded that immunity is finite, and increased herd-level immunity brought about by the use of a vaccine is unlikely to succeed over the long term if initiated without meaningful changes in husbandry and hygiene.
- Feeding prebiotics or oligosaccharides may be beneficial.

Clostridium perfringens—**Enterotoxemia**

Etiology

Enterotoxemia caused by *C. perfringens* type C is a commonly fatal disease that occurs in dairy and beef calves. Enteric disease caused by types A, B, and D has been reported in calves but is far less common. Neonates are most commonly affected, although disease losses in older calves (usually ≤3 months of age) can be significant. *C. perfringens* type A is a gram-positive anaerobic bacterium that is part of the normal intestinal flora of vertebrates. Intake of large quantities of soluble carbohydrate and/or protein is considered a risk factor for the development of type C enterotoxemia; the organism undergoes explosive growth under such conditions, creating a "superinfection" of the enteric lumen and producing exotoxins (termed major lethal toxins) that cause the majority of damage to host tissues. The exact reason for infection often is difficult to determine in sporadic cases but usually can be linked to "pushing" calves nutritionally when endemic problems are observed in a herd. Feeding of large volumes of milk or milk replacer, especially in the form of large meals, appears to be a common triggering factor. Heavy grain feeding, foraging on grain crops, sudden access to high-quality forage, or overfeeding following a period of hunger are also considered risks.

Beta toxin is the principal major lethal toxin of type C, although variable amounts of alpha toxin are produced by this organism. Beta toxin induces necrosis of enterocytes in the small intestine, thereby allowing toxin access to the deeper layers of the gut wall, which creates extensive submucosal necrosis and intraluminal hemorrhage. Alpha toxin is a phospholipase that destroys lecithin within host cell membranes and membranous organelles. Terminally, multisystemic signs of disease can result from absorption of the major lethal toxins and from other gut-origin toxins and/or organisms from the damaged gut into the bloodstream.

Beta toxin is a protein that is inactivated by exposure to trypsin. Thus the lethal effects of beta toxin may be exacerbated in neonates because of either low pancreatic trypsin production or the presence of trypsin inhibitors in colostrum. When calves ingest large volumes of milk or concentrate, the calf's pancreatic enzymes may be sufficiently diluted to prevent inactivation of beta toxin; alternatively, the organism may proliferate to a degree that the massive amounts of toxin released simply exceed the limited amount of trypsin in the gut.

Clinical Signs

Signs of enterotoxemia are acute or peracute and consist of colic, abdominal distention, dehydration, depression, and diarrhea. Sudden death or such rapid progression of signs that the calf is not observed to be ill before death can occur in peracute infections. Colic and abdominal distention usually precede diarrhea, and although the feces are loose, they are never as voluminous or watery as those found in calves with ETEC or salmonellosis. Feces in some enterotoxemia calves contain obvious blood and mucus (Figure 6-11). Acute cases characterized by abdominal distention and colic may mimic intestinal obstructions unless diarrhea develops to rule out

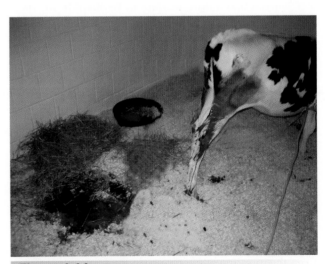

Figure 6-11

A 5-week-old Holstein with acute and severe hemorrhagic enteritis caused by *C. perfringens* type C. The calf recovered after intensive therapy with IV administered antibiotics (penicillin and ceftiofur), IV fluids, clostridium antitoxin, blood transfusion, flunixin meglumine, gastroprotectants, and transfaunation.

obstruction. Ballottement of the right lower quadrant reveals increased fluid in the small intestine. Progressive dehydration, depression, abdominal distention, and shock ensue unless intensive therapy is instituted. Neurologic signs are observed occasionally in the terminal stages of fatal cases of type C enterotoxemia. Affected calves usually have been in excellent condition and are often reported to have been vigorous eaters.

Ancillary Data

Blood work seldom is helpful or specific in enterotoxemia patients. Hemoconcentration is a given, but the leukogram and serum chemistry may be normal. In subacute cases, the serum albumin may be low because of intestinal losses and some loss into the peritoneal cavity. Hyperglycemia and glycosuria have been purported to be diagnostic but are more indicative of *C. perfringens* type D in lambs—not cattle. Any stressful disease may result in hyperglycemia and glycosuria in neonatal ruminants, and these findings are not pathognomonic for enterotoxemia in calves.

Acid-base and electrolyte data are not dramatically abnormal. Enterotoxemia calves *do not* usually have a severe metabolic acidosis as calves severely affected with acute ETEC or *Salmonella* tend to have.

Diagnosis

Other than the physical signs, there are few clues to assist in the diagnosis of enterotoxemia. For fatal cases, necropsy findings often are quoted as diagnostic. However, they seldom are, and necropsy is used primarily to rule out other diseases. In field situations, it may be impossible to obtain meaningful samples and have them reach a diagnostic laboratory in time to be helpful. All dead animals have some *C. perfringens* in their intestines, so the relative numbers and toxin types must be assessed to diagnose accurately the type of *C. perfringens* present and attach significance to the organism. Intestinal enzymes tend to break down alpha and beta toxins within hours of death. *C. perfringens* type A may proliferate in the gut and invade tissues within a short period after death—especially in warm weather. In fact, postmortem enteric proliferation of *C. perfringens* type A may be so extensive that it masks the presence of type C when luminal contents are cultured. The absolute diagnosis of enterotoxemia caused by type C organisms requires culturing *C. perfringens* from the gut, genotyping to determine that the isolate is type C, demonstration of gross or histologic lesions, and, if available, testing to identify beta toxin from the intestine of fatal cases. In the less common type B and type D enterotoxemias in cattle, absolute diagnosis requires demonstration of epsilon toxin of type D in addition to identification of the organism by culture and genotype. Genotypic analysis is usually performed by multiplex PCR (mPCR), although mouse protection testing can also be used.

Calves with acute enterotoxemia must be diagnosed primarily based on clinical signs of colic, abdominal distention with fluid distention of the small intestine, dehydration, diarrhea, and a rapidly progressive course. Ancillary data, if available, can help rule out other differential diseases. Progressive shock secondary to abomasal perforation with diffuse peritonitis can be ruled out by transabdominal ultrasound and paracentesis. Acid-base and electrolyte determinations on venous blood and fecal cultures help rule out ETEC and acute salmonellosis because enterotoxemia calves seldom have a profound metabolic acidosis.

Feces or enteric contents may be cultured and assayed for toxins. Toxin identification is laborious and difficult because the toxins are labile and may be rapidly degraded. Proper sampling, storage, and shipment to a qualified laboratory are necessary.

Treatment

Supportive treatment requires IV fluids (crystalloids and colloids such as Hetastarch 5 to 10 ml/kg) with appropriate electrolytes and glucose to rehydrate the calf. Ideally IV potassium or sodium penicillin (44,000 U/kg IV every 6 hours) should be given for the first 24 to 48 hours of therapy but can then be replaced by procaine penicillin (44,000 U/kg IM every 12 hours) if the calf is improved. Calves that are in shock may also be given dexamethasone or flunixin meglumine (0.5 to 1.1 mg/kg IV) as one-time treatments.

Resolution of clinical signs is gradual and slow. Abdominal distention sometimes takes days to resolve, and diarrhea tends to be sporadic rather than voluminous. Recovering calves have variable appetites primarily based on their degree of abdominal distention and hydration status. Recovery in successful cases may require fluid and antibiotic support for up to 7 days. Progressive intestinal ulceration and subsequent perforation have been observed as an occasional complication in recovering calves. Therefore repeated use of nonsteroidal and steroidal drugs is contraindicated to avoid further damage to the intestinal tract. Prolonged ileus and failure of abomasal emptying may evolve as a problem in recovering calves. If conservative therapy with IV fluid support and antibiotics fails to resolve this problem and the patient becomes more distended after drinking milk or electrolytes, metoclopramide (0.1 to 0.25 mg/kg SQ every 8 to 12 h or as a continual infusion) may be helpful to increase abomasal emptying and relieve abdominal distention. Administration of histamine antagonists may also be considered as described by Ahmed et al in calves with poor abomasal emptying as a means of trying to increase luminal pH and lessen the chances of mucosal ulceration (cimetidine 50 to 100 mg/kg orally every 8 hours, ranitidine 10 to 50 mg/kg orally every 8 hours or preferably ranitidine 1.5 mg/kg IV every 8 hours). Antitoxins are available commercially, and although they may be of use early in the course of the disease, efficacy of these products is difficult to determine. Blood and/or plasma transfusions may be needed due to intestinal damage.

Control

Presentation of excessive amounts of starch, sugar, or soluble protein into the stomach and/or intestine is considered pivotal in the development of enterotoxemia; thus all potential influences on this pivotal event must be considered when formulating a preventive plan. Evaluation of ration net energy, fiber content and forage length, bunk space, animal hierarchy within a pen, feeding frequency, the rate and magnitude of changes in ration between successive production groups, and feed mixing practices is essential to identify and correct problems with carbohydrate overload and/or slug feeding. Prevention of enterotoxemia in calves requires consideration of environmental or management factors that may trigger ingestion of larger than normal volumes of milk or replacer. Decreasing the volume of milk fed per feeding by increasing the frequency of feedings has met with some success. Milk and milk replacer should be fed at or near body temperature to prevent induction of ileus. For pasture-fed animals, turnout onto a new pasture should be very gradual (e.g., day 1, 15 minutes of grazing; day 2, 30 minutes; day 3, 1 hour; day 4, 2 hours, and so on).

Vaccination with *C. perfringens* toxoids is indicated for herds that have experienced sporadic or endemic enterotoxemia. When successful diagnostic tests confirm a specific type, toxoids obviously should contain that type. When specific types have not been identified, types C and D toxoid usually are suggested because type C is the most commonly identified in calf enterotoxemia.

All dry cows and heifers should be vaccinated twice, 2 to 4 weeks apart (or according to manufacturer's recommendations); thereafter yearly boosters should be given 1 month before calving; and calves should be vaccinated with the same vaccine at 8 and 12 weeks of age. Immunization of neonatal calves has been utilized for enterotoxemia control in problem herds. However, no change in antibody titers to *C. perfringens* toxins has been demonstrated in immunized calves (immunized at ~7 weeks of age) or lambs (immunized twice up to 6 weeks of age) that received colostrum from vaccinated dams.

Type A Enterotoxemia and Abomasitis

Etiology

Sporadic cases of enterotoxemia associated with *C. perfringens* type A have been reported in calves. Abomasitis, abomasal tympany and bloat, and ulceration of the abomasum have also been linked to *C. perfringens* type A. It is uncertain whether the *Clostridium* organism is

the cause of this condition, and *C. septicum*, *Salmonella*, and most recently *Sarcina* sp. have been implicated.

Abomasitis is a sporadic disorder of neonatal to weanling calves, lambs, and kids. This disease is characterized by diffuse, hemorrhagic to necrotizing inflammation of the abomasal mucosa, frequently involving the deeper layers of the abomasal wall in severe or chronic cases. Intramural emphysema and edema of the abomasal wall may be present. Abomasal ulceration and perforation may occur in a subset of affected animals.

A variety of putative etiologies for this disease exist, including primary bacterial or fungal infection, immunosuppression, and pica; trauma from coarse feed or trichobezoars; and vitamin/mineral deficiencies. In 1987, investigators at Kansas State University detected *C. perfringens* types A and E in stomach contents of affected calves and the following year reproduced the disease experimentally by intraruminal inoculation of *C. perfringens* type A in calves. The ability of this organism to produce gas is considered to contribute to the gastric dilation and intramural emphysema evident in affected animals. More recently *S.* Typhimurium DT104 was isolated from the abomasal wall of midwestern veal calves with abomasitis. Although authors of earlier case reports associated copper deficiency with abomasitis and abomasal ulcers in beef calves, Roeder and colleagues demonstrated that, in the absence of copper deficiency, abomasitis could occur spontaneously and be induced experimentally. Thus although copper deficiency may act as a contributory factor for abomasitis and enteric disease of calves, it does not appear to be a requisite factor for either condition.

Clinical Signs

Clinical signs include lethargy, abdominal tympany, colic, bruxism, fluid distention of the stomach, diarrhea, and death. Although the number of case studies on abomasitis is few, on review of the available literature, the case fatality rate appears to be very high (75% to 100%). Typically significant signs of tympany and colic precede diarrhea, which is usually low in volume.

Treatment

Treatment of enterotoxemia caused by *C. perfringens* type A is similar to that used for types C or D. Antitoxin for types C and D has unknown efficacy in treatment of type A cases. For abomasal tympany or abomasitis, IV fluid therapy, plasma therapy, parenteral antibiotic therapy, and antitoxin administration as for enterotoxemia are warranted in the initial medical management. Orogastric tube passage and decompression may be helpful in some cases; elevation of the calf's forequarters while the tube is placed may be helpful in releasing gas. Oral antibiotics such as penicillin or tetracycline may be helpful in reducing the rate of intraluminal gas production. Decompression of the abomasum via percutaneous ventral abomasocentesis has been described, and intraluminal injection of antibiotics could be performed after decompression. Laxatives appear to be of limited benefit in such cases, and large doses of magnesium oxide/hydroxide laxatives are likely contraindicated because they may exacerbate metabolic alkalosis seen in early stages of the disease, induce hypermagnesemia, and simply pull more fluid into the gut lumen.

A large, right-sided tympanic resonance in an ill calf may be a case of abomasal or cecal volvulus, and surgical exploration is indicated if initial medical management does not result in resolution of tympany. Similarly, a left-sided tympanic resonance may reflect left displacement of the abomasum (LDA), and given the apparent high rate of ulceration of the abomasum associated with LDA in calves, surgical exploration is warranted in cases that do not respond to medical management. Abomasotomy may be indicated for refractory cases of abomasal tympany. Abomasotomy allows for removal of luminal foreign bodies such as hairballs and removal of putrefying milk, both of which may prevent a satisfactory response to medical management.

Prevention

In dairy calves, poor milk hygiene, intermittent feeding of large volumes of milk, and feeding cold milk or milk replacer, often via bucket, have been empirically incriminated as potential contributory factors for abomasal tympany, ulceration, and abomasitis. Epidemiologists at The Ohio State University are currently conducting a practitioner survey study on abomasitis and abomasal tympany, and potential preventive strategies for this disease may be forthcoming. Anecdotal reports indicate that increasing the frequency of milk or milk replacer feeding and decreasing the volume fed at each feeding, as well as maintaining milk or replacer at body temperature until it is fed, may reduce the incidence and severity of this condition. A vaccine (*Clostridium perfringens* type A toxoid, Novartis Animal Health, Larchwood, IA) that induces high antibody titers against alpha toxin, a primary virulence factor of *C. perfringens* type A, has recently been released into the U.S. market for prevention of diseases in cattle caused by this organism. As a dry cow vaccine, this product may increase colostral titers against alpha toxin, but the efficacy of this product in reducing calfhood diseases caused by *C. perfringens* type A is currently undetermined.

Other Possible Infectious Causes of Calf Diarrhea

Table 6-3 lists other possible infectious causes of diarrhea that have been documented in calves.

Diarrhea and Emaciation Caused by Milk Replacer Feeding

Etiology

There has been a great deal of change in composition and formulation of modern day milk replacers compared with early milk replacers produced during the 1950s and 1960s. Like adult cow rations, milk replacers may be formulated on a least-cost basis for ingredients—especially those comprising the crude protein fraction because this is the most expensive component.

TABLE 6-3 Other Reported Infectious Causes of Calf Diarrhea (Significance of These Organisms Is Unknown)

Organism	Signs	Treatment	Reference
Giardia	Often no signs. High morbidity, low mortality. Diarrhea in 2- to 12-wk-old calves	Fenbendazole 15 mg/kg bwt for 3 days	Claerebout E, et al: New therapeutic approaches to Cryptosporidiosis and Giardiosis. In *ACVIM Proceeding*, 2006.
Campylobacter sp. (*jejuni, fecalis,* or *coli*)	Generally no disease. Diarrhea with blood and mucus	IV and oral fluids. Tetracycline or erythromycin	Morgan JH, Hall GA, Reynolds J: The association of *Campylobacter* species with calf diarrhea. In *Proceedings: 14th World Congress on Diseases Cattle*, 1986, pp. 325-330.
Clostridium difficile	Possible diarrhea in calves <2 wk of age, although experimental inoculation did not cause diarrhea	Supportive	

Milk proteins have been the preferred source of proteins for milk replacers, and pasteurized skim milk powder (low heat prepared and then spray dried) is ideal. Unfortunately the price of skim milk has risen to a point where it is no longer economically possible to include it as the total source of proteins in most milk replacers. Most milk proteins are now derived from whey protein concentrate, dried whole whey, dried whey products that are byproducts of cheese manufacturing with casein and fat extracted, and/or spray-dried plasma (often from other species, e.g., porcine).

Other protein sources such as modified soy protein, soy protein concentrate, soy protein isolate, and special processed soy flour also have been utilized. Special processing of these soy protein sources by heat or chemical is necessary to deter allergic gastroenteritis in calves ingesting these. Such processing reduces antinutritional factors (ANFs) in soy proteins and allows a soluble product. Moreover, soy proteins seldom are fed as the entire protein source and often comprise less than 50% of total protein, thus allowing their inclusion and successful use for milk replacer protein sources.

The total protein content of a milk replacer should be a minimum of 20%, with most current minimal recommendations being 22%. Milk proteins should compose as much of the protein as possible, and processing of the proteins should not damage the nutrient by subjecting it to high temperatures or other factors.

Fat content of milk replacers is another source of controversy between feed companies and nutritionists. Countless feeding trials have been conducted to show that each company's product is the perfect feed. However, in northern climates, there is no question that a 20% or higher fat content is best based on field observations.

The fiber level in milk replacers is a rough correlation to plant origin sources of protein in some instances. With the advent of acceptable soy protein sources, however, fiber levels cannot be the sole means of evaluation. Early milk replacers with soy flour or other soy source added could be judged somewhat by crude fiber because each 0.1% crude fiber suggested 10% of the protein to be of plant origin. Inclusion of modified soy protein, soy protein concentrate, and soy protein isolate, however, does not increase the fiber content significantly. Therefore crude fiber is not of great value when evaluating current milk replacer protein content.

Yet another controversial aspect of milk replacer feeding involves physiologic "clotting" in the calf abomasum. Milk fed by conventional means causes reflex esophageal groove closure and diversion into the abomasum rather than forestomach. In the abomasum, milk quickly is separated into a casein and milk fat coagulum and a liquid component, whey. Chymosin (rennin) and pepsin in the presence of calcium and hydrochloric acid assist this separation. The whey, which contains lactose, protein, immunoglobulins, and minerals, passes into the duodenum for digestion, whereas the casein/fat coagulum is digested slowly. For many years, it was thought that milk replacers had to "clot" in the abomasum or else they were inferior and caused diarrhea and poor growth. Because only milk or skim milk feeds have casein and whey components, tests for clotting were most applicable to those milk replacers with skim milk as the source of protein. In essence, tests for clotting were designed to detect skim milk origin whey proteins that had been heat denatured by excessive temperatures during processing or drying and therefore would not clot. Because most current milk replacers have a high composition of whey protein or soy-origin protein, they do not clot, yet appear to be well digested.

In addition to the composition of milk replacers, practitioners should be familiar with the common errors associated with milk replacer feeding. The amount of milk replacer fed may or may not be enough for maintenance and growth of suckling calves. Similarly the dilution may be too great or the owner may be skimping because of economic pressures. Replacer should be reconstituted at approximately 12.5% solids (similar to whole milk) and fed at least twice daily for a total of *at least* 10% to 12% body weight. Cold weather extremes and northern winter housing *will* necessitate higher volumes or a third or fourth feeding each day. Some manufacturers do not recommend enough milk replacer to meet maintenance *and* growth requirements. Therefore recommended total amounts may be erroneous. Another problem with some milk replacers is the high sodium content, which may cause neurologic signs if free water is unavailable!

In the past, it has been commonplace for newborn calves to receive colostrum until 3 to 4 days of age and then be switched to replacer or whole milk. This is no longer so frequently practiced, and milk replacer may be fed as early as day 2 of life in many settings. Yet another common feeding error for farmers using milk replacer is not increasing the amount fed as the calf ages. In other words, the calf receives 1 cup of milk replacer in 2 quarts of water twice daily at 4 days of age and is still being fed the same amount at 4 weeks of age. Only through a step-by-step discussion with the owner and by careful observation can the veterinarian detect and correct some calf feeding problems.

High-quality calf starter grains can mask the effect of a poor-quality milk replacer; some authors believe that up to 50% to 75% of calf weight gain before weaning may result from high-quality calf starter intake. Milk replacers containing antibiotics or decoquinate are advertised widely, but their value is difficult to assess because studies yield contradictory results.

Calf diarrhea, emaciation, or both can result from errors in milk replacer feeding. The preceding discussion lists some of the common problems in milk replacer composition and feeding. The true "etiology" of milk replacer–related calf mortality varies but would include:

- Poor-quality milk replacer (i.e., one with less than 22% protein, 20% fat, or poor-quality or overprocessed protein source)
- Feeding at the wrong dilution
- Feeding the wrong amount (usually not enough)

Clinical Signs

Calves suffering malnutrition from poor-quality milk replacer appear thin, have dull hair coats with patchy alopecia, usually have diarrhea that coats their perineum, tail, and hind legs, and are hungry. Affected calves have a normal or subnormal temperature unless an opportunistic infection (e.g., pneumonia) causes a fever in the terminal stages. Calves have no body fat and are weak. Owners complain about calf mortality that usually occurs at 3 to 6 weeks of age and attribute death to diarrhea. Calves may die suddenly but often remain hungry and willing to nurse even if recumbent 1 to 2 days before death. All calves in the preweaning group look thin. The owner may report that the calves look good for the first week but then seem to deteriorate. Calves that survive to weaning often do well on high-quality solid feeds and regain condition.

Ancillary Aids

If calves are dying as early as 3 weeks of age, enteric pathogens and parasites must be ruled out by submission of either fecal samples from live animals or feces and gut samples from necropsy samples. It may be necessary to assess blood selenium and vitamin E values from calves that become recumbent. Total protein values may be low because of persistent low protein intake or fecal losses associated with enteritis, a result of poor-quality protein sources. Blood work is normal unless a stress leukogram exists. Assessment of adequacy of passive transfer is also prudent.

Necropsy confirms malnutrition based on serous atrophy of fat in the epicardial grooves, omentum, and perirenal areas. Gut contents are often fluid, reflecting either poor digestion of nutrients in the cachectic state or opportunistic, secondary enteric infections of the compromised host. Pneumonia may be present as a concurrent condition.

Diagnosis

Diagnosis usually can be made by inspection of the calves coupled with a careful history and evaluation of the milk replacer and feeding procedures. Differential diagnoses include infectious causes of diarrhea, coccidiosis, and selenium deficiency. Calves that are less than 3 weeks of age require careful consideration of infectious enteric bacterial, viral, or protozoan pathogens, whereas older calves between 3 weeks of age and weaning require consideration of coccidiosis and salmonellosis. The owner will be adamant that an infectious disease is responsible because so many calves appear to be affected by ill thrift.

Improper preparation and mixing are occasional factors that augment malnutrition. Careful reading of the instructions on milk replacers and/or consultation with a nutritionist affiliated with the manufacturer may reveal that mixing at hot temperatures (104 to 106° F) is required for complete solubilization of fat in the replacer; subsequent cooling to body temperature is necessary for acceptance by the calf. In such cases, greasy residue may be detected in the mixing vessel as well as in the bottles or buckets following ingestion by the calf.

Inspection of the whole group of calves is very helpful—especially when the veterinarian routinely observes the calves at monthly visits. The sight of a whole group of malnourished but hungry and bright nursing calves in a barn that usually has well-conditioned calves almost guarantees that the owner has switched to a new (cheaper) milk replacer. Calves "eat until they die" and appear hungry even though they are in poor condition. Necropsy of fatal cases confirms serous atrophy of fat and allows other diseases to be ruled out following submission of appropriate samples.

Prevention

Correction and prevention merely require the feeding of a high-quality milk replacer at proper dilution and in proper quantities. The owner must be convinced that milk replacer is not the place to save pennies. In fact, given the increased costs associated with calf losses in such cases, it can be stated that the most expensive milk replacer a producer can buy is often the cheapest one. Milk replacer is never as good as whole milk for calves; therefore whenever possible, owners should be encouraged to feed calves whole milk that is at least 22% crude protein and 20% crude fat (dry matter basis) unless there is a problem with Johne's disease, *Salmonella*, *Mycoplasma*, or leukosis in the herd. Milk discarded because of antibiotic residues is not ideal and should not be fed to group-housed calves. It carries an increased risk for transmission of several contagious, infectious diseases unless pasteurization is performed. Many owners need to reassess the costs of feeding milk versus milk replacer because feeding proper quantities of high-quality milk replacer may be nearly as expensive as whole milk and can never be as good a diet. Use of a pasteurizer for feeding waste milk to calves has been shown to be of economic benefit on larger dairies. Pasteurization of waste milk is worthy of consideration for those operations that routinely produce calves for sale as replacement stock because milk-borne transmission of infectious agents of concern (e.g., *Mycoplasma* spp.) may be reduced.

Soured colostrum and pickled colostrum provide other excellent sources of feed for calves, but their storage problems and potential for spreading pathogens frequently discourage farmers from using these feeds.

If the veterinarian has made a diagnosis of diarrhea and emaciation due to milk replacer issues and feeding of pasteurized whole milk cannot be done, the following instructions can be followed:

1. Ensure adequate colostral feeding to ensure passive transfer of immunoglobulins during the first 12 hours of life.
2. Feed colostrum for the first 3 days of the calf's life at 10% to 12% body weight, but only if sure the cow is not shedding *M. paratuberculosis* or *M. bovis*.
3. Begin feeding a high-quality milk replacer on day 4 at 10% body weight:
   • Minimum 22% protein—most or all of milk origin if possible
   • Minimum 20% fat
   • Minimal crude fiber
4. After the first week, quantity can gradually be increased to maintain 10% to 12% body weight intake.
5. Be sure dilution factors for milk replacer are correct to mimic the total solids of milk.
6. All calves should have fresh water and a high-quality calf starter available *at all times*. Feed starter in small amounts initially until the calf begins to eat well enough that the starter does not spoil in the feeder. High-quality hay can be available in small quantities starting at 2 weeks of age.

7. Regularly monitor the preparation and feeding temperature of milk replacer.

An excellent calf starter, adequate feed intake, and good management may mask the effects of a poor-quality milk replacer. This is why some farms seem to have "starving" calves on a specific milk replacer, whereas others seem to achieve acceptable growth with the same product.

Summary for Neonatal Calf Diarrhea (<14 Days of Age)—Diagnostic Protocol
Table 6-4 gives a diagnostic plan for herd neonatal diarrhea problems.

Coccidiosis
Etiology
Coccidiosis has become one of the most serious problems encountered in raising dairy calves when the calves are grouped and housed in mini free stall barns equipped with lock-in head gates. This style of management currently is very popular because it decreases labor requirements.

Although up to 20 species of *Eimeria* may infect cattle, *E. bovis* and *E. zuernii* are considered the major pathogenic species. Sporulated oocysts that are infective for calves and cattle arise from oocysts passed in the feces of cattle with patent infections. Moisture and cool conditions are conducive to sporulation, whereas

TABLE 6-4 Diagnostic Plan for Workup of Herd Neonatal Diarrhea Problems (<14 Days of Age)

Management	Patient

I. Assess success of passive transfer on at least two or three consecutive affected calves
  A. T. P. and/or GGT
  B. Specific immunoglobulin level on serum from affected calves
II. Discuss management of dry cow
  A. Vaccines
  B. Housing
  C. Calving area (cleaned and so forth)
  D. Colostrum and how fed
  E. Are affected calves from primiparous or multiparous dams or both?
III. Statistics on morbidity/mortality in calves
IV. What are calves fed after initial colostrum?
	I. Feces collected immediately after onset of diarrhea to diagnostic lab on at least two or three consecutive affected calves
	  A. Bacterial
	  —*E. coli* (type and sensitivity) *Salmonella* (type and sensitivity)
	  —*Clostridium perfringens* (relative numbers + is toxin present?)
	  B. Viral—EM, ELISA
	  —Isolation possibly
	  —Rule out BVDV by buffy coat isolation from blood
	  C. Parasitic—*Cryptosporidium*
	  —Coccidia
	  —Giardia
	II. Serum and whole blood
	III. Acid/base and electrolytes
	IV. Hydration status
	V. Body condition

Generalities

1. If FPT, ignore *E. coli* unless same organism confirmed also on non-FPT calves.
2. Whenever possible, more than one calf should be sampled before blaming the whole herd problem on a single isolate.
3. Only fresh cases are worth sampling.
4. If patient older than 2 weeks, consider poor replacer rather than infectious diseases.

extreme heat and dryness are detrimental. Oocysts can remain viable for more than 1 year in favorable conditions that include moisture and absence of temperature extremes. Fecal contamination of feedstuffs, water, or hair coats allows ingestion of infective oocysts by cattle. Conditions that favor fecal contamination of feed and water exist when calves are grouped in mini free stalls or bedded packs. Calves may ingest feces containing oocysts from feed bunks that become contaminated when calves come running up to the bunk when being fed and then splash manure into the bunk or waterers, from calves licking themselves and ingesting feces or fecal-stained hair, or from browsing on a contaminated bedded pack under the roofed area of the housing unit.

Coccidia are quite host-specific intracellular parasites that complete both the asexual and sexual phases of reproduction within the host, but, as mentioned previously, sporulation occurs outside the host. Ingested sporulated oocysts excyst in the host, release sporozoites that invade host cells (central lacteals of ileal villi for *E. bovis*, connective tissue cells of ileal lamina propria for *E. zuernii*), and grow to schizonts (meronts) that release merozoites that then infect epithelial cells in the cecum and colon. Second-generation schizonts then form in these cells and subsequently release merozoites that begin the sexual phase of the reproductive cycle by invading yet another host epithelial cell and become microgamonts (male) or macrogamonts (female). Microgamonts release microgametes that seek host cells containing macrogametes (matured macrogamont); fertilization takes place; and a zygote forms and matures to an oocyst that then is released by rupture of the host cell. Invasion of cells and subsequent release of merozoites and oocysts incite varying degrees of pathology to the epithelium of the cecum and colon of affected calves. The magnitude of enteric pathology appears to be related to the dose of oocysts ingested. Small doses of ingested oocysts may result in inapparent infection and eventual induction of immunity. Large doses are more likely to result in clinical disease.

Oocysts are observed in feces (patent infection) approximately 17 to 20 days following infection with *E. bovis* and 16 to 17 days with *E. zuernii*. The numbers of oocysts in the feces do not always correspond with the degree of enteric pathology or clinical signs because even asymptomatic animals may shed fairly large numbers of oocysts. Conversely, some calves become severely ill before the majority of protozoa complete their life cycle and produce oocysts; therefore fecal oocyst counts may be relatively low despite the serious pathology present in the large intestine.

Recovered calves are thought to be relatively immune to reinfection by the same species of *Eimeria* but at risk for infection by other species. Factors that have a negative influence on the calves' immune competence enhance the pathogenicity of coccidia. Therefore calves exposed to coccidia oocysts and simultaneously subjected to stress, poor nutrition, exogenous corticosteroids, concurrent inflammatory diseases, or acute or persistent BVDV infection would likely show severe signs of coccidiosis.

Clinical Signs

Classical textbook signs of acute coccidiosis in calves include diarrhea containing mucus and blood, tenesmus, depression, and reduced appetite. Rectal prolapse may occur secondary to proctitis and prolonged tenesmus. Affected calves appear dehydrated, thin, and have poor hair coats. Milder cases merely show mild diarrhea without systemic signs and many cases are subclinical.

In fact, the textbook signs of acute coccidiosis seldom occur in dairy calves. The predominant signs of coccidiosis in group-raised dairy calves are loose manure, poor condition, poor growth rates, and poor hair coats (Figure 6-12). The feces seldom contain blood or mucus and tend to have a pea soup consistency. Feces stain the perineum, tail, and hocks of typical cases. Although most calves in the group are infected, only those with severe infection show dramatic signs. Coccidiosis is a perfect example of the "weak sister" law in parasitology—this law states that when a group of animals are parasitized, the most seriously affected bring attention to the problem and act as a signal that the entire group needs treatment. Dairy calves and heifers occasionally show textbook signs of blood- and mucus-stained feces, tenesmus, and inappetence. Tenesmus can be severe and sufficient to prevent the patient from concentrating on eating or drinking.

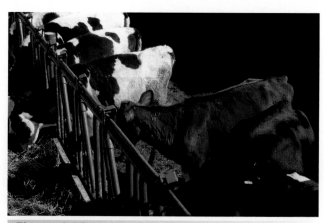

Figure 6-12

Typical signs of coccidiosis in dairy calves. Some of the calves are well grown and have normal hair coats, whereas others (especially the heifer that is not in a lock-in stanchion) are undergrown, have a rough, dry unshed hair coat, and are thin. Many have looser feces than normal for their diet, and the hindquarters are stained by loose feces.

Coccidiosis is a major disease in group-raised dairy calves and heifers. Heifers raised in confinement groups require prophylactic treatment for coccidiosis, or growth rates can be severely compromised. The age of onset for clinical signs varies. Theoretically it is possible that calves will show signs by 3 weeks of age based on life cycles of *E. zuernii* and *E. bovis*. Fortunately this seldom occurs unless newborn calves are put in contaminated environments such as group housing arrangements or hutches that have not been cleaned since previous occupancy by infected calves. In general, coccidiosis becomes a problem for dairy calves at weaning when they are grouped. Weaning and grouping of calves that were previously housed individually induce stress. This stress, combined with an environment that fosters fecal contamination of feedstuffs, water sources, and hair coats, creates an ideal situation for coccidiosis. Therefore clinical signs of coccidiosis are most commonly seen in 8- to 16-week-old calves raised in mini free stall or automatic lock-in facilities. Occasional outbreaks have been observed in 12- to 18-month-old heifers as well and rarely in milking age animals. It would be assumed that older animals showing signs of coccidiosis had never developed resistance to the *Eimeria* sp. involved.

Morbidity is higher than expected because many infected animals remain subclinical or show mild signs. Mortality is low unless the problem is neglected, if severe oocyst loads exist, or if concurrent disease affects the coccidiosis patients.

Nervous coccidiosis has been well described in Canada and the northern United States. Although this form has been observed primarily in beef calves, it may occur in dairy calves as well. Heavy loads of coccidia coupled with severe winter weather seem to be contributing factors to nervous coccidiosis. Affected calves can show a variety of neurologic signs, including (but not limited to) severe tremors, nystagmus, and recumbency. Opisthotonos may be observed and confuse the diagnosis with that of polioencephalomalacia. The mortality rate is high for calves with nervous coccidiosis.

Diagnosis

Clinical signs coupled with fecal flotation to confirm high numbers of coccidia allow a positive diagnosis. The diagnostic limitations of fecal oocyst numbers must be kept in mind:

1. Diarrhea may precede the highest oocyst counts by a few days in acute cases because merozoite damage to the colonic epithelium may cause diarrhea before full patency and maximal oocyst shedding to occur. In other words, an animal severely affected by coccidiosis may have relatively low or even zero oocyst counts on a given fecal sample. Necropsy and histopathology may be necessary to confirm the diagnosis in such cases.
2. Nonpathogenic species of coccidia may artificially elevate oocyst counts as they traverse the intestinal tract.
3. Healthy animals may have oocysts in their feces.

In general, oocyst counts of >5000/g of feces are considered significant when coupled with clinical signs. Several calves should be sampled to confirm the diagnosis because severely affected groups of calves tend to show higher oocyst counts as a population.

The major differential diagnoses are salmonellosis, BVDV infection, endoparasitism as a result of nematodes, and poor nutrition. These diseases should be ruled out when response to treatment for coccidiosis fails to correct the problem. Nervous coccidiosis dictates a much broader differential diagnosis, including polioencephalomalacia, *Histophilus somni (Haemophilus somnus)* meningoencephalomyelitis, lead poisoning, and many other neurologic diseases. A CSF tap would be an essential test to rule in or out some of the differential diagnoses.

Calves that die from acute, severe coccidiosis may or may not have gross pathologic lesions in the cecum and colon. Severe infections may cause a diphtheritic membrane from sloughed mucosa, blood, and fibrin. Whole blood clots occasionally are found in the colon, and the mucosa of the cecum, colon, and rectum may be thickened. Small white spots (schizonts) may be apparent on close inspection of the mucosa of the ileum or colon. Microscopic lesions mainly reflect colonic damage secondary to second-generation schizonts and sexual phases. Inflammation, sloughing of epithelial cells, cellular infiltrates, and alteration of the appearance of infected epithelial cells to a less columnar shape may be observed. Schizonts of *E. bovis* tend to be located in the villous tips, whereas *E. zuernii* schizonts are located adjacent to the muscularis layer.

Treatment and Prevention

Treatment and prevention of coccidiosis in calves entail orally administered coccidiostatic or coccidiocidal agents, some of which also are used as prophylactic treatment when exposure of calves to coccidia is likely. Amprolium, monensin, lasalocid, and decoquinate are the drugs used most commonly to treat groups of affected or at-risk calves. These drugs are added to feed or water at the rates listed in the chart (Table 6-5).

Ionophores such as monensin and lasalocid are fed continuously in many calf-raising operations where coccidiosis is known to exist; the same is true for decoquinate. Manufacturer's warnings, dosages, and withdrawal times must be observed and are subject to change. Decoquinate is not toxic to young calves, but ionophores may be. Although various sulfa drugs were the first treatments for coccidiosis in animals, they are not used at present except to treat small groups or individual calves so sick they may not be eating or drinking

TABLE 6-5   Drugs that Aid in Prevention and Treatment of Coccidiosis

Drug	Name	Use	Dose
Amprolium	Corid*	Prophylactic	5 mg/kg body weight (bwt) for 21 days
		Therapeutic	10 mg/kg bwt for 5 days
Monensin	Rumensin†	Prophylactic	16.5-33.0 g/ton feed continuously, or
			1.0 mg/kg bwt for 28 days
Lasalocid	Bovatec‡	Prophylactic	1 mg/kg bwt continuously
Decoquinate	Deccox§ (several products available)	Prophylactic	0.5 mg/kg bwt for 30 days
Sulfamethazine		Therapeutic	140 mg/kg bwt loading dose, then
			70 mg/kg bwt for 5-7 days
Sulfadimethoxine	Several products available	Therapeutic	55 mg/kg bwt loading dose, then
			27.5 mg/kg bwt for 5-7 days

*Corid (amprolium), Merial Ltd., Duluth, GA.
†Rumensin 60 (monensin sodium), Elanco Animal Health, Greenfield, IN.
‡Bovatec (lasalocid), Alpharma, Inc., Fort Lee, NJ.
§Deccox (decoquinate), Alpharma, Inc.

well enough to ingest therapeutic dosages of drugs added to their feed or water. When sulfa drugs are used for treatment, it is beneficial to treat simultaneously with amprolium at treatment levels. Individual calves that are severely dehydrated may require supportive fluids and, rarely, blood transfusions if colonic hemorrhage has been severe. Tenesmus may be so severe and persistent as to require epidural anesthesia to allow the calf or heifer to rest, eat, and drink.

Although the aforementioned drugs are used widely for prophylaxis in calves at risk for coccidiosis, they should not be thought of as the only means of control. Management practices that allow dirty environments, manure buildup, feeding on ground level, feed and water contaminated by manure, and crowding should be corrected. If calves are kept in a clean environment, manure should be scraped away daily to prevent "splashing" of feces into bunks, troughs, waterers, and all over calves' bodies. If premises are cleaned and disinfected between consecutive groups of calves, the risk of coccidiosis is lowered tremendously. Unfortunately many farmers would rather rely on a drug placed in the feed than do the required cleaning. Many of the coccidiostats are only effective for as long as fed, so calves become at risk if medicated feed is discontinued. Therefore anticoccidial drugs usually are included in the ration from weaning through breeding age rather than based on manufacturer's recommendations (e.g., 30 days). Increasingly, calf starters and milk replacers including coccidiostats are being marketed for dairy calves. Although these drugs may not be necessary in preweaned calves, it is possible that clinical coccidiosis could occur as early as 2 to 3 weeks of age. Although the rumen is poorly developed in the neonatal calf, lasalocid fed from day 1 improved gain and also counterbalanced coccidial infection (experimentally induced) before weaning. Certainly if management conditions allow preweaning coccidiosis, mixed infections of the gastrointestinal tract would be possible in the 2- to 4-week-old calf. *C. parvum*, rotavirus, coronavirus, *E. coli*, or *Salmonella* sp. could be involved. Obviously mixed infections could worsen the pathology.

Nematodes

Etiology

Intestinal nematodes are an important concern for pastured calves and growing heifers. Although current trends make pasturing of young dairy calves and heifers uncommon, consideration of intestinal parasite burdens is worthwhile for confined heifers and essential for growing heifers on pasture. A basic understanding of parasites' life cycles and the geographic incidence of the various intestinal parasites is essential when making recommendations to owners. Pastured heifers require planned parasite control programs that include management and anthelmintic components.

The major nematode parasites of the abomasum include *Ostertagia ostertagi*, *Trichostrongylus axei*, and *Haemonchus placei*. *O. ostertagi* (brown stomach worm) is the most important nematode in cattle because of its ability to undergo hypobiosis or arrested development of the L4 stage within the abomasum of infected young cattle. Arrested larvae reside in the lumen of gastric glands during seasons of the year that would likely interfere with the parasites' existence outside the host. Therefore larvae acquired during late fall and early winter at temperatures found in northern climates persist in the host as inhibited larvae for weeks to months before maturing in late winter and spring. In southern temperate zones, larvae acquired during the spring become inhibited and finally mature in late summer or early fall. The biologic purpose of *O. ostertagi* hypobiosis is to avoid exposure of eggs and larval stages to weather not conducive to survival of the parasite. Therefore harsh winters are avoided in the north, as are hot dry summers in southern zones. In the abomasal wall, hypobiotic larvae are apparently not targeted by the immune system for elimination, even in previously exposed adult cattle. When arrested larvae emerge from the abomasal glands, they tend to do so with a vengeance that creates severe abomasal pathology and illness known as ostertagiasis type II. Maturation and emergence of large numbers of inhibited L4 larvae cause acute anorexia, weight loss, hypoproteinemia, and severe diarrhea as a result of abomasal mucosal injury, increased abomasal pH because of parietal cell dysfunction, and hyperplasia. The mortality rate is high, although prevalence usually is low. The resultant greatly thickened and nodular abomasal wall has caused pathologists to describe the gross lesion as "Moroccan leather" in appearance. Because ostertagiasis type II occurs in the late winter and spring in northern zones and late summer or fall in southern areas, parasites may not be considered as the cause of illness in affected heifers. Inhibited larvae also are resistant to many commonly used anthelmintics. Ostertagiasis type I is more classically typical of nematode infections because pastured heifers acquire significant loads of larvae that mature to adults over approximately 3 weeks. Type I infections occur during peak pasture seasons and can result in diarrhea, weight loss, hypoproteinemia, or simply poor weight gain.

H. placei and other species found less commonly in cattle also possess the ability to undergo hypobiosis to avoid temperature extremes detrimental to survival outside the host. *H. placei* is pathogenic as a result of blood sucking that can lead to severe anemia.

T. axei may cause injury to the abomasal mucosa that leads to hypoproteinemia, altered digestion and defense mechanisms, and diarrhea. *Gangylonema* spp. also live in the abomasum and forestomach but are not thought to be major pathogens. Small intestinal nematodes include other *Trichostrongylus* spp., *Cooperia* spp., *Nematodirus helvetianus*, *Bunostomum phlebotomum*, *Toxocara vitulonum*, and several other parasites. *Bunostomum phlebotomum* and the *Cooperia* spp. are bloodsuckers that damage the intestinal mucosa and create anemia. *N. helvetianus* is an extremely hardy, weather-resistant parasite that causes diarrhea in cattle when present in great numbers.

Large intestinal nematodes include *Oesophagostomum radiatum*, *Chabertia ovina*, *Trichuris discolor*, and *Trichuris ovis*. *O. radiatum* causes multiple inflammatory reactions in the cecum and colon of cattle. This inflammation, subsequent nodule formation, and hemorrhage cause inflammatory bowel disease that result in diarrhea, weight loss, and hypoproteinemia in heavily parasitized animals. Subsequent long-term pathology and full or partial immunity allow *O. radiatum* nodules to become necrotic or calcified. These chronic lesions are grossly apparent in the bowel serosa and are responsible for the parasite being labeled the "nodular worm." Intussusceptions sometimes occur at the site of chronic *O. radiatum* lesions, and therefore pathologists theorize that the lesions may disrupt or alter normal intestinal motility.

Trichuris spp. occasionally are identified as the cause of severe diarrhea in heifers. *Trichuris* spp. are known as "whipworms" and concentrate in the cecum of cattle hosts.

The aforementioned nematodes all possess pathogenicity of varying degrees to young animals or mature animals not previously exposed to parasites. Pastured animals, especially those pastured on lands that are grazed every year, are at risk. The first pasture season of an animal's life presents the greatest risk. Thereafter, partial or full immunity develops to protect animals during their adult years. Fortunately anthelmintics are available to counteract these parasites. Anthelmintics used appropriately, combined with pasture management, allow dairy heifers to be pastured successfully. All authorities agree that parasites are detrimental to calves and heifers—especially those on pasture. Much controversy exists, however, when the topic of worming adult dairy cattle is discussed. Natural immunity (at least for cows that grazed pasture and acquired exposure to parasites as heifers) should protect adult cattle previously exposed to parasites. Attempts to demonstrate milk yield difference between wormed and nonwormed dairy cattle have given mixed results, and much debate exists on the relative merits of adult cow deworming.

Clinical Signs

As with any parasitic infestation or infection, overt clinical signs may be present only in a few animals within a group. However, all animals in the group will harbor parasite loads. Mild nematode levels simply deter normal growth and gain rates in heifers without causing clinical signs of disease. Moderate levels of nematodes cause some animals in the group to show variable amounts of diarrhea, weight loss, poor hair coats, decreased appetite, hypoproteinemia, and anemia. Heavy nematode levels cause acute appearance of these signs and a greater prevalence of animals showing signs within the group. Appetite depression is consistent, responsible for weight loss or lack of weight gain, and, as yet, is unexplained. The predominant types of nematodes in each herd will dictate the signs observed. For example, in ostertagiosis type II, acute hypoproteinemia, severe diarrhea, and inappetence would be observed in some animals within the group, and the time of year would not coincide with atypical parasitic problem. If *Haemonchus* spp., *Bunostomum* spp., or *Cooperia* spp. predominates, anemia could be the major sign.

Ancillary Data

Anemia caused by blood loss and hypoproteinemia characterized by hypoalbuminemia are the major abnormalities detected on complete blood count and serum biochemistry. Abomasal pH increases as acid production decreases secondary to parietal cell dysfunction. Pepsinogen is not activated completely to pepsin, a proteolytic enzyme, because this activation requires a low abomasal pH. Therefore increased plasma pepsinogen levels may be demonstrated when severe abomasal pathology exists as a result of *O. ostertagi* or less commonly *T. axei*. Few, if any, veterinary diagnostic laboratories in North America routinely offer serum pepsinogen analysis on a commercial basis, however. Eosinophilia may or may not be present in WBC differentials and is not an essential aid to diagnosis. Fecal flotation and larval culture provide the definitive diagnostic tools. Very severe, acute infections with profuse diarrhea may have significant electrolyte losses of Na^+, Cl^-, HCO_3^-, and K^+.

Diagnosis

A definitive diagnosis requires identification of worm eggs or larvae in the feces of cattle having signs consistent with nematodiasis and ruling out other infections or toxic diseases. When diarrhea is a major sign, salmonellosis, BVDV infection, coccidiosis, and toxicities that result in diarrhea must be ruled out.

Treatment and Control

Minimizing pasture contamination by parasite eggs and larvae is a major portion of parasite control for dairy heifers. Heifers should be wormed before turnout and then at 3 and 6 weeks following turnout (or 3 and 8 weeks after turnout if ivermectin is used). This schedule helps to reduce recently ingested worm burdens before mature females begin to contaminate pastures with eggs, and the second treatment should kill ingested overwintered larvae that contaminate the pasture. The two-treatment program helps prevent the dramatic L3 load that generally occurs in northern climate pastures during late summer and early fall. Migration of L3 from manure to herbage occurs earlier during wet summers than dry ones, whereas L3 loads tend to peak in the fall in northern climates. Although it may be ideal to select an anthelmintic specifically directed against the major nematodes present on each farm, it is more practical to select broad-spectrum anthelmintics that kill most types of nematodes. Available anthelmintics for nonlactating or nonbreeding age dairy cattle are listed in Table 6-6. Label recommendations and changes in status of approval may occur with any of the drugs listed in this table. Therefore the practitioner should always verify

that label approval exists for dairy animals. Pasture rotation with worming before movement to new pasture is another management tool seldom practiced with dairy operations because of limited acreage.

Although worming and parasite control are definitely beneficial to pastured heifers, the economic benefits of worming adult lactating dairy cows are controversial. Worming programs for lactating cattle may be justified if the cattle are pastured for a significant time each year. Worming would primarily benefit first calf heifers and newly acquired cattle that perhaps had not been pastured as heifers—thus not likely to have parasite resistance. Dairy herds with a high percentage of first calf heifers *and* utilizing pasture for a portion of the year probably can justify anthelmintic treatment of lactating cattle.

Economic justification may be lacking for use of anthelmintics in lactating cows from totally confined herds whose heifers never are pastured. Available anthelmintics for lactating dairy cattle are listed in Table 6-7.

Trematodes

Etiology and Signs

Liver flukes are a greater problem in beef than dairy cattle, but certain geographic areas harbor flukes and their intermediate hosts, thereby representing risks for pastured dairy heifers and cows. *Fasciola hepatica* is found in certain areas in the Gulf Coast and western United States. Cattle, along with sheep, are the primary definitive hosts of *F. hepatica* and shed eggs with feces. Eggs require a moist environment to hatch miracidia, which find a snail intermediate host. Following a complicated reproductive cycle in the snail, the parasite eventually produces metacercaria, which are ingested by the host. Metacercaria invade the duodenum, and immature flukes then penetrate the gut and seek out the liver, where they penetrate the capsule, migrate in the parenchyma, and eventually reside in the bile ducts. This wandering through the gut and liver parenchyma creates a great deal of pathology, which in heavy infestations may cause hypoproteinemia, anemia, reduced appetite, peritonitis, clostridial diseases such as bacillary hemoglobinuria (*C. hemolyticum*), or black disease (*C. novyi*).

Fascioloides magna, the deer liver fluke, is a large fluke that can infect cattle and sheep. The fluke is found along the Gulf Coast, the Great Lakes region, and the northwestern United States. Although cattle can be infected, the resulting parenchymal cyst does not allow egg release, thus making cattle dead-end hosts. In deer, the natural host, thin-walled parenchymal cysts are formed that allow eggs to emerge into bile ducts. *F. magna* is particularly vicious in sheep because continued migration without encystment is the rule. Because infections are not patent in cattle, liver condemnation or gross

TABLE 6-6 Anthelmintics Approved for Nonlactating Dairy Animals (Data Assembled from Information Given on Manufacturer's Labels)

Drug	Dose	Slaughter Withdrawal Time (days)	Spectrum/Comments
Albendazole	10 mg/kg PO	27	Gastrointestinal nematodes, including hypobiotic *Ostertagia* L4, lungworms, *Moniezia* (tapeworms), adult liver flukes *(Fasciola)*
			Not for use in female dairy cattle of breeding age; potentially teratogenic if administered in early pregnancy
Doramectin injectable	200 µg/kg SQ	35	Gastrointestinal nematodes, including hypobiotic *Ostertagia* L4, lungworms, grubs, sucking lice, mites
			Not for use in female dairy cattle of breeding age or in veal calves
Doramectin (pour-on)	500 µg/kg topically	45	Gastrointestinal nematodes, including hypobiotic *Ostertagia* L4, lungworms, grubs, sucking and biting lice, mites
			Not for use in female dairy cattle of breeding age or in veal calves
Eprinomectin (pour-on)	500 µg/kg topically	0	Gastrointestinal nematodes, including hypobiotic *Ostertagia* L4, lungworms, grubs *(Hypoderma)*, sucking and biting lice, mites, and horn flies
			Effective when applied to wet cattle
Fenbendazole	5 mg/kg PO	8-13 (depending on product)	Gastrointestinal nematodes (adult), lungworms
	10-15 mg/kg PO	8-13 (depending on product)	Gastrointestinal nematodes, including hypobiotic *Ostertagia* L4, lungworms, tapeworms
Ivermectin (injectable)	200 µg/kg SQ	35	Gastrointestinal nematodes (adult and larvae), including hypobiotic *Ostertagia* L4, *Dictyocaulus* (lungworm), grubs *(Hypoderma)*, sucking lice, and mites
			Not for use in female dairy cattle of breeding age or in veal calves
Ivermectin (pour-on)	500 µg/kg topically	48	Gastrointestinal nematodes, including hypobiotic *Ostertagia* L4, *Dictyocaulus* (lungworm), grubs *(Hypoderma)*, sucking and biting lice, mites, and horn flies
			Not for use in female dairy cattle of breeding age or in veal calves
Levamisole	Varies with formulation	7 days	Gastrointestinal nematodes (adult), lungworms
			Not for use in female dairy cattle of breeding age
Moxidectin (injectable)	200 µg/kg SQ	21 days	Gastrointestinal nematodes (adult and larvae), including hypobiotic *Ostertagia* L4, *Dictyocaulus* (lungworm), grubs *(Hypoderma)*, sucking lice, and mites
			Not for use in female dairy cattle of breeding age or in veal calves
Moxidectin (pour-on)	500 µg/kg topically	0	Gastrointestinal nematodes, including hypobiotic *Ostertagia* L4, *Dictyocaulus* (lungworm), grubs *(Hypoderma)*, sucking and biting lice, mites, and horn flies
			Not for use in veal calves
Morantel tartrate	0.44 g/ 100 lb PO	14 days	Gastrointestinal nematodes (adult)
Oxfendazole	4.5 mg/kg PO	7 days	Gastrointestinal nematodes, including hypobiotic *Ostertagia* L4, lungworms, tapeworms
			Not for use in female dairy cattle of breeding age
Clorsulon	7 mg/kg	8 days	*Fasciola hepatica* adults and late immature larvae
Clorsulon and Ivermectin	1 ml/110 lb SQ	49 days	Gastrointestinal nematodes (adult and larvae), including hypobiotic *Ostertagia* L4, lungworms, *Fasciola hepatica* adults, grubs *(Hypoderma)*, sucking lice, and mites
			Not for use in female dairy cattle of breeding age or in veal calves

TABLE 6-7 Anthelmintics Approved for Lactating Dairy Cattle (Assembled from Manufacturer's Labels)

Drug	Dose	Withdrawal Period for Slaughter and Milk (days)	Spectrum
Eprinomectin (pour-on)	500 μg/kg topically	Meat = 0 Milk = 0	Gastrointestinal nematodes, including hypobiotic *Ostertagia* L4, lungworms, grubs (*Hypoderma*), sucking and biting lice, mites, and horn flies Effective when applied to wet cattle
Fenbendazole	5 mg/kg PO	Meat: 8-13 (depending on product) Milk: 0	Gastrointestinal nematodes (adult), lungworms
Morantel tartrate	0.44 g/100 lb PO	Meat = 14 Milk = 0	Gastrointestinal nematodes (adult)
Moxidectin (pour-on)	500 μg/kg topically	Meat = 0 Milk = 0	Gastrointestinal nematodes, including hypobiotic *Ostertagia* L4, lungworms, grubs (*Hypoderma*), sucking and biting lice, mites, and horn flies

postmortem lesions are the major consequences of *F. magna* infection.

Dicrocoelium dendriticum occurs in many geographic regions around the world and in a few areas in the northeastern United States (including the central New York region of our practice) and Canada. The life cycle is complex, with both the land snail (*Cionella lubrica*) and the black ant (*Formica fusca*) necessary for transmission back to a definitive host, such as cattle, sheep, goats, horses, pigs, and people. Metacercariae (in ants) ingested by host cattle penetrate the duodenum and directly enter the bile ducts where they usually cause little detectable illness. However, heavy infestations can occasionally inflame or obstruct biliary ductules and the gallbladder. Most cases are self-limiting.

Fasciola gigantica is limited to tropical regions and will not be discussed here.

Paramphistomum, the rumen fluke, is thought not to be highly pathogenic in the United States but can cause illness in tropical zones. Ingested metacercariae may encyst in the duodenum or migrate to the duodenum wall where they stay for weeks before migrating upstream to become adults in the rumen and reticulum. Acute paramphistomiasis, which is rare in the United States, refers to duodenal pathology created by large populations of wandering and invading immature flukes.

Diagnosis

Identification of fluke eggs in the feces is possible for *F. hepatica* and *D. dendriticum*. *Paramphistomum* spp. eggs can be confused with *F. hepatica*, especially because both are operculated, but *F. hepatica* eggs are slightly smaller and stained yellow. Routine sampling of feces from 10 to 15 at-risk animals is indicated when *F. hepatica* is suspected. An ELISA serologic test also has been devised to diagnose *F. hepatica* lesions. Necropsy specimens are very helpful whenever fluke infestations are suspected.

Treatment

Table 6-6 also lists the available drugs to counteract fluke infestation in nonlactating dairy heifers. Albendazole, clorsulon, and clorsulon-ivermectin are effective against adult and late immature *F. hepatica*. Albendazole is effective against *F. magna* and *D. dendriticum*. Control measures include avoidance of pastures harboring intermediate hosts or killing intermediate hosts such as snails with molluscicides. Veterinarians practicing in endemic fluke regions should be familiar with diagnosis and control measures if their clients pasture heifers.

Cestodiasis

Moniezia benedeni is the small intestinal tapeworm of cattle and is thought to be nonpathogenic. Oribatid mites are the intermediate hosts, and following ingestion of infective cysticercoids by cattle, the worms mature over 2 months and then are shed spontaneously several months later. Treatment with albendazole is effective when necessary. Other tapeworms such as *Taenia saginata*, the beef tapeworm of humans, *Taenia hydatigena* (adults in dogs), and *Echinococcus granulosus* are not major parasites of dairy cattle and will not be discussed here.

Cryptosporidium muris

Cryptosporidium muris causes gastric cryptosporidiosis in young and adult cattle. The organisms, which have larger oocysts than *C. parvum*, are found in the peptic glands of the abomasum. The significance of these organisms is unknown, but infection apparently causes hypertrophy or thickening of the abomasum and the mucosal folds within. The same author has identified the organism by histopathology, fecal flotation, and acid-fast staining of fecal smears.

Papular Stomatitis

Etiology

A parapoxvirus indistinguishable from the virus of pseudocowpox and also possibly related to the contagious ecthyma virus of sheep and goats is the cause of papular stomatitis in calves. The disease is spread by contact between infected and noninfected calves or common feeding devices or containers. The virus is quite contagious in young calves and also can cause lesions on the skin of humans working with calves. Such zoonotic infection creates lesions similar to the milker's nodules of pseudocowpox in people. Papular stomatitis virus lesions on the muzzle and in the oral cavity of calves frequently are confused with erosions caused by BVDV. It was first described in the United States in 1960.

Signs

A raised papule on the muzzle or nares is the most commonly observed lesion because of the external nature of the lesion (Figure 6-13). Papules on the palate, tongue, or lips probably are more common but are less likely to be observed (Figure 6-14). Although red and raised on the external mucosa, the lesions may appear crusty or brownish-yellow in the oral cavity and have roughened edges (Figure 6-15). Oral cavity lesions may be flat and therefore confused with erosions. Some papules develop a necrotic white center that sloughs, leaving an ulcerated area within the raised papule. Papular stomatitis lesions may cause an affected calf to show mild salivation and reluctance to nurse or eat. Such signs usually lead to

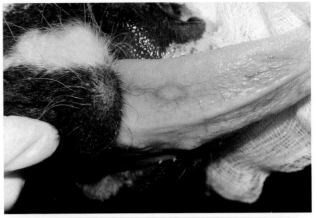

Figure 6-14

Circular papular stomatitis lesions on the ventrum of a calf's tongue.

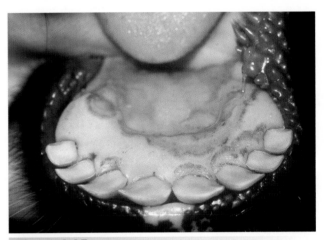

Figure 6-15

Papular stomatitis lesions caudal to the incisor teeth and ventral to the tongue in a calf. The lesions are brownish-yellow in color, slightly raised, and have rough edges.

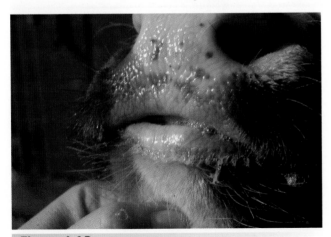

Figure 6-13

Typical raised circular lesions of papular stomatitis on the muzzle and lips of a calf.

examination of the oral cavity and subsequent diagnosis. Many, if not most, cases are asymptomatic and go undiagnosed.

Calves from several weeks to several months of age are most commonly affected, but the disease has also been observed in older growing cattle. Lesions also occur in the esophagus and forestomach mucosa but are only detected in those locations during necropsy examination. Such lower alimentary lesions may be confused with infectious bovine rhinotracheitis (IBR)– or BVDV-induced lesions.

Severe illnesses or immunodeficiencies frequently allow extensive proliferation of papular stomatitis virus and subsequent advanced lesions. When such severe lesions occur, they are clinically suspected to be BVDV infections. In fact, concurrent BVDV infection in immunocompetent calves or poor-doing BVDV-PI calves will greatly accentuate papular stomatitis lesions when the virus is present. Similarly, IBR virus and chronic bacterial infections predispose to worsening of existing papular stomatitis virus. Clinical errors are most common, however, when BVDV-PI calves with a superinfection with cytopathic (CP)-BVDV or chronic concurrent diseases develop amplification of papular stomatitis lesions. Most spontaneous, uncomplicated papular stomatitis lesions resolve within several weeks in immunocompetent animals and are diagnosed by inspection. Severe cases may require biopsy and viral culture to differentiate the lesions from BVDV. Intracytoplasmic eosinophilic inclusions are typical in the cytoplasm of degenerating cells.

Although the disease may be fatal, most early reports that cited extensive lesions and fatalities probably represented concurrent BVDV infections.

Treatment and Prevention

No specific treatment or method of prevention exists other than to minimize spread by housing calves separately and not using common feeding devices or buckets.

INFECTIOUS DISEASES OF THE GASTROINTESTINAL TRACT—ADULTS

Actinobacillosis

Etiology

Actinobacillus lignieresii, a gram-negative pleomorphic rod, is a normal commensal organism in the oral flora of cattle. Injuries to the oral mucosa or skin that become contaminated with *A. lignieresii* may develop soft tissue infection characterized by an initial cellulitis that evolves into a classical pyogranulomatous infection that can be confused with neoplasia or actinomycosis. Sulfur granules, which are yellow-white cheesy accumulations containing the organism, develop in pus or pyogranulomatous soft tissue lesions associated with *A. lignieresii* infection.

"Wooden tongue," a soft tissue infection of the tongue of cattle, is the classical example of *A. lignieresii* infection in cattle, but soft tissue granulomas developing around the head, neck, or other body areas are common as well. Granulomas of the esophagus, forestomach, and occasionally other visceral locations also are possible. Lymphadenitis, lymph node abscesses, and infectious granulomas originating from lymph nodes may follow soft tissue infections of the oral cavity or pharynx. Extremely fibrous feed material has been incriminated as the cause of mucosal injury that allowed opportunistic *A. lignieresii* infection as a herd problem in dairy heifers. Direct inoculation of the organism into mucosal wounds can occur in the oral cavity, esophagus, and forestomach. Inoculation probably occurs from oral secretions or saliva when soft tissue wounds of the skin are infected at sites distant from the oral cavity.

Signs

Acute wooden tongue in cattle appears as a diffusely swollen, firm tongue that fills the oral cavity. Firm or fluctuant intermandibular swelling usually accompanies the inflammatory enlargement of the tongue (Figure 6-16). Salivation is observed, and the swollen tongue may protrude from the oral cavity. Anorexia is relative or complete because the tongue has reduced mobility and may be injured by the teeth if chewing is attempted. Fever is present in acute infections but frequently absent in subacute or chronic cases. Distended salivary ducts appearing as ranulae may be observed ventral to the tongue.

Chronic wooden tongue lesions consist of pyogranulomatous masses and fibrosis of the tongue. Weight loss and salivation are common in chronically infected cattle.

Atypical *A. lignieresii* infection is characterized by granulomas, pyogranulomas, or lymph node abscesses. Serous or mucoid nonodorous pus may drain from abscessed infections. Granulomas are raised, red, fleshy to firm in consistency, and contain sulfur granules. Granulomas may occur in the oral cavity, esophagus, forestomach, or other visceral locations. In addition, external granulomas have been observed in the nares, eyelids, face, pharyngeal region, neck, limbs, and abdomen (Figure 6-17). Infection of abomasopexy toggles or sharp incision sites also has produced granulomas (Figure 6-18).

Diagnosis

Excision or biopsy of granulomas to provide material for bacterial culture and histopathology is the only means to confirm a diagnosis of *A. lignieresii*. Clinical

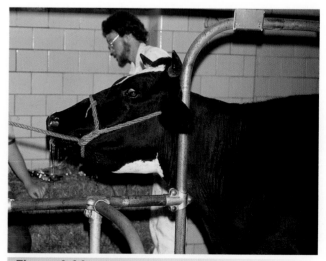

Figure 6-16

Acute wooden tongue with intermandibular cellulitis and salivation.

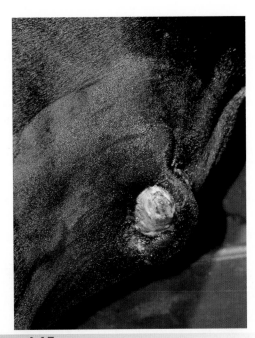

Figure 6-17

Atypical actinobacillosis granuloma in the jugular furrow of a cow secondary to a perivascular administration of concentrated dextrose solution.

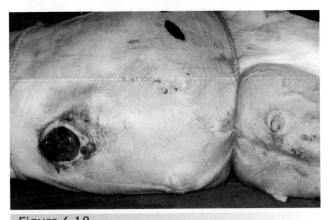

Figure 6-18

Actinobacillosis granuloma at the site of an abomasopexy incision.

appearances and the presence of sulfur granules are suggestive of diagnosis but not specific because the masses must be differentiated from actinomycoses, botryomycosis, neoplasia, parasitic or foreign body granuloma, and exuberant granulation tissue. Acute wooden tongue can be diagnosed by aspiration of fluid-distended salivary ranulae, the tongue itself, or intermandibular phlegmon when present. Aspirates are submitted for cytology and culture. Chronic wooden tongue lesions are best diagnosed by biopsies submitted for both culture and histopathology.

Treatment

Wooden tongue and other lesions of *A. lignieresii* respond to systemic sodium iodide therapy. IV sodium iodide (20% solution) is an extremely irritating preparation that should be administered IV only by a veterinarian. IV sodium iodide is administered at a dose of 70 mg/kg body weight. This dose is repeated at 2- to 3-day intervals until iodism occurs. Alternatively, oral organic iodide can be fed (1 oz/450 kg body weight, daily) following initial IV therapy until iodism occurs. Signs of iodism include serous lacrimation, seromucoid nasal discharge, and scaly dandruff-like skin appearing on the face and neck of treated cattle. For acute wooden tongue lesions, response to iodine therapy is usually dramatic. Subacute lesions respond more slowly, and chronic lesions carry a guarded prognosis. Sulfonamides, tetracycline, or ampicillin also may be useful and can be used alone or in conjunction with iodine therapy for severe *A. lignieresii* infections of the tongue.

Treatment of *A. lignieresii* granulomas consists of debridement or debulking (if the involved anatomic area allows surgical intervention), coupled with medical therapy as outlined previously. Recurrent or severe lesions can be treated with combined therapy as discussed previously. Cryosurgical treatment has been combined with surgical debulking of some *A. lignieresii* granulomas and appears most effective when mushrooming granulomas attached to a narrow skin base are selected for therapy.

The exact reason that iodides are effective in *A. lignieresii* infection is not known. Suggested mechanisms include penetrance into granulation tissue and destruction of organisms, simple decrease in the granulomatous response, and combinations of activity against *A. lignieresii* and the granulomatous inflammatory response. Iodides are unlikely to cause abortion in cattle, although some commercially available preparations of injectable sodium iodide are labeled with a warning that forbids their use in pregnant cattle.

Actinomycosis

Actinomyces bovis, a gram-positive filamentous organism (Figure 6-19) that can assume many forms, is the cause of lumpy jaw in cattle and occasionally causes granulomatous infection in other areas of the body. In young cultures, diphtheroid organisms are observed, but in older cultures and crushed preparations of sulfur granules obtained from pus, the organism may be filamentous, branching, coccoid, club-shaped, or diphtheroid. Infection with *A. bovis* typically results in formation of "sulfur granules" in pus or infected tissue. These so-called sulfur granules contain large numbers of the organism. In older literature, the term actinomycosis implied granulomatous infections containing sulfur granules and did not differentiate *A. lignieresii* or staphylococcal infections from those caused by *A. bovis*.

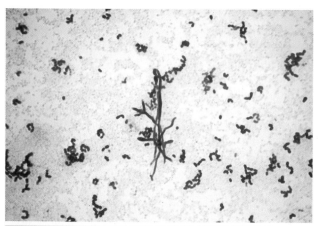

Figure 6-19

Gram stain of aspirate from lumpy jaw lesion. Gram positive branching filamentous rods are characteristic of *Actinomyces bovis*.

The organism is difficult to culture to the degree necessary for bacterial susceptibility testing. This fact contributes to the dearth of scientific information regarding the appropriate therapy for lumpy jaw in cattle. Many other species of *Actinomyces* have been studied in people, and comparative information from these studies suggests that *A. bovis* is much more resistant to antibiotic therapy than human isolates such as *Actinomyces israeli*.

Lumpy jaw is a debilitating disease of cattle resulting from infection of the mandible or maxilla by *A. bovis*. The organism has been described as a normal inhabitant of the oral flora and digestive tract of cattle. It is assumed that infection of bones and teeth occurs following injury to the oral mucosa by fibrous feeds or dental eruption (this may be a reason that lumpy jaw seems most common in young adult cattle) and subsequent inoculation of *A. bovis*. The organism also may penetrate around the alveoli of the teeth or contaminate skin wounds in common feed and water troughs. Dr. Rebhun observed one herd with an epidemic of lumpy jaw, with 7 of 60 cows affected. The point source cow had a large, draining, lumpy jaw lesion, and all cows ate silage twice daily from a feed bunk made of coarse boards. Discharge of the organism from the point source cow certainly contaminated the sideboards and bunk. Whether the organism had gained access through the oral cavity, injury to the oral cavity by wood splinters, or skin puncture from wood slivers on the sideboards could not be ascertained. Lumpy jaw usually is a sporadic infection but, as in the aforementioned herd, can be an epidemic or endemic herd problem.

Rarely *A. bovis* causes infectious granulomas on soft tissues similar to those caused by *A. lignieresii*. Granulomas caused by *A. bovis* have been identified in the trachea, testes, and digestive tract.

Clinical Signs

Early *A. bovis* infections of the mandible or maxilla appear as warm, painful swellings consisting of distinct edema overlapping a firm, painful, bony swelling (Figure 6-20). Such early infections easily could be confused with a traumatic injury. Over a period of weeks, however, bone enlargement becomes obvious and soft tissue edema much less apparent. Salivation and some difficulty in eating may be observed, but inappetence and weight loss seldom are a problem in early cases. Once the infection is established in bone, the swelling becomes hard and painful (Figures 6-21 to 6-23). Severe

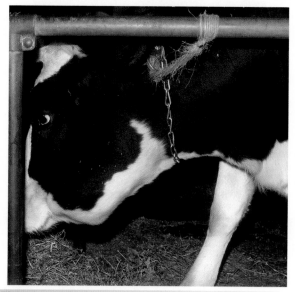

Figure 6-20

Early lumpy jaw lesion consisting of an edematous soft tissue swelling overlying a painful, firm, bony swelling on the mandible.

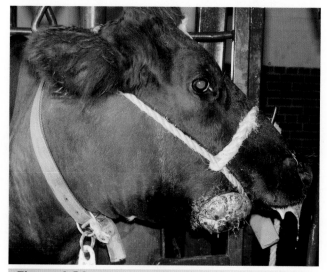

Figure 6-21

Severe *A. bovis* infection of the mandible with ulceration of the skin and granulomatous proliferation.

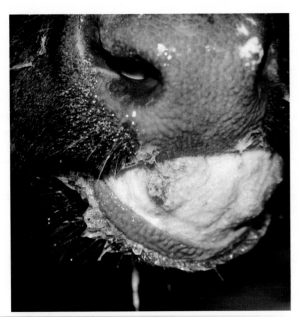

Figure 6-22

Actinomycosis of the mandibular symphysis region in a cow.

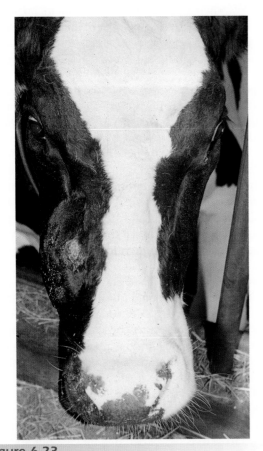

Figure 6-23

Actinomycosis of the maxilla.

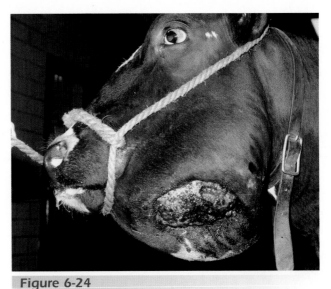

Figure 6-24

Advanced lumpy jaw with draining tracts.

cases will have distortion of the teeth anchored in the affected bone when the mouth is examined. External swelling is merely the "tip of the iceberg" as established by skull radiographs that confirm severe osteomyelitis with multifocal radiolucencies caused by rarefaction of bone. Pyogranulomatous infection of bone and associated soft tissues evolves in untreated cases, and these animals will have granulomas develop at the site of draining tracts through the skin or into the oral cavity (Figure 6-24). Because of distortion, malocclusion, or loss of teeth, eating becomes more difficult for severely affected cows. Salivation, reduced appetite, hesitant attempts to chew, and dropping food from the mouth may be observed. Oral mucosal or tongue lacerations may be apparent. Draining tracts discharge copious quantities of serous or mucopurulent pus that should be considered infectious to other cows.

Diagnosis

Absolute diagnosis requires a tissue core biopsy or fluid aspirate to identify the causative organism. Core biopsies also allow histologic confirmation. Radiographs confirm osteomyelitis with multiple radiolucent zones and proliferation of periosteal bone (Figure 6-25). Radiographs also help differentiate lumpy jaw from bony neoplasia, tooth root infections, fractures, sequestra, and, when the maxilla is involved, sinusitis.

Treatment

Recommended treatment for lumpy jaw usually includes sodium iodide, but this treatment is often not effective and should be considered an adjunct, at best, to appropriate antibiotic therapy.

Discussion of treatment also must allow for the tremendous variation in severity of osteomyelitis caused by *A. bovis*. Basketball-sized lesions are unlikely to respond

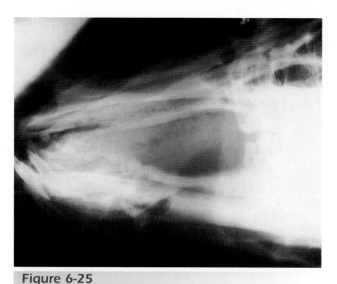

Figure 6-25

Skull radiograph of cow affected with advanced lumpy jaw. Osteomyelitis and characteristic multifocal radiolucencies are present.

to any therapy, whereas early lesions may be resolved successfully by several protocols. Therefore treatment is best instituted early. Long-term antibiotic therapy is necessary for well-established infections, and this fact makes owners reluctant to treat cows that do not appear ill and are still producing well. Ironically when this same untreated cow eventually becomes ill as the lesion enlarges, many owners will then want something to be done.

Streptomycin or penicillin-streptomycin combinations have been the drugs of choice for lumpy jaw; unfortunately streptomycin and penicillin-streptomycin combinations no longer are available for use in cattle in North America. Therefore other treatments will need to be considered. In one comparative study, erythromycin was active against *A. bovis* when mean inhibitory concentration (MIC) of 0.06 to 0.12 was achieved. Therefore erythromycin may be a good choice. Isoniazid can be used at 10 to 20 mg/kg orally every 24 hours for 30 days, and rifampin can be used at 20 mg/kg orally every 24 hours for 30 days or used at 5 to 10 mg/kg orally every 24 hours and combined with procaine penicillin at 22,000 U/kg SQ every 24 hours for 30 days. Isoniazid may cause abortion, should be used with caution in pregnant cattle, and represents extra-label drug use in the United States. Because antibiotic therapy necessitates prolonged administration and may involve extra-label use of drugs, the implication of such therapy should be discussed with owners before instituting therapy.

Current recommendations include penicillin 22,000 U/kg once daily and sodium iodide IV (30 g/450 kg) administered once or repeated at 2- to 3-day intervals until iodism occurs. Alternatively, organic iodides can be fed at 30 g/450 kg body weight once daily until iodism occurs. Duration of therapy is dependent on the severity

of the lesion and response to therapy. Recently we have also been injecting antibiotic-coated (penicillin or erythromycin) beads into the lesion. Long-term antibiotic therapy has resulted in a surprising cure in a few advanced cases.

Surgery has been suggested and still is used by some as treatment for lumpy jaw of the maxillae. Surgical debulking or removal of large pyogranulomas projecting from the skin of advanced cases may reduce the size of the lesion. Surgical debulking may incite severe hemorrhage. In addition, the affected bone may be further compromised or fractured if overzealous debridement and curettage are performed. Once again, the external swelling or masses are just the tip of the iceberg. Loose teeth may require extraction, and fistulous tracts may be flushed with iodine solution as ancillary aids.

Vesicular Stomatitis

Etiology

Vesicular stomatitis virus (VSV) causes lesions that may be indistinguishable from those of foot-and-mouth disease (FMD) in cattle and pigs. Horses also may be infected with VSV, whereas FMD does not occur in horses. The causative virus of VSV is a member of the genus *Vesiculovirus* in the family *Rhabdoviridae*, and two distinct serotype groups—Indiana and New Jersey types—are recognized. Each of these major types may be further subdivided into subtypes. The New Jersey VSV type tends to be more pathogenic in cattle. VSV is considered endemic in parts of South America, Central America, and the southwestern United States. In recent years, many livestock operations in the intermountain West have been quarantined following detection of VSV infection in cattle and/or horses. VSV usually occurs during the summer and fall, but one large epidemic developed during the late fall and early winter in California during 1982 and 1983. The general trend for cases to occur in the summer and fall is suggestive of an arthropod vector. Recent attention has focused on a species of midge, *Culicoides sonorensis*, as a likely vector for VSV because viral replication in multiple tissues of this insect has been documented following experimental VSV infection. Ingestion of infected grasshoppers has also been shown to induce infection in cattle. Other insects, such as blackflies and sandflies, may act as mechanical vectors for transmission among animals. Many different animals can be infected by VSV, including sheep, goats, wildlife, birds, and insects.

During outbreaks, the virus spreads rapidly from infected animals through secretions and aerosol transmission. Intact skin is not penetrated by VSV, but abrasions or injuries allow infection through the skin and may explain the spread of teat lesions through infected herds by milking machines. When epidemics occur, morbidity is high—especially in dense populations of animals—but mortality usually is low.

Clinical Signs

After VSV is introduced to susceptible animals, clinical signs of varying intensity occur. Classical signs include salivation, fever, lameness, and teat lesions. Fever may precede the more obvious signs because viremia is short-lived. Blanched lesions of the oral mucosa, coronary band, and teats evolve into vesicles that rupture and then slough the involved mucosa to leave denuded surfaces. Within the oral cavity, the lips, tongue, gums, or other areas may be involved. Obvious problems with mastitis occur when teat lesions are widespread. Many animals in some outbreaks have minimal or subclinical lesions that escape detection. Once the disease is signaled by a few animals with obvious lesions, physical examination of other animals on the premises frequently will reveal small erosions or ulcers resulting from earlier infection. As with many diseases, severity of disease varies greatly based on serotype of VSV, density of the population infected, concurrent diseases, and other factors. Many of these signs cannot be distinguished from FMD lesions.

People working with VSV-infected animals or with VSV in laboratories can become infected asymptomatically or develop signs of fever, muscular aches and pains, and possible lip blisters.

Infected cattle usually recover; mortality rates are low. However, economic losses resulting from decreased production are profound. Oral lesions cause infected cows to eat less, thereby affecting production. Lameness, if present, further deters appetite and access to feed. Teat lesions represent the most disastrous consequence of VSV because mastitis can easily follow incomplete "milk-out" as a consequence of the painful teat lesions. Therefore although mortality of the natural disease is low, the cull rate and economic losses can be catastrophic to dairy farmers.

Diagnosis

Whenever a diagnosis of vesicular stomatitis is possible, state and federal regulatory veterinarians should be alerted for help in diagnosis and ruling out FMD.

Treatment and Control

Common sense measures such as milking cows with teat lesions last, using aggressive disinfection practices in the milking parlor, reducing animal density, attempting isolation of clinical cases, and reducing stress are the only means of treatment. Softened feeds may be more easily ingested by affected animals. Secondary bacterial infections of lesions may necessitate occasional use of antibiotics.

Control measures and containment must be left to regulatory veterinarians. On Colorado dairies that experienced repeated annual outbreaks, the rate and scope of spread on infected dairies have been curtailed when aggressive insect control measures were initiated soon after detection of the disease. Humans working with infected cattle should wear gloves and perhaps masks.

Bluetongue

Bluetongue (BTV) is an *Orbivirus* transmitted by *Culicoides* gnats from infected to noninfected ruminants. BTV is almost uniformly asymptomatic in cattle. Cattle and wild ruminants are thought to be reservoirs of BTV, whereas sheep suffer a more apparent clinical disease characterized by fever, edema, excessive salivation, frothing, and hyperemia of the nasal and buccal mucous membranes. These acute signs in sheep progress to crusting, erosions, and ulcers of the mucous membranes. In addition, affected sheep are lame, resulting from both coronitis and myositis. Pregnant ewes infected with BTV may abort, resorb, or subsequently give birth to lambs with congenital anomalies such as hydranencephaly, cerebellar lesions, spinal cord lesions, retinal dysplasia, and other ocular anomalies or skeletal malformations. The aforementioned clinical signs for sheep summarize a "classical" case, but BTV can be subclinical in sheep and cattle.

In fact, tremendous variation in clinical manifestations and consequences are possible following BTV infection. One reason for this variation is the multitude of BTV serotypes (at least 24) that have been identified. In addition, there are at least nine serotypes of epizootic hemorrhagic disease viruses—a similar orbivirus that primarily affects whitetail deer but can affect cattle causing BTV-like signs—that have been identified. In the United States, four to five BTV serotypes and two epizootic hemorrhagic diarrhea virus (EHDV) serotypes have been identified. BTV-positive cattle are not found in the northeastern United States unless the cows were transported from other regions.

Control of the disease is difficult for several reasons:
1. The biologic vector, *Culicoides* spp., is difficult to control, and the virus may overwinter in the larval form of these insects.
2. Infection in cattle, goats, and possibly other wild ruminants can remain subclinical, but infected hosts can act as reservoirs of disease. Sheep are the major species to show clinical signs of disease.
3. Multiple serotypes require specific testing rather than group antigen testing for best detection.
4. Some strains of BTV may cause only subclinical infections in cattle—thereby not arousing clinical suspicion of disease.

Transmission of virus from infected to susceptible animals by *Culicoides* sp. has been studied and results in seroconversion. Laboratory or experimental infections in cattle usually do not result in clinical illness, but some reports of field outbreaks describe obvious clinical illness with signs similar to those in sheep with BTV. Therefore even though most BTV in cattle is thought to be subclinical, certain husbandry or environmental conditions or strains of BTV in field outbreaks appear capable of causing clinical disease. Sunlight may enhance or worsen the clinical signs when sheep are infected with BTV.

Clinical Signs

Most cattle infected with BTV are asymptomatic. When clinical signs are observed in field outbreaks, mucosal and skin lesions predominate. Hyperemia and oral vesicles that ulcerate may involve the mucous membranes of the mouth or tongue. The muzzle may undergo similar vesicular changes that lead to a "burnt" appearance with a dry cracked skin that may slough. Salivation is common, and swelling of lips may occur. Fever is present. Stiffness or lameness is common as a result of both myositis and coronitis. Coronary band hyperemia, ulceration, necrosis, exudates, or sloughing may occur. The skin of the neck and withers may become thickened, exudative, and painful. Therefore depending on the clinical signs demonstrated, the differential diagnosis for a bovine case of BTV infection might include BVD, vesicular stomatitis, FMD, malignant catarrhal fever (MCF), IBR, rinderpest, and bovine papular stomatitis. Cattle infections with EHDV are thought to be rare but can cause signs and fetal consequences similar to BTV. Obviously given the overlap of clinical signs of some BTV infections in cattle with important foreign animal diseases, regulatory officials must be contacted following detection of such lesions.

Reproductive consequences are rare in infected cattle but include fetal death, fetal resorption, abortion, persistent infection of immunotolerant fetuses, and congenital defects such as hydranencephaly, skin disorders, ocular disorders, and skeletal lesions. Infected bulls may become temporarily sterile. Cattle infections with EHDV are thought to be rare but can cause signs and fetal consequences similar to BTV.

Most cattle with clinical signs recover but may carry the virus for prolonged periods, and others suffer prolonged lameness or poor condition.

Diagnosis

Clinical signs aid diagnosis and require differentiation from photosensitization, BVDV, MCF, IBR, VSV, and FMD. If sheep reside on the premises, clinical signs may be obvious. Regulatory veterinarians should be consulted immediately when BTV is suspected because the differential diagnoses include exotic diseases.

Absolute diagnosis can be achieved by BTV isolation from heparinized blood, fetal specimens, spleen, or bone marrow. Samples should not be frozen. In an experimental challenge study, BTV could be isolated from the blood of infected cattle for up to 49 days postinoculation; however, infected cattle maintained a level of viremia infective for *Culicoides* spp. for a maximal duration of 3 weeks.

Caution should be used in interpreting these results, however, because different strains of BTV may behave differently in cattle. Monoclonal FA, virus neutralization, or molecular probes may identify serotypes of virus isolated from blood or tissues. The blood of infected cattle remains positive for viral nucleic acids on PCR for a much longer duration (nearly 4 months) than for virus isolation.

An outer-coat protein, VP2, is responsible for causing virus-neutralizing antibody against BTV and EHDV in infected animals. Inner-core protein VP7 is a serogroup-specific antigen as are the nonstructural proteins NS1 and NS2. The older complement fixation tests and serum neutralization antibody tests primarily detected group antigens. An immunodiffusion test has also been used, but currently a competitive ELISA is recommended. The ELISA test is quantitative and is serotype-specific through incorporation of monoclonal antibody.

In utero infection resulting in persistent infection of immunotolerant animals can be confirmed only by viral isolation—probably best performed by collecting precolostral blood so that maternal passive antibody in colostrum does not confuse the situation. Precolostral blood for ELISA testing may allow diagnosis of in utero infection and seroconversion of immunocompetent fetuses with or without congenital anomalies. For adult cattle, virus isolation or paired ELISA tests on serum to confirm an increasing titer are required for diagnosis.

Treatment

If clinical cases even exist, treatment would be symptomatic. Affected cattle should be kept out of sunlight if possible.

Control

As previously mentioned, control is extremely difficult. Regulatory veterinarians should be consulted. Although a stable positive serum antibody titer only indicates past infection, the economic implications of a positive titer are profound. Export markets, embryo transfer potential, sale of bulls to bull studs, and sale of semen to various markets are negated by positive BTV antibodies in healthy cattle. Geographic incidence of BTV antibodies varies greatly, with serologic evidence of infection in the Northeast being quite rare but relatively common in the southern states, Great Plains, and West.

Pharyngeal Trauma

Etiology

Natural or iatrogenic pharyngeal trauma commonly results in gastrointestinal and respiratory consequences in affected cattle. Coarse or fibrous feeds, awns, and metallic foreign bodies occasionally cause pharyngeal punctures or lacerations, but the most common cause of pharyngeal trauma in dairy calves and cattle is iatrogenic injury. Inappropriate, rough, or malicious use of balling guns, paste guns, esophageal feeders, magnet retrievers, Frick speculums, and stomach tubes are the usual causative instruments. Failure of laypeople to lubricate implements, judge appropriate depth of the oral cavity, or hold the animal's head and neck straight when administering oral medication are the most common errors. Purely rough or sadistic treatment also is common.

Acute pharyngeal injury or trauma can have many sequelae. Small punctures may have few acute consequences but eventually result in cellulitis or pharyngeal abscesses. Most acute injuries result in both local and systemic effects. Local effects include pain, reluctance or inability to swallow, salivation, and cellulitis. Systemic effects reflect damage to vagal nerve branches in the pharynx. Such nerve damage can affect rumen motility, eructation, swallowing, and predispose to inhalation pneumonia. Bloat resulting from failure of eructation reflects direct or inflammatory injury to vagal nerve branches controlling the complex act of eructation, which requires coordinated activity of larynx, pharynx, and proximal esophageal muscle.

Often cattle that suffer pharyngeal injuries had primary illnesses, the treatment of which included administration of oral medications. Therefore early clinical signs of pharyngeal injury may be thought to represent failure of response or worsening of the primary condition. Pharyngeal trauma is common in dairy cattle and is underdiagnosed as a cause of illness.

Clinical Signs

The chief complaint in cattle with pharyngeal trauma is anorexia and a suspected abdominal disorder that has not responded to medication (including orally administered medications). Direct tissue trauma is quickly complicated by cellulitis or phlegmon of the retropharyngeal tissue. Clinical signs usually include salivation, a "sore throat" as evidenced by an extended head and neck, fever, fetid breath, soft tissue swelling in the throat latch, and localized or diffuse pharyngeal pain (Figure 6-26). Most cattle are unable or unwilling to eat. Dysphagia may be present in severe cases and may lead to dehydration because of inability to drink. Other gastrointestinal signs caused by varying amounts of direct or indirect damage to vagal nerve branches may occur; these include bloat, rumen stasis, or signs of vagus indigestion. Megaesophagus is an infrequent complication. Respiratory complications include nasal discharge associated with dysphagia, inspiratory stridor, and inhalation pneumonia. Subcutaneous emphysema is present in some patients as air is sucked into the retropharyngeal area and dissects subcutaneously. Although subcutaneous emphysema sometimes is limited to the retropharyngeal area, usually air dissects down the neck and reaches the thorax or locations further caudal.

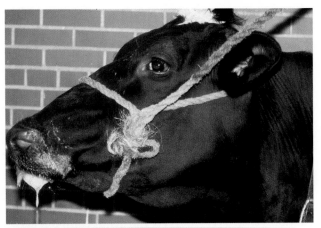

Figure 6-26

Anxious expression, extended head and neck, salivation, and soft tissue swelling in the throat latch region of a cow with pharyngeal trauma.

Pharyngeal trauma usually only occurs in one animal in the herd, but herd epidemics have been associated with mass medication (Figure 6-27).

Diagnosis

Frequently the clinical signs, coupled with a manual examination of the oral cavity to palpate the pharyngeal laceration, are sufficient for diagnosis. Most injuries are in the caudal pharyngeal region dorsal to the larynx. Severe lacerations also may damage the soft palate or proximal esophagus. Administered boluses or magnets may still be embedded in the retropharyngeal tissues in some cases. An oral speculum and focal light examination also may allow a view of pharyngeal injuries.

Endoscopy and radiology are very helpful ancillary aids, especially when a manual examination of the oral

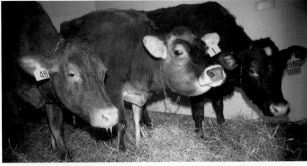

Figure 6-27

Three representative Jersey cows from a herd with an epidemic of pharyngeal trauma associated with mass medication delivered by an owner. Salivation, extended head and neck because of sore throats, anxious or depressed appearance, dyspnea, inhalation pneumonia, bloat, and subcutaneous emphysema occurred to varying degrees in the affected cattle.

cavity is inconclusive or when the size of the animal—as with a calf—precludes manual examination. Endoscopy usually allows a view of pharyngeal injuries, but diffuse swelling of the pharynx, larynx, and soft palate sometimes interferes with this procedure. Radiographs are diagnostic of pharyngeal trauma in most cases because air densities and radiolucent retropharyngeal tissues are readily apparent. Pharyngeal foreign bodies and embedded boluses or magnets also are apparent with radiographs (Figure 6-28).

Treatment

Broad-spectrum antibiotics, analgesics, and supportive measures such as IV fluids are the major components of therapy for pharyngeal trauma. Whenever possible, it is best to avoid *any* oral medications. However, sometimes gentle passage of a stomach tube to provide an economical means to hydrate a patient with dysphagia is necessary. Most small pharyngeal lacerations respond to antibiotics such as ceftiofur (2.2 mg/kg IM every 24 hours), tetracycline (9 mg/kg, IV every 24 hours), ampicillin (6.6 to 11.0 mg/kg IM or SQ every 12 hours), or other broad-spectrum combinations. Penicillin is not a good initial choice because it seldom is able to control the expected mixed infection. Judicious use of analgesics such as flunixin meglumine (0.5 to 1.1 mg/kg IV every 24 hours) aids patient comfort, relieves the "sore throat," and may allow an earlier return of appetite. Resolution of dysphagia, when present, is an important positive prognostic sign because the patient can now drink effectively and hydrate herself. Resolution of fever

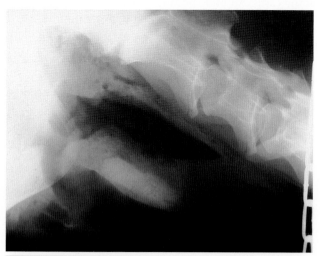

Figure 6-28

Radiograph of the pharyngeal region of a cow that suffered pharyngeal trauma, laceration, and foreign body deposition of a sulfa bolus delivered with a balling gun. A large radiolucent area and tissue emphysema are apparent ventral to the cervical vertebrae, and the bolus can be seen embedded between the air density dorsally and the trachea.

is another positive prognostic sign but may be misleading if temperature decreased because of concurrent therapy with nonsteroidal antiinflammatory drugs (NSAIDs).

Nursing procedures and ensuring access to fresh clean water and soft feeds such as silage or gruels of soaked alfalfa pellets are helpful. In severe cases, placement of a rumen fistula may be necessary to allow for direct placement of mashes or liquids directly into the rumen, thereby bypassing the damaged and painful tissues. Antibiotic therapy should be continued 7 to 14 days or longer depending on response to treatment and healing of the pharyngeal wound. Foreign bodies, boluses, or magnets embedded in retropharyngeal locations must be removed.

Prognosis is good for most cases but is guarded for cattle having large lacerations, soft palate lacerations, proximal esophageal lacerations, inhalation pneumonia, and vagus indigestion.

Prevention

Veterinarians should educate laypeople on how to safely administer oral medications. Stomach tubes, speculums, esophageal feeder tubes, and balling guns should be inspected after each use to identify any sharp edges or "burrs" that may incite future injury. Proper size speculums, tubes, and so on should be based on the animal's size and not "one size fits all."

Alimentary Warts

Etiology

Papillomas and fibropapillomas are observed sporadically in the oral cavity, esophagus, and forestomach of dairy cattle. Oral lesions may occur on the hard palate, soft palate, or tongue. Bovine papilloma virus (BPV) of various types is the suspected cause of these lesions. The genome of BPV2 has been found in such lesions, but the complete virus itself may not be present. These lesions tend to be present in adult animals rather than calves. BPV2 has also been demonstrated in association with urinary bladder tumors in cows with chronic enzootic hematuria.

Jarrett and co-workers have also found a high incidence of papillomas and carcinomas of the upper alimentary tract and forestomach in cattle ingesting bracken fern in Scotland. A BPV labeled BPV4 has been identified in these lesions.

Signs

Papillomas and fibropapillomas of the mouth, esophagus, and forestomach create no clinical signs unless they interfere with eructation. Occasional warts at the cardia or distal esophagus act as a ball valve to interfere with eructation and cause chronic or recurrent bloat, leading to signs of vagus indigestion (Figure 6-29). Such lesions

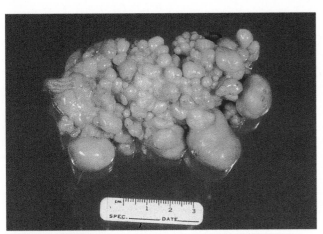

Figure 6-29

A fibropapilloma that was surgically removed via rumenotomy from a 2-year-old cow with chronic bloat.

may be precursors for carcinomas, but this has not been proven except when associated with the ingestion of bracken fern.

Diagnosis

Inspection, endoscopic biopsy, and histopathology are the means of diagnosis. Rumenotomy may be necessary to confirm lesions at the cardia.

Treatment

Lesions are not treated except when discovered during rumenotomy in cattle with failure of eructation. In such cases, removal is curative.

Salmonellosis

Etiology

Much of the discussion regarding salmonellosis has been addressed in the section on calf diarrhea. *Salmonella* sp. causes enterocolitis that varies tremendously in severity in adult cattle. Septicemic salmonellosis may result in abortion or shedding of the causative organism into milk. The organism also may be found in milk secondary to environmental contamination and subsequent mastitis. This latter route appears to be typical of *S.* Dublin mastitis and possibly to lesser degrees for other types.

Salmonella spp. are facultative intracellular organisms that can hide in macrophages, be distributed along with these cells, and occasionally cause bacteremia following invasion of the intestine. Fecal-oral infection is the most common route of infection, but other mucous membranes can be invaded by some serotypes. Following ingestion of *Salmonella* organisms, a cow may or may not become clinically ill. Factors that determine pathogenicity include:

1. Virulence of the serotype
2. Dose of inoculum
3. Degree of immunity or previous exposure of host to this serotype
4. Other stressors currently affecting the host

The first two factors relate to the serotype of *Salmonella* involved. Because more than 2000 serotypes have been described, it is not surprising that a great deal of variation exists in the clinical signs, prevalence, morbidity, and mortality. Because *Salmonella* spp. often act as opportunistic pathogens, management, nutritional, and environmental factors that adversely impact the cow's defenses are often at play when the disease becomes problematic on a given operation.

Salmonellosis was primarily a sporadic disease in dairy cattle in the northeastern United States until the 1970s. A single cow within a herd may develop the disease secondary to septic metritis, septic mastitis, BVD, or other periparturient disorders. Infection seldom spreads to other cows. However, in recent decades, larger herds and increased use of free stall housing have changed the clinical epidemiology of salmonellosis, such that herd outbreaks with variable morbidity and mortality are now the rule. Free stall housing creates a nightmarish setting for diseases such as salmonellosis that are spread by fecal-oral transmission. Stressors include such things as concurrent infection with other bacterial or viral pathogens, transportation, parturition, poor transition cow management, gastrointestinal stasis or disturbance of the gastrointestinal flora by recent feed changes, heat or cold, and recent anesthesia or surgery.

Another contributing factor to herd infections is contaminated ration components fed to dairy cattle. Protein source supplements and animal byproduct components may be contaminated with *Salmonella* sp. Improperly ensiled forages that fail to reach a pH <4.5 can harbor *Salmonella* sp. Birds shedding *Salmonella* can contaminate cut forages or feed bunks to infect adult cattle. This latter pathogenesis has been suspected in several herd outbreaks of type E, but birds also could transmit other types of *Salmonella* by acting as either biological or mechanical vectors. Farm implements used to handle manure or haul sick or dead animals can be a very efficient means of spreading *Salmonella* if these are used to haul feed, bedding, or healthy animals. The spreading of liquid manure on fields in addition to no-plow planting of crops has caused an increase in forage contamination.

Herd epidemics with an acute onset and high morbidity should be investigated as point source outbreaks of feed or water contamination. Chronic, endemic problems may represent spread of infection by carrier cattle to susceptible or stressed herdmates who then propagate the herd problem by shedding large numbers of organisms in feces during acute disease. It is not unusual to have a herd outbreak in lactating cows without an outbreak in young calves or vice versa.

In the northeastern United States, types B, C, and E are responsible for most herd endemics. Most type B isolates are *S.* Typhimurium of varying virulence and antibiotic susceptibility. Type C includes *S.* Newport and *S.* Litchfield. Type E usually is *S.* Anatum. In general, types B and C *Salmonella* are more virulent than type E, but because of the multitude of existing serotypes, it is impossible to generalize further. Type D, most of which are *S.* Dublin, are common in the western United States. A summary of the typical characteristics of diseases induced by the various serogroups is presented earlier in this chapter in the section on salmonellosis in calves.

S. Dublin is largely host adapted to cattle, whereas other types are nonhost adapted. A particularly frightening characteristic of *S.* Dublin infection is that infected cows remain carriers for a long time or even forever. Some shed consistently, others intermittently, and others are "latent" carriers that shed only when stressed. *S.* Dublin also causes mastitis, which tends to be subclinical and persistent. Mastitis caused by *S.* Dublin is thought to originate from environmental contamination of the udder by feces from infected cattle rather than septicemic spread to the udder. Infection of calves by *S.* Dublin is common in the western United States and has begun to appear in the eastern and midwestern United States. Infected calves shed large numbers of organisms, frequently are septicemic, and have respiratory signs coupled with fever that confound the diagnosis and mislead veterinarians unfamiliar with this disease. Other than *S.* Dublin–infected cattle, most cattle infected with nonhost-adapted serotypes such as *S.* Typhimurium are thought to shed the organism for less than 6 months. However, latent carriers or chronic infection may occur occasionally, and chronic *S.* Typhimurium mastitis has been documented following an enteric epidemic.

Salmonella spp. are capable of attachment to, and destruction of, enterocytes. Pathogenic serotypes gain access to the submucosal region of the distal small intestine and colon where their facultative intracellular characteristics guard them against normal defense mechanisms of naive cattle. From this location, the organisms enter lymphatics and may commonly create bacteremia in calves. As with most facultative intracellular bacteria, the host's cell-mediated immune system is essential for effective defense. Diarrhea caused by *Salmonella* sp. is primarily of inflammatory origin with lesser contributions (in some serotypes) by secretory mechanisms. Because mucosal destruction occurs, maldigestion and malabsorption contribute to the diarrhea, and protein loss into the bowel is significant when virulent strains infect cattle. Severe inflammation of the colon is common with resultant fresh blood in the feces or dysentery.

Clinical Signs

As in calves with salmonellosis, adult cattle infected with *Salmonella* sp. have enteric disease of greatly varied severity. Type E organisms usually cause mild diarrhea, dehydration, fever for 1 to 7 days, and a clinical situation that resembles winter dysentery in that affected cattle appear neither severely dehydrated nor toxic. As a rule, fresh blood is seen less commonly in the feces of type E infections than in type B and C infections. However, the same type E organisms may overwhelm cattle stressed by concurrent infections or metabolic disease caused by altered defense mechanisms or preexisting acid-base and electrolyte abnormalities.

Fever and diarrhea are expected in salmonellosis consistently, although fever may be absent or have preceded the onset of diarrhea by 24 to 48 hours. This prodromal fever has been confirmed in hospitalized animals that acquired nosocomial salmonellosis. These patients were found to have fever without any signs of illness 24 to 48 hours before developing diarrhea subsequently confirmed as *Salmonella* types B or C. Fever ranges from 103.0 to 107.0° F (39.4 to 41.7° C) and correlates poorly with other clinical signs as regards severity of illness. However, detection of fever in sick or apparently healthy cows during a herd outbreak is an extremely important aid to diagnosis of an infectious disease rather than a dietary indigestion. Diarrhea is consistent, at least in animals with clinical disease, and may appear as loose manure, watery manure, loose manure with blood clots, or dysentery (Figure 6-30). Endotoxemia and dehydration accompany diarrhea when virulent strains are encountered or when enteric invasion and bacteremia exist. Anorexia usually accompanies the onset of diarrhea and may be transient in mild cases or prolonged in patients with severe diarrhea and endotoxemia. Feces from cows with types B and C salmonellosis often are foul-smelling, containing blood and mucus. Whenever diarrhea with fresh blood and

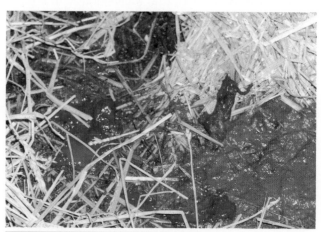

Figure 6-30

Fresh blood clots mixed with feces of a cow that had a type C *Salmonella* sp. enterocolitis.

mucus is observed in cattle, salmonellosis should be considered. Recently fresh cows are very susceptible to infection during herd epidemics, and errors in transition cow management often amplify the impact of disease on these cows. Environmental factors such as heat stress tend to amplify the clinical signs and increase morbidity and mortality. Recording temperatures in apparently healthy cows during a herd outbreak may confirm fevers in some that are about to develop diarrhea or may represent subclinical infections. Concurrent infection with *Salmonella* sp. and BVDV following the purchase of herd additions can lead to devastating mortality. Dr. Rebhun observed one herd with this combination of acute infections that lost 35 of 130 adult cattle within 7 days (Figure 6-31). The usual mortality rate in herd outbreaks of S. Typhimurium is approximately 5% to 10%.

Abortions are common, especially when serotypes B, C, or D cause infection and can occur for several reasons:

1. Septicemia with seeding of the fetus and uterus causing fetal infection and death
2. Endotoxin and other mediator release that cause luteolysis via prostaglandin release and apparent alteration in hormonal regulation of pregnancy
3. High fever or hyperthermia brought about by concurrent fever and heat stress during hot weather

Cows may abort at any stage of gestation, but as with many causes of abortion, expulsion of 5- to 9-month fetuses are most likely to be observed by dairy personnel.

Salmonella sp. may be found in the milk of infected cattle. With types B, C, and E organisms, this contamination of milk may represent septicemic spread of the organism to the mammary gland, environmental fecal contamination of the milk and milking equipment, or both. Herds infected with S. Dublin have chronic mastitis in a percentage of cows infected by this organism. Mastitis caused by S. Dublin may be subclinical, and environmental contamination of quarters has been shown to be a more likely cause than septicemic spread to the udder. Occasional cows have chronic mastitis with *Salmonella* spp. other than S. Dublin. Quarters that shed organisms and feces from infected cows create major public health concerns for farm workers and milk consumers. Contaminated milk is a major risk for the entire dairy industry and reasons enough to investigate every herd outbreak of diarrhea in dairy cattle with appropriate diagnostic tests. Whereas proper pasteurization reliably eliminates the organism from milk, raw milk should not be consumed.

Diarrhea and illness caused by salmonellosis are common in farm workers and families whenever herd outbreaks occur. It is the veterinarian's obligation to inform clients and workers regarding the public health dangers of salmonellosis and to direct sick farm workers or family members to physicians for treatment.

Ancillary Aids and Diagnosis

Hematology and acid-base electrolyte values are valuable ancillary aids for individual or valuable cattle but are seldom diagnostic because of the great variation in clinical illness. Fecal cultures are the "gold standard" of diagnosis, and samples from several patients in the early stages of the disease should be submitted to a qualified diagnostic laboratory. Isolates should be typed and antibiotic susceptibility determined. Unlike salmonellosis in horses, *Salmonella* spp. can usually be cultured from even a "watery" fecal sample from cattle with salmonellosis.

Peracute salmonellosis associated with virulent serovars tends to create a neutropenia with degenerative left shift in the leukogram and metabolic acidosis with Na^+, K^+, and Cl^- values all lowered in affected adult cattle. Elevations in PCV, blood urea nitrogen (BUN), and creatinine can be anticipated in those patients with severe diarrhea. Total protein values initially may be elevated because of severe dehydration but are just as likely to be normal or low because albumin values decrease quickly as a result of the severe protein-losing enteropathy. BUN and creatinine may be elevated simply because of prerenal azotemia or because of acute nephrosis resulting from septicemia/endotoxemia.

Just as fever precedes the onset of diarrhea in some patients, so may the expected neutropenia with left shift. This has been documented in some cattle that acquire nosocomial hospital infections, although it is unlikely to be detected in field outbreaks because cattle yet unaffected with diarrhea seldom are sampled. Cattle with less than overwhelming acute salmonellosis may

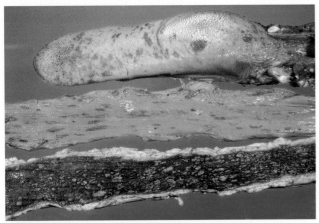

Figure 6-31

Necropsy specimens from a cow having concurrent BVDV and salmonellosis. The tongue (top) shows multiple BVDV erosions; the esophagus (middle) shows multifocal linear BVDV erosions; and the colon (bottom) shows severe inflammatory colitis with mucosal necrosis caused by salmonellosis. *(Photo courtesy Dr. John M. King.)*

have neutropenia, normal WBC numbers, or neutrophilia. Recovering cattle tend to have a neutrophilia.

Sodium, potassium, and chloride tend to be low in most cattle having severe or prolonged diarrhea. As mentioned, peracute severe salmonellosis will result in metabolic acidosis as a result of massive fluid loss and endotoxic shock, but most adult cattle with nonfatal diarrhea do not develop significant acidosis.

Differential diagnosis of salmonellosis in adult cattle is brief if limited to diseases causing fever and diarrhea. BVDV infection and winter dysentery would be the primary differentials. Herds with serotypes such as type E causing relatively mild signs of fever and diarrhea require differentiation from winter dysentery (depending on the time of year), BVDV infection, and indigestions. Herds suffering mortality associated with very virulent type B or C infections must be differentiated from BVDV infection. For cases of more chronic diarrhea, subacute ruminal acidosis, internal parasites, Johne's disease, eosinophilic enteritis, lymphosarcoma, chronic peritonitis, and copper deficiency should be considered. Viral isolation should be attempted from the buffy coat of ethylenediaminetetraacetic acid (EDTA) blood samples or necropsy specimens to rule out BVDV infection and fecal cultures from multiple patients or necropsy samples evaluated for presence of *Salmonella* sp. Infections caused by *Campylobacter* sp. and *Yersinia* sp. occasionally have been reported in adult cows with fever and diarrhea. The significance and disease incidence associated with these organisms are unknown.

Classical gross necropsy lesions of diffuse or multifocal diphtheritic membranes lining the region of mucosal necrosis in the distal small bowel and colon are present in subacute and chronic cases. In peracute cases, however, minimal gross lesions other than hemorrhage and edema may exist within the involved bowel and enlarged mesenteric lymph nodes. The more acute the death, the less likely gross lesions will be observed. Fibrin casts sometimes are found in the gallbladder and are considered pathognomonic for salmonellosis by some pathologists.

Treatment

Supportive treatment with IV fluids is necessary for patients that have anorexia, depression, and significant dehydration. Individual patients may be treated aggressively following acid-base and electrolyte assessment. However, outbreaks in field settings seldom allow extensive ancillary workup, and fluid therapy is administered empirically. Use of balanced electrolyte solutions such as lactated Ringer's solution is sufficient for most cattle. Cattle having severe acute diarrhea and >10% dehydration are likely to have metabolic acidosis and may require supplemental bicarbonate therapy. For example, a 600-kg patient judged to be 10% dehydrated and mildly acidotic (base excess = −5.0 mEq/L) should

receive 60 L of balanced fluids for correction of dehydration. Rehydration alone may decrease the lactic acid and correct the metabolic acidosis. (The only times that bicarbonate therapy is absolutely needed for correction of acidosis in dairy cattle are for severe rumen acidosis, enterotoxigenic *E. coli*, or other enteric infections causing excessive production of D-lactate.) If balanced electrolyte fluid therapy does not correct the metabolic acidosis, the cow may need to be treated with bicarbonate. This hypothetical cow has 200 kg or L of ECF (0.3 [ECF] × 600), and the base deficit of −5.0 mEq/L implies that each liter of her ECF is in need of 5.0 mEq/L HCO_3^-. Thus 1000 mEq $NaHCO_3$ (0.3 × 600 × 5) could be added just to make up the existing deficit, and more $NaHCO_3$ would likely be necessary to compensate for anticipated continued losses. This example readily highlights the feeling of helplessness that veterinarians and herd owners experience when a virulent serotype causes serious dehydration in more than a few cows. Placement of a catheter in an auricular vein may prevent catheter damage from head catches, a common problem with jugular catheters on dairies. Auricular or jugular vein catheter placement may allow for repeated administration of IV fluids and repeated IV administration of flunixin meglumine. Hypertonic saline (7.5 times normal) administered at 3 to 5 ml/kg followed by 10 to 20 gallons of oral electrolyte solution, either consumed voluntarily or given by orogastric tube, is a highly practical method of fluid resuscitation in a field setting. This method has become commonplace and is a time- and labor-efficient way of addressing dehydration in grade cattle. Administration of hypertonic saline into smaller-diameter veins, such as the auricular vein, may result in phlebitis and catheter failure. When multiple animals merit oral fluid administration during an outbreak of salmonellosis or any other enteric disease, or if the same equipment is to be used for drenching of other cattle, laypeople should be aggressively educated as to the possibility of cross-contamination and the need for disinfection between uses. As a crude rule of thumb, cattle that show no voluntary interest in drinking following rapid IV administration of 3 to 5 ml/kg of 7.5 times normal saline solution should provisionally be given at best a guarded prognosis and are mandatory candidates for large-volume oral fluid drenching.

Oral fluids and electrolytes may be somewhat helpful and much cheaper than IV fluids for cattle deemed to be mildly or moderately dehydrated. The effectiveness of oral fluids may be somewhat compromised by malabsorption and maldigestion in salmonellosis patients but still should be considered useful. Cattle that are willing to drink can have specific electrolytes (NaCl, KCl) added to drinking water to help correct electrolyte deficiencies.

Antibiotic therapy is controversial. Its opponents warn of the potential for emergence of resistant strains that may present great risk for people and animals in the future. Evidence for this phenomenon is sparse except for long-term feed additive antibiotics, and one could argue that other species, including humans, represent similar risks when treated with antibiotics. Further opposition states that systemic antibiotics prolong the excretion of *Salmonellae* in the feces and may not shorten the clinical course of purely enteric disease. However, discerning those animals with infection limited to the gut wall from those animals with gut wall *and* systemic infection is never easy.

Proponents of antibiotic therapy remind us that salmonellosis frequently induces bacteremia (although this is most common in calves), thereby risking septicemic spread of the organism. Clinical differentiation of septicemia versus endotoxemia without septicemia is not easy unless localized infection appears in a joint, eye, the meninges, or lungs. In other words, clinicians can seldom accurately predict all salmonellosis patients that are truly septicemic. In addition, appropriate antibiotic therapy reduces the total number of organisms shed into the environment by counteracting septicemic spread that allows all bodily secretions, not just feces, to harbor the organism. These points should be considered by veterinarians and probably dictate against the use of antibiotics in salmonellosis patients having mild to moderate signs (e.g., low grade fever, diarrhea, and mild dehydration). Except for valuable cattle that are seriously ill with salmonellosis, systemic antibiotics are seldom administered to adult cows with salmonellosis in the Cornell Hospital.

Therefore antibiotics are sometimes used when patients appear moderately to severely ill and show signs of fever, dehydration, and profuse diarrhea or dysentery. These patients usually have elevated heart and respiratory rates, are weak, and appear endotoxemic or septicemic. Given the unpredictable nature of antimicrobial susceptibility of *Salmonella*, antimicrobial therapy should be guided by culture and susceptibility results. Withdrawal periods should be observed for any nonlabel usage of antibiotics. Antibiotics should be continued 4 to 7 days in patients that are improving.

NSAIDs, especially flunixin meglumine, may be helpful for "antiendotoxic" effects and blockage of various mediators of inflammation and shock. Cattle may be started on 1.1 mg/kg body weight IV every 24 hours and then tapered to 0.50 mg/kg body weight every 24 hours, or the medication may be discontinued after 1 to 2 days. If repeated IV administration is not practical, SQ administration is vastly preferred over IM administration, which may result in marked muscle damage. Overdosage or administration of repeated doses of flunixin may cause abomasal or renal pathology, and IM administration may induce myoglobin release that augments the renal adverse effects. Corticosteroids are contraindicated except as a *one-time* dose of water-soluble corticosteroid

for a gravely ill patient in shock. Prednisolone sodium succinate is preferred in this instance.

Isolation of patients with salmonellosis is ideal, albeit difficult, in field settings. Whenever possible, cattle with diarrhea should be confined to an area of the barn away from the rest of the herd. Workers must be educated regarding mechanical transmission of infected feces and other discharges from infected to uninfected cattle. Workers should also be educated regarding the zoonotic implications inherent with salmonellosis.

Prevention and Control

Herd epidemics appear to be increasing in frequency based on confirmed isolations from multiple cow outbreaks identified from New York and the rest of the northeastern United States. Conditions that contribute to an increasing incidence of epidemic salmonellosis include larger herd size, more intensive and crowded husbandry, and the trend for free stall barns with loose housing, which contributes to fecal contamination of the entire premises. Other major contributing factors include the use of feedstuffs that may be contaminated with *Salmonella* sp. and spreading contaminated manure on unplowed fields. Outbreaks caused by types C and E *Salmonellae* have been caused by contaminated feed components, and type E also has been spread by birds that are carriers of the organism.

When salmonellosis has been confirmed in a herd, the following control measures should be considered:
1. Conduct an epidemiologic investigation to help determine the source.
   - Commodities barn/feed storage and handling: Inspect and document source(s), and obtain samples of commodities for culture. Are there other dairies in the area with similar problems? Who hauls the feed onto the farm, and in what? Is this vehicle or trailer used solely for feed transport (not animals, bedding, or manure)? On the farm, how is the feed handled? Is the feed-hauling equipment used for other purposes (e.g., carcass hauling, bedding removal)? Are there other animals or a large population of birds with exposure to the feeds?
   - Water sources: Is there likely fecal contamination? What are the containers used to haul water to pastured cattle, and how/by whom are they handled?
   - Manure handling: Equipment used and destination? What is the flow pattern of flush water? Are the personnel involved in manure handling later handling animals or their feed? Is the manure being spread on unplowed crop fields? Flow patterns of labor, vehicles, water, bedding, and movement of sick and healthy cattle on the dairy should be critiqued.

- Introduction of new animals: Are newly purchased animals quarantined and cultured? How are cattle taken to shows handled on return? Has bulk tank milk been tested for BVD?
- Management of cows in the sick pen and maternity pen: Too often, these two sets of cattle are managed and housed together, creating ideal circumstances for infection of fresh cows and heifers. Physical separation and careful allocation of personnel and equipment to each group should be reviewed.

2. Isolate obviously affected animals to one group if possible.
3. Treat severely affected animals.
4. Institute measures to minimize public health concerns.
   - No raw milk should be consumed.
   - Workers and milkers should wear coveralls, disposable or rubber boots, gloves, and perhaps masks when milking or cleaning barns. Workers and milkers should be encouraged to wash well after work or before eating. Disinfectant footbaths should be placed at exits and entrances to the barn and parlor (for humans and beast), and these footbaths should be maintained regularly.
5. Physically clean the environment, improve hygiene, and disinfect premises (see also the section on calf salmonellosis). Pressure spraying to physically remove organic matter is very helpful before disinfection. Because removal of organic debris is incomplete on some surfaces, use of a disinfectant that retains its activity in organic debris and that has documented efficacy against *Salmonella* is optimal. Because shedding is likely to occur from recovered cattle for some time, ongoing efforts at improved hygiene are in order. In particular, protect dry cows and disinfect maternity areas.
6. Following resolution of the outbreak or crisis period, a mastitis survey should be conducted that includes bulk tank surveillance. If any *Salmonellae* are recovered, culture of the whole herd is indicated to identify carrier cows that should be culled immediately. For *S.* Dublin outbreaks, all cattle should be screened by milk culture and, if available, serologic testing performed to detect carriers that should be culled.

If an epidemic continues despite all of the above guidelines, autogenous bacterins may be considered. Although efficacy and safety of autogenous bacterins are (justifiably) questioned, many practitioners have claimed excellent results when all other measures fail to stop ongoing endemic infections when freshening cows become ill, abortions continue to appear, or calves continue to become ill because of salmonellosis. At the time of this writing, a new siderophore receptor/porin vaccine derived from *S.* Newport has just become licensed in the United States for use in dairy cattle

(SRP vaccine, Agri-Labs, St. Joseph, MO). It remains to be seen what impact this product will have on salmonellosis in the modern dairy industry. The efficacy of J-5 vaccines in salmonellosis control in adult cattle is unknown; in a large field trial, J-5 immunization of calves did not affect survival to 100 days. Unfortunately it is difficult to evaluate the efficacy of vaccines used to control endemic salmonellosis in field settings because improvement may be attributed to the vaccine but influenced by herd immunity or alterations in management. (For a further discussion of vaccinations for salmonellosis, see the section on calf salmonellosis.)

Prevention is best accomplished by maintaining a closed herd and culturing new feed additives and components before using them in the ration.

Hemorrhagic Bowel Syndrome (Jejunal Hemorrhage Syndrome)

Hemorrhagic bowel syndrome (HBS) is a newly emerging, highly fatal intestinal disease that has been recognized most frequently in adult dairy cows in the United States. Recently reports of HBS in Canadian dairy and beef cattle have been published. Other names given to HBS include jejunal hemorrhage syndrome, bloody gut, dead gut, and clostridial enteritis. HBS is characterized by sudden, progressive, and occasionally massive hemorrhage into the small intestine, with subsequent formation of clots within the intestine that create obstruction. Affected areas of the intestine become necrotic, and affected cows appear to suffer from the combined effects of blood loss, intestinal obstruction, and devitalization of bowel. The disease is seen most commonly in adult dairy cows early in lactation, although cases occasionally occur in late lactation or the dry period.

Etiology

The cause of HBS is currently unknown, and no consistent predisposing factor has been identified. The majority of HBS cases occur during the first 4 months postpartum. In a large survey of American dairy producers, the median parity for cows affected by HBS was reported to be the third lactation, and the median number of days in milk for affected cows was 104 days. During this period, dairy cows experience physiologic stress associated with peak milk yield. In addition, the rations fed during this stage of production are rich in energy and protein and fiber-depleted relative to rations fed later in lactation. These factors have been proposed to place cows at greater risk for HBS, but the events that lead up to the development of this disease remain undetermined.

The gross and histologic features of HBS have been described in a few reports. Gross lesions are usually segmental or multifocal in distribution in the small intestine, primarily in the jejunum with occasional involvement of the duodenum or ileum. Affected segments show purple or red discoloration of the intestinal wall, with distention of affected segments caused by intraluminal casts or clots of blood (Figures 6-32 and 6-33). The intestine orad to these lesions may be distended with fluid and gas, indicating obstruction of affected segments. Fibrin accumulation on the surface of affected intestine may be evident, and affected

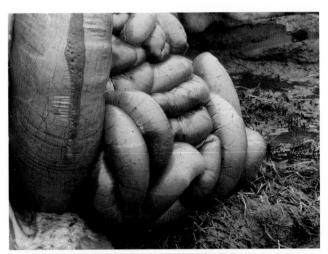

Figure 6-32

Fresh field autopsy performed within minutes of death on a mature Holstein cow with HBS. Note the purplish discoloration and gas production throughout the small intestine. There was diffuse jejunal involvement with death occurring as a result of blood loss.

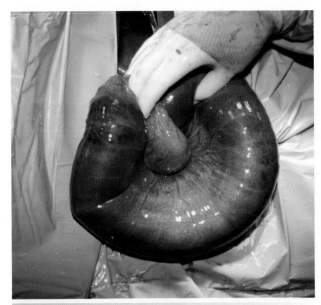

Figure 6-33

Intraoperative picture of mature Brown Swiss cow with HBS. In contrast to the cow in Figure 6-29, this animal demonstrated the rather more common involvement of just a segment of jejunum with a blood clot obstructing an approximately 12-inch section of bowel. *(Photo courtesy Dr. Liz Santschi.)*

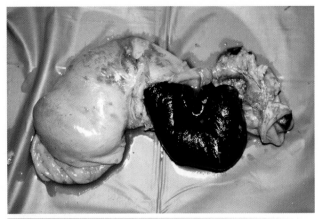

Figure 6-34

Resected section of jejunum cut open to show tenacious intraluminal blood clot from an adult Holstein with HBS.

segments may rupture antemortem or postmortem. The blood clot in affected segments is often tenaciously attached to the mucosa, and manual removal of the clot often results in "peeling off" of the surrounding mucosa (Figure 6-34). On histologic examination of affected bowel, HBS appears to be a segmental, necrohemorrhagic enteritis, with submucosal edema, mucosal ulceration, transmural hemorrhage, and neutrophil accumulation evident in affected areas. Sloughing of mucosa in affected areas may also be present.

Several reports indicate an association between *C. perfringens* type A and HBS. This association is based on the following observations: (1) affected cows have positive fecal cultures for this organism; (2) *C. perfringens* type A can be readily isolated in heavy growth from blood clots in the jejunum of affected cows; (3) there is microscopic evidence of intestinal necrosis associated with a dense intraluminal population of large, gram-positive bacteria; and (4) other enteric pathogens associated with hemorrhagic enteritis are rarely identified in tissues or enteric contents of affected cows. In addition, based on anecdotal evidence, reduced monthly incidence of HBS has occurred following administration of an autogenous *C. perfringens* vaccine to adult cows on certain dairies. At present, data from controlled studies are not available for evaluation of the effect of such vaccines on the incidence of this disease.

C. perfringens is a large, gram-positive, anaerobic bacillus that is considered to be ubiquitous in the environment and in the gastrointestinal tract of most mammals. The rate of isolation of the organism from the gastrointestinal tract of cattle may be enhanced by high grain diets. Genetic classification of *C. perfringens* is performed by mPCR. Type A usually produces alpha toxin, although different isolates may produce different quantities of this toxin. Alpha toxin is a calcium-dependent phospholipase that is capable of cleaving phosphatidylcholine in eukaryotic cell membranes. Additionally, the recently discovered beta2 toxin may be produced by *C. perfringens* type A. Beta2 toxin is also a lethal toxin, and strains of *C. perfringens* with the *cpb2* gene produce variable amounts of beta2 toxin in vitro.

In two studies, *C. perfringens* type A and/or type A + beta2 was isolated from feces and/or intestinal contents of 28 of 32 cows with HBS. These bacteriologic findings are concordant with those of other reports. In the past, veterinary microbiologists have been reluctant to consider *C. perfringens* type A as an important disease-causing pathogen of livestock because this organism is part of the normal flora of the cow's intestine. Furthermore, this organism proliferates rapidly in the intestine after death, making isolation from necropsy specimens of questionable diagnostic significance. Because *C. perfringens* types A and A + beta2 can be isolated from the gastrointestinal tract of apparently healthy animals, the diagnostic significance of isolation of these organisms from animals with enteric disease is increased if the corresponding toxins can be detected in gastrointestinal contents or blood. In a recent study, *C. perfringens* types A and A + beta2 were isolated from multiple sites of the intestinal tract of HBS cows at a significantly higher rate than unaffected herdmates (cows with LDA). In addition, intraluminal toxin production was demonstrated in the intestine of HBS cows but not in the intestine of control herdmates with LDA.

It is unclear at present whether enteric proliferation of and intraluminal toxin production by *C. perfringens* type A occur as part of the primary insult to the intestine, or if these processes occur secondary to another disease or triggering factor. Hemorrhage into the intestine from another cause could, in theory, initiate secondary proliferation of the ubiquitous *C. perfringens* because this organism is likely to rapidly multiply when large quantities of soluble protein or carbohydrate is presented to the intestine. In other words, blood certainly could act as a very rich culture medium for this organism. Once the organism proliferates, however, the toxins that it releases during rapid growth could contribute to the degradation of the intestinal wall that is so characteristic of HBS. This destruction of the intestinal wall in sections of the gut affected by HBS is likely to contribute to the subsequent shock and peritonitis that is evident in so many affected cows.

Investigators at Oregon State University have focused on characterizing the role of *Aspergillus fumigatus*, a fungus that can be found in livestock feeds. Genetic material of this fungal agent can be detected in the blood and intestine of affected cattle but not in unaffected cattle. Two hypotheses can be presented regarding the possible participation of *A. fumigatus* in HBS: (1) as a primary contributor to the intestinal lesion; or (2) as an agent that impairs the cow's immune system, thereby facilitating or inciting whatever disease process

triggers HBS. Anecdotal reports suggest that the incidence of HBS can be reduced on dairies following the introduction of a feed supplement (Omnigen AF, Prince Agri Products, Quincy, IL) into the ration. Controlled studies on the efficacy of this product for HBS prevention are pending. This product has recently been demonstrated to improve certain indicators of immune function in the WBCs taken from immunosuppressed sheep.

Clinical Signs

Cows are rapidly debilitated by the combined effects from sudden and massive hemorrhage into the small intestine. As a result, affected cows may simply be found dead or dying. A rapid pulse and rapid respiratory rate are commonly found in affected animals, and the mucous membranes are pale. The cow's extremities are often cool, and the rectal temperature is often below normal; the loss of blood into the intestine and the resulting shock contribute to these findings. In this sense, affected cows can resemble milk fever cases. Unlike milk fever, however, the feces of affected cows are dark, tarlike, and may contain dark red to black clots of digested blood (Figure 6-35). As clots form in the affected segments of the intestine, the intestine often becomes obstructed, causing some cows to show abdominal distention, reduced fecal output, and signs of colic. Glucose can often be detected in the urine of affected cows, indicating a severe stress response.

When viewed from behind, the abdominal contour is typically round or pear-shaped in the standing animal. Progressive distention is often appreciated in the lower right abdomen, presumably resulting from accumulation of multiple loops of blood-filled small intestine in the ventral abdominal cavity. Scattered, low-pitched

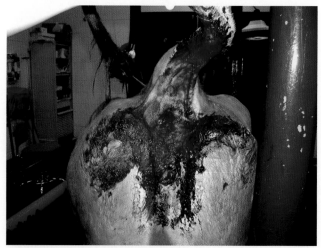

Figure 6-35

Perineum of mature Brown Swiss cow demonstrating the admixture of fresh and digested blood clots typical of HBS.

"pings" may be evident in the lower right abdomen. This progressive abdominal distention distinguishes cases of HBS from cases of bleeding abomasal ulcer. Occasionally motility is reduced throughout the gastrointestinal tract, and affected cows can appear bloated. In our experience, rectal examination often does not reveal distended loops of intestine because the blood-filled segments of intestine seem to sink to the ventral abdomen, thereby becoming beyond the reach of the examiner. However, small intestinal distention was palpable per rectum in six of eight cows in a Canadian study.

Ultrasonography can be used to visualize intestinal distention and clot formation within loops of affected bowel. A 3.5- or 5.0-MHz, sector- or linear-array probe is placed on the abdominal wall at the lower aspect of the right side. Dilated loops of intestine can often be seen, and on occasion, material consistent with the appearance of clotted blood can be seen within the distended loops (Figure 6-36).

Differential diagnoses include intussusception, intestinal volvulus, enteritis, and abomasal ulcer. Cows with an abomasal ulcer may show melena and shock but rarely develop the progressive abdominal distention characteristic of HBS. Cattle with enteritis continue to pass significant quantities of feces, particularly following treatment with fluids and calcium salts, whereas cattle with HBS usually do not. Further, once hydration, electrolyte balance, and normocalcemia are restored by fluid therapy, cattle with enteritis typically show resolution of any mild abdominal distention that might have developed as a result of ileus. Differentiation of HBS from intussusception and intestinal volvulus requires exploratory laparotomy.

Treatment

Successful treatment of this disease is difficult. Occasional, anecdotal reports exist of successful treatment with fluids, laxatives, antiinflammatory drugs, and antibiotics; however, it appears that such treatment successes are quite rare. Cows treated with medical support alone almost inevitably develop ileus, intestinal necrosis (tissue death) with subsequent peritonitis, and shock. Death of affected cattle occurs within several hours to 1 to 2 days after the onset of clinical signs.

At surgery, multiple inflamed segments of jejunum, ileum, or rarely duodenum are found. The serosal surface of affected segments is often dark purple to black in color. The affected segments of intestine are friable and turgid with luminal blood, and the casts of clotted blood within the lumen of the intestine impart a gelatin-like feel to the affected bowel (Figure 6-37). Involvement of multiple segments of jejunum and/or ileum is frequently found, which eliminates the option for intestinal resection and anastomosis. Techniques for surgical management of HBS cases to date include manipulation of the affected intestine so as to break down the obstructing clots, enterotomy and removal of the offending clots, and resection and anastomosis of affected segments. Common reasons for poor surgical outcome include discovery of multiple segments of nonviable bowel, septic peritonitis, and bowel rupture during intestinal manipulation. Also, if the initial surgical procedure is completed successfully, affected cows may develop repeated clotting and recurrent obstruction of the intestine after surgery. Of 22 cows affected

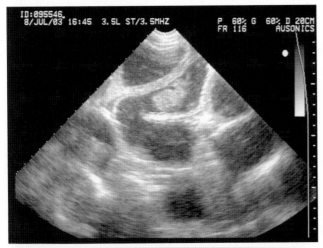

Figure 6-36

Transabdominal ultrasound image of lower right quadrant of a cow with HBS, demonstrating variably distended loops of small intestine and one small, nonadherent, hyperechoic intraluminal blood clot.

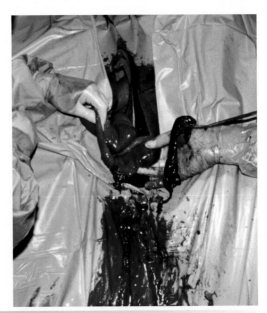

Figure 6-37

Intraoperative image of enterotomy site being used to manually remove and massage obstructing blood clots out of the jejunum in a cow with HBS. *(Photo courtesy Dr. Ryland Edwards.)*

with HBS presented to a university veterinary hospital over a 3-year period, only 5 (23%) survived; four of these survivors were treated surgically. In other studies, treating HBS cases with surgery, medical management, or both has resulted in little success.

Prevention

Preventive strategies for HBS remain somewhat speculative at present, given the lack of understanding about the pathogenesis of this disease. In addition, controlled studies on the clinical efficacy and economic impact of particular preventive measures have not been completed. Nonetheless, potential risk factors for clostridial overgrowth in the intestine of ruminants have been identified in previous studies, and strategies to reduce those risks might, at least in theory, provide benefits in HBS control. Similarly, the potential role of pathogenic fungi in HBS warrants careful consideration when designing preventive strategies. In short, until more refined information regarding the cause of HBS is published, it may be best to first consider all proposed causes or risk factors (e.g., bacteria, fungi, and reduced host disease resistance) and take measures to mitigate these potential risk factors. In so doing, one should consider: (1) identifying and correcting management and environmental factors that might impair cow immunity, (2) performing a careful partial budget analysis of the cost of specific preventive measures, and (3) deciding on which specific corrective measure(s) might be most justified for a particular dairy.

To begin, a thorough analysis of transition and fresh cow management should be performed to identify problems with cow comfort, hygiene, nutrition, and disease control that might impact disease resistance during the apparent period of greatest risk for HBS, which is the first 3 to 4 months of lactation. Ration formulation and mixing should be reviewed as well, with due consideration given to such issues as effective fiber and soluble carbohydrate content and their potential dietary influences on gut flora. Feed bunk and pen management should be carefully critiqued to ensure that feed intake is consistent; efforts should focus on identifying and correcting management problems that cause "slug feeding" (e.g., pen overcrowding, poor parlor throughput, and infrequent feeding) and that predisposes to subacute rumen acidosis. Silage management, commodity storage, and feed preparation should be examined to determine whether spoilage and mold formation are problematic. Because these critical areas impact numerous facets of cow health other than HBS, identification and correction of problems in these areas will likely provide an overall benefit to cow health. Finally, potential use of feed additives or vaccines directed against specific, potential contributory pathogens should be considered carefully, with the costs of the proposed interventions and their potential

efficacy weighed against the prevalence and costs of the disease.

Bovine Virus Diarrhea

Etiology and Background

The disease commonly referred to as bovine virus diarrhea (BVD) was first described by Olafson et al in 1946. This initial disease was highly infectious, contagious, and imparted high mortality. The causative organism was later isolated and so began the prolific long-term research into this pathogen of cattle. The initial clinical descriptions of BVD by Fox were of a severe disease characterized by high fever, diarrhea, mucosal lesions, and leukopenia. However, throughout the period of 1950 to 1975, the disease was largely disregarded in parts of the United States—including the northeast—because serologic surveys suggested that most adult cows had serum neutralization titers against BVDV. These results were interpreted to mean that BVDV frequently infected cattle as a subclinical or mild infection and was of little clinical significance. A direct consequence of this thinking was a nearly complete lack of interest in vaccination of dairy cattle against BVDV. The major clinical evidence of BVDV during the years 1950 to 1975 was sporadic subacute or chronic infection in one or more heifers on a farm. These affected animals usually were between 6 and 24 months of age; they developed diarrhea, typical mucosal lesions, fever, weight loss, and survived in poor condition for a variable time before death. Because of the sporadic appearance of such cases, these animals were thought to be immunodeficient and therefore susceptible to BVDV. This theory was tenable for single-case infections but became less believable when four to six heifers on one farm developed similar signs because the likelihood of multiple immunodeficient animals on one farm seemed small.

During that time, the use of modified-live BVDV (ML-BVDV) vaccines occasionally preceded the development of signs of BVD in a group of heifers by 1 to 4 weeks. Although this further discouraged the use of BVDV vaccines, it was explained as an unfortunate circumstance and likely that the heifers had already been incubating field virus. These subacute or chronic cases—usually in heifers—were often called "mucosal disease" because of the easily observable oral erosions and gastrointestinal lesions often found at necropsy, as well as the characteristic clinical signs of fever, weight loss, and diarrhea. Virologic limitations at many diagnostic laboratories during this period added further confusion to the disease clinically referred to as BVD or mucosal disease. Diagnosis was based primarily on serum neutralization titers and FA procedures on tissue samples rather than viral isolation. Current knowledge helps explain why so many of these clinically obvious BVD patients had low or nonexistent serum neutralization (SN) titers against

BVDV. Further, the FA techniques used were poor tests that gave erratic results. Therefore in many cases over this time period, a textbook example of clinical BVD could not be confirmed as BVDV infection.

Reproductive and fetal consequences of the virus were studied during these years (1950 to 1975), and the implications of BVDV in reproductive failure were questioned clinically but seldom confirmed. The virus was shown to be a potential cause of abortion and congenital anomalies such as cerebellar hypoplasia and ocular defects. Absolute diagnosis of BVDV infection as a cause of clinical reproductive, gastrointestinal, or other system disease was made difficult by limited laboratory capabilities.

The past 20 years have brought both a wealth of research regarding the virus and the reemergence of BVDV as a major pathogen in cattle. The virus had been classified as a pestivirus within the *Togaviridae* family because of similarities with hog cholera virus and the virus of Border disease. Recent reclassification finds BVDV as a member of the genus *Pestivirus* within the family *Flaviviridae*. BVDV is classified in vitro into one of two "biotypes," cytopathic (CP-BVDV) or noncytopathic (NCP-BVDV), based on how each biotype affects cell cultures. CP-BVDV causes vacuolation and death of certain cell lines within days of inoculation into cell culture, whereas NCP-BVDV inoculation into cell culture results in inapparent infection. NCP-BVDV is the more prevalent biotype in cattle. It serves as the parent virus from which, following genetic recombination, CP-BVDV arises.

In addition, a multitude of "strains" or *heterologous isolates* exist within each of the BVDV biotypes. The exact number of strains or genetic variation in the virus is not known, but the implications regarding clinical variations and effective immunization against these multiple strains constitute the major current concerns for BVDV. Further, the strain of virus used to complete a research study may or may not have implications for cattle exposed to a heterologous strain in the "real world." Some strains may be capable of causing congenital anomalies, whereas others cause severe gastrointestinal injury. Therefore the strain chosen for study may have a profound outcome on the study results.

Through genetic sequencing, BVDV can be further classified according to one of two major genotypes (commonly called "types"): 1 and 2. Type 1 strains are considered the classic genotypes banked since the 1950s. Type 2 BVDV was first detected by genetic sequencing of isolates from severe clinical cases in adult cattle and calves in the northeastern United States and eastern Canadian provinces in 1993 to 1994. There are currently 11 recognized subgenotypes of BVDV type 1 (designated 1a, 1b, 1c, and so on) and two subgenotypes of type 2. Viral isolates within a given subgenotype are closely related in nucleotide sequence, sharing >90% sequence homology. Although severe clinical disease was characteristic of the outbreak of type 2 BVDV in the early 1990s, it should be emphasized that virulent strains of type 1 exist.

Perhaps the most important discovery about BVDV has been the identification and explanation for cattle persistently infected (PI) with BVDV. Animals with BVDV-PI and having little or no SN antibody against the homologous strain were recognized and later produced experimentally by infecting fetuses between 40 and 120 days gestation with NCP-BVDV. These workers were able to cause the PI state by directly infecting fetuses in seropositive dams (58 to 125 days) or infecting seronegative dams carrying fetuses (42 to 114 days) with NCP-BVDV. For unknown reasons, PI cannot be caused by experimental challenge with CP-BVDV.

A brief review of the PI condition is warranted here. Fetuses that are exposed to NCP-BVDV between the approximate ages of 40 and 125 days gestation may become PI with this strain of virus. These animals are immunotolerant of that NCP strain because they consider those viral antigens to be self. Such PI fetuses have several potential outcomes: being born normal and growing to adulthood normally; being born apparently normal but succumbing to disease before 1 year of age; or being born weak, small, or dead. However, if a PI animal is challenged by a heterologous CP-BVDV, severe disease may ensue, and in such instances, PI animals usually succumb with signs of acute, subacute, or chronic BVD. Apparently the immunotolerance of the PI animal to its homologous NCP-BVDV renders it unable to mount functional immunologic defenses against certain CP-BVDV strains. This scenario of infection by CP-BVDV in NCP-BVDV-PI animals was assumed by many previous researchers to be the only way animals could get the characteristic "mucosal disease" or fatal clinical BVD. Further, this "superinfection" of PI animals by CP-BVDV strains appeared to explain the outbreaks of BVD that followed use of modified-live BVDV vaccines.

More recent studies have shown that animals that develop naturally occurring BVDV-PI often harbor antigenically similar CP and NCP viruses. Genetic studies of these viruses have revealed that insertion of novel RNA into the NCP-BVDV can cause conversion into the CP-BVDV biotype. In other words, a PI animal may develop fulminant CP-BVDV infection from genetic reassortment of its own virus, from transfer of genetic material from a heterologous strain to its own virus, or from exposure to an entirely novel CP or NCP strain. In those instances, classic "mucosal disease" may develop in the PI animal.

"Mucosal disease" is often considered as a separate entity from "BVD" by clinicians and researchers. Dr. Rebhun believed strongly that mucosal lesions do not dictate a separate, uniformly fatal entity that is necessarily distinct from BVD, and that signs of BVD follow the biologic bell-shaped curve. True, it has been proven that certain CP-BVDV strains can cause superinfection of PI animals, resulting in fatal disease. This fatal disease may follow an acute, subacute, or chronic course and is frequently characterized by fever, diarrhea, weight loss, mucosal ulcerations of the gastrointestinal tract, digital lesions, and/or dermatologic lesions. However, clinical experience has shown that naive cattle can have mucosal lesions caused by NCP-BVDV infection, yet subsequently survive and form SN titers against this strain. Clinical experience also has shown that fatal BVD has occurred solely as a result of virulent strains of NCP-BVDV and that PI animals are not the only animals that die when exposed to certain CP- or NCP-BVDV. In short, the presence of mucosal lesions is not predictive of death or survival, nor of the PI status. Although the signs of BVD may be more obvious or more profound in superinfected PI than in non-PI animals, the same disease is present.

Similarly it has been tempting to be "clear-cut" when explaining temporal variation in consequences of fetal exposure to BVDV. Exposure to infected semen may prevent implantation or result in embryonic failure (for reasons that are unclear) until the dam develops immunity against the virus. Infection of the fetus before day 40 may or may not result in fetal death or infertility. Some work suggests embryonic death is likely during this time, but some cattle (or some cattle infected with some strains of virus) can conceive despite acute infection created by oral or IV routes.

Fetuses that are infected with NCP-BVDV before 125 days of gestation are at risk for PI. Fetuses exposed to NCP-BVDV strains between 90 and 180 days may also develop congenital anomalies such as cerebellar hypoplasia, ocular lesions, and many other problems. Because of the overlap between possible PI and congenital lesions, a calf born with a congenital lesion may be either PI or possess a precolostral titer against the BVDV that infected it in utero. Fetuses exposed to NCP-BVDV after 180 days of gestation are thought to either form antibodies against the virus and survive or be aborted. CP-BVDV strains apparently do not cause PI when pregnant seronegative cows are infected before fetal immunocompetence. Fetal infection by CP-BVDV may cause fetal death, abortion, or the subsequent birth of healthy calves having precolostral antibodies against the infecting CP-BVDV. Congenital lesions may also result from in utero CP-BVDV infections.

The major concern raised by PI animals is constant dissemination of virus because these animals remain a reservoir of BVDV within the herd and shed large amounts of virus in secretions and excretions. Although non-PI herdmates can be vaccinated against BVDV, potential risk to fetuses and young calves remains a concern for herds harboring PI animals. Put simply, PI animals may shed so much virus that the finite immunity in herdmates can be overwhelmed, resulting in

infection of non-PI, immunocompetent, and previously exposed and/or immunized herdmates. Exposure of pregnant herdmates to asymptomatic PI animals is a well-established means of perpetuating endemic BVD infection in both dairy and beef herds.

PI explains many heretofore confusing aspects of clinical problems created by BVDV but does not explain the profound variations and patterns of clinical disease caused by BVDV. This variation is more likely explained by multiple strains of NCP-BVDV and CP-BVDV, some of which appear to have a degree of organ specificity. Obviously previous exposure of cattle to BVDV through natural exposure or vaccination, other diseases that exist concurrent to BVDV exposure, age and genetics of the cattle, and the strain of BVDV all have a great influence of the clinical picture created when a group or herd of cattle are exposed. There is no question, however, that within each herd having detectable clinical disease associated with BVDV, the specific clinical signs of disease are repeatable. For example, herds with abortions as a common finding will continue to see abortion, and herds with calves affected with congenital lesions will continue to see such calves without necessarily having cows affected with high fever and diarrhea. Other herds will experience high calf mortality associated with BVDV, and yet others will have recently fresh cows developing high fevers. Thus it is unusual to see multiple clinical situations within a single herd experiencing disease caused by BVDV. A specific "set" or pattern of signs is more typical, and clinicians never should underestimate the ability of BVDV infection to assume multiple appearances. Future research may allow further distinction of BVDV strains capable of producing specific clinical signs such as thrombocytopenia, specific congenital anomalies, abortions, or gastrointestinal disease. The disturbing implications of multiple BVDV strains—each possibly possessing individual pathogenicity—center on the consequential potential need for vaccines that can protect cattle and their fetuses against the heterogenous array of BVD viruses.

Clinical Signs

A multitude of clinical signs are possible in cattle exposed to BVDV. Frequently it is emphasized that most naive cattle or calves experimentally infected with BVDV show little if any evidence of illness yet seroconvert and develop neutralizing antibodies against the infecting strain of BVDV. Such subclinical infection and absence of overt disease also may occur in field situations. However, many other factors such as age of the animal, concurrent diseases or stresses, relative exposure, dosage, strain and biotype of BVDV, herd and individual cow immune status from previous exposure to BVDV via natural or vaccination means, and presence or absence of PI cattle in the herd must be considered in field situations. As discussed previously, herds experiencing clinical disease because of BVDV will tend to establish a specific pattern of signs rather than variable signs. Clinicians must keep an open mind when considering BVDV as a cause of disease because the signs may be so variable. New signs of BVDV continue to emerge and will continue to do so as more strains evolve. Much of the current experimental work with BVDV has been done with a limited number of strains. These laboratory strains may or may not cause signs similar to wild or field strains. Certain field strains seem capable of causing specific clinical signs. For example, a field strain of NCP-BVDV (genotype 2) found to cause thrombocytopenia was able to create thrombocytopenia in experimentally infected cattle. However, it is obvious that not all strains of BVDV cause thrombocytopenia.

The reported dearth of clinical signs in cattle acutely infected with BVDV is further questioned now that many references to support this theory are quite dated. In addition, the strains responsible for subclinical infections as evidenced by these serologic surveys may or may not be as prevalent currently as they were 20 to 30 years ago. Clinical signs will be described based on field outbreaks that have been confirmed as BVDV infections.

Acute Illness

Classical signs of fever and diarrhea are possible in naive but immunocompetent calves or adult cattle infected with certain strains of BVDV. Fever and depression usually precede the onset of diarrhea by 2 to 7 days, and fever is frequently biphasic. This biphasic fever starts as high fever (105.0 to 108.0° F/40.6 to 42.2° C) that diminishes over several days only to recur 5 to 10 days after the original fever. Diarrhea and gastrointestinal erosions may be observed during or after the second fever spike, or the patient may recover without showing further signs. Oral erosions will be present in only 30% to 50% of the infected cattle, so *absence of oral erosions does not rule out BVDV.* Outbreaks of BVDV are most common in 6- to 10-month-old heifers but in naive populations could occur at any age. A high incidence of clinical disease (mostly high fever) has been seen in recently fresh cows being reintroduced into the milking herd that had a PI animal.

Initial clinical signs in addition to fever include slight to moderate depression and reduced appetite and production. Cattle with very high initial fever often show tachypnea and may be erroneously diagnosed as having a "viral pneumonia." The tachypnea usually is simply a physiologic response to allow loss of heat caused by fever. If a second fever wave occurs, the clinical signs tend to worsen as appetite and milk production plummet. If gastrointestinal lesions develop, the cow's appetite is completely suppressed. *Few diseases cause the severe degree of anorexia apparent in acute BVDV patients with fever, diarrhea, and gastrointestinal lesions.*

Oral erosions and digital lesions (described below) are the only "lesions" of BVDV visible to clinicians seeking signs of the disease. Because many, if not most, acutely infected cattle show lesions in neither area, clinicians must maintain an index of suspicion based on other signs (e.g., fever, diarrhea) and examine as many affected animals as possible. In some herds having this form of BVDV, only recently fresh cows develop signs, and these affected fresh cows are observed sporadically rather than as an epidemic. Morbidity and mortality levels vary with the classical acute illness but usually range from 10% to 30%. Occasional catastrophic outbreaks with much higher mortality rates are still encountered in naive or highly stressed groups of cattle. When present, oral erosions are much less obvious than those observed in pathology texts or in chronic or classic mucosal disease (Figure 6-38). Focal or multifocal erosions can occur anywhere in the oral cavity and are most common on the hard or soft palates. Hyperemia and erosive changes on the papillae near the lip commissures are sometimes apparent. The papillae may be blunted, shortened, or simply have erosions on the apical portion, causing these areas to appear much more pink or red than the bases (Figure 6-39). Erosions at the gingival area adjacent to the incisor teeth may

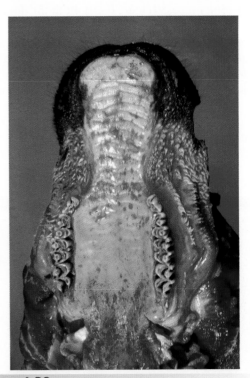

Figure 6-38

Extensive erosion on the soft and hard palate regions of a heifer that died from chronic BVDV infection. This heifer was persistently infected with BVDV. Oral erosions in most field cases of BVDV infection involving naive cattle are not this dramatic or extensive. *(Photo courtesy Dr. John M. King.)*

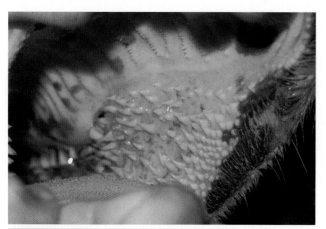

Figure 6-39

Hyperemia and erosion of the mucosa of the papillae near the lip commissures of an acutely infected naive cow. The papillae in the middle of the region are eroded, inflamed, and more pink or red than unaffected papillae. Such papillae may or may not appear "blunted."

occur but sometimes are difficult to interpret because of the natural pink appearance of the gingiva adjacent to the teeth. Close inspection of this area will distinguish sloughing epithelium and erosions from the normal healthy pink mucosa (Figure 6-40). Both the dorsal and ventral surfaces of the tongue should be examined carefully for ulcers (Figure 6-41). Slight to moderate salivation may be observed in cattle with oral erosions, and grinding of the teeth may indicate pain caused by other gastrointestinal lesions. Digital lesions are infrequent in adult cattle experiencing acute BVDV infection, but, when present, they appear as coronary band hyperemia, exudation and erosion, or interdigital erosions. Lameness is a distinct sequela to such lesions. The character

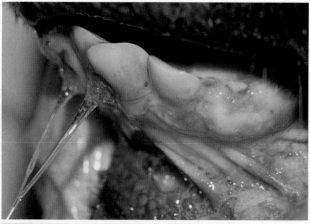

Figure 6-40

Distinct erosions of the mucosa adjacent to the incisor teeth of an acutely infected cow from a herd outbreak of BVDV.

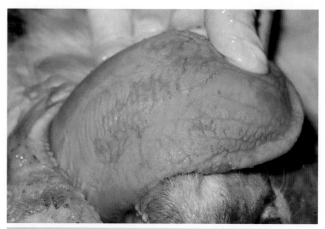

Figure 6-41

Erosions on the ventral surface of the tongue in a superinfected PI-BVDV heifer.

of the feces in BVDV patients with diarrhea varies from simply loose to watery, and blood or mucus may be apparent in severe cases or in those having thrombocytopenia. Tenesmus may develop secondary to profuse diarrhea and rectal irritation and may be confused with signs of coccidiosis. Leg edema and dermatitis may be noticeable in some PI animals.

Immunocompetent seronegative cows exposed to strains of BVDV capable of causing classical acute signs usually seroconvert and survive. However, some seronegative non-PI cows exposed to these viruses become seriously ill and may die. Some NCP-BVDV strains possess sufficient pathogenicity to kill adult, immunocompetent, seronegative cattle. This fact was highlighted by the 1994 epidemic of BVD in Ontario and the northeastern United States. Therefore a cow or calf does not have to be PI to be killed by a field strain of BVDV. Fatal consequences of BVDV (other than superinfection of PI animals) can occur directly as a result of BVDV-induced thrombocytopenia with subsequent hemorrhage, electrolyte, fluid, and protein losses caused by severe diarrhea, and other causes. Most commonly, however, fatal consequences of BVDV are secondary to opportunistic pathogens creating concurrent infection during BVDV viremia. Even immunocompetent healthy cattle suffer profound alterations in cellular defense mechanisms during the time between onset of BVDV infection and humoral antibody production or recovery. Most healthy cattle exposed to BVDV infection survive this time uneventfully, but less fortunate ones may develop pneumonia, mastitis, metritis, or other bacterial infections while viremic. Temporarily altered cellular immunity affects lymphocytes neutrophils, macrophages, and may predispose to bacteremia or alter clearance of circulating microbes. The clinical consequence of this temporary lapse in cellular defenses is an inability of such patients to overcome routine infections. Cattle infected with BVDV experimentally may or may not be exposed to other routine infections, whereas cattle naturally infected with BVDV are subject to multiple stresses and infections. During the period of viremia and altered cellular defense, dairy calves and cows may succumb to IBR virus, other enteric pathogens (especially *Salmonella* sp.), bacterial mastitis, bacterial pneumonia, and other infections. High mortality has been observed when BVDV and *Salmonella* sp. concurrently infect groups of calves or cows. Recently assembled herds or purchased groups of replacement heifers may trigger severe disease by introducing a new strain of BVDV to a resident herd. Immune responsiveness returns to normal as BVDV infection wanes and serum neutralization titers against the virus increase. Therefore seronegative immunocompetent cattle infected with BVDV do not have any residual or permanent immunodeficiency following resolution of the infection and seroconversion. Both increased severity of concurrent disease and lack of responsiveness to conventional therapy for that disease may be seen during the window of time that a patient is viremic with BVDV. Concurrent infections such as IBR or pneumonia caused by *Mannheimia haemolytica* in animals viremic with BVDV may be so severe as to mask the underlying BVDV because signs of illness or postmortem lesions incriminate respiratory pathogens as the cause of illness. Failure of these more obvious infections to respond to conventional therapy should raise the index of suspicion regarding BVDV infection. For example, a severe outbreak of *M. haemolytica* pneumonia masked underlying BVDV in a herd that had recently added 20 replacement heifers. Cultures obtained from affected cattle from tracheal wash and necropsy confirmed *M. haemolytica* sensitive to several antibiotics. The indicated antibiotics had been used to treat affected animals, but the expected clinical response was not obtained. Mucosal lesions subsequently were found in a few of the fatal cases, and a NCP-BVDV was isolated from the blood buffy coat of several affected animals.

In addition to altered cellular immune responsiveness, acute BVDV usually causes a leukopenia characterized by lymphopenia and sometimes neutropenia. Therefore not only are WBC functions diminished but also their absolute numbers are as well. Leukopenia increases the risk of opportunistic bacterial infection, and neutropenia seems to be associated with increased severity of concurrent diseases.

BVDV also attacks lymphoid tissues such as the spleen, lymph node germinal centers, and Peyer's patches and can infect lymphocytes and macrophages (Figure 6-42).

Combining all the aforementioned negative effects on host immunity helps explain why some non-PI cattle die during acute BVDV infection. Some would argue that these cattle in fact die from *Mannheimia* sp., *Salmonella* sp., or whatever secondary infection overwhelms

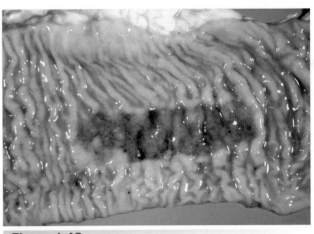

Figure 6-42

Necrosis of Peyer's patch in necropsy specimen of fatal BVDV infection. *(Photo courtesy Dr. John M. King.)*

the animal during the transient altered immunity caused by acute BVDV infection rather than from BVDV itself. The net effect, however, is mortality, and some BVDV strains can kill or contribute to the death of seronegative, immunocompetent, adult cattle.

Thrombocytopenia associated with type 2 acute BVDV infection has been observed in adult dairy cattle, dairy calves, and veal calves. Although platelet counts <100,000/μl are abnormal, clinical evidence of bleeding seldom is observed unless the platelet count is <50,000/μl. Conditions such as stress, injections, trauma, or insect bites that may contribute to clinical signs of bleeding in thrombocytopenic clinical patients may not be present in experimental models. Thrombocytopenia associated with bleeding causes blood loss anemia, which is highly fatal unless treated with fresh whole blood transfusions. Thrombocytopenia occurs as a result of viral infection and destruction of megakaryocytes in bone marrow. Dysfunction of circulating platelets may contribute to clinical signs of impaired coagulation. Field outbreaks of acute BVDV with thrombocytopenia are characterized by one or more of the affected cattle having signs of epistaxis, bloody diarrhea, bleeding from injection or insect bite sites, ecchymoses and petechial hemorrhages on mucous membranes, or hematoma formation (Figure 6-43). Not all infected cattle show signs of bleeding, and the magnitude of thrombocytopenia varies greatly. In addition, inapparent infection with subsequent seroconversion may occur in some herdmates. However, when bleeding is associated with other clinical signs such as diarrhea, fever unresponsive to antibiotics, gastrointestinal ulceration, and leukopenia, then BVDV should be strongly suspected. Platelet counts and isolation of BVDV from mononuclear cells in whole blood confirm the diagnosis. Other causes of bleeding can be ruled out by coagulation panels, including assessment of fibrin degradation products.

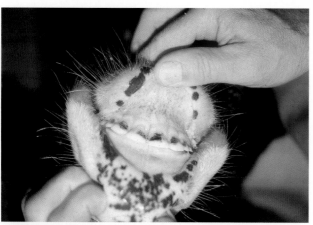

Figure 6-43

Petechiation and severe intestinal bleeding (PCV 10) in an 8-month-old heifer having thrombocytopenia associated with acute BVDV infection. After a blood transfusion, the heifer recovered.

Acute BVDV infection of naive, non-PI calves may cause inapparent infection with seroconversion or clinical signs that include fever and diarrhea of varying severity. The greatest risk for calves with acute BVDV infection is concurrent infection with other enteric or respiratory pathogens. Transient reduction of cellular immune function and defense mechanisms during BVDV viremia predispose to and worsen concurrent infection. Therefore diarrheic neonatal calves (<2 to 3 weeks of age) can have acute BVDV infection masked by identification of encapsulated *E. coli*, *Salmonella* sp., rotavirus, coronavirus, or *C. parvum* (Figure 6-44). Similarly calves up to several months of age may have overt respiratory disease caused by *Mannheimia* sp., *H. somni*, or respiratory viruses that are isolated from tracheal wash or necropsy specimens. In all of these situations, concurrent BVDV

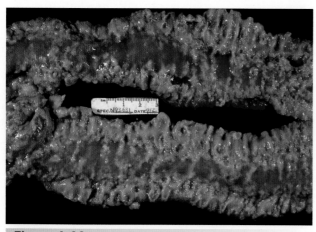

Figure 6-44

Concurrent *S.* Typhimurium and BVDV-induced intestinal lesions in a neonatal calf. *(Photo courtesy Dr. John M. King.)*

should be suspected when the severity of disease, morbidity, and mortality seem excessive for the identified pathogens. Naive, non-PI calves born to seropositive cows should acquire passive antibody protection against homologous strains for 3 to 12 months. However, this passive protection may or may not protect against heterologous strains and may not be protective if calves receive less than adequate amounts of colostrum. In addition, overwhelming exposure to BVDV may override any passive protection in some instances. Seronegative calves are at risk at all times. Whenever severe calf mortality associated with enteric or respiratory pathogens occurs, BVDV should be considered and ruled in or out by viral isolation from blood, necropsy tissue samples, or tracheal wash samples.

Persistent Infection

PIs caused by NCP-BVDV arise from fetal infections occurring before 125 days of gestation. Such calves are born seronegative and PI if the dam is PI. Alternatively, a PI calf can be born to a non-PI, immunocompetent dam—the sole requirement is BVDV infection that creates viremia in the dam of sufficient magnitude to cause transplacental infection. PI calves may be transiently seropositive if the dam (PI or not) was infected during pregnancy and passed antibodies to the calf through colostrum; PI dams may generate colostral antibody titers to heterologous strains of BVDV.

Calves may appear normal at birth, grow normally, and become productive members of the herd. This situation is perhaps the most frightening because such PI cattle are not easily detected and continue to harbor and shed homologous BVDV through body secretions. Apparently healthy PI cattle also reliably reproduce PI offspring that subsequently act as reservoirs of infection for herdmates. PI calves or cattle that are clinically normal may develop signs of acute or chronic ("mucosal disease") BVD if exposed to heterologous strains of CP-BVDV through natural exposure, administration of modified live BVDV vaccines, or genetic recombination of their homologous BVDV strain. In fact, the source of RNA that causes conversion to CP from NCP biotype may even be derived from the RNA of the animal's own cells.

At one time, it was assumed that all heterologous strains of BVDV would cause fatal infections in PI cattle because such cattle would not recognize these strains as foreign. It also was assumed that CP-BVDV strains were necessary to cause disease in PI animals because many workers found both CP- and NCP-BVDV in cattle having chronic or mucosal disease. Not all heterologous strains of BVDV cause PI animals to develop illness, however. Experimental inoculation of PI cattle with certain CP-BVDV strains not only may fail to produce disease but also may be associated with seroconversion against the heterologous CP-BVDV and continued failure of seroconversion against the homologous NCP-BVDV. This situation and that of the PI calf that attains passive-colostrum origin antibodies from its dam constitute two reasons that a PI animal could have serum-neutralizing antibodies against BVDV.

Apparently healthy PI animals often remain in the herd, produce PI offspring, and represent significant sources of perpetuating infection for herdmates and fetuses. Some PI calves are born weak, small, or die shortly after birth. Weak calves that survive generally succumb to enteric or respiratory pathogens within the first few weeks of life. Clinical signs and gross necropsy findings may not suggest BVDV infection, and death is attributed to enteritis or pneumonia of varying causes. This clinical scenario allows BVDV to escape detection unless blood or tissue samples are submitted for viral isolation or antigen detection. Some workers have observed domed skulls and finer-than-normal maxillary shape ("deer noses") in PI calves that are weak, small at birth, and often do not thrive (Figure 6-45).

The intermediate clinical view for PI calves falls somewhere between the apparently healthy PI calf that remains healthy, and the calf that is obviously weak, small, or nonviable at birth. This intermediate type is apparently normal at birth but dies before 2 years of age. The cause of death in such PI animals is variable. Recurrent or chronic infections are the hallmark of these calves. Enteritis, pneumonia, ringworm, pinkeye,

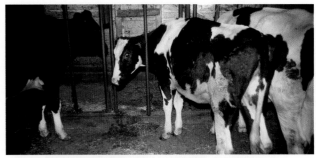

Figure 6-46

BVDV-PI yearling heifer that is stunted and has not grown well. The heifer is stanchioned between two healthy herdmates of the same age.

ectoparasites, or endoparasites may affect such calves, and they may persist or respond poorly to therapy. Unexplained pneumonia and/or diarrhea in a single growing heifer on a farm should arouse a suspicion of PI in that animal. Poor growth and stunting compared with herdmates is obvious in these PI animals (Figure 6-46). Because chronic bacterial, parasitic, or fungal infections typify many of the PI calves in this category, the integrity of immune responses must be questioned. Although PI animals initially were thought to have complete immunocompetence except for the "self" BVDV that they harbor, complete immunocompetence seems unlikely in all cases. There may be a variable expression of cellular or secretory immunity, and other factors, such as the exact time of in utero infection and the strain of NCP-BVDV, may play roles in relative immunocompetence. At least some PI animals appear to have reduced lymphocyte and neutrophil function.

In addition to apparently heightened susceptibility to a variety of opportunistic pathogens, PI animals in this category can succumb to superinfection with CP-BVDV (Figure 6-47), as discussed previously for classical mucosal disease. In fact, PI animals in this category (e.g., chronic disease, poor-doers, less than 2 years of age) compose the majority of "classic BVD," "chronic BVD," or "mucosal disease" cases. Signs of BVD tend to be profound with diarrhea, poor condition, dehydration, mucosal lesions, and sometimes leg edema (Figure 6-48) and skin and digital lesions. The course of disease is highly variable—some cases die rapidly, whereas others linger on as poor-doers. The major differential diagnoses for chronic poor-doer BVDV-PI animals are bovine leukocyte adhesive deficiency (BLAD) and chronic internal abscessation because all of these conditions yield similar gross clinical appearances.

Congenital Lesions

Some BVDV infections may only become apparent after the birth of calves with congenital lesions. Once again, the individual *pattern of disease* or *set of signs* within a specific herd may be unique to that herd. Adult cattle

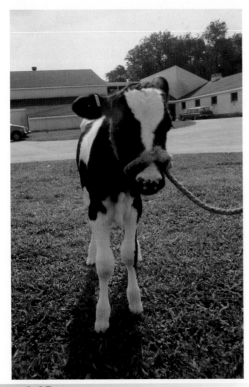

Figure 6-45

A 6-week-old BVDV-PI calf with poor growth and abnormally developed skull.

may experience subclinical infection that results in abortion or congenital anomalies such as cerebellar hypoplasia, cataracts, retinal and optic nerve degeneration, hydranencephaly, hypomyelinogenesis, brachygnathism, varying degrees of hairlessness, and other congenital lesions (Figures 6-49 to 6-51; see also Figure 12-15). It must be mentioned here that BVDV is not responsible for all congenital cataracts; there are many other causes. Although a plethora of types of congenital lesions are possible, only one or two may appear in a

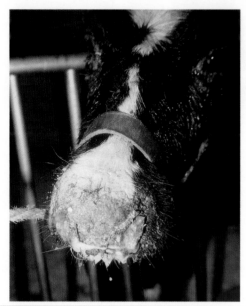

Figure 6-47

"Classic" mucosal disease in a 6-month-old heifer. After contact with "outside" cattle, an entire group of replacement heifers developed fever, diarrhea, and dermatitis, but this heifer that was a PI animal was the only one that died.

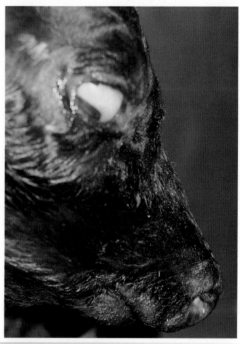

Figure 6-49

Brachygnathism in a calf associated with in utero BVDV infection.

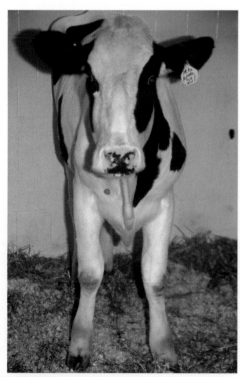

Figure 6-48

A 12-month-old heifer with persistent fever and edema of all four legs caused by vasculitis and BVDV-PI.

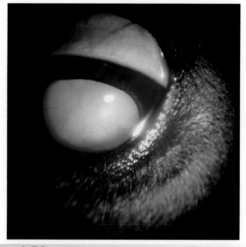

Figure 6-50

Diffuse cataract (bilateral) in a calf that was infected by BVDV during the mid-trimester of gestation.

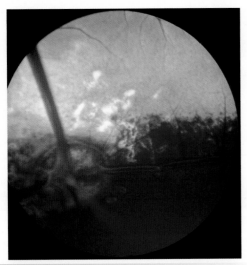

Figure 6-51

Optic nerve degeneration and chorioretinal scarring apparent as hyperreflective zones dorsal to the optic disc in a calf infected by BVDV during the mid-trimester of gestation.

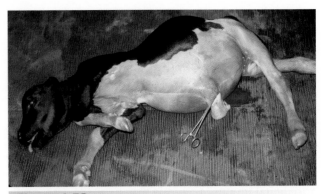

Figure 6-52

Aborted fetus from a BVDV-infected cow.

single herd and will be repeated in affected calves born over a period of weeks or months. Usually several consecutive calves are affected with the same type of congenital lesion. For example, in a herd that Dr. Rebhun investigated, brachygnathism and cataracts typified the congenital lesions, whereas in other herds, other ocular lesions or cerebellar hypoplasia may predominate. The strain of infecting BVDV certainly may play a role in determining the anatomic area of congenital defects because some strains seem to possess a degree of organ specificity. Both CP and NCP strains are capable of inducing fetal anomalies. Most congenital lesions are thought to indicate in utero infection between days 75 to 150 of gestation. Overlap between this time and the period for persistent infection (40 to 125 days) exists. Therefore calves born with congenital lesions may be PI or may be seropositive in precolostral blood samples depending on exactly when the in utero infection occurred and whether NCP or CP BVDV caused the congenital lesion. Calves with congenital lesions should be tested to determine whether they are PI—especially if the congenital lesions are not life threatening and the owner would like to keep the animal.

Reproductive Signs

In addition to fetal congenital defects, BVDV may cause a variety of reproductive consequences. Abortion always is a possibility when in utero BVDV infection occurs (Figure 6-52). Abortion has been observed or caused (experimental infections) at most stages of gestation with CP-BVDV and is possible in the midtrimester or last trimester as a result of NCP-BVDV. Fetuses may be infected several weeks or months before abortion in

some instances. Mummification also is possible following in utero BVDV infection.

Perhaps the greatest concerns for future BVDV research revolve around effective protection of the fetus from BVDV. The temporal relationships among PI, congenital lesions, and, to a lesser degree, abortion or mummification seem to have been worked out. However, the consequences of early in utero fetal infection (0 to 40 days) are not as well known.

Acutely infected immunocompetent bulls and PI bulls shed BVDV in semen. Insemination with infected semen will cause infection and subsequent seroconversion in seronegative cattle. Cattle infected by such semen tend not to conceive until establishing immunity and seroconversion. Oophoritis has been detected several weeks following experimental infection, and ovarian dysfunction may be responsible for the impaired fertility seen in some infected cow populations. Semen is a possible source of infection for herds and probably has been the occasional cause of reduced fertility and other BVDV problems in herds. Frozen semen also has been shown to be capable of BVDV transmission to susceptible cattle. Although PI bulls may have detectable abnormalities of semen, these are not consistent, and standard semen testing should not be used in lieu of viral isolation or antigen detection to identify infected bulls. Some immunocompetent (non-PI) bulls may shed the virus in the semen for an extended time. Most commercial bull studs now routinely screen incoming bulls for PI status or virus shedding before semen collection for AI purposes.

Intrauterine infusion of BVDV at the time of insemination was shown to cause susceptible cows to have early reproductive failure, low pregnancy rates, high return rates, and seroconversion. Reproductive failure appeared as a result of failure of fertilization. However, when either seronegative or seropositive cattle were infected orally or nasally rather than intrauterine, conception was not affected. Thus the consequences of maternal exposure to BVDV at the times of breeding, fertilization, implantation, or early gestation remain somewhat unknown when infection by routes other than intrauterine occur.

Fluids containing BVDV-contaminated fetal bovine serum used for embryo transfer also can serve as a source of infection in susceptible cattle and reproductive failure. The potential consequences of PI embryo donors or PI recipients currently dictate testing of animals to be used for these purposes in embryo transfer.

Diagnosis

In classic cases with fever, diarrhea, mucosal lesions, and digital lesions, diagnosis may be made with confidence based on the clinical signs. Unfortunately this represents a distinct minority of the cases. Clinicians must remember that even in epidemic acute disease <50% of infected cattle may have detectable lesions on clinical examination. In addition, because most cattle infected by strains of BVDV have subclinical or mild infections, signs suggestive of BVDV may be absent. Specific physical examination findings are limited to oral mucosal lesions and digital lesions. Such lesions may be obvious in superinfected PI animals having all of the signs of severe BVD ("mucosal disease") but may be subtle or absent in seronegative animals experiencing acute BVDV infection. Mucosal lesions also may lag behind nonspecific early signs of fever, depression, and reduced milk production. Whenever BVDV infection is suspected, a methodical examination of the oral cavity—aided by focal light illumination—is essential if subtle erosions are to be found. Lesions can be in any area of the oral cavity, but focal erosions of the hard and soft palates, tongue erosions, erosions at gingival border of the incisor teeth, and blunted hyperemic papillae that are eroded at the tip are most commonly seen. Digital lesions are even less common than oral mucosal lesions in field outbreaks of BVDV. When present, coronitis and interdigital erosions are most common. Laminitis usually is observed only secondary to chronic coronitis in PI animals suffering superinfection. Although not widely practiced, endoscopy to see the esophageal mucosa might allow detection of typical linear erosions that are quite common in both acute and chronic infections.

Persistence of high fever or biphasic high fever occurring over more than 7 days is found in many acute BVDV infections. Initially the affected animal may not appear seriously ill and may be thought to have a "respiratory virus." If, however, fever persists and is unresponsive to antibiotics, these same cattle may show more overt anorexia, depression, and dehydration after several days. Diarrhea and mucosal lesions are more common at this time. Few diseases of dairy cattle cause the profound and complete anorexia observed in BVDV-infected cattle having mucosal and gastrointestinal lesions. Oral erosions, esophageal erosions, forestomach erosions, and lower gastrointestinal lesions contribute

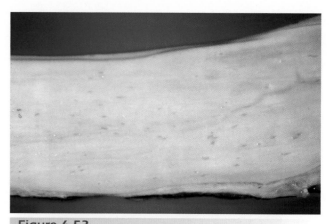

Figure 6-53

Multifocal linear erosions of the esophageal mucosa caused by acute BVDV infection.

to patient pain, discomfort, and subsequent anorexia (Figure 6-53). Salivation and bruxism also may be observed in these patients.

Bleeding associated with fever and diarrhea in several calves or cows should raise the suspicion of thrombocytopenia associated with acute BVDV infection; it necessitates confirmation of both BVDV infection through isolation and thrombocytopenia through taking platelet counts. Similarly herd reproductive problems such as abortions, mummified fetuses, or dramatically reduced conception rates should be grounds for ruling BVDV in or out as a potential cause. Congenital malformations or lesions in one or a series of calves born within a few weeks or months also should dictate BVDV as part of the differential diagnosis.

Laboratory work may suggest BVDV infection but is not reliable as a sole diagnostic aid. For example, leukopenia characterized by lymphopenia is present in most calves and cattle suffering acute infection with BVDV. Many of these animals are neutropenic as well. Fever of unknown origin coexisting with persistent leukopenia should raise suspicion of acute BVDV but could be mimicked by other diseases.

Without question, the most difficult cases of BVDV infection occur when acute BVDV breaks out concurrently with other pathogens such as *Mannheimia* sp. pneumonia, *Salmonella* sp. enterocolitis, or viral respiratory infections such as IBR or BRSV. In such outbreaks, morbidity and mortality may be exceedingly high, and physical findings and lesions at necropsy are predominated by the non-BVDV diseases. Cattle with acute BVDV infection may have had little time to develop pathognomonic gross lesions consistent with BVDV before dying from their concurrent diseases because the transient immune suppression of cellular defense mechanisms during acute BVDV infection frequently predisposes to concurrent opportunistic infection and alters normal immune responses to these opportunists. Necropsy findings in such cases identify overwhelming bronchopneumonia (*Mannheimia* sp.) respiratory pathology consistent with IBR or BRSV, or severe enterocolitis caused by *Salmonella* sp. Lesions consistent with BVDV infections may be absent or only present in a minority of the fatal cases. The temptation for the clinician and pathologist is to accept these gross lesions as sufficient evidence of the primary cause and thus fail to submit samples for viral isolation.

Similarly some PI calves or yearlings that are chronic poor-doers and have chronic pneumonia, ringworm lesions, chronic or intermittent diarrhea, chronic parasitism, chronic pinkeye, or other lesions that have not responded to conventional therapy may be written off as having illness caused by the more obvious bacterial infection if viral lesions are not present or missed. Once again, diagnostic testing to demonstrate the presence of BVDV in the animal is essential for positive diagnosis.

Although high mortality calf diarrhea outbreaks are more typically caused by *E. coli*, rotavirus, coronavirus, cryptosporidium, and *Salmonella* sp., occasional outbreaks may have concurrent BVDV infection, and viral isolation should be a part of the diagnostic material submitted from both live and necropsied calves in such cases. The differential diagnosis for BVDV infection is lengthy and depends somewhat on the clinical signs present in the affected herd. Acute infections characterized by diarrhea and fever must be differentiated from salmonellosis and other causes of enteritis by bacterial fecal cultures and blood cultures. Abortion epidemics must be differentiated from other bacterial, viral, and protozoan causes of abortion. When hemorrhages are present along with signs of fever and diarrhea, BVDV must be differentiated from bracken fern intoxication, disseminated intravascular coagulation (DIC), or other coagulopathies and certain mycotoxicoses.

Other mucosal diseases such as BTV and vesicular diseases—both endemic and exotic—must be considered in unusual cases and may necessitate consultation with federal regulatory veterinarians if confusion exists as to the definitive diagnosis.

Concurrent bacterial, viral, or parasitic diseases may confuse or mask the presence of BVDV infection. Whenever multiple animals fail to respond to conventional therapy for suspected or confirmed bacterial infection, the possibility of BVDV infection should be investigated. Weak or unthrifty PI calves must be differentiated from bacterial septicemia, selenium deficiency, and enteric pathogens. The source of illness in chronic "poor-doers" or unthrifty PI calves or yearlings with multiple problems must be differentiated from BLAD, chronic internal abscesses, malnutrition, parasitism, and chronic pneumonia or enteritis.

Because of the variability in clinical signs of BVDV infection, the only absolute proof of BVDV infection is diagnostic testing to demonstrate the presence of virus in tissues or blood. Tracheal wash samples may contain virus in some live calves, and tissues such as intestine, lymph nodes, spleen, and lung may demonstrate virus on necropsy specimens. The presence of virus in blood can be confirmed through submission of whole blood samples for viral isolation from the buffy coat or for detection of viral genetic material through PCR. Antigen-capture ELISA (AC-ELISA), which detects virus in serum, can also be used on adults and calves over 6 months of age. AC-ELISA is considered less reliable in younger calves because colostral antibody may bind to the virus in the blood and limit the ability of antibodies on the ELISA plate to bind to, and therefore detect, the virus. Further, AC-ELISA may not be able to detect the low levels of viremia in some acute infections, so this test may lack sensitivity relative to other viral detection methods for acute cases. In young calves with colostral antibodies against BVDV, PCR on whole blood is the preferred diagnostic test. Alternatively, skin biopsy (usually ear notches) in formalin or kept cold in saline (check with the diagnostic laboratory) can be submitted for immunohistochemical staining, virus isolation, AC-ELISA, or PCR. Ear notch testing is the preferred test for PI animals because virus antigen is consistently found in the ear skin of those animals at any age. In acute infection of immunocompetent adults, detectable viremia persists for up to 2 weeks. On rare occasions, acutely infected, immunocompetent animals may remain viremic up to 30 to 40 days. The period of viremia tends to be much shorter in subclinically infected animals.

Serology, despite limitations in PI animals, may be helpful when seroconversion can be demonstrated following illness; many animals possess titers >512 following a recent herd epidemic. Paired sera can be obtained at a 14-day interval from animals with clinical signs and/or their penmates; serologic testing for both type 1 and type 2 BVDV should be performed. Obviously serum titers representing neutralizing antibody levels may be greatly influenced by vaccinations and natural infection. Antibody titers from recently infected, immunocompetent animals are often indistinguishable from vaccination-induced titers.

Positive viral isolation coupled with low or nonexistent neutralizing antibody levels suggest acute infection (immunocompetent animal) or persistent infection with BVDV (immunotolerant animal). Generally, immunocompetent animals will seroconvert and clear viremia within 2 to 4 weeks, whereas PI animals remain viremic with low or nonexistent titers to the homologous strain.

PI animals can be detected by virus isolation or PCR performed on whole blood, and skin biopsies can be submitted for immunohistochemistry, virus isolation, AC-ELISA, or PCR. A positive result on any of these tests may simply reflect acute infection in a normal animal, so PI status is technically confirmed by repeat testing and detection of the virus 3 to 4 weeks after the initial positive result. Animals confirmed as PI should be culled or well isolated from the remainder of the herd because they serve as a constant source of high viral challenge for their herdmates. Again, on occasion, acutely infected, immunocompetent (non-PI) animals can remain viremic for 30 to 40 days. Delaying the second test for 6 weeks may be preferred if the tested animals are of particularly high value; in such cases, false incrimination of an animal as PI would result in significant financial loss. Such animals should be considered PI until proven otherwise by the second test and well isolated from their herdmates. Methods for screening the herd for PI animals are discussed further below in the section on prevention.

Treatment

Cattle with mild clinical disease associated with acute BVDV infection do not require specific therapy but should be offered fresh feed and water and not be subjected to any exogenous stress, transport, or vaccinations. Cattle with specific problems such as diarrhea may require oral or IV fluid therapy if continued diarrhea coupled with relative or absolute anorexia causes dehydration. Clinically ill animals (i.e., those with fever, depression, diarrhea, and dehydration) should be subjected to no extraneous stress and may benefit from prophylactic bactericidal antibiotics to minimize the potential for opportunistic bacterial infections such as pneumonia. Calves with acute BVDV infection are more likely to require supplemental fluids and electrolytes.

In cattle with clinical evidence of bleeding caused by thrombocytopenia, benefit may be derived from fresh whole blood transfusions. Usually 4 L of whole fresh blood collected from a BLV-negative, non-PI-BVDV donor is adequate unless blood loss has caused life-threatening anemia. Other affected cattle in these herds with thrombocytopenic strains of BVDV may merely be observed if clinical bleeding is not apparent. Such cattle should not be subjected to surgical procedures, parenteral injections, or crowding and should have insect populations controlled to avoid multiple insults that could cause clinical bleeding. Clinical bleeding seldom occurs unless platelet counts are $<50,000/\mu l$ and trauma to skin or tissues is excessive. Diarrhea may become bloody in some patients in these herds because inflammatory gastrointestinal lesions may sufficiently irritate the colon to cause bleeding.

Despite the fact that most acute BVDV infections are subclinical, this does not hold true for all field epidemics, and some immunocompetent animals do develop severe illness as a result of acute infection with various BVDV strains and thus may benefit from symptomatic therapy. Acute BVDV can be fatal to immunocompetent calves and adult cattle. Death caused by BVDV does not implicitly confirm superinfection of PI animals. This is especially true when complications such as thrombocytopenia or secondary bacterial or viral infections befall an immunocompetent cow with transiently depressed cellular immune responses resulting from acute BVDV infection.

Corticosteroids and NSAIDs are contraindicated in cattle suffering acute BVDV infection because both categories of drug further predispose to digestive tract erosion and ulceration. Animals that are ingesting feed and water can be treated with judicious doses of aspirin as an antipyretic, but even aspirin reduces cytoprotective prostaglandins in the gastrointestinal tract and kidney to some degree.

Prevention

Effective control of BVDV infection in dairy cattle requires four fundamental steps:
- Improvement of herd immunity through immunization
- Identification and removal of PI animals within the herd
- Screening of new animals for PI status before introduction into the herd
- Implementation of biosecurity practices to prevent fetal exposure to BVDV; in other words, prevention of future PI animals

1. *Improvement of herd immunity through immunization*
The goals of a BVDV immunization program on dairies include (a) prevention or reduction in severity of acute disease in adults and young stock; (b) prevention or reduction of the rate of fetal infection in pregnant heifers and cows; and (c) enhancement of colostral immunity for protection of newborns. Two fundamental challenges to effective vaccination for BVDV exist. First, the broad antigenic diversity of BVDV makes it difficult to create a vaccine that induces immunity to all of the potential strains that a herd may encounter over time. Second, the massive amounts of virus shed by PI animals may result in infection even in immunized cattle. The importance of this second issue cannot be overemphasized. Exposure to viremic animals compromises any effort at complete protection of a herd through immunization, and elimination of PI animals from the herd is *the vital step* in BVDV control.

As of 2004, more than 180 United States Department of Agriculture (USDA)-licensed BVDV vaccines were commercially available. The practitioner must choose between modified-live and inactivated (killed products). Both have advantages and disadvantages, summarized below:

MLVs—advantages:
- Activation of cellular and humoral immunity
- Long duration of immunity
- Good, albeit incomplete, fetal protection; greater than inactivated vaccines

MLVs—disadvantages:
- Potential for transient immunosuppression

- Potentially unsafe for administration to pregnant cattle (not for all products—some have documented safety for use in pregnant animals)
- Colostrum-derived antibodies may block immune response in calves
- Potential for transient ovarian infection and transient impairment of fertility (not to be used in cattle immediately before breeding)
- May induce acute disease in PI cattle—this should not be a deterrent to use, however.
  Inactivated (killed) vaccines—advantages:
- Not immunosuppressive
- No risk of fetal or ovarian infection (safe for administration to pregnant cattle and immediately before breeding)
  Inactivated (killed) vaccines—disadvantages:
- Primarily activate the humoral immune response (less cell-mediated immunity)
- Require more frequent administration (boostering)
- Shorter duration of immunity
- Variable fetal protection (field versus vaccine strain heterogeneity may limit efficacy)

In the past, MLV vaccines were suspected of inducing clinical disease, including persistent infection, because of insufficient attenuation of the virus used in the product and/or live virus contamination of vaccine reagents. With greater testing procedures available for extraneous virus testing, as well as higher standards for reagents such as fetal bovine serum for cell culture systems, the risk of live virus contamination of MLV has been greatly reduced over the past. To ensure that these precautions are used for a given product, safety data and quality control procedures for vaccine production should be requested from manufacturers of MLV vaccines.

A single recommendation for vaccination for dairy herds is unlikely to be uniformly accepted as optimal. This likely reflects different practitioners having different experiences with a variety of different vaccines. It is likely that this variation in professional opinion is because practitioners have been observing a variety of BVDV strains challenging a variety of herds over time. The following guidelines are recommended by us and others:

  Replacement heifers (separated from pregnant cows and heifers): Immunize with a MLV product, ideally containing type 1 and type 2 strains, at 5 to 6 months of age and again 60 days before breeding. This schedule allows replacement heifers to receive two doses of vaccine before they become pregnant and limits potential problems caused by transient ovarian infection by vaccine virus.

  Adult cows: Administer a MLV vaccine with a label claim for safety in pregnant cattle, once annually 2 to 4 weeks before breeding.

Immunosuppression following MLV BVDV vaccination has been documented, so immunization should be timed to occur during periods of relatively low stress and low pathogen challenge.

If killed products are to be used, manufacturer's recommendations should be followed regarding the timing of the priming and booster immunization; the interval for these immunizations is typically 2 to 3 weeks. To maximize antibody spectrum, a product containing inactivated type 1 and type 2 virus should be used, or at least one giving demonstrative cross protection against both. Cows and heifers should receive a booster immunization before breeding, in midgestation/midlactation, and for lactating animals, again at dry-off. Killed products may be optimal for administration to newly purchased, pregnant heifers and cows of unknown previous vaccination status.

Adequately vaccinated cattle should impart passive antibody protection to calves through colostrum—at least against homologous strains of BVDV. This passive protection probably dissipates between 3 and 8 months of age in most instances. Therefore the timing of initial active immunization of calves against BVDV is somewhat controversial. If killed products are used, calves born to vaccinated cows should probably be vaccinated three times—at 12, 14, and 18 weeks of age. Manufacturer's recommendations as regards appropriate intervals between dosing should be followed, but *all* calves or older cattle of questionable immune status must be vaccinated at least twice to establish primary immunity. Semiannual boosters are then recommended.

Modified live vaccines are more likely to be blocked by maternal-derived (colostral) antibody in calves, so delaying administration of the first dose until 5 to 6 months is recommended. If protection of younger calves is desired, killed products may be administered at an interval determined by the label.

A common error in vaccination programs is to give a single killed vaccine to first-calf heifers that have never received previous adequate primary immunization. Management deficiencies allow this mistake to occur more commonly than we realize. Do not assume that dairy farmers have "done it right" and always make directions for use clear-cut when selling vaccine to owners. With more widespread use of computerized records, documentation of proper timing of immunization can be implemented by making BVDV vaccination a recorded "health event" for all cattle.

As dairies become larger, the gap between management and the cow-side worker has widened. What the manager perceives to be the standard operating procedure for vaccination and what occurs when cows and calves are vaccinated may be vastly different. Therefore it is imperative the veterinarian take an active role in training workers on proper vaccine storage, handling, and administration. Personal observation of immunization practices often allows the veterinarian to detect and quickly correct problems. Because labor forces on dairies may turn over rapidly, repeated training sessions on this topic are often required. When necessary, the veterinarian should be willing to assume the role of long-term educator of the workforce.

2. *Identification and removal of PI animals from the herd*

The prevalence of PI animals is thought to vary greatly from dairy to dairy. Data from a few large prevalence studies indicate that PI cattle typically represent approximately 2% or less of the cattle population. Because the virus may be transmitted vertically, even closed herds may have PI animals.

In the past, serologic screening of the herd after immunization was used to attempt to identify PI animals—the concept was these animals, being immunotolerant to BVDV, would tend to have low titers, and low-titered animals could then be targeted for testing by virus isolation to confirm PI status. However, in light of the fact that PI animals may mount an immune response to heterologous field or vaccine strains, this method is unlikely to accurately identify all PI animals and is not currently endorsed.

Tests that detect the presence of virus in the live animal are considered necessary for accurate identification of the PI state. Initially all animals in the herd, regardless of age or apparent health status, should be included for testing. Tests include virus isolation or PCR on whole blood and AC-ELISA, IHC, PCR, or virus isolation on skin biopsies. AC-ELISA should not be used on calves under 6 months of age, owing to potential problems with colostrum-derived antibody interference with viral detection. To prevent confusion between acutely viremic immunocompetent animals and PI animals, it may be necessary to repeat testing on any positive animal 3 to 4 weeks (or, for valuable animals, 30 to 40 days) after the first positive test.

To reduce testing costs on large numbers of animals, certain laboratories offer testing on pooled samples—for example, skin biopsies from multiple animals can be placed together in saline, and PCR can be run on the pooled sample to detect the presence of BVDV. Alternatively, composite milk samples can be pooled together and checked for the presence of virus by PCR or virus isolation. Bulk tank samples or string samples can also be used to screen large numbers of lactating cows. Current recommendations state that pooled milk samples should represent fewer than 400 animals to optimize chances of detection of PIs. It is best to check with the regional veterinary diagnostic laboratory for the preferred number of samples to be pooled, shipment requirements, and so on. Obviously a positive result on a pooled sample would require follow-up testing of the constituent individuals to identify the viremic or PI animal(s).

On rare occasions, infected bulls may shed virus only in the semen. Therefore to cover this rare, yet complication-rich scenario, bulls that test negative for virus in blood or skin biopsy should ideally have their semen screened by virus isolation or PCR.

Ethical considerations regarding the fate of PI animals are worthy of mention. Sale of animals known to be PI at livestock auctions is simply unethical because these animals serve as virus-producing machines that expose many other animals, causing potentially devastating disease on the farms of the unknowing purchasers. The most ethical practice is to euthanize these animals on the premises, although otherwise healthy animals may be considered for slaughter. To our knowledge, no studies currently exist on the persistence of BVDV in properly composted carcasses, but data on the survivability of viruses related to BVDV indicate that long-term environmental persistence is unlikely. Alternatively, carcasses of PI animals can be removed from the premises for rendering.

Once all animals in the herd have been tested and PI animals removed, testing should focus on the calves born to gestating, non-PI females. Once these calves have been tested and PIs removed, testing should focus on new introductions, show animals, semen and embryos, and heifers raised off-site (see numbers 3 and 4 below). The producer must understand, however, that introduction of a novel strain of BVDV onto a farm may result in fetal infection in non-PI, pregnant females, warranting eventual testing of their offspring.

3. *Screening of new animals for PI status before introduction into the herd*

Reducing risk of introduction of BVDV is best accomplished by avoiding the purchase of untested cattle. Without question, the greatest disasters resulting from acute BVDV have followed the purchase of assembled cattle from sales to increase herd size. These purchased animals may be PI. Alternatively, they may be acutely infected—in either case, they represent sources of new virus to the herd. In addition, if newly purchased cows and/or heifers were exposed to BVDV and became viremic in early pregnancy, they may be carrying PI fetuses. Therefore for optimal herd protection, purchased adults should be tested before introduction into the herd; later, *the offspring that they were carrying at the time of purchase* should be tested for PI status because PI calves can be born to immunocompetent dams. Whenever possible, new herd introductions should be tested and well isolated from the remainder of the herd for 4 to 6 weeks—during this period, any PI animals in the group of new introductions can be identified and removed, and any acutely infected animals can be given adequate time to recover. Any contact between isolated new introductions and the remainder of the herd, even at fence lines, should be avoided during this period.

Tests to detect virus should be used on newly purchased cattle. Virus isolation, PCR, immunohistochemistry, or AC-ELISA on blood or skin biopsies can be used. Pooling of samples can be considered when large numbers of animals are to be introduced (see number 2 above). Collection of samples for testing for other diseases in newly purchased stock (e.g., Johne's disease, *Mycoplasma* spp. mastitis) can be performed at the same time.

4. *Implementation of biosecurity practices to prevent fetal exposure to BVDV*

Fetal infection leading to the PI state is a critical control point because PI animals represent a massive source of viral challenge for the herd. Even with good vaccination practices, all immunity is finite, and overwhelming viral challenge could theoretically lead to transplacental passage of virus even in immunized, pregnant females. Therefore protection of pregnant cows and heifers from exposure to high viral challenge is a critical goal of BVDV control within a herd biosecurity program.

Contact with cattle outside the herd should be eliminated or minimized, even at fence lines. Cows and heifers in the first trimester of pregnancy should be considered the most susceptible to creation of the fetal PI state. These animals should be located on the farm in the area that is most protected from contact with outside cattle, new introductions, and show cattle. Pen allocation and pen milking sequence should be critiqued and, if necessary, changed to maximize protection of these animals. Contact of these animals with ill cattle should be minimized whenever possible.

Heifers raised and bred at heifer-raising operations warrant particularly careful scrutiny in a BVDV control program. Heifers from multiple herds are often raised on such operations, and viral challenge from PI animals or acute BVDV infections on that operation could easily induce fetal infection in pregnant heifers. Therefore young heifers should be tested before transport to heifer-raising operations; if this is not feasible, prompt testing after arrival on such operations is warranted. In addition, all calves born to heifers raised off-site should be considered potential PI animals and tested after birth.

Cattle taken to shows should be considered another source of novel virus on a farm. In the ideal world, show cattle should be tested and confirmed to be non-PI before being taken to shows or sales—this is simply a good ethical practice intended to protect other animals and producers. Show cattle should also be well immunized to limit the likelihood of them developing acute infection while off the premises. Given the shortcomings of vaccines in protecting against the tremendous number of strains of BVDV, even well-vaccinated show cattle should be considered potentially exposed to novel BVDV at shows or sales and ideally kept isolated from the home herd for 4 to 6 weeks on return. If exposed at shows, pregnant show cows and heifers may experience viremia of sufficient magnitude to induce fetal infection, and their calves should be subsequently tested for PI status.

Most reputable sources of semen, embryos, and fetal calf serum have BVDV testing strategies in place. However, nothing should be taken for granted, and the individuals or companies providing bull semen and/or embryos should be requested to provide documentation of their current control programs and quality control measures on reagents. Control of BVDV in embryo and semen production operations has been recently reviewed. In short, acutely or persistently infected bulls, embryo donors, and embryo recipients are potential animal sources of BVDV. Animals within these populations that shed large amounts of virus may cause fetal infection in others, so BVDV testing of all animals with which bulls, embryo donors, and embryo recipients come in contact during semen/embryo collection, transfer, and pregnancy is necessary. Rarely, infected bulls may shed virus only in semen (i.e., test negative on blood or skin IHC), and semen testing by PCR or virus isolation is considered optimal. All animal-origin reagents used in embryo transfer or in vitro fertilization (including semen and oocytes) should be screened for the presence of BVDV.

Winter Dysentery

Etiology

The etiologic agent responsible for winter dysentery has remained elusive for as long as the disease has existed. In the northern hemisphere, the disease is characterized by explosive herd outbreaks of diarrhea between the months of October and April. *Campylobacter fetus jejuni* long was suspected as a cause, but Koch's postulates never were confirmed. MacPherson, however, was able to infect susceptible cattle using filtered feces from infected cows and therefore believed a virus was involved. Bovine coronavirus has been demonstrated in feces and colonic epithelium of affected cattle, and the same strain that causes diarrhea in calves has been used to experimentally create winter dysentery in adult cows. In Europe, Breda virus (Torovirus) has been associated with winter dysentery outbreaks.

Winter dysentery is of economic importance primarily because of production losses both during the acute outbreak and because some cows do not return to previous production levels for the remainder of that lactation. Death losses are minimal but do occur—almost always in first-calf heifers that develop hemorrhagic diarrhea.

The disease is highly contagious and can spread easily from an affected herd to unaffected herds via fomites—both inanimate and animate. Veterinarians, milk tank drivers, inseminators, salespeople, and other farm visitors frequently are blamed for spreading the disease. Newly purchased cattle and cattle attending shows during the fall, winter, or early spring also can be infected and instigate a herd outbreak. Herds experiencing winter dysentery subsequently appear immune for 2 to 3 years, based on clinical impressions that many herds have an outbreak every third year. Relative age-related resistance is observed, but this protection is incomplete. Cattle infected for the first time tend to have more severe clinical signs than those previously affected.

Clinical Signs

Signs include acute diarrhea in 10% to 30% of the cows within a herd, followed by similar signs in another 20% to 70% of the animals within the ensuing 7 to 10 days. The diarrhea is explosive and appears semi-fluid, dark brown in color, has a pea-soup consistency, is malodorous, and forms bubbles as puddles of manure are formed. Most affected cows have decreased appetite, production losses of 10% to 50%, and become mildly to moderately dehydrated. Some develop cool peripheral parts and sluggish rumen motility suggestive of hypocalcemia. Severely affected animals—especially first lactation cattle experiencing the disease for the first time—have hemorrhagic enterocolitis with dysentery and fresh blood clots in the feces. Tenesmus may be present in these animals, and blood loss anemia may develop. A soft moist cough is apparent in several of the affected animals, but the lungs auscult normally in these cattle. Fever usually precedes clinical signs by 24 to 48 hours, and experienced clinicians will detect fever in apparently healthy herdmates that have not yet developed diarrhea. Fevers are mild, ranging from 103.0 to 105.0° F (39.44 to 40.56° C). Some cattle have mild fever 103.0 to 104.0° F (39.44 to 40.0° C) accompanying the onset of diarrhea. Herd production decreases commensurate with incidence and severity of disease. Affected cows, especially those in mid or late lactation, may never return to previous production levels for the remainder of their current lactation.

Diagnosis

Winter dysentery must be differentiated from dietary diarrhea, coccidiosis, BVDV, and salmonellosis. Dietary diarrhea seldom causes fever and usually is associated with feed changes. Coccidiosis can cause diarrhea, dysentery, whole blood clots, and tenesmus in heifers and first lactation cows but seldom affects multiparous cows. Fecal smears and flotation allow a diagnosis of coccidiosis. Usually BVDV infection causes leukopenia, higher fever, more prolonged disease, and could be ruled out by viral isolation and paired serum samples. The most likely differential diagnosis is salmonellosis caused by type E or mildly pathogenic types of B or C *Salmonella* spp. Salmonellosis of these types can cause fever—frequently preceding the onset of diarrhea—and a variable number of animals may develop diarrhea that contains blood, fibrin strands, or mucus. A neutropenia with left shift in the leukogram would suggest acute salmonellosis but is not a constant finding. Fecal

culture obtained from several acute cases is the only way to rule out salmonellosis.

Confirmation of the presumptive diagnosis requires demonstration of bovine coronavirus in feces by electron microscopy, ELISA, or PCR. Immunohistochemical staining of colonic tissue may be used on necropsy specimens in acute cases.

Treatment

For most affected cattle, supportive treatment with oral astringents remains the time-tested mode of therapy. Occasional high-producing cattle require parenteral calcium solutions to counteract secondary hypocalcemia or treatment of ketosis secondary to reduced appetite. Oral fluids and electrolytes may be necessary for moderately dehydrated cattle. All cattle should have access to salt and to fresh water.

Severely dehydrated cows occasionally require IV fluid therapy, and first-calf heifers that become anemic because of blood loss require fresh whole blood transfusions in some instances. Cattle with tenesmus may necessitate epidural anesthesia to allow rest and reduce rectal and colonic irritation.

Treatment usually is only necessary for 1 to 5 days, by which time most affected cows have recovered their appetites and normal manure consistency. Unfortunately the disease often dwindles through the herd for 7 to 14 days, such that new cases are still appearing at a time when most cattle are recovered. Although there is no proven efficacy to preventive measures, practicing sound herd biosecurity regarding new herd introductions and show cattle may reduce the likelihood of outbreaks (see descriptions in section on BVDV). Further, disinfected boots and equipment should be required for all visitors to a dairy, as well as clean outer garments. The efficacy of immunization with commercially available coronavirus vaccines is currently unknown.

Campylobacter jejuni

Etiology

Campylobacter jejuni, formerly *Vibrio jejuni*, is a gram-negative, curved to spiral motile rod capable of causing enterocolitis in many species, including humans, in which the organism is one of the major causes of bacterial enterocolitis. *C. jejuni* may be present in the normal intestinal flora of many domestic animals and people but is found with greater incidence in diarrhea patients. Because of its ubiquitous nature, the significance of isolation of *C. jejuni* from diarrheic feces sometimes is hard to interpret. However, isolation of *C. jejuni* coupled with failure to isolate other pathogens such as *Salmonella* sp., *Clostridium* sp., or enteric viruses should be considered significant.

Diarrhea and other clinical signs vary from inapparent or mild to fulminant and may be influenced by concurrent diseases, stress, inoculum, strain of *C. jejuni*, other enteric pathogens, and other factors. This variation is highlighted by the reported profound differences observed between experimental infection of gnotobiotic calves and experimental infections of calves with normal gastrointestinal flora. Gnotobiotic calves had mild catarrhal enteritis with minimal clinical signs, whereas fever, chronic diarrhea for up to 2 weeks, and some degree of dysentery were observed in nongnotobiotic calves. Although most experimental infections have been completed in calves, adult cattle are thought to be susceptible as well. Infection in people can occur at any age.

The strain of *C. jejuni* and other factors may influence the site of colonization within the intestine, but most strains affect both the small intestine and colon. *C. jejuni* produces a cholera-like enterotoxin that is an important component of pathogenicity. The organism is mucosa associated but does not appear to be invasive—at least in experimental studies.

Clinical Signs and Diagnosis

Mild or inapparent cases yield little or no detectable signs. Clinical patients with severe signs of diarrhea, fever, dehydration, anorexia, cessation of milk production, and dysentery tend to be sporadic or only represent a low percentage of cattle within a herd. Adult cows and calves are at risk.

The signs are nonspecific and require differentiation from those indicating salmonellosis, coccidiosis, BVDV infection, and other enteric pathogens. Isolation of *C. jejuni* from diarrheic feces and ruling out other enteric pathogens are essential for diagnosis. Enterocolitis resulting from *C. jejuni* seldom is confused with winter dysentery because of low morbidity in the former contrasted with high morbidity in the latter. Salmonellosis represents the primary differential diagnosis.

Treatment

Calves or cattle with severe diarrhea or dysentery may require 7 to 14 days for recovery. Some diarrhea may persist despite improved vital signs in recovering patients. Oral or IV fluids may be required, and it is best to select fluids following blood acid-base and electrolyte analysis. In humans, antibiotics such as erythromycin, tetracycline, and aminoglycosides are most effective, whereas penicillin, ampicillin, cephalosporins, and trimethoprim-sulfa combinations appear ineffective. Antibiotic susceptibilities are not known for *C. jejuni* infections in cattle and would be best determined by fecal culture and susceptibility results.

Control

Because animals and animal products, such as unpasteurized milk and improperly cooked meat, usually are blamed for *C. jejuni* enterocolitis in humans, a positive diagnosis of *C. jejuni* diarrhea in cattle justifies public health concerns. Infected cattle may throw off the infection over several weeks or may remain carriers. Obviously many cattle (and people) are asymptomatic carriers so that wide-scale herd testing serves no purpose. However, veterinarians should advise caution in handling infected cattle and avoidance of unpasteurized milk on farms where the problem is confirmed. *C. jejuni* will grow in milk and may arrive in milk from a septicemic spread but is more likely to contaminate milk because of environmental contact.

Enterotoxemia in Adult Dairy Cattle

Etiology

Enterotoxemia thought to be caused by *C. perfringens* has been observed as a sporadic cause of acute death in adult dairy cattle. Some herds have had endemic problems with more than one cow being found dead or agonal over a few months. Premonitory signs are not observed, and, as in calves, the condition is believed to be related to diets exceptionally rich in protein and energy. *C. perfringens* organisms present in the intestinal tract take advantage of such rich diets and proliferate to produce excessive exotoxins—especially beta-toxin. Although *C. perfringens* and toxin have been identified from acute necropsy specimens in adult cattle, it is not known whether a particular strain of the organism is responsible for the adult cow disease.

Signs

Signs are minimal, and most affected cows are found down, agonal, or already dead. Diarrhea may be observed or the animal simply may have abdominal distention, colic, and depression. Another clinical syndrome is one that causes fever, anorexia, small-volume diarrhea, and death, with severe abomasal edema found at necropsy.

Diagnosis

Fresh necropsy specimens must be obtained if *C. perfringens* is suspected as a cause of acute death. Necropsy lesions, as in calves infected by *C. perfringens* type C, may be minimal but might include small intestinal fluid distention, serosal hemorrhages, and an edematous mesentery. Feces and small intestinal content should be cultured for *C. perfringens;* if possible, luminal contents should be tested for the presence of toxins. Samples should be transported in a cooled but unfrozen state. A complete necropsy to rule out other causes of acute death is imperative because the diagnosis of *C. perfringens* enterotoxemia is made by exclusion of other diseases such as peracute, virulent salmonellosis.

Treatment and Control

Treatment is seldom possible, but if specific *C. perfringens* organism and toxins are identified, vaccination with appropriate toxoids would be indicated.

Malignant Catarrhal Fever

Etiology

MCF has been observed in domestic and wild ruminants worldwide and is caused by a group of gamma herpesviruses. It is a severe lymphoproliferative disease characterized by high fever, corneal edema, mucosal erosions, and lymph node enlargement in clinically affected animals. Lymphocytic vasculitis of a variety of tissues is the classic microscopic lesion. Many ruminant species and pigs are susceptible to MCF viruses, and losses have been incurred on dairies, feed lots, ranches, game farms, zoos, and deer meat-raising facilities. In Africa, the causative agent has been isolated and identified as alcelaphine herpesvirus-1 (AHV1). The term alcelaphine relates to the subfamily of *Bovidae, Alcelaphinae,* in which wildebeest, hartebeest, and topi are classified. These species are thought to be the reservoir. The virus apparently is highly cell associated but can be spread during stress such as parturition or shipment and may be free in fetal fluids or young of wildebeest. At those times when the virus is released, it becomes infectious for cattle.

In other parts of the world, including the United States, MCF is termed "sheep-associated" because sheep appear to be the most likely reservoir of infection. Ovine herpesvirus type 2 (OvHV2) has been identified from ruminants with MCF using PCR, and seroconversion of cattle with MCF to OvHV2 can be demonstrated using competitive inhibition ELISA (CI-ELISA). However, the virus has not yet been isolated and grown in tissue culture, so this virus is currently considered a likely, but not definitive, cause of the disease. Sheep-associated MCF occurs in cattle, bison, pigs, deer, elk, and moose.

Most sporadic or epidemic MCF in cattle has been associated with proximity to sheep. Infection is widespread in North American sheep, and ovine infection is almost always asymptomatic. Cattle and sheep do not have to interact or be in common pastures for the disease to appear. Cases can be observed at any time of year. In addition, some cattle that develop MCF have no historical direct or indirect exposure to sheep. Asymptomatic, persistent infections with OvHV2 in cattle may occur, and these infections may or may not develop into clinical MCF. Hence, the incubation period for this disease has been difficult to ascertain, with infected cattle developing disease weeks to months after exposure. This may explain why some cases do not seem linked to exposure to sheep. In a recent study, most dairy cattle exposed to OvHV2 under natural conditions (close proximity to a sheep feed lot) developed asymptomatic infection rather than overt signs of MCF.

Clinical Signs

Most cattle affected with MCF have dramatic clinical signs of multisystemic inflammatory disease. A great deal of variation is possible, however, and has caused many authors to categorize MCF based on predominant signs. Such categorization is difficult because significant overlap and intermediary clinical situations occur frequently. Sporadic cases are most common in cattle, but herd epidemics have been described in several areas of the United States.

Fever is common in all cases and is high (105.0 to 108.0° F/40.56 to 42.2° C). Peracute, acute, chronic persistent, and chronic intermittent cases all have fever that usually persists as long as signs are observed. Lymphadenopathy is another finding that is common to most cases. All other signs result from a severe vasculitis that affects many organs but may affect some organs more than others in individual patients. Vasculitis is profound and histologically associated with lymphocytic infiltrates that occasionally can be so extensive as to suggest lymphoreticular neoplasia. Vasculitis affects the gastrointestinal tract, central nervous system, eyes, urinary system, liver, skin, upper respiratory tract, and other areas.

Peracute cases may die within 1 to 2 days because of overwhelming viremia and vasculitis of all major organs and yet have minimal clinical signs other than fever, lymphadenopathy, depression, and prostration. Terminal neurologic signs are possible as a result of central nervous system vasculitis.

The classical "head and eye" form of MCF is most common in sporadic cases. This form is characterized by persistent high fever (105.0 to 108.0° F/40.56 to 42.22° C), lymphadenopathy, severe nasal and oral mucosal lesions, ocular lesions, and remarkable depression (Figure 6-54). In acute cases, extensive mucosal lesions may make it appear as though the animal has had its mucous membranes burned. Frequently the muzzle and

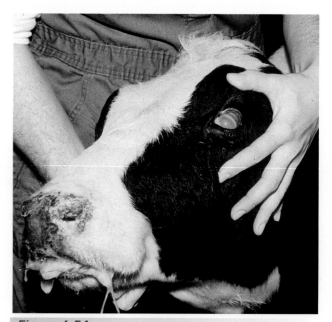

Figure 6-54

Adult Holstein cow with the head and eye form of MCF.

large regions of the oral mucosa appear hyperemic and have a blanched necrotic epithelium that sloughs to leave erosions and ulcers if the patient survives long enough for this to occur. The muzzle may appear dried or sunburned, and the superficial epithelium subsequently may slough away. Sloughing of the nasal mucosa may result in diphtheric crusts that occlude the airways. Salivation and copious nasal discharge are typical findings. On occasion, oral and nasal lesions are present in the caudal aspects of the mucosal surfaces, out of visual range during physical examination.

Bilateral ophthalmitis results from vasculitis throughout the eyes that spares only the choroid in most cases. Corneal edema is the most common lesion and occurs because of inflammatory changes and exudative cellular deposits on the corneal endothelium that disrupt this layer, thereby allowing overhydration of the corneal stroma. The corneal edema typically begins at the limbus within 2 to 5 days after the onset of fever. The corneal edema then rapidly spreads to the center of the cornea. This centripetal spread of edema distinguishes the ocular features of MCF from contagious keratoconjunctivitis (pinkeye). A severe anterior uveitis, scleritis, conjunctivitis, and retinitis usually coexist. As in other regions of the body, mononuclear cell infiltrates appear in the eyes. Depression is profound because of central nervous system vasculitis, and CSF confirms a dramatic inflammation characterized by increased protein values and mononuclear cell pleocytosis. Other neurologic signs are possible. Skin lesions and inflammation of the coronary bands and horn basal epithelium also are possible in those patients that survive more than a few days. The clinical course for most "head and eye" MCF cattle is 48 to 96 hours, although some cases may survive for a longer time and a few had even been reported to survive.

Acute MCF also may cause severe enterocolitis with diarrhea being a predominant sign. Such cases also are febrile and can have some degree of mucosal lesions, ocular lesions, and other organ involvement. This "enteric form" is again a relative designation because patients frequently have other detectable lesions in addition to diarrhea. However, severe diarrhea may be the most apparent sign and thus may confuse the diagnosis of MCF with BVDV, rinderpest, or other enteric diseases. In bison, enteric signs tend to predominate in acute cases.

Mild forms of MCF also have been observed. The broad spectrum of potential and observed clinical signs in MCF also makes it likely that some cattle suffer subclinical mild disease, recover, and respond immunologically to the causative virus. Although previously considered to be a highly fatal disease, up to 50% of MCF cases may survive the acute disease to either recover or become chronic cases.

A rare acute form of the disease presents as a severe hemorrhagic cystitis with hematuria, stranguria, and polyuria. Cattle having this form of acute infection have high fever and only survive 1 to 4 days. Although the most striking clinical signs are limited to the urinary system, histologic evidence of vasculitis and lymphocytic infiltration are generalized on necropsy study.

Chronic MCF is characterized by a long clinical course—usually weeks—of high fever, erosive and ulcerative mucosal lesions, bilateral uveitis, papular or hyperkeratotic skin lesions, lymphadenopathy, and digital lesions (Figures 6-55 and 6-56). Mucosal lesions tend to be severe, slough tissue, and cause salivation and inappetence (Figure 6-57). Some chronic cases recover only to relapse weeks to months later. Such cases appear healthy between episodes, but recurrence of fever and mucosal, ocular, and skin lesions is debilitating. It is rare for chronic MCF cattle to recover completely and survive.

Diagnosis

Given the wide variability of possible clinical signs of MCF in cattle, differential diagnosis could include many diseases. Head and eye lesions could be confused with severe IBR respiratory and conjunctival infections because corneal edema can occur in some severely affected IBR conjunctivitis cases. However, IBR usually is epidemic and affected animals have characteristic mucosal plaques present on the palpebral conjunctiva and nasal mucosa. Most mucosal diseases such as BVDV, BTV, VSV,

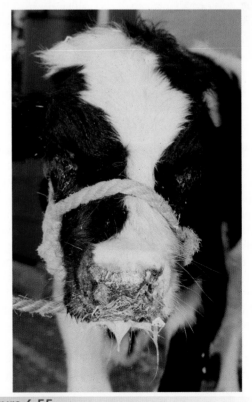

Figure 6-55

A 6-month-old Holstein bull with chronic MCF.

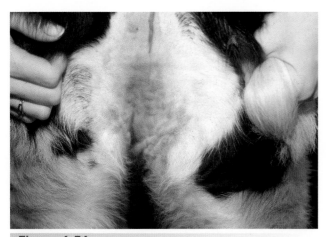

Figure 6-56

Papular dermatitis in the escutcheon region in a calf with chronic MCF.

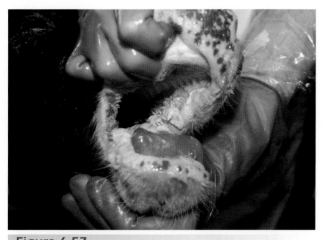

Figure 6-57

Chronic necrotic oral and lingual lesions in a yearling heifer with chronic recurrent MCF.

and FMD may need to be considered depending on the duration, location, and severity of signs. Cattle having severe diarrhea but minimal mucosal lesions could be confused with BVDV or rinderpest infections.

Acute bracken fern intoxications, bacillary hemoglobinuria, and other causes of hematuria may be considered in acute MCF characterized by hemorrhagic cystitis. Acute or subacute mucosal lesions that cause sloughing of muzzle epithelium could be confused with primary or secondary (hepatic) photosensitization.

When ocular lesions are present in MCF patients, the diagnosis is made easier because none of the other mucosal diseases cause severe uveitis and ophthalmitis. As mentioned, IBR conjunctivitis can have corneal edema in severe cases, but intraocular inflammation does not occur with IBR. There are no ocular lesions in acute or chronic postnatal BVDV infections. The acute mucosal lesions of MCF also are unique in classic cases. The oral

mucosa is diffusely inflamed and appears as though the patient drank boiling water. The muzzle mucosa appears burnt, crusty, or eroded in these same patients. Unfortunately these classic mucosal lesions do not occur in all MCF patients, and patients with multifocal erosions or ulcers can be more difficult to differentiate from those with BVDV and other mucosal diseases.

High fever (105.0 to 108.0° F/40.56 to 42.22° C) that persists through the entire clinical course is characteristic of most acute MCF cases. Chronic MCF cases also will have persistent fever that may or may not be as high as that found in acute cases.

Nervous signs suggest a diagnosis of MCF because central nervous system involvement is rare with other mucosal diseases. However, high fever and terminal prostration are common in fatal cases of most mucosal diseases and could be confused with neurologic signs.

Clinical diagnosis of MCF is best supported by CSF analysis. The characteristic CSF mononuclear cell pleocytosis and elevated protein value found in MCF patients is useful whenever the patient's clinical signs dictate consideration of differential diagnoses. Confirmation of sheep-associated MCF requires demonstration of viral genome in the blood through PCR analysis of white cells obtained from a whole blood (EDTA) sample. Depending on the primers used, PCR for OvHV2 is specific for that virus and will not detect the genome of AHV1. Alternatively, CI-ELISA can be used to detect MCF antibodies, but this test may not be positive at the time of initial clinical signs. CI-ELISA detects antibodies to both OvHV2 and AHV1 and cannot currently distinguish between wildebeest- and sheep-associated MCF.

Histopathology allows detection of pathognomonic diffuse vasculitis with lymphocytic infiltrates in many organs, including the gastrointestinal tract, urinary tract, liver, adrenals, central nervous system, skin, and eyes. Necrotizing vasculitis is present in lymphoid tissues.

Prevention

Prevention of MCF centers on limiting exposure to infected wildebeest and sheep. Airborne transfer of OvHV2 is suspected to occur over a distance of more than 70 meters, so segregation of cattle from sheep by greater distances may be protective. For cattle and bison herds, Callan recommends a separation distance of 1 mile from sheep. Carrier (asymptomatically infected) cattle may be identified by CI-ELISA on serum and PCR on whole blood. The CI-ELISA test detects seroconversion in exposed individuals that may, owing to varying viral loads in blood, be intermittently negative by PCR on whole blood. Alternatively, acutely infected animals may be positive on PCR but negative on CI-ELISA owing to the delays inherent in generation of an immune response. Therefore application of both tests may provide optimal sensitivity for detecting infected cattle. Although OvHV2 DNA can be detected in milk, nasal secretions, and ocular secretions of asymptomatic and clinically affected cattle, this viral DNA appears to be cell-associated and does not pose a significant risk for horizontal transmission. Transmission from cattle or bison to other animals has not been demonstrated and is considered likely to be a rare event, if it occurs at all.

Johne's Disease (Paratuberculosis)

Etiology

M. avium subspecies *paratuberculosis* (MAP), the cause of paratuberculosis—better known as Johne's disease—is an acid-fast, gram-positive, intracellular bacterium. The organism is extremely hardy and can remain viable in the environment for up to 1 year, given sufficient moisture and cool temperatures. Extremes of heat and dryness decrease viability.

Johne's disease is a chronic insidious disease of cattle characterized by a majority of subclinical infections with no evidence of infection. Debilitated animals having chronic diarrhea, weight loss, and hypoproteinemia during the terminal stages of the disease represent a small minority of infected animals (<5%). Typically infection occurs most commonly through fecal-oral contamination during the early perinatal period. Infected fecal material is ingested by calves either when nursing the dam or by licking environmental materials contaminated with manure. Older calves have a more variable outcome following infection, and larger doses of MAP are required to cause infections that lead to later onset of clinical signs. Furthermore, young adult or adult cattle seem to have even greater age-related resistance. However, this resistance is relative rather than absolute, and some experimental infections of older calves and adults have been reported. Factors including concurrent diseases, genetics, environment, and other stressors may contribute to increased susceptibility to infection. Although difficult to define, certain breeds and genetic lines within these breeds have been thought to be susceptible to Johne's disease. Guernseys, for example, appear to have inherent susceptibility. Unfortunately it is difficult to separate true genetic weakness from massive exposure to organisms in infected herds.

In addition to the fecal-oral route of infection, in utero infection of fetuses harbored by infected dams is possible with an estimated 25% of fetuses from dams with clinical signs infected in utero.

Similarly, infected macrophages in milk from infected cows have been suggested as a source of infection for calves. The percentage of infected cows that shed *M. paratuberculosis* in milk varies with the stage of infection. In utero and milk containing MAP occur more commonly in heavy shedders and cattle with clinical signs of Johne's disease. Semen and reproductive tracts from infected bulls also have yielded *M. paratuberculosis,* but semen rarely appears to be a source of infection. Infection of susceptible calves may occur throughout the small intestine with less colonization of the large intestine. The ileum is commonly believed to be the most predisposed site, but in some cattle the ileum may have little or no MAP, whereas the mid-jejunum will be heavily colonized. Following initial uptake of MAP by the macrophages in the mucosa, the organism elicits a granulomatous response in the mucosa extending to the submucosa. Over time, MAP spreads to the regional lymph nodes and eventually becomes systemic in advanced stages of the disease. The extent of infection varies greatly among individual cattle. In addition, the incubation period is extremely long, often requiring 2 to 3 years up to 10 years in some cases from time of infection to the development of clinical signs. Several points deserve emphasis.

1. Most infected cattle never develop clinical signs before being culled from the herd. Factors that contribute to clinical disease versus asymptomatic infection are not known but probably include organism dose, age at infection, nutrition, concurrent diseases, stresses, and genetics. Infected cattle shed MAP in their manure and transmit the disease to herdmates by MAP contamination of the environment. Herd infection prevalence varies from 20% to 100% in heavily infected herds. Despite this rather high incidence of infection, it is unusual to see clinical signs in more than 5% to 10% of adult cows in the herd per year. Johne's disease has been shown to persist in some herds for more than 10 years with no overt clinical signs of infection.

2. It is widely accepted that cattle that develop clinical signs shed large numbers of organisms and represent the greatest threat to contaminate the environment. Recently described super-shedders may shed MAP in higher concentrations (1 to 5 million CFU/g of manure) than cattle with clinical disease. Potentially these animals represent the greatest source of environmental contamination and reservoir for possible transmission to herdmates. Most super-shedders are asymptomatic with no evidence of diarrhea or weight loss, yet excrete huge numbers of MAP organisms into the environment.

3. Passive shedding of MAP may occur when noninfected cattle ingest manure contaminated forage or water. With a super-shedder in the herd, ingestion of as little as 5 ml of manure contamination in forage may result in passive shedding and give rise to a positive fecal culture for a previously uninfected cow. The risk of misclassification of such cattle must be considered when control programs include fecal cultures of all adult animals. Recent experience suggests this phenomenon may represent 50% of all culture-positive cattle in the herd when a super-shedder is present.

Because most infected cattle are asymptomatic and clinical cases may have decreased production and be culled before a final diagnosis is made, the true incidence of Johne's disease is hard to estimate. The 1996 National Animal Health Monitoring Survey (NAHMS) estimated 20% of dairy herds were infected. In herds with more than 400 cows, the prevalence increased to 40%. Current unofficial estimates suggest more than 75% of dairy herds in the United States are infected with MAP, with an individual dairy cow prevalence of between 5% and 10% depending on method of detection.

Regional surveillance of Pennsylvania and, indirectly, other areas of the northeastern United States confirmed a dairy cow prevalence of up to 7.3% in many areas. With ever increasing dairy herd size, largely attributed to purchase of cows of unknown status, the herd prevalence will continue to increase. In herds in which 10% of the culled cows have clinical Johne's disease, the average loss exceeds $220 per cow or $22,000 for a herd with 100 milk cows. Without question, this disease is of tremendous economic importance to the entire cattle industry and especially to the dairy industry.

Clinical Signs

Although most cattle infected with MAP remain asymptomatic, cattle with clinical signs signal the diagnosis and alert both veterinarian and herd owner to the possibility of a herd-wide problem. However, if the cow with clinical signs was purchased, the magnitude of the herd problem may not be as extensive. Clinical signs consist of chronic diarrhea, progressive wasting and loss of condition, and eventually ventral pendent edema, especially in the submandibular area as a result of hypoproteinemia. Temperature and vital signs are normal. The diarrhea classically has been defined as pea soup in consistency and often forms bubbles because of the rather liquid consistency. However, given today's laxative diets, the diarrhea observed in a Johne's disease patient is best described as looser compared with herdmates. Initially the manure of an infected cow is formed but loose, then becomes pea soup-like, and finally, in advanced cases, a very watery consistency. Appetite and attitude remain normal in early cases, but milk production and body condition deteriorate because of progressive protein loss. Abomasal displacement is another observed complication in cattle with moderate to severe Johne's disease. The exact cause of displacement is unknown, but gastrointestinal stasis caused by hypocalcemia and reduced dry matter intake may contribute to the condition.

Moderate to advanced clinical cases have obvious weight loss characterized by muscle wasting, a poor dry hair coat, significant production losses, dehydration, and reduced feed intake—particularly high-energy feedstuffs (Figure 6-58). Ventral edema is apparent but may vary in the anatomic area involved. Intermandibular,

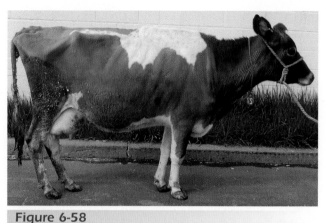

Figure 6-58

Jersey cow affected with Johne's disease. Poor condition, a dry hair coat, and fecal staining of the hind quarters and tail are apparent.

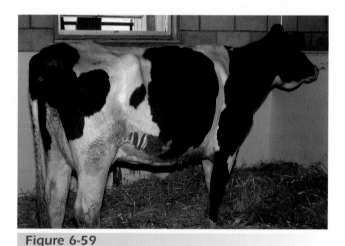

Figure 6-59

Four-year-old Holstein cow with submandibular edema (bottle jaw) and weight loss caused by Johne's disease. Diarrhea was minimal. The diagnosis was confirmed by right flank laparotomy and ileal lymph node biopsy.

brisket, ventral, udder, and lower limb edema all are possible (Figure 6-59). The pea soup-like or liquid manure seen in advanced cases stains the tail, perineum, and hind limbs. It will stain the rear quarters if the tail switches liquid feces onto the quarters, flanks, and gluteal region.

Despite loose manure, loss of body condition, and diminished milk production, cows with Johne's disease do not appear seriously ill until the terminal stages when finally the appetite is markedly reduced. Occasionally cattle have diarrhea intermittently rather than continually, but this is unusual. We have also observed cows with Johne's disease with obvious diarrhea that spontaneously reverted to apparently normal manure after shipment to our hospital for diagnosis. Whether stress associated with shipment or a change in diet is responsible for this temporary improvement in fecal consistency is unknown.

Clinical signs develop only after a prolonged incubation period and usually appear between 2 and 5 years of age. However, signs have been observed in heifers less than 12 months of age and in mature cows up to 8 to 10 years of age (Figure 6-60). If several 2-year-old heifers in a herd develop clinical signs of diarrhea, this would suggest a rather heavy dose of MAP at an early age, whereas clinical signs in 5- to 7-year-old cows would suggest a much lower dose of MAP or older age at the time of exposure. Thus age of onset of clinical signs will assist the astute clinician as to the severity of the herd problem. Age of onset is probably affected by many factors, such as dose and duration of exposure to infectious organisms, nutrition, genetics, concurrent diseases or stresses, and other factors. The clinical impression that signs frequently develop following the onset of lactation in the first, second, or third lactations suggests lactational stress may be sufficient to amplify subclinical signs and hypoproteinemia to a clinical state. It also is possible that this observation is simply a reflection of closer monitoring of appetite, production, and body condition in lactating animals as opposed to heifers or dry cows. Lactation stress is not a prerequisite to the development of clinical signs, as proven by bulls and steers having clinical Johne's disease. Interestingly, some severely affected bulls and steers with Johne's disease have developed abomasal displacements during the advanced stages of disease.

Many cattle with signs of Johne's disease are culled because of poor production before a diagnosis of Johne's disease is confirmed or suspected. This is especially common in free stall operations in which an individual cow's manure consistency may not be as obvious as it would be in conventional housing and individual stalls. Cattle with clinical or subclinical infection also may have higher cull rates than uninfected herdmates because of mastitis and reproductive failure. Other studies

have found a higher cull rate and reduced production but less mastitis in infected versus noninfected herdmates. Increased mastitis and reproductive failure may be partially explained by hypoproteinemia, negative energy and protein balance, stress, and poor condition.

Diagnosis

Cattle with advanced signs of Johne's disease are easily suspected of having the disease because of diarrhea, hypoproteinemia, production loss, weight loss, and overall deterioration of condition. The only abnormalities detected routinely in serum biochemistry are hypoalbuminemia, hypoproteinemia, and occasionally hyperphosphatemia (>7 mg/dl). Clinical Johne's disease must be differentiated from chronic parasitism, coccidiosis, chronic salmonellosis, toxicities, intestinal neoplasia, heart failure, glomerulonephropathies, renal amyloidosis, eosinophilic enteritis, and chronic BVD infections.

Confirmation of a clinical diagnosis of Johne's disease should focus on the agar gel immunodiffusion- (AGID), ELISA, or PCR test. Typically more than 85% of cattle with clinical Johne's disease will be positive on either the ELISA or AGID test. Nearly 100% should be positive when using a robust PCR test. Each of these tests has a turnaround time of less than 1 week, often 2 to 3 days. Fecal cultures are the most sensitive test but have a much longer turnaround time from submission to final result (12 to 16 weeks for solid media culture and 30 to 42 days for liquid media culture). The gold standard diagnosis is culture of ileum, ileocecal lymph nodes, or other mesenteric lymph nodes for cattle with clinical Johne's disease. This technique has been used to identify Johne's disease-infected cattle at slaughter houses and to gather epidemiologic data regarding prevalence of the disease. Although harvesting ileocecal lymph nodes constitutes an invasive procedure for clinical patients, extremely valuable or individually purchased cows suspected of having Johne's disease may warrant invasive techniques to diagnose the condition definitively, especially when the herd has not been known to have Johne's disease in the past. A right flank exploratory laparotomy is performed to harvest a full-thickness 1.0-cm wedge of ileum and an ileocecal lymph node (Figures 6-61 and 6-62). The ileal biopsy and half of the lymph node are submitted for culture and histopathology, including a Ziehl-Neelsen stain. The remaining half of the lymph node is used for impression smears that are stained for acid-fast organisms. An absolute diagnosis usually is possible from the impression smears, but if this fails or is questionable, the histopathology generally confirms or denies the diagnosis without the prolonged delay associated with cultures.

For asymptomatic infected cows, the sensitivity of all Johne's disease diagnostic tests is much reduced compared with cattle with clinical signs. Specificity of fecal

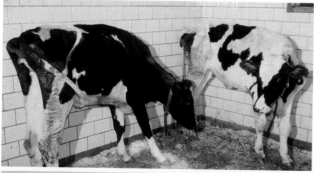

Figure 6-60

A pair of 18-month-old Holstein heifers with advanced Johne's disease. These heifers were representative of an age-grouped epidemic involving 12- to 24-month-old heifers on a single farm. This would imply extremely heavy environmental contamination with *M. paratuberculosis.*

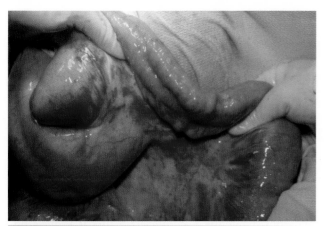

Figure 6-61

Thickened, edematous ileum and visibly distended lymphatics on the serosal surface in a cow showing early signs of Johne's disease. A rapid definitive diagnosis was established by biopsy of the ileum and ileocecal lymph node.

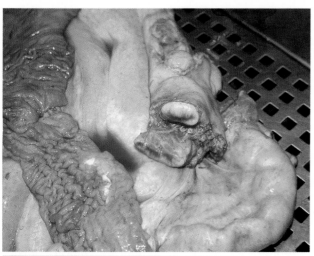

Figure 6-62

Necropsy view of thickened ileum and edematous (cut) ileocecal lymph node from a cow with advanced Johne's disease.

cultures usually has been estimated to be 100%, although recent work confirms that passive excretion of MAP may occur in heavily contaminated environments. Positive fecal cultures in noninfected cows may occur as the result of "pass-through" when super-shedders are present in the herd. Up to 50% of the positive fecal cultures may be the consequence of one or more super-shedders in the herd. Several USDA-licensed ELISA tests are available and commonly used today. The overall ELISA sensitivity for detection of Johne's disease is estimated at 25% as reported by the National Johne's Working Group. The sensitivity of fecal culture was estimated to be 40%. Cattle in the eclipse phase, before

onset of fecal shedding are typically negative on all tests for Johne's disease. In an attempt to determine whether such cattle are infected, testing older animals in the herd of origin with pooled fecal cultures or testing environmental manure samples by reverse transcriptase-PCR are good strategies. Because ELISA tests are not 100% specific, fecal samples for all ELISA-positive cattle should be submitted for culture or PCR testing. Overall, approximately one third of fecal samples from ELISA-positive cattle are culture positive. Some herd owners are choosing to do fecal cultures on all adult cattle in the herd, especially those owners who have made the requisite management changes designed to reduce transmission of Johne's disease within the herd. Laboratory testing in the absence of management changes to reduce the risk of transmission is not recommended.

No currently available diagnostic test will detect all infected cattle; thus repeated, usually annually, testing is necessary to detect infected cattle. Thus a negative test for Johne's disease should not be construed as proof of a noninfected animal, but only as data that suggest that if MAP infection was present, it was not detectable at that time. A more sound epidemiological approach would be testing of adult cattle in the herd using pooled or environmental manure samples. Recent reports suggest pooled fecal samples (five samples/pool) and composite environmental manure samples provide excellent tools to detect herd infections, and that if these tests are negative they indicate the herd is at low risk for Johne's disease. Both of these testing scenarios have been incorporated into the National Johne's Herd Status program.

Gross and histological lesions obtained at necropsy or slaughter facilities are extremely helpful to render an absolute diagnosis. Mild clinical cases may have a thickened edematous ileum with distended lymphatics on the serosal surface. Thickening of the mucosal surface and a raised corrugated appearance is typical. Moderate to advanced cases have obvious thickening and edema of the ileum with marked corrugation of the mucosal surface (see Figure 6-62). Lymphatic distention is obvious on the serosal surface of the ileum, and the ileocecal lymph nodes, as well as other mesenteric lymph nodes, are enlarged and edematous on cut sections. Lesions may be present in the cecum and colon of advanced clinical cases and can extend orad from the ileum to more proximal regions of the small intestine. Although MAP may be isolated from other organs such as the liver, uterus, or fetus in some advanced cases, gross lesions consisting of granuloma formation are rare in these organs, and truly disseminated infections having gross lesions are very rare. However, disseminated infections detected by culture of MAP from lymph nodes such as the prescapular, prefemoral, supramammary, or popliteal lymph nodes do occur in cattle with clinical disease. Aortic calcification has been observed in advanced cases.

Histopathology confirms a granulomatous enterocolitis with macrophages and epithelioid cells in the submucosa and lower mucosa. Ziehl-Neelsen staining confirms the presence of MAP in the intestine and lymphatics. However, culture of these same tissues has a much greater sensitivity to detect MAP than does histopathology.

Treatment

Although treatment seldom is attempted, therapeutic options do exist for valuable animals that may justify the expense and the continued exposure risk these cattle may represent for transmission to herdmates.

Clofazimine and isoniazid have both been used to successfully alleviate clinical signs of MAP infection in cattle and small ruminants. Although the drugs reduce fecal shedding, the infection persists despite daily therapy. Typically treated animals will gain weight, have improved manure consistency, and plasma protein levels are restored within a few weeks. Continued daily therapy is necessary to maintain the animal free of clinical signs. Isoniazid (20 mg/kg orally, once daily) has been used either alone or in conjunction with rifampin (20 mg/kg orally, once daily). As with clofazimine, however, the infection is only suppressed, not cured despite an improved clinical picture. Isoniazid is the most economical choice but may require adjunctive therapy with rifampin to achieve clinical improvement. All therapy for Johne's disease involves extralabel drug use, requires prolonged (i.e., months-long) treatment, precludes use of milk or meat for human consumption, and is expensive. Unless isolation of the patient is possible, treated cattle continue to shed MAP and pose a risk to infect herdmates.

Control

Once a diagnosis of Johne's disease has been confirmed, the herd owner must be counseled regarding the economic implications and options for control or eradication of the disease. Economic considerations extend beyond the loss of clinical cases to increased cull rates in subclinical cases; fear of dissemination of disease to noninfected herds through sale of infected but apparently normal calves or cattle; risks inherent to embryo transfer; and decreased productivity. Currently states offer Johne's disease programs to aid control and support testing costs of the herd to detect infected cattle. All federally supported Johne's disease programs require that a Johne's disease–certified veterinarian does a herd risk assessment and a herd management plan before funds are available to support the diagnostic testing.

Although difficult, eradication of the infection from a herd requires intensive and repeated use of fecal cultures on all animals older than 24 months of age for many years. All clinically suspicious cattle should be culled immediately or tested by AGID or ELISA. If positive on either of these tests, the animals should be culled. Calves

should be born in disinfected, cleaned maternity areas and removed from the dam immediately. Calves should be raised completely separately—preferably on a separate farm—from the adult cattle. All calves should be fed colostrum from ELISA-negative, or better, fecal culture–negative cows. The purchase of replacement animals from herds of unknown Johne's disease status continues to represent the greatest risk to introduce or reintroduce Johne's disease to the herd. Minimizing fecal contamination of feedstuff, water, pastures, and exposure of calves to adult cow feces is essential and must be evaluated on an individual herd basis. Equipment used for manure removal or that could be contaminated by manure must remain separate from feeding implements and the calf environment.

Although these principles for eradication are straightforward, they may not be practical or affordable in some instances. Compromises in eradication may allow "control" but do not eliminate the disease and continue to compromise sale opportunities for purebred herds.

Vaccines for Johne's disease have been used in Europe, Australia, and several states in the United States. In the United States, a licensed killed vaccine is available, but its use is limited to infected herds, and approval by the state veterinarian is required. The herd must be tuberculin test negative. If approved for use in a specific herd, the herd owner must agree to have all calves vaccinated before 35 days of age. Each calf must have an ear tattoo and a special ear tag that signifies a Johne's disease vaccinate. The vaccine is administered SQ in the brisket and frequently predisposes to a local abscess over the next few months or years. The vaccine should be used in conjunction with management changes to reduce the incidence of infection in herds. However, the vaccine does not prevent infection, but vaccinated cattle shed fewer organisms in their manure. Most importantly, the vaccine prevents clinical signs in nearly all vaccinated cattle. Because premature culling from the herd because of Johne's disease infection is the major economic loss attributable to Johne's disease, the vaccine is considered highly efficacious by herd owners who have years of experience with Johne's disease. Other disadvantages for vaccine use include concern regarding interpretation of tuberculin reactions and accidental self-inoculation of the vaccine by veterinarians.

Foreign Animal Disease

Mucosal diseases such as BVDV, BTV, MCF, and VSV require differentiation from foreign animal diseases that threaten livestock in the United States (Table 6-8). Extreme vigilance is necessary to prevent entrance of those diseases to this country, and consultation with regulatory state or federal veterinarians is imperative whenever confusion exists. Because a great deal of overlap is possible for the clinical signs present in domestic and

TABLE 6-8 Foreign or Exotic Animal Diseases Affecting the Gastrointestinal Tract

Disease	Cause	Clinical Signs	Major Differential Diagnosis	Diagnosis	Reference
Foot and mouth disease (Aftosa)	FMDV = genus Aphtovirus, family Picorniviridae	Fever, salivation, lipsmacking, lameness, teat lesions	Vesicular stomatitis	Call regulatory veterinarians	Kahrs RF: *Viral diseases of cattle*, Ames, IA, 1981, Iowa State University Press.
(Aphthous fever)	7 distinct serotypes with multiple subtypes	Vesicles progressing to erosions and ulcers of oral mucosa, nasal mucosa, interdigital space, coronary band, teats Abortion	BVDV Bluetongue Malignant catarrhal fever Rinderpest	Fluid from vesicles Oropharyngeal fluid Tissues Paired sera	Sutmoller, P: Vesicular diseases. In Committee on Foreign Animal Diseases, editors: *Foreign animal diseases*, Richmond, VA, 1992, United States Animal Health Association.
Rinderpest (cattle plague) (Peste bovine)	RV = genus Morbillivirus, family Paramyxoviridae	*Peracute*—high fever, death	BVDV	Call regulatory veterinarians	Kahrs RF: *Viral diseases of cattle*, Ames, IA, 1981, Iowa State University Press.
	1 major serotype with field strains possessing variable pathogenicity	Classic fever, mucous membrane congestion, necrosis, and subsequent erosion	Malignant catarrhal fever Vesicular stomatitis Foot and mouth disease	Samples best obtained from febrile animals with mucosal lesions (early cases)	
		Mucous membrane lesions cause salivation, ocular discharge	Salmonellosis Bluetongue	Serologic testing Viral isolation	Seek B, Cook R: Rinderpest. In Committee on Foreign Animal Diseases, editors: *Foreign animal diseases*, Richmond, VA, 1992, United States Animal Health Association.
		Severe hemorrhagic diarrhea and tenesmus start several days after mucosal lesions Dehydration, death Subacute or atypical-lower mortality, greater difficulty in distinguishing from differential diagnosis	Arsenic poisoning		

foreign mucosal diseases, positive diagnosis including appropriate serologic and virologic confirmation is essential.

Liver Abscess

Etiology

Abscesses of the liver occur at all ages in cattle. In calves, liver abscesses are often the result of omphalophlebitis, whereas in older cattle they most often are secondary to reticulorumenitis. In feed lot cattle, it is well recognized that the change from pasture to a high concentrate ration causes a rapid increase in rumen fermentation and organic acid production, which may result in erosion and inflammation of the rumen epithelium. Metastasis of bacteria from the inflamed and necrotic rumen wall to the liver occurs via the portal vein. In dairy cattle, similar failure of adaptation of rumen fermentation may occur at the onset of lactation when there is an abrupt increase in the energy content of the diet. Liver abscesses also may occur as a result of traumatic reticulitis. The most common organisms isolated from hepatic abscesses are *Fusobacterium necrophorum* and *Arcanobacterium pyogenes*. Streptococci and staphylococci also may be isolated from mixed cultures.

Clinical Signs

Local, circumscribed liver abscesses are characteristically silent clinically and are not associated with systemic abnormalities or with hepatic dysfunction. Such abscesses are found incidentally during the postmortem examination of slaughtered cattle and are of importance economically because of the condemnation of affected livers.

Liver abscess, when located adjacent to the vena cava, may distort the vessel wall and cause phlebitis and thrombosis. Septic thromboembolism from the vena cava may cause a respiratory syndrome characterized by cough, dyspnea, and/or pulmonary hemorrhage that is described in Chapter 4. In a postmortem series of 6337 slaughtered cattle, liver abscesses were found in 368 (5.8%), and of these, 24% were located in the craniodorsal aspect of the liver with the potential for causing vena caval thrombosis.

Liver abscesses may be associated with constitutional abnormalities that include fever, anorexia, weight loss, and reduced milk production. Neutrophilic leukocytosis and significant increases in serum globulin and fibrinogen are characteristic. Growth of a liver abscess near the common bile duct may obstruct bile flow and may result in clinical signs and laboratory abnormalities associated with impeded flow of bile (see below). Liver abscess also has been recognized as a cause of vagal indigestion.

Ultrasonographic examination of the liver is a valuable diagnostic procedure for determining the location of the abscess(es) and for evaluating prognosis and response to therapy (Figures 6-63 and 6-64). The lesions may vary in diameter from a few centimeters to more than 20 cm. Characteristically they may be visualized in three or four adjacent intercostal spaces, and needle aspiration may not be necessary for diagnosis. On rare occasion a large liver abscess can be seen on radiographs displacing the diaphragm (Figure 6-65, *A* to *C*).

Treatment

When liver abscesses are recognized clinically and their location identified, it is possible to consider antibiotic therapy and/or surgical drainage. The decision regarding

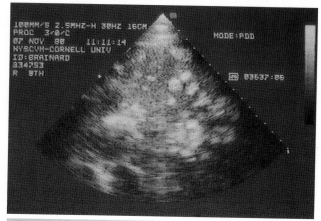

Figure 6-63

Transabdominal sonogram of the liver in a mature cow with multiple hyperechoic abscesses. The hyperechoic appearance suggests dense purulent exudate, decreasing the chances of successful treatment.

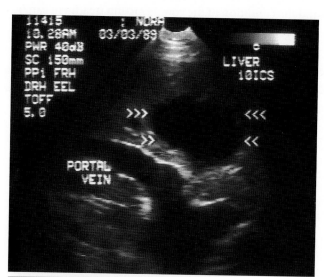

Figure 6-64

Transabdominal sonogram of the liver in a 3-year-old Holstein cow with weight loss and diminished production. A single large hypoechoic abscess can be seen, and the cow recovered following 1 month of systemically administered penicillin treatment.

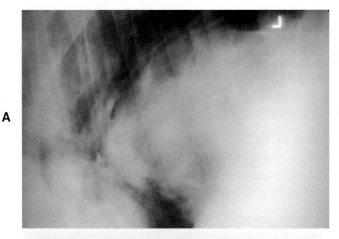

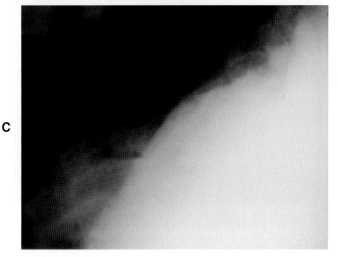

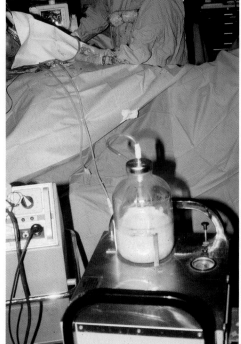

Figure 6-65

A, Thoracic radiographs of a 14-month-old Holstein heifer showing a very large mass (liver abscess) displacing the diaphragm. **B,** The liver abscess was drained. **C,** Radiographs repeated after drainage.

drainage of liver abscesses depends on the size, location, and the condition of the cow. Penicillin treatment can be successful in some cows with smaller, hypoechoic abscesses, but relapses often occur unless treatment is for 4 or more weeks. Even with surgical drainage, relapses may occur. Prognosis for treatment of liver abscesses that have caused clinical signs is guarded and is least favorable for large and hyperechoic abscesses. Successful surgical treatment of a liver abscess that caused vagal indigestion has been described.

Bile Duct Obstruction and Cholangitis

Intrahepatic cholestasis is observed in lactating cattle with severe fatty liver during the periparturient period and is described in Chapter 14. Extrahepatic cholestasis is caused by obstruction of bile flow from choleliths within the common bile duct or by obstruction of flow in the common bile duct as a result of external mechanical pressure exerted on the common bile duct by liver abscesses, by extensive adhesions in the area of the cystic and common bile ducts, or by smaller inflammatory lesions of the common duct near the hilus or the duodenal papilla (see video clip 13).

The characteristic sterility of the biliary tract is maintained by the continued production and flow of bile into the intestine. Partial or complete obstruction of bile flow predisposes to ascending infection of the biliary tract by intestinal microorganisms. Infection of the biliary tree causes cholangitis and may result in significant alterations in the physical characteristics of bile, including the accumulation of inspissated products of inflammation and of precipitated bile constituents (bile acids, cholesterol, and even stone formation) (Figure 6-66), which further impedes the flow of bile.

The clinical signs of extrahepatic bile duct obstruction and cholangitis include malaise, colic, fever, icterus with orange-colored urine (Figure 6-67), and, in some cases photodermatitis (Figure 6-68) secondary to retention of phylloerythrin. Abnormal laboratory findings consist of leukocytosis, hyperbilirubinemia, bilirubinuria, and elevations in serum globulin and fibrinogen, bilirubin, and in the serum activities of SDH, AST, AP, and GGT. Ultrasonographic findings in cows with extrahepatic cholestasis include severe dilatation of the gallbladder, the cystic and common duct, and other major intrahepatic bile ducts. Dilatation of the gallbladder is not specific because in all anorectic cows, the gallbladder may

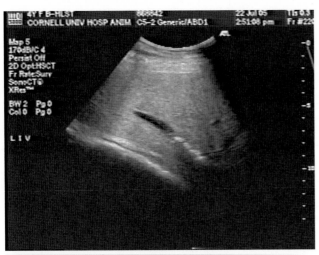

Figure 6-66

Abdominal sonogram of an adult Holstein hospitalized because of anorexia and mild colic. The cows' GGT was 1500 IU/L. Stones are observed in the intrahepatic ducts. There was a marked clinical improvement within 3 days of initiating therapy with penicillin, IV fluids, flunixin meglumine, and forced feeding.

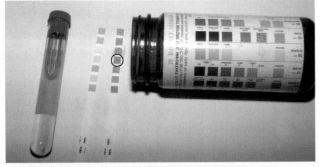

Figure 6-67

A sample of urine collected from an adult cow with icteric membranes, fever, anorexia, depression, and hepatogenous photosensitization of the muzzle. The cow responded well to symptomatic treatment similar to Figure 6-66. The urine is orange and positive on Multi-strip examination for bilirubin. Circled square is positive test. Untested strip to the left.

be distended. The diagnostic findings for extrahepatic cholestasis, however, were dilatation of the cystic and common bile ducts and of the major intrahepatic bile ducts (see video clip 14).

A case of cholelithiasis with cholestasis has been reported by Drs. Rebhun and Cable that was clinically similar to those in which bile duct obstruction was caused by external mechanical pressure on the common bile. A laparotomy was performed, and concretions 1 to 3 cm in diameter were palpated in the gallbladder. The choleliths in the gallbladder were crushed manually, and

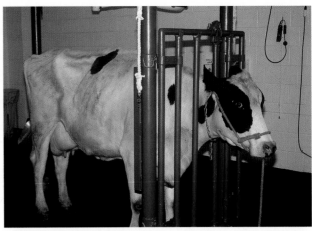

Figure 6-68

The cow in Figure 6-67 with pronounced hyperemia (photosensitive dermatitis) of the muzzle.

the material was massaged through the distended cystic and common ducts, into the duodenum, and on into the jejunum. Following the procedure, there was significant improvement in clinical condition and in liver function tests, although the improvement was transient.

A clinical syndrome of unknown etiology has been observed that is clinically similar to that described above but in which there is no laparotomy evidence of extrahepatic cholestasis. The clinical signs and laboratory test results are similar. When force-fed for a few days and treated with penicillin for at least 1 month, there has been gradual improvement in clinical signs and laboratory abnormalities return to normal (see Figures 6-67 and 6-68).

Primary hepatic neoplasms are unusual in cattle but could cause obstruction of bile flow and should be considered in cows with both icterus and photosensitization. In a necropsy series of 66 primary bovine hepatic neoplasms, 40 were classified as hepatocellular carcinomas, 10 as hepatocellular adenomas, and 10 as cholangiocellular tumors. Less frequently observed primary tumors of the liver in this series included hemangiosarcoma, hemangioma, fibroma, and Schwannoma. In the postmortem examination of the livers of 24,169 slaughtered cattle, primary liver tumors of hepatocellular origin were identified in 22 (0.09%). In a third series of 1.3 million livers of cattle examined at slaughter, 36 had primary liver tumors of which 13 were classified as primary hepatocellular neoplasms and 21 as cholangiocarcinomas.

The clinical signs of cattle associated with primary hepatic neoplasms have not been extensively described. The expected clinical signs would be those associated with the growth of an expanding hepatic mass or with metastasis to the lung or to the spleen, both of which have been observed at necropsy. If the tumor obstructs bile flow, then icterus and photosensitization would be

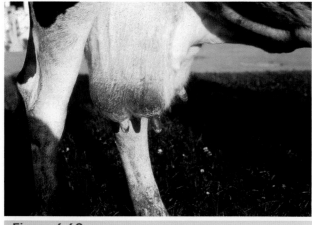

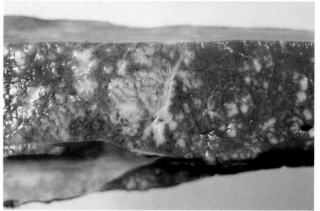

Figure 6-69

A, An 8-year-old Holstein cow with weight loss, inappetence, and photosensitization, which is best seen on the teats and udder. **B,** The cow had a cholangiocarcinoma.

expected (Figure 6-69, *A* and *B*). Dermatitis caused by photosensitization is frequently most severe on the teats and muzzle, although it may be more generalized (Figure 6-70). Ultrasonography should be of value in locating and otherwise assessing the location and prognosis of primary liver tumors.

Hepatic Insufficiency Associated with Sepsis

A syndrome of hepatic insufficiency has been described in lactating cattle following acute septic mastitis or metritis in which the initial clinical signs were compatible with endotoxemia. Subsequent clinical signs included anorexia, weight loss, reduced milk production, and, in one case, photodermatitis. In addition to increased serum activities of liver enzymes, the cows had remarkable delays in the sulfobromophthalein (BSP) plasma clearance test. Liver biopsies showed hepatocellular vacuolization or necrosis that was attributed to the effects of endotoxemia associated with acute systemic infection. Similar hepatic injury has been reported in humans following endotoxic shock. Five such cases were treated by force-feeding and with other symptomatic support. Three of the cows responded satisfactorily to therapy, one failed to respond, and the fifth cow was lost to follow-up evaluation. Based on these observations, it is important to consider the possibility of hepatic injury in the initial management of cows with postpartum sepsis and in the longer term management when there is a sluggish response to therapy of the acute disease. If there is a history of prolonged antimicrobial therapy, intestinal and hepatic mycosis must also be considered (Figure 6-71).

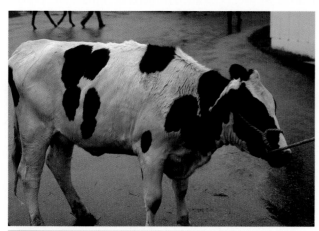

Figure 6-70

Hepatogenous photosensitization caused by a suspected hepatotoxin.

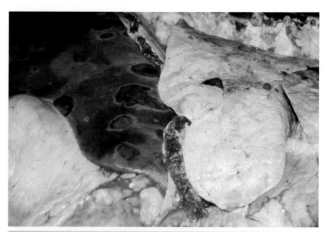

Figure 6-71

The liver from a 6-year-old Holstein that had intestinal (forestomach and abomasum) and hepatic aspergillosis secondary to generalized sepsis and treatment with broad-spectrum antibiotics.

RECOMMENDED READINGS

Abutarbush SM, Carmalt JL, Wilson DG, et al: Jejunal hemorrhage syndrome in 2 Canadian beef cows, *Can Vet J* 45:48-50, 2004.

Abutarbush SM, Radostits OM: Jejunal hemorrhage syndrome in dairy and beef cattle: 11 cases (2001 to 2003), *Can Vet J* 46:711-715, 2005.

Acres SD: Enterotoxigenic *Escherichia coli* infections in newborn calves: a review, *J Dairy Sci* 68:229-256, 1985.

Ahmed AF, Constable PD, Misk NA: Effect of orally administered cimetidine and ranitidine on abomasal luminal pH in clinically normal milk-fed calves, *Am J Vet Res* 62:1531-1538, 2001.

Alcaine SD, Sukhnanand SS, Warnick LD, et al: Ceftiofur-resistant *Salmonella* strains isolated from dairy farms represent multiple widely distributed subtypes that evolved by independent horizontal gene transfer, *Antimicrob Agents Chemother* 49:4061-4067, 2005.

Allison MJ, Robinson IM, Doughtery RW, et al: Grain overload in cattle and sheep: changes in microbial populations in the cecum and rumen, *Am J Vet Res* 39:181-185, 1975.

Al-Mashat RR, Taylor DR: Production of diarrhoea and dysentery in experimental cakes by feeding pure cultures of *Campylobacter fetus* subspecies *jejuni*,*Vet Rec* 107:459-464, 1980.

Anderson BC: Gastric cryptosporidiosis of feeder cattle beef cows and dairy cows, *Bov Pract* 23:99-101, 1988.

Ares-Mazas E, Lorenzo MJ, Casal JA, et al: Effect of a commercial disinfectant ('Virkon') on mouse experimental infection by *Cryptosporidium parvum*, *J Hosp Infect* 36:141-145, 1997.

Arthington JD, Jaynes CA, Tyler HD, et al: The use of bovine serum protein as an oral support therapy following coronavirus challenge in calves, *J Dairy Sci* 85:1249-1254, 2002.

Audet S, Crim R, Beeler J: Evaluation of vaccines, interferons, and cell substrates for pestivirus contamination, *Biologicals* 28:41-46, 2000.

Bellamy J, Acres SD: A comparison of histopathological changes in calves associated with K99- and K99+ strains of enterotoxigenic *E. coli*, *Can J Comp Med* 47:143-149, 1983.

Berchtold JF, Constable PD, Smith GW, et al: Effects of intravenous hyperosmotic sodium bicarbonate on arterial and cerebrospinal fluid acid-base status and cardiovascular function in calves with experimentally induced respiratory and strong ion acidosis, *J Vet Intern Med* 19:240-251, 2005.

Berghaus RD, McCluskey BJ, Callan RJ: Risk factors associated with hemorrhagic bowel syndrome in dairy cattle, *J Am Vet Med Assoc* 226:1700-1706, 2005.

Bertone A, Rebhun WC: Tracheal actinomycosis in a cow, *J Am Vet Med Assoc* 185:221-222, 1984.

Besser TE, Gay CC: Septicemic colibacillosis and failure of passive transfer of colostral immunoglobulin in calves, *Vet Clin North Am: Food Anim Pract* 1:445-459, 1985.

Besser TE, Gay CC, Pritchett L: Comparison of three methods of feeding colostrum to dairy calves, *J Am Vet Med Assoc* 198:419-422, 1991.

Besser TE, Lejeune JT, Rice DH, et al: Increasing prevalence of Campylobacter jejuni in feedlot cattle through the feeding period, *Appl Environ Microbiol* 71:5752-5758, 2005.

Besser TE, McGuire TC, Gay CC, et al: Transfer of functional immunoglobulin G (IgG) antibody into the gastrointestinal tract accounts for IgG clearance in calves, *J Virol* 62:2234-2237, 1988.

Bettini G, Marcato PS: Primary hepatic tumours in cattle. A classification of 66 cases, *J Comp Pathol* 107:19-34, 1992.

Bezek DM, Mechor GD: Identification and eradication of bovine viral diarrhea virus in a persistently infected dairy herd, *J Am Vet Med Assoc* 201:580-586, 1992.

Bistner SI, Rubin LF, Saunders LZ: The ocular lesions of bovine viral diarrhea-mucosal disease, *Pathol Vet* 7:275-285, 1970.

Blanchard PC: Sampling techniques for the diagnosis of digestive disease, *Vet Clin N Am Food Anim Pract* 16:23-36, 2000.

Bolin SR, Grooms DL: Origination and consequences of bovine viral diarrhea virus diversity, *Vet Clin N Am: Food Anim Pract* 20:51-68, 2004.

Bolin SR, McClurkin AW, Cutlip RC, et al: Severe clinical disease induced in cattle persistently infected with noncytopathic bovine viral diarrhea virus by superinfection with cytopathic bovine viral diarrhea virus, *Am J Vet Res* 46:573-576, 1985.

Bonneau KR, DeMaula CD, Mullens BA, et al: Duration of viraemia infectious to *Culicoides sonorensis* in bluetongue virus-infected cattle and sheep, *Vet Microbiol* 88:115-125, 2002.

Booth AJ, Naylor JM: Correction of metabolic acidosis in diarrheal calves by oral administration of electrolyte solutions with or without bicarbonate, *J Am Vet Med Assoc* 191:62-68, 1987.

Borriello SP, Carman RJ: Clostridial diseases of the gastrointestinal tract in animals. In Borriello SP, editor: *Clostridia in gastrointestinal disease*, Boca Raton, FL, 1990, CRC Press, pp. 195-221.

Borzacchiello G, Iovane G, Marcante ML, et al: Presence of bovine papillomavirus type 2 DNA and expression of the viral oncoprotein E5 in naturally occurring urinary bladder tumours in cows, *J Gen Virol* 84(Pt 11):2921-2926, 2003.

Bowne JG, Luedke AJ, Jochim MM, et al: Bluetongue disease in cattle, *J Am Vet Med Assoc* 153:662-668, 1968.

Braun U: Ultrasound as a decision-making tool in abdominal surgery in cows, *Vet Clin North Am Food Anim Pract* 21:33-35, 2005.

Braun U, Gotz M, Guscetti F: Ultrasonographic findings in a cow with extrahepatic cholestasis and cholangitis, *Schweiz Arch Tierheilkd* 136:275-279, 1994.

Braun U, Pospischil A, Pusterla N, et al: Ultrasonographic findings in cows with cholestasis, *Vet Rec* 137:537-543, 1995.

Braun U, Pusterla N, Wild K: Ultrasonographic findings in 11 cows with a hepatic abscess, *Vet Rec* 137:284-290, 1995.

Brownlie J: The pathogenesis of mucosal disease. A dual role for bovine viral diarrhea virus. In: *Proceedings 2nd University of Nebraska Mini-Symposium on Veterinary Infectious Diseases—Bovine Viral Diarrhea Virus: New Challenges for the New Decade*, Lincoln, NE, May 19, 1990.

Brownlie J, Clarke MC, Howard CJ: Experimental production of fatal mucosal disease in cattle, *Vet Rec* 114:535-536, 1984.

Bruer AN: Actinomycosis of the digestive tract in cattle, *Vet J* 3:121-122, 1955.

Bruner DW, Gillespie JH: *Hagan's infectious diseases of domestic animals*, ed 8, Ithaca, NY, 1988, Comstock Publishing Associates.

Bueschel DM, Jost BH, Billington SJ, et al: Prevalence of cpb2, encoding beta2 toxin, in *Clostridium perfringens* field isolates: correlation of genotype with phenotype, *Vet Microbiol* 94:121-129, 2003.

Cable CS, Rebhun WC, Fortier LA: Cholelithiasis and cholecystitis in a dairy cow, *J Am Vet Med Assoc* 211:899-900, 1997.

Callan RJ: Malignant catarrhal fever: recent findings. Proceedings 19th Annual Forum, *Amer Coll Vet Int Med* 19:336-338, 2001.

Callan RJ: Unpublished data, Fort Collins, CO, 2006.

Campbell SG, Cookingham CA: The enigma of winter dysentery, *Cornell Vet* 68:423-441, 1978.

Campbell SG, Whitlock RH, Timoney JF, et al: An unusual epizootic of actinobacillosis in dairy heifers, *J Am Vet Med Assoc* 166:604-606, 1975.

Carlson SA, Stoffregen WC, Bolin SR: Abomasitis associated with multiple antibiotic resistant *Salmonella enteritica* serotype *typhimurium* phagetype DT104, *Vet Microbiol* 85:233-240, 2002.

Carter G, Chengappa M, Roberts AW: *Clostridium. Essentials of veterinary microbiology*, Media, PA, 1995, Williams and Wilkins, pp. 134-137.

Castrucci G, Frigeri F, Ferrari M, et al: The efficacy of colostrum from cows vaccinated with rotavirus in protecting calves to experimentally induced rotavirus infection, *Comp Immun Microbiol Infect Dis* 7:11-18, 1984.

Chigerwe M, Dawes ME, Tyler JW, et al: Evaluation of a cow-side immunoassay kit for assessing IgG concentration in colostrum, *J Am Vet Med Assoc* 227:129-131, 2005.

Cho KO, Halbur PG, Bruna JD, et al: Detection and isolation of coronavirus from feces of three herds of feedlot cattle during outbreaks of winter dysentery-like disease, *J Am Vet Med Assoc* 217:1191-1194, 2000.

Cho KO, Hasoksuz M, Nielsen PR, et al: Cross-protection studies between resporatory and calf diarrhea and winter dysentery coronavirus strains in calves and RT-CR and nested PCR for their detection, *Arch Virol* 146:2401-2419, 2001.

Clark MA: Bovine coronavirus, *Br Vet J* 149:51-70, 1993.

Cobbold RN, Rice DH, Davis MA, et al: Long-term persistence of multidrug-resistant Salmonella enterica serovar Newport in two dairy herds, *J Am Vet Med Assoc* 228:686-692, 2006.

Constable PD: Antimicrobial use in the treatment of calf diarrhea, *J Vet Intern Med* 18:8-17, 2004.

Corapi WC, French TW, Dubovi EJ: Severe thrombocytopenia in young calves experimentally infected with noncytopathic bovine viral diarrhea virus, *J Virol* 63:3934-3943, 1989.

Coretese V: Bovine vaccines and herd vaccination programs. In Smith BP, editor: *Large animal internal medicine*, ed 3, St. Louis, 2002, Mosby.

Coria MF, McClurkin AW: Specific immune tolerance in an apparently healthy bull persistently infected with bovine viral diarrhea virus, *J Am Vet Med Assoc* 172:449-451, 1978.

Craig TM: Treatment of external and internal parasites of cattle, *Vet Clin N Am: Food Anim Pract* 19:661-678, 2003.

Current WL: Cryptosporidiosis, *J Am Vet Med Assoc* 187:1334-1338, 1985.

Davidson HP, Rebhun WC, Habel RE: Pharyngeal trauma in cattle, *Cornell Vet* 71:15-25, 1981.

de Graaf DC, Vanopdenbosch E, Ortega-Mora LM, et al: A review of the importance of cryptosporidiosis in farm animals, *Int J Parasitol* 29:1269-1287, 1999.

de la Rosa C, Hogue DE, Thonney ML: Vaccination schedules to raise antibody concentrations against epsilon toxin of *Clostridium perfringens* in ewes and their triplet lambs, *J Anim Sci* 75:2328-2334, 1997.

Dennison AC, Van Metre DC, Callan RJ, et al: Hemorrhagic bowel syndrome in adult dairy cattle: 22 cases (1997-2000), *J Am Vet Med Assoc* 221:686-689; erratum 221:1149, 2002.

Dennison AC, Van Metre DC, Morley PS, et al: Comparison of the odds of isolation, genotypes, and in vivo production of major toxins by *Clostridium perfringens* obtained from the gastrointestinal tract of dairy cows with hemorrhagic bowel syndrome or left displaced abomasum, *J Am Vet Med Assoc* 227:132-138, 2005.

de Verdier KK: Enhancement of clinical signs in experimentally rotavirus infected calves by combined viral infections, *Vet Rec* 147:717-719, 2000.

Donis RO: Bovine viral diarrhea: the unraveling of a complex of clinical presentations, *Bov Proc* 20:16-22, 1988.

Dougherty RW, Habel RE, Bone HE: Esophageal innervation and eructation reflex in sheep, *Am J Vet Res* 19:115-118, 1958.

Dougherty RW, Hill KJ, Campeti FL, et al: Studies of the pharyngeal and laryngeal activity during eructation in ruminants, *Am J Vet Res* 23:213-219, 1962.

Drolet BS, Campbell CL, Stuart MA, et al: Vector competence of *Culicoides sonorensis* (Diptera: Ceratopogonidae) for vesicular stomatitis virus, *J Med Entomol* 42:409-418, 2005.

Dubovi EJ: Personal communication [to W.C. Rebhun], Ithaca, NY, 1993.

Elitok B, Elitok OM, Pulat H: Efficacy of azithromycin dihydrate in treatment of cryptosporidiosis in naturally infected dairy calves, *J Vet Intern Med* 19:590-593, 2005.

Embury-Hyatt CK, Wobeser G, Simko E, et al: Investigation of a syndrome of sudden death, splenomegaly, and small intestinal hemorrhage in farmed deer, *Can Vet J* 46:702-708, 2005.

Ernst JV, Benz GW: Intestinal coccidiosis in cattle, *Vet Clin North Am: Food Anim Pract* 2:283-291, 1986.

Espinasse J, Viso M, Laval A, et al: Winter dysentery: a coronavirus-like agent in the faeces of beef and dairy cattle with diarrhoea, *Vet Rec* 11:385, 1982.

Ewaschuk JB, Naylor JM, Palmer R, et al: D-lactate production and excretion in diarrheic calves, *J Vet Intern Med* 18:744-747, 2004.

Ewoldt JM, Anderson DE: Determination of the effect of single abomasal or jejunal inoculation of Clostridium perfringens type A in dairy cows, *Can Vet J* 46:821-824, 2005.

Farrell CJ, Shen DT, Wescott RB, et al: An enzyme-linked immunosorbent assay for diagnosis of *Fasciola hepatica* infection in cattle, *Am J Vet Res* 42:237-240, 1981.

Fayer R, Morgan U, Upton SJ: Epidemiology of *Cryptosporidium*: transmission, detection, and identification, *Int J Parasitol* 30:1305-1322, 2000.

Fayer R, Santin M, Xiao L: *Cryptosporidium bovis* n. sp. (Apicomplexa: Cryptosporidiiae) in cattle (*Bos taurus*), *J Parasitol* 91:624-629, 2005.

Firehammer BD, Myers LL: *Campylobacter featus* subspecies *jejuni*: its possible significance in enteric disease of calves and lambs, *Am J Vet Res* 42:918-922, 1981.

Fleenor WA, Stott GH: Hydrometer test for estimation of immunoglobulin concentration in bovine colostrum, *J Dairy Sci* 63:973-977, 1980.

Fossler CP, Wells SJ, Kaneene JB, et al: Herd-level factors associated with isolation of Salmonella in a multi-state study of conventional and organic dairy farms I. Salmonella shedding in cows, *Prev Vet Med* 70:257-277, 2005.

Fowler ME: Recent calf milk replacer research update. In *Proceedings: American Association Bovine Practitioners Convention*, vol 2, 1992, pp. 168-175.

Fubini SL, Ducharme NG, Murphy JP, et al: Vagus indigestion syndrome resulting from a liver abscess in dairy cows, *J Am Vet Med Assoc* 186:1297-1300, 1985.

Garmory HS, Chanter N, French NP, et al: Occurrence of *Clostridium perfringens* beta2-toxin amongst animals, determined by using genotyping and subtyping PCR assays, *Epidemiol Infect* 124:61-67, 2000.

Georgi JR: *Parasitology for veterinarians*, ed 4, Philadelphia, 1985, WB Saunders, pp. 62-72.

Gibbs EPJ: Bluetongue—an analysis of current problems, with particular reference to importation of ruminants to the United States, *J Am Vet Med Assoc* 182:1190-1194, 1983.

Gibbs EPJ. Bluetongue disease, *Agri-Practice* 4:31-38, 1983.

Gibbs HC, Herd RP: Nematodiasis in cattle: importance, species involved immunity, and resistance, *Vet Clin North Am: Food Anim Pract* 2:211-224, 1986.

Gibert M, Jolivet–Reynaud C, Popoff M: Beta$_2$ toxin, a novel toxin produced by *Clostridium perfringens*, *Gene* 203:65-73, 1997.

Giles N, Hopper SA, Wray C: Persistence of salmonella-typhimurium in a large dairy herd, *Epidemiol Infect* 103:235-242, 1989.

Gillespie JH, Bartholomew PT, Thomson RG, et al: The isolation of non-cytopathic virus diarrhea from two aborted fetuses, *Cornell Vet* 57:564-571, 1967.

Givens MD, Waldrop JG: Bovine viral diarrhea virus in embryo and semen production systems, *Vet Clin N Am: Food Anim Pract* 20:21-38, 2004.

Godden S, Frank R, Ames T: Survey of Minnesota veterinarians on the occurrence of and potential risk factors for jejunal hemorrhage syndrome in adult dairy cows, *Bov Pract* 35:97-103, 2001.

Goldman L, Ausiello D: Campylobacter enteritis. In Wyngaarden JB, Smith LH Jr, editors: *Cecil textbook of medicine*, ed 22, Philadelphia, 2004, WB Saunders.

Goodger WJ, Thurmond M, Nehay J, et al: Economic impact of an epizootic of bovine vesicular stomatitis in California, *J Am Vet Med Assoc* 186:370-373, 1985.

Grahn TC, Fahning ML, Zemjanis R: Nature of early reproductive failure caused by bovine viral diarrhea virus, *J Am Vet Med Assoc* 185:429-432, 1984.

Griesemer RA, Cole CR: Bovine papular stomatitis, *J Am Vet Med Assoc* 137:404-410, 1960.

Grooms D, Baker JC, Ames TR: Diseases caused by bovine virus diarrhea virus. In Smith BP, editor: *Large animal internal medicine*, ed 3, St. Louis, 2002, Mosby, pp. 707-714.

Grooms DL: Reproductive consequences of infection with bovine viral diarrhea virus, *Vet Clin N Am: Food Anim Pract* 20:5-19, 2004.

Grooms DL, Brock KV, Ward LA: Detection of bovine viral diarrhea virus in the ovaries of cattle acutely infected with bovine viral diarrhea virus, *J Vet Diagn Invest* 10:125-129, 1998.

Haggard DL: Bovine enteric colibacillosis, *Vet Clin North Am: Food Anim Pract* 1:495-508, 1985.

Haines DM, Chelck BJ, Naylor JM: Immunoglobulin concentrations in commercially available colostrum supplements for calves, *Can Vet J* 31:36-37, 1990.

Hamdy FM, Dardiri AH, Mebus C, et al: Etiology of malignant catarrhal fever outbreak in Minnesota. In *Proceedings: 82nd US Animal Health Association*, 1978, p. 248.

Hammerberg B: Pathophysiology of nematodiasis in cattle, *Vet Clin North Am: Food Anim Pract* 2:225-234, 1986.

Hand MS, Hunt E, Phillips RW: Milk replacers for the neonatal calf, *Vet Clin North Am: Food Anim Pract* 1:589-609, 1985.

Hansen DE, Thurmond MC, Thorburn M: Factors associated with the spread of clinical vesicular stomatitis in California dairy cattle, *Am J Vet Res* 46:789-795, 1985.

Hasoksuz M, Hoet AE, Loersch SC, et al: Detection of respiratory and enteric shedding of bovine coronaviruses in cattle in an Ohio feedlot, *J Vet Diagn Invest* 14:308-313, 2002.

Hebeller HF, Linton AH, Osborne AD: Atypical actinobacillosis in a dairy herd, *Vet Rec* 73:517-521, 1961.

Hendrick SH, Kelton DF, Leslie KE, et al: Efficacy of monensin sodium for the reduction of fecal shedding of *Mycobacterium avium* subsp. *paratuberculosis* in infected dairy cattle, *Prev Vet Med* 75:206-220, 2006.

Herd RP, Heider LE: Control of internal parasites in dairy replacement heifers by two treatments in the spring, *J Am Vet Med Assoc* 177:51-54, 1980.

Herd KP, Heider LE: Control of nematodes in dairy heifers by prophylactic treatments with albendazole in the spring, *J Am Vet Med Assoc* 186:1071-1074, 1985.

Heuschele WP: Malignant catarrhal fever. In Committee on Foreign Animal Diseases, editors: *Foreign animal diseases*, Richmond, VA, 1992, United States Animal Health Association.

Holland RE: Some infectious causes of diarrhea in young farm animals, *Clin Microbiol Rev* 3:345-375, 1990.

Holloway NM, Tyler JW, Lakritz J, et al: Serum immunoglobulin G concentrations in calves fed fresh colostrum or a colostrum supplement, *J Vet Intern Med* 16:187-191, 2002.

Holmberg SD, Osterholm MT, Senger KA, et al: Drug-resistant Salmonella from animals fed antimicrobials, *N Engl J Med* 311:617-622, 1984.

Hornick RB: Salmonella infections other than typhoid lever. In Wyngaarden JB, Smith LH Jr, editors: *Cecil's textbook of medicine*, ed 18, Philadelphia, 1988, WB Saunders.

Howard TH, Bean B, Hillman R, et al: Surveillance for persistent bovine viral diarrhea virus infection in four artificial insemination centers, *J Am Vet Med Assoc* 196:1951-1955, 1990.

Jamaluddin AA, Carpenter TE, Hird DW, et al: Economics of feeding pasteurized colostrum and pasteurized waste milk to dairy calves, *J Am Vet Med Assoc* 209:751-756, 1996.

Jarrett WFH, Campo MS, Blaxter ML, et al: Alimentary fibropapilloma in cattle. A spontaneous tumor, nonpermissive for papillomavirus replication, *J Nat Cancer Inst* 73:499-504, 1984.

Jarrett WFH, et al: Papilloma viruses in benign and malignant tumors of cattle, *Cold Spring Harbor Conference on Cell Proliferation*, 1980, pp. 215-222.

Jeong WI, Do SH, Sohn MH, et al: Hepatocellular carcinoma with metastasis to the spleen in a Holstein cow, *Vet Pathol* 42:230-232, 2005.

Kahrs R: Effect of bovine viral diarrhea on the developing fetus, *J Am Vet Med Assoc* 163:877-878, 1973.

Kahrs R, Atkinson G, Baker JA, et al: Serological studies on the incidence of bovine virus diarrhea, infectious bovine rhinotracheitis, bovine myxovirus, parainfluenza-3, and Leptospira pomona in New York State, *Cornell Vet* 54:360-369, 1964.

Kahrs RF: Rotavirus associated with neonatal diarrhea, In Kahrs RF, editor: *Viral diseases of cattle*, ed 2, Ames, IA, 2001, Iowa State University Press, pp. 239-246.

Kahrs RF: *Viral diseases of cattle*, ed 1, Ames, IA, 1981, Iowa State University Press.

Kahrs RF, Scott FW, de Lahunte A: Congenital cerebella hypoplasia and ocular defects in calves following bovine viral diarrhea-mucosal disease infection in pregnant cattle, *J Am Vet Med Assoc* 156:1443-1450, 1970.

Katayama SI, Matsushita O, Minami J, et al: Comparison of the alpha-toxin genes of *Clostridium perfringens* type A and C strains: evidence for extragenic regulation of transcription, *Infect Immun* 61:457-463, 1993.

Kelling CL, Steffen DJ, Cooper VL, et al: Effect of infection with bovine viral diarrhea virus alone, bovine rotavirus alone, or concurrent infection with both on enteric disease in gnotobiotic calves, *Am J Vet Res* 63:1179-1186, 2002.

Kelling CW: Evolution of bovine viral diarrhea virus vaccines, *Vet Clin N Am: Food Anim Pract* 20:115-129, 2004.

Kendrick JW, Franti CE: Bovine viral diarrhea: decay of colostrum-conferred antibody in the calf, *Am J Vet Res* 35:589-591, 1974.

Kenney DG, Weldon AD, Rebhun WC: Oropharyngeal abscessation in two cows secondary to administration of an oral calcium preparation, *Cornell Vet* 83:61-65, 1993.

Ketelsen AT, Johnson DW, Muscoplat CC: Depression of bovine monocyte chemotactic responses by bovine viral diarrhea virus, *Infect Immun* 25:565-568, 1979.

Kimball A, Twiehaus MJ, Frank ER: *Actinomyces bovis* isolated from six cases of bovine orchids: a preliminary report, *Am J Vet Res* 15:551-553, 1954.

Kingman HE, Paven JS: Streptomycin in the treatment of actinomycosis, *J Am Vet Med Assoc* 118:28-30, 1951.

Kirkpatrick MA, Kersting KW, Kinyon JM: Case report—Jejunal hemorrhage syndrome of dairy cattle, *Bov Pract* 35:104-116, 2001.

Knight AP, Messer NT: Vesicular stomatitis, *Compend Contin Educ Pract Vet* 5:S517-S534, 1983.

Koopmans M, van Wuijckhuise-Sjouke L, Schukken YM, et al: Association of diarrhea in cattle with torovirus infections on farms, *Am J Vet Res* 52:1769-1773, 1991.

Kumper H: A new treatment for abomasal bloat in calves, *Bov Pract* 29:80-82, 1995.

Lechtenberg KF, Nagaraja TG: Hepatic ultrasonography and blood changes in cattle with experimentally induced hepatic abscesses, *Am J Vet Res* 52:803-809, 1991.

Lee KM, Gillespie JH: Propagation of virus diarrhea virus of cattle in tissue culture, *Am J Vet Res* 18:952-953, 1957.

Lerner PI: Susceptibility of pathogenic actinomycetes to antimicrobial compounds, *Antimicrob Agents Chemother* 5:302-309, 1974.

Li H, Shen DT, O'Toole D, et al: Investigation of sheep-associated malignant catarrhal fever virus infection in ruminants by PCR and competitive inhibition enzyme-linked immunosorbent assay, *J Clin Microbiol* 33:2048-2053, 1995.

Lilley CW, Hamar DW, Gerlach M, et al: Linking copper deficiency with abomasal ulcers in beef calves, *Vet Med* 80:85-88, 1985.

Lofstedt J, Dohoo IR, Duizer G: Model to predict septicemia in diarrheic calves, *J Vet Intern Med* 13:81-88, 1999.

Lorenz I: Influence of D-lactate on metabolic acidosis and on prognosis in neonatal calves with diarrhoea, *J Vet Med A Physiol Pathol Clin Med* 51:425-428, 2004.

Lucchelli A, Lance SE, Bartlett PB, et al: Prevalence of bovine group A rotavirus shedding among dairy calves in Ohio, *Am J Vet Res* 53:169-174, 1992.

Luedke AJ, Jones RH, Jochim MM: Transmission of bluetongue between sheep and cattle by *Culicoides variipennis*, *Am J Vet Res* 28:457-460, 1967.

MacPherson LW: Bovine virus enteritis (winter dysentery), *Can J Comp Med* 21:184-192, 1957.

Maddox C, Hattel A, Drake T, et al: *Clostridium perfringens* type A strains recovered from acute hemorrhagic enteritis of adult lactating dairy cattle (abstract), *Proceedings of the 42nd Annual Meeting, American Association of Veterinary Laboratory Diagnosticians*, San Diego, 1999, p. 51.

Malmquist WA: Bovine viral diarrhea-mucosal disease: etiology, pathogenesis, and applied immunity, *J Am Vet Med Assoc* 152:763-768, 1968.

Malone JB Jr: Fascioliasis and cestodiasis in cattle, *Vet Clin North Am: Food Anim Pract* 2:261-275, 1986.

Manteca C, Daube G, Pirson V, et al: Bacterial intestinal flora associated with enterotoxaemia in Belgian Blue calves, *Vet Microbiol* 81:21-32, 2001.

Manteca C, Jauniaux T, Daube G, et al: Isolation of *Clostridium perfringens* from three calves with hemorrhagic abomasitis, *Rev Med Vet* 152:637-639, 2001.

Markham RJF, Ramnaraine ML: Release of immunosuppressive substances from tissue culture cells infected with bovine viral diarrhea virus, *Am J Vet Res* 46:879-883, 1985.

McClurkin AW, Bolin SR, Coria MF: Isolation of cytopathic and noncytopathic bovine viral diarrhea virus from the spleen of cattle acutely and chronically affected with bovine viral diarrhea, *J Am Vet Med Assoc* 186:568–569, 1985.

McClurkin AW, Coria MF, Cutlip RC: Reproductive performance of apparently healthy cattle persistently infected with bovine viral diarrhea virus, *J Am Vet Med Assoc* 174:1116-1119, 1979.

McClurkin AW, Littledike ET, Cutlip RC, et al: Production of cattle immunotolerant to bovine viral diarrhea virus, *Can J Comp Med* 48:156-161, 1984.

McDonough PL: Epidemiology of bovine salmonellosis. In *Proceedings of the 18th Annual Convention of American Association Bovine Practitioners*, 1985, pp. 169-173.

McGuirk SM: Colostrum: quality and quantity. In *Proceedings of the XVII World Buiatrics Congress*, vol 2, 1992, pp. 162-167.

McGuirk SM, Collins M: Managing the production, storage, and delivery of colostrum, *Vet Clin N Am: Food Anim Pract* 20:593-603, 2004.

McLauchlin J, Amar C, Pedraza-Diaz S, et al: Molecular epidemiological analysis of *Cryptosporidium* spp. in the United Kingdom: results of genotyping *Cryptosporidium* spp. in 1,705 fecal samples from humans and 105 fecal samples from livestock animals, *J Clin Microbiol* 38:3984-3990, 2000.

Mebus CA, Newman LE, Stair EL: Scanning, electron, light and immunofluorescent microscopy of intestine of gnotobiotic calf infected with calf diarrhea coronavirus, *Am J Vet Res* 36:1719-1725, 1975.

Mebus CA, Underdahl NR, Rhodes MB, et al: Calf diarrhea (scours): reproduced with a virus from a field outbreak, *Univ Nebr Res Bull* 233:2-15, 1969.

Mechor GD, Gröhn YT, VanSaun RJ: Effect of temperature on colostrometer readings for estimation of immunoglobulin concentration in bovine colostrum, *J Dairy Sci* 74:3940-3943, 1991.

Meer R, Songer JG: Multiplex polymerase chain reaction assay for genotyping *Clostridium perfringens*, *Am J Vet Res* 58:702-705, 1997.

Meyling A, Jensen AM: Transmission of bovine virus diarrhoea virus (BVDV) by artificial insemination (AI) with semen from a persistently infected bull, *Vet Microbiol* 17:97-105, 1988.

Miller HV, Drost M: Failure to cause abortion in cows with intravenous sodium iodide treatment, *J Am Vet Med Assoc* 172:466-467, 1978.

Milne MH, Barrett DC, Mellor DJ, et al: Clinical recognition and treatment of bovine cutaneous actinobacillosis, *Vet Rec* 148:273-274, 2001.

Moon HW, McClurkin AW, Isaacson RE, et al: Pathogenic relationship of rotavirus, *Escherichia coli*, and other agents in mixed infections in calves, *J Am Vet Med Assoc* 173:577-583, 1978.

Morley PS, Morris N, Hyatt DR, et al: Evaluation of the efficacy of disinfectant footbaths as used in veterinary hospitals, *J Am Vet Med Assoc* 226:2053-2058, 2005.

Motiwala AS, Li L, Kapur V, et al: Current understanding of the genetic diversity of *Mycobacterium avium* subsp. *Paratuberculosis*, *Microbes Infect* 8:1406-1418, 2006.

Muller-Doblies UU, Li H, Hauser B, et al: Field validation of laboratory tests for clinical diagnosis of sheep-associated malignant catarrhal fever, *J Clin Microbiol* 36:2970-2972, 1998.

Nagarja TG, Chengappa MM: Liver abscesses in feedlot cattle: a review, *Anim Sci* 76:287-298, 1998.

Naylor JM: Neonatal ruminant diarrhea. In Smith BP, editor: *Large animal internal medicine*, ed 3, St. Louis, 2002, Mosby, Inc., pp.352-381.

Naylor JM: Severity and nature of acidosis in diarrheic calves over and under one week of age, *Can Vet J* 28:168-173, 1987.

Neitz WO, Riemerschmid G: The influence of solar radiation on the course of bluetongue, *Onderstepoort J Vet Res* 20:29-55, 1944.

Niilo L: *Clostridium perfringens* in animal disease: a review of current knowledge, *Can Vet J* 21:141-148, 1980.

Niilo L: *Clostridium perfringens* type C enterotoxemia, *Can Vet J* 29:658-664, 1988.

Norman LM, Hohenboken WD, Kelley KW: Genetic differences in concentration of immunoglobulin G_1 and M in serum and colostrum of cows in serum of neonatal calves, *J Anim Sci* 53:1465-1472, 1981.

Nunamaker RA, Lockwood JA, Stith CE, et al: Grasshoppers (Orthoptera: Acrididea) could serve as reservoirs and vectors of vesicular stomatitis virus, *J Med Entomol* 40:957-963, 2003.

Nydam DV, Mohammed HO: Quantitative risk assessment of Cryptosporidium species infection in dairy calves, *J Dairy Sci* 88:3932-3943, 2005.

Ogilvie TH: The persistent isolation of *Salmonella typhimurium* from the mammary gland of a dairy cow, *Can Vet J* 27:329-331, 1986.

Olafson P, MacCallum AD, Fox FH: An apparently new transmissible disease of cattle, *Cornell Vet* 36:205-213, 1946.

O'Sullivan EN: Two-year study of bovine hepatic abscessation in 10 abattoirs in County Cork, Ireland, *Vet Rec* 145:389-393, 1999.

Palotay JL: Actinobacillosis in cattle, *Vet Med* Feb:52-54, 1951.

Panciera RJ, Thomas RW, Garner FM: Cryptosporidial infection in a calf, *Vet Pathol* 8:479-484, 1971.

Parish SM, Evermann JF, Olcott B, et al: A bluetongue epizootic in northwestern United States, *J Am Vet Med Assoc* 181:589-591, 1982.

Parreno V, Bejar C, Vagnozzi A, et al: Modulation by colostrum-acquired antibodies of systemic and mucosal antibody responses to rotavirus in calves experimentally challenged with bovine rotavirus, *Vet Immunol Immunopathol* 100:7-24, 2004.

Peek SF, Hartmann FA, Thomas CB, et al: Isolation of Salmonella spp from the environment of dairies without any history of clinical salmonellosis, *J Am Vet Med Assoc* 225:574-577, 2004.

Pellerin C, van den Hurk J, Lecompte J, et al: Identification of a new group of bovine viral diarrhea virus strains associated with severe outbreaks and high mortalities, *Virology* 203:260-268, 1994.

Perdrizet JA, Rebhun WC, Dubovi EJ, et al: Bovine virus diarrhea—clinical syndromes in dairy herds, *Cornell Vet* 77:46-74, 1987.

Perry GH, Vivanco H, Holmes I, et al: No evidence of *Mycobacterium avium* subsp. *paratuberculosis* in *in vitro* produced cryopreserved embryos derived from subclinically infected cows, *Theriogenology* 66:1267-1273, 2006.

Perryman LE, Kapil SJ, Jones ML, et al: Protection of calves against cryptosporidiosis with immune bovine colostrum induced by a *Cryptosporidium parvum* recombinant protein, *Vaccine* 17:2142-2149, 1999.

Petit L, Gibert M, Popoff M: *Clostridium perfringens*: toxinotype and genotype, *Trend Microbiol* 7:104-110, 1999.

Pettit HV, Ivan M, Brisson GJ: Digestibility and blood parameters in the preruminant calf fed a clotting or nonclotting milk replacer, *J Anim Sci* 66:986-991, 1988.

Phillips RW: Fluid therapy for diarrheic calves: what, how, and how much, *Vet Clin North Am: Food Anim Pract* 1:541-562, 1985.

Plowright W: Malignant catarrhal fever, *J Am Vet Med Assoc* 152:795-806, 1968.

Pohlenz J, Moon HW, Cheville NF, et al: Cryptosporidiosis as a probable factor in neonatal diarrhea in calves, *J Am Vet Med Assoc* 172:452-457, 1978.

Popísil Z, et al: Decline in the phytohaemagglutinin responsiveness of lymphocytes from calves infected experimentally with bovine viral diarrhoea-mucosal disease virus and parainfluenza 3 virus, *Acta Vet Brno* 44:360-375, 1975.

Potgieter LND, McCracken MD, Hopkins FM, et al: Comparison of the pneumopathogenicity of two strains of bovine viral diarrhea virus, *Am J Vet Res* 46:151-153, 1985.

Powers JG, Van Metre DC, Collins JK, et al: Evaluation of ovine herpesvirus-2 infections, as detected by competitive inhibition ELISA and polymerase chain reaction assay, in dairy cattle without signs of malignant catarrhal fever, *J Am Vet Med Assoc* 227:606-611, 2005.

Pritchett LC, Gay CC, Besser TE, et al: Management and production factors influencing immunoglobulin G_1 concentration in colostrum from Holstein cows, *J Dairy Sci* 74:2336-2341, 1991.

Pritchett LC, Gay CC, Hancock DD, et al: Evaluation of the hydrometer for testing immunoglobulin G$_1$ in Holstein colostrum, *J Dairy Sci* 77:1761-1767, 1994.

Puntenney SB, Wang Y, Forsberg NE: Mycotic infections in livestock: recent insights and studies on etiology, diagnostics, and prevention of hemorrhagic bowel syndrome, *Proceedings, Southwest Animal Nutrition Conference, University of Arizona, Department of Animal Science,* Tucson, AZ, 2003, pp. 49-63.

Pyorala S, Laurila T, Lehtonen S, et al: Local tissue damage in cows after administration of preparations containing phenylbutazone, flunixin, ketoprofen, and metamizole, *Acta Vet Scand* 40:145-150, 1999.

Qi F, Ridpath JF, Berry ES: Insertion of a bovine SMT3B gene in NS4B and duplication of NS3 in a bovine viral diarrhea virus genome correlate with the cytopathogenicity of the virus, *Virus Res* 57:1-9, 1998.

Quilez J, Sanchez-Acedo C, Avendano C, et al: Efficacy of two peroxygen-based disinfectants for inactivation of *Cryptosporidium parvum* oocysts, *Appl Environ Microbiol* 71:2479-2483, 2005.

Radostits OM: Clinical examination of the alimentary system—ruminants. In Radostits OM, Mayhew IG, Houston DM, editors: *Veterinary clinical examination and diagnosis,* London, 2000, WB Saunders, pp. 409-468.

Radostits OM, Gay C, Blood DC, et al: *Veterinary medicine. A textbook of the diseases of cattle, sheep, pigs, goats and horses,* ed 7, Philadelphia, 1989, Bailliere Tindall [with contributions by Arundel JH, Gay CC]. (The latest edition in the 9th edition.)

Radostits OM, Stockdale PH: A brief review of bovine coccidiosis in Western Canada, *Can Vet J* 21:227-230, 1980.

Ramsey HA: Non-milk protein in milk replacers with special emphasis on soy products, Presented at the Annual Meeting American Dairy Science Association 1982.

Rebhun WC, French TW, Perdrizet JA, et al: Thrombocytopenia associated with acute bovine virus diarrhea infection in cattle, *J Vet Intern Med* 3:42-46, 1989.

Rebhun WC, King JM, Hillman RB: Atypical actinobacillosis granulomas in cattle, *Cornell Vet* 78:125-130, 1988.

Reggiardo C, Kaeberle ML: Detection of bacteremia in cattle inoculated with bovine viral diarrhea virus, *Am J Vet Res* 42:218-221, 1981.

Ridpath J, Bolin S: Differentiation of types Ia, Ib, and 2 bovine viral diarrhea virus (BVDV) by PCR, *Mol Cell Probes* 12:101-106, 1998.

Roberts SJ: Winter dysentery in dairy cattle, *Cornell Vet* 47:372-388, 1957.

Rodak L, Babiuk LA, Acres SD: Detection by radioimmunoassay and enzyme-linked immunosorbent assay of coronavirus antibodies in bovine serum and lacteal secretions, *J Clin Microbiol* 16:34-40, 1982.

Roden LD, Smith BP, Spier SJ, et al: Effect of calf age and *Salmonella* bacterin type on ability to produce immunoglobulins directed against *Salmonella* whole cells or lipopolysaccharide, *Am J Vet Res* 53:1895-1899, 1992.

Roeder BL, Chengappa MM, Nagaraja TG, et al: Experimental induction of abomasal tympany and abomasal ulceration by intraruminal inoculation of *Clostridium perfringens* type A in neonatal calves, *Am J Vet Res* 49:201-207, 1988.

Roeder BL, Chengappa MM, Nagaraja TG, et al: Isolation of *Clostridium perfringens* type A from neonatal calves with ruminal and abomasal tympany, abomasitis, and abomasal ulceration, *J Am Vet Med Assoc* 190:1550-1555, 1987.

Rood J, McClane B: *The Clostridia, molecular biology and pathogenesis,* San Diego, 1997, Academic Press, pp. 153-160.

Ross CE, Dubovi EJ, Donis RO: Herd problems of abortions and malformed calves attributed to bovine viral diarrhea, *J Am Vet Med Assoc* 185:429-432, 1986.

Ross CE, Rebhun WC: Megaesophagus in a cow, *J Am Vet Med Assoc* 188:623-624, 1986.

Roth JA, Bolin SR, Frank DE: Lymphocyte blastogenesis and neutrophil function in cattle persistently infected with bovine viral diarrhea virus, *Am J Vet Res* 47:1139-1141, 1986.

Runnels PL, Moon HW, Matthews PJ, et al: Effects of microbial and host variables on the interaction of rotavirus and *Escherichia coli* infections in gnotobiotic calves, *Am J Vet Res* 47:1542-1550, 1986.

Sahal M, Karaer Z, Yasa Duru S, et al: Cryptosporidiosis in newborn calves in Ankara region: clinical, haematological findings and treatment with Lasalocia-NA (article in German), *Dtsch Tierarztl Wochenschr* 112:203-208, 210, 2005.

Saif LJ, Redman DR, Smith KL, et al: Passive immunity to bovine rotavirus in newborn calves fed colostrum supplements from immunized or nonimmunized cows, *Infect Immun* 41:1118-1131, 1983.

Saif LJ, Smith L: Enteric viral infections of calves and passive immunity, *J Dairy Sci* 68:206-228, 1985.

Saliki JT, Dubovi EJ: Laboratory diagnosis of bovine viral diarrhea virus infections, *Vet Clin N Am: Food Anim Pract* 20:69-83, 2004.

Sanchez J, Dohoo I, Leslie K, et al: The use of an indirect Ostertagia ostertagi ELISA to predict milk production response after anthelmintic treatment in confined and semi-confined dairy herds, *Vet Parasitol* 130:115-124, 2005.

Sattar SA, Jacobsen H, Rahman H, et al: Interruption of rotavirus spread through chemical disinfection, *Infect Control Hosp Epidemiol* 15:751-756, 1994.

Schlafer DH, Scott FW: Prevalence of neutralizing antibody to the calf rotavirus in New York cattle, *Cornell Vet* 69:262-271, 1979.

Scott FW, Kahrs RF, De LahunteA, et al: Virus induced congenital anomalies of the bovine fetus: I. cerebellar degeneration (hypoplasia), ocular lesions and fetal mummification following experimental infection with bovine viral diarrhea-mucosal disease virus, *Cornell Vet* 63:536-560, 1973.

Selim SA, Cullor JS, Smith BP, et al: The effect of *Escherichia coli* J5 and modified live *Salmonella* dublin vaccines in artificially reared neonatal calves, *Vaccine* 13:381-390, 1995.

Sinks GD, Quigley JD III, Reinemeyer CR: Effects of lasalocid on coccidial infection and growth in young dairy calves, *J Am Vet Med Assoc* 200:1947-1951, 1992.

Smith BP: Personal communication, 2006.

Smith BP: Salmonellosis in ruminants. In *Large animal internal medicine,* ed 3, St. Louis, 2002, Mosby, pp. 775-779.

Smith BP: Understanding the role of endotoxins in gram-negative septicemia, *Vet Med* 81:1148-1161, 1986.

Smith BP, Dilling GW, Roden LD, et al: Aromatic-dependent *Salmonella dublin* as a parenteral modified live vaccine for calves, *Am J Vet Res* 45:2231-2235, 1984.

Smith BP, Oliver DG, Singh P, et al: Detection of *Salmonella dublin* mammary gland infection in carrier cows using an ELISA for antibody in milk or serum, *Am J Vet Res* 50:1352-1360, 1989.

Smith BP, Reina-Guerra M, Hoiseth SK, et al: Aromatic-dependent *Salmonella typhimurium* as modified live vaccines for calves, *Am J Vet Res* 45:59-66, 1984.

Smith HW: A laboratory consideration of the treatment of *Actinobacillus lignieresii* infection, *Vet Rec* 63:674-675, 1951.

Smith RH, Wynn CF: Effects of feeding soya products to preruminant calves, *Proc Nutr Soc (London)* 30:75A, 1971.

Smithlie LK, Modderman E: BVD virus in commercial fetal calf serum and normal and aborted fetuses, In *Proceedings: 18th Annual Meeting American Association Veterinary Laboratory Diagnosis,* 1975, pp. 113-119.

Snodgrass DR, Fahey KJ, Wells PW, et al: Passive immunity in calf rotavirus infections: maternal vaccination increases and prolongs immunoglobulin G$_1$ antibody secretion in milk, *Infect Immun* 28:344-349, 1980.

Snodgrass DR, Stewart J, Taylor J, et al: Diarrhea in dairy calves reduced by feeding colostrum from cows vaccinated with rotavirus, *Res Vet Sci* 32:70-73, 1982.

Snodgrass DR, Terzolo HR, Sherwood D, et al: Aetiology of diarrhea in young calves, *Vet Rec* 119:31-34, 1986.

Snyder DE, Floyd JG, DiPietro JA: Use of anthelmintics and anticoccidial compounds in cattle, *Compend Contin Educ Pract Vet* 13:1847-1860, 1991.

Sockett DC, Brower AI, Porter RE, et al: Hemorrhagic bowel syndrome in dairy cattle: preliminary results from a case control study. In *Proceedings, 47th Annual Conference, American Association of Veterinary Laboratory Diagnosticians*, Greensboro, NC, 2004, p. 37.

Songer JG: Clostridial diseases of small ruminants, *Vet Res* 29:219-232, 1998.

Songer JG: Clostridial enteric diseases of domestic animals, *Clin Microbiol Rev* 9:216-234, 1996.

Songer JG: *Clostridium perfringens* type A infection in cattle. In *Proceedings, 32nd Annual Convention, American Association of Bovine Practitioners*, 1999, pp. 40-44.

Speer CA, Scott MC, Bannantine JP, et al: A novel enzyme-linked immunosorbent assay for diagnosis of *Mycobactyerium avium* subsp. *paratuberculosis* infections (Johne's disease) in cattle, *Clin Vaccine Immunol* 13:535-540, 2006.

Spier SJ, Smith BP, Cullor JS, et al: Persistent experimental *Salmonella dublin* intramammary infection in dairy cows, *J Vet Intern Med* 5:341-350, 1991.

Stockdale PH, Niilo L: Production of bovine coccidiosis with *Eimeria zuernii*, *Can Vet J* 17:35-37, 1976.

Stott JL: Bluetongue and epizootic hemorrhagic disease. In Committee on Foreign Animal Diseases, editors: *Foreign animal diseases*, Richmond, VA, 1992, United States Animal Health Association.

Sulaiman IM, Xiao L, Yang C, et al: Differentiating human from animal isolates of *Cryptosporidium parvum*, *Emerg Inf Dis* 4:681-685, 1998.

Swarbrick O: Atypical actinobacillosis in three cows, *Br Vet J* 123:70-75, 1967.

Sweeney RW, Divers TJ, Whitlock RH, et al: Hepatic failure in dairy cattle following mastitis or metritis, *J Vet Intern Med* 2:80-84, 1988.

Sweeney RW, Uzonna J, Whitlock RH, et al: Tissue predilection sites and effect of dose on *Mycobacterium avium* subs. *paratuberculosis* organism recovery in a short-term bovine experimental oral infection model, *Res Vet Sci* 80:253-259, 2006.

Sweeney RW, Whitlock RH, McAdams S, et al: Londitudinal study of ELISA seroreactivity to *Mycobacterium avium* subsp. *paratuberculosis* in infected cattle and culture-negative herd mates, *J Vet Diagn Invest* 18:2-6, 2006.

Takahashi E, et al: Epizootic diarrhoea of adult cattle associated with a corona-like agent, *Vet Microbiol* 5:151-154, 1980.

Tennant B, Ward DE, Braun RK, et al: Clinical management and control of neonatal enteric infections of calves, *J Am Vet Med Assoc* 173:654-660, 1978.

Terzolo HR, Lawson GHK, Angus KW, et al: Enteric campylobacter infection in gnotobiotic calves and lambs, *Res Vet Sci* 43:72-77, 1987.

Timoney JF, Gillespie JH, Scott FW, et al: *Hagan and Bruner's microbiology and infectious diseases of domestic animals*, ed 8, New York, 1988, Cornell University Press.

Tompkins T: Milk replacer options, *Large Anim Vet* January:24-29, 1993.

Tompkins T, Drackley JK: Clotting factor in bovine preruminant nutrition. In *Proceedings: XVII World Buiatrics Congress*, vol 2, 1992, pp. 176-181.

Tompkins T, Jaster EH: Preruminant calf nutrition, *Vet Clin North Am: Food Anim Pract* 7:557-576, 1991.

Torres-Medina A, Schlafer DH, Mebus CA: Rotaviral and coronaviral diarrhea, *Vet Clin North Am: Food Anim Pract* 1:471-493, 1985.

Trainin Z, et al: Oral immunization of young calves against enteropathogenic E. coli. In *Proceedings: XI International Congress on Diseases of Cattle*, 1980, p. 1313.

Traven M, Naslund K, Linde N, et al: Experimental reproduction of winter dysentery in lactating cows using BCV—comparison with BCV infection in milk-fed calves, *Vet Microbiol* 81:127-151, 2001.

Troxel TR, Gadberry MS, Wallace WT, et al: Clostridial antibody response from injection-site lesions in beef cattle, long-term antibody response to single or multiple doses, and response in newborn beef calves, *J Anim Sci* 79:2558-2564, 2001.

Tsunemitsu H, Smith DR, Saif LJ: Experimental inoculation of adult dairy cows with bovine coronavirus and detection of coronavirus by RT-PCR, *Arch Virol* 144:167-175, 1999.

Tyler JW, Hancock DD, Wilson L, et al: Effect of passive transfer status and vaccination with Escherichia coli (J5) on mortality in commingled dairy calves, *J Vet Intern Med* 13:36-39, 1999.

Tyler JW, Parish SM, Besser TE, et al: Detection of low serum immunoglobulin concentrations in clinically ill calves, *J Vet Intern Med* 12:40-43, 1999.

Tyler JW, Steevens BJ, Hostetler DE, et al: Colostral IgG concentrations in Holstein and Guernsey cows, *Am J Vet Res* 60:1136-1139, 1999.

Udall DH: *The practice of veterinary medicine*, ed 6, Ithaca, NY, 1954, published by the author, p. 624.

Underdahl NR, Grace OD, Hoerlein AB: Cultivation in tissue culture of a cytopathogenic agent from bovine mucosal disease, *Proc Soc Exp Biol Med* 94:795-797, 1957.

Uzal FA, Blanchard P, Songer G, et al: Studies on the so-called "clostridial enteritis" of cattle (abstract). In *Proceedings, 43rd Annual Meeting, American Association of Veterinary Laboratory Diagnosticians*, Birmingham, AL, 2000, p. 15.

Van Campen H: personal communication, 2006, Fort Collins, CO.

van Schaik G, Stehman SM, Jacobson RH, et al: Cow-level evaluation of a kinetics ELISA with multiple cutoff values to detect fecal shedding of *Mycobacterium avium* subspecies *paratuberculosis* in New York State dairy cows, *Prev Vet Med* 73:221-236, 2005.

Vance HN: A survey of the alimentary tract of cattle for *Clostridium perfringens*, *Can J Comp Med Vet Sci* 31:260-264, 1967.

Voges J, Horner GW, Rowe S, et al: Persistent bovine pestivirus infection localized in the testes of an immunocompetent, non-viraemic bull, *Vet Microbiol* 61:165-175, 1998.

Walz PH, Bell TG, Steficek BA, et al: Experimental model of type II bovine viral diarrhea virus-induced thrombocytopenia in neonatal calves, *J Vet Diagn Invest* 11:505-514, 1999.

Walz PH, Steficek BA, Baker JC, et al: Effect of experimentally induced type II bovine viral diarrhea virus infection on platelet function in calves, *Am J Vet Res* 60:1396-1401, 1999.

Wang YQ, Puntenney SB, Forsberg NE: Identification of the mechanisms by which OmniGen-AF, a nutritional supplement, augments immune function in ruminant livestock. In *Proceedings, Western Section, American Association of Animal Science*, 2004, p. 55.

Ward GM, Roberts SJ, McEntee K, et al: A study of experimentally induced bovine viral diarrhea-mucosal disease in pregnant cows and their progeny, *Cornell Vet* 59:525-539, 1969.

Warnick LD, Kanistanon K, McDonough PL, et al: Effect of previous antimicrobial treatment on fecal shedding of *Salmonella enterica* subsp. *Enterica* serogroup B in New York dairy herds with recent clinical salmonellosis, *Prev Vet Med* 56:285-297, 2003.

Washburn KE, Step DL, Kirkpatrick JF, et al: Bluetongue and persistent bovine viral diarrhea virus infection causing generalized edema in an adult bull, *J Vet Intern Med* 14:468-469, 2000.

Watts TC, Olsoh SM, Rhodes CS: Treatment of bovine actinomycosis with isoniazid, *Can Vet J* 14:223-224, 1973.

Weaver DM, Tyler JW, Barrington GM, et al: Passive transfer of colostral immunoglobulins in calves, *J Vet Intern Med* 14:569-577, 2000.

Weaver LD: Malignant catarrhal fever in two California dairy herds, *Bov Pract* 14:121-127, 1979.

Weldon AD, Moise NS, Rebhun WC: Hyperkalemic atrial standstill in neonatal calf diarrhea, *J Vet Intern Med* 6:294-297, 1992.

White DM, Wilson WC, Blair CD, et al: Studies on overwintering of bluetongue viruses in insects, *J Gen Virol* 2:453-462, 2005.

Whitmore HL, Zemjanis R, Olson J: Effect of bovine viral diarrhea virus on conception in cattle, *J Am Vet Med Assoc* 178:1065-1067, 1981.

Williams JC, Corwin RM, Craig TM, et al: Control strategies for nematodiasis in cattle, *Vet Clin North Am: Food Anim Pract* 2:247-260, 1986.

Williams JC, Knox JW, Marbury KS, et al: *Osterlagia ostertagi*: a continuing problem of recognition and control, *Anim Nutr Health* March:42-45, 1985.

CHAPTER 7

Skin Diseases

Danny W. Scott

INFECTIOUS DISEASES

Papillomatosis (Fibropapillomas, "Warts")
Etiology

Papillomas are the most common tumors in dairy cattle; fortunately most papillomas are benign and self-limiting. Animals between 6 and 24 months seem most at risk for warts, and previous incidence of the tumors gives an individual a degree of immunity. Papillomas are well documented to be caused by bovine papilloma virus (BPV) types 1 through 6. These viruses have some common antigenic components but do not have good immunologic cross-reactivity. BPV1 and especially BPV2 cause typical warts on the head, neck, trunk, and legs of young cattle (Figure 7-1). A "typical" wart means

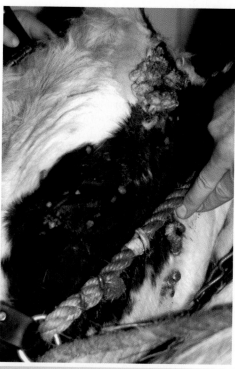

Figure 7-1

Multiple small fibropapillomas on the eyelids, masseter region, and a large fibropapilloma originating at the dehorning site.

that a true fibropapilloma exists histopathologically. These masses usually are cauliflower-like, rough, or crusty-surfaced skin lesions that are colored white to gray. Some appear flatter, gray, and have a broad-based skin attachment. Others have a pedunculated base. The virus infects the basal cells of the epithelium, and as these cells eventually reach the surface, large quantities of virus are available to contaminate fomites and the environment. Therefore warts tend to become endemic rather than occur sporadically. Stanchions, feed bunks, neck straps, brushes, halters, pens, and back rubs all become coated with virus. Abrasion of the skin caused by mild trauma from sharp objects (e.g., nails, splintered wood, barbed wire, and bolt ends) allows inoculation of the virus into skin and will increase the incidence in a group of calves. Epidemic and endemic situations also have been associated with dehorning (Figure 7-2), ear tagging, and the use of tattooing devices or emasculatomes when disinfection of a common instrument has not been performed. This is especially true when laypeople perform the aforementioned procedures. Insects also have been suspected of spreading or inoculating the virus into skin, but this remains difficult to prove.

Cattle with large multiple warts that do not regress probably have concurrent deficient cell-mediated immunity (Figure 7-3) or some other immunodeficiency such as persistent infection with bovine virus diarrhea virus (BVDV) or bovine leukocyte adhesion deficiency (BLAD). Genital fibropapillomas caused by BPV1 are commonly found on the penis of young bulls, on the teats, and occasionally in the vagina of heifers.

Atypical warts that tend to persist for years have been associated with BPV3 infections. Young and mature animals may be affected, and the lesions are multiple low, flat, and annular, with fingerlike or frondlike projections that are papillomas with epithelial proliferation but lack dermal fibrosis. These lesions are not raised as noticeably as BPV1 or BPV2 warts and may simply be interspersed with normal-haired skin.

Alimentary warts involving the esophagus, forestomach, and oral cavity are thought to be associated with BPV4. Although cattle with alimentary fibropapillomas

295

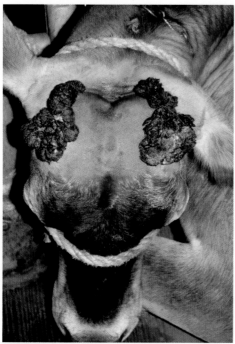

Figure 7-2

Large bilateral fibropapillomas in a Jersey calf representative of an epidemic occurrence following dehorning by a layperson.

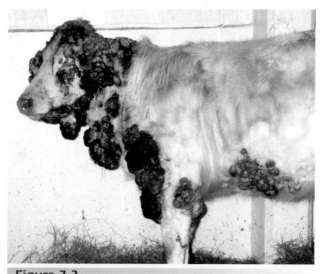

Figure 7-3

Multiple large warts that failed to regress over a 6-month period in a heifer.

are asymptomatic, occasionally fibropapillomas interfere with effective eructation, resulting in signs associated with vagal indigestion. Malignant transformation of BPV4-induced alimentary lesions to carcinomas is also possible and is a much greater risk when carcinogens such as bracken fern compose a major portion of the diet.

BPV4, as well as BPV1 and BPV2, may contribute to urinary bladder tumors in cattle consuming bracken fern at pasture. This condition, known as enzootic hematuria, can be life threatening to affected cattle.

BPV5 causes so-called "rice-grain" teat fibropapillomas, probably the most common form of teat wart seen in dairy cattle in the United States. (This virus is discussed further in Chapter 8). It is spread by milking procedures and machines that predispose to teat chapping or minor teat abrasions. Similarly BPV6 has been shown to cause papillomatous frondlike lesions on the skin of the udder.

Signs

Signs usually are obvious for skin papillomas, but flat wide-based gray warts occasionally may be misdiagnosed as crusty ringworm lesions. Lesions tend to be multiple and mainly occur in facial, neck, shoulder, and trunk locations. Lesions limited to a common anatomic area in most infected animals may help identify the cause of infection. This is especially easy for eartag and dehorning wounds, for example. Fly irritation, myiasis, and bleeding are common problems associated with large cauliflower-like warts during warm weather. Hemorrhage may be life threatening in those rare cattle with huge, multiple warts over a large portion of the body.

Penile warts in young bulls may interfere with breeding and can spread the virus to cows naturally serviced or to other bulls from artificial vaginas that are not routinely disinfected. Bleeding from the penis or sheath following collection or service is the usual owner complaint concerning affected bulls. Heifers with vaginal fibropapillomas frequently go undetected unless the mass becomes large.

Alimentary warts seldom are observed clinically except during oral examination, esophageal endoscopy, or rumenotomy. The lesions commonly are observed during gross postmortem examination.

Enzootic hematuria leads to obvious hematuria and dysuria or stranguria in affected cattle on pastures containing bracken fern.

Although teat lesions of fibropapillomas (BPV1, BPV2), rice-grain lesions (BPV5), or papilloma (BPV6) may be observed in individual cattle, they frequently become endemic in a herd. Warts may interfere with effective milking or be irritated by milking but seldom cause serious problems unless they occur at the teat end. Interference with effective milkout and mastitis are risks for cattle having teat end warts.

Diagnosis

Clinical signs are sufficient for diagnosis in most instances. Atypical lesions may require biopsy and histopathologic study. Gross sectioning of surgically excised fibropapillomas also is suggestive because epidermal proliferation over dermal fibroplasia is obvious on cut sections.

Treatment

Because skin warts usually are self-limiting within 1 to 12 months, treatment seldom is necessary. However, the variable duration of warts (up to 12 months) before self-cure causes owners to request treatment, particularly in young show cattle. In addition, various treatments, vaccines, and quack medications have gained acceptance because owners attribute eventual resolution of warts to treatment with these products, rather than to a spontaneous cure. Commercial or autogenous vaccines have been used extensively. Unfortunately they suffer from some major deficiencies:

1. Vaccines tend to be used for treatment rather than prevention.
2. The strains of virus used in commercial products may not be homologous with those causing the clinical warts in specific anatomic locations.
3. When used as treatment, no way exists to prove the vaccines more efficacious than a time-related natural cure.

Vaccination may be helpful when used as a preventive measure to decrease the risk of penile warts for bull calves assembled in bull studs or in herds with a high incidence of warts.

"Emergency treatment" is a frequent owner request during the summer months when heifers are to be shown in cattle shows. This frustrating situation results from regulations forbidding animals with warts to be shown for fear of contagion. Veterinarians are pressured into doing "something" to resolve lesions quickly, and this may be impossible.

Many treatments, such as surgical removal or crushing of individual warts, have been tried in an effort to stimulate the cell-mediated immunity that is most important to eventual resolution of the problem. In addition, autogenous bacterins injected intradermally or subcutaneously (SQ), levamisole, and other products have been tried. The success of these techniques is not known. Cryosurgery on selected tumors may be used both to destroy the tumor and to stimulate cell-mediated immunity to cause rejection of other tumors in the same animal. I have found this technique most useful in severe epidemics of warts following dehorning by laypeople in which each affected heifer has bilateral warts overlying the skin of the dehorning wounds.

Prevention is the best form of treatment and includes identification of likely fomites and contaminated or sharp structural devices that can be removed or corrected. In addition, surgical instruments, tattooing implements, and dehorners should be sterilized or disinfected with virucidal solutions between uses.

Penile fibropapillomas in bulls require careful surgical dissection followed by cryosurgery of the base of the wart. A double freeze-thaw-freeze gives the best results. Although the tumor base should be frozen to at least −30.0° C, it is difficult to use thermocouples to monitor temperature in this tissue, so subjective ensurance of adequate freezing by viewing the ice ball may be necessary. Pedunculated penile warts are much easier to treat and less likely to recur than those with a broad base. Vaginal fibropapillomas requiring treatment are rare. When necessary, excision at the base or cryosurgery may be successful. Vaginal warts may have extremely vascular stalks, and ligatures are sometimes necessary to prevent severe hemorrhage during removal.

Flat or rice-grain teat warts seldom are removed, but raised fibropapillomas or papillomas on the teat or teat end that mechanically interfere with milking may have to be removed flush with the skin by scissors.

Individual cattle with large multiple warts that persist indefinitely probably have deficient cell-mediated immunity. This may be a genetic fault or be associated with medical problems such as persistent infection with BVDV or previously bovine leukocyte adhesion deficiency (BLAD). This problem, when unrelated to either persistent infection with BVDV or BLAD, seems more common in beef cattle (especially Herefords) than in the dairy breeds.

Dermatophytosis ("Ringworm")

Etiology

Dermatophytosis or ringworm is extremely common in dairy calves and may occur in adult cows as well. *Trichophyton verrucosum* is the most common pathogen, with lesser instances of *Trichophyton mentagrophytes* and other dermatophytes. Calves over 2 months of age through yearling stage are most commonly affected. This coincides with the ages of young dairy animals that are grouped rather than managed individually. The causative organisms are extremely hardy and survive on inanimate objects, bedding, and soil for months after cattle have been removed. Concentration or grouping of young cattle—especially during the winter months—leads to an increased incidence in herds having the problem. It is not unusual to find yearly epidemics in heifers on farms that have had ringworm in the past. Conversely, herds that do not have clinical ringworm seem to remain free of the problem unless new animals that are infected are introduced. Adult cattle may experience severe infections as well. These outbreaks tend to occur during the winter months and frequently follow infected freshening heifers being introduced into the milking herd. Although adult cows that had ringworm when calves have been assumed to be "immune for life," the existence of outbreaks in adult cattle raise serious questions as to the longevity of immunity following natural exposure.

Dermatophytes affect the keratinized layers of skin thanks to toxins and allergens with resultant exudation, crusting, and alopecia. Fungal organisms themselves do not invade tissue and survive best when they provoke little host inflammatory reaction. Lesions tend to be oval or circular and are often multifocal. Incubation requires 1 to 4 weeks, and lesions persist for 1 to 3 months in most circumstances. Infection by contact is accelerated by mechanical irritation of the skin by contaminated objects. Stanchions, neck straps, halters, milking straps for old-fashioned bucket milking machines, brushes or curry combs, chutes, and other devices may spread infection through a group of cattle. Chronically ill, unthrifty, poorly nourished, or acutely ill cattle will show diffuse or rapidly progressive lesions compared with herdmates. This may imply either cellular or humoral factors that contribute toward worsening of dermatophytosis. Calves persistently infected with BVDV and calves with BLAD are examples of animals that frequently have severe ringworm lesions, whereas healthy herdmates remain either unaffected or have only mild lesions. Adult cows or heifers with typical ringworm lesions may progress to diffuse lesions when stressed by acute severe infections such as pneumonia or peritonitis. Exogenous corticosteroids will worsen existing ringworm lesions.

Lack of sunlight also has been proposed as a contributing cause because animals penned indoors seem to have a higher incidence. This theory also led many veterinarians to administer vitamins A and D as a treatment. However, the appearance of ringworm in both calves and adult cows during the summer months seems to diminish the importance of sunlight in prevention or cure.

Signs

Round or oval areas of crusting and alopecia that range from 1.0 to 5.0 cm in diameter are typical for ringworm in calves. Early lesions may appear raised because of serum oozing or secondary bacterial pyoderma underlying the crust (Figure 7-4). In calves, the periocular region, ears, muzzle, neck, and trunk are most usually affected, but lesions may occur anywhere (Figures 7-5 and 7-6). Head and neck lesions are common because lock-ins, stanchions, or neck straps become contaminated and help spread the disease. Posts or beams that are used for scratching may provide an area that infects the trunk in a group of heifers. The escutcheon is another area that frequently is affected with one or more lesions. Skin lesions may be painful but are rarely pruritic.

In adult cattle, the lesions may be anywhere on the body but often appear on the trunk and neck, with fewer cows showing the typical facial lesions found in calves. In addition to oval and circular lesions, larger geographic lesions of ringworm occasionally appear in adult cattle.

During ringworm outbreaks in adult cattle, individual cows that experience unassociated systemic illness may show dramatic worsening of their ringworm lesions.

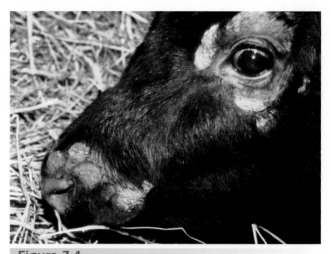

Figure 7-4

Raised, crusted lesions of ringworm involving the facial and periocular region of a Holstein calf.

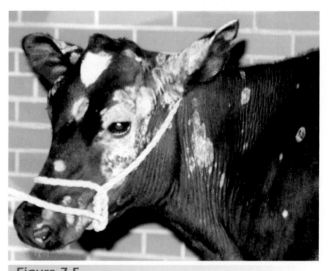

Figure 7-5

Multifocal ringworm lesions that appear as dry, crusted areas of alopecia of the head, neck, and shoulders in a Holstein heifer.

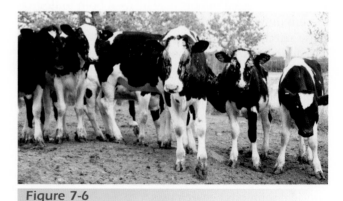

Figure 7-6

Epidemic ringworm in a group of Holstein yearlings. *(Photo courtesy Dr. Pam Powers.)*

Ketotic cattle treated with corticosteroids also will show worsening of the ringworm condition. Adult cattle also may have lesions on the udder, skin of the flank, or hind limbs that increase the risk of zoonotic disease because these lesions occur where milkers come into contact with the animals. Lesions of ringworm in milkers or handlers of infected cattle are a common occurrence. Ringworm is the most common example of a zoonosis in cattle practice.

Diagnosis

Cultures of hair from the peripheral zone of a lesion on selective media such as dermatophyte test medium, scrapings of lesions for mineral oil or potassium hydroxide preps, or skin biopsies can be used to confirm the diagnosis, but clinical signs usually suffice. Early lesions may be sufficiently raised in appearance to mimic warts or other lesions, but careful examination will differentiate them.

Treatment

Although hundreds of products have been used to treat ringworm in cattle, few have been shown to be efficacious. The self-limiting nature of ringworm infection in most cattle that are otherwise healthy makes it difficult to assess how much, if at all, the treatment helped natural healing. Controlled studies are essential for any product to be proven as efficacious against ringworm.

Treatment often is requested because of zoonotic potential or because an affected heifer or cow has been selected to go to a show or a sale. Animals with ringworm, as with warts, are ineligible for admission to shows or sales. This latter situation often leads to the sudden "emergency" status of ringworm even though it has been present on the animals for months.

Before discussing various treatments, one must realize the magnitude of the labor required to treat hundreds of ringworm lesions in a group of calves, heifers, or cows. The failure of treatment and lack of owner interest in it are simply based on the sometimes impossible task of catching, restraining, and treating groups of heifers. Treatment more often involves selected animals that need to be "cured" so they can enter a fair or a show. Owners who are willing to treat their calves also should be educated about disinfection and prevention.

Topical treatments that probably are efficacious are:
1. Lime sulfur 2% to 5% (Orthorix; Lym Dyp, Ortho Garden Supply)
2. 0.5% Sodium hypochlorite (Clorox)
3. 0.02% Enilconazole (Imaverol); not currently available in the United States

Numbers 1 through 3 are applied as a spray or dip daily for 5 days, then once weekly until cured.

Topical treatments that may be effective for limited lesions or selective treatment of a few animals:

1. Numbers 1 through 3 of the above applied or sprayed topically.
2. 3% to 5% thiabendazole paste applied once or twice daily.
3. Miconazole or clotrimazole cream once or twice daily.

Systemic treatment that probably is efficacious:
1. Griseofulvin 20 to 60 mg/kg orally for 7 or more days. Griseofulvin is *not* approved for use in cattle.

Systemic treatments that may be efficacious:
1. Sodium iodide 20% solution—150 cc per 450 kg intravenously (IV)—repeat in 3 to 4 days
2. Vitamins A and D—only indicated if animals have been kept completely out of sunlight. Efficacy never proven.

For best results, animals that are treated with any of the aforementioned products should first have their lesions scraped or brushed to remove the infective crusts. Clipping also may be helpful but risks spread of the infection. Remember that brushes, curry combs, and clippers used on infected animals should be cleaned and disinfected. Workers handling the cattle should wear gloves or wash thoroughly following handling of the animals with an iodophor or tincture of green soap.

Disinfection of premises and fomites offers the best opportunity to avoid future outbreaks. Physical cleansing and pressure spraying can be followed with lime sulfur or Clorox disinfection. Premises should be allowed to dry and supplied with new bedding. Only animals without detectable lesions should be reintroduced.

Vaccines have been developed in some parts of the world and have been reported to be efficacious; however, they are not available in the United States.

Dermatophilosis ("Rain Scald")

Etiology

Dermatophilosis, also called Streptothricosis or rain scald, is a common skin infection of cattle and other large animals caused by *Dermatophilus congolensis*. Moist environmental conditions and long hair coats predispose to contagious infection by *D. congolensis*. Rain and snow that wet hair coats and cause matting present the greatest opportunity for infection. In addition to moisture and long hair, physical damage to the skin seems to be necessary because *D. congolensis* is thought not to be able to invade healthy skin. Depending on the region and time of year, external parasites such as flies and lice may sufficiently injure skin and also help spread the infection. Other sources of skin injury include abrasions from scratching, rubbing, or licking and moist dermatitis that develops under wet matted hair.

D. congolensis probably is part of the normal skin flora in some cattle and is known to proliferate in a moist environment. Cattle that are highly stressed by illness, transient or long-standing alterations of their immune status, or treated with corticosteroids may develop severe lesions.

Heifers that are housed outside and some herds of adult cattle that have access to outdoor environments each day are most at risk for dermatophilosis.

Signs

In animals housed outdoors, a crusty dermatitis along the topline represents the classical distribution of dermatophilosis. Animals with short hair coats may have a folliculitis with mild raised crusts and tufts of hair, whereas more classical cases with long hair coats have thick tufts of matted hair and crusts that can be plucked off to expose a thick, yellow-green pus on the skin and attachment areas of crust. Pink areas of dermis may be apparent after removal of crusted tufts of hair (Figure 7-7).

Cattle that have access to farm ponds, deep mud, or lush wet pastures may develop lesions on the lower limbs and muzzle rather than the classical dorsal distribution. Bulls may develop the lesions on the skin of the scrotum, and occasionally cows develop lesions on the udder and/or teats (see Chapter 8).

Dermatophilosis that becomes widespread or covers more than 50% of the body surface may be fatal. Fortunately severe dermatophilosis is rare in the United States but remains a serious cause of cattle mortality in tropical climates, where greater heat and humidity coupled with more profound insect loads exist (Figure 7-8). Death may occur in severe cases as a result of debility, discomfort, protein loss, and septicemia.

Animals with long hair coats, crusts of matted hair with underlying pus, and a dorsal distribution, especially over the gluteals, loin, and withers, are easily diagnosed

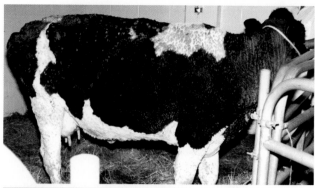

Figure 7-8

Unusually severe dermatophilosis in a single Holstein cow from a New York herd. A heavy summer fly load apparently contributed to the diffuse spread of the organism in this cow. That no other herdmates were affected and that the disease occurred during July both were unusual in this case.

by physical examination. Animals with short hair coats that have signs of folliculitis or lesions on the extremities may present a difficult differential diagnosis that includes staphylococcal folliculitis, viral infections, zinc-responsive dermatoses, dermatophytosis, and immune-mediated dermatoses.

Diagnosis

When pus can be found underneath plucked tufts of hair or on the bottom of the detached tuft, it provides an excellent diagnostic specimen for direct microscopic examination. Smears may be examined with Gram stain, new methylene blue, or Diff-Quik (Baxter Healthcare) to look for chains of branching and multiseptate coccoid bacteria resembling hyphae and clumps of gram-positive coccoid cells arranged in characteristic parallel rows ("railroad tracks"). When pus cannot be found, diagnosis is made more difficult. Crusts may be ground up and made into smears for microscopic examination, but the most helpful techniques remain skin biopsy and culture. Histopathology may show folliculitis, intracellular edema of keratinocytes, and surface crusts with alternating layers of keratin and leukocytic debris (palisading crust); the organisms may be observed in crusts or other locations. Gram stain used on sections may highlight the organisms more so than standard hematoxylin and eosin.

Treatment

Treatment is difficult and time consuming. In wet or damp, cold environments, the thought of bathing large numbers of cows to treat the condition is dismissed quickly by most owners. Infections often resolve spontaneously over several weeks if affected animals can be kept dry. In addition to keeping the animals dry, it is helpful to remove tufts of crusted hair or to clip matted

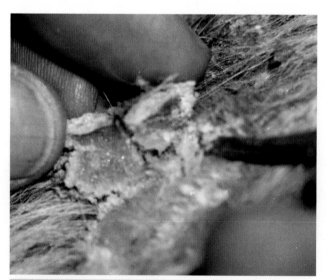

Figure 7-7

A crusted tuft of hair being removed from a cow infected with dermatophilosis. Although the underside of this tuft appears somewhat dry, more typical cases will have a thick pus evident.

hair to reduce the numbers of organisms present. Whenever possible, combining grooming with an iodine or chlorhexidine shampoo is an excellent treatment. Unlike ringworm, dermatophilosis lesions seldom are focal enough to be treated individually. Therefore overall grooming or clipping usually is necessary. Clippers, combs, and other grooming equipment must be thoroughly disinfected before reuse with chlorhexidine, iodophors, or bleach to prevent cross-contamination. The rational treatment of the disease also is complicated by the fact that in the winter animals may need as much hair as possible to survive outdoors. Unless there is an opportunity for indoor housing, owners are reluctant to clip hair. Systemic therapy with penicillin or oxytetracycline is highly efficacious and can be life saving for animals with diffuse disease. Therefore standard treatment recommendations include:

1. Topical—whatever is practical
   Grooming to remove crusts is very helpful
   Clipping long hair, if possible
   Iodine shampoos, if possible
2. Systemic—intramuscular (IM) penicillin twice daily dosed at 20,000 U/kg twice daily for 5 to 7 days, or IM long-acting oxytetracycline dosed at 20 mg/kg once

Human infections with *D. congolensis* are possible, and veterinarians should advise handlers to wear gloves and wash themselves with iodophor soaps after handling or treating affected cattle.

Other Cutaneous Diseases Caused by Infectious Agents

Numerous bacterial, fungal, viral, and protozoal infections may produce dermatologic lesions. An in-depth discussion of these diseases—especially their noncutaneous manifestations—is beyond the scope of this chapter, but a listing of these disorders is provided in Table 7-1.

NEOPLASTIC DISEASES

Lymphosarcoma (Lymphoma)

Etiology

Lymphosarcoma may involve the skin in the classic "skin form" of lymphosarcoma, wherein affected cattle usually are serologically negative for antibodies against the bovine leukemia virus (BLV), or as sporadic skin tumors associated with lymphadenopathy and other organ involvement with the adult form of lymphosarcoma that occurs in BLV-positive animals.

The skin form of lymphosarcoma usually occurs in cattle 6 to 24 months of age and is a progressive disease causing multifocal skin tumors. Lymphadenopathy may accompany the skin lesions. The skin form of lymphosarcoma is observed in all breeds but is most

common in Holsteins. This may simply reflect the number of Holsteins in the United States. Genetic predisposition has not been demonstrated, and association with BLV has not been confirmed. Skin tumors caused by lymphosarcoma in adult cattle are uncommon compared with tumors in more typical target organs (e.g., abomasum, heart, uterus, retrobulbar area, and lymph nodes) but may reach sizeable proportions in some affected cattle.

Signs

Diffuse nodular skin masses (1.0 to 10.0 cm in diameter) develop over the neck and trunk of young cattle with the skin form of lymphosarcoma. Lesions are initially dermal or subcutaneous, and the overlying skin appears normal. However, alopecia, crusting, hyperkeratosis, and ulceration develop with time. The tumors may become numerous enough to obliterate any normal skin spaces between them (Figure 7-9). Tumors may occur on the skin over any portion of the body. Peripheral lymph nodes are usually enlarged. The heifer or young cow seems otherwise healthy at the onset. However, over a period of 6 to 12 months, affected animals become uncomfortable because of the tumor burden, and visceral masses may develop. Fly and other insect irritation can be intense during warm weather, causing bleeding from the enlarging nodular tumors, which may have become alopecic (Figure 7-10). Most cases are BLV negative.

In adult cattle with lymphosarcoma, singular or multiple skin tumors may appear along with typical signs of lymph node enlargement and target organ lesions. Skin tumors in this form are larger, often plaquelike, and may be on the neck, chest or trunk, or eyelids. Physical examination usually identifies other lesions or locations of lymphosarcoma.

Fine needle aspirates or skin biopsies are the best means of definitive diagnosis for lymphosarcoma.

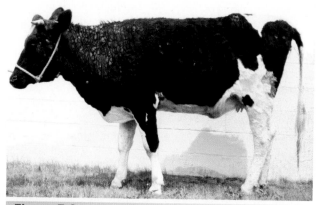

Figure 7-9

The skin form of lymphosarcoma in an 18-month-old Holstein heifer.

TABLE 7-1   Miscellaneous Bacterial, Fungal, Viral, and Protozoal Disorders of the Skin

Disorders	Signs
Bacterial disorders	
Abscess	Any age; anywhere on body; fluctuant, subcutaneous, often painful; especially *Arcanobacterium pyogenes*
Actinobacillosis ("wooden tongue")	Adult; single or multiple nodules and abscesses; especially face, head, and neck; *Actinobacillus lignieresii*
Actinomycosis ("lumpy jaw")	Adult; firm, variably painful, immovable swellings with nodules, abscesses, and draining tracts; especially mandible and maxilla; *Actinomyces bovis* and *A. israelii*
Bacterial pseudomycetoma ("botryomycosis")	Adult; single or multiple crusted nodules and ulcers on udder; *Pseudomonas aeruginosa*
Cellulitis	Adult; marked swelling and pain with variable exudation and draining tracts; especially leg (*Staphylococcus aureus* or *A. pyogenes*) or face, neck, and brisket (*Fusobacterium necrophorum*, *Bacteroides* spp., *Pasteurella septica*)
Clostridial cellulitis	Any age; acute onset and rapidly fatal; poorly circumscribed, painful, warm, pitting, deep swellings progressing to necrosis and slough with variable crepitus; especially leg (*Clostridium chauvoei*; "black leg") or head, neck, shoulder, abdomen, groin, and following tail docking (*C. septicum*, *C. sordelli*, *C. perfringens*; "malignant edema")
Corynebacterium pseudotuberculosis granuloma	Adult; single or multiple subcutaneous abscesses and ulcerated nodules; anywhere on body (especially head, neck, shoulder, flank, and thigh)
Farcy	Adult; firm, painless subcutaneous nodules with enlarged and palpable lymphatics; anywhere on body (especially head, neck, shoulder, legs); *Mycobacterium senegalense*
Impetigo	Adult; pustules, erosions, and crusts on udder, teats, ventral abdomen, medial thighs, vulva, perineum, and ventral tail; nonpruritic and nonpainful; *S. aureus*
Necrobacillosis	Adult; moist, necrotic, ulcerative, and foul-smelling lesions anywhere on body (especially axillae, groin, udder, between digits); *F. necrophorum*
Nodular thelitis	Adult; painful papules, plaques, nodules, and ulcers on teats and udder; *Mycobacterium terrae* and *M. gordonae*
Opportunistic mycobacterial granuloma	Adult; single or multiple nodules, often in chains with enlarged and palpable lymphatics; especially distal leg; *Mycobacterium kansasii*
Staphylococcal folliculitis and furunculosis	Adult; tufted papules, crusts, and alopecia; anywhere on body (especially rump, tail, perineum, distal legs, neck, face); nonpruritic; *S. aureus*, occasionally *S. hyicus*
Ulcerative lymphangitis	Adult; firm to fluctuant nodules, often with enlarged and palpable lymphatics, usually unilateral on distal leg, shoulder, neck, or flank; especially *A. pyogenes*, *C. pseudotuberculosis*, and *S. aureus*
Fungal disorders	
Phaeohyphomycosis	Multiple ulcerated, oozing nodules over rump and thighs (*Dreschlera rostrata*) or pinnae, tail, vulva, and thighs (*D. spicifera*)
Malassezia otitis externa	Ceruminous to suppurative otitis externa; predominantly *Malassezia sympodialis* in summer and *M. globosa* in winter; organism may also cause udder dermatitis
Viral disorders	
Cowpox (orthopoxvirus)	Typical pox lesions and thick, red crusts; usually confined to teats and udder, but occasionally medial thighs, perineum, vulva, and scrotum
Pseudocowpox (parapox virus)	Edema, pain, orange papules, dark red crusts (especially in "ring" or "horseshoe" shape); usually teats and udder, but occasionally medial thighs, perineum, and scrotum
Bovine popular stomatitis (parapoxvirus)	Typical pox lesions on muzzle, nostrils, and lips, especially on calves; occasionally flanks, abdomen, hind legs, scrotum, prepuce, and teats
Bovine lumpy skin disease (capripox virus)	Acute onset of papules and nodules, progressing to necrosis, slough, ulcer, and scar; especially tail, head, neck, legs, perineum, udder, and scrotum

TABLE 7-1   Miscellaneous Bacterial, Fungal, Viral, and Protozoal Disorders of the Skin—cont'd

Disorders	Signs
Infectious bovine rhinotracheitis (bovine herpesvirus 1)	Erythema, pustules, necrosis, and ulceration of muzzle, vulva, and rarely perineum and scrotum
Herpes mammillitis (bovine herpesvirus 2)	Acute swollen, tender teats, and udder skin progressing to vesicles, sloughing, and ulceration and crusting
Pseudolumpy skin disease (bovine herpesvirus 3)	Similar in appearance and distribution to true lumpy skin disease but more superficial
Herpes mammary pustular dermatitis (bovine herpesvirus 4)	Vesicle and pustules on lateral and ventral aspects of udder
Malignant catarrhal fever (alcelaphine herpes virus 1, wildebeest; ovine herpesvirus 2, sheep)	Erythema, scaling, necrosis, ulceration, and crusting of muzzle and face, and occasionally udder, teats, vulva, and scrotum; variable coronitis
Pseudorabies (porcine herpesvirus 1)	Intense, localized, unilateral pruritus; especially head, neck, thorax, flank, and perineum
Bovine virus diarrhea (pestivirus)	Erosions of muzzle, lips, and nostrils, and occasionally vulva, prepuce, coronet, and interdigital space; rarely crusts, scales, and alopecia on perineum, medial thighs, and neck
Foot-and-mouth disease (aphthovirus)	Vesicles and bullae, painful erosions and ulcers in mouth and on muzzle, nostrils, coronet, interdigital space, udder, and teats
Vesicular stomatitis (vesiculovirus)	Vesicles, painful erosions and ulcers in mouth and on lips, muzzle, feet, and occasionally prepuce, udder, and teats
Rinderpest (morbillivirus)	Erythema, papules, oozing, crusts, and alopecia over perineum, flanks, medial thighs, neck, scrotum, udder, and teats
Bluetongue (orbivirus)	Edema, dryness, cracking, and peeling of muzzle and lips; ulcers and crusts may be seen on udder and teats
Protozoal disorders	
Sarcocystosis	Loss of tail switch; variable alopecia of pinnae and distal legs
Besnoitiosis	Warm, painful swellings on distal legs and ventrum, skin then becomes thickened, lichenified, alopecic, and may fissure, ooze, scale, and crust

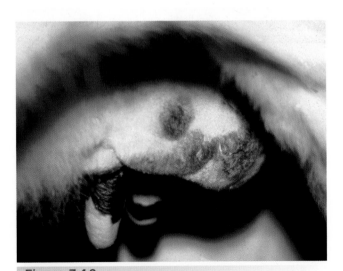

Figure 7-10

A 4-year-old Holstein with the cutaneous form of lymphosarcoma involving the udder.

Although advanced cases of the skin form are unlikely to require diagnostics, early cases with fewer lesions may require differentiation from other neoplasms and diseases such as urticaria and infectious or sterile granulomas.

Treatment

Although corticosteroids may reduce the size of tumors or result in short-term remission, it is impractical to treat cattle with lymphosarcoma because the tumors can never be fully controlled, and the animal will suffer a prolonged course or complications as a result of the medication.

Angiomatosis

Angiomatosis, although uncommon, is a cause for concern to owners of affected cattle because of the friable nature of the skin masses that predisposes to repeated bouts of hemorrhage that are dramatic given the small size (1.0 to 2.5 cm) of the tumors. Affected cattle tend to be mature with the average age reported to be 5.5 years.

The soft, pink or reddish masses are located on the dorsum over the withers, back, and loin. They may be singular or multiple and are always fragile. Treatment is by surgical removal. I have seen one Holstein cow with angiomatosis that had the lesion spontaneously resolve over 12 months, but generally it is better to remove the masses, lest insect irritation during the summer cause repeated hemorrhage.

Lipomatosis (Infiltrative Lipoma)

A rare condition in dairy cattle that may represent a hamartoma involving fat, lipomatosis appears as enlarging masses in the facial area or heavy muscles of the hind limbs (Figure 7-11). The masses may be so large as to interfere with function (e.g., mastication or respiration). They are fluctuant and soft on palpation, but attempts at fluid aspiration yield nothing. Fine needle aspirates or biopsy provides the diagnosis. No treatment exists because surgical removal is impossible as a result of infiltration of the fatty mass into musculature.

Squamous Cell Carcinomas

Squamous cell carcinomas are the most common malignant skin tumors of dairy cattle. Skin at mucocutaneous junctions such as the eyelids and vulva in cattle lacking pigment in these locations are at greatest risk. Cows that are mostly white or any cows with nonpigmented, mucocutaneous regions may be affected. Holsteins are the most common dairy breed I have observed to have squamous cell carcinomas, but this probably is because of the larger numbers of Holsteins compared with other breeds. Ayrshires, Guernseys, and

Milking Shorthorn cattle also may be at risk, depending on pigment patterns. There are two major reasons the overall incidence of squamous cell carcinoma in dairy cattle is less than in beef cattle:
1. Dairy cattle in the United States seldom experience as much sunlight as pastured beef cattle.
2. Fewer dairy cattle reach or exceed the age of greatest risk (7 to 9 years) because of culling for other reasons.

Sunlight, age, genetics, and infections with BPV are all factors in the occurrence of squamous cell carcinoma in cattle.

In addition to mucocutaneous junctional areas, squamous cell carcinoma occasionally may arise from chronically irritated skin wounds via tissue metaplasia. Brand keratomas occasionally transform into squamous cell carcinomas. Aged cattle with squamous cell carcinoma of the udder or ear tips also have been observed.

Signs
Clinical signs of a pink, cobblestone, raised or ulcerated mass arising from a depigmented area of skin are pathognomonic for squamous cell carcinoma (Figure 7-12). Frequently a white or yellow "cake frosting" of necrotic material covers the pink, highly vascular tumor surface, and an anaerobic or necrotic odor is detectable. Heavy purulent discharges make the tumors greatly attractive to flies and maggots. Biopsies are preferable to cytology for definitive diagnosis.

Treatment
Treatment may be easy or may be impossible based on the size of the tumor, its anatomic location, and the lack or presence of obvious metastases to regional lymph nodes.

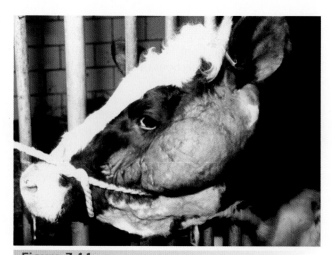

Figure 7-11

Lipomatosis of the facial muscles in a yearling Holstein heifer.

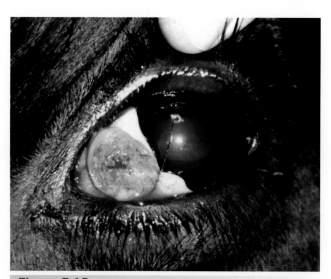

Figure 7-12

Squamous cell carcinoma of the nictitans in a Holstein cow.

Small squamous cell carcinomas are amenable to many treatment modes such as cryosurgery, radiofrequency hyperthermia, radiation, immunotherapy, or even sharp surgery. Each tumor must be evaluated by anatomic location, how much tissue may be destroyed without loss of tissue function (e.g., an eyelid), and expense of treatment. Treatment is addressed in detail in Chapter 13. In general, cryosurgery, radiofrequency hyperthermia, and radiation are the best treatments for small tumors and allow preservation of critical normal structures. Immunotherapy, especially with intratumor injections of Bacillus Calmette Guérin (BCG) or other mycobacterial cell wall products, will risk future tuberculosis tests being positive but may be helpful in large tumors. Other topical or intralesional treatments that are used in horses for sarcoids could be beneficial but no reports are available. Regional lymph nodes should be palpated and biopsied if they appear enlarged or firm, thus possibly indicating metastasis. Metastases have been reported to occur in about 10% of squamous cell carcinomas, but clinically, obviously neglected or large tumors are more likely to metastasize than early or small lesions.

Other Cutaneous Neoplasms and Nonneoplastic Growths

A number of neoplastic and nonneoplastic growths occur in the skin of cattle. A listing of these uncommon to very rare disorders is provided in Table 7-2.

ALLERGIC OR IMMUNE-MEDIATED DISEASES

Urticaria, Angioedema, and Anaphylaxis

Etiology

Urticaria, angioedema, and anaphylaxis are the most obvious clinical consequences of hypersensitivity reactions or "allergic" reactions. Urticaria (hives) appears as skin wheals or mucous membrane swellings as a result of dermal edema (Figure 7-13). Angioedema tends to imply larger swelling or plaques of edema that involve subcutaneous tissue. Anaphylaxis is the life-threatening extreme manifestation of these hypersensitivity reactions, and its rapid onset causes severe respiratory and cardiovascular signs resulting from smooth muscle contraction and vascular alteration. Anaphylaxis usually is fatal unless attended immediately and may or may not have urticaria and angioedema associated with it. A plethora of drugs, feeds, and other stimuli may evoke hypersensitivity reactions in calves and adult cattle. The exact immunologic phenomenon or type of hypersensitivity reaction (types I through IV) is sometimes difficult to determine, but most probably represent type I and type III hypersensitivity reactions. Type I hypersensitivities are IgE mediated,

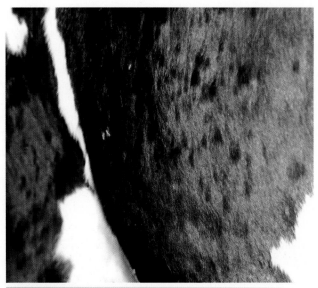

Figure 7-13

Urticaria on the thorax and flank of an adult Holstein cow. Raised tufts of hair appear over painful areas of dermal edema. These lesions appeared within 20 minutes following an IM injection of ampicillin.

whereas type III are associated with immune complexes. Type I hypersensitivities cause mast cell and basophil degranulation with subsequent release of histamine, leukotrienes, prostaglandins, and other mediators. Type I reactions probably provoke most ruminant causes of urticaria, angioedema, and anaphylaxis. Type III reactions may include some drug-induced causes, but this conclusion is largely speculative.

In dairy cattle, most cases of urticaria, angioedema, and anaphylaxis result from injections of various products, including antibiotics, vaccines, whole blood, lidocaine, and IV fluids. Insect bites occasionally cause urticaria and angioedema but seldom anaphylaxis. Milk allergy is another important cause of urticaria, angioedema, and anaphylaxis that ranges from mild to severe in individual patients. Milk allergy is observed in cattle (any breed but more commonly Channel Islands breeds) at drying off or when delays in milking occur either accidentally or intentionally when showing or selling cattle. Alpha-casein appears to be the milk protein that causes type I hypersensitivity in these cows.

Virtually any antibiotic can cause sporadic hypersensitivity reactions. Penicillin, tetracycline, ampicillin, various sulfonamides, and streptomycin have been incriminated. It is important to differentiate procaine reactions from true hypersensitivity to penicillin when procaine penicillin has been given. Many owners and veterinarians interpret the relatively common procaine reactions as penicillin hypersensitivity, and this is wrong. Cattle with procaine reactions may still be safely given penicillin.

Vaccines are the most common cause of anaphylaxis. Although serum origin products are used less frequently,

TABLE 7-2   Miscellaneous Neoplastic and Nonneoplastic Growths

Basal cell tumor	Adult to aged; solitary firm to fluctuant nodule; often alopecic and ulcerated; anywhere on body; benign
Trichoepithelioma	Adult to aged; solitary firm to fluctuant nodule; often alopecic and ulcerated; anywhere on body; benign
Sebaceous adenoma	Adult to aged; solitary nodule; anywhere on body (especially eyelid); benign
Sebaceous adenocarcinoma	Adult to aged; solitary nodule; anywhere on body (especially jaw); malignant
Epitrichial (apocrine) adenoma	Adult to aged; solitary nodule; tail; benign
Fibroma	Adult to aged; solitary, firm or soft, dermal or subcutaneous nodule; anywhere on body (especially head, neck, shoulder); benign
Fibrosarcoma	Adult to aged; solitary, firm or soft, dermal or subcutaneous nodule; anywhere on body (especially head, neck); malignant
Hemangioma	Adult to aged animals develop solitary, firm to soft, red to blue to black dermal nodules; anywhere on body (especially head, legs); benign; multiple lesions occur congenitally or in animals less than 1-year-old; may be accompanied by widespread internal lesions
Hemangiosarcoma	Adult to aged; solitary nodule, often necrotic, ulcerated, and bleeding; anywhere on body (especially leg); malignant
Hemangiopericytoma	Adult to aged; solitary nodule, anywhere on body (especially jaw); benign
Lymphangioma	Congenital or animals less than 1-year-old; solitary soft nodule; anywhere on body (especially leg, brisket); benign
Myxoma	Congenital to aged; solitary soft nodule; anywhere on body (especially pinna, leg); benign
Myxosarcoma	Adult to aged; solitary nodule; anywhere on body; malignant
Neurofibroma (Schwannoma; neurofibromatosis)	Congenital to adult; usually multiple firm papules and nodules; unilateral or bilateral; anywhere on body (especially muzzle, face, eyelids, neck, brisket); benign
Lipoma	Adult to aged; solitary subcutaneous nodule; anywhere on body (especially trunk); benign
Mast cell tumor	Adult to aged animals develop solitary or multiple papules and nodules that are often alopecic, erythematous, and ulcerated; anywhere on body; multiple lesions can be present congenitally on calves; 60% of animals with widespread lesions have metastases
Melanocytic neoplasms	All ages (>50% of cases in cattle <18 months old); about 80% of lesions are benign (melanocytoma), and 20% are malignant (melanoma); usually solitary dermal to subcutaneous nodules, gray-to-black in color, firm to fluctuant; anywhere on body (especially leg)
Dermoid cyst	Congenital; solitary nodule; especially dorsal midline of neck, eyelid, and periocular area; benign
Branchial cyst	Congenital; solitary firm to fluctuant swelling in ventral neck area; benign
Cutaneous horn	Adult to aged; hornlike hyperkeratosis, usually overlies squamous cell carcinoma or papilloma

many "antisera" are still available on the market, and these are especially dangerous as causes of both immediate and delayed hypersensitivity reactions. Polyvaccines have gained favor in the cattle industry, and it is not unusual to give a single shot that contains antigens of four viruses, five serotypes of leptospirosis, and a vehicle. Reactions to such polyvaccines make determining the causative antigen difficult. Strain 19 Brucella vaccine occasionally has caused either immediate or delayed hypersensitivity reactions. A rare reaction involves the larynx, causing severe laryngeal edema within 24 hours of strain 19 vaccine. Although some vaccines are more notorious than others as causes of anaphylaxis,

any vaccine may cause occasional reaction. Various gram-negative bacterins containing slight amounts of bacterial-origin endotoxin can induce reactions that mimic anaphylaxis through a genetic sensitivity—especially in Holsteins. This theory may explain why reactions are seen in some herds but not in others.

Whole blood or plasma may cause skin hypersensitivity reactions when administered IV. Transfusion reactions are possible because of genetic blood types or too rapid administration. IV fluids, especially formulated fluids, occasionally cause hives and angioedema. This is most likely a result of contaminants, cleaning chemicals incompletely rinsed from large fluid jugs, or endotoxin.

Hypoderma larvae that are killed in situ have caused anaphylactic reactions or reactions to toxins that mimic anaphylactic reactions. Feeds certainly may cause hypersensitivity reactions in individual cattle.

Signs

With urticaria, skin wheals or "hives" appear in variable numbers anywhere on the body within minutes to hours of the antigenic stimulus. Most commonly, these 1.0- to 10.0-cm raised areas of skin appear round or oval, but smaller urticarial swellings may resemble multiple fly bites or areas of raised hair. In cattle, concurrent swelling of mucous membranes and mucocutaneous junctions is very common, so that marked swelling of the eyelids, lips, vulva, or anus may appear. Some cows have swelling in only one location, whereas others have marked skin lesions and mucocutaneous junctional swelling. Other signs include trembling, salivation, mild rumen tympany, and diarrhea. Abortion and/or renal failure may occur within 1 week following a severe hypersensitivity reaction. Although animals with urticaria may be anxious and painful, they are not in a life-threatening situation unless pulmonary or laryngeal edema develops. With anaphylaxis, however, life-threatening vascular and smooth muscle effects occur rapidly—often before urticaria or angioedema even appear on the skin. Depression, dyspnea, anxiety, and hair coat standing on end are early signs of anaphylaxis. Later signs include salivation, pulmonary froth at the muzzle, severe dyspnea, and collapse.

Treatment

Removal of the offending antigen or subsequent avoidance is the long-term goal of treatment, but more immediate needs are to stop the hypersensitivity reaction from injuring the host. When urticaria or angioedema is present but the animal displays no dyspnea, antihistamines and nonsteroidal antiinflammatory agents with or without corticosteroids are indicated for treatment. If the animal is pregnant or has an infectious medical problem, however, corticosteroids should be avoided. When corticosteroids are used, 100 to 500 mg of methylprednisolone sodium succinate or 40 mg of dexamethasone is adequate for adult cattle. Antihistamines and flunixin meglumine should be used at standard dosages. Treatment may need to be repeated at 8- to 12-hour intervals for one or two additional treatments.

Adult cattle with dyspnea or any sign of respiratory distress should receive epinephrine (1 to 5 ml at 1:1000 dilution IV or 4 to 8 ml IM or SQ) in addition to the aforementioned drugs. If laryngeal edema is judged to be life threatening to the patient, a tracheostomy may be required, and if pulmonary edema is severe, furosemide (0.5 to 1.0 mg/kg IV) may be indicated.

Because cattle suffering from milk allergy should be milked out immediately, they may not be able to be immediately dried off (Figure 7-14). This is variable because some cattle only show one or a few bouts of milk allergy, whereas others can be very difficult to dry off. Some cows with milk allergy are culled.

Allergies to feeds or feed components are difficult to diagnose specifically and tend to be sporadic rather than endemic. Individual cows may show urticaria and angioedema (especially of vulva and anus) when exposed to high levels of corn or wheat (this must be differentiated from "estrogenic mycotoxins"). However, today's dairy cattle feeds are so complex that determination of the exact antigen would be similar to searching for "a needle in the haystack." Prevention is difficult when vaccines are causative because all avoidance of vaccines would be disastrous to cattle health. However, certain vaccines that seem to cause a high incidence of anaphylactic reaction should be avoided and a safe product sought through discussion with colleagues. Calves less than 6 months of age seem most susceptible to anaphylaxis from polyantigen vaccines. Whether this represents residual passive immunity, direct antigenic reaction, genetic-mediated endotoxin sensitivity to small amounts of bacterial endotoxins in bacterins, or reaction to vehicles is not known. Veterinarians vaccinating cattle always should have epinephrine and other treatments for anaphylaxis available. Veterinarians who sell cattle vaccine for owner administration may consider selling epinephrine to avoid medicolegal entanglements if anaphylaxis should occur in one or more of the cattle.

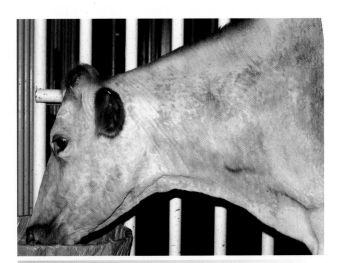

Figure 7-14

Urticaria over the neck and head that developed suddenly in an excellent Guernsey cow that had been dried-off the night before (milk allergy). The cow was treated with SQ administered antihistamines, and the hives resolved. The cow was 7.5 months pregnant, and steroid administration would have been contraindicated!

Contact Dermatitis

Contact dermatitis may be irritant, resulting from extreme concentration of a contacting agent, or allergic, wherein even small concentrations incite a hypersensitivity reaction. Irritant causes include chemicals added to bedding (coarse limestone) and disinfectants or teat dips used on teats and udders. Strong iodine solutions, concentrated chlorine bleach, concentrated chlorhexidine, and teat dips that have separated into layers because of freezing all have caused irritant contact dermatitis. Certain light-skinned cows appear to develop contact dermatitis when at pasture, but this may be difficult to differentiate from sunburn in some instances. Soaps or disinfectants that are not thoroughly rinsed off following preparation of the perineum during dystocia or vaginal examination are another source of contact dermatitis to the skin of the perineum, tail, and mucous membranes of the vulva and rectum. Fly sprays and other chemicals may evoke a contact dermatitis if applied in excess or if applied under a bandage.

Calves frequently develop an irritant contact dermatitis when fed milk replacer from a bucket. Alopecia develops at the muzzle, nose area, and ears, but the skin itself does not seem to be inflamed beyond occasional erythema. Some cases may have *Dermatophilus* infections at this site. Urine and fecal scalding are very common in calves that are kept in poorly cleaned pens or have prolonged recumbency because of systemic illness or musculoskeletal disease. The perineum, ventrum, and hind legs show alopecia and a pink-red erythematous skin in areas of alopecia. Calves with chronic diarrhea may show scalding of the tail, perineum, and medial hind limbs. Adult cows suffering prolonged recumbency may develop urine and fecal scalding as well.

Allergic contact dermatitis is less common than irritant contact dermatitis and may be seen in response to plants, bedding, and perhaps insects. Allergic contact dermatitis usually is limited to one animal, whereas irritant contact dermatitis frequently affects multiple cows in the herd. Avoidance, dilution, or replacement of causes of irritant contact dermatitis constitutes the treatment. For cattle with allergic contact dermatitis, a careful history may give the most useful insight into possible causes in the form of new bedding or recent exposure to pasture, among other sources. If a cause can be determined, avoidance is the only practical treatment.

DAMAGE FROM PHYSICAL AGENTS

Thermal Injury

Sunburn

Etiology. Ultraviolet rays, a form of shortwave radiation, may cause thermal injury to the skin of lightly pigmented cattle exposed to intense or prolonged sunlight.

The skin of the teats and udder may become sufficiently burned to make milking painful to the cow. Resultant difficulty in milking, failure to milk out completely, and mastitis are all clinical consequences. Teat skin, being hairless, is most at risk. Burning may be worse on the lateral teat surfaces in cows with well-conformed udders but is generalized in cows with pendulous udders. Maximal burning occurs when cows are recumbent. Once burned, blisters, chafing, peeling, and dryness of the affected skin will be present for 1 to 2 weeks. During this time, other irritants such as teat dips may slow healing. Colonization of the dry cracked teat skin by environmental organisms risks clinical mastitis outbreaks as well. Lightly pigmented haired skin on the dorsum also will be erythematous but is seldom burned.

Treatment. Avoidance of direct sunlight by turning cows out in the early morning or evening is one alternative. Topical treatment with lanolin or aloe-based emollient ointments may soothe affected skin. Severely burned cows, such as down cows exposed to prolonged periods of direct sunlight, may require more intensive therapy.

Fire Injuries (Barn, Brush)

Thermal injury caused by flames is long-wave radiation damage classified based on the depth of the skin injury. First-degree burns involve only the superficial layers of the epidermis, whereas second-degree burns involve the entire epidermis. Blisters resulting from fluid accumulations between the stratum granulosum and basal layers are common in second-degree burns. Eschars are produced by severe second-degree and third-degree burns. Third-degree burns damage dermis and epidermis and destroy hair follicles. Fourth-degree burns extend through skin to destroy fascia, muscle, tendons, and other tissues deep to the skin.

Burns tend to be most severe on the dorsum in barn fires (Figure 7-15) and on the ventrum in brush fires.

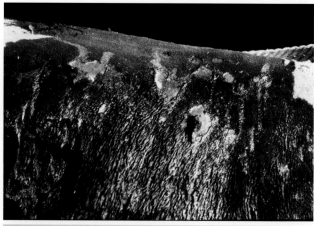

Figure 7-15

Acute second- and third-degree burns on the dorsum of a yearling Holstein bull that had been in a barn fire.

Depending on the animals' surroundings, facial burns also are common.

Thermal injuries caused by fire are associated with much more than skin pathology. Shock, dehydration, elevated catecholamine levels from extreme stress, electrolyte shifts caused by cellular destruction, smoke inhalation, and decreased resistance to local and systemic infections are only a few of the potential medical problems in burn patients. The profound anxiety, fear, and stress associated with fire itself affect surviving cattle. They may be apprehensive in addition to being in pain from burns.

The full extent of thermal injury often is impossible to predict immediately. Large areas of skin on the dorsum may appear warm with hair loss but apparently intact skin; later full-thickness skin may slough off the back (Figure 7-16). The development of blisters, fluid separation of epidermis and dermis, and especially eschars may not appear until several days following the injury. Eschars feel leathery, firm, taut, and often in cattle have underlying fluid that is subject to infection by opportunistic bacteria. Eschars eventually will slough.

Wound or burn infection is common in cattle, and *Pseudomonas aeruginosa* is the most common organism to establish infection. The normal skin defense mechanisms (e.g., epidermis, sebum) are injured or destroyed following second-degree or worse burns. Thus opportunistic bacteria from the normal skin flora or environment may be able to colonize the skin, fluid in blisters, or tissue and fluid under eschars. Infection under eschars is a common problem in cattle in which large areas of dorsal skin are burned.

Signs. The signs are dramatic and suffice for diagnosis. The odor of burnt hair lingers around affected animals and the whole area of the fire. Individual surviving animals should be assessed as to extent of skin injury, extent of other injury or smoke inhalation, and likelihood of survival. Pain may be minimal or not present in deeper burns because of loss of innervation, but this is a poor means of assessment because simple edema may cause reduced sensation.

Burns that involve large areas of skin on the dorsum and sides are likely to heal poorly and require lengthy treatment. Facial burns, muzzle encrustation, and dyspnea should alert the clinician to upper and lower airway damage by heat and smoke. Burnt teats that will not withstand milking indicate a grave prognosis because mastitis is inevitable regardless of other skin damage. Badly burned feet may slough claws. Facial burns involving the cornea may lead to permanent stromal opacities even after reepithelialization.

Unfortunately emotionalism makes it difficult for the veterinarian to be objective and predict which, if any, surviving animals have a reasonable prognosis. Many times, owners want to "do everything" to save survivors only to complain weeks later when ongoing complications and wound care require immense effort despite the prognosis for the animals remaining poor. It is imperative to warn clients during the highly emotional aftermath of fire that badly burned survivors will not only look worse later (after the skin sloughs) but also that they may never again be productive.

Treatment. Immediate treatment consists of assessing surviving cattle for systemic needs, burn needs, and likelihood of survival and future productivity. By circumstance, this must be done in a chaotic, emotion-filled environment. Immediate treatment includes:

1. Overall assessment of survivors—recumbent, obviously badly burned, suffering animals should be euthanized;
2. Individual surviving cattle may benefit from mild sedation that allows better evaluation of systemic and local injuries;
3. Cool water can be run through a hose to cool all burned cattle in the immediate phase of treatment; and
4. Treat for shock, smoke inhalation, and dehydration if necessary.

Following the immediate treatment, individual cattle that are to be treated for burns should again be gently hosed with running water to remove charred hair, crusts,

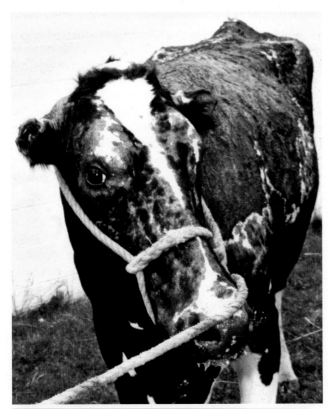

Figure 7-16

Adult Holstein cow that had been burned in a barn fire 1 month earlier. Skin sloughing was caused by third-degree burns over the dorsum.

and debris. First-degree burns should be coated with silver sulfadiazine 1% cream (Silvadene, Marion Laboratories). Initial blisters should be allowed to remain in place for 1 to 2 days on second-degree burns. Ruptured blisters should be débrided, the underlying tissue gently cleansed with Betadine scrub (Purdue), and silver sulfadiazine ointment applied under loosely applied moist gauze, if possible.

Second- and third-degree burns may be managed by occlusive dressings (closed) or by eschar, which is Mother Nature's coating of burnt tissue overlying the wound. In cattle and other large animals, it is difficult for either of these techniques to be used. Closed treatment with dressings may be impossible because of the anatomic location and size of skin burns. Eschars seldom stay in place long enough to allow complete epithelialization or remain so intact that bacteria do not invade the underlying tissue. The environment of large animals is not conducive to good burn management because of the constant potential for contamination of wounds. Loosely woven gauze and petroleum jelly are a good combination for either occlusive dressings or dressings laid over large areas of burns to prevent desiccation and continued fluid loss from the tissue. Heat loss and fluid loss are ongoing problems for animals with large areas of thermal injury. This also is true even when an eschar covers the injured area.

Eschars over large second- or third-degree burns should be left undisturbed unless separation of the healthy skin/eschar border becomes apparent or if infection is likely under the eschar. Infection of fluid under the eschar leads to fever and malaise, as well as a detectable fluctuation in the area of the burn.

Regardless of the treatment method used, the goal is epithelialization. Complete epithelialization should be possible with mild second-degree burns but may require skin grafts for severe second-degree and virtually all third-degree burns. Silvadene treatment to protect the wounds against opportunistic bacteria (especially *Pseudomonas* sp.), gentle washing, and moisture holding occlusive or semiocclusive dressings are indicated until such time that skin grafting is indicated. Lanolin or aloe-based products also may be helpful when incorporated into wound care to prevent drying of the skin or epithelial edges. Fragile layers of epithelium bridging large skin burns may be subject to cracking because of desiccation or excessive motion. Scratching or licking at burns can lead to delayed healing or self-mutilation in some cows. In one recent case, I treated a Holstein cow injured in a barn fire in which pruritus and consequent licking became so intense that sedation was necessary.

Supportive therapy includes analgesics, daily nursing care, as clean an environment as possible, and adequate nutrition. Corticosteroids are never indicated unless used during the immediate postfire treatment for smoke inhalation. Systemic antibiotics are not as effective as topical dressings for most burn wounds. However, large areas of eschar formation over the dorsum that present a high risk of infection may benefit from systemic antibiotics in large animals. Broad-spectrum coverage is indicated if systemic antibiotics are deemed necessary. The negative side effect is further patient discomfort caused by injections.

Skin grafting can be performed for third-degree burns once a healthy bed of granulation tissue covers the wound. Pinch grafts are most commonly used, and success rates vary because of difficulties encountered in aftercare of the grafts. Problems include physical and bacterial contamination of the graft site—especially on large dorsal burns, failure of graft to take, and self-induced trauma or scratching. Skin for grafts may be obtained from healthy areas on the patient.

Frostbite

Etiology. Excessive exposure of tissue to cold or windchill may cause frostbite. Mild frostbite leads to blanching of the tissue and reduced sensation followed by painful erythema, scaling, and alopecia. Severe frostbite leads to dry gangrene, anesthesia, and eventual sloughing. The most commonly affected areas are the extremities such as ear tips, tails, teats, scrotum, and lower limbs. Neonates and animals with reduced peripheral circulation because of systemic illness are at much greater risk for frostbite.

Extremities that become wet and are then subjected to severe environmental cold are at risk of frostbite. This is especially true for cows milked in milking parlors that are discharged to the free stall environment before teat dip solutions have dried on the teats. Similarly, neonatal calves housed in hutches may show superficial muzzle sloughing from frostbite caused by the rapid freezing of milk or milk replacers on the muzzle following feedings. Frostbite seldom is encountered in healthy animals when environmental temperatures are greater than 10.0° F (−12.22° C). Frostbite is not unusual when temperatures reach 0° F (−17.78° C) or windchill lowers the cold level to less than 0° F (−17.78° C). Unhealthy animals that are suffering decreased perfusion to extremities are at greater risk of frostbite even at higher environmental temperatures. Heifers with severe periparturient udder edema and subsequent reduced perfusion to the teats are at great risk of frostbitten teats when temperatures are less than 0° F (−17.78° C).

Treatment. If the condition is noticed promptly, the animal should be moved to an area where refreezing is not possible, and the frostbitten tissues should be thawed rapidly using water at a temperature of 105.0 to 111.0° F (40.5 to 43.9° C). Rapid warming is more painful than slow warming but leads to less cellular destruction in the affected tissue. Lanolin or aloe ointments should be applied and the animal kept protected from subnormal temperatures until healing occurs. Tissue having suffered frostbite once is more susceptible to the problem in the future.

Severe frostbite leads to dry gangrene and sloughing of tissue. The edges of healthy and gangrenous tissue should be kept clean, protected, and allowed to slough naturally. Daily checks for infection under the sloughing skin should be performed. Systemic antibiotics and tetanus immunization may be indicated for cattle with extensive frostbite.

Gangrene

Etiology

Gangrene implies necrosis and sloughing of tissue. Moist gangrene is found when lymph and venous vessels are obstructed. Dry gangrene occurs when arterial blood supply is lost but venous and lymph vessels remain intact. Moist gangrene usually is associated with infection, whereas dry gangrene is sterile. Classical examples of toxic causes of dry gangrene include ergotism and fescue foot. Ingestion of the sclerotium of the fungus *Claviceps purpurea*, which can contaminate seed grains, is the cause of ergotism. Chronic ingestion of contaminated grain and the toxic alkaloids associated with this fungus lead to small arterial dysfunction and decreased arterial blood supply to extremities. Similarly toxins from molds contaminating tall fescue grass are thought to be responsible for "fescue foot," a dry gangrene of the extremities observed in cattle, mostly calves, having chronic access to tall fescue pasture or hay. Cold weather may contribute to the severity or incidence of gangrene with these fungal toxins.

These classic examples of toxic causes of gangrene are rare in dairy cattle because of modern management systems. More common causes of gangrene in dairy cattle include:
1. Pressure necrosis—encircling bands, wires, strings, or adhesive tape may cause necrosis in extremities. A common example is the intentional application of elastrator bands to the tails of dairy cattle to dock tails. Far more common, however, is local pressure over bony prominences that results in decubital sores. These are areas of moist gangrene that become infected and slough following chronic impingement on venous and lymph return. Decubital sores are the most common cause of spontaneous gangrene in calves and cows. Prolonged recumbency, musculoskeletal lesions that cause extended periods in recumbency, and poor bedding of concrete surfaces increase the likelihood of decubital sores. Internal pressure caused by severe cellulitis occasionally may cause gangrene of skin, and internal pressure (edema) plus chafing are responsible for udder sores in adult cattle.
2. Thermal injury—burns of all types and frostbite
3. Snake bite—regional problems
4. Vasculitis—unusual cause in cattle
5. Infectious diseases that cause thrombosis, septic thrombosis, or thromboemboli. Most commonly young calves with septicemia may slough extremities as a result of gram-negative organisms such as *Salmonella* sp. Cattle with clostridial myositis certainly have skin gangrene at the site of muscular infection if they survive long enough for this to be detected. Septic mastitis that results in gangrenous mastitis with sloughing of skin plus the teat and gland occasionally occurs as a result of *Staphylococcus aureus*, anaerobes, or *Escherichia coli* infections. Herpes mammillitis infections frequently cause geographic necrosis of the skin of the udder or teats, and it is not unusual for an entire teat to slough because of dry gangrene.

Signs

With moist gangrene, the area that eventually will slough becomes swollen, discolored, edematous, and infected. A necrotic odor is apparent. Moist gangrene occurs in pressure or decubital sores and in septic infarction of venous return in systemic states. The latter condition is most common in calves and causes a moist fetid swelling around the coronary band before sloughing of the hoof or digit. Moist gangrene also has been observed with gauze or adhesive tape tail wraps inadvertently left on tails after surgery. Although dry gangrene is expected with encircling pressure, the tape or gauze appeared to exert lesser but sufficient pressure to cause moist gangrene. Gangrene caused by encircling band pressure is best exemplified by elastrator bands placed on scrotums or tails. Accidental encircling bands such as rubber jar rings, washers, strings, wires, or twine occasionally are found in encircling areas of necrosis on an extremity.

Gangrenous mastitis first appears as a red or reddish-blue cool discoloration of a teat and the adjacent skin over the gland. Within hours, a blue or blue-black hue predominates, and the skin may become moist as necrosis proceeds.

Ergotism and fescue foot cause dry gangrene of the lower limbs, tail, ear tips, teats, and scrotum (Figure 7-17). Antecedent blue or blue-red alopecic skin appears before the lesions dry; it becomes leathery, insensitive, cold, and mummified and shows sloughing. Frostbite appears in a similar manner, and teats that slough secondary to herpes mammillitis also appear as dry gangrene.

Treatment

Gangrene implies irreversible necrosis of the involved skin. However, in some instances, the core of tissue in an extremity has not lost its blood supply, even though the skin has. If diagnosed early, some encircling bands may be removed in time to save the extremity. Gangrenous mastitis requires rapid action to amputate or incise the

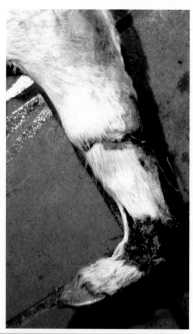

Figure 7-17

Dry gangrene of the distal hind limb in a calf.

teat and allow escape of secretions, organisms, and toxins. Prognosis for life remains guarded. Treatment of frostbite has been discussed. When moist gangrene is present, necrotic tissue should be allowed to drain and slough naturally. Similarly, dry gangrene establishes its own plane of dissection and is best left to separate naturally. Systemic antibiotics may be more indicated for those with severe moist gangrene than dry. Tetanus prophylaxis always is indicated, and two doses of tetanus toxoid 2 weeks apart are the best means of protecting the cow during sloughing of tissue. Fly control is necessary to avoid myiasis in patients with gangrenous wounds.

Lameness and neurologic signs may be observed in some cattle with ergotism before the appearance of sloughing digits or extremities. Once dry gangrene appears, it may be too late to save the animal, but the obvious treatment is to discontinue feeding the toxin-containing feed whenever ergotism or tall fescue toxicity is diagnosed.

Photosensitization

Photosensitization occurs when a photodynamic substance enters the skin and is acted on by sufficient ultraviolet light to activate inflammation or create a photochemical reaction that releases energy, causing subsequent skin damage (Box 7-1). The absorption of ultraviolet light of specific wavelengths and sufficient duration to activate photodynamic substances primarily occurs in light or nonpigmented regions of skin and is especially noticeable where the skin is both nonpigmented and has few hairs. Areas of mucocutaneous

junctions and patches of white hair are the most common sites of photosensitization in cattle.

Primary photosensitization implies that a photodynamic agent or metabolite reaches the skin through the circulation following ingestion or parenteral administration. Other primary photodynamic agents merely require contact with the skin.

Most causes of primary photosensitization are plants such as St. John's wort (*Hypericum perforatum*), buckwheat (*Fagopyrum esculentum*), and various types of rape, trefoil, and clover. Chemical causes of primary photosensitization also exist, with phenothiazine being the classic example. Tetracyclines, sulfonamides, and other drugs also have been incriminated as chemicals capable of causing primary photosensitization.

Photosensitization also may occur secondary to liver disease (hepatogenous) and aberrant pigment synthesis as occurs in porphyria. In hepatogenous photosensitization, liver function has been reduced to such a degree that phylloerythrin levels in the blood are exceedingly high and allow this metabolite to act as a photodynamic agent.

Hepatogenous causes of photosensitization reflect excessive blood levels of phylloerythrin, a metabolite of chlorophyll. Phylloerythrin normally is conjugated within the liver and excreted in bile. Liver or biliary pathology interferes with this normal metabolism to varying degrees. As blood levels of phylloerythrin increase, dermal levels of phylloerythrin eventually increase to a threshold level necessary for photosensitization.

Although severe hepatobiliary pathology predisposes all large animals to secondary photosensitization, many cattle with severe hepatic or biliary and hepatic pathology do not show photosensitization. This probably results from confinement away from sunlight. Hepatotoxic plants are the most common cause of hepatogenous photosensitization in cattle. Pyrrolizidine alkaloids (*Senecio* spp., *Crotalaria* spp.), blue-green algae, *Panicum* sp., some *Brassica* spp., and many other plants have the potential to cause hepatic injury. Molds such as *Aspergillus* sp., *Fusarium* sp., and *Pithomyces* sp. produce hepatotoxic mycotoxins and thereby predispose to photosensitization as well.

Diffuse infection or neoplasia of the liver also may predispose to hepatogenous photosensitization, but these causes are rare in dairy cattle. Liver flukes, a hepatic abscess that obstructs bile flow, or necrotic hepatitis following bacterial toxemia may result in hepatogenous photosensitization. It is very rare for hepatic lipidosis to cause photosensitization in dairy cattle!

Bovine erythropoietic porphyria (bovine congenital porphyria), also known as "pink tooth," is an autosomal recessive trait in many breeds of cattle and is a disease to be remembered when cattle are sold or sent to bull studs. It is of primary concern in Holsteins, but cases have been observed in Ayrshires and Shorthorns.

Box 7-1   Causes of Photosensitization

Primary photosensitization

Plants
St. John's wort (*Hypericum perforatum*)
Buckwheat (*Fagopyrum esculentum, Polygonum fagopyrum*)
Bishop's weed (*Ammi majus*)
Dutchman's breeches (*Thamnosma texana*)
Wild carrot (*Daucus carota*)
Spring parsley (*Cymopterus watsonii*)
Prairie lily (*Cooperia pedunculata*)
Smartweeds (*Polygonum* spp.)
Perennial ryegrass (*Lolium perenne*)
Burr trefoil (*Medicago denticulata*)
Alfalfa silage

Chemicals
Phenothiazines, thiazides, acriflavines, rose Bengal,
   methylene blue, sulfonamides, and tetracyclines

Hepatogenous photosensitization

Plants
Burning bush, fireweed (*Kochia scoparia*)
Ngaio tree (*Myoporum* spp.)
Lechuguilla (*Agave lechugilla*)
Rape, kale (*Brassica* spp.)
Coal oil brush, spineless horsebrush (*Tetradynia* spp.)
Moldy alfalfa hay
Sacahuiste (*Nolina texana*)
Salvation Jane (*Echium lycopsis*)
Lanta (*Lantana camara*)
Heliotrope (*Heliotropium europaeum*)
Ragworts, groundsels (*Senecio* spp.)
Tarweed, fiddleneck (*Amsinckia* spp.)
Crotalaria, rattleweed (*Crotalaria* spp.)

Millet, panic grass (*Panicum* spp.)
Ganskweed (*Lasiopermum bipinnatum*)
Verrain (*Lippia rehmanni*)
Bog asphodel (*Narthecium ossifragum*)
Alecrim (*Holocalyx glaziovii*)
Vuusiektebossie (*Nidorella foetida*)
Athanasia trifurcata
Asaemia axillaris

Fungi
Pithomyces chartarum (especially rye)
Anacystis spp. (blue-green algae in water)
Periconia spp. (Bermuda grass)
Phomopsis leptostromiformis (lupins)
Fusarium spp. (moldy corn)
Aspergillus spp. (stored feeds)

Infections
Leptospirosis
Liver abscess
Parasitic liver cysts (flukes, hydatids)
Rift Valley fever

Neoplasia
Lymphosarcoma
Hepatic carcinoma

Chemicals
Copper, phosphorus, carbon tetrachloride,
and phenanthridium

Aberrant Pigment Synthesis Photosensitization
Erythropoietic porphyria
Protoporphyria

The basic defect concerns the porphyrin structure of hemoglobin. Affected cattle are deficient in uroporphyrin III cosynthetase, a necessary enzyme for proper formation of hemoglobin. Therefore uroporphyrin and coproporphyrin accumulate and are deposited in bones, teeth, skin, urine, and other tissue as secretion. Accumulations of these porphyrin metabolites in the skin predispose to photosensitization. Affected animals also have an anemia as a result of a variety of red blood cell problems, such as reduced life span, delayed maturation in bone marrow, and hemolysis.

Bovine protoporphyria is an autosomal recessive trait associated with decreased heme synthetase (ferrochelatase) levels. Increased levels of protoporphyrin accumulate in blood and tissues. Protoporphyria is distinguished clinically from erythropoietic porphyria by the absence of anemia and discoloration of teeth and urine.

In addition to the aforementioned primary and secondary causes of photosensitization, occasional sporadic cases of photosensitization are observed in individual cattle having none of the known primary or secondary causes. Usually these cattle have been on pasture of clover or alfalfa, but the exact cause is never known and liver function is normal (Figure 7-18).

Signs
Signs of photosensitization include edema, erythema, vesicles, dermal effusions, and skin necrosis. These are quickly followed by crusting, ulcerations, and sloughing of leathery, necrotic patches of skin. Lesions are generally confined to nonpigmented regions of the body and are more severe on those areas receiving the most sunshine and ultraviolet light. Affected cattle are uncomfortable because of the pain associated with photosensitization, and pruritus may be a prominent sign.

Cattle with severe hepatic diseases and hepatogenous photosensitization also may show jaundice, but this is neither specific nor pathognomonic. Cattle with advanced

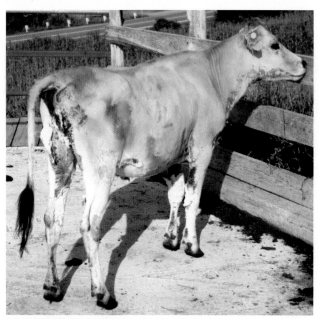

Figure 7-18

Jersey heifer with photosensitization of unknown cause. The heifer had been on pasture, was the only animal affected, recovered fully following confinement, and subsequently became a productive cow.

hepatic diseases usually are very ill with inappetence, decreased milk production, and weight loss.

Cattle affected with bovine erythropoietic porphyria show photosensitization, red or brownish-red urine, brownish-red or pink teeth, anemia, and stunting or poor growth rates. Ultraviolet examination of teeth and urine with a Wood's lamp reveals an obvious orange or red fluorescence.

Diagnosis

Clinical signs usually suffice for diagnosis of photosensitization, but establishment of the cause of photosensitization may be difficult. Serum biochemistry with specific requests for tests for liver disease such as gamma glutamyl transferase, aspartate aminotransferase, abdominal paracentesis, sorbitol dehydrogenase, and function tests (e.g., conjugated bilirubin) should be requested on all animals showing photosensitization unless the etiology is quickly established to be a primary photosensitization or porphyria. Liver or biliary disease and porphyria should be ruled out in all cases suspected to be primary photosensitization, and the causative primary agent should be sought. In hepatogenous photosensitization, hepatotoxic plants must be searched for and identified in pastures or forage; ultrasound and liver biopsies may be helpful in categorizing the type of hepatobiliary disease.

Confinement of dairy cattle limits both the risk for and the clinical signs associated with primary photosensitization and many of the hepatogenous causes as well. However, farm ponds (blue-green algae) and pastures still exist on many farms, and forages also may be contaminated with potentially causative agents.

Cattle suspected to have erythropoietic porphyria have greatly elevated blood and urine levels of uroporphyrin I and coproporphyrin I.

Treatment

Treatment of primary photosensitization includes removing the animals from exposure to sunlight and avoidance or removal of the causative plant or chemical from the environment. If secondary bacterial dermatitis develops in areas of photosensitized skin, systemic antibiotics may be necessary. Sloughing skin may need to be débrided, and surveillance for myiasis is indicated. The prognosis is fair to good unless extensive skin loss has occurred.

Treatment of hepatogenous photosensitization requires specific and supportive measures to benefit the hepatobiliary disease and removing affected animals from sunlight. When multiple animals are affected because of toxins or poisonous plants, identification of the causative agent and avoidance is necessary to reduce further incidence of disease. Prognosis is poor for hepatogenous photosensitization patients because most have severe hepatic or hepatobiliary disease. No treatment exists for bovine erythropoietic porphyria other than keeping affected animals out of sunlight. However, affected animals should be culled and specific recommendations made to breed organizations regarding the carrier status of both dams and sires of affected cattle.

Congenital and Inherited Skin Diseases

Numerous congenital and inherited skin conditions have been described in cattle. Because of the relative infrequency of these diseases and the excessive number of them, only a brief description of those diseases most likely in dairy herds is included in Table 7-3.

MISCELLANEOUS DISEASES OF CATTLE

Anagen Defluxion

Widespread loss of hair over the neck, trunk, limbs, and, to a lesser degree, the head that leaves healthy skin occasionally develops in calves that have recently been severely ill with high fever resulting from pneumonia, septicemia, or severe diarrhea (Figure 7-19). This condition in the past has been called telogen defluxion (effluvium); however, telogen defluxion describes a delayed shedding of hair 2 to 3 months following a stressful disease or incident. Anagen defluxion occurs within days of the calf's illness as a result of injury to the anagen portion of hair growth. Frequently it coincides with clinical improvement

---

TABLE 7-3   Congenital and Inherited Disorders of the Skin

Disorder	Inheritance and Signs
Lethal hypotrichosis	Holstein-Friesians; autosomal recessive; sparse hair coat present only on muzzle, eyelids, pinnae, tail, and pasterns
Semihairlessness	Ayrshires; autosomal recessive; sparse hair coat of coarse, wiry hairs
Viable hypotrichosis	Guernseys, Jerseys, Holsteins, autosomal recessive; hair present only on legs, tail, eyelids, and pinnae
Hypotrichosis and missing incisors	Holstein-Friesians; autosomal dominant; hypotrichosis on face and neck; lack 4 to 6 incisors
	Friesian crosses; x-linked, incomplete penetrance; generalized hypotrichosis and absent incisors
Streaked hypotrichosis	Holstein-Friesians; sex-linked dominant in females; hypotrichosis in vertical streaks over hips and sometimes sides and legs
Tardive hypotrichosis	Friesians; sex-linked recessive in females; hypotrichosis of face, neck, and legs begins at 6 weeks to 6 months of age
Inherited epidermal dysplasia ("baldy calf syndrome")	Holstein-Friesians; autosomal recessive; absent horn buds and elongated, narrow pointed hooves: generalized thinning of hair coat and patchy areas of scale, crust, and thickened and wrinkled skin; begins at 1 to 2 months of age; tips of pinnae curl medially; ulcers and crusts on carpi, hocks, and stifles
Color-related follicular dysplasias	Black and white or tan ("buckskin") and white Holsteins; normal at birth, but hypotrichosis and scaling develop in the black or tan areas
Ichthyosis	Mild form in Holsteins and Jerseys; autosomal recessive; generalized hyperkeratosis and hypotrichosis at birth or within a few weeks. Severe form in Friesians and Brown Swiss; autosomal recessive; generalized alopecia, hyperkeratosis, thickening, and fissuring at birth; ectropion and eclabium; dead at birth or within a few days
Cutaneous asthenia ("dermatosparaxis," "Ehlers-Danlos syndrome")	Holstein-Friesians; autosomal recessive, variable degrees of loose skin, cutaneous fragility and hyperextensibility
Epidermolysis bullosa ("epitheliogenesis imperfecta")	Holsteins, Jerseys, Ayrshires; autosomal recessive; vesicles, bullae, and ulcers in oral cavity, distal legs, pressure points, and pinnae; at birth or within a few days
Hereditary zinc deficiency ("inherited parakeratosis" "Adema disease," "lethal trait A46")	Holstein-Friesians; autosomal recessive; erythema, scale, crust, and alopecia of face, distal legs, and mucocutaneous areas begin at 4 to 8 weeks of age; dark hair coat often fades, especially periocularly ("spectacles")
Lymphedema	Ayrshires; autosomal recessive; variable degrees of edema of hind legs, and sometimes the front legs, tail, prepuce, pinnae, and face

---

of the primary condition but causes great concern as to the calf's prognosis. The skin remains healthy, assuming the calf is provided good nursing care and bedding. Hair growth recommences within weeks, and recovery is complete if the primary disease fully resolves.

The condition needs to be differentiated from vitamin C–responsive dermatosis (Figure 7-20), urine and fecal scalding, and inherited hypotrichoses (see Table 7-2).

Urine or Fecal Scalding

Although best discussed with contact irritant dermatitis, urine and fecal scalding occasionally leads to large areas of alopecia that are confused with inherited hypotrichoses, anagen defluxion, and nutritional dermatoses. Calves or cows that are forced to lie in filthy or urine-drenched stalls for prolonged periods because of protracted recumbency, musculoskeletal diseases, metabolic diseases, or simple poor husbandry are at risk for urine and fecal scalding. Large areas of skin over pressure points, the hind limbs, and the ventrum may lose hair and appear pink or pink-red as a result of chemical irritation by urine and feces. This skin remains intact and nonulcerated unless inadvertent trauma or pressure necrosis associated with prolonged recumbency ensues. Similarly many calves and occasionally adult cattle with severe diarrhea will develop alopecia and pink-red irritated skin in the perineum,

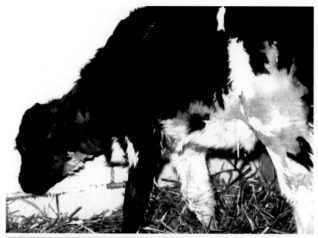

Figure 7-19

Anagen defluxion in a 2-week-old Holstein calf that was recovering from severe diarrhea, hypoproteinemia, and fever caused by *E. coli*. Widespread alopecia and easily broken hair were present.

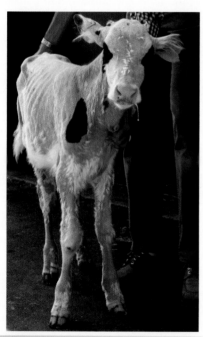

Figure 7-20

A 6-week-old Holstein calf with vitamin C-responsive dermatosis.

tail, and caudal aspect of the hind limbs from fecal-contact irritant dermatitis. Adult cattle with tail paralysis secondary to sacral or coccygeal injury also are at risk because they cannot effectively raise their tail when defecating or urinating.

Treatment consists of gently washing and cleaning affected areas with mild soap, drying, and providing dry bedding. Recumbent animals should be moved several times daily to allow dry bedding to be placed beneath them. Soothing and drying ointments, such as zinc oxide, may be applied to denuded areas of skin. Recovery is complete if the primary condition resolves. Cattle with sacral nerve injuries causing permanent tail paresis or paralysis may require continual care or tail amputation.

Leukotrichia and Leukoderma

Leukotrichia and leukoderma are acquired depigmentations of hair and skin, respectively, that develop following traumatic or inflammatory insults to the skin. In cattle, leukotrichia is commonly observed in the neck region corresponding to pressure and irritation from calves being tied with baling twine or tight neck straps of any type. Management systems that keep young calves and heifers tied with baling twine have a high incidence of this lesion appearing as a rather circumferential ring of white hair in the midcervical region. Leukotrichia appears during calfhood and may remain in the adult, depending on the degree of damage to melanocytes in the area. Leukotrichia also may appear in areas of skin previously injured by decubital sores, lacerations, thermal injuries, and tumors (usually large papillomas). Leukoderma probably implies such a drastic reduction in melanocytes that the skin remains depigmented. Burns, freeze brands, cryosurgery, deep full-thickness wounds, and other skin injuries may result in leukoderma in cattle. No practical treatment exists, and tattooing seldom is indicated for leukoderma because cosmetics rarely are of concern.

Alopecia Areata

Alopecia areata is a rare autoimmune dermatosis. Anagen hair follicle antigens are the targets of cell-mediated and humoral autoimmune responses. There are no apparent age, sex, or breed predilections.

Lesions may be solitary or multiple and consist of annular-to-oval areas of alopecia (Figure 7-21). The

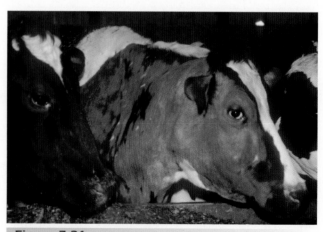

Figure 7-21

Alopecia areata in a Holstein cow.

exposed skin appears normal. Lesions most commonly occur on the face, neck, brisket, and shoulder. Spontaneous regrowth of hair often features hairs that are lighter in color and smaller in size than normal. Affected cattle are healthy otherwise.

Diagnosis is confirmed by skin biopsy. Animals with one or a few lesions may spontaneously recover over the course of a year. Animals with widespread lesions usually do not recover. Successful treatment has not been reported.

PARASITIC DISEASES

Hypodermiasis (Warbles) (Grubs)

Etiology

The warble or heel flies of cattle are *Hypoderma lineatum* and *Hypoderma bovis*. *H. lineatum* lay eggs on the heels of the forelegs and dewlap, whereas *H. bovis* lay eggs on the hindquarters and loin area. The adult flies of *H. bovis* frighten cattle because of a bumblebee-like noise they make. Cattle may become extremely anxious and frightened when beset by these flies. Cattle frequently run wildly ("gadding") from the flies and may injure themselves or run through fences during this panic. This behavior can be observed in pastured cattle during the late spring and early summer in the northeastern United States. Geographic and climatic conditions cause the life cycle of these parasites to vary as to specific time of year for the appearance of various stages.

Eggs hatch within 1 week, and first instar larvae burrow through the skin, aided by proteolytic enzymes. Further migration ensues with *H. lineatum* larvae eventually reaching the submucosa of the caudal third of the esophagus and *H. bovis* larvae reaching the epidural adipose tissue between the dura mater and periosteum of the thoracolumbar vertebrae. The esophagus and spinal canal usually are reached by the larvae in approximately 4 weeks and are known as the "winter resting sites" where the larvae spend 2 to 4 months. Mature first instar larvae of *H. bovis* and *H. lineatum* arrive at their "spring resting site" in the subcutaneous tissue of the back during the late winter or spring. Again, this time will vary based on climatic and latitude conditions. At this site, they establish a breathing hole and molt to a second instar phase. During this molting, the visible subcutaneous swellings in the back of affected cattle appear. A second molt to the third instar larvae occurs within 1 month after completion of the first molt. The third instar larvae eventually leave the warble, drop to the ground, pupate in the soil for 1 to 2 months, and finally emerge as adult flies that live less than 1 week.

Warbles are more common in first-calf heifers than older cows because of age-related resistance to the parasite.

Economic losses as a result of hypodermiasis occur for several reasons:

1. Frightened cattle on pasture cannot eat or gain weight at normal rates when being attacked by adult flies.
2. Major economic losses occur because of hide injury and meat trim from warbles. This is a major economic loss in beef cattle more than dairy cattle.
3. Occasional complications occur, including esophageal and spinal injuries from larvae killed too late in the life cycle by insecticides (see Treatment section), toxic or anaphylactic reactions caused by grubs being killed inside a warble, and cosmetic defects associated with warbles in show or sale animals.

Signs

Clinical signs of adult fly activity can be observed when pastured cattle run wildly about the pasture. Some even bellow in fright as they try to escape *H. bovis* adults. The only other obvious clinical sign is the "warble" itself on the back of affected cattle. Individual cattle may have only one swelling or as many as several hundred. Air holes are visible and further clarify the diagnosis.

Treatment

Treatment starts with fly control measures to minimize the environmental factors that propagate fly numbers. Heifers at pasture should be treated with fly repellents (e.g., dust bags) to minimize the irritation of flies. Specific treatment with systemic insecticides should be performed routinely on dairy heifers. The exact time of year for treatment varies with climate and latitude, but this information is readily available from regional extension agencies. In the northeastern United States, for example, treatment for early *Hypoderma* sp. larvae occurs between October 15 and November 15, after frosts have ended the fly season but before the larvae have reached a large size. Adult lactating cows should not be treated because they have a lower incidence of infestation as a result of age-acquired immunity and to avoid the complications of the entire issue of milk residues. Heifers may be treated during routine fall handling for vaccinations. Heifers due to freshen within several months should not be treated.

Because chemical formulations and approvals change constantly, recommendations must be based on currently available products that are allowed for dairy cattle. Always read the label! Pour-on products such as eprinomectin (Eprinex Pour-On, Merial) and moxidectin (Cydectin Pour-On, Fort Dodge) currently are approved for dairy cattle with no milk discard time issues.

Local reactions at the sites of first instar larvae occasionally are observed following treatment. These reactions are much more likely if treatment is delayed beyond the proper time within a geographic area because the larvae are larger. Adverse reactions with *H. lineatum* larvae include esophageal inflammation that may result in chokelike signs of salivation, bloat, and inability to eat. Adverse reactions with *H. bovis* larvae include temporary or permanent paralysis caused by aberrant migration or simple inflammation in the extradural region of the thoracolumbar spinal cord. Reports of "paralysis" are widely debated, and very few factual references exist as to the pathology that causes signs of paralysis. Many of these reactions may have been caused by drug toxicities rather than host/parasite interactions. The use of larvicidal insecticides late in the first instar life cycle may cause reactions to the dying larvae that appear as severe swelling along the topline. The same reaction has occurred when larvae in warbles have been accidently killed by crushing or by owners attempting to "squeeze" the larvae out of an airhole. Such reactions may result from larval toxins and proteases or may be an immune-mediated reaction caused by both cellular and humoral immune responses that have evolved as the parasite migrates through the host. Occasional "anaphylactic" reactions with toxemia or death of the cow have occurred following crushing of a larva in a warble. No reference specifically and factually explains whether such reactions are anaphylactic or are caused by the release of potent toxins from the dead larvae. In either event, owners should be warned not to interfere with the natural life cycle of *Hypoderma* spp. once subcutaneous lesions in the back appear.

Although vaccination against *Hypoderma* spp. has been attempted, no commercially available vaccines are currently available in the United States.

Louse Infestation

Etiology

Louse infestation in cattle seldom is thought of as a significant deterrent to weight gain or production, but this has not been my experience. Sucking lice, such as *Haematopinus eurysternus*, *Solenopotes capillatus*, and *Linognathus vituli*, and biting lice, such as *Bovicola bovis* (*Damalinia bovis*), can reach high levels of infestation during winter in northern climates. Longer hair coats, cooler skin and environmental temperatures, and confinement aid in propagation of lice during winter. Lice are host specific, spending their entire life cycle on the host; moreover, each species of louse has a favorite location on the host's body. Sunlight and heat are great deterrents to reproduction and survival of lice. Thus shorter hair coats, exposure to direct sunlight, and high environmental temperatures in summer tend to depress the louse population naturally. Age-specific resistance does not appear significant in cattle in response to louse infestation. Biting lice feed on skin debris and prefer the dorsum and flank region. Sucking lice prefer the head, neck, withers, axillae, and ventrum. However, when louse populations are extensive, the parasites can be found anywhere on the body. Lice, as is true of many parasites, are likely to have the greatest

negative effect on animals subjected to poor nutrition, other diseases, overcrowding, and other stresses. Severe infestation with fleas (*Ctenocephalides felis* [cat flea]) may occur in calves, but anemia, weakness, and weight loss are the predominant clinical signs.

Signs

Pruritus, restlessness, and excessive licking are the major signs of louse infestation in cattle (Figure 7-22). Mild infestations are not likely to result in clinical signs that owners observe, but large numbers of lice definitely interfere with growth of calves and production in dairy cattle. Cattle with heavy infestations are made uncomfortable or irritable by the parasites and spend a great deal of time rubbing against inanimate objects and licking themselves. Heavy infestation of sucking lice in young calves or animals kept under poor husbandry conditions may result in blood loss anemia. Louse infestations often are detected by the "weak sister" principle of parasitology. That is, one or a few animals will show obvious clinical signs caused by severe infestation when in fact a herd problem exists. Signs are most apparent in the winter when longer hair coats and lower environmental temperatures contribute to heavy louse infestation.

Lick marks created by the tongue in response to pruritus that resemble the marks left by a wet paintbrush are classic on calves and cows with louse infestations (Figure 7-23). Lick marks are present over the sides, flanks, dorsum, hindquarters, and wherever the animal can reach if not confined (Figure 7-24). Stanchioned cattle are very restless because their restraint limits their ability to lick or scratch. They tend to "rattle" the stanchions and rub vigorously back and forth or up and down in the stanchion, causing areas of hair loss on the neck and shoulders. Dr. Francis Fox described excessive "rattling" of stanchions as one of the cardinal signs of

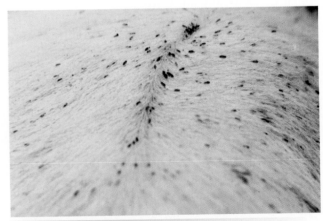

Figure 7-22

Heavy louse infestation in a Holstein calf. The calf was hypothermic, causing the lice to move from the skin surface to become more obvious in the hair coat than normal.

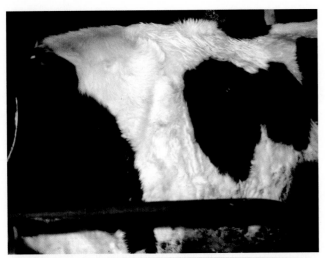

Figure 7-23

Lick marks on the dorsum, thorax, and flank of a Holstein infested with lice.

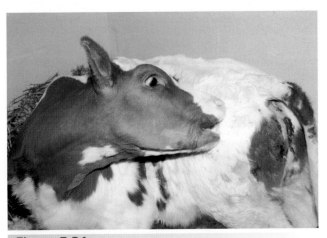

Figure 7-24

Severe pruritus in a calf infested with lice.

heavy louse infestation in stanchioned cattle. Self-induced alopecia and excoriations are common, and generalized scaling may be observed. Hairballs may be more common in calves with louse infestation as a result of chronic licking.

Diagnosis

Diagnosis is made by observing clinical signs and finding lice during the physical examination. Usually a penlight and careful separation of the hair is sufficient for identification. Areas that appear most disturbed by licking or rubbing are excellent locations to examine. The neck, dorsum, and gluteal regions frequently harbor sufficient numbers of lice to allow early diagnosis. Another tremendous aid to diagnosis is clipping hair. I have found this to be a dramatic means to demonstrate lice in our hospital and also in the field when cattle are clipped in preparation for abdominal surgery. Lice are

apparent as brown "dots" that do not wash away easily. Hundreds or thousands may be observed in some heavily infested cattle when the abdomen is clipped before paramedian or flank surgery.

Cattle that have died or are hypothermic as a result of shock may have lice leave the skin and appear in large numbers on the external hair coat. This abandonment of the host has been compared with "rats leaving the sinking ship."

Treatment

Individual treatment seldom is warranted because heavy infestation in one or a few cattle indicates a herd problem. Treatment of all animals and the environment is indicated whenever significant numbers of lice are identified. Only products approved for dairy cattle should be used. Eprinomectin and moxidectin pour-ons are approved, effective, and have no milk discard time issues. Several pyrethrin or permethrin preparations and coumaphos products are available for appropriate use in dairy cattle and calves. These products may be used as sprays or powders. All bedding should be cleared away, the barn sprayed, and all animals treated as a blitz treatment. Repeat treatment in 2 to 4 weeks or as indicated by manufacturers of selected products should follow. Herds having annual problems should be treated in the fall before peak louse numbers. Housed cattle should be clipped whenever possible to prevent excessively long hair coats that foster increased numbers of lice.

Flies

Fly control contributes greatly to cow comfort and production. Excessive numbers of flies not only irritate cows and farm workers but may represent vectors of infectious keratoconjunctivitis, environmental causes of mastitis through teat end injury, dermatophilosis, papillomatosis, and other infectious diseases. Mosquitoes, *Culicoides* spp., tabanids, horn flies (*Haematobia*), blackflies (*Simulium*), stable flies (*Stomoxys calcitrans*), and others are all capable of being annoying and causing painful bites and skin injury to cattle. *Phormia regina* (black blowflies) are blowflies that lay eggs in wounds causing subsequent maggot infestation. Calliphorids (blue blowflies) may lay eggs on dead animal or plant material and cause fly-strike in some geographic areas of the world. *Cochliomyia hominivorax*, the true screw worm that feeds on living flesh, requires regulatory vigilance to prevent return of this parasite to the United States from Mexico. *Musca domestica*, a filth fly, may mechanically transmit pathogens but does not bite. Mosquitoes, blackflies, tabanids, and *Culicoides* reproduce prolifically when nearby water allows fertile breeding grounds. Stable flies, horn flies, and *Musca* spp. lay eggs in manure, so poor husbandry or dirty yards contribute to increased numbers of these pests. All these insects reach peak numbers during the summer months.

Every farm has fly problems to some degree, and control is frequently frustrated by limited labor and management procedures to deter excessive fly numbers. However, the brevity of this section should not be interpreted as a lack of significance regarding the importance of flies as an irritant to cattle. Flies create a tremendous negative impact on cow comfort and subsequent productivity.

Signs

The clinical signs of excessive flies and other biting insects in cattle include restlessness, irritability, decreased feed intake, decreased production, and painful skin papules, wheals, or crusts. One simply has to enter the cows' environment to appreciate and experience the problem. On a warm summer day, it may be impossible to perform a thorough physical examination on a cow that is being bitten by large numbers of flies because of her discomfort and irritability.

Diagnosis is made by observation of the cattle and their environment.

Treatment

Management practices that reduce fly breeding areas are of primary concern in prevention and treatment of excessive fly numbers. Draining swamps, stagnant water, or ponds may reduce mosquitoes, tabanids, and *Culicoides*. Blackflies usually require moving water or fast-flowing streams as breeding grounds. Stable flies, *Musca* sp., and horn flies can be reduced by cleaning away manure from barns, barnyards, and collection or feeding areas. Dead animals, placentas, and surgically removed tissue should be discarded rather than left for blowflies, and wounds should be attended daily to avoid blowflies and subsequent maggots.

Insecticides and larvicides comprise the treatment options that most owners use—sometimes in lieu of management procedures—to reduce fly numbers. Sprays for premises and insecticides to be used on cattle should be labelled specifically for use on dairy cattle and on dairy premises. Some premise sprays are designed for use in barns when the cattle are not present. Chemical toxicities are possible if cattle are sprayed directly with sprays intended only for use on the premises. Barns should be sprayed early in the season rather than at the peak of fly populations.

Self-applicating dust bags for cattle should contain only approved substances for lactating cows. Fly baits should be placed in areas where cattle cannot ingest them. Feed-additive insecticides such as stirofos may reduce filth flies (*Musca* sp., *Stomoxys calcitrans*, and blowflies) by killing fly larvae in manure but should not be used unless specifically labeled for use in dairy cattle.

Insecticide-impregnated ear tags may be used in heifers or nonlactating animals as a deterrent to face flies (*Musca autumnalis*), which are the major vectors of infectious bovine keratoconjunctivitis. These same ear tags may also help control horn flies (*Haematobia irritans*), and thereby reduce "fly worry" and irritation caused by these pests. Eprinomectin and moxidectin pour-ons are approved and effective for horn fly control and have no milk discard time issues.

Tick-Borne Diseases

Ticks represent important vectors of disease that also cause parasitic irritation, damage to hides, and great economic loss in some cattle-raising areas of the world. Seldom are cattle the only host for the ticks that will be discussed; each species of tick varies in life cycle, host range, and time periods for blood feeding. Various soft-bodied ticks (*Argasidae*) and hard-bodied ticks (*Ixodidae*) parasitize cattle. Ticks tend to be less host-specific than lice. Specific ticks that are disease vectors for cattle will be discussed further in the section on infectious diseases.

Signs

Painful bites that heal poorly or become secondarily infected are a major problem for cattle infested with ticks. Damage to hides is an economic concern when beef cattle are affected with large numbers of ticks. Irritation, anxiety, and decreased feed consumption and growth rates are symptomatic of painful infestation with ticks and other ectoparasites.

In addition to these localized signs, the potential for spread of infectious diseases is unique for ticks. Cattle diseases such as anaplasmosis can be spread easily by ticks, and because ticks are not highly host specific, ticks in cattle may represent a threat to human health because of the many infectious diseases they carry.

Diagnosis

Identification of ticks on cattle or confirmation of tick-borne disease in cattle suffices for diagnosis.

Treatment

Treatment is difficult and expensive because it is labor intensive. In addition, various life stages of some ticks may not occur on the animal. Chemical dips, sprays, pour-on and spot-on products, and ivermectin products have been used to control ticks. Ticks have developed resistance to many acaricides, and new products will continue to appear on the market. Dips have produced the best means of application in the past, but newer chemicals and innovative delivery systems (e.g., slow-release, spot-on products) may reduce the labor necessary for treatment. Obviously tick infestations are more likely in pastured and range cattle than confined dairy cattle. However, in many areas of the United States, dairy cattle are at risk for tick infestation and subsequent tick-borne problems. Products selected for acaricides must be approved for use in dairy cattle.

Genetic resistance to ticks appears in Zebu cattle *(Bos indicus)* and Zebu-cross cattle. This fact has allowed the beef industry in regions with heavy tick populations to breed cattle requiring less tick treatment.

Mange

Chorioptic Mange

Etiology. Chorioptic mange is the most common mange to cause clinical signs in dairy cattle. *Chorioptes bovis* feeds primarily on epidermal debris and is host adapted. The mite has a life cycle that requires 2 to 3 weeks and is completed on the host. The length of time that *C. bovis* mites can survive off the host has been debated, but this seldom is of major concern if adequate treatment is provided.

The major problems observed in dairy cattle affected with clinically apparent chorioptic mange are discomfort, pruritus, agitation, and subsequent interference with feed intake and maximal production. Calves seldom are affected clinically, and the disease tends to occur in mature milking cows in affected herds. Sporadic cases may be observed, but it is more common to have 10% to 20% of the herd showing mild lesions. The greater the percentage of clinically apparent lesions, the greater the effect is on herd milk production.

Chorioptic mange appears more common during the winter months. This may reflect biologic activity of the mites, environmental factors, longer hair coats, confinement causing increased density of cattle during winter, or other factors. The disease may regress spontaneously during warmer months, and residual mite populations are thought to concentrate in the pastern or lower digital skin during this time.

Signs. Pruritus characterized by restlessness, treading, violent swishing of the tail, and rubbing of the tail and perineum against stationary objects is prominent in moderate to severe cases. Skin lesions with alopecia and crusting may be apparent in the ischiatic fossa, tail head, perineum, caudal udder, medial thigh, or scrotum (Figure 7-25). Papules and erythema of the infested skin may be prominent—especially if the cow has been scratching against solid objects. Very heavy crusts on the tail head or between the tail head and pin bones are common with mild to moderate infestations and frequently are observed during routine rectal palpations for reproductive purposes. Similar lesions of the skin of the digit also may be observed but are less common than the aforementioned lesions in dairy cattle.

Diagnosis. The clinical signs are very diagnostic, but definitive diagnosis requires skin scrapings to identify *C. bovis* mites specifically. Important differentials include lice and the reportable manges—sarcoptic and psoroptic.

Treatment. As with other ectoparasites, many insecticides are available to kill *C. bovis*, but few are approved for dairy cattle. Coumaphos (0.03%) applied as a spray

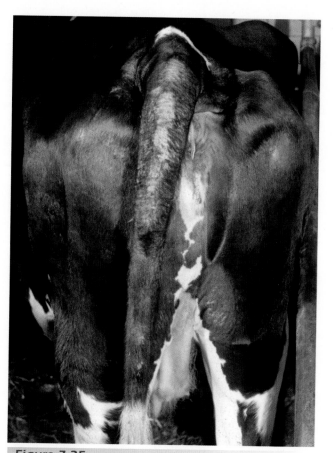

Figure 7-25

Chorioptic mange lesions on the tail head, tail, perineum, medial thigh, and udder.

according to approved concentrations for dairy cattle is very effective when two applications at 2-week intervals are completed. Lime sulfur (2%) applied once weekly for four treatments also is effective. Eprinomectin and moxidectin pour-ons are approved, effective, and have no milk discard time issues. All cattle in the herd should be treated rather than just those showing obvious dermatologic signs. It also is helpful to use a curry comb to remove heavy crusts before the insecticide treatment, although this increases the labor necessary for herd control. Treatment should be coordinated with complete removal of bedding and cleaning of the environment for best results.

Demodectic Mange

Demodectic mites are considered normal inhabitants of hair follicles and sebaceous glands of cattle but seldom cause clinical signs of disease. The *Demodex* mites of cattle are host specific and require no time off the host to complete their life cycle. Demodectic mite infestation of calves is thought to occur naturally through contact with the dam during the first few days of life. Dairy calves often have very little exposure to the dam following birth, and this may decrease transmission. Other forms of transmission are uncommon. Because most cattle with demodectic mites are asymptomatic, those with symptoms may have genetic or immunologic defects allowing the host-parasite relationship to be altered.

Signs. Palpable nodules and papules over the neck, withers, shoulder, and flank regions characterize the infestation. The number and size of these lesions vary, but most are 0.5 to 1.0 cm in diameter and covered with normal hair (Figure 7-26). Pruritus and other clinical signs are not apparent. Clinical signs of crusting, folliculitis, drainage, or ulceration constitute possible advanced lesions and occasionally are observed. *Demodex bovis* and an unclassified species are found around the eyelids and body skin. *Demodex ghanensis* has been found primarily around the eyelids in cattle.

Diagnosis. The diagnosis can be confirmed by deep skin scrapings or expressing exudate harboring mites from lesions for microscopic examination and confirmation of *Demodex* sp. Because of the follicular location of demodectic mites, other causes of folliculitis (e.g., dermatophytes, staphylococci, and *Dermatophilus*) must be considered. Asymptomatic cases also may appear similar to insect bites.

Treatment. Treatment usually is not necessary. This is fortunate because control of clinical demodectic mange always is difficult at best and would be more so in dairy cattle, given the limited insecticides approved for lactating cows. Individual cattle with overt dermatologic disease caused by *Demodex* sp. should be assessed for immunologic compromise or genetic weakness.

Sarcoptic Mange

Etiology. A reportable disease in dairy cattle, sarcoptic mange causes dramatic clinical signs and production losses when introduced into a dairy herd. *Sarcoptes* spp.

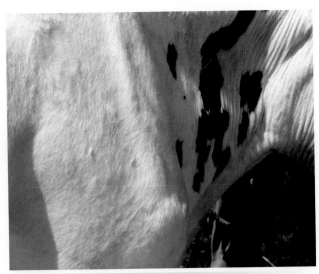

Figure 7-26

Demodectic mange in a Holstein. Small raised hair tufts are apparent on the shoulder region and thorax.

mites burrow in the upper skin layers, feed on fluids and debris, and females reproduce to worsen the condition. The life cycle requires approximately 2 weeks and is completed on the host. Cattle may acquire the disease by direct contact with infested cattle or contact with inanimate objects that have been used for rubbing by infested cattle. *Sarcoptes* spp. mites can only survive for several days off the host and are susceptible to dryness.

Although *Sarcoptes* spp. affecting various domestic species closely resemble each other, parasitologists debate the idea of a common species with adaptation to various hosts versus separate *Sarcoptes* spp. for each host species. Regardless, when examined microscopically, the sarcoptic mites from cattle (*Sarcoptes scabiei* var. *bovis*) will appear very similar to those found on other species. Transient, superficial sarcoptic mite infestations may occur in humans working with cattle affected with sarcoptic mange.

Signs. Profound pruritus characterizes sarcoptic mange. Lesions may appear anywhere, but the tail, neck, brisket, shoulders, rump, and inner thighs are common sites. Papules, crusts, alopecia, abrasions, and thickening of the skin are observed in affected areas of skin. Pruritus causes biting, licking, and excessive rubbing on inanimate objects. Self-induced lacerations and skin abrasions are common because cattle occasionally will rub on sharp objects or persist in rubbing until abrasions occur. Dr. Francis Fox was consulted and diagnosed sarcoptic mange in a free stall herd in which affected cattle bowed gates so badly through rubbing that all divider gates had been destroyed.

The obvious effects of this intense pruritus are decreased productivity because affected cattle have reduced feed intake, fail to show heats, lose weight, and have dramatic decreases in production. Untreated animals may become debilitated, and death as a result of secondary diseases and overall debility is possible.

Diagnosis. Clinical signs and deep skin scrapings that identify mites, eggs, and fecal debris are required for diagnosis. Sarcoptic mites are notorious as being difficult to find, but multiple deep scrapes and persistence usually allow positive diagnosis.

Treatment. Call regulatory veterinarians; this is a reportable disease. For lactating cattle, 2% lime sulfur heated to 95.0 to 105.0° F (35.0 to 40.5° C) is used as a dip or spray. No withdrawals are required when this product is used on dairy cattle, but treatment may need to be repeated at 10- to 14-day intervals. Eprinomectin pour-on is approved, effective, and has no milk discard time issues. Doramectin (Dectomax Pour-On, Pfizer Animal Health) is approved and effective but cannot be used in female dairy cattle *more than* 20 months old.

Psoroptic Mange

Etiology. Another reportable disease of dairy cattle, psoroptic mange is similar to sarcoptic mange in that severe pruritus characterizes the disease. Psoroptic mites live on the skin surface, feed on serum and lymph fluids, and require 2 to 3 weeks for a complete life cycle from egg to egg-laying female. Psoroptic mites live off the host better than sarcoptic mites and may survive 1 month or more in the environment under certain conditions. The mites survive best off the host during winter and worst during hot, dry summer periods. Similar to sarcoptic mange, psoroptic mange may be spread by both direct and indirect means—that is, contaminated common scratching posts, environment, and so on.

Signs. Intensive overwhelming pruritus accompanying generalized skin lesions with papules, crusts, abrasions, and alopecia are the main signs. Although skin lesions may appear anywhere, the withers and tail head and then later the back and sides are typical locations. The skin becomes thickened and appears wrinkled with time. Pruritus is so severe that affected cattle can think of little else. Therefore weight loss and production loss are profound. Neglected cattle become weak, emaciated, often develop secondary infections, and may die.

Diagnosis. The clinical signs and skin scraping to identify the causative mites, *Psoroptes ovis*, constitute proof of diagnosis.

Treatment. Call regulatory veterinarians; this is a reportable disease. Available treatments are as for sarcoptic mange. Lime sulfur 2% heated to 95.0 to 105.0° F (35.0 to 40.5° C) is an approved dip or spray for lactating dairy cattle. Moxidectin pour-on is approved, effective, and has no milk discard time issues. Doramectin pour-on is approved and effective but cannot be used on female dairy cattle *more than* 20 months old.

Stephanofilariasis

Etiology
Stephanofilaria stilesi is the common cause of a filarial dermatitis on the ventral midline of cattle in the United States. Adults live in the dermis, and microfilariae are ingested by the horn fly, *H. irritans*. Microfilariae develop into infective larvae during a 2- to 3-week time period spent in the fly and then are injected into the skin of cattle when the fly feeds.

Signs
Dermatitis on the ventral midline consists initially of serum exudate, crusts, and papules. Chronicity leads to alopecia, skin thickening, and hyperkeratosis. The usual site is between the brisket and umbilicus, but extensive lesions may extend more cranially or caudally. Lesions occasionally are observed on the udder. Pruritus causes affected cows to attempt to scratch their belly while partially recumbent. Cows may rise to their knees and rock the brisket and ventral abdomen fore and aft in an effort to relieve the itching sensation associated with dermatitis.

Diagnosis
Clinical signs coupled with skin biopsies provide the best means of establishing a definitive diagnosis. Cross-sections of adult worms may be observed in hair follicles when biopsies are examined histologically. Microfilariae and eosinophils may be found in the dermis.

Treatment
Approved treatments for stephanofilariasis are not available for lactating cattle. Topical avermectins are useful for nonlactating cattle, but appropriate withdrawal times should be observed for any products used for this purpose.

Fly-Strike from Maggots (*Calliphorine myiasis*) (Blowflies)

Etiology
Many species of blowflies are capable of causing fly-strike in domestic animals. Several species of calliphorids (blue blowflies) and *P. regina* (black blowfly) are the major blowflies in North America. The flies are at peak numbers during spring, early summer, and fall. Adult flies may travel several miles in search of food and egg-laying sites. Dead carcasses, rotten meat or plant material, and necrotic wounds attract adult flies. *P. regina* probably is the primary blowfly to cause fly-strike in cattle wounds in the United States, but different calliphorids predominate in other regions of the world.

Females lay eggs in wounds such as those caused by dehorning, castration, or trauma. Occasionally fly-strike occurs in exposed placentas, the umbilicus of newborn calves, and necrotic or lacerated vulvas following dystocia. Recumbent calves with diarrhea are at risk for fly-strike around the diarrhea-soaked anus, perineum, and tail. Calves or cattle that have had corneal perforations, sunken eyes, and phthisis bulbi secondary to pinkeye may have fly-strike in the affected orbit (Figure 7-27).

In warm weather, blowfly eggs hatch to maggots in 1 to 3 days. If both warmth and moisture are present, eggs may hatch in less than 12 hours. The maggots persist, and the odor of the wound attracts more blowflies.

Toxemia secondary to myiasis seems to occur more commonly in young calves but also may develop in adult cattle. Although many animals infested with maggots have primary diseases, maggots seem to contribute to anorexia, depression, and debility. The exact pathophysiology for this "toxemia" or depressant effect of maggots on the host is not understood. The true screw worm, *C. hominivorax*, currently has been eradicated from the United States but is a constant threat to Texas with subsequent risk of spread into the rest of the United States again. True screw worms penetrate and feed on living flesh in wounds. Calliphorine maggots secrete proteolytic enzymes to digest and liquefy host tissue (usually necrotic) but do not feed on living tissue. If maggots are found in living flesh,

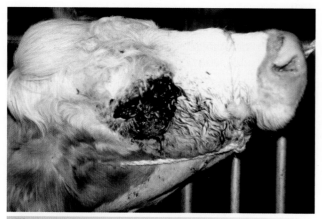

Figure 7-27

Maggots in the orbital region of a cow with a neglected orbital squamous cell carcinoma.

true screw worm infestation should be ruled out by laboratory identification of the maggot species.

Signs

Signs are grossly obvious to the eyes and nose of the examiner. A sickening necrotic odor accompanies the disturbing sign of maggots moving within the wound. Secondary bacterial infections of the wounds may contribute to the odor and probably contribute to attraction of blowflies. Sometimes it is difficult to assess the degree of illness associated with the primary problem of the animal versus the degree of illness associated with the maggots. Neonatal calves are at greatest risk of death because the primary diseases (e.g., diarrhea, white muscle disease, and septicemia) that weaken the calf usually are very serious, and maggots add an additional "toxic" component.

Treatment

The wound must be clipped, cleaned, débrided if necessary, and the maggots killed. Clipping the hair is very important for wounds on haired tissue because this procedure will greatly deter future fly-strike; moist matted hair creates an ideal fly-strike environment. The wound may be lavaged with warm water and pine oil (1 oz pine oil/32 oz water), or an insecticide may be sprayed on to destroy the maggots. Coumaphos 0.25% may be sprayed locally on the maggots, but application should not be overdone in calves, lest toxicity occur. Wounds in nonlactating animals and calves should be treated with topical insecticide sprays or ointments. These products also should be used prophylactically to protect fresh wounds at risk for fly-strike.

Lactating cattle require careful selection of insecticides such that only approved products are used. Prevention of maggots is much easier than treatment; therefore fly control and diligent cleaning and protection of cattle wounds during the fly season are imperative. Wound ointments containing fly repellents or insecticides should be used routinely during the fly season. Fly smears are applied in a circle around the wound rather than to open tissue to minimize the potential for chemical absorption and toxicity, especially in calves.

Miscellaneous Parasitic Causes of Dermatologic Disease

Other parasites are occasional causes of skin lesions in cattle in the United States and abroad (Table 7-4).

Miscellaneous Physical, Chemical, and Nutritional Causes of Dermatologic Disease

Many physical insults, chemical toxicoses, and nutritional imbalances involving minerals and vitamins directly or indirectly cause skin lesions. Although most of these conditions are rare in dairy cattle because of confinement and ration surveillance, some of the major toxicoses and deficiencies are listed in Tables 7-5 and 7-6. Details of these conditions—particularly their

TABLE 7-4 *Miscellaneous Parasitic Skin Disorders*	
Disorder	**Signs**
Psorergatic mange	Subtle degrees of patchy alopecia and scaling with little or no pruritus, especially over dorsum; *Psorergates bos*
Onchocerciasis	Asymptomatic subcutaneous nodules over brisket, hip, and stifle *(Onchocerca gibsoni)*; shoulder, stifle, hip *(O. gutturosa)*; udder, scrotum *(O. ochengi)*
Parafilariasis	Nodules that discharge a bloody exudate; especially neck, shoulder, trunk: *Parafilaria bovicola*; spring and summer
Pelodera dermatitis	Pruritic, papular dermatitis of ventral abdomen and thorax, medial and lateral thighs, udder, and teats; *Pelodera strongyloides*
Rhabditic otitis externa	Bilateral, painful, odiferous, suppurative otitis externa; *Rhabditis bovis*
Raillietia otitis externa	Bilateral suppurative, painful otitis externa; *Raillietia auris*

TABLE 7-5 Miscellaneous Physical and Chemical Disorders of the Skin

Disorder	Description
Amanita toxicosis	Eating mushroom *Amanita verna*; papules, vesicles, and necrotic foci around tail base and perineum
Arsenic toxicosis	Dry, dull, easily epilated hair coat progresses to alopecia and exfoliative dermatitis
Chlorinated naphthalene toxicoses	Progressive scaling, hyperkeratosis, thickening, fissuring, and alopecia beginning on the withers and neck
Dermatitis, pyrexia, and hemorrhage syndrome	Pruritic, papulocrustous dermatitis on head, neck, tail head, perineum, and udder
Foreign bodies	Papules, nodules, abscesses and draining tracts; especially legs, hips, muzzle, and ventrum
Hairy vetch toxicosis	Pruritic papules, plaques, oozing, crusts, and alopecia; begins on tail head, udder, and neck, and progresses to face, trunk, and legs
Hematoma	Acute onset, fluctuant, subcutaneous; especially stifle, ischial tuberosity, tuber coxae, perineum, ventral abdomen, lateral thorax, and point of shoulder
Hyalomma toxicosis ("sweating sickness")	Erythema, edema, oozing, foul smell on pinnae, face, neck, axillae, flank, and groin; lesions are painful; matted hair coat is easily epilated leaving erosions and ulcers
Intertrigo	Variable degrees of erythema, edema, and oozing; junction of lateral aspect of udder and medial thigh
Iodism	Scaling—with or without alopecia—especially dorsum, neck, head, and shoulders
Mercurialism	Progressive, generalized alopecia
Mimosine toxicosis	Gradual loss of long hairs (e.g., tail switch) and variable hoof dysplasias
Oat straw toxicosis	Papules, plaques, and fissures on udder, hindquarters, lips, muzzle, and vulva
Polybrominated biphenyl toxicosis	Abscesses and hematomas over back, abdomen, and hind legs; alopecia and lichenification over lateral thorax, neck, and shoulders; hoof dysplasias
Selenium toxicosis	Progressive loss of long hairs, coronitis, and hoof dysplasias
Snake bite	Progressive edema, pain, and discoloration with variable necrosis and sloughing; especially nose, head, and legs
Stachybotryotoxicosis	Necrotic ulcers in mouth and on lips and nostrils
Subcutaneous emphysema	Soft, fluctuant, crepitant, subcutaneous swelling; especially neck and trunk
Vampire bat bite	Multiple bleeding, crusted ulcers; especially dorsum and legs

TABLE 7-6 Miscellaneous Nutritional Disorders of the Skin

Disorder	Signs
Cobalt deficiency	Rough, brittle, faded hair coat
Copper deficiency	Rough, brittle, faded hair coat with variable excessive licking; periocular hair coat fade and hair loss ("spectacles")
High-fat milk replacer dermatosis	Alopecia and scaling of muzzle, periocular area, base of pinnae, and legs
Iodine deficiency	Newborn calves; generalized alopecia and thick, puffy skin (myxedema)
Riboflavin deficiency	Generalized alopecia and rough, brittle, faded hair coat
Selenium deficiency	Dermatitis over rump and tail base
Vitamin A deficiency	Rough, dry, faded hair coat and generalized seborrhea
Vitamin C-responsive dermatosis	Calves; scaling, alopecia, erythema, petechiae and ecchymoses beginning on the head and/or legs
Zinc-responsive dermatitis	Scaling and erythema progress to crusting and alopecia; face, pinnae, mucocutaneous junctions, pressure points, distal legs, flanks, and tail head; pruritus may be intense or absent

noncutaneous features—are beyond the scope of this chapter, and Tables 7-5 and 7-6 only include their dermatologic features. Several plants and toxins causing photosensitization and gangrene already have been discussed in other sections of this chapter.

SUGGESTED READINGS

Andre-Fontaine G, Bouisset S, Ganiere JP, et al: Photosensibilisation leptospirosique: mythe ou réalité, *Point Vét* 20:247, 1988.

Andrews AH, Blowey RW, Boyd H, et al: *Bovine medicine. Diseases and husbandry of cattle*, ed 2, Oxford, England, 2004, Blackwell Sciences.

Barth D, Hair JA, Kunkle BN, et al: Efficacy of eprinomectin against mange mites in cattle, *Am J Vet Res* 58:1257, 1997.

Duarte ER, Batista RD, Hahn RC, et al: Factors associated with the prevalence of Malassezia species in the external ears of cattle from the State of Minas Gerais, Brazil, *Med Mycol* 41:137, 2003.

Gourreau JM, Scott DW, Cesarini JP: Les tumeurs mélaniques cutanés des bovines, *Point Vét* 26:785, 1995.

Griffiths IB, Done SH: Citrinin as a possible cause of the pruritus, pyrexia, haemorrhage syndrome in cattle, *Vet Rec* 129:113, 1991.

Harper P, Cook RW, Gill PA, et al: Vetch toxicosis in cattle grazing Vicia villosa ssp dasycarpa and V. benghalensis, *Aust Vet J* 70:140, 1993.

House JC, George LW, Oslund KL, et al: Primary photosensitization related to the ingestion of alfalfa silage by cattle, *J Am Vet Med Assoc* 209:1604, 1996.

Howard JL, Smith RA: *Current veterinary therapy. Food animal practice*, ed 4, Philadelphia, 1999, WB Saunders.

Jubb TF, Vassallo RI, Wroth RH: Suppurative otitis in cattle associated with ear mites (Raillietia auris), *Aust Vet J* 70:354, 1993.

Jubb TF, Malmo J, Morton JM, et al: Inherited epidermal dysplasia in Holstein-Friesian calves, *Aust Vet J* 67:16, 1990.

Kahrs RF: *Viral diseases of cattle*, ed 2, Ames, IA, 2001, Iowa State University Press.

Lonneux JF, Nguyen TQ, Delhez M, et al: Efficacy of pour-on and injectable formulations of moxidectin and ivermectin in cattle naturally infected with Psoroptes ovis, *Vet Parasitol* 69:319, 1997.

Machen M, Montgomery T, Holland R, et al: Bovine hereditary zinc deficiency: lethal trait A46, *J Vet Diagn Invest* 8:219, 1996.

Milne MH, Barrett DC, Mellor DJ, et al: Clinical recognition and treatment of bovine cutaneous actinobacillosis, *Vet Rec* 148:273, 2001.

O'Toole D, Fox JD: Chronic hyperplastic and neoplastic lesions (Marjolin's ulcer) in hot-brand sites in adult beef cattle, *J Vet Diagn Invest* 15:64, 2003.

Panciera RJ, McKenzie DM, Ewing PJ, et al: Bovine hyperkeratosis: historical review and report of an outbreak, *Compend Cont Educ* 15:1287, 1993.

Radostits OM, Gay CC, Blood DC, et al: *Veterinary medicine. A textbook of the diseases of cattle, sheep, pigs, goats and horses*, ed 10, Philadelphia, 2007, WB Saunders.

Rooney KA, Illyes EF, Sunderland SJ, et al: Efficacy of a pour-on formulation of doramectin against lice, mites, and grubs of cattle, *Am J Vet Res* 60:402, 1999.

Scott DW: *Large animal dermatology*, Philadelphia, 1988, WB Saunders.

Scott DW, Anderson WI: Bovine cutaneous neoplasms: literature review and retrospective analysis of 62 cases (1978 to 1990), *Compend Cont Educ* 14:1405, 1992.

Scott DW, Gourreau JM: Alopecia areata (pelade) chez les bovines, *Point Vét* 22:671, 1990.

Scott DW, Gourreau JM: Fibromes, fibrosarcomes et mastocytomes cutanés chez les bovines, *Point Vét* 24:539, 1992.

Scott DW, Gourreau JM: La dermatite à Pelodera strongyloides et l'otite externe à Rhabditis bovis chez les bovines, *Méd Vét Québec* 23:112, 1993.

Scott DW, Gourreau JM: La folliculite et la furonculose staphylococciques des bovines, *Point Vét* 23:79, 1991.

Scott DW, Gourreau JM: Les tumeurs des vaisseaux sanguins cutanés chez les bovines, *Point Vét* 28:941, 1996.

Scruggs DW, Blue JK: Toxic hepatopathy and photosensitization in cattle fed moldy alfalfa hay, *J Am Vet Med Assoc* 204:264, 1994.

Thorel MF, Morand M, Fontaine JJ, et al: Bovine nodular thelitis: a clinicopathological study of 20 cases, *Vet Dermatol* 1:165, 1990.

Wu W, Cook ME, Chu FS, et al: Case study of bovine dermatitis caused by oat straw infected with Fusarium sporotrichoides, *Vet Rec* 140:399, 1997.

Yeruham I, Perl S, Orgad U: Congenital skin neoplasia in cattle, *Vet Dermatol* 10:149, 1999.

Yeruham I, Friedman S, Perl S, et al: A herd level analysis of a Corynebacterium pseudotuberculosis outbreak in a dairy cattle herd, *Vet Dermatol* 15:315, 2004.

Yeruham I, Perl S: Melanocytoma and myxoma—tumours of the limbs in cattle, *Berl Munch Tierärztl Wschr* 115:425, 2002.

Yeruham I, Yadin H, Haymovich M, et al: Adverse reaction to FMD vaccine, *Vet Dermatol* 12:197, 2001.

CHAPTER 8

Diseases of the Teats and Udder

Lisle W. George, Thomas J. Divers, Norm Ducharme, and Frank L. Welcome

The udder of a dairy cow consists of four separate glands suspended by medial and lateral collagenous laminae. The medial laminae are more elastic, especially cranially, than the lateral laminae and are paired. Caudally, the medial laminae are more collagenous and originate from the subpelvic tendon. The lateral laminae are multiple, inserting at various levels of mammary tissue, and originate from the subpelvic tendon caudally and external oblique aponeurosis cranially. The medial and lateral laminae provide udder support that is essential for udder conformation and for solid attachment to the ventral body wall. The external pudendal artery constitutes the major blood supply to the udder; the artery courses through the inguinal canal along with the pudendal vein and lymph vessels to supply the craniolateral portion of the mammary gland. Caudally, the internal pudendal artery branches into the ventral perineal artery at the level of the ischiatic arch and courses caudally to the vulva, along the perineum to the base of the rear quarters. The caudal superficial epigastric vein (subcutaneous abdominal vein or milk vein) is the major venous return from the mammary gland. Located superficially along the ventral abdomen, it courses cranially to the "milk well" where it enters the abdomen to join the internal thoracic vein, draining first into the subclavian vein, and finally into the cranial vena cava. Lymph drainage moves dorsally and caudally to the superficial inguinal (mammary, supramammary) lymph nodes, which can be palpated by following the rear quarter dorsally until it ends, then palpating deep just above the gland along the lateral laminae. Although the prefemoral (subiliac) lymph nodes that are located in the aponeurosis of the external abdominal oblique muscle, approximately 15 cm dorsal to the patella, are not strictly drainage lymph nodes of the udder, they should be palpated as part of the routine physical examination of cattle. Because of their regional proximity and combined lymphatic drainage with the supramammary lymph nodes into the medial iliac lymph nodes, many cows with mastitis have obvious lymphadenopathy of the prefemoral lymph nodes, and they are easily palpable.

UDDER

Premature Development

Premature symmetric development of the udder in calves and heifers has been associated with chronic estrogenic stimulation resulting from cystic ovaries, feedstuffs containing excessive estrogens, and the mycotoxin zearalenone. In some cases, udder development is accompanied by vulvar swelling. When the more common etiology of ingesting feed containing estrogenic substances has occurred, multiple heifers within a group are typically affected, and successful resolution of the mammary development requires removal of the contributing feed material. Idiopathic symmetric udder development in individual heifers is occasionally encountered when no obvious endocrinologic or intoxicant cause can be elucidated. Asymmetric gland enlargement in group-reared heifers should always raise suspicion of mastitis secondary to cross-sucking.

Breakdown or Loss of Support Apparatus

Breakdown of either the lateral or the medial udder supports can occur. Medial laminae breakdown causes the medial longitudinal groove between the left and right halves of the udder to disappear and causes the teats to project laterally. Loss of lateral support laminae causes the halves of the udder to project ventrally to the level of the hocks or lower. Occasionally cows lose fore udder support such that the forequarters appear detached from the ventral abdominal wall, and a hand may be inserted between the skin covering the glandular tissue and the ventral body wall. Similarly loss of rear udder attachment tends to make the rear udder pendulous without clearly defined udder attachment and obvious stretching of the skin in the escutcheon region. In the latter condition, the rear quarters no longer appear to curve up to the escutcheon but simply hang.

All these various deficiencies in udder support predispose to udder edema, teat and udder injuries, and mastitis. Edema is worsened by the pendulous nature of the udder, reduced venous and lymphatic return, and trauma. Injuries to the teat and udder in cows with pendulous udders (Figure 8-1) result from environmental trauma that includes contact of the udder with flooring when the cow is recumbent and direct damage from claws and dewclaws or from being stepped on by neighboring cows. Mastitis is predisposed to by environmental contamination of the teats and udder, teat injuries that affect milkout, and imperfect milkout caused by persistent edema in the floor of the udder. In some cows—especially those with severe loss of median support—it may not be possible to attach a milking machine claw simultaneously to seriously deviated teats. The result often is mastitis or culling because of milking difficulties. In addition, purebred cattle that are classified are discriminated against in classification score if these undesirable mammary characteristics are present.

Etiology of udder breakdown is complex and consists of genetic, nutritional, and management factors. Although udder breakdown is largely thought of as a problem in multiparous cows, in herds that approach an average of 25,000 lb per lactation, breakdown of the udder may occur at earlier ages.

No treatments exist for the ligament ruptures. Prevention of the condition is also problematic because other than genetic selection and control and prompt treatment of excessive parturient edema little else can be done.

Hematomas

Etiology

Self-induced trauma as a result of awkward efforts to rise or lie down and external trauma from butting or kicking by other cows are theorized as the causes of udder hematomas, but injuries from these sources seldom are confirmed. Caudal udder hematomas originating in the escutcheon region may represent thrombosis and/or rupture of the perineal vein because they tend to occur during the dry period. Udder hematomas, regardless of cause, are dangerous because blood accumulates subcutaneously, allowing massive blood loss. In addition, the exact location of the bleeding often is impossible to determine clinically because of the extensive venous plexus. Surgical attempts at finding the bleeding vessel are often futile and may lead to excessive blood loss.

Signs

Soft tissue swellings immediately cranial to the udder are most common in lactating dairy cattle (Figure 8-2), whereas extreme swelling in the escutcheon region ventral to the vulva and dorsal to the rear quarters is more common in dry cows (Figure 8-3). The swelling may be fluctuant, soft, or firm, depending on the amount of blood causing the distention; usually it is painless and cool. Rare instances of hematomas

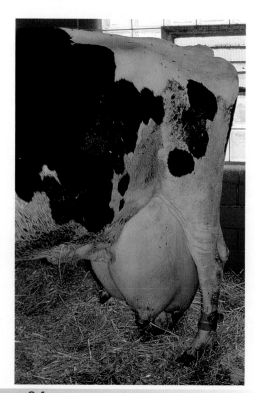

Figure 8-1

Mature cow with pendulous udder.

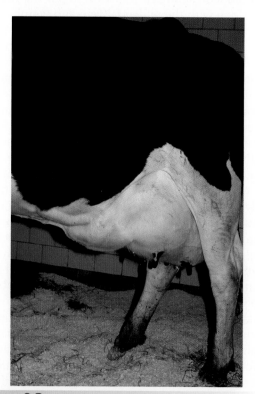

Figure 8-2

Udder hematoma apparent as soft tissue swelling cranial to the udder. The hematoma also has infiltrated the medial laminae to separate the forequarters pathologically.

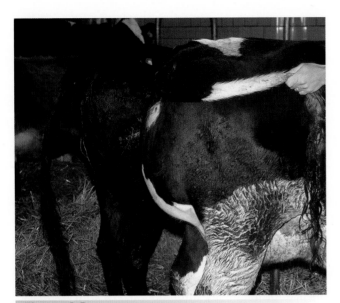

Figure 8-3

Udder hematoma caudodorsal to the rear quarters in a dry cow.

between the base of the udder and ventral body wall also have been encountered.

Progressive enlargement of the swelling coupled with progressive anemia signal a guarded prognosis for cattle affected with udder hematomas. Signs of anemia include pallor of the mucous membranes and teats (if nonpigmented skin), elevated heart and respiratory rate, and weakness. Cattle with udder hematomas that progressively enlarge may die over 2 to 7 days.

Diagnosis

Progressive fluctuant swelling adjacent to the udder coupled with progressive anemia and absence of fever usually are sufficient for diagnosis. Ultrasound may be used to confirm the presence of a fluid-filled mass but does not always make a definitive diagnosis on its own. Ultrasonographic distinction between an abscess and a hematoma can be valuable because clinical experience suggests that aspiration of a hematoma, even under controlled and aseptic conditions, will frequently be associated with subsequent abscess formation. Ultrasonographic evidence of gas shadowing within an encapsulated mass should be taken as proof of an abscess, but mixed echogenicity images can be obtained with both abscesses and hematomas. Abscesses tend to be warm, painful, and may cause fever in the affected cow. Seromas are unusual adjacent to the udder but would give similar signs of swelling. However, seromas usually do not enlarge as much as a hematoma in this location, and progressive anemia would not be expected with a seroma.

In confusing cases, an aspirate under sterile condition may be needed to differentiate hematoma from an abscess or seroma. Clinicians should be reluctant to aspirate known hematomas for fear of introducing

infection or disturbing pressure equilibrium that might allow further bleeding.

Treatment

For management of mammary gland hematomas, box stall rest and close monitoring of the animal at 12- to 24-hour intervals are important components of therapy. Complete blood counts (CBCs) and coagulation panels may be indicated to rule out bleeding disorders. Flunixin and other nonsteroidal antiinflammatory drugs (NSAIDs) should be withheld during the period of active hemorrhage.

In general, bleeding disorders of cattle are rare and are unlikely causes of udder hematomas. Occasionally consumptive thrombocytopenia may occur in cows with udder hematomas. Cows that experience hemorrhage sufficient to reduce packed cell volumes (PCVs) to 10% to 12% and have a heart rate exceeding 100 beats/min and a respiratory rate in excess of 60 breaths/min require a whole blood transfusion of 5 to 8 L. Platelet-rich whole blood from a healthy donor (negative for bovine leukemia virus [BLV], bovine virus diarrhea virus [BVDV], bluetongue virus, anaplasmosis, and Johne's disease) is important if anemia becomes severe.

Stabilization of the size of the hematoma and other clinical signs are positive prognostic indicators, whereas progressive anemia and enlargement of the hematoma despite therapy are negative indicators. Affected cows should be separated from herdmates to avoid further trauma. *Incision of udder hematomas to arrest bleeding is unrewarding, may exacerbate bleeding, and therefore is contraindicated.* Stabilized udder hematomas eventually resorb, but some may abscess and drain by 4 weeks because of pressure necrosis of overlying skin. When drainage occurs, large necrotic clots of blood and serosanguineous fluid drain from the area. Surgical debridement of naturally draining hematomas is not indicated except in chronic cases (>4 weeks) with abscessation, in which case ultrasound guidance should be considered. The condition does not recur once fully resolved. Udder asymmetry, abnormal teat deviation, and persistent residual edema are common sequelae to udder hematoma and abscess resolution, and although these are of limited economic impact in a grade cow, they may be a considerable frustration for the owners of show and pedigree cows.

Abscesses

Etiology

Udder abscesses may appear anywhere in the mammary tissue or adjacent to the glands. Frequently skin puncture with subsequent abscessation is suspected when obvious abscesses appear in quarters having completely normal secretion and no evidence of mastitis. Endogenous abscesses can form secondary to mastitis with abscessation, as is typical of mastitis caused by *Arcanobacterium pyogenes.*

However, this discussion will be confined to udder abscesses requiring percutaneous drainage, and discussion of mastitis origin abscesses will be addressed in the mastitis section.

Most udder abscesses harbor typical contaminants such as *A. pyogenes* or staphylococci, but occasionally other organisms may be involved.

Abscesses appear as firm, warm swellings that may be either distinct or indistinct from gland parenchyma (Figure 8-4). Palpation of the swelling may be painful to the affected cow. Milk from the affected quarter usually is normal, and the abscesses tend to be well-encapsulated.

Diagnosis

Physical signs usually are sufficient for diagnosis, but ultrasonography or aspiration may be indicated if the owner is impatient regarding diagnosis and therapy. Ultrasound may be beneficial to diagnosis and treatment of udder abscesses because flocculent material may be observed, and major vessels overlying the lesion may be located if aspiration and drainage are necessary. A thick capsule around the abscess is usually observed.

Treatment

A conservative approach usually is rewarded by eventual natural rupture and drainage of the abscesses in 2 to 8 weeks. This has been standard treatment because practitioners fear lancing anything in the udder because of the extensive blood supply to the entire organ. Conservative treatment probably still is the safest. The only risk from conservative therapy is the same for neglected abscessation in other tissues—that is, chronic antigenic stimuli that may predispose to glomerulonephritis, amyloidosis, or bacteremia, which may cause endocarditis or other infectious disease.

Therefore the practitioner may be pressured by owners of valuable or show cattle to encourage early drainage. Ultrasound and aspiration are indicated before draining, as discussed previously.

Following natural or surgical drainage, the abscess cavity should be flushed daily with dilute antiseptics or saline, and the drainage hole should be kept open, lest premature closure allow the abscess to reform. Usually antibiotic treatments are unnecessary.

Thrombophlebitis and Abscessation of the Milk Vein. Thrombophlebitis of the mammary vein is an occasional complication of venipuncture at this site (Figure 8-5). This vessel seems attractive for the intravenous (IV) administration of pharmaceuticals, particularly in pit parlors and for producers for whom its size and accessibility make it a less challenging alternative compared with the jugular or coccygeal veins. However, the consequences of mammary thrombophlebitis with respect to udder symmetry and future production are sinister enough that it should never be used in show or valuable individual cows. It should only be used under considerable duress even in grade cattle. Abscesses may develop secondary to phlebitis from the use of contaminated needles or subsequent to hematoma formation when vascular damage and perivascular leakage occur as the cow resists the procedure. As with all cases of thrombophlebitis there is a risk of embolic spread, potentially causing endocarditis or nephritis. If treatment is initiated immediately following the inciting attempted venipuncture, antiinflammatory and antimicrobial therapy is indicated. However, veterinary attention is often only sought after abscessation has already occurred, at which time the goal of therapy should be surgical drainage followed by antimicrobial therapy. It can be challenging to avoid significant blood loss when lancing such abscesses because of the highly vascular nature of the region, and ideally the procedure should be performed under ultrasound guidance. The

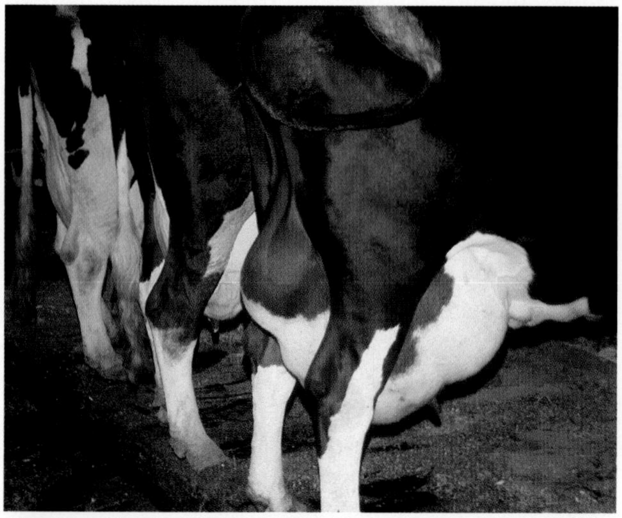

Figure 8-4

Udder abscess associated with the left rear quarter.

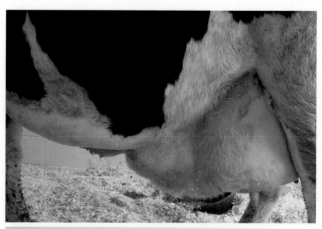

Figure 8-5

Mature Holstein with mammary thrombophlebitis subsequent to repeated oxytocin injection to facilitate milk let down. Note edema cranial to forequarters.

bacterial species implicated include the common pyogenic anaerobes, and antimicrobial therapy should include beta-lactam antibiotics. Treatment of valuable cattle may include rifampin under appropriate extra-label drug use guidelines.

Udder Cleft Dermatitis

Etiology
Udder sores are foul-smelling areas of moist dermatitis that result from pressure necrosis of skin associated with periparturient udder engorgement and edema. Common locations include the skin reflection between the medial thigh and dorsal attachment of the lateral udder, on the ventral midline immediately adjacent to the median septum of the foreudder, and on the median septum of the udder—either between the forequarters or in the fold that is centered between the four quarters.

Pressure necrosis associated with udder edema is enhanced by frictional injury and chafing with limb and udder movement. The abraded skin oozes serum, which, coupled with the omnipresent skin hair, leads to moist dermatitis. Finally, opportunistic anaerobic bacteria such as *Fusobacterium necrophorum* and *A. pyogenes* invade and propagate under crusts, scabs, and necrotic skin. The organisms cause the smell that distresses milkers each time they get close to the udder—hence the name "udder rot." Chorioptic mange mites and *Malassezia* spp. have been incriminated in some cases.

Signs
A fetid odor similar to that found in septic metritis or retained placenta emanates from areas of moist dermatitis in the groin area or more commonly the ventral median area of the udder. Skin necrosis may be mild or severe. In the worst cases, large patches of skin (10 to 30 cm in length) may be peeled off. Matted hair, scabs, and necrotic skin are present (Figure 8-6, *A* and *B*). Myiasis may occur in warm weather. In some first-calf heifers, groin infections can be so severe that lameness may occur.

Diagnosis
The combination of necrotizing fold dermatitis and malodorous discharge in a postpartum cow is sufficient for the diagnosis of udder fold dermatitis.

Treatment
Although the principles of treatment are straightforward, client compliance may be lacking because of time constraints, and udder cleft dermatitis is not treated on larger dairies.

For dairies that request therapy, a commercially available topically applied wound spray (Granulex Aerosol Spray, Pfizer Inc., Exton, PA) consisting of a mixture of castor oil, balsam of Peru, and trypsin has been successfully by field veterinarians for the treatment of udder cleft dermatitis. The spray is marketed for administration

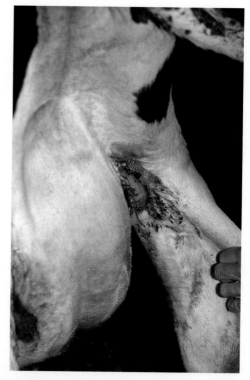

A

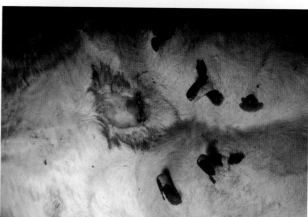

B

Figure 8-6

A, Necrotic udder sore in the right groin inguinal area of a first-calf heifer that had bilateral lesions. **B,** Necrotic udder sore between the forequarters of a cow positioned in dorsal recumbency in preparation for abomasopexy.

in humans and has been effective for treatment of decubitus in bedridden patients. Other compounded remedies have been recommended for the treatment of udder cleft dermatitis, but given the current drug compounding regulations of the U.S. Food and Drug Administration (FDA), these formulations cannot be recommended for use in food-producing animals. Patients that have developed cleft fold pyodermas secondarily to udder edema should be treated with diuretics (furosemide, 1 mg/kg) to reduce edema and anaerobiosis in the skin of the mammary gland. Diuretics are calciuretic and kaluretic, so during diuretic treatment of postpartum cows, calcium status should be monitored, and if the cow shows weakness, lassitude, and cold extremities, she should be given IV calcium gluconate and 100 g of potassium chloride orally.

The prognosis in cases of udder cleft pyoderma is excellent, but healing time may be prolonged for months in untreated cases. If the inguinal lesions are causing severe lameness, surgical debridement can speed healing.

Udder Dermatitis

Etiology
Udder dermatitis may be associated with a multitude of chemical, physical, and microbiologic causes.

Chemical causes of udder dermatitis include irritants in bedding such as hydrated lime, ammonia from urine, copper sulfate, or formaldehyde from foot baths.

Physical causes of udder skin inflammation include sunburn, frostbite, and pressure necrosis caused by decubitus. Lesions of photosensitization may appear on the sun-exposed, nonpigmented skin of teats and the udder.

Staphylococci and streptococci occasionally cause a diffuse miliary folliculitis or pustular dermatitis named "udder impetigo." Rarely *Dermatophilus congolensis* affects the skin of the udder, but this tends to occur as part of a severe generalized infection. Disseminated infections of *Trichophyton verrucosum* may affect the skin of the udder. Viral lesions of the skin of the udder include herpes mammillitis (see the discussion of Teat Skin Infections), BVDV, bovine bluetongue virus infection, and malignant catarrhal fever (MCF).

Signs
Signs vary with specific etiology of the lesions. Chemical and physical teat skin dermatitis is characterized by extreme erythema, swelling, and evidence of pain. Vesicles may be present in extreme cases associated with irritant chemicals. The skin of the teats and the udder may be involved. Serum oozing and slight matting of the hair may be apparent.

Sunburned teat skin of dairy cattle has a similar appearance to that found in other species, and the cow may show evidence of sunburn in other locations. Affected skin is warm, painful, and may have vesicles or bullae caused by burns on nonhaired skin near the teat-udder junction. Multiple cows in the herd may show signs simultaneously and resent milking procedures because of painfully burned skin. Signs may be present on only one side of the udder if the cow preferentially lies on one side. Frostbite occurs during extreme winter cold—mostly in free stall barns and mostly in periparturient cows with udder edema that already compromises tissue circulation. Patchy areas of skin on the teats and udder become cool, discolored, swollen, and then turn leathery and completely cold. Frostbite must be differentiated from herpes mammillitis.

Other physical causes of udder dermatitis include photosensitization, which again would be apparent because of signs in other depigmented regions of skin and known exposure to sunshine.

Pressure necrosis or decubital sores from extended periods of recumbency occur mostly in cattle with very pendulous udders but may also occur in downer cattle or lame cows that lie down more than normal. Such sores often are located where the medial hock makes contact with the udder. Lesions initially are reddened, ooze serum, and then slough, leaving a necrotic crater-like lesion in the udder.

The clinical signs of infectious dermatitis vary with the causative agent. Staphylococcal dermatitis causes a diffuse folliculitis with small raised tufts of hair joined with dry or moist exudate. Pustules may be apparent in the worst cases. Usually only one or a few cows in the herd are affected, but occasionally outbreaks of pustular dermatitis have been observed. *D. congolensis* may appear as larger confluent areas of folliculitis with dry or moist crusts that hold tufts of hair together. Plucking these tufts of hair or crusts may reveal purulent material on the underside of the crust or adjacent skin. Cows with dermatophilosis on the skin of the udder usually have other obvious *Dermatophilus* lesions.

T. verrucosum lesions on the udder are circular or patchy alopecic areas that are 1.0 to 10.0 cm in diameter. Most lesions have crusts as observed in ringworm lesions in other locations, but some lesions may appear as moist alopecic regions as a result of the paucity of hair in certain regions of the udder. Other areas of ringworm infection usually are identified during inspection of the cow. Herpes mammillitis lesions coexist on the skin of the teats and udder. Recognition of bullae or vesicles in early cases is imperative to diagnosis.

Herpes mammillitis (bovine herpes virus 2 [BHV2]) most often occurs in first-calf heifers, and usually more than one animal will be affected. Another herpesvirus, BHV4, the DN599 strain of BHV that has been isolated from the respiratory tract of cattle, may be capable of causing pustular mammary dermatitis. Multiple vesicles and pustules from 1.0 to 10.0 mm in diameter have been observed on the udder of lactating cows, and lesions have been observed in farm workers.

Treatment
Treatment for chemical dermatitis only requires gentle washing of the udder with warm water and removal of the offending agent from the cow's skin. Individual cows may be sensitive to a chemical despite the majority of cows in the herd being exposed to the same chemical yet remaining unaffected. Warm water cleansing of the udder to remove residual chemical followed by application of aloe or lanolin products is recommended.

Physical causes of dermatitis are best treated by preventing further exposure to the specific physical cause and by symptomatic therapy. Sunburned cows must be kept inside or provided shade if at pasture. Cool water compresses followed by aloe or lanolin ointments to deter skin cracking and peeling caused by dryness are helpful. Udder supports may help prevent sunburn. Frostbite is best prevented by therapy for excessive udder edema and keeping periparturient cows well bedded for warmth. Periparturient cows in free stalls during extreme cold are at greatest risk because free stall beds usually are poorly bedded for warmth. Once frostbite has occurred, careful sharp debridement of necrotic tissue and protection against further injury are the only potentially effective treatments.

Pressure necrosis or decubital sores are treated by providing soft bedding for cows that spend more time than normal recumbent and minimizing udder edema. Extremely pendulous udders are at greater risk for decubital sores. Treatment of decubital sores requires gentle cleansing and debridement following by the application of Granulex spray. Decubital sores may require weeks or months to heal.

Photosensitization must be treated by avoiding further sunlight, applying cleansing lesions, debriding necrotic skin, and determining the cause of photosensitization.

Microbiologic causes of udder skin dermatitis are managed according to the specific cause. Staphylococcal folliculitis is treated by clipping the hair on the udder, washing gently with povidone iodine scrub solutions, rinsing with water, and drying. Washing and rinsing should be done once or twice daily. Antibiotics generally are not necessary. Filthy environmental contributing factors should be eliminated.

D. congolensis infections should be treated by clipping the hair of the udder followed by removal of all crusts through gentle washing with povidone iodine scrubs and drying. In those with severe or generalized dermatophilosis, penicillin (22,000 IU/kg body weight, once or twice daily, intramuscularly [IM]) may be necessary for 5 to 7 days in addition to local therapy.

Ringworm lesions can be managed by clipping the hair on the udder (especially if it is long or filthy) followed by topical application of chlorine bleach diluted 50:50 with water, miconazole, or clotrimazole ointments to the lesions once or twice daily. Care should be taken such that antifungal medications do not contaminate milk during milking procedures.

No specific treatment exists for udder lesions resulting from herpes mammillitis or other dermatopathic viruses.

Edema

Etiology

Udder edema, also known as "cake," may be physiologic or pathologic. Physiologic udder edema begins several weeks before calving and is more prominent in heifers preparing to have their first calf. Many questions remain

unanswered as regards the etiology of udder edema. Genetic factors certainly exist, and bull stud services sometimes grade production sires by probability of udder edema in their female offspring. Individual cows with severe or pathologic edema should be examined to rule out medical considerations that could contribute to ventral or udder edema. Some conditions to consider include cardiac conditions, caudal vena caval thrombosis, mammary vein thrombosis, and hypoproteinemia resulting from one of a number of diseases. Physical examination and serum chemistry screens may be helpful in the evaluation of such individuals.

Postparturient metritis has been associated with persistence of physiologic or pathologic udder edema by some owners and veterinarians. The pathophysiology of this relationship is unknown.

When many cows in a herd have either severe physiologic udder edema or pathologic udder edema, herd-based causes must be considered. Although feeding excessive grain to dry cows and early lactation cows has long been discussed as a cause of such endemic udder edema problems, feeding trials do not support this theory Similarly, high protein diets do not seem to be directly involved. Currently, excessive total dietary potassium and sodium are considered possible culprits in herd-wide udder edema problems. Total intake of potassium may be excessive in some instances when high quality alfalfa haylage constitutes a major portion of the ration. Forages harvested from land that is fertilized repeatedly with manure are becoming an increasing problem because of their high potassium content. One article recommends no more than 227 g/day/head of potassium in heifers. Similarly sodium levels may be excessive when considering total available sodium in the basic ration, water, and mineral additives plus or minus free choice salt.

Hypoproteinemia and especially low albumin fractions in affected cows also may contribute to udder edema. Metabolic profiles need to be performed to assess this possibility and determine the origin.

Signs

Physiologic udder edema may start in the rear udder, fore udder, in the left or right half of the udder, or symmetrically in all four quarters. Edema tends to be most prominent in the rear quarters and floor of the udder (Figure 8-7). Cows with moderate to severe udder edema usually have a variable degree of ventral edema extending from the fore udder toward the brisket.

Udder edema pits and associated ventral edema may be soft and fluctuant or firm and pitting. Physiologic edema increases up to calving and then begins to gradually resolve over 2 to 4 weeks.

Pathologic edema persists longer than physiologic edema. Pathologic edema may be present for months following parturition or for the entire lactation. The tendency for pathologic edema is increased in cows with

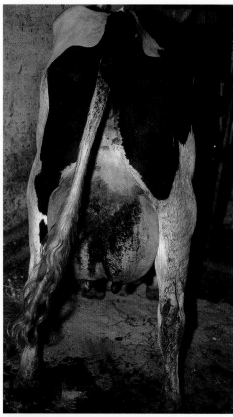

Figure 8-7

Forced abduction of the hind limbs is obvious because of severe udder edema in this first-calf heifer.

breakdown of udder support structures, and conversely pathologic udder edema may contribute to breakdown of udder support structures. Therefore severe edema may affect a cow's longevity and classification in some instances.

Pronounced udder edema interferes with complete milkout because it causes the affected cow discomfort, and milking may accentuate that discomfort. In addition, interstitial edema in the mammary glands may cause pressure differentials that interfere with normal production and let down of milk. Therefore chronic or pathologic edema may have a negative effect on the lactation potential because cattle never reach their projected production. Interference with complete milkout resulting from pain, as well as mechanical or pressure influences, also may lead to postmilking leakage of milk in cows with severe udder edema. This translates into an increased risk of mastitis.

Cows with udder edema do not act ill but may be uncomfortable or painful because of the swollen, edematous udder swinging as they move or from constantly being irritated by limb movement as they walk. In addition, when resting, the cow may tend to lie in lateral recumbency with the hind limbs extended to reduce body pressure on the udder.

Diagnosis

Diagnosis is based on inspection, palpation, evaluation of milk secretions to rule out mastitis, and ruling out conditions such as udder abscess or hematoma. Pitting edema should be present, especially on the floor of the udder. Pitting edema may be evident over the entire udder in severe cases, and ventral edema frequently coexists in these instances.

Treatment

Treatment of individual preparturient or postparturient cows is indicated when edema has the potential to break down the udder support structure. Treatment also is indicated for preparturient cows having severe udder edema associated with leakage of milk from one or more teats.

Diuretics constitute the principal treatments for udder edema. Preparturient treatment of cattle with furosemide (0.5 to 1.0 mg/kg body weight) as an initial treatment followed by decreasing dosages of furosemide once or twice daily for 2 to 4 days is commonly used. Salt restriction should be considered. Premilking may be indicated in preparturient cows with severe udder edema that are leaking milk. This must be an individual decision based on the owner's experience with premilking. Obviously if the option of premilking is selected, the newborn calf will require colostrum from another cow. Although premilking is controversial, some owners of show cattle swear by the technique to preserve udder conformation. Udder supports also may be helpful if fitted properly.

A word of warning about furosemide—urinary losses of calcium may be sufficient to increase the risk of periparturient hypocalcemia, and this should be anticipated in multiparous cows receiving multiple doses of the drug.

Parturient and postparturient cows judged to need treatment for udder edema may receive either furosemide or dexamethasone-diuretic combinations orally.

Individual cows may respond to one product better than the other, but this is impossible to predict. Furosemide seems to work well in some herds, whereas the dexamethasone-diuretic combination is superior in others. When considering dexamethasone-diuretic combinations, the veterinarian should first rule out contraindications to corticosteroid use. Udder supports and salt restriction may or may not be practical but should be considered. Nursing procedures including udder massage, more frequent milking, and mild exercise are helpful but labor intensive. Metritis should be ruled out or treated.

In herds with endemic udder edema, nutritional consultations are imperative to evaluate anion-cation balance. Total potassium, total sodium, and serum chemistry to profile affected and nonaffected cows should be performed. Diets with anionic salt supplementation and those with added antioxidants may show some tendency to diminish udder edema in affected herds. Water and availability of free choice salt or salt-mineral combinations should be included in the nutritional evaluation.

Hemorrhage into a Gland

Etiology

Hemorrhage into one or more glands is common at parturition in cows with severe udder edema or pendulous udders that have been traumatized by hind limb movement and awkward posture during recumbency. Milk from one or more quarters contains blood and may appear as pink, red, or reddish-brown with blood clots. Generally this condition clears within four to eight milkings and is not a major problem. Cows with bloody milk should be watched closely for mastitis because blood provides an excellent growth medium for bacteria.

As opposed to the usually innocuous parturient hemorrhage described previously, severe hemorrhage involving one or more quarters occasionally is observed in dairy cattle during lactation. The cause is unknown, but nonspecific trauma usually is suspected. Thrombocytopenia has been confirmed in some but not all of these cows, and when it is identified, it is not known whether it was as cause or effect.

Signs

The chief complaint for a cow with intramammary hemorrhage is persistent blood-stained milk from one or more quarters. Anemia may develop if extensive bleeding continues to occur over several milkings. The milk usually is red rather than pink, and blood clots are obvious. Large intraluminal clots occasionally plug the papillary duct, causing difficulty in milkout.

Diagnosis

The clinical signs of intramammary hemorrhage are sufficiently diagnostic, but laboratory work should be performed to assess thrombocyte numbers. Coagulation profiles that may be used to incriminate specific bleeding disorders are frequently unreliable in cattle. Specific causes of intramammary hemorrhage are seldom identified. Intramammary hemorrhage may increase the risk for mastitis.

Treatment

Decisions for appropriate therapy are difficult because of the likelihood of iatrogenic complications. An apparently obvious solution is to stop milking the affected quarters—thereby stopping further blood loss and allowing pressure to build up in the gland to deter further bleeding. However, this approach may provoke such severe blood clotting in the ductules, gland cistern, and teat cistern that future milking is impossible. On the other hand, once- or twice-a-day milking usually allows blood clots to be stripped out but causes more blood loss and may allow continued bleeding from whatever vessel is leaking. Generally reduction of milking frequency (usually to once daily) has been considered to be an optimal management for intramammary hemorrhage. Blood clots that form may be stripped out as they form and do not ruin future potential. If this approach does not resolve the problem within several days, a decision to stop milking and risk severe cisternal clots must be considered to save the cow.

Thrombocytopenia and other coagulation defects should be excluded as causes of the hemorrhage. When thrombocytopenia or severe anemia (PCV, <10%) exists, an immediate fresh whole blood transfusion from a donor that is uninfected by BLV, BVDV, bluetongue virus, anaplasmosis, and Johne's disease should be administered. Approximately 4 to 6 L of blood should be transfused at a single time. Blood transfusion also may become necessary regardless of cause if the cow's anemia becomes severe enough to warrant transfusion.

MAMMARY TUMORS

Except for fibropapillomas (warts), mammary tumors in dairy cattle are rare. Lymphosarcoma is the most common and will be considered below under a separate heading. Relatively few dairy cows live to an old age, but those that do still have a very low incidence of mammary tumors. Both squamous cell carcinomas and mammary gland adenocarcinomas have been observed in older dairy cattle (≥15 years). Fibropapillomas (warts) are more common on the skin of the teats but also may appear on the skin of the udder. Many other sporadic tumors, including fibromas, fibrosarcomas, and papillary adenomas, have been reported.

Lymphosarcoma

Lymphosarcoma is the most common tumor to appear within the gland and associated lymph nodes in dairy cattle. Focal and diffuse infiltration of the gland with lymphosarcoma and rarely adenocarcinoma has been observed (Figure 8-8, *A* and *B*). The mammary gland is hardly ever the only site of lymphoma infiltration, however. Usually tumor masses in other target organs or lymph nodes supersede mammary involvement. Affected glands may merely appear edematous rather than firm, and secretions may appear normal. Diffuse lymphocytic infiltration of the udder may appear similar to the diffuse mild edema that develops in hypoproteinemic cattle. The mammary lymph nodes (superficial inguinal) may be enlarged because of lymphosarcoma or chronic inflammation and should routinely be palpated during physical examination.

Juvenile tumors of the mammary gland have been observed in two heifers referred to our clinic. Surgical extirpation of these masses was performed before udder

A

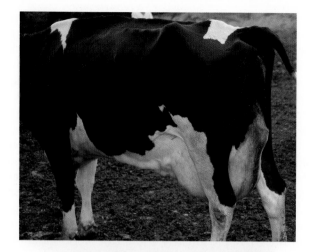

B

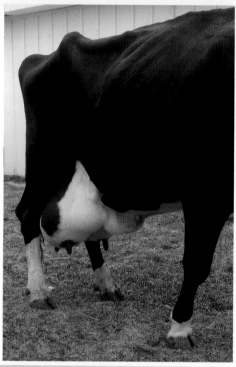

Figure 8-8

A, A mature Holstein affected with lymphosarcoma. The right supramammary lymph node is markedly enlarged and appears as a firm swelling in the dorsal aspect of the right rear mammary gland. The cow also had diffuse infiltration of the mammary gland and cardiac neoplasia. **B,** A 14-year-old Holstein with mammary gland adenocarcinoma. There was diffuse neoplastic involvement of the gland. *(Photo courtesy R.H. Whitlock.)*

development. Juvenile tumors found to be fibromas associated with the teat also have been recognized in two yearling heifers.

Signs

Affected cows have a varied clinical presentation ranging from focal enlargement to diffuse and massive udder enlargement. Some squamous cell carcinomas are ulcerated, firm, and pink with a malodorous smell. Precursor papilloma or epithelioma masses may have been observed by the owner. Fibropapillomas or warts are obvious and are of little concern.

Juvenile tumors of the gland cause an obvious enlargement that may be confused with mastitis in the undeveloped udder.

Diagnosis

Biopsy or aspirate of a suspicious mass is essential for diagnosis. Biopsy of the gland may be performed if diffuse lymphosarcoma is suspected. Commercial true-cut biopsy needles work very well for mammary gland biopsies, and the procedure is safe.

Treatment

Juvenile tumors of the gland may be excised, but prognosis for production in the affected gland must be guarded. However, in the two juvenile gland tumors observed by Dr. Rebhun and in the two reported teat skin fibromas in yearlings, long-term follow-up evaluation indicated that all glands that had undergone surgery were functional at first calving. Squamous cell carcinomas may be treated according to severity. Cryosurgery may suffice in early stages of the disease, but udder amputation may be required in advanced cases. Treatment for lymphosarcoma is rare and generally of limited success.

Udder Amputation

Hemimastectomy or radical mastectomy is rarely performed in cattle. Indications for this in valuable or pet cattle would be neoplasia, chronic incurable mastitis, and/or suspensory apparatus failure that causes the udder to sag and be persistently traumatized (Figure 8-9). Individual animals that undergo udder amputation must be in good general condition. Significant blood loss can occur with udder amputation because of the vascularity of the mammary gland. Cattle with septic mastitis or in poor physical condition should not undergo udder amputation until their physical condition is significantly improved.

The cow must be placed in dorsal recumbency and preferably under general anesthesia. A fusiform skin incision is made to facilitate subsequent skin closure. Therefore the lateral incisions must extend to the junction between the middle third and dorsal third of the udder to allow sufficient skin for closure under minimal tension. Following skin incision, the dissection is first directed toward the inguinal canal where the pudendal arteries and then vein are ligated. The procedure is repeated on the contralateral side. Using curved Mayo scissors, the loose fascia on the proximal aspect of both lateral laminae is incised starting cranially and extending caudally until the left and right perineal arteries and veins are located and double ligated. To minimize systemic blood loss (through retention in the

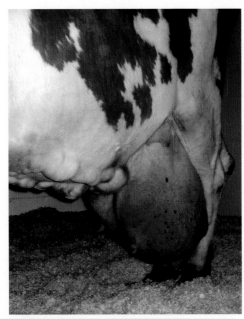

Figure 8-9

Red and White Holstein with severely "dropped" udder that had successful amputation.

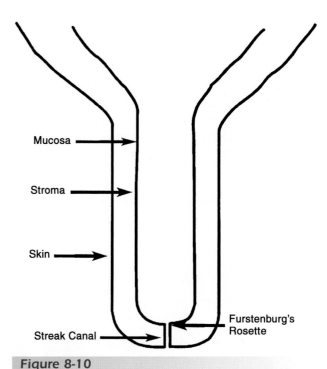

Figure 8-10

Schematic of the bovine teat to illustrate the basic anatomic terms used in this chapter.

mammary gland), the caudal superficial epigastric veins are ligated last. The lateral laminae are then sharply transected and dissection extended on the dorsal aspect of the mammary gland to complete the excision.

Before closure, one should attempt to control the extent of postoperative seromas by placing two, 2.5-cm Penrose drains in the space between the ventral abdominal fascia and the subcutaneous tissues on either side of the midline along the ventral abdomen. Stab incisions are used to create portals for the drains to exit on either side of the incision and secured to the skin using a single interrupted suture to avoid accidental drain removal.

Closure is performed in three layers. The subcutaneous tissue is closed in two layers using no. 2 absorbable suture material (such as chromic catgut or polyglactin 910) in a simple continuous pattern. Every 2 or 3 cm, the subcutaneous sutures should penetrate the abdominal fascia to reduce dead space. The skin is closed in a forward interlocking pattern with a nonabsorbable material (such as polyamide), and a stent is sutured over the incision to help diminish the tension on the incision.

TEAT DISEASE

The tissue layers in the teats of dairy cattle include skin, inner fibrous, stroma, and mucosa. Stroma is a vascular and muscular layer containing veins that drain to the large subcutaneous venous plexus at the juncture of teat and udder. The inner fibrous layer is a thin membrane that is interposed between the mucosa and the stroma (Figure 8-10).

The papillary duct (teat canal) or streak canal is the exit for milk from the teat sinus or cistern and is surrounded by the teat sphincter muscle. The papillary duct and sphincter muscle represent a significant component of the defense mechanism against mastitis, and they are the most frequently injured portions of the teat.

The streak canal in the healthy state acts both as a valvular obstruction to milk flow and as a unique deterrent to ascending infection of the gland. The canal is lined with keratin as a result of a specialized stratified squamous epithelium arranged longitudinally. Keratin in the papillary duct binds bacteria and then desquamates to form a plug with antimicrobial activities that may deter bacterial entrance.

Congenital Anomalies

Etiology and Signs

Supernumerary teats are the most common congenital abnormality, which is likely heritable in dairy cattle. There has been little genetic selection away from this trait in heifers simply because it is not reported back to artificial insemination stud services and because the problem is so easily treated. Supernumerary teats are extremely common in certain lines of cattle—especially Guernseys. Usually one to four extra teats is observed, although more can occur. Generally the supernumerary teats are placed caudal to the rear quarter teats or between the rear and forequarter teats. These "extra" teats require treatment, lest functional glands evolve that would likely become infected because they cannot be milked effectively. Such infections provide a chronic source of infection for other quarters in the herd.

Supernumerary teats that are joined to one of the four major teats have been called webbed or "Siamese" teats. These may appear as distinct teats or only as small raised areas on the wall of one of the major teats (Figure 8-11, A to D). Although these teats frequently have a separate gland of their own, they may communicate with the teat or gland cistern of the major teat (Figure 8-12). In either case, these joined teats require special treatment and careful differentiation from simple supernumerary teats, lest future production of the gland be compromised.

Keratinized corns or keratomas on the teats of heifers have been recognized. These structures are tightly adherent to the teat end, grow progressively, and their physical weight stretches and elongates the affected teat (Figure 8-13).

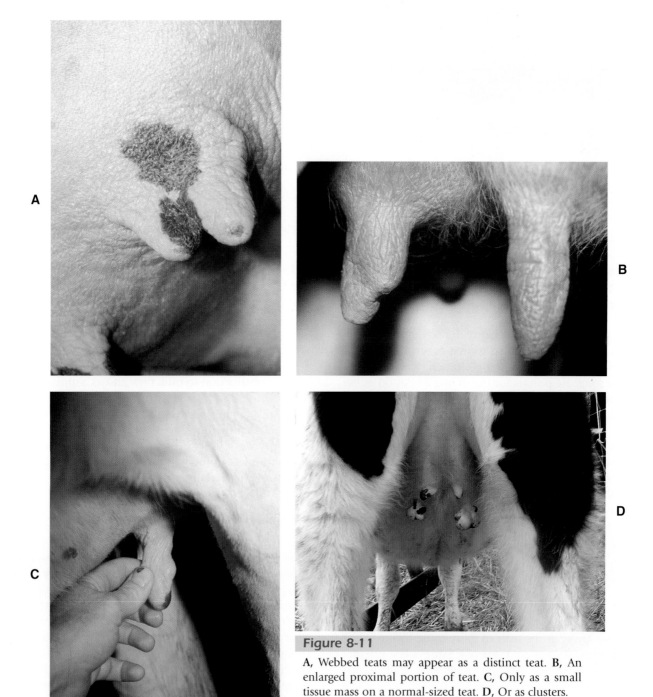

Figure 8-11

A, Webbed teats may appear as a distinct teat. B, An enlarged proximal portion of teat. C, Only as a small tissue mass on a normal-sized teat. D, Or as clusters.

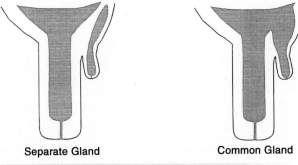

Separate Gland   Common Gland

Figure 8-12

Co-joined supernumerary teats may communicate with a separate gland or the gland of the major teat.

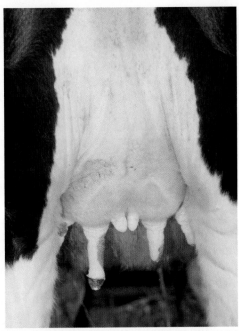

Figure 8-13

Keratin corn on the left hind teat of a heifer.

Juvenile tumors of the skin adjacent to the teats of two heifers have been described and were found to be a fibroma and a fibrosarcoma.

Diagnosis

Diagnosis of supernumerary teats, Siamese teats, and keratinized corns simply requires inspection. Supernumerary teats cojoined to a major teat require more careful consideration and treatment, but if identified in calfhood, the treatment is the same. Tumors associated with the teat require biopsy to allow definitive diagnosis.

Treatment

Heifer calves should be examined for the presence of supernumerary teats at a routine time during the first 8 months of life. Most veterinarians perform this examination when vaccinating 4- to 8-month-old calves for brucellosis. Following restraint of the heifer, the supernumerary teats are grasped and cut off with scissors at the point where the skin of the teat meets the skin of the udder. A suitable antiseptic is applied to the wound following removal, but sutures generally are not used except when a cosmetic appearance is required immediately. Care must be exercised when removing supernumerary teats, lest a true teat be removed accidentally.

If confusion exists as to which teats are the true ones, the heifer should be allowed to grow for a few months and then be rechecked. It is important, however, to force owners to check for supernumerary teats when the heifers are young so that surgical removal is easier for both the animal and the veterinarian. Removing supernumerary teats on a 2-year-old heifer that is already springing can be difficult and unpleasant for all involved parties.

Supernumerary teats cojoined to a major teat (webbed teats) need to be repaired surgically rather than just snipped off. The repair should be performed when the teat is large enough to be manipulated easily and then sutured. Many surgeons prefer to operate on animals at approximately 8 months of age. Aseptic technique is essential because infection of the future mammary gland is a major risk. Following an 8- to 12-hour fast, the heifer is sedated with xylazine (4 to 5 mg/kg/100 lb body weight, IV), tied in dorsal recumbency, and the hair is clipped from the udder near the extra teat. Following routine preparation, a fenestrated drape is placed, and the supernumerary teat is excised by scalpel or scissors. This excision is nearly flush with the skin of the main teat but should leave enough skin to close the wound (Figure 8-14). After excision, the mucosa of the rudimentary teat should be closed with fine synthetic absorbable suture (e.g., Monocryl, Ethicon, Johnson & Johnson, Somerville, NJ), such as 3-0 or 4-0. The skin and stroma are sutured as a single layer using interrupted vertical mattress sutures or alternatively closed with individual layers. Many suture materials are suitable for stroma and skin closure, but absorbable sutures such as 3-0 or 4-0 Vicryl (Ethicon, Johnson & Johnson, Somerville, NJ) or Monocryl are

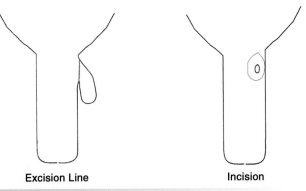

Excision Line   Incision

Figure 8-14

Schematic illustration of excision line for co-joined supernumerary teat (*left*) and outline of a resultant incision (*right*). The inner circle in the incision represents mucosa, and the outer circle indicates skin.

popular because they do not require subsequent removal and associated restraint. Antibiotics such as IM penicillin (22,000 IU/kg) should be administered preoperatively and for 2 to 3 days postoperatively.

When surgery is done at this early age, it does not matter whether the ancillary teat has a separate gland. If, however, surgery is delayed until after the first lactation, surgical repairs may become considerably more complicated because of the need to connect separate gland cisterns to the major teat.

Keratin corns or keratomas may be surgically dissected from the teat ends, but simpler means of therapy exist. A light teat bandage held on the teat by adhesive tape may be used to moisten the keratinized material, and the keratinized material may be gently separated from the teat itself after several days of soaking. Saline, lanolin and aloe mixtures, and ichthammol ointment have all been used successfully to soften keratin corns and allow subsequent removal.

Successful removal of tumors associated with the teat has been described. Future production was not destroyed in these animals; nonetheless a guarded prognosis is justified.

Teat-End Injuries

Etiology

Teat ends are the most common site of mammary injury in dairy cattle and are the most common reason for owners to seek veterinary consultation regarding the teats of dairy cattle. Teat-end injuries may affect the sphincter muscle, the streak canal, or both. Injuries to the teat end are caused by the digit or medial dewclaw of the ipsilateral limb of the affected cow or by injury from neighboring cows stepping on the teat. Teat-end injuries are more common in cows with pendulous udders or in those that have lost support laminae. Acute injuries cause inflammation, hemorrhage, and edema within the distal teat stroma and sphincter muscle. Subsequent soft tissue swelling in the teat end mechanically interferes with proper milk release from the streak canal. In addition, the streak canal epithelium and keratin may be disrupted, crushed, lacerated, partially inverted into the teat cistern, or partially inverted from the teat end. Occasional distal membranous obstruction occurs as a result of teat injuries followed by local fibrosis (Figure 8-15). Obvious laceration of the distal teat skin may be present but frequently is not. When present, lacerations tend to be at the teat end. Degloving injuries to the teat end are also occasionally encountered subsequent to claw or limb trauma when the teat becomes trapped against solid flooring. Repeated or chronic teat-end injury leads to fibrosis of the affected tissues, granulation tissue at the site of any mucosal or streak canal injury, and continued problems with milkout. Subclinical teat-end injury has been associated with defective milking machine

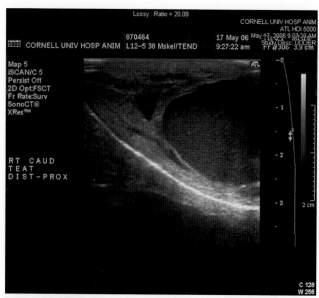

Figure 8-15

Sonogram of the distal aspect of the teat made with a linear 12.5-MHz probe (distal to the left). A focal occlusion at the distal aspect of the teat cistern is identified as a 3-mm band of tissue. The rosette of Furstenberg and the streak canal (thin hyperechoic line at the tip of the teat) are normal. *(Courtesy Dr. Amy Yeager, Cornell University.)*

functions such as increased vacuum pressures or overmilking.

In addition to traumatic injuries, teat-end ulceration is a common problem that may involve individual cows or be endemic in certain herds. Crater-like ulcers filled with dried exudate and scabs make milkout very difficult and predispose to mastitis. Many causes, including irritation from teat dips, excessive vacuum pressure, and mechanical abrasions have been suggested, but the exact cause of the lesion often is difficult to ascertain.

Signs

Painful soft tissue swelling of the distal teat is the cardinal sign of acute teat-end injury. The skin may be hyperemic or bruised (Figure 8-16). The cow resents any handling or manipulation of the teat end and objects to being milked. A combination of mechanical interference with milkout and pain-induced reluctance to let down milk predisposes to incomplete milkout from affected quarters. Mastitis is the feared and frequent sequela to incomplete milkout in cows with teat-end injuries. The cow is further predisposed to mastitis if the physical defense mechanism of the streak canal is compromised.

Chronic teat-end injury often includes a history of acute injury followed by continued difficulty in milking. Palpation of the teat end allows detection of fibrosis in the sphincter muscle or granulation tissue dorsal to the streak canal and sphincter muscle at the ventral-most portion of the teat cistern. Pain is not as apparent with chronic teat-end injuries as in acute cases.

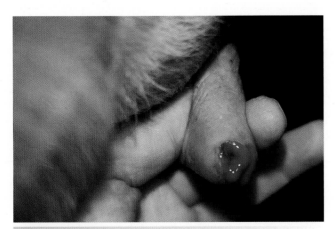

Figure 8-16

Acute teat-end injury showing diffuse swelling and a blood clot extruding from the streak canal.

Treatment

Treatment of acute teat-end injuries should address both the injury and any management factors that might lead to further injury, such as overcrowding, lack of bedding, and milking machine problems.

Treatment considerations must be acceptable and logical to the milkers because the milkers are responsible for any ongoing treatment. Milkers also are subject to the end results of the cow's pain caused by manipulation of the acutely injured teat. Unless one has milked cows, it may not be apparent exactly how difficult it is to remain patient when being kicked at by cattle that object to having injured teats handled. Client compliance necessitates empathy for the patient, as well as the people responsible for milking the cow. Advice regarding patient restraint, minimizing pain, and preventing mastitis must be included in any treatment regimen.

The best treatments for acute teat-end injury include symptomatic antiinflammatory therapy and reducing further trauma to the teat end. Each injury must be assessed individually. If milkout is simply reduced but not prevented, milkers sometimes use dilators of various types between milkings to stretch the sphincter muscles, thus allowing machine milkout. If milkout is difficult, it is best to avoid further machine milking and to utilize a teat cannula to effect milking twice daily when the other quarters are machine milked. If cannulas are used, the milker must exert extreme care to avoid exogenous inoculation of the teat cistern with microbes. Therefore the teat end must be cleaned gently, and alcohol must be applied before introducing the sterile cannula. Usually a disposable 1-in plastic cannula is used for this purpose. After complete milkout, the teat end is dipped as usual and a repeat dip performed in 10 minutes. Alternatively, some practitioners recommend indwelling plastic cannulas that may be capped between milkings. Several types are available commercially. In addition to facilitating milkout, these indwelling cannulas act as dilators

that may reduce the possibility of streak canal adhesions or fibrosis. Teat dilators impregnated with dyes are not favored because they seem to induce chemical damage to the steak canal. However, many owners use such dilators anyway (Figure 8-17). Wax and silicone teat inserts that may retain patency with less iatrogenic mastitis are commercially available. The wax insert is recommended for initial use, but it disintegrates after several days. Insertion of silicone rubber inserts after the wax has disintegrated is recommended. The inserts have comparable efficacy and antibacterial properties. Both inserts are readily available in the United States. Alternatively, milk can be drained from the gland, intramammary antibiotics infused, a wax teat insert (Figure 8-18) placed in the teat, followed by icing and bandaging the teat with no further milkout for 2 to 3 days.

Nursing care is helpful but unfortunately is often not available on modern dairy farms. Soaking the injured teat with concentrated Epsom salts in a cup of warm

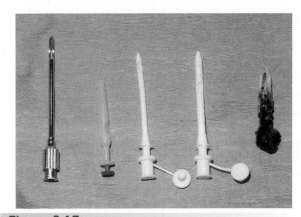

Figure 8-17

Teat cannulas and dilators.

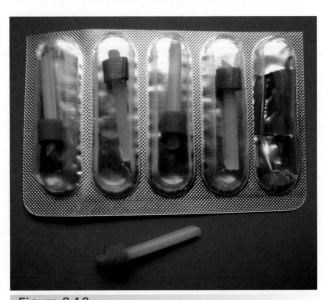

Figure 8-18

NIT natural teat inserts.

water for 5 minutes twice daily helps reduce edema and inflammation. It is most important to avoid further trauma to the teat end and to minimize the risks for developing mastitis. Therefore avoidance of machine milking is indicated for at least several days whenever possible.

Problems that have been associated with teat-end lesions include crusts, necrosis, ulceration (Figure 8-19), and mastitis. All result in continued pain to the patient and mechanical interference with milkout as a result of scab or exudate buildup. Gentle soaking in warm dilute Betadine solution (Purdue Pharma, Cranbury, NJ) followed by removal of crusts or exudate aids complete milkout. Teat injury predisposes the cow to mastitis, particularly infections with gram-positive organisms.

Gradual return to normal milking is hoped for in 3 to 7 days following acute teat-end injury. Subacute or chronic injuries that continue to interfere with milkout may necessitate surgical intervention. Surgery should be avoided in acute teat-end injury because any sharp injury to an already damaged sphincter muscle and streak canal only serves to worsen the acute inflammation and hemorrhage, as well as the ensuing fibrosis. If milk flow is still obstructed after edema has resolved, examination should determine site of injury, fibrosis, or granulation tissue obstruction. Granulation tissue at the most dorsal aspect of the streak canal or most ventral part of the teat cistern is common. Fibrosis of the sphincter musculature also is very common. Instrument manipulation or sharp surgery on the teat end is then indicated. Wax inserts should be used to decrease stricture.

Before surgical intervention, the quarter should be full of milk. Experienced owners will not milk out the affected quarter before the veterinary visit, but if they have forgotten and done so, the cow should be given 20 units of oxytocin IV to fill the quarters. Without adequate milk

in the quarter, it is impossible to assess how much the obstruction has been relieved.

For surgical correction of obstructed teat ends, the teat should be washed, cleaned, and disinfected with alcohol (Box 8-1). The cow should be restrained and/or sedated before surgery. A teat bistoury or knife, preferably one with a small single cutting edge and blunt tip, should be used. The aim of this procedure is to relieve the stricture in the streak canal through two to four angled cuts made at 90-degree intervals (Figure 8-20, A and B). The cuts are made into the dorsal sphincter muscle but tapered so as *not* to cut the distal sphincter or teat end. We prefer the use of a Larsen teat blade because it allows a better control of the dept of the cut and facilitates the creation of a tapered incision. These radial incisions release the sphincter and frequently are the only treatments required. Some veterinarians use wax inserts to reduce hemorrhage following this procedure and to diminish subsequent inflammation and swelling that may impede milkout.

A Moore's teat dilator also has been used for sphincter muscle fibrosis. This instrument is inserted into

Box 8-1	Preparation for Teat Surgery or Treatment

Infusion of quarter or placement of cannula
Wash and completely clean teat and base of udder with mild soap or disinfectant
Dry
Alcohol swab teat end carefully
Treat or cannulate with sterile devices
Alcohol swab teat end carefully
Apply teat dip used by owner

Surgical manipulation through the teat canal
Restrain and/or sedate cow
Wash and completely clean teat and base of udder with soap or disinfectant
Dry or alcohol swab until dry
Ring block base of teat if prolonged manipulation anticipated
Alcohol swab teat end carefully
Perform procedure with sterile or cold-sterilized/disinfected instruments
Alcohol swab and teat dip (unless the owner is to strip quarter frequently)

Surgical thelotomy or repair of full-thickness lacerations and fistulae
Decide on position (standing, tilt table, dorsal recumbency), means of restraint, and required sedation
Aseptic technique including clipping hair on udder, surgical preparation, ring block of base of teat, and fenestrated drapes are indicated
Sterile instruments
Preoperative and postoperative antibiotics

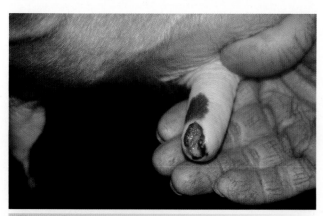

Figure 8-19

Chronic teat-end injury with an ulcerative bed of granulation tissue ringed by crusted edges. This type of wound repeatedly produces a crusty scab that interferes with effective milkout and is an extremely common sequela to acute teat-end injuries.

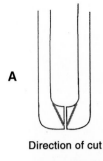

A

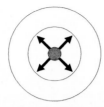

Direction of cut

Top view of sphincter from inside of teat showing 4 quadrant cuts

B

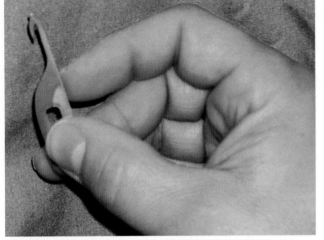

Figure 8-20

A, Schematic illustration of teat knife incisions required to relieve sphincter muscle fibrosis. **B,** Preferred teat bistoury for radial cut for treatment of streak canal fibrosis. Note cutting edge is in the acute angle and thus allows control of the depth of the incision. In addition, if the operator flexes his/her wrist while pulling distally, only the proximal half of the streak canal will be incised.

the teat following routine preparation and advanced slowly to stretch the sphincter muscle without sharp surgery.

Masses of granulation tissue in the streak canal can act as an obstruction between the canal and teat cistern. They are generally a result of injury to the rosette of Furstenberg. These masses or growths are generally removed with the aid of a Hug's teat tumor extractor. This instrument can be opened to allow excessive tissue to be grasped and cut off by the sharp edge of the extractor. It is a commonly used teat instrument, but care should be taken not to excise excessive surrounding healthy mucosa when removing granulation or fibrous tissue. The collateral mucosal damage associated with the blind use of the teat tumor extractor frequently results in recurrence of the stenosis. To precisely remove diseased tissue, and leave adjacent healthy tissue undisturbed, thelotomy with sharp incision is indicated (see teat-cistern obstructions). Minimally invasive fiberoptic theiloscopy in combination with electrosurgery is preferable, but the equipment is expensive, although it leads to improved

long-term outcomes. The equipment is available from the Karl Storz Company (Charlton, MA).

Occasional instances of prolapsed streak canal mucosa are observed following crushing teat-end injuries. This tissue should be cut off flush with the teat end and then gently probed with a teat cannula to replace any everted tissue back into position in the streak canal.

Most veterinarians initially are too cautious and conservative when treating teat-end fibrosis. Experience is necessary to know "how much to cut" to allow not only short-term results but also to avoid subsequent reoperation because of recurrence of the problem. If in doubt, it is best to be conservative because the procedure always can be repeated. Most experienced veterinarians not only want to see a reduced resistance to hand milkout but also a slight dripping of milk immediately postoperatively. This dripping usually subsides as sphincter tone improves following resolution of dilatation associated with surgical instrumentation.

Repeated self-induced teat-end trauma to a specific teat dictates evaluation of the cause. Foot-induced trauma may be detected by smearing dye on the medial dewclaw and observing the teats for dye transmission onto the teat. In this case, removal of the medial dewclaw may help prevent injury in the future. Cows with pendulous udders that suffer repeated teat-end injuries usually have to be culled.

Teat-end necrosis or ulceration is difficult to manage because buildup of scab material in the crater-like ulcer recurrently interferes with milking. Gentle soaking and mechanical removal of the scabs are necessary for milkout. A mild teat dip with glycerin or lanolin for softening is indicated in these patients. Some require surgical manipulation if continued irritation or overmilking damages the sphincter muscle or dorsal streak canal. When teat-end necrosis is observed in more than one cow in a herd, the milking machinery and procedures should be examined carefully to rule out excessive vacuum pressure and physical or chemical irritants in teat dip or bedding (Figure 8-21).

Acquired Teat-Cistern Obstructions

Etiology

Teat-cistern lesions resulting in obstructed milk flow may be focal or diffuse. Most teat-cistern obstructions result from proliferative granulation tissue, mucosal injury, or fibrosis—all secondary to previous teat trauma. Occasional cases have no history of previous acute injury. Focal and diffuse lesions in the cistern cause an increasing degree of flow restriction that interferes with effective milk delivery to the streak canal during machine milking. With ultrasound examination, obstruction at the junction of the gland and teat cistern can be visualized (Figures 8-22 and 8-23). This type of obstruction leads to slow refill of the teat cistern such that they

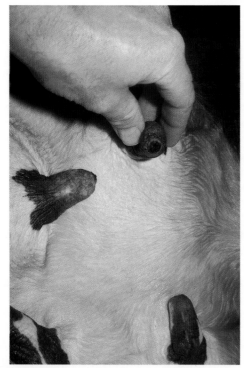

Figure 8-21

Chronic proliferative teat-end lesions caused by excessive vacuum pressure or overmilking. Such lesions are hyperkeratotic or proliferative, circular, and tend to be present in more than one quarter in each affected cow. The problem usually appears in multiple cows within the herd.

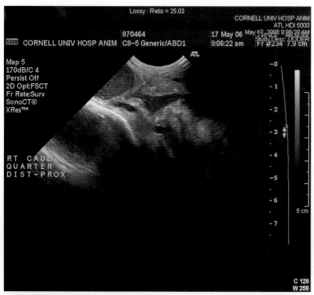

Figure 8-22

Sonogram of the junction of the teat and gland cistern made with a convex 8.5-MHz probe (distal is to the left). At this location, the lumen abruptly narrows from 2 cm to 3 mm because the wall of the teat is thick and irregular. Also, a 3-mm thick band of tissue occludes the lumen of the teat cistern. (*Courtesy Dr. Amy Yeager, Cornell University.*)

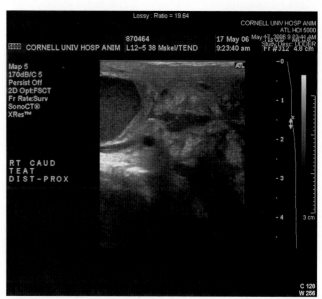

Figure 8-23

Sonogram of the junction of the teat and gland cistern made with a linear 12.5-MHz probe (distal is to the left). The high-resolution image demonstrated the 7-mm-thick, irregular, hyperechoic scar tissue in the wall of the very narrow region of the sinus. Also, a 3-mm-thick band of tissue occludes the teat cistern. (*Courtesy Dr. Amy Yeager, Cornell University.*)

cannot be milked by machine. However, they can be milked by teat cannula or siphon. In addition to fixed lesions, floating objects known as "milk stones" or "floaters" may cause problems in milkout because they are pulled into the teat and mechanically interfere with milking. These floaters may be completely free or may be attached to the mucosa by a pedunculated stalk. Mucosal detachments also are encountered secondary to external teat trauma. The detached mucosa folds onto the opposite teat wall, causing a valve effect as milking progresses. Submucosal hemorrhage or edema from previous trauma is thought to cause detached mucosa; the problem may not be apparent until resolution of the submucosal fluid allows the detached mucosa to become mobile within the cistern.

"Pencil" obstructions that fill part or the entire teat cistern usually are caused by mural and mucosal trauma that creates adhesions obliterating part or the entire teat cistern. The lesions may be mucosal adhesions or, more often, granulation tissue bridging areas of mucosal tissue that adheres itself to the opposite wall of the lumen. Pencil obstructions may follow diffuse teat injury that causes the entire teat to be swollen with severe stromal edema and hemorrhage. Palpation of pencil obstructions reveals a longitudinal (vertical) firm mass that appears to obstruct the teat cistern. Most severe lesions involve fibrosis of the gland cistern (Figure 8-24, *A* and *B*).

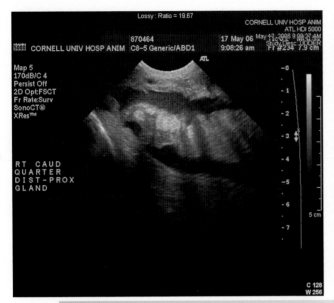 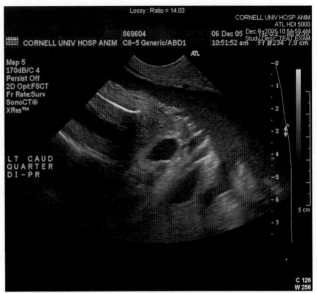

Figure 8-24

A, Sonogram of the distal aspect of the gland cistern made with a convex 9.5-MHz probe (distal is to the left). The gland cistern is diffusely narrow (1 cm in diameter) because the wall is thick as a result of soft tissue swelling (fibrous tissue or edema). The gland cistern is the hypoechoic lumen located in the near field; the anechoic lumen in the far field is a normal vein. **B,** For comparison, sonogram of the distal aspect of a normal gland cistern made with a convex 9.5-MHz probe (distal is to the left). Teat (0.7-cm diameter) and gland (2.5 cm in diameter) cisterns are normal. *(Courtesy Dr. Amy Yeager, Cornell University.)*

Signs

Depending on the individual lesion, teat-cistern obstructions cause partial, intermittent, or complete interference with milk flow during hand and machine milking. Focal lesions tend to cause partial or intermittent milk flow disturbance because of the valve effect they create. Similarly floaters may lead to intermittent cessation of milk flow. If the floater is completely free, it will only cause obstruction after sufficient milkout allows the floater to enter the teat cistern from the gland cistern. Floaters occur primarily in recently fresh cows from the release of sterile fibrous or granulomatous masses and concretions that had resided in mammary ductules. However, floaters or milk stones occasionally may develop in cows further advanced into lactation. Palpation of the teat and hand milking to determine the degree of obstruction are necessary for diagnosis. These conditions usually are not painful to the patient unless they have been caused by recent trauma.

Focal detachment of mucosa after injury leads to intermittent or gradual obstruction as milking progresses. Palpation of the detached mucosa can be appreciated best during hand milking when the mucosa is felt to "slip" between the fingers and thumb as milk is expressed from the teat. This sensation is similar to that felt while slipping fetal membranes for pregnancy diagnosis.

Diffuse teat swelling from recent injury may collapse the available teat cistern such that the teat feels turgid, swollen, and is painful to the cow (Figure 8-25). No

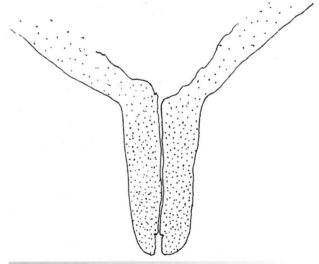

Figure 8-25

Schematic illustration of acute, diffuse teat swelling. Notice that the stroma is diffusely infiltrated, and sharp instrument manipulation of the teat lumen therefore is contraindicated.

distinct mass can be felt in the teat cistern, and passage of a 2- to 3-in stainless steel teat cannula allows milk to be obtained from the gland cistern.

Pencil obstructions are palpated as firm longitudinal masses in the teat cistern. They may fill part or the entire teat cistern (Figure 8-26). Sometimes the lesion extends into the gland cistern. Milk flow is severely altered, and

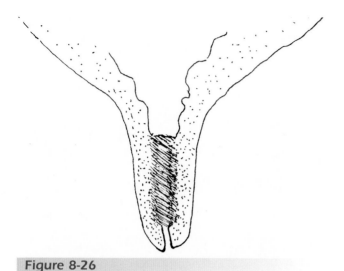

Figure 8-26

Schematic illustration of pencil obstruction.

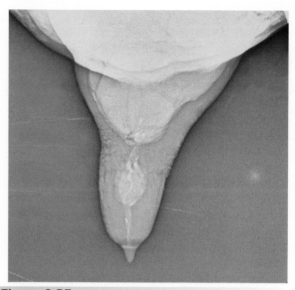

Figure 8-27

Positive contrast study showing a distinct obstructive lesion in the teat canal. (*Photo courtesy Dr. Normand Ducharme.*)

passage of a teat cannula may be met with resistance as the cannula grates against granulation or fibrous tissue. Passage of the teat cannula is similar to passing an insemination pipette through a cervix. Pencil obstructions may occur after known trauma, overly aggressive surgical approaches to focal obstruction, or following injury or infection during the dry period.

Diagnosis

In the past, diagnosis was reached by history, palpation, and probing with teat cannulas. Current methods for evaluating teat obstructions include ultrasound, radiographs, xeroradiographs, and contrast radiographic studies. Radiographic contrast studies can be obtained by injecting 10 ml of an iodine-based radiopaque material into the teat and gland cistern and then radiographing the teat and ventral gland cistern (Figure 8-27). In our experience, ultrasound examination is the most practical diagnostic aid for evaluation of patency of the teats and gland cistern (see video clips 15 and 16). It is best performed before milking because the absence of milk in the teat cistern will cause an apposition of the mucosal lining, giving the false appearance of stenosis (see video clips 17 to 19). Teat and gland cistern obstruction can be readily identified because their lumen is compromised. One has to be careful not to cause deformation of the teat and gland cistern with the probe, and therefore the teat should be examined with minimal pressure. A complete examination is done by transverse and longitudinal imaging.

Treatment

Each cow with teat-cistern obstruction must be evaluated individually for treatment options. Conservative therapies such as drying the quarter off or continued milking with a teat cannula are possibilities for any cisternal obstruction that prevents machine milking. However, the loss of production associated with drying off these

quarters and the likelihood that the obstruction will still be present in the next lactation may not make drying off an attractive option to the owner. Continued milking with a cannula may be an alternative to maintain productivity and allow further time for healing in acute or subacute cisternal obstructions. The negative side of continued cannula use is the risk of mastitis. Cows with focal or diffuse cisternal obstructions that are near the end of lactation should be dried off to rest the injured area and then examined after 4 weeks to evaluate whether the lesion is better, worse, or unchanged.

Treatment for focal cisternal obstruction may be provided by either open or closed teat surgery. If closed surgery is chosen, the veterinarian must be careful that instrument manipulations do not worsen the condition through excessive damage to the teat mucosa. Overly aggressive instrumentation with teat knives or Hug's tumor extractors can destroy healthy mucosa and results in more granulation tissue, further fibrosis, and membranous adhesions. Well-demarcated fibrous cisternal obstructions are the best candidates for closed surgical removal using a tumor extractor or bistoury. Acute or subacute focal cisternal obstructions should not be approached in a closed teat. Open surgery (thelotomy) has the following major advantages: it allows a view of the lesion; more exacting dissection of the lesion is possible; and mucosal defects can be closed or oversewn with healthy mucosa. Open thelotomy is performed as follows. The cow is sedated and placed in dorsal (preferable) or lateral recumbency. Local anesthetic is applied at the base of the teat (ring block). After aseptic preparation of the teat, a metal cannula is inserted through the streak canal into the teat cistern. Using a no. 15 or 10 Parker-Kerr blade, a skin incision is made opposite the lesion (in show cows, the incision is placed medially). The incision is started proximally on the teat cistern but distal to the base of the teat because one wants to avoid the annular venous plexus. The incision then is extended distally but stops proximal to the streak canal. It is critical that the incision does not extend into the streak canal or proximally into the annular venous plexus at the base of the teat. The incision is extended into the teat cistern, and the obstruction is addressed: the detached mucosa is reattached by suturing to the adjacent mucosa; the granulation tissue is removed and the adjacent mucosa sutured to cover the defect; or the granulation tissue is removed and an implant placed to prevent recurrence of granulation tissue. Closure is obtained by reapposing the mucosa of the teat cistern using a simple continuous pattern (penetrating the mucosa) using 4-0 absorbable monofilament suture. If only a larger-size suture is available, the submucosa is reapposed using a continuous Cushing pattern (it is important with a suture larger than 4-0 that the mucosa is not penetrated). The stromal tissue is reapposed using a 0-0 absorbable suture, again using a simple continuous pattern. The skin is closed with a monofilament suture using a simple interrupted pattern.

With thelotomy as described above, although the risk is small, there is a potential for teat fistula formation if wound repair fails. In addition, lack of confidence and experience in open-teat surgery may discourage the practitioner. Both open and closed surgery techniques also predispose to infection of the quarter.

Currently open thelotomy performed by an experienced surgeon offers the best chance for correction of focal cisternal obstructions and prevention of recurrence. This is because open thelotomy permits surgical resolution of the mucosal defect after removal of focal lesions, including those that cannot be fully bridged with mucosa.

Floaters can be removed by slowly and patiently dilating the streak canal and sphincter muscle with a small pair of mosquito forceps. Usually this takes 5 to 8 minutes. Before dilating the streak canal, the quarter is hand milked until the floater enters the teat cistern and can be held there. Once the sphincter muscle stretches sufficiently to allow entrance of the mosquito or an alligator forceps, the floater may be grasped and removed through the streak canal. Many times, the floater can be "milked out" without any manipulations inside the teat cistern once the sphincter muscle has been stretched adequately. The veterinarian may open the jaws of the hemostat to stretch the streak canal while exerting firm milking pressure to the dorsal teat cistern to cause a jet of milk to eject the floater. Alternatively, if the floater is in the streak canal, it can be forced out by slowly rolling two smooth syringe cases down the teat. Regardless of the procedure, following removal, the teat should be iced for 20 minutes at least three times on the day of the

procedure and appropriate antiinflammatory therapy administered depending on the degree of suspected trauma. Following removal, the quarter should be treated prophylactically with antibiotics or watched carefully for signs of mastitis. The streak canal and sphincter return to normal function 24 to 48 hours after being dilated.

Mucosal detachments or tears that impede milkout are best treated by drying the quarter off or by open thelotomy. Closed-teat instrumentation may increase mucosal injury in the cistern or lead to granulation tissue in areas of mucosal detachment. Open surgery allows the mucosa to be repaired and "tacked down" to the underlying stroma in areas of detachment. If an open approach is used, after the teat incision is done, the tissue underneath the mucosa is debrided, and the mucosa is then brought back into its original site. Detached mucosa is then sutured to the adjacent secured mucosa using no. 4-0 monofilament absorbable suture using a simple continuous pattern.

Diffuse swelling of the teat associated with recent injury should be managed medically. Severe edema, hemorrhage, and inflammation within the stromal tissues cause the cistern to be swollen shut. There may or may not be associated mucosal injury. Surgery or instrument manipulation is contraindicated, lest the mucosa be further damaged. Epsom salt soaks and lanolin/aloe ointments to protect the teat should be used immediately. If a stainless steel teat cannula passes easily through the teat cistern to the gland cistern, it can be used to allow twice-daily milkout. If a cannula cannot be passed easily, the quarter should be dried off or consideration given to open surgery and implant placement.

Diffuse pencil obstruction of the cistern is best treated by open surgery and implantation of silicone or polyethylene tubes unless the owner elects to dry off the quarter. Closed manipulation or surgery with sharp instruments is contraindicated and will only worsen existing damage. Much has been learned about diffuse teat-cistern obstructions because open-teat surgery has been more widely used. The ability to see the gross pathology and obstruction within the cistern has been a great education and has encouraged veterinarians to devise new surgical techniques. Although prognosis for diffuse teat-cistern obstructions (pencil obstructions) remains guarded, many successes have been recorded thanks to specific surgical intervention either with or without implants. An implant technique initially reported by Donawick has been modified and used by Ducharme. This technique uses thelotomy to identify gross pathology, surgical opening of the teat sinus, and implantation of a Silastic tube into the teat sinus before surgical closure of the wound. Sterile Silastic silicone medical tubing with an inside diameter of 7 mm and an outer of 10 mm is measured during thelotomy and placed into the teat cistern. The distal end of the tube abuts against the distal end of the teat cistern, and the proximal end of the tube is fenestrated and lies

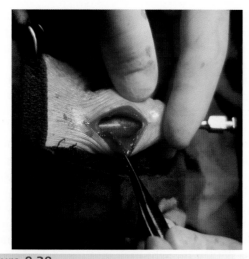

Figure 8-28

Sterile Silastic silicone tubing implant being placed in a teat having a pencil obstruction. *(Photo courtesy Dr. Normand Ducharme.)*

flush with the junction of the gland cistern (Figure 8-28). Two or three polypropylene nonabsorbable 2-0 sutures are placed parallel to the long axis of the teat to secure the tubing to the teat stroma. It is important to anchor the tubing well and yet to take care not to distort or malposition the tubing while placing anchor sutures. This is done by placing the securing sutures with a teat cannula placed through the streak canal into the tubing, serving as a rigid implant and thus maintaining proper alignment. Following standard closure of the teat and removal of the cannula, machine milking is instituted. If this is unsuccessful, the cow may temporarily require a teat cannula for milking or flushing with sterile saline to free blood clots from the implant. Occasional cows require the use of wide-bore milk liners to effect milkout because of the increased thickness or diameter of the teat.

The tubing is left in place permanently unless it loosens or breaks away from the teat cistern. Complications may include an increased incidence of mastitis, lower long-term milking success, and abnormal milking times when compared with teats requiring thelotomy without implants. However, despite the risks of complication, this technique currently is the best hope for preservation of teat function in cattle with diffuse cisternal obstructions. Before the introduction of these techniques, most diffuse cisternal obstructions resulted in permanent drying off or in a hopeless prognosis for the affected quarter. With careful case selection, 50% or more of diffuse cisternal obstructions may be helped by implants and allow completion of the lactation. Implant techniques are unlikely to help cows with combined diffuse teat-cistern obstructions and gland cistern obstruction or fibrosis. In addition, implant techniques are contraindicated if mastitis has already complicated the teat injury.

Fistulas

Etiology

Teat fistulas may be congenital or acquired secondary to full-thickness teat injuries that enter the teat cistern. Congenital teat fistulas are a smaller variant of webbed or Siamese teats and often are not detected until lactation begins (Figure 8-29). Congenital teat fistulas may communicate with the teat cistern of the major teat but usually represent outflow from a separate gland.

Acquired teat fistulas may occur following accidental full-thickness wounds, lacerations, or surgical thelotomy. Ineffectual closure or breakdown of the mucosal layer is thought to cause most fistulas in surgically repaired teat injuries.

Leakage of milk from fistulas predisposes the gland to infection. Even when the fistula represents a separate gland, infection is undesirable because the major quarter may be exposed to contagious organisms by leakage of mastitic milk from the fistula. Leakage of milk from acquired fistulas may unbalance the udder and be unsightly for show cattle. Depending on the location of the fistula on the teat, machine milking may or may not provide effective milkout.

Signs

Congenital fistulas usually are not observed in calves but become apparent in bred heifers or after freshening when milk is noticed to leak from the wall of the teat. A small raised area of skin may be present around the fistula, but this skin usually is less prominent than that observed in a webbed teat. Acquired teat fistulas have a history of teat injury or surgery penetrating into the teat cistern followed by leakage of milk from the scar or incision. Acquired teat fistulas have obvious scar tissue around the fistula and often are larger in diameter than congenital fistulas.

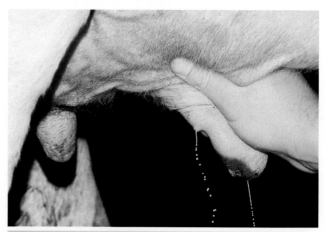

Figure 8-29

Congenital teat fistula that was not apparent until lactation started. Milking causes milk to escape from the fistula and the streak canal.

Diagnosis

Diagnosis is obvious based on clinical signs. For congenital lesions, dye injected into the fistula followed by milkout of the major teat or contrast radiography may be indicated to determine whether one or two glands are present. New methylene blue (10 to 30 ml) may be used for dye injection into the fistula. Milking of the major teat then allows differentiation of fistulas (or webbed teats) that have their own accessory gland (no dye in milk) or have a common gland with the major teat (dye in milk).

Treatment

Surgical repair of fistulas is identical to repair of webbed or Siamese teats. When webbed teats are repaired in calves, determining the presence of an accessory gland is impractical and unnecessary because complete closure will ensure eventual pressure atrophy of the accessory gland. Congenital fistulas that attach to accessory glands rather than to the gland of the major teat but are not detected until the onset of lactation may be managed in two ways:

1. Surgical repair (see Figure 8-14) as performed in calves and nonmilking gland. This approach disregards the accessory gland and relies on pressure atrophy of the accessory gland. This technique is best performed during the dry period to allow 4 full weeks of healing before the next lactation. This technique may also result in some unbalancing of the udder as the accessory gland atrophies. This may make the affected quarter somewhat slack.

2. Surgical repair through thelotomy. The common wall between the two glands is removed, and the mucosa of each gland is sutured over the defect again using 4-0 absorbable suture. This allows a communication to be established between the teat cistern of the major teat and the cistern of the fistula. This technique is only recommended if the fistula is discovered after calving and initiation of lactation. The advantages of this technique are preservation of milk production from the accessory gland (which may be almost as large as the "major" gland in some cattle) and cosmetic appearance of the quarter. The disadvantages are that greater technical skills are required to establish communication of the cisterns and to suture mucosa to preserve the communication.

The technique for repair of fistulas is well accepted and includes elliptical incision around the fistula, debridement of necrotic or fibrous tissue (in acquired fistulas), dissection of the mucosal layer, exacting closure of the mucosal defect, and routine teat closure as described under closure of thelotomy. Teat cannulas are used as guides to allow accurate incision and dissection of the fistula (Figure 8-30, A through D). Acquired fistulae with severe cicatricial fibrosis are very difficult because tissue compliance and healing are negatively influenced. This is especially problematic in fistulae that are very distal in the teat cistern near the teat sphincter. The size of the elliptical incision should be sufficient to allow removal of the fistula and associated fibrous tissue but not so large as to interfere with ease of closure. Previous dogma suggested the best time for repair of teat fistulas was during the dry period. This allowed several weeks for tissue repair without concern of endogenous milk pressure or exogenous milking pressure being felt on the incision. More recent reports seem unconcerned about this advantage. It may still be preferable to perform closure during the dry period after the udder is completely slack and the cow still has 3 to 4 weeks before freshening.

Fine 4-0 absorbable suture material (3-0 if performed during the dry period) placed in continuous fashion is preferred for mucosal closure in a continuous Cushing's pattern. Surgeon preference dictates suture material and pattern for stromal and skin closure. Generally 3-0 polyglactin 910 or other absorbable material such as Monocryl is used for stroma in interrupted fashion, and interrupted 2-0 or 3-0 nonabsorbable sutures such as polypropylene are used in the skin. Some surgeons close the stroma and skin in one layer with interrupted 2-0 or 3-0 nonabsorbable sutures in a vertical mattress fashion. Sutures are placed closer together than in other areas of skin closure in the hope of more uniform closure pressure. Although not successful in our hands, some surgeons have used tissue adhesives for fistula closure and full-thickness teat lacerations. Skin staples or Michel wound clips also have been used, mainly for skin repair. If fistulas are repaired during lactation, it may be wise to use indwelling teat cannulas that are left open to prevent endogenous pressure on the incision until healing is complete; however, the use of these should be balanced by legitimate concerns for introducing mammary pathogens. If inserted, indwelling milk tubes should be changed daily, or alternatively, silicone (SIMPL) or wax (NIT) inserts may be used. Wax inserts deteriorate after several days and can be replaced by silicone inserts. Both insert types are commercially available in the United States. The inserts have been shown to improve surgical results in lactating cattle.

Lacerations

Etiology

Trauma from the patient's hind foot or medial dewclaw, trauma by a neighboring cow, or lacerations from barbed wire or other sharp objects may induce teat lacerations. Lacerations may involve skin only, skin and stroma, or enter the teat cistern following mucosal laceration. All lacerations are problematic because of mechanical interference with teat cup placement, milkout, and pain to the patient. Associated mucosal damage, avulsion, or detachment may lead to focal or diffuse cisternal obstruction. Full-thickness lacerations are considered emergencies

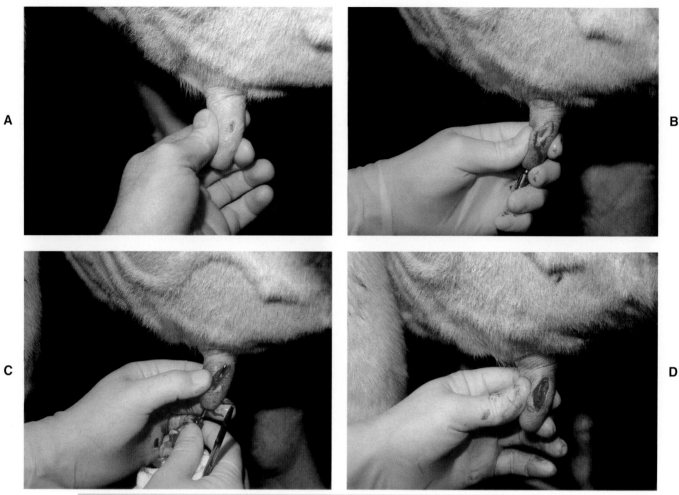

Figure 8-30

Appearance of an acquired teat fistula and subsequent surgical repair in a dry cow. **A,** Fistula surrounded by fibrotic cicatricial tissue. **B,** Elliptical skin incision. **C,** Teat cannula protruding from mucosal defect following en bloc resection of elliptical skin piece and fistula tract. **D,** Mucosal closure with continuous absorbable suture.

and require repair of all layers to avoid mastitis or fistula formation.

Degloving injuries peel away a circumferential amount of skin on the distal teat (Figure 8-31). Teat flaps are created by incomplete removal of skin on the teat. Although flaps of skin may be created by any horizontal laceration of the teat, the term teat flap usually is reserved for a lesion that extends through skin, stroma, and a portion of the sphincter muscle (Figure 8-32). The streak canal is often transected, but a portion of the streak canal and sphincter remains proximal to the laceration and suffices for sphincter tone, barring future injury.

Lacerations may be vertical, horizontal, or circumferential. Depth of laceration and duration of time since injury are important determinants when surgical repair is considered. The more acute the injury, the more likely surgery will be successful, and the less likely infection has occurred in the wound or the quarter.

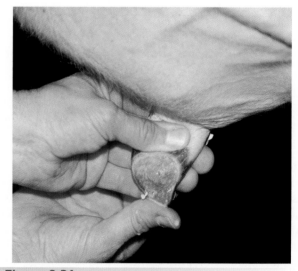

Figure 8-31

Degloving injury.

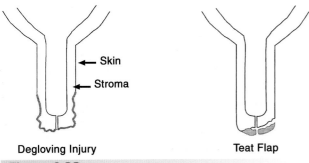

Figure 8-32

Schematic illustration of degloving and teat flap lacerations.

Signs

These are obvious in most cases of teat laceration. The injured teat is swollen, bleeding, and the cow resents any handling of it. Regardless of depth, teat lacerations may cause sufficient swelling to interfere mechanically with teat cup placement, cause pain during milking, lead to incomplete milkout, and predispose to mastitis. Full-thickness lacerations may be obvious because of milk leak but sometimes are plugged with fibrin and blood clots that mask the extent of the lesion. Teat flaps often appear to have milk leaking out of the teat cistern (Figure 8-33, *A*). In fact, the distal flap of tissue is so swollen as to suggest laceration above the sphincter. Fortunately close examination of the wound will often reveal functional streak canal and sphincter muscle above (dorsal) to the swollen flap.

Diagnosis

The clinical signs and careful cleansing of the wound to allow detailed evaluation of depth suffice for diagnosis. The cow may need to be restrained or sedated to allow cleansing and inspection of the wound.

Treatment

Owners neglect many superficial teat lacerations but tend to call veterinarians when the lacerations enter the cistern or cause mechanical interference with milking. Similar to lacerations anywhere on the body, teat lacerations are best approached as soon after injury as possible. Repair of teat lacerations involving only skin and stroma may be performed with sutures, wound clips, or cyanoacrylate products. Before repair (see Box 8-1), careful cleansing of the wound is essential, and gentle debridement with a no. 15 scalpel blade is helpful. In general, vertical lacerations heal better than horizontal or circumferential ones. Flaps that transect the streak canal should be clipped off with scissors because repair of the transected streak canal is impossible (Figure 8-33, *B* and *C*).

Full-thickness lacerations that enter the cistern are sutured similarly to the repair of teat fistulas described previously. All principles are identical to repair of a surgical wound into the cistern, but in the words of

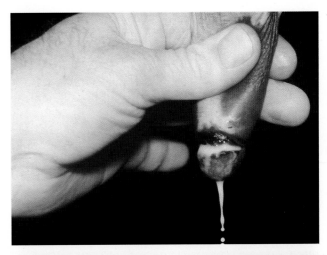

A

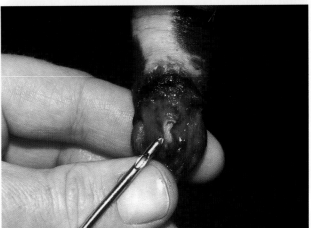

B

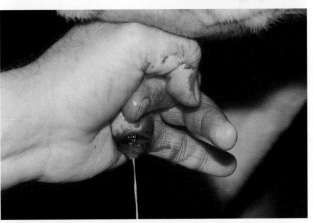

C

Figure 8-33

Teat flap laceration. **A,** Milking appears to cause milk to leak from the teat cistern. **B,** Eversion of the lacerated flap confirms the presence of remaining streak canal and sphincter muscle proximal to the flap. **C,** Removal of the flap restores teat function.

Dr. Bruce Hull, Professor of Large Animal Surgery at the Ohio State University, "the wound is made with a manure-laden foot rather than a sterile scalpel." This statement helps explain the frustration and failures that are part of full-thickness repairs. Small details make large differences. Careful debridement, aseptic technique, carefully placed sutures, and absolute closure of the mucosal layer are all important (see closure of fistula or thelotomy). Use of indwelling cannulas following surgery will help decrease internal pressure on the wound. The cannula should be left open to drain continually for several days. Systemic antibiotics are used for 3 to 5 days, and the quarter is infused with antibiotics following repair.

Blind Quarters and Membranous Obstructions

Etiology

Blind quarters appear to be laden with milk at freshening but are nonpatent. Congenital or acquired lesions that impair milk flow from the gland cistern cause blind quarters. Complete teat-cistern obstruction may be congenital, acquired before first lactation, or acquired as a diffuse cisternal obstruction or pencil obstruction during the dry period.

Degeneration of the gland cistern and connecting ducts is the most common lesion found in freshening heifers that have either small amounts or no milk from a quarter that appears to be of normal size. The condition is thought to be caused by intramammary infection or blunt trauma during calfhood. Such infections can be initiated by aggressive nursing of incompletely weaned heifers. At the time the blind quarter is identified, mastitis is usually not present in the affected quarter.

Signs

Anticipated quantities of milk cannot usually be obtained from the affected quarter. The teat usually feels flabby and meaty rather than turgid, as expected in normal milk filling. Palpation of the teat may suggest diffuse obstruction in cases in which congenital or acquired cisternal obstruction is present, and palpable fibrosis may extend dorsally toward the gland cistern.

Diagnosis

Careful probing of the teat cistern and gland cistern with a 3- or 4-in (7.5 to 10.0 cm) teat cannula allows detection of membranous or fibrous obstructions at the base of the gland cistern. This technique also allows assessment of any teat-cistern obstruction and permits milk to be obtained for examination. If the diagnosis is still in question following probing of the quarter or if surgical treatment is contemplated, ultrasound examination is recommended. If the lesion extends proximally so that no gland cistern is detected on ultrasound, treatment is not possible at this time. It is important to establish the presence and productivity of the glandular tissue before any heroic attempts at surgical fenestration, lest the latter be completely futile.

Treatment

Treatment of fibrous or membranous obstructions at the base of the gland cistern is not likely to be successful. Fenestration of single membranes at the junction of the teat and gland cisterns has been successful rarely, but most surgical interventions are unsuccessful. Treatment of teat obstruction is as described in diffuse teat-cisternal obstruction. Temporary or permanent teat implants offer the best success rates for heifers and cows that have normal glands and gland cisterns. Success rates of 50% or more are likely for this type of teat obstruction when implants are used.

Stenosis or atresia of the teat end is treated by slow dilation of the streak canal when the canal can be seen or by sharp puncture of the apparent dimple at the teat end when a streak canal cannot be identified. Usually a sharp 14-gauge needle is directed into the teat lumen at the apparent dimple that correlates with where the streak canal should have been. After needle puncture, the stenosis can be opened further with a bistoury.

Leaking Teats

Etiology and Signs

Many cows leak milk just before normal milking times because of intramammary pressure; this is considered normal or physiologic. However, constant leaking of milk and that which occurs at times other than milking or that affects show potential is considered abnormal.

Generally milk leaking is more common in previously injured teats. The injury has disturbed normal sphincter tone or integrity of the teat end by fibrosis or loss of tissue so that leaking occurs.

Diagnosis

Only the history and physical inspection of the teat are required for diagnosis. The teat may be probed to assess the streak canal diameter but seldom is this necessary.

Treatment

Injecting about a drop of Lugol's iodine solution with a tuberculin syringe at four equidistant spots in the sphincter muscles has been reported to correct leaking in approximately 50% of the cases.

Skin Lesions

Viral Causes

Bovine Papillomavirus

Etiology. Bovine papillomavirus (BPV) may induce papillomas (BPV6) or fibropapillomas (BPV1 and BPV5). The most common lesion in dairy cattle is the flat "rice-grain" fibropapilloma caused by BPV5. Frond-shaped warts on the teat or udder are usually caused by DNA types BPV1 or BPV6 and appear to have more epithelial projections. These latter types are most problematic when they occur on teat ends. Warts are contagious and spread primarily by milking machines and milkers' hands that carry the virus, which then infects the skin in areas of abrasions. There is increasing evidence that BPV DNA can be found even in normal, healthy bovine skin using more sensitive modern, molecular techniques. Viral and host-specific factors that dictate when and to what extent individual cattle develop papillomas or how and why BPV2 is involved in the carcinogenesis of bladder wall tumors are still uncertain.

Signs. Flat or rice-grain fibropapillomas generally are multiple, may involve one or several teats, and tend to spread through a herd (Figure 8-34). Fibropapillomas do not cause problems unless the teat end is involved. Florid warts that appear as classical papillomas or fibropapillomas with epithelial projections may be more clinically significant. These warts may be large enough to cause some mechanical interference with teat cup placement, and larger growths may become torn, causing pain to the cow and bleeding. Warts at the teat end sometimes interfere with effective milkout and always predispose to mastitis because of environmental contaminants. Herds with endemic instances of this type of wart can be extremely frustrating because means to stop spread are limited. Teat warts are extremely common in dairy cattle.

Diagnosis. If signs are not pathognomonic, excisional biopsy is confirmatory. Some specialized laboratories are able to identify subtypes of BPV through molecular techniques.

Treatment and Prevention. Usually no treatment is required for rice-grain (BPV5) flat lesions unless they interfere with milkout at the teat end. Snipping off frondlike BPV1 and BPV6 warts is commonly necessary, especially when the lesions are near the teat end. Whenever large numbers of cattle are affected, freezing of the warts by application of a steel rod chilled to liquid nitrogen

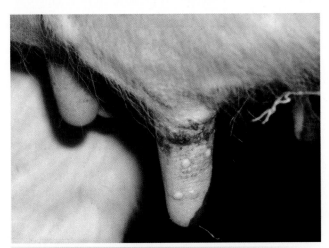

Figure 8-34

Flat "rice-grain" fibropapillomas on the skin of a teat. The abrasion on the proximal teat skin is unrelated.

temperature will be curative. Salicylic acid (10%) and fig tree latex applied every 5 days has also been shown to be effective.

Virucidal teat dips may be indicated when faced with a herd endemic problem as a result of BPV. Chlorhexidine would be one example, and Udder-Gold (American Breeders Service Division, W. R. Grace and Co., DeForest, WI) is also thought to have antiviral properties. Milking affected cows last makes good sense but is difficult in free stall barns. Minimizing trauma to the skin of teats also may decrease incidence. This is accomplished primarily by improving bedding, good milking technique, and the use of nonirritating teat dip.

Because of the current concerns about transmission of prions among cattle, autogenous vaccines cannot be recommended.

Although most warts are thought to disappear spontaneously by 3 to 6 months, this is not always the case in teat warts, which may persist for years.

The use of common utensils during udder washing and drying should be avoided; udders should be washed and dried with individual paper towels before milking.

Herpes Mammillitis

Etiology. BHV2 causes skin lesions of both the teat and udder. The disease is known as herpes mammillitis and has its highest incidence in first-calf heifers joining herds where the virus has persisted in recovered older cattle. Introduction of BHV2 into a naive herd through replacement stock may cause lesions in cows of any age. Outbreaks usually begin in autumn and continue sporadically through the winter. Incidence varies but will be higher in a naive herd than in the typical situation of a mixture of immune adult cattle but susceptible first-calf heifers. Annual incidence is possible on endemic farms. The exact means of spread is unknown because rather deep inoculation of the virus into the teat wall is required for experimental reproduction of the disease. Several authors suggest an insect mode of transmission, but this theory does not coincide with the peak seasonal (fall-winter) incidence. Until further work denies the possibility, milking equipment and personnel should be suspected in the transmission of BHV2.

Signs. Types of early lesions vary but may include vesicles, edematous plaques, and serum crusts. Initially vesicles form on the skin of the teat and udder, and the skin appears edematous. However, the vesicles quickly rupture, so they may not be observed. Within 1 to 2 days, erythema, serum oozing, crusting, and ulceration of the skin predominate (Figure 8-35). Sizes of lesions range widely from a few millimeters to several inches in diameter and vary in number in infected cattle. After several days, dense crusts and dark-colored scabs cover the ulcerations and persist for 10 to 14 days until healing begins. Sometimes the entire teat becomes necrotic (Figure 8-36). Regardless of the size of individual lesions, the affected cow resents handling of the teats and udder, does not milkout well,

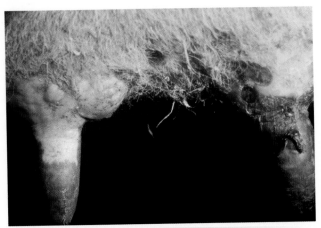

Figure 8-35

Herpes mammillitis. Vesicles are present on the skin of the teat-gland junction at left, and ulcers and crusts are present on the teat and gland to the right.

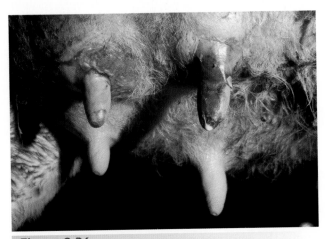

Figure 8-36

Severe herpes mammillitis. A large ulcer is present on the skin above the right hind teat, and the right front teat is sloughing.

and frequently develops mastitis. This is especially true for first-calf heifers, which tend to develop the infection shortly after freshening and have not fully acclimated to being milked. The lesions are the most severe skin lesions of the teat and udder seen in dairy cattle. Multiple skin lesions, especially in first-calf heifers and beginning in autumn, should alert the veterinarian to the diagnosis of herpes mammillitis. Up to 50% of affected heifers may subsequently be lost or sold for salvage because of mastitis. Calves that nurse affected cows may develop oral lesions. Concurrent, severe udder edema can make the clinical presentation of BHV2 mammillitis catastrophic in first-calf heifers.

Diagnosis. Clinical signs, history, and diagnostic laboratory tests help confirm diagnosis. If vesicles are observed in very early cases, fluid should be aspirated into a syringe and submitted for viral culture. Other useful tests include biopsy of early skin lesions and the edges of ulcers to look for intranuclear inclusions that help differentiate the disease from pseudocowpox (intracytoplasmic inclusions) and syncytia formation. Some laboratories may offer serology because infection does confer detectable serum antibodies. Natural infection is thought to impart resistance for at least 2 years.

Treatment. There is no effective treatment for BHV mammillitis. Supportive measures include careful milking to minimize mastitis, application of softening creams to the teat lesions, use of iodophor teat dips to inactivate the virus, and milking affected animals last. Individual paper towels should be used for washing and drying udders during milking. Live vaccines prepared from the vesicular fluid of early lesions from herdmates injected away from the udder probably may work well but are difficult to obtain and administer. There is no evidence to corroborate the use of either killed or modified live BHV1 vaccines to confer protection against herpes mammillitis. Dietary measures to control udder edema in first-calf heifers during the winter months in endemic herds make intuitive sense and can lessen lesion severity.

Pseudocowpox

Etiology. The cause of pseudocowpox lesions on the teats of cattle is a member of the genus *Parapoxvirus* within the family *Poxviridae*. The pseudocowpox virus is very similar to the papular stomatitis virus and the virus that causes contagious ecthyma (orf) in sheep and goats. Pseudocowpox causes painful papules, vesicles, and denuded circular raised areas that heal under a thick scab. This feature helps to differentiate pseudocowpox from the cowpox or vaccinia viruses, which are orthopoxviruses (and may be the same virus) and tend to cause ulcerative lesions. Cowpox or vaccinia are extremely rare and currently may not be present in the United States. When cowpox or vaccinia is present, cows usually have become infected from a milker recently vaccinated against smallpox with the vaccinia virus. By comparison, pseudocowpox is common in dairy cattle.

Signs. Lesions occur on the teats and ventral udder. Individual lesions consist of multiple white papules that erupt and then are covered by a thick scab. The lesions may be 1.0 to 2.5 cm in diameter and circular or horseshoe shaped (Figure 8-37, *A* and *B*). Once the lesion heals under the scab, it becomes proliferative and raised rather than ulcerated (Figure 8-38). Lesions usually heal within 2 to 3 weeks but may become chronic for unknown reasons. Lesions are painful in early but not in the advanced stages. Pseudocowpox virus is spread by milking equipment and milkers' hands. New infections slowly appear in the herd over several weeks, then may disappear for a time, and then recur. Some outbreaks do not seem to end for months. Milker's nodules may be reported on the hands or other skin areas

A

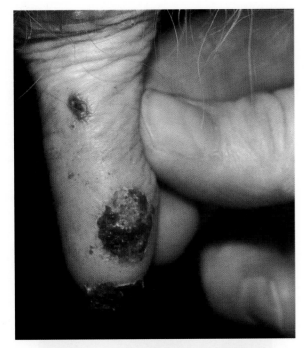

B

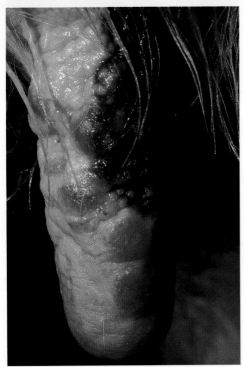

Figure 8-37

A, Pseudocowpox lesions covered by thick scabs.
B, Earlier lesion of pseudocowpox with papules.

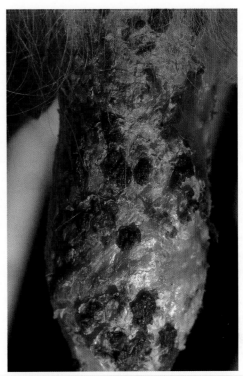

Figure 8-38

Chronic lesions of pseudocowpox.

Diagnosis. Because of the public health significance of pseudocowpox and the similarity to cowpox or vaccinia and exotic diseases, it is best to make a definitive diagnosis through viral isolation from tissue or vesicular fluid, or else electron microscopy should be performed on vesicle fluid. Standard histopathology of a biopsy specimen may show intracytoplasmic inclusions, but this will not identify the exact poxvirus. Cattle should be examined for other mucosal disease lesions if illness accompanies the teat lesions because pseudocowpox is not associated with systemic illness. There have been several outbreaks of teat lesions resembling pseudocowpox in cattle for which a definitive diagnosis could not be reached.

Treatment. There is no specific treatment for pseudocowpox. Efforts to reduce teat abrasions and to milk affected cows last may or may not be possible. It is not known which teat dips, if any, may control the virus, but those likely to be virucidal (chlorhexidine and chlorous acid-chlorine dioxide) could be tried. Milkers should be instructed to wear gloves to prevent infection and to avoid contact with scabs because the virus is extremely hardy and resistant to environmental destruction. Individual paper towels should be used for washing and drying udders.

Vesicular Stomatitis

Etiology. The rhabdovirus that causes vesicular stomatitis (VSV) has been identified in the southern United States. An Indiana and a New Jersey strain apparently are distinct virus types. Antigenic forms of both of these

of milkers working with the herd. The major complication for infected cows is mastitis, but the incidence of mastitis and severity of lesions with pseudocowpox are much less than with herpes mammillitis. Calves sucking affected cows may develop lesions indistinguishable from papular stomatitis.

strains have been isolated from clinical cases during epidemics in the southwestern United States in the late 1990s and early 2000s. Although the exact means of transmission is unknown, insect vectors are suspected because of the typical spring/summer incidence of disease. Transmission of the Indiana strain of VSV has been confirmed experimentally using the biting midge *Culicoides sonorensis.* The virus has also been isolated from several other insect species, including blackflies and sand flies. VSV is infectious for horses and swine, as well as cattle, and has caused an influenza-like disease in people. Clinical signs are very similar to those of foot-and-mouth disease; therefore regulatory agencies should be notified whenever the disease is suspected so that appropriate samples to confirm the diagnosis and rule out exotic diseases may be obtained.

Signs. In dairy cattle, the disease may either be sporadic or epizootic. Serologic studies during recent North American outbreaks suggest that the majority of infections in cattle are subclinical. Oral lesions consisting of vesicles and sloughing tissue coincide with vesicles on the teats. Occasional cows show lesions on the coronary bands and interdigital areas. Mastitis secondary to refusal to let down milk and pain induced by milking is common. Milking mechanisms may spread the disease. Fever may be present but is transient and can be overlooked. Salivation, anorexia, and lip smacking are observed.

Diagnosis. When signs consistent with VSV are present in cattle, state and federal regulatory agencies should be notified to assist in appropriate sample submission and quarantine procedures. Appropriate samples to submit include the epithelium of surface vesicles, vesicular fluid, swabs of lesions, and serum. Virus isolation, antigen-capture enzyme-linked immunosorbent assay, and polymerase chain reaction tests for viral RNA are the tests that confirm the diagnosis. Exclusion of other exotic vesicular diseases is important but typically performed under the guidance of the administering regulatory officials.

Treatment. Treatment is supportive and usually will be dictated by the appropriate regulatory officers. People working with the animals or diagnostic material should be warned concerning the zoonotic potential of the disease.

Other Viral Infections. Although rare or not present in the United States, the viruses of foot-and-mouth disease and rinderpest may cause herd epidemics of teat lesions. If there is reasonable doubt about the diagnosis, consultation with regulatory veterinary services should be considered.

BVDV occasionally causes teat lesions that are characterized by hyperkeratosis, fissuring, and erosive dermatitis.

Some herds have endemic or even epidemic disease affecting the teats, udder, and/or legs for which no etiology can be proven (Figure 8-39).

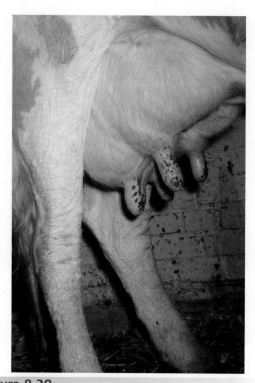

Figure 8-39

Teat lesions and dermatitis of the legs in an adult cow. Etiology was unproven.

MCF can cause vasculitis in any tissue, and some cattle with MCF have multiple raised papules on the skin of the udder but seldom on the teats.

Bacterial Causes

Staphylococci (Udder Impetigo). Multiple small pustules and papules on the udder sometimes involve the dorsal aspect of the teat or the entire teat in herds with udder impetigo. This disease has been discussed under causes of udder dermatitis. Diagnosis is confirmed by culture of the organism and ruling out other causes. Chlorhexidine and Udder-Gold may be helpful dips in these herds, and udders may need to be clipped and cleaned gently with antiseptics. Filthy environments or bedding should be identified and corrected.

Chemical and Physical Causes

Etiology. Irritating dips or udder washes may produce teat dermatitis during cold weather and low relative humidity. Teat dips that lack glycerin or emollients may contribute to the problem. Teat dips that have been frozen and then thawed may separate into dermatopathic components. Chemicals such as fly sprays, lime or limestone in bedding, and sanitizers for milking machines are other potential chemical teat irritants.

Causes of physical teat injuries include sunburn, frostbite, direct trauma, periparturient edema, and insect bites. Sunburn and photosensitivity may be severe in lightly pigmented cattle and in cows with udder edema or pendulous udders. Similarly frostbite tends to be more likely in cattle with severe periparturient edema, especially first-calf heifers. Compromised circulation of blood as a result of severe edema predisposes to frostbite of the teats when temperatures reach 0.0° F (−17.78° C) or lower. Wind chill also may contribute to frostbite. Obviously this problem is usually limited to free stall cows or cows housed outdoors. Trauma has been discussed (teat obstructions). Photosensitization is rare but certainly can affect nonpigmented skin on the teats and udder. Primary and secondary causes of photosensitization must be considered in dairy cattle, and porphyria is a genetic disease that may lead to photosensitization. In today's management systems, it is possible that some animals may never have enough exposure to sunlight to show signs of photosensitization. Photosensitization of the skin of the teats and udder following induction of calving by corticosteroids has been reported. The frequent use of automatic milking machines has caused an increase in circular muscular hypertrophy of the teat sphincter muscle.

Signs. Signs that are associated with physical and chemical teat injuries include erythema, blistering or chapping, and pain. Once again, pain leads to a vicious cycle of resentment that is manifested by kicking off equipment and milkers, incomplete milkout, leaking milk, and finally to an increased incidence of environmental mastitis. Sunburn appears just as in humans, with generalized redness to nonpigmented skin and blisters or vesicles in severe cases of teat injury. Skin cracks may appear after 2 to 3 days because of necrosis resulting from ultraviolet irradiation. Frostbite initially appears as extremely pale cold swelling of one or more teats. As the skin begins to slough, the teat becomes more swollen, erythematous or blue, and painful; the skin becomes leathery and dry. In severely frostbitten teats, the entire teat becomes leathery, black, and eventually sloughs. Small patches of frostbite-damaged skin slough, leaving an ulcerated surface. Signs of frostbite must be differentiated from those of herpes mammillitis because dark sloughing scabs on teats and udder may be present in both diseases.

Bites from the stable fly (*Stomoxys calcitrans*) can contribute to teat injuries and increase the incidence of staphylococcal mastitis, particularly in heifers. Therefore a high incidence of staphylococcal mastitis in calving first-calf heifers should raise concern about fly control.

Photosensitization may lead to erythema, necrosis, and sloughing of exposed nonpigmented skin (Figure 8-40). Generally the lesions are more severe on the lateral aspect of the teats and udder. Absence of lesions of pigmented skin aids in the diagnosis of photosensitization. Sloughs frequently occur in other areas besides the skin of the teats and the udder. Cattle with congenital

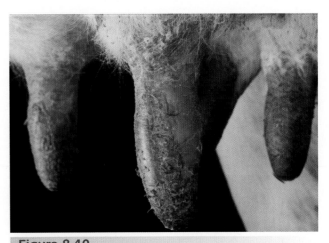

Figure 8-40

Photosensitization of the nonpigmented skin of the teats and udder.

porphyria may have discolored dentine named "pink tooth" and urine that fluoresces under ultraviolet light. Cattle with secondary photosensitization caused by hepatic disease may be jaundiced. Cattle that have eaten photosensitizing plants but are free of liver disease appear healthy except for the skin necrosis.

Treatment. Treatment is different for each condition. The use of chemical irritants should be discontinued. Assess all teat dips for their ingredients, and discard any freeze-damaged products or dips that do not contain skin protectants. Treatment of affected cattle is symptomatic and includes lanolin or aloe ointments and protection of irritated tissues from sunlight.

Frostbite may be treated by tepid water soaks to restore circulation slowly and soften the skin. The damage usually has been done by the time diagnosis is made, however. Therefore putting the cow in a warm area and protecting any injured skin with lanolin creams constitute the best treatment for the majority of affected cattle. Leathery skin should be allowed to separate naturally unless infection develops subcutaneously or the leathery darkened skin interferes with machine milking.

Excessive fly bites or retrospective suspicion of fly bites caused by endemic mastitis in freshening heifers should be approached through fly control using pyrethrin-based insecticides, baited fly traps, and fly paper. Seldom is fly control as much a problem as environmental or management factors that allow a buildup of mud and manure.

Photosensitization must be treated by removal of affected animals from exposure to sunlight and determination of the cause of photosensitization. Primary photosensitization is best treated by avoidance of the causative chemical or toxin coupled with avoidance of sunlight. Secondary photosensitization caused by liver pathology from toxins or individual disease requires consideration, and porphyria should be considered and ruled out.

MASTITIS

To simplify an extremely complex topic, mastitis will be broken down into *contagious* organisms that colonize the mammary gland and can be spread by milking machines and milkers, and *environmental* pathogens that do not normally infect the mammary gland but can do so when the cow's environment, the teats and udder (or injuries thereof), or the milking machine is contaminated with these organisms and they gain access to the teat cistern.

Common contagious organisms include *Streptococcus agalactiae, Streptococcus dysgalactiae, Staphylococcus aureus,* and *Mycoplasma* sp. Environmental organisms include *Escherichia coli, Klebsiella pneumoniae, Enterobacter aerogenes, Serratia* sp., *Proteus* sp., *Pseudomonas* sp., and other gram-negatives, coagulase-negative staphylococci, environmental streptococci, yeast or fungi, *Prototheca, A. pyogenes,* and *Corynebacterium bovis.*

From a therapeutic perspective, it is also helpful to consider where (i.e., 1-3) the highest concentration of the infectious organisms may be, because this consideration is helpful in determining likelihood of successful treatment with intramammary therapy, duration of therapy needed, and whether systemic antibiotics may be needed:

1. Milk and lining epithelial cells (*S. agalactiae,* coagulase-negative *Staphylococcus* spp., and *S. dysgalactiae*)
2. Deep tissue of the gland (*S. aureus, Streptococcus uberis,* and *A. pyogenes*)
3. Simultaneous infection of the udder and other body organs (coliforms).

Contagious organisms are spread by milking procedures, contaminated machinery, and the hands of milkers. *S. agalactiae* is the classic example of this group of bacteria because it is highly contagious and an obligate inhabitant of the mammary gland. Although it does not invade the glandular tissue to cause fibrosis and abscesses as does *S. aureus, S. agalactiae* colonizes epithelial surfaces and results in subclinical mastitis or intermittent clinical signs of mastitis. *S. dysgalactiae* is not as contagious as *S. agalactiae* but is similar in the means by which it spreads in a herd. *S. aureus* is probably the worst of the contagious bacterial organisms because it causes chronic, deep infections of the mammary glands and is extremely difficult to cure. Most contagious organisms cause new infections within the first 2 months of lactation. Contagious bacterial organisms are capable of causing subclinical mastitis that results in decreased production. Estimates of financial losses as a result of subclinical mastitis are frequently quoted or estimated in lay and veterinary publications. Although exact financial figures are subject to debate, anyone connected with the dairy industry realizes that there is significant economic loss associated with chronic, subclinical mastitis. These losses include unrealized production, costs of medication and discarded milk, and imposed milk-quality penalties based on high somatic cell counts (SCCs) or bacterial plate counts. It is estimated that every doubling of SCC greater than 50,000 cells/ml results in a loss of approximately 0.5 kg/milk/day. Proper hygiene during udder preparation and milking, postmilking dipping of teats, segregation or culling of infected cows, appropriate treatment of clinical cases, regular milking machine maintenance, and dry cow therapy are key points in the control of contagious bacterial organisms.

Mycoplasma mastitis may be impossible to cure unless self-cure occurs. Therefore the aforementioned procedural efforts to reduce new infections become even more important, and segregation or culling of infected cows is essential.

Environmental organisms can best be discouraged by clean bedding, clean housing, avoidance of wet environments including mud and manure packs, proper udder preparation, only milking *dry* udders, fly control, decreasing teat-end injuries, and implementation of proper milking procedures. Teat dipping and dry cow therapy have less impact on the environmental bacteria, but teat sealants are moderately effective. Coagulase-negative staphylococci possess traits of both environmental and contagious pathogens. Although they are not normal inhabitants of the mammary gland, they commonly colonize the skin of the teat, the teat end, teat injuries, and the hands of milkers. Therefore they can be mechanically spread and present major risks for cows with teat-end injuries. They also have been shown to infect teat ends following fly bites and therefore may be a major cause of heifer mastitis. It is uncertain how gram-positive organisms gain entrance into the udder of prepartum heifers. They are presumed to enter via the teat end and are generally the same strains found on the heifer's udder or in mastitic milk from lactating cows. The incidence of prepartum infections in some herds may exceed 30%. A single intramammary infusion with an appropriate antibiotic, such as pirlimycin, 10 to 14 days before freshening can reduce the infection rate. Environmental organisms that invade the mammary gland result in clinical mastitis that may be peracute or acute. Some of these organisms are also capable of establishing chronic infection of the gland. Environmental organisms first must be present in the cow's environment and then be given an opportunity to invade the udder and overcome the normal defense mechanisms of the teat and udder to establish infection.

The dry period is considered an important time for new intramammary infections with environmental pathogens such as *S. uberis* and *E. coli.* In many cows, multiple organisms (e.g., *S. uberis, E. coli,* and/or coagulase-positive staphylococci) may be cultured from the same gland during the dry period, suggesting a synergy between them. This differs from *Corynebacterium* infections, which often exist as the only isolate. The proportion of quarters from which positive cultures involving major bacterial pathogens may be obtained increases from 3.8% at the end of lactation to 15.6% just before calving. If dry cow therapy and the use of teat sealants are not incorporated, this increase in mammary infection during the dry period may be as high as 20%.

Contagious Causes

Streptococcus agalactiae

Etiology. An obligate agent of the mammary gland, *S. agalactiae* is a contagious cause of mastitis within a herd. Sloppy milking procedures promote the spread of this organism, whereas hygienic procedures control its spread. Mastitis is largely subclinical with occasional acute flareups. Therefore the major losses associated with *S. agalactiae* are in lost production and financial penalties levied for violative SCCs. The bacteria do not cause mammary gland abscesses but permanently decrease productivity in infected glands in chronic infections. Young calves fed mastitic milk containing *S. agalactiae* and housed in common pens have a high incidence of *S. agalactiae* mastitis at freshening. This probably results from calf suckling.

Herd mastitis caused by *S. agalactiae* even with low or moderate prevalence causes profound elevations in SCCs that quickly affect milk quality tests in the bulk tank. Herd problems with *S. agalactiae* should therefore be suspected whenever there is a rapid and unexplained increase in bulk tank SCCs.

Signs and Diagnosis. Cows seldom show systemic illness as a result of *S. agalactiae* mastitis but can be febrile during the initial infection and with intermittent flareups. Infection can be suspected by finding abnormalities in the milk during strip plate or California mastitis test (CMT) evaluation. Absolute diagnosis must depend on culture because the signs as regards strip plate (clots, flakes) and CMT are nonspecific. Culture techniques to confirm *S. agalactiae* use the CAMP test that highlights the ability of Lancefield group B streptococci to lyse in the presence of staphylococcal beta-toxin.

Treatment. Although all authorities recognize that penicillin, cloxacillin, erythromycin, and cephalosporins all have excellent success in curing *S. agalactiae* mastitis, great debates regarding "when, and who, to treat" have ensued.

Dry cow therapy with 100,000 U of penicillin G or cloxacillin should cure 90% or more of infected quarters. Therefore dry cow therapy is an integral part of *S. agalactiae* control. However, dry cow therapy cannot address the immediate problems presented by infected cows in lactation that are causing high SCCs in tank milk or resulting in warnings from the milk plant.

When cultures confirm *S. agalactiae* in problem herds, management and antibiotic therapy must be considered.

The following represent some general guidelines for the approach to *S. agalactiae* mastitis in problem herds:

1. Milking procedures to discourage spread of contagious organisms must be practiced (i.e., backflushing or dipping in disinfectant of milking machine claws is indicated; use of teat dips postmilking; checks for proper functioning and use of milking equipment should be initiated). There should be no common washing or drying cloths.
2. Dry cow therapy is imperative to treat infections and minimize new intramammary infections during the dry period. *S. agalactiae* tends to infect early in the dry period.
3. Cattle in early and mid-lactation should be treated using intramammary and systemic penicillin G. Such lactating cow therapy has been shown to return profits in the form of increased production that outweighs drug and discarded milk cost.

Although some studies suggest not treating cows in late lactation because of a lack of economic benefit, leaving these cows untreated means that a source of infection remains. Therefore unless milking procedures are definitely corrected, new or repeat infections are likely when some infected quarters are left untreated. Thus controversy exists regarding treating all infected cows ("blitz technique") or only those in early or mid-lactation.

Lactating cow therapy must be based on bacteriological cultures of individual quarter or composite samples of all cows. SCCs or indirect measures of SCCs *are not* a good basis for the absolute diagnosis and subsequent therapy. There is too much overlap between SCC numbers in cows with chronic infections caused by a variety of contagious organisms and cows that have recovered from a variety of mastitis causes. Therefore not all cows with high SCCs have infections. Conversely some clinically infected quarters may have fairly low SCCs.

Clear differentiation of "old versus new" intramammary infections is imperative when evaluating *S. agalactiae* incidence in a herd. Persistence of infection may mean ineffective treatment, whereas new intramammary infections mean poor control measures. New intramammary infections dictate further management of milking hygiene, teat dipping, and dry cow therapy.

Streptococcus dysgalactiae

Etiology. Although contagious, *S. dysgalactiae* tends to have a lower prevalence in affected herds than that observed with *S. agalactiae* infections and may become overtly clinical (abnormal milk, swollen quarter) earlier than is typical for *S. agalactiae*. Injured teat ends and improper milking hygiene promote the spread of the organism within the herd.

Signs and Diagnosis. Signs are nonspecific. Subclinical cases may be suspected when clots and flakes are observed in forestrippings or when a positive CMT is detected. Clinical cases have mild fever and a swollen, warm, doughy quarter with abnormal secretion. Definitive diagnosis requires culture.

Treatment. Similar to *S. agalactiae*, *S. dysgalactiae* responds well to penicillin, cloxacillin, and cephalosporins. The same principles of treatment listed for *S. agalactiae* are pertinent to control of this organism. Special attention should be directed to milking and management practices that decrease teat-end injuries.

Staphylococcus aureus

Etiology. Once established within a herd, *S. aureus* is difficult, if not impossible, to eliminate. Chronic infections, resistance to antibiotics, and difficulty in diagnosis typify the organism. *S. aureus* is not an obligate organism of the mammary gland and may also colonize unhealthy skin on the teat or udder, vagina, tonsils, and other areas of the body. However, the major source of infection is secretion from infected quarters spread by the hands of milkers and milking equipment.

Calves acquire infection with *S. aureus* from suckling following the feeding of mastitic milk. Heifers 3 months of age and older may acquire *S. aureus* infections by fly-bite irritation of the teat end and vector transmission of *S. aureus* by flies. This and a dirty environment may contribute to a high incidence of *S. aureus* mastitis in freshening heifers and will severely damage milk production.

Subclinical infections are the rule, but acute mastitis or recurrent flareups are more common with *S. aureus* than the contagious streptococci. Infection with *S. aureus* is chronic, and self-cures are rare. In addition to decreased productivity, infected glands suffer permanent parenchymal damage with fibrosis and microabscess formation.

S. aureus commonly acquires resistance to antibiotics. Incomplete killing of the bacterium by penicillin and cephalosporin drugs may give rise to L-forms, which regrow after cessation of antibiotic therapy. L-forms are cell wall-deficient variants that may not grow on standard culture media. Single cultures before antibiotic therapy are considered to have a satisfactory sensitivity for most bacterial causes of mastitis except in *S. aureus* infections, for which the sensitivity may be less than 75%! Therefore misleading negative cultures may erroneously suggest clinical cure following antibiotic therapy, and subsequent clinical relapses may be erroneously thought to be a new infection. Such regrowth explains relapses after apparent cures. The production of L-forms occurs following exposure of *S. aureus* to beta-lactam drugs. Phagocytes do not provide effective defenses against L-forms. Freezing and thawing of milk samples may allow improved culture detection as intracellular organisms are released from phagocytes.

Signs. Signs in subclinical infections may be mild and nonspecific and include abnormal milk (e.g., clots, flakes, and/or watery secretion) observed on strip plate and positive CMT. The ability to predict the causative organism of mastitis based on appearance of the milk has been shown to be poor in several field studies. Acute

or peracute mastitis is not unusual with *S. aureus*, however. Clinically infected glands have intermittent acute attacks usually noticed by the owner. During acute flareups or initial infection, the affected cow may be febrile, have a swollen, painful, warm quarter, and show a slightly reduced appetite. Secretion tends to be creamy or purulent with alternating serum-like secretion interspersed with clots, flakes, or creamier secretion. The character of the secretion is in no way pathognomonic for any specific intramammary organism.

Peracute *S. aureus* occurs most commonly in recently fresh cows or in cows suffering initial infection. Peracute infection causes systemic illness characterized by high fever (105.0 to 107.0° F/40.56 to 41.67° C), depression, inappetence, and a hard, swollen, painfully inflamed quarter. Affected cows may become lame because of inflammation and pain in the affected gland. Gangrenous mastitis is the worst example of peracute *S. aureus* mastitis. Gangrenous changes occur most frequently in postpartum cows. Although other organisms such as anaerobes are capable of causing gangrenous mastitis, *S. aureus* is the most frequent cause of gangrenous mastitis in dairy cattle. Signs of toxemia worsen when gangrene develops, and the greatly swollen, firm quarter changes color from pink to red to purple to blue within a few hours. Affected cattle have tachycardia, gradually diminishing fever, profound toxemia, depression, and inappetence. The quarter develops a purplish discoloration, becomes cold, and may develop intrafascicular emphysema. A line of demarcation between healthy and gangrenous skin usually is apparent on the skin of the udder (Figure 8-41, *A* and *B*). Later the skin becomes necrotic and sloughs (Figure 8-41, *C*). The secretion is serosanguineous, indicating the presence of vascular disturbance. The alpha-toxin of *S. aureus* that is dermonecrotic and vasoconstrictive is thought responsible for the tremendous tissue damage associated with gangrenous infection. Other toxins and leukocidin may contribute as well. Compromised defense mechanisms in the recently fresh cow may further predispose to such overwhelming infection.

Heifers freshening with chronic *S. aureus* mastitis usually have ricelike clots or pus in the secretion from the infected quarter or quarters. The quarters are firm, edematous, and warm, but because of periparturient edema, may be difficult to identify as infected by observation or palpation.

Chronic *S. aureus* mastitis results in palpable fibrosis of the mammary gland. Although many cows are suspected of having chronic *S. aureus* infections based on abnormal milk or acute flareups, others remain subclinical and escape detection. Palpation of the mammary glands can be a helpful sign and also can point out the obvious permanent damage to productivity. Chronic subclinical infections remain a major reservoir of *S. aureus* and a major risk to uninfected herdmates.

Diagnosis. Strip plate evidence of creamy or puslike secretion from forestrippings and a history of recurrent

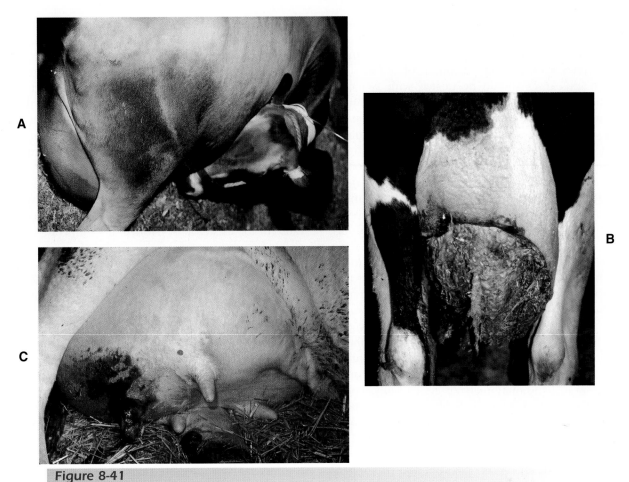

Figure 8-41

A, Gangrenous mastitis of the right hindquarter caused by *S. aureus* in a Jersey cow; notice the distinct discoloration of part of the gland. **B,** Sharp line of demarcation between healthy and necrotic tissue in a cow that had survived the acute stages of gangrenous mastitis. **C,** Gangrenous mastitis of the right hindquarter caused by *S. aureus* in a recently fresh cow.

bouts of mastitis may suggest *S. aureus* mastitis, but definitive diagnosis requires culture of the coagulase-positive organisms. Approximately 75% of *S. aureus* infections are identified by single quarter samples. The sensitivity of cultural isolation can be increased to 94% and 98% by sampling two or three times, respectively.

Increases in bulk tank SCC and standard plate counts (SPCs) are not sensitive indicators of a *S. aureus* herd problem. Up to 50% of the cows in a herd may be infected by *S. aureus* before bulk tank SCC or SPCs become alarmingly elevated. This is in distinct contrast to *S. agalactiae* herd infections, in which even a few heavily shedding infected cows may dramatically increase the bulk tank SCC and SPCs. Therefore SCCs and CMT results are not as reliable as individual quarter cultures in the diagnosis of *S. aureus* mastitis. However, cows with linear SCC scores above 4.5 are the best candidates for individual quarter samples to detect contagious mastitis organisms such as *S. aureus*.

Treatment. Treatment of *S. aureus* mastitis includes both lactation therapy for acute mastitis flareups and dry cow therapy. Acute flareups require treatment during lactation to reduce the shed of large numbers of bacteria and somatic cells into bulk tank milk. Unfortunately the true cure rate with lactation therapy is probably less than 40%. Reasons for the low cure rate during lactation include using the wrong drug, using a reduced dosage or compromised length of treatment, resistant strains of the organism, decreased activity of the drug because of the environment in the mammary gland (pH, biofilm production by the staphylococcus, inflammatory debris, high SCC), and inability of the drug to reach the organism (intracellular location of *S. aureus,* existence of abscesses and fibrotic lesions containing organisms). The inability of a drug to reach the organism is partially related to duration of infection; bacteriological cure rates for newly acquired infections (<2 weeks) may be as high as 70%. Younger cows (<48 months) have also been shown to have higher cure rates (81%) than cows >96 months (55% cure rate). Early lactation infections are cured better than infection in other stages of lactation, and cows with only one quarter infected are two times more likely to be cured than cows with multiple quarter infections. Cure rates are higher for front quarters compared with hindquarters and also decrease with increasing SCC and duration of infection. The most significant treatment factor affecting cure is treatment duration, but economics often mitigates against protracted antimicrobial use.

Gangrenous cases should be treated with systemic antibiotics (extra-label doses of ceftiofur or tetracycline), fluids, and flunixin. If the teat is purple, it should be removed with an emasculator or emasculatome to allow drainage of the necrotic quarter.

There may be an advantage to combined systemic and local therapy that is continued for up to 5 days when treating clinical, nongangrenous *S. aureus* mastitis. Penicillin has been used systemically in several studies with success, but results suggest that antibiotic selection based on culture and sensitivity results may have the best chance of cure when using a combination of systemic and local therapy. Penicillin resistance is the best documented antimicrobial resistance demonstrated by *S. aureus*, but the prevalence of penicillin-resistant strains from bovine mastitis cases appears to have decreased in recent years in the United States. Similarly combination therapy utilizing either ceftiofur or pirlimycin has resulted in greater cure rates than either drug given alone just intramammary or systemically. Local therapy alone is highly unsuccessful to effect clinical cure but may yield clinical improvement or remission that masquerades as a cure to the owner. Extra-label use of intramammary products (e.g., three tubes per treatment) may provide higher cure rates but have prolonged withdrawal times. The success of therapy is related to not only choosing the right antibiotic but also to the duration and extent of the mastitis and the immune status of the cow.

Culture and susceptibility testing of *S. aureus* quarters are indicated, and antibiotics selected for local treatment should be used at least four times at 12-hour intervals or as directed. Cloxacillin and approved cephalosporins are most commonly used for local treatment of lactation flareups. Pirlimycin is also frequently used in cattle with gram-positive mastitis. Milkers should handle the teats of infected cows carefully to minimize spread of infection. Infected cows to be treated should be milked last or at least have mandatory backflushing or dipping of teat cups and milking machine claws into disinfectants. Iodine sanitizers may be used for disinfection of milking machines when diluted to a final iodine concentration of 200 ppm; the shell and claws are dipped before and after milking an infected cow. Teat dip may be used before and after milking. Because the infected cow's milk is not going into the tank, the extra iodine in milk caused by these procedures is not a problem. This same technique can be used prophylactically for fresh cows or heifers that are thought to be at high risk for mastitis based on concurrent diseases, uterine discharges, and the like.

Dry cow therapy for *S. aureus* is reported to be much more successful at curing infection than lactation therapy.

Wide-ranging estimates of cure percentages exist, and some authorities believe that 80% to 85% of *S. aureus* quarters may be cured by dry cow therapy with benzathine cloxacillin or other antibiotics. Higher percentage estimates of success seem hard to believe given the long list of potential reasons for failure mentioned in the discussion of lactation therapy. Less dilution of the drug, longer duration of the drug within the udder, and fewer opportunities for the bacteria to form biofilms and L-forms during the dry period may account for the greater success rate of dry cow therapy. Concerns remain as to what determined "cure" in these studies. A negative posttreatment culture may or may not indicate success because of the existence of L-forms, intermittent shedding, or low but persistent numbers of intracellular organisms. Given the apparent success of dry cow therapy as treatment for *S. aureus*, all quarters in infected herds should be treated at dry off and a teat seal applied. Selection of the appropriate dry cow formulation should be made following assessment of antibiotic sensitivity of the predominant *S. aureus* strains in that herd. Dry cow therapy is also helpful in reducing new intramammary infection during the early part of the dry period by both *S. aureus* and *S. agalactiae*. Thus dry cow therapy helps reduce existing intramammary infection and decreases the incidence of new intramammary infection. Dry cow therapy has also been used for heifers before calving when high incidences of *S. aureus* exist in freshening heifers. Autogenous and commercial bacterins have been advocated and used for chronic *S. aureus* mastitis in problem herds. Commercial bacterins may or may not contain the same strain of *S. aureus* that exists on the farm in question. Further, more than one strain may be present on a given farm experiencing *S. aureus* mastitis. Autogenous bacterins may be somewhat helpful in decreasing new infections, but they do not clear existing infections. Systemic immunization during the dry period may be more effective than during lactation and mainly induces IgG$_1$ immunoglobulin, helps neutralize toxins, and may improve opsonization. Local immunization (of mammary lymph nodes) may be more dangerous as regards delayed hypersensitivity reactions but would be expected to generate more IgA and IgM and to improve cell-mediated defenses. Recent work also suggests that immunized heifers are significantly *less* likely to develop *S. aureus* mastitis. Bacterins may be incorporated into the control scheme for *S. aureus* problem herds but should never be substituted for improved milking management. It is hoped that improved vaccines for prevention of *S. aureus* will be available in the future.

Dry off of affected quarters and culling cows are the last components of treatment and control of *S. aureus* mastitis. Valuable brood cows that cannot be cured and cannot be culled can be dried off permanently or have the affected quarters killed. Culling of problem cows that are chronically infected may be necessary for the sake of milk quality control and reducing the risk of new intramammary infections. Veterinarians and producers need to be aware of the inverse relationship between duration of infection and the likelihood of cure when selecting individual cows for treatment in endemic or high prevalence herds, lest unrealistic expectations regarding cure rates be established.

The future may hold significant hope for treatment of *S. aureus* without antibiotic therapy. Interest in nonantimicrobial treatment of *S. aureus* mastitis has in part been fueled by the limited efficacy of traditional treatments combined with the growth of the organic dairy business. Bacteriocins that are natural bactericidal proteins are being produced by molecular techniques and marketed for treatment of *Streptococcus* and *S. aureus* mastitis and for use in teat dips. Lysostaphin, originally isolated from *Staphylococcus simulans,* has been reproduced by recombinant techniques and used in clinical trials. Nisin, another bacterial peptide originally isolated from *Lactococcus lactis,* has been reproduced by similar techniques and may be marketed soon. Immunomodulating cytokines, including various interleukins, also have shown promise (experimentally) as a nonantibiotic mode of therapy for *S. aureus.* Combination cytokine and antibiotic therapy may improve the bactericidal efficacy of certain antibiotics. Other immunomodulators such as beta-1, 3 glucan have either unproven efficacy or have shown no benefit in small clinical trials. It is possible in the future that transgenic cows may be developed, expressing antibacterial endopeptidase in the mammary gland, which enhances resistance to mastitis.

Calves should not be fed unpasteurized mastitic milk, and heifers should be raised in clean, dry environments where fly control can be maintained to reduce the incidence of *S. aureus* colonization of teat canals with subsequent infection of developing glands.

Mycoplasma Mastitis

Etiology. *Mycoplasma bovis* is the most common cause of mastitis caused by *Mycoplasma* spp., but up to 11 other species have been isolated from milk in various parts of the United States. Historically *Mycoplasma californicum* has been a common isolate in California, but it has been identified in many other states, including New York. *Mycoplasma* spp. cause herd endemics of acute mastitis that subsequently evolve into chronic mastitis. Following acute attacks, cattle may show chronic mastitis, intermittent acute flareups, or have subclinical infection requiring culture confirmation. Mastitis may occur in only one quarter but frequently appears in two or more quarters in each affected cow. Much of the current evidence suggests that herd outbreaks occur via horizontal transmission, most likely from asymptomatic carriers. The possibility of internal transmission to the udder from other internal organs within an asymptomatic cow also challenges the view that *Mycoplasma* is purely contagious from cow to cow

and spread in an identical fashion to other contagious causes of mastitis, such as *S. aureus* and *S. agalactiae,* which are predominantly spread during milking.

M. bovis may be found on mucous membranes and secretions from the respiratory and urogenital tracts. Infection may be introduced by a purchased animal from an infected herd or may appear spontaneously following mechanical transmission of organisms by contaminated workers. Isolates that include *M. bovis, Mycoplasma dispar, Mycoplasma bovirhinis, Mycoplasma bovigenitalium, Mycoplasma canadense, Mycoplasma alkalescens,* and *M. californicum* have been isolated from single herds. *Mycoplasma* populations usually are highest in calves and heifers. Clinical signs of *Mycoplasma* infection including respiratory disease, otitis interna/media, arthritis, or reproductive problems may or may not be obvious or reported in problem herds, but *Mycoplasma* spp. can be cultured from the respiratory or reproductive tract in young cattle and adults. Therefore although purchase of infected cattle represents a risk of introduction of *Mycoplasma* mastitis, perhaps the greater risk is chance contamination transmission and spread of the organisms from infected nasal, urogenital, or joint secretions to the udder, most likely from animals without evidence of clinical disease. Following infection of one cow, the disease spreads as a contagious mastitis. Fresh cows appear to be at greater risk than cows in mid-lactation. Cold, wet seasons also may increase the incidence of infection because the organisms may persist longer in the environment.

Signs. Acute mastitis in one or more quarters of a cow is the usual history. The affected quarters are warm, swollen, and firm. Secretions are variable in appearance. Early secretions may be watery and have flakes of "sandy material," but this is not observed in many cases. The secretion may evolve over several days to a tannish serous-like material, clots, flakes, or pus. Although acute *Mycoplasma* mastitis is associated with fever (103.0 to 105.5° F/39.44 to 40.83° C), affected cows may not appear ill. Some acutely infected cows may be slightly off feed, perhaps associated with fever. Milk production decreases dramatically in those with acute *Mycoplasma* mastitis but may not be obviously reduced in subclinical cases.

Acute mastitis involving multiple quarters and swollen, painful joints occurring in several cows within a short period should alert the veterinarian to the possibility of *Mycoplasma* mastitis. The signs are less suggestive in chronic *Mycoplasma* mastitis, for which subclinical infections predominate. Intermittent acute flareups will be present but may not be as dramatic as the signs of acute *Mycoplasma,* especially when the organism is first introduced into a herd. Generally by the time a diagnosis of *Mycoplasma* mastitis is confirmed, at least 10% of the herd is already infected.

Arthritis, lameness, reproductive problems, calf pneumonia and/or otitis interna/media, and adult cow respiratory diseases may be other owner complaints when procuring a history in herds with *Mycoplasma* mastitis. These other diseases may or may not be associated with *Mycoplasma* spp. Frequently the existence of multiple health problems more likely indicates management deficiencies and overcrowding of cattle. Increased incidence of *Mycoplasma* respiratory disease and arthritis has been confirmed in several herds that were monitored for several years because of *Mycoplasma* mastitis. The fact that occasional outbreaks of *Mycoplasma* sp. mastitis occur in the absence of new purchases and herd additions reinforces the view that some cattle can remain asymptomatic carriers for extended periods. The introduction of bred heifers, reared off farm or purchased commercially, appears to be a particularly common antecedent event to acute herd outbreaks of *Mycoplasma* mastitis.

Diagnosis. Definitive diagnosis of *Mycoplasma* mastitis requires isolation from milk. Most *Mycoplasma* will not grow on culture media that is routinely used to identify bacterial pathogens. Therefore *Mycoplasma* mastitis should be suspected when obvious mastitis is present, bacterial culture yields negative results, and antibiotic treatment has failed to improve the signs. Special media such as Hayflick's medium incubated at 37.0° C and kept in 10% CO_2 are necessary for culture of *Mycoplasma* sp. *Mycoplasma* is shed in great quantities in milk, and consequently culture of bulk tank milk may be used as a sensitive method for early identification of infection in a few cattle. Following growth of *Mycoplasma* sp., speciation is indicated and requires an indirect immunoperoxidase assay or fluorescent antibody (FA) technique performed by a competent laboratory. *Mycoplasma* may be grown following freezing of milk.

Identification of specific species may assist an epidemiologic investigation of predisposing factors that contributed to the *Mycoplasma* mastitis problem. In addition, one saprophytic organism, *Acholeplasma laidlawii*, is a fairly common contaminant of tank milk and should not be thought of as a cause of mastitis.

Treatment. Approved antibiotics are ineffective against *Mycoplasma* mastitis. Macrolide and tetracycline antibiotics that are used to treat *Mycoplasma* infection in other organ systems have not been successful against *Mycoplasma* mastitis. Fluoroquinolones are legal in Europe for mastitis treatment and would be the preferred treatment. It is not legal to use fluoroquinolones in dairy cattle in North America.

Because of the lack of therapeutic options, culling all infected cattle should be considered. Cows that continue to have clinical mastitis and agalactia are easier for an owner to cull than cows that apparently recover and continue to produce milk. Because of the high number of cattle that are affected initially, culling of as many as 10% or more of a herd may be required. This is seldom acceptable to an owner. Lag times between collection of milk

samples and positive identification of infected cattle following milk culture allow new infections to occur. Therefore when more cows become positive based on follow-up cultures, the owner becomes discouraged, having already culled "all" positive cows based on initial culture. Owner compliance with culling is much more likely if only a few cows are infected. Segregation of infected and noninfected cattle has been practiced in California and other states when large numbers of cattle are infected and owners are unwilling or economically unable to cull all infected cattle.

Control. The goal of *Mycoplasma* control is the identification of infected animals and their isolation and segregation from uninfected herdmates. Once *Mycoplasma* has been identified in a herd, quarter samples from all cows should be submitted for culture, all cows should be dipped with 1% iodine dips after milking, milking claws and teat cups should be rinsed with 30 to 75 ppm iodine and sanitized or backflushed with the same solution between cows, and all milking procedures should be evaluated carefully.

Following results of the quarter cultures, infected cattle should be culled or segregated from the noninfected herdmates. Cultures should be collected from all quarters of the remaining cows monthly, and new positives should be identified and culled. After herd cultures are negative, milk filters should be cultured monthly, and aggressive quarter culturing and culling programs should be reinitiated if *Mycoplasma* is reisolated. Ideally infected milk should not be fed to calves, but pasteurization has become an attractive option for some larger dairies. There are differences in the thermal resistance patterns of different *Mycoplasma* species, so when waste milk is pasteurized before feeding to calves, periodic quality control checks of pasteurization equipment are critical. Submitting pasteurized milk samples as fed to calves for routine bulk tank testing, to include specific *Mycoplasma* culture, is an important part of the preventative calf health program on those larger dairies that pasteurize waste milk.

Infected cows may recover from acute infections and become productive, but others develop chronic mastitis or lameness. The frequency of long-term carriers and shedding from milk of recovered cattle is unknown. Infection with one species of *Mycoplasma* does not confer immunity against other species. In addition, active immunity to a single species is likely to be short lived. One report concerning *M. bovis* showed that cattle that recovered from *Mycoplasma* mastitis were resistant to reinfection in all quarters for 55 days and were resistant in previously infected quarters for 180 days, but they became susceptible to reinfection in all quarters by 1 year following initial recovery.

A vaccine for *M. bovis* is commercially available, both as a licensed product and produced on a custom basis; however, the efficacies of the products are not well established. Further use in field settings will determine the eventual usefulness for control of the infection in cattle. The wide variation in antigenicity between different species and strains of *Mycoplasma* does not bode well for cross-protection against all of the currently encountered *Mycoplasma* spp. for the prevention of mastitis, arthritis, or respiratory disease.

Environmental Causes of Mastitis

Streptococcus uberis and Other *Streptococcus* spp. (Non-*agalactiae*)

Etiology. *S. uberis* is ubiquitous throughout the farm environment because of fecal, salivary, and nasal contamination by cows harboring the organism in their rumen, vagina, external genitalia, mouth, and skin of the teats and udder. Poor cleansing and preparation of the udder before milking predispose to mastitis caused by *S. uberis* as with other environmental pathogens. It is the most prevalent environmental *Streptococcus* sp. associated with clinical mastitis. Most infections occur early in lactation or late in the dry period, although failure to use dry cow treatment may allow earlier infection during the dry period. Injuries to the teat or chapping of the teat skin encourages colonization of the skin by *S. uberis* and increases the risk of infection. There is an increased incidence of infection in the winter months. It is more common in older multiparous cows than first- or second-lactation animals.

Signs and Diagnosis. Acute mastitis with swelling, edema, and firmness of the affected quarter are nonspecific signs observed in those with *S. uberis* mastitis. Fever, malaise, and varying degrees of inappetence may be associated with the mastitis. The secretion tends to have clots and flecks present and is more watery than normal, but the gross appearance of the milk is too nonspecific to allow an etiologic diagnosis to be made (Figure 8-42). Lack of

Figure 8-42

Milk clots on a strip plate from a cow with mastitis. Almost any etiologic agent could cause a similar appearance to the milk. It is difficult to predict causative agent from appearance of the milk!

specificity of the clinical signs mandates bacteriologic culture for differentiation of *S. uberis* from other environmental streptococci. Subclinical cases are more common than clinical cases, especially in late lactation, and cause high SCCs and bacteria counts in the bulk tank milk.

Treatment. Penicillin, cloxacillin, ampicillin, and cephalosporins are effective against most *S. uberis* infections. Erythromycin and pirlimycin are frequently used but have lower in vitro susceptibility. Tetracycline also is reported to work very well against *S. uberis* but not against other environmental streptococci. Clinical cure during lactation may be more difficult than during the dry period. For example, extended-duration intramammary treatment with ceftiofur (5 or 8 days of treatment instead of the standard 2-day treatment) may confer a significant increase in bacteriologic cure rates. Some environmental streptococci (non-*agalactiae*) are extremely resistant to antibiotics and require antibiotic sensitivity testing to best determine specific treatments. It appears that persistence of *S. uberis* mastitis in the face of antibiotic treatment is more often the result of antimicrobial resistance of the original strain than a result of reinfection with new ones, reinforcing the need for initial microbiologic testing to include susceptibility patterns in the face of an outbreak. Reinfection is common when cattle have teat or teat-end lesions that allow skin colonization by these organisms. It may be helpful in severe cases to combine systemic erythromycin or penicillin administration with intramammary treatment for a period of 3 to 5 days. Herds in which *S. uberis* and other environmental streptococci have been identified as causes of mastitis should have the environment of the cows evaluated, and if organic bedding is heavily contaminated switching to sand may be helpful, although it may also become contaminated with environmental organisms unless properly cleaned and/or replaced. Particular attention should be paid to the environment of the dry cows because infections are more common in the dry period. Milking procedures should also be reviewed because improper procedures may damage the teats and increase susceptibility. Routine dry cow antibiotic treatment should be used, and for herds with persistent problems, prelactation therapy may decrease infection rate. Teat dipping should routinely be used, but for environmental *Streptococcus* spp. infections, it may not be as important for control as dry cow therapy.

Coagulase-Negative Staphylococci

Etiology. Coagulase-negative staphylococci are normal flora of the skin of the teat and external orifice of the streak canal. Factors that contribute to teat skin irritation or injury increase the numbers of coagulase-negative staphylococci at these locations. Bulk milk may be heavily contaminated with coagulase-negative staphylococci if milking procedures are inadequate, hygiene is poor, teat skin is irritated, and postmilking teat dips are not used. These organisms are commonly cultured from the milk of prepartum and first-calf heifers. Older cows may also be infected but at a lower incidence, supporting the efficacy of dry cow and lactation therapy in resolving the udder infection.

Mastitis resulting from these organisms (*Staphylococcus xylosis, Staphylococcus warneri,* and *S. simulans*) creates subclinical mastitis that results in decreased production and elevated SCC in infected glands. The increased SCC tends not to represent as dramatic an effect on bulk tank numbers as seen in contagious *S. agalactiae* outbreaks. In fact, up to 50% of the herd may be infected before the bulk tank SCC causes great concern. Loss of production can occur, especially when a significant percentage of the herd is infected. Mastitis caused by coagulase-negative staphylococci is reported to be common, with some sources claiming that it is the most common intramammary infection in many herds. Infections most commonly occur during early and late lactation or in the dry period if dry cow therapy is not used.

Calves 3 to 9 months of age can develop staphylococcal mastitis from contamination by mastitic milk or by contaminated flies that feed on injured teat ends.

Signs. Other than latent decreased production, positive CMT results, and elevated SCCs, no clinical signs exist that specifically identify coagulase-negative *Staphylococcus.* Heifers freshening with mastitis should be suspected to have coagulase-negative staphylococcal infection.

Diagnosis. Culture of individual quarters from all cows is essential to identification, treatment, and prevention of further new intramammary infection. Individual cow SCC (or linear score), bulk tank SCC, and bacterial cultures or counts may assist initial diagnosis but are not sufficient for detection, treatment, and control.

Treatment and Control. Improved milking hygiene, correction of milking machine problems, postmilking teat dipping with iodine teat dips, and dry cow therapy are very effective in the control of coagulase-negative staphylococci. Obvious causes of teat skin irritation should be eliminated. Wet milking or poor udder preparation are notorious problems in producing high numbers of coagulase-negative staphylococci in bulk tank milk and a high incidence of mastitis resulting from these organisms.

Antibiotic therapy may be used during lactation if the cow is sufficiently early in lactation that treatment costs are outweighed by production losses if left untreated. Dry cow therapy is also indicated in herds with a high percentage of intramammary infection as a result of these organisms. Antibiotic therapy should be based on sensitivity reports, with antibiotics having efficacy against beta-lactamase-positive organisms preferred. Iodine teat dips have been reported to be superior to other chemicals, and backflushing milking machine claws will reduce spread of the organism.

Calves should not be fed mastitic milk—especially if kept in common calf pens. Heifers should be kept in clean, dry environments, and fly control should be emphasized to decrease staphylococcal infection before calving. If there is a herd problem with coagulase-negative *Staphylococcus* in heifers at freshening, treatment with a cephalosporin or pirlimycin 1 to 2 weeks before freshening may be indicated.

Arcanobacterium pyogenes (Formerly *Corynebacterium* and *Actinomyces pyogenes*)

Etiology. *A. pyogenes* causes "dry cow" or "summer" mastitis. Infection is extremely purulent, and abscessation of affected glands is common. Most, but not all, infections occur during the dry period, and the incidence of infection is increased during the dry period by unhygienic environments. Because *A. pyogenes* is a common skin organism of cattle, it is routinely isolated from abscesses and wounds in a variety of tissues. The organism may be spread by flies and fly bites of the teat end during summer months but can occur year-round in some operations. Teat injury may predispose to *A. pyogenes* and other gram-positive infections. Most infections begin after the udder has been dry for 2 weeks or more. Epidemics with up to 25% of the dry cows being affected are possible.

A. pyogenes infection of the gland in heifer calves has been reported in England and in warm-weather zones of the United States. Affected calves were at pasture during the summer months and ranged in age from 5 to 22 months. The degree of damage to infected glands based on future productivity was not reported. Fly control reduced further incidence of disease.

Signs. Swelling of the infected quarter usually is acute and results in a very firm or hard, inflamed, painful gland or glands. Fever and inappetence may accompany acute infection. Cattle that are closely observed may have a less severe and gradual inflammation of the infected gland. Therefore "acute" cases may in fact be well advanced when finally recognized and represent fulminant abscessation of a longer-standing, subacute or chronic infection. Cows having truly acute infections are febrile and have firm inflamed quarters and watery secretion with thick clots or ricelike clumps in the secretion. *Cows with subacute or chronic infections do not appear ill systemically but have extremely hard, greatly swollen glands with toothpaste-like or thick malodorous pus as the major secretion.* Milking the affected quarter may be difficult because of the viscosity of the secretions. Abscesses may appear in chronic cases and are located anywhere in the gland. Such abscesses eventually drain percutaneously through the skin of the udder (Figure 8-43) with typical discharge and odor associated with *A. pyogenes.* Most chronically infected glands are ruined by the infection. Dry cows with *A. pyogenes* occasionally may abort because of toxemia and fever in acute cases. Occasionally *A. pyogenes* will be isolated from a recurrent or chronic case of mild clinical mastitis in a cow with a history of coliform

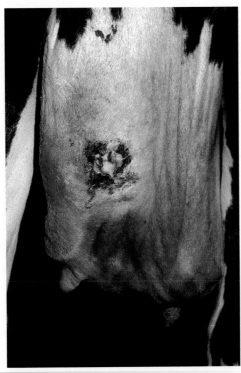

Figure 8-43

Arcanobacterium pyogenes mastitis causing a firm, swollen left rear quarter in a dry cow. A draining abscess is apparent.

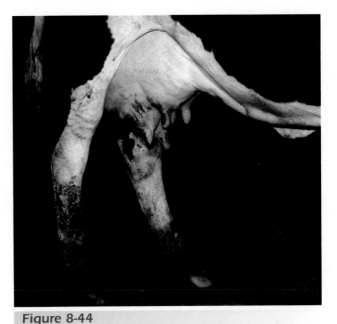

Figure 8-44

Arcanobacterium pyogenes mastitis of both rear quarters in a dry cow. Notice that the cow has been kept in a filthy environment as evidenced by dried mud on the udder and rear legs.

mastitis or mastitis caused by some other primary pathogen. The presumed pathogenesis in these cases is vascular damage, tissue infarction, and subsequent colonization of necrotic or compromised mammary tissue from pyogenic foci elsewhere in the body or via the teat.

Diagnosis. Diagnosis is confirmed by culture of secretion from the quarter.

Treatment. Although the prognosis is guarded, early recognition of *A. pyogenes* mastitis before abscessation offers the best opportunity for resolution. Before intramammary administration of antimicrobials, infected quarters must be milked out completely.

Penicillin also should be administered systemically (22,000 U/kg IM, twice daily) for a minimum of 1 week. Penicillin should be infused into the quarter once or twice daily using approved lactational intramammary products. Most cattle that improve require 7 to 14 days of antibiotic therapy. Cattle that do not improve eventually develop draining udder abscesses and cease lactating in the infected quarters. Gradual softening of the infected quarter is the desired response. Other signs of improvement include reduced size of the gland and a more fluid secretion. Prevention of *A. pyogenes* mastitis revolves around provision of clean, dry environments for nonlactating cows and heifers, frequent observation of dry cow's udders for evidence of overt swelling or asymmetry, fly control, and aseptic administration of dry cow treatments. Although dry cow preparations certainly

discourage *A. pyogenes* infections, careless administration of dry cow products may introduce *A. pyogenes* to the teat cistern. Although protective against introduction of some mastitis pathogens, dry cow formulations would be ineffective in conditions of overwhelming bacterial challenge (Figure 8-44). Cure rates have been so low historically for *A. pyogenes* mastitis that practitioners have frequently elected to attempt to dry off the affected quarter or chemically sterilize it using solutions containing iodine, chlorhexidine, or formaldehyde. In some cases, attempted dry off or chemical sterilization meets with the identical outcome as the natural progression of the disease, namely, abscessation and spontaneous drainage from the skin of the affected quarter.

Coliform Mastitis

Etiology. The lactose-fermenting gram-negative rods such as *E. coli*, *Klebsiella* sp., and *Enterobacter* sp. are the causative organisms of coliform mastitis. Coliform mastitis is familiar to all bovine veterinarians because of the mortality associated with the infection in dairy cattle and because farmers call on veterinarians to treat coliform mastitis more often than any other type of mastitis. Coliform mastitis also is the subject of heated debate regarding proper therapeutics, drug residues, and drug withdrawal times. *E. coli*, *Klebsiella* sp., and *Enterobacter* sp. will be referred to collectively as coliforms in this discussion unless a specific point needs to be made.

Coliform mastitis is a classic example of an environmental cause of mastitis. Management factors that contribute to a buildup of coliforms increase the risks of coliform mastitis. Deep mud in barnyards greatly increases the likelihood of coliform organisms contaminating the udder. Summer heat and humidity contribute to multiplication and persistence of coliforms in the environment such that the incidence of coliform mastitis usually is increased during the summer months. However, because of the widespread use of free stall housing for cattle, the damp barn environment present in free stalls predisposes to coliform mastitis, regardless of seasonality. Contact of the teat end with retained fetal membranes may also increase the risk of coliform infection.

Sawdust bedding, especially when wet, has been known to harbor high levels of coliforms. Epidemics of *Klebsiella* mastitis have been associated with the use of wet sawdust. Within days of being placed as bedding and although still appearing clean, fresh sawdust may harbor 10^7 coliform/g, and it has been shown that even 10^6 coliform/g of bedding increases the risk of coliform mastitis. Kiln-dried sawdust may be better but is harder, and more expensive, to obtain. Straw bedding would seem to be a better choice than sawdust, and inorganic bedding materials such as sand and crushed limestone will reduce the environmental exposure to coliform bacteria still further. In terms of both cow health and comfort, sand should be viewed as a preferable bedding material for free stall housing. Any advantage of specific types of bedding, however, is negated by lack of daily maintenance because any bedding material will continue to accumulate coliform bacteria, although some simply do it faster than others. An advantage of sand is that it is pushed out of the free stall bed by the cows more slowly than sawdust. However, if beds are not picked and scraped free of manure daily, coliform counts will quickly increase. Recycling of sand is becoming an attractive economic option for larger free stall dairies that use this bedding material. It appears that properly recycled sand does not carry forward high-risk gram-negative bacterial populations in bedding, although persistence of environmental streptococci may be an issue. The addition of hydrated lime to bedding has been helpful in many barns but is labor intensive and, if too concentrated, can initiate skin irritation.

Cows are at greater risk for coliform mastitis in the immediate postpartum period than at other stages of the lactational cycle. Cows in herds with low somatic cell counts experience the highest incidence of clinical mastitis within the first 30 days of lactation. Udder edema, incomplete milkout, hemorrhage into the gland, sprinkling cows with water, and leaking milk between milkings are important contributing factors to coliform mastitis in fresh cows. Leaking of milk allows environmental mastitis pathogens to enter the teat cistern and gland. Concurrent metabolic diseases such as hypocalcemia that cause the cow to remain recumbent also may increase the exposure to environmental coliforms. Other concurrent diseases in

the postpartum period, such as hepatic lipidosis or retained placenta, may depress neutrophil function and alter the intramammary defenses. Neutrophils may respond to infection of the gland at a slower rate in recently fresh cows than in those in mid-lactation.

Dry cows exposed to heavy numbers of environmental coliforms may become inapparently infected until the periparturient period. Indeed, rates of new intramammary infections caused by coliforms are greater during the dry period than during lactation. Dry cows are at greatest risk for infection just after drying off and just before calving, when intramammary lactoferrin concentrations are lowest. Coliform mastitis is most frequently seen in herds in which contagious causes of mastitis have been controlled. The reasons for this association are unclear; however, the high rate of intramammary infections in herds with poor mastitis control probably results in high SCCs in a large proportion of cows. High concentrations of intramammary neutrophils have been shown to deter coliform mastitis via the rapid engulfment of coliforms gaining access to the quarter. Milking procedures and teat-end injuries are important contributing factors to coliform mastitis. In some herds with a low level of contagious mastitis, coliforms are not only the most common cause of clinical mastitis but also may be the most common organism cultured from the milk of subclinical cases. The common presentation of severe, peracute disease allied with the fact that it is a potentially fatal disease heightens producer and veterinarian awareness of this form of mastitis over most others.

Poor udder sanitation before milking is an obvious problem. Similarly failure to dry teats and udder before milking or use of contaminated wash water for udder disinfection contributes to outbreaks of coliform mastitis. Mechanical or procedural milking problems such as vacuum fluctuations leading to squawking or drop off can reverse milk flows at the teat end that inject coliform-contaminated milk droplets into the teat end and streak canal. High bulk tank coliform counts indicate poor udder preparation, too much filth in the environment, or both, but do not necessarily correlate with the incidence of coliform mastitis.

Teat-end injuries caused by abrasive surfaces, skin chafing, excessive milking vacuum, overmilking, injuries, infections, and irritants all predispose to colonization of glandular tissues by coliforms. These injuries also cause pain, which leads to incomplete milkout, and a tendency to leak milk between milkings and a predisposition toward coliform infection.

Coliforms multiply rapidly by 16 hours after entering the streak canal and overcoming local resistance mechanisms. The bacteria are destroyed by phagocytosis and intracellular killing in phagocytes. However, in the course of bacterial lysis, the release of endotoxin initiates a cascade of inflammatory mediators, which in turn leads to the local and systemic signs of coliform mastitis. The endotoxin-induced mediator cascade is complicated and involves both the cyclooxygenase and lipoxygenase pathways. Inflammatory mediators including histamine, serotonin, and eicosanoids are activated or are released during the process. Production of prostaglandins such as $PGF_{2\alpha}$ and PGE_2 and thromboxane B_2 has been detected in cows with coliform mastitis. Oxygen free radicals probably are produced during acute coliform infections because studies have shown a reduced incidence of severity of coliform mastitis in herds that have adequate vitamin E and selenium levels. Endotoxins cause rumen stasis and ileus and delay calcium absorption from the gut. In addition, the inappetence reduces calcium intake in the face of continued calcium drain from lactation.

Hypokalemia can be a major contributing cause to weakness or recumbency in cows with coliform mastitis. The electrolyte disturbance is thought to occur by a combination of decreased potassium consumption, decreased potassium absorption from the gut, and ileus-related metabolic alkalosis. Clinical signs associated with coliform mastitis probably become apparent after bacterial levels have peaked and the inflammatory cascade is maturing.

The efficient bactericidal activities of neutrophils that have been recruited by the liberated endotoxins may explain the inability of clinicians to isolate coliforms from some acutely infected quarters. Delaying collection of milk for culture or previous treatment further contributes to negative cultures. Freezing of milk samples may increase the sensitivity of bacteriologic culturing by releasing bacteria that are engulfed in phagocytes that would have been killed normally. Cattle can spontaneously clear the intramammary coliform infection as early as 10 days; however, some chronic infections do occur. The role of host (cow) factors in deciding whether a cow will develop severe systemic illness and potentially die appears to be more important than that of pathogen-specific factors in coliform mastitis. Gram-negative bacterial isolates associated with even fatal disease do not belong to the more virulent strains of *E. coli*, such as enterotoxigenic *E. coli* or enteropathogenic *E. coli*. Undoubtedly the size of the inoculum plays a role, and therefore the level of environmental contamination on the farm is an important control point, but the metabolic and immunologic status of the transition cow are very important factors in deciding the prevalence and severity of new, coliform intramammary infections in dairy cattle.

Chronic cases of coliform mastitis once were thought to be rare but now have been routinely confirmed in at least 10% of infected quarters. Chronically infected quarters may be nonproductive or may have subclinical mastitis with intermittent flareups that mimic other causes of acute mastitis. Unfortunately spontaneous cure is difficult for the cow that has been chronically infected. Many cows die as a result of coliform mastitis,

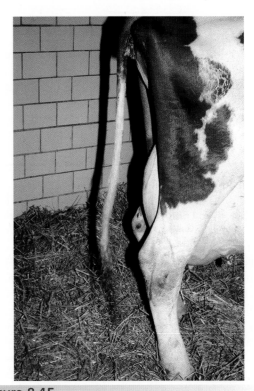

Figure 8-45

A Red and White Holstein cow with chronic coliform mastitis and a "rock hard" right rear quarter. On postmortem examination the gland had infarction.

not only because of lipopolysaccharide (endotoxin) and its effects but also from deep infection of the gland. Also somewhat neglected by research is the cow that has chronic active infection or infarction in the infected mammary gland (Figure 8-45). These cows do not recover spontaneously and certainly do not have sterile quarters. Coliform mastitis-associated bacteremia may be present in up to 40% of severely infected cows, sometimes causing uveitis, arthritis, meningitis, or tenosynovitis associated with their illness.

Clinical Signs. Acute or peracute inflammation of a quarter accompanying systemic signs of illness typifies coliform mastitis in dairy cattle. Affected quarters are warm and swollen. The degree of "firmness" varies, with some cows having only doughy or edematous quarters, whereas others are very firm. Peracute inflammation may cause subtle swelling of the quarter in some periparturient cows that may mask the inflammation-related edema. Regardless of the degree of swelling, the secretion in coliform mastitis (acute) is more watery than that in unaffected quarters. The typical secretion is described as "serum-like" or "watery" by most experienced clinicians and is best detected by first stripping normal milk from an unaffected quarter onto a black-colored plate, then milking secretions from the affected quarter onto the normal milk. Watery milk is easily detected under reflected light. Intramammary subcutaneous and intrafascicular emphysema may be detected in some coliform-affected quarters.

In addition to the local signs in the affected quarter, the cow has systemic illness (Figure 8-46). Owners first notice inappetence and depression. Rectal temperatures ranging between 104.0 and 107.0° F (40.0° and 41.67° C) occur in acute cases of coliform mastitis. Cows with concomitant recumbent periparturient hypocalcemia may be hypothermic rather than febrile. Additional signs from endotoxemia, hypocalcemia, and mediator cascade include inappetence, fever, rumen stasis, tachycardia, tachypnea, diarrhea, weakness, and dehydration. Some affected cows will shiver and have their hair stand on end as early nonspecific signs that are associated with fever and endotoxemia. Ophthalmic consequences of the toxemia associated with coliform mastitis may include scleral injection, miosis, hypopyon, and hyphema. Cows may become recumbent from the profound weakness resulting from the combination of electrolyte disturbance, hypocalcemia, and the endotoxemia. Recumbency worsens prognosis and may interfere with detection of the mastitis. *The udders of all recumbent cattle, especially those in the early periparturient period, should be examined to exclude the possibility of coliform mastitis.*

Systemic complications include musculoskeletal injuries secondary to recumbency, laminitis, metabolic disorders such as hypocalcemia, hypokalemia, and shock

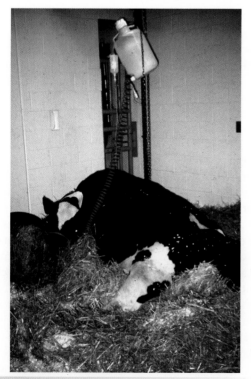

Figure 8-46

Cow with severe toxemia caused by *Klebsiella* mastitis. The individual was recumbent, severely dehydrated, and acidemic.

with lactic acidosis, and multiple organ system failures such as acute renal or hepatic failure. Disseminated intravascular coagulation and thrombocytopenia occasionally are observed. Leukopenia and neutropenia associated with coliform mastitis predispose affected cows to other infections such as metritis, pneumonia, and infection in other quarters of the udder. Patients that have been treated with high doses of dexamethasone have developed fatal bacterial or fungal septicemia. Overuse of NSAIDs combined with disruption of the rumen microflora may result in abomasal ulceration.

Rarely cattle with peracute coliform mastitis have developed lactic acid indigestion following ingestion of large meals of high-moisture corn. In those cases, the profound rumen stasis from endotoxemia was thought to contribute to malfermentation of the grain.

The severity of endotoxic signs varies tremendously in cattle with coliform mastitis. Infections by *Klebsiella* sp. cause the most dramatic and persistent signs of endotoxemia of all coliforms. Many cattle affected with acute coliform mastitis that subsequently was confirmed as resulting from *Klebsiella* sp. remained anorectic, depressed, and weak for up to 7 days, regardless of the rate of therapeutic response.

Diagnosis. In peracute and acute coliform mastitis, the combination of local and systemic signs is a highly reliable indicator of the diagnosis. The most specific signs of coliform mastitis include serum-like secretion, swollen and hard quarter, tachypnea, tachycardia, fever, weakness, and shivering. Although these signs are not absolute, they probably are even more specific when the cow resides in a herd with an overall low SCC, is living in a wet, damp, or dirty environment, or has recently freshened.

The importance of careful examination of the milk with a black strip plate cannot be overemphasized. Plates should be examined under reflected lighting to detect subtle changes that may occur early during coliform mastitis.

Tests based on increased milk pH are used for the detection of coliform mastitis in Europe, but such tests are less available in the United States. A CBC may also suggest coliform mastitis because the acute infection and endotoxemia frequently result in a degenerative left shift, with leukopenia, neutropenia, and band neutrophils observed.

Definitive diagnosis can be achieved through bacteriologic cultures of milk. Freezing and thawing the samples before inoculation onto media increases the sensitivity of the test but could also kill some sensitive bacteria. Lack of culture sensitivity despite preculture freezing and thawing is probably the result of phagocytosis and destruction of the causative organisms by mammary gland phagocytes before collection.

Treatment. Treatment of coliform mastitis has been controversial because of the administration of extra-label drugs without specific knowledge of antibiotic withdrawal times and the lack of controlled therapeutic trials under rigorous, blinded conditions. Many experimental studies of coliform mastitis emphasize that infection resolves spontaneously as a result of the inflammatory neutrophilic influx into the gland and that most clinical signs simply represent the effects of endotoxins and other mediators of inflammation on the cow. Although these studies suggest that antibiotics may not be a necessary component of treatment, they are counterbalanced by the high mortality rate from coliform mastitis. It is impossible, clinically, to distinguish signs that are associated with persistent infection from those of persistent endotoxemia, and furthermore continued signs of endotoxemia may imply continued persistence of infection. Even knowing about these studies, the practicing veterinarian may not wish to withhold antibiotic therapy when faced with a greatly distressed or litigious owner whose valuable cow becomes gravely ill with coliform mastitis. Although the majority of experimental studies demonstrate that antibiotic therapy confers no benefit on induced coliform mastitis, there are a smaller number of studies that do show favorable outcomes when severe field cases are treated with antibiotics such as ceftiofur. These findings, taken with the repeated demonstration of true bacteremia in a proportion of cows with naturally occurring coliform mastitis, are strong arguments in favor of systemic antibiotic administration. The pros and cons of antibiotic therapy, albeit controversial, should be understood by bovine practitioners. The pharmacology and likely benefits or risks associated with each antibiotic should be known (see Pharmacology discussion). Currently approved antibiotics for use in lactating cattle are listed in Table 8-1. Antibiotics should be at least considered as therapy for coliform mastitis to ensure complete elimination of the infection and avoidance of chronic infection, and should be used in severe cases.

Studies that report antibiotic susceptibility of gram-negative bacteria causing mastitis have been reported, and the accumulated data from these studies and reviews combined with more recent culture and antibiotic sensitivity results indicate the following:
1. Gentamicin, amikacin, third-generation cephalosporins, and ticarcillin-clavulanic acid work against most coliforms in vitro
2. Polymyxin B and cephalothin work against 60% to 80% in vitro
3. Tetracycline, ampicillin, neomycin, and kanamycin work against 40% to 80% in vitro

Inflammation and serum leakage into the gland increase the pH of the milk to nearly physiologic levels (7.2), which inhibits diffusion of some alkaline drugs into the gland tissue. Inflammation, cellular debris, and decreased ability to diffuse drugs throughout the quarter diminish the effectiveness of antibiotics—especially intramammary antibiotic infusions. Therefore the pharmacology of each drug considered, regardless of antibiotic

sensitivity results, must be evaluated. By and large, weak acids are better choices for intramammary administration for the treatment of clinical mastitis, whereas the weak bases achieve better tissue levels when given systemically. Macrolide antibiotics and potentiated sulfonamides, when given systemically, establish high milk/plasma ratios in healthy cattle because these drugs are weak bases. Tetracycline attains a fair to good milk/plasma ratio when given systemically. Penicillin and ampicillin, weak acids, attain limited ratios in the milk of a healthy cow following parenteral administration. Systemic ceftiofur and the aminoglycosides have the poorest distribution in mastitis patients.

Results of studies examining experimental and natural coliform mastitis treatments are highly confusing. In one field study, no apparent benefit resulted when systemic gentamicin was used in the treatment of coliform mastitis. The reported success in cows treated systemically with gentamicin (to which the organisms were sensitive) was no better than in cows treated systemically with erythromycin, even though the causative organisms were resistant to erythromycin, or in nontreated controls. All quarters in this study were treated with cephalothin, regardless of the systemic antibiotic chosen. This differs from another study that demonstrated a beneficial effect of ceftiofur treatment in cows with severe coliform mastitis. It is no wonder that most practitioners develop an individual or clinic-based approach to the therapy of coliform mastitis in the field based on their own experiences. It has become increasingly important that treatment decisions are made within the framework of federally regulated drug approvals and with due diligence with respect to residue avoidance, especially when extra-label drug use is performed.

Many practitioners use oxytetracycline HCl systemically when treating coliform mastitis. Although the likelihood of sensitivity of the organism to oxytetracycline is only moderate, distribution of the drug to the udder should be good, and the drug may provide some antiinflammatory properties within the udder. Nephrotoxic effects may occur in dehydrated cows treated with oxytetracycline. It is impossible to recommend one treatment because of geographic differences in bacterial populations, resistance patterns of coliform organisms present on each farm, and many other factors. Culture and sensitivity results should be obtained for isolates from each farm to better determine appropriate antibiotic therapy when faced with an acute coliform mastitis.

New antibiotics such as florfenicol, a derivative of chloramphenicol that is not associated with aplastic anemia, and the fluoroquinolones such as norfloxacin are experimental drugs that have been shown to have good distribution via systemic and intramammary routes for bovine mastitis. Despite the therapeutic efficacy of the fluoroquinolones against coliforms, the U.S. FDA has prohibited the use of those drugs in dairy production

TABLE 8-1   Drugs Used in Lactating and Nonlactating Cows

Active Ingredient	Milk Withholding Time*	Meat Withholding Time*
Lactating Cows		
Approved Drugs for Injectable Use		
Amoxicillin trihydrate	96 hr	25 days
Ampicillin	48 hr	6 days
Ceftiofur sodium		
EXCEDE	None	13 days
EXCENEL	None	3 days
NAXCEL	None	4 days
Erythromycin	72 hr	2-14 days
Penicillin G (procaine)	48 hr	4-10 days
Sulfadimethoxine	60 hr	5 days
Approved Drugs for Intramammary Use		
Amoxicillin trihydrate	60 hr	12 days
Ceftiofur hydrochloride	72 hr	2 days
Cephapirin (sodium)	96 hr	4 days
Cloxacillin (sodium)	48 hr	10 days
Erythromycin	36 hr	14 days
Hetacillin (potassium)	72 hr	10 days
Novobiocin	72 hr	15 days
Penicillin G (procaine)	60-84 hr	4-15 days
Pirlimycin	36 hr	9 days
Salicylic acid	48 hr	None
Nonlactating Cows		
Approved Drugs for Intramammary Use		
Ceftiofur	None if treatment 30 days or more before calving	16 days
Cephapirin (benzathine)	72 hr postcalving	42 days
Cloxacillin (benzathine)	None	28-30 days
Dihydrostreptomycin sulfate with procaine penicillin	96 hr postcalving	60 days
Erythromycin	36 hr postcalving	10 days
Novobiocin	72 hr postcalving	30 days
Penicillin G (procaine)	24-96 hr postcalving	14-60 days

Depending on drug type. Any deviation from label instructions is extra-label use. Milk should be routinely tested for antibiotic residues.

animals. One study has suggested that intramammary florfenicol treatment of cows with coliform mastitis had no advantage over intramammary cloxacillin therapy. However, the study did not determine whether the florfenicol when delivered systemically would have a beneficial effect on the survival rate of endotoxemic cattle. Florfenicol is also not approved for lactation-age dairy cows.

Obviously the dosage, vehicle, degree of inflammatory debris or plugging of milk ductules, and nature of the secretion may alter patterns of distribution (Figure 8-47). New formulations will continue to appear on the market following testing, and it is hoped that the pharmacokinetics and efficacy of approved drugs will be further evaluated. Although most farms harbor a multitude of coliforms, culture and antibiotic sensitivity results from previous cases of coliform mastitis should be catalogued for individual farms to provide background data that may be useful in selecting initial therapy for future cases.

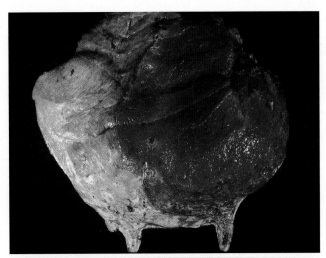

Figure 8-47

Necropsy view of a fatal chronic coliform infection showing a large infarcted zone in the infected gland. Methylene blue was administered IV before euthanasia. It is apparent that neither IV nor local therapy can counteract the walled-off infection in such cases.

Every cow with coliform mastitis should be evaluated individually as to present and future productive and genetic value before a decision to treat with antibiotics is made. Cows of marginal economic or emotional importance may best be culled before initiation of potentially expensive therapy. Prolonged residues in meat and milk as a result of extended use of antibiotics should be avoided unless the cow is deemed valuable enough to live or die on the farm and salvage for meat is not an option. If the cow's life is in jeopardy and extra-label drugs or dosages are deemed necessary to save the cow, the owner and practitioner are responsible for ensuring adequate withdrawal time. Because of fear of residues, antibiotic therapy often is not used or compromised by lack of intensity, reduction in dosages, or shortened duration of treatment. All these factors not only limit the potential for successful treatment but also increase the likelihood of chronic infection or resistant organisms. Although many cases of coliform mastitis are life-threatening, the destruction of glandular tissue is generally less than what occurs with gram-positive infections, and if the cow survives and quickly clears the infection (with or without antibiotics), return to near maximum production may be possible in the next lactation.

Supportive measures are extremely important for a successful therapeutic outcome in cases of coliform mastitis. Supportive therapy should be administered regardless of the decision for or against antibiotic therapy. Frequent milking out of the affected quarter has previously been considered the most valuable nursing procedure. The philosophy behind frequent stripping was that it removed organisms, endotoxins, and mediators of inflammation, as well as neutrophils and macrophages whose products further foster inflammation. Historically stripping every 1 or 2 hours has been advocated, but that has now been refuted with respect to outcome, and current guidelines call for stripping no more than every 4 to 6 hours even in peracute cases. Too frequent stripping may cause the teat sphincter to remain open, allowing other organisms to gain entrance. Chronic cases may also benefit from stripping. Oxytocin (20 IU) may be administered systemically to facilitate milk let down and to remove accumulated endotoxin from the quarter. Alternatively, one or more calves may be placed in a box stall with the affected cow to nurse the quarters frequently.

NSAIDs should be used in an effort to block the prostaglandin-mediated inflammation associated with lipopolysaccharide endotoxemia. Flunixin meglumine is the most potent of these drugs in common use and may be given initially at 0.5 mg/kg every 12 hours, IV for two to three treatments, and then tapered to 0.25 mg/kg at 8- to 12-hour intervals. Aspirin, although not approved for use in lactating cattle, has been used at 1.0 grain/kg at 12-hour intervals as an alternative. It is important to realize that the NSAIDs have been shown to be most effective when administered prophylactically. Obviously, however, in clinical practice, their use is never prophylactic because clinical signs only appear after endotoxemia already has occurred. Nevertheless, NSAIDs are most effective when administered early in the course of the disease. NSAIDs should be used cautiously because they are potentially toxic to the gastrointestinal tract and kidneys. Abomasal ulceration is the most frequent gastrointestinal complication of overdosage, prolonged use, or employment of these drugs (especially flunixin meglumine) in very dehydrated patients. Renal papillary necrosis and renal infarcts may develop in cattle treated with NSAIDs, and dehydration of the patient increases the risk of renal problems. Therefore IV or oral fluids should be administered to correct existing dehydration whenever NSAIDs are used in critically ill patients.

Corticosteroid use in coliform-affected cattle is controversial. Some clinicians use intramammary corticosteroids such as 10 to 20 mg of dexamethasone as a one-time treatment. Other clinicians administer 10 to 40 mg of dexamethasone systemically. Although corticosteroids may alleviate the inflammatory cascade, they present risk of chronic infection and deter defense mechanisms. Corticosteroids should never be used as maintenance therapy, and "shock" dosages, such as 100 to 200 mg of dexamethasone, have been suggested by some clinicians but should be considered as being very dangerous to cattle. A low-dose, one-time treatment may be acceptable in nonpregnant dairy cows with coliform mastitis, but high-dose or continued treatment is contraindicated.

IV fluid therapy is indicated whenever dehydration is obvious or when appetite or water consumption is depressed by the disease. Balanced electrolyte solutions such as lactated Ringer's solution usually are the best choice, but severely affected cattle that show signs of shock coincident with acidemia may require replacement bicarbonate therapy as well. Although metabolic alkalosis is the most common acid-base disturbance in off-feed cattle, peracute/acute coliform mastitis is one of the few common illnesses in adults that is often associated with metabolic acidosis. If the patient shows profound weakness, an acid-base and electrolyte panel should be submitted to guide further fluid and electrolyte replacement. Many clinicians use hypertonic saline (1 to 3 L IV) as therapy for dehydrated, endotoxic patients, but it is important to remember that there needs to be follow-up administration of large-volume IV or, more practically, oral fluids following the infusion of such hypertonic solutions.

Calcium should be administered to all multiparous cows that develop coliform mastitis because of the likelihood of clinical or subclinical hypocalcemia. In cattle with coliform mastitis that are able to stand, calcium is more safely administered subcutaneously or diluted in 5 to 10 L of IV fluids. Cattle that are recumbent may require careful and slow IV administration.

Antihistamine therapy also is controversial. Many authors comment that no true indication exists for the use of antihistamines, but some experimental studies confirm the presence of increased concentrations of histamines in the milk of cattle with coliform infections. These studies have been taken to indicate the potential therapeutic benefits of antihistamine therapy in coliform-infected cattle. Counteraction of oxygen free radicals using antioxidant drugs including dimethyl sulfoxide (DMSO) cannot be recommended because of the lack of FDA approval of the compound for use in food-producing animals and the lack of proven efficacy. In fact, DMSO is illegal and should not be used in cattle. Other nursing procedures include packing the quarter in ice or snow and application of an udder support. It is of interest to note that recombinant bovine somatotrophin (BST) administration appears to confer a production benefit during the remainder of lactation for cows that have suffered from coliform mastitis. The increase in production is not as significant in cows with severe coliform mastitis compared with those with milder clinical disease but is also paralleled by a quicker return to normal milk composition.

Cows with persistent anorexia may require repeated treatment with IV or oral fluid supplementation, rumen transfaunations and feeding of slurries with alfalfa pellets, rumen bypass fats, and probiotics to reestablish rumen function.

Implementation of a single protocol for treatment of coliform mastitis in dairy cattle seems futile because of the varying economic factors, the severity differences among cows, availability of approved drugs, intended

future of the patient, and past experiences of the attending veterinarian. Therapeutic guidelines are offered in Tables 8-1 and 8-2 and Box 8-2. Culture and antibiotic sensitivity testing should be completed in all cases.

Prevention. Other than implementation of good milking management and the provision of a hygienic, clean environment, no reliable specific prevention for coliform mastitis currently exists. However, attempts at prevention of the disease, or at least, the reduction of severity of the endotoxemia through the use of *E. coli* J-5 vaccine is indicated. Currently the J-5 strain of *E. coli*, which is an R-mutant strain possessing core antigens similar to other coliform organisms, has been shown to be effective in decreasing severe disease from coliform infections in cattle. Briefly, an *E. coli* J-5 bacterin has been used to immunize dairy cattle and has resulted in decreased incidence of coliform mastitis in vaccinates versus controls in the same herds. Use of J-5 bacterin has also been shown to be of economic benefit in well-managed herds. The vaccine is licensed for administration to dairy cattle at 7 and 8 months of gestation and then a third time around 2 weeks postpartum. Regardless of the efficacy of the J-5 vaccine, bacterins must not be used as an excuse for poor management or dirty conditions. No vaccine can counteract overwhelming environmental contamination or poor milking procedures.

Other Gram-Negative Bacterial Causes

Etiology. *Pseudomonas* spp. and *Serratia* spp. occasionally cause mastitis in dairy cattle. Infections may be epidemic, sporadic, or endemic within a herd. Epidemics

TABLE 8-2	Extra-Label Drugs
Drug	**Dosage**
Extra-Label Intramammary Drugs*	
Gentamicin	300-500 mg in 250 ml sterile saline
Amikacin	400-600 mg in 250 ml sterile saline
Polymyxin B	500,000 U in 60 ml sterile saline
Ticarcillin	1000 mg in 100 ml sterile water or other approved diluent
Ticarcillin-clavulanic acid	1000 mg diluted in 100 ml sterile water or other approved diluent
Extra-Label Systemic Drugs	
Ampicillin	12-22 mg/kg twice daily
Oxytetracycline	7.5-12 mg/kg twice daily
Gentamicin	6.6 mg/kg daily
Amikacin	20 mg/kg daily
Ceftiofur	3-4 mg/kg twice daily

*Extra-label dosages of even approved intramammary products would include any deviation from label recommendations.

Box 8-2	**Therapy for Cattle Having Coliform Mastitis (antibiotic usage must be considered as ancillary to the other suggested treatments)**

Treatment for coliform mastitis with minimal systemic signs

A. Strip out quarter frequently for first day ± oxytocin prior to stripping
B. Administer calcium subcutaneously
C. Administer intramammary therapy following first and last milkout of the day, and leave in for 4 hours or until first morning milking (ceftiofur or aminoglycoside, plus polymyxin B)
D. If improvement in 24 hours, continue A and C or administer some intramammary drug twice daily for six to eight total treatments. (The decision as to milk out frequently or treat quarters twice daily will be made based on how much secretion is obtained via frequent stripping. If secretion is obtained with each stripping, it is beneficial to continue 4 times/day strippings and treat intramammary at night. If little or no secretion is obtained because of agalactia, twice-daily treatment following milking-time stripping is indicated.)

Coliform mastitis with moderate systemic signs

A. Strip out quarter frequently ± oxytocin prior
B. Administer flunixin 0.3 mg/kg three times daily
C. Administer calcium subcutaneously
D. Assess and correct hydration deficits
E. Administer intramammary therapy as above
F. Systemic antibiotics: the systemic drug should be the same drug as used intramammary or one that attains good distribution to the udder following systemic administration

G. If improvement within 24 hours, continue stripping intramammary and systemic antibiotics at least 3 days

Coliform mastitis with severe systemic signs and endotoxemia

A. Strip out quarter frequently following oxytocin injection
B. Administer flunixin 1.0 mg/kg once daily
C. Administer calcium subcutaneously if standing or very slowly intravenously if recumbent
D. Administer 20 to 40 L balanced intravenous fluids or 2 to 3 L hypertonic saline, and consider submission of blood acid-base and electrolytes to guide fluid therapy
E. Administer intramammary antibiotics as discussed above
F. Administer systemic antibiotics as discussed above
G. Consider ancillary drugs such as antihistamine, intramammary corticosteroids or dexamethasone 30 mg IM (once only); do not use in late pregnancy
H. Continue to address fluid needs, and consider feeding via stomach tube twice daily

Chronic or intermittent coliform mastitis with minimal systemic signs

A. Following completion of culture and antibiotic sensitivity results, treat quarter for at least eight consecutive times following milking, or select appropriate dry cow formulation to treat when dry

of *Pseudomonas* mastitis have been associated with contaminated wash hoses and water supplies in milking parlors. Water tanks, hoses, and pipeline connectors should be suspected as harboring *Pseudomonas* sp. whenever cases of this type of mastitis are diagnosed. Antibiotics or sublethal concentrations of sanitizers may allow proliferation of *Pseudomonas* sp. or the development of resistant strains phenotypically expressing glycocalyx or slime. Contaminated udder infusion vials, cannulas, or syringes are other common sources of *Pseudomonas* sp. Filthy environments and lack of udder preparation may predispose to mastitis by *Pseudomonas* sp. as well.

Although sporadic infection from *Pseudomonas* sp. is possible because of poor management and milking procedures, herd epidemics usually have a point source that frequently is contaminated teat dip.

Serratia, another opportunistic environmental pathogen, may also survive in chlorhexidine digluconate and quaternary ammonia products. The agent does not

survive in recommended concentrations of iodine or chlorhexidine acetate. Contaminated infusion devices and intramammary infusions are another source of *Serratia* infections.

Signs. *Pseudomonas* sp. causes acute, necrotizing, endotoxic mastitis. The affected quarter remains very hard, swollen, and warm. The secretion is serum-like or blood-tinged and often contains clots. Following initial infection, the quarter may remain hard and agalactic or may improve somewhat but remain clinical with clots or pus in the secretion. Chronic mastitis with intermittent clinical flareups or subclinical infection is also possible. Somatic cell values are elevated in herd outbreaks.

Serratia liquefaciens or *Serratia marcescens* cause a chronic subclinical or clinical mastitis that has no unique signs. Secretion tends to be serous with clots. A high SCC and several new intramammary infections may be the only signs. Persistent infection is likely once *Serratia* sp. has colonized the mammary gland.

Diagnosis. Both organisms require culture because signs are nonspecific. Environmental samples and milking equipment (e.g., teat dip cups, wash hoses) should be cultured as well, once these organisms have been identified in a herd.

Treatment. Treatment of *Pseudomonas* sp. rarely is successful because of tissue necrosis within the gland, the resistance of the bacterium to antimicrobials, the tendency of the bacterium to become septicemic, and the difficulties of penetrating the udder by antimicrobials. Chronic infections may appear to improve clinically, but infected cattle usually shed *Pseudomonas* sp. for the remainder of their lives. Treatment of a valuable cow should be based on results of cultures and sensitivity tests because of the antibiotic resistance associated with *Pseudomonas* sp. Sterilization of a *Pseudomonas*-infected quarter is unlikely, even with large doses of antimicrobials. When obvious chronic mastitis or agalactia is present, affected cattle should be culled.

Treatment of *Serratia* sp. should be based on culture and sensitivity results for cows deemed valuable enough to treat. Because mastitis resulting from *Serratia* sp. tends to be chronic, treatment should be intense and continue for several days to yield the best chance of success. Many cows may spontaneously resolve the infection. Cows that remain culture positive after treatment should receive an appropriate dry treatment medication. Treatment needs to address the source of infection in endemic situations. An epidemiologic investigation and cultures from possible fomites should be completed.

Yeast Mastitis

Etiology. Yeast mastitis is most commonly caused by *Candida* spp. The yeast infects the mammary gland iatrogenically through contaminated infusion cannulas, syringes, or multidose mammary infusion solutions. Yeast mastitis almost always is secondary to a primary acute bacterial mastitis that required treatment by the owner. Persistent swelling of the gland and abnormal secretion finally force the owner to seek veterinary advice.

Yeast grows very well in the presence of some antibiotics. Therefore continued use of antibiotics or combinations of antibiotics by the owner in an effort to cure this "resistant" infection only perpetuates the yeast infection. Corticosteroids worsen the condition. Yeasts reside on the mucosal lining and cause inflammation from this location.

Signs. Yeast infections produce a diffusely swollen doughlike quarter. The affected cow may have fever (103.0 to 106.0° F/39.44 to 41.11° C) but does not appear severely depressed or endotoxic. Cows with high fever may be depressed and partially anorectic, but the majority of infected animals remain alert and appetent. Invariably the owner of a cow with yeast mastitis relays a history of chronic mastitis (1 to 3 weeks duration) that has not responded to therapy with a variety of intramammary antimicrobials.

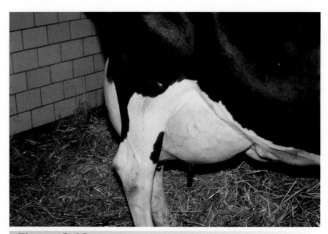

Figure 8-48

Swollen udder on a cow with yeast mastitis in all four glands.

The degree of swelling in yeast-infected quarters varies but is often dramatic (Figure 8-48). Edema and moderate inflammation create a doughy consistency. Because the glandular parenchyma is not infected, the quarter seldom feels "hard." The secretion varies from almost normal milk that is slightly watery to one with clots or flakes. The secretion from an infected gland may change appearance from day to day.

Diagnosis. The chronic history, appearance of the infected gland, and good systemic condition of the affected cow suggest the diagnosis. A stained smear of milk from the quarter or culture provides definitive diagnosis (Figure 8-49).

Treatment. Spontaneous cure will occur in most cows affected with yeast mastitis if all antibiotic therapy is stopped and the affected quarters are milked out four or more times daily. Resolution of the infection usually takes 2 to 6 weeks. Despite the likelihood of spontaneous cures, owners need reassurance of success to resist the temptation to try yet another antibiotic. A variety of antifungal or antiyeast preparations have been used to treat yeast mastitis. Miconazole, nystatin, and iodine in

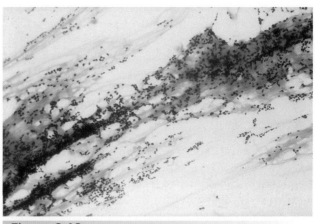

Figure 8-49

Gram stain of milk culture from the cow in Figure 8-48.

ether preparations have been used, but it is difficult to evaluate success of any therapy because of the high rate of spontaneous cure.

Prevention should be addressed whenever yeast mastitis is diagnosed. Although most cases are sporadic, endemic incidence has been observed as a result of contaminated multidose mastitis formulations. Client education is essential whenever iatrogenic problems occur in intramammary therapy.

Other Agents

Aspergillus spp. and other opportunistic fungi gain access to the udder through the same mechanisms as *Candida*. Severe, potentially fatal mastitis has been documented in association with *Trichophyton beigelii* in the United States. Nocardia, a partially acid-fast bacterium, has been isolated rarely from cattle. Little is known regarding spontaneous cure, treatment, or prognosis. Culture is essential for definitive diagnosis. Antimicrobial treatment would necessitate miconazole, clotrimazole, ketoconazole, or other antifungal drugs, but efficacy data for these drugs are lacking, and some may be illegal for use in cattle. Those cows with hard quarters and persistent fever should have the gland killed if it is desirable for the cow to stay in the herd.

Cryptococcus neoformans has been reported to cause mastitis and represents a public health risk if contaminated raw milk is consumed.

Prototheca Spp.

Etiology. Cattle can develop mastitis when infected by the algae *Prototheca* spp. *Prototheca zopfii* is most common, but *Prototheca wickerhamii* and *Prototheca trispora* also have been identified from infected glands. *Prototheca* spp. are widespread in the environment and are found routinely in mud, feces, water, stagnant ponds, and other locations. Most reports of protothecal mastitis appear to be from tropical or subtropical environments. *Prototheca* spreads within a herd as an environmental pathogen. The agent has been isolated from the environment of farms that have never had a clinical case of *Prototheca* mastitis. Therefore management, milking procedures, or contaminated intramammary infusions probably initiate *Prototheca* mastitis. When ingested, *Prototheca* spp. pass through the intestinal tract intact and contaminate the environment. Persistent long-term enteric infections with fecal shedding in herdmates after removal of infected animals have been reported. Public health concerns exist to some degree because infections have been reported in immunocompromised humans. Unpasteurized milk should not be consumed from dairies that harbor cattle with protothecosis.

Signs. Affected mammary glands have watery secretions and are firm. There are usually no systemic signs of *Prototheca* sp. infection. Milk production from infected quarters is greatly decreased. The affected cattle do not respond to intramammary antimicrobial

therapy. SCCs are increased. Subclinical infections have been documented.

Diagnosis. Definitive diagnosis of *Prototheca* mastitis requires microscopic identification and culture of the organism. Tissue biopsy and histopathology of infected glands have demonstrated that the organism invades cells and glandular parenchyma. Therefore as opposed to yeast that simply affect the mucosa, *Prototheca* infections are tissue-invasive and unlikely to resolve. Definitive identification of the alga in tissue is possible because it appears round or ovoid (2 to 15 μm in diameter), forms endospores by mitosis, and does not have budding forms or pseudomycelia.

Treatment. Treatment fails to improve or only transiently improves the secretion.

Cows with *Prototheca* should be culled. Management for prevention of *Prototheca* mastitis should include improved milking procedures, mechanical cleaning and disinfection of water supplies and feed troughs, and fencing cattle from algal concentrations in mud holes, ponds, and irrigation ditches. The algae are usually disseminated through the environment, making source identification and successful eradication difficult.

Corynebacterium bovis

Although little is known about this organism, it occasionally is cultured from individual quarters and bulk tank samples. The organism has been shown to colonize teat skin and the streak canal or teat canal. There appears to be minimal mastitis or true infection of the gland, but SCCs can be slightly elevated. The isolation of *C. bovis* from milk cultures basically indicates poor teat dipping procedures or products. Effective teat dipping, coupled with dry cow therapy, should correct the problem.

Clostridium perfringens type A

Clostridium perfringens type A is a rare cause of gangrenous mastitis in first-calf heifers. The heifers are acutely ill from septicemia, and the udder is discolored and has a crepitant feel because of the gas production. It should be noted that gas in the udder is not pathognomonic for *C. perfringens* because other causes of gangrenous mastitis, including *S. aureus*, *Pseudomonas aeruginosa*, *Corynebacterium*, and *A. pyogenes*, can have palpable gas in the udder. Additionally, some cows with coliform mastitis have palpable gas in the udder; it is unclear if this is a superinfection with anaerobic bacteria or if it occurs from unusually frequent stripping action allowing air to enter the udder.

Diagnosis. First-calf heifers with acute gangrenous mastitis and large amounts of crepitus in the udder are likely candidates for the diagnosis. Gram stain of the milk will reveal large numbers of large gram-positive rods. Anaerobic cultures will confirm the diagnosis.

Treatment. The treatment is three pronged: administration of high levels of penicillin both systemically and intramammary, shock treatment (fluids, flunixin), and drainage of necrotic tissue via teat removal or incision into necrotic skin and udder. With aggressive early treatment, the prognosis for survival is good, but future production from the affected quarter is unlikely.

CAUSES REQUIRING PUBLIC HEALTH CONCERN (TABLE 8-3)

Detection and Monitoring for Udder Health

Complete mastitis surveillance requires a combination of cowside and laboratory tests. Although not all herds require all available tests, the veterinarian should be familiar with the tests that supplement physical examination of the udder and may detect subclinical mastitis.

Cowside Tests

Strip Plate or Cup. A black-colored strip plate is invaluable in detecting abnormal secretions in forestrippings. Although flakes and clots may be palpable or obvious on other surfaces, subtle serum-like or watery milk can best be detected by mixing with milk from other quarters on the black background with surface illumination. Large milking parlors may have black floor tiles placed strategically under the cow's udder to evaluate forestrippings for incidence of gross mastitis. The problem with this technique is that forestripped milk hitting the floor will spray or spatter, making it difficult to pool the milk as one can do by gently stripping into a strip plate. In addition, this spraying of milk may spread contagious organisms.

California Mastitis Test. The CMT qualitatively estimates the amount of DNA in milk secretions. The concentrations of DNA and white blood cells (WBCs) in milk are directly correlated. The CMT reagent lyses the cells and gels the DNA. The amount of gel formation can be used to estimate the numbers of WBCs in the milk sample. The test is subjectively read as negative, trace, +1, +2, and +3; these scores equate well with somatic cell levels as listed in Table 8-3. The CMT is most helpful in detecting subclinical mastitis and, although accurate, serves little purpose in acute clinical mastitis.

A CMT will tend to have a high score in recently fresh cows and in cows at the end of lactation just before dry off. A CMT is also elevated in secretions from cows whose milk production has decreased precipitously because of illness. For example, cows in peak lactation that become acutely ill as a result of traumatic reticuloperitonitis may

---

TABLE 8-3 Causes of Mastitis That Require Public Health Concern

Organism	Means of Infection of Udder	Signs	Diagnosis	Treatment and Control
Salmonella dublin*	Environmental contamination by feces of carrier cows most likely Possible result of septicemic spread to udder	Usually subclinical and chronic (≥6 mo) Increased somatic cell count may be present Steroids may cause acute clinical flareup	ELISA (IDETEK Inc., San Bruno CA) performed on serum or milk to detect antibodies in carrier cows Culture milk and feces	None. Detection and culling of carriers should be performed to avoid milk contamination Prohibit drinking of raw milk
Listeria monocytogenes	Septicemic spread to udder usually Possible environmental contamination by feces of cows ingesting *L. monocytogenes*	Neurologic signs Abortions Subclinical	Only diagnostic signs appear in neurologic form Culture	Prohibit drinking raw milk Pasteurization of milk regardless of intended use
Brucella abortus	Septicemic spread to udder	Abortions	Serology Culture	Prohibit drinking raw milk Regulatory intervention
Staphylococcus spp. producing enterotoxin†	Contagious or environmental	Subclinical ± acute flareups Elevated somatic cell count	Culture Culture of bulk tank raw milk	Inadequate refrigeration or prolonged storage should be avoided Pasteurization essential Do not drink raw milk

TABLE 8-3 Causes of Mastitis That Require Public Health Concern—cont'd.

Organism	Means of Infection of Udder	Signs	Diagnosis	Treatment and Control
Nocardia asteroides‡§	Contaminated intramammary multiple-dose vials, syringes, or cannulas Environmental contamination by infected secretions	Acute mastitis in recently fresh cows with fever and hard quarters Mild or subclinical mastitis in cows further into lactation. These cows then may develop acute, severe mastitis following their next freshening or may remain chronically infected with subclinical or intermittent acute flareups. Fibrosis of the gland is progressive in most infected cattle, and some cows develop pyogranulomatous reactions in infected quarters. This may lead to fistulas or draining abscesses.	Culture	Treatment seldom successful Identification and culling of infected cows Do not drink raw milk
Cryptococcus neoformans (rare) ‖	Contaminated intramammary products	Acute mastitis and mammary lymph node enlargement Thick gray-white secretion	Culture Stained smears Udder biopsy	Cull affected cows Do not drink raw milk

*From Spier SJ, et al: Persistent experimental Salmonella dublin *intramammary infection in dairy cows,* J Vet Intern Med *5:341–350, 1991.*

†From Cullor JS, Tyler JW, Smith BP: Disorders of the mammary gland. In Smith BP, editor: Large animal internal medicine, *St. Louis, 1990, CV Mosby.*

‡From Sears PM: Nocardial mastitis in cattle: diagnosis, treatment, and prevention, *Compend Contin Educ Pract Vet 8:F41–F46, 1986.*

§From Linquist WE: Nocardial mastitis—a case report, *unpublished observations, Ithaca, NY, 1979.*

‖From Blood DC, Radostits OM: Veterinary medicine. A textbook of the diseases of cattle, sheep, pigs, goats and horses, *ed 7, Philadelphia, 1989,* Baillière Tindall [*with contributions by JH Arundel and CC Gay*].

have milk production plummet acutely. Although these cows do not have mastitis, based on normal udder palpation and strip plate evaluation, the CMT will be positive. The high CMT scores represent a failure of fluid milk production to dilute the somatic cells.

Because results of the CMT are interpreted subjectively, discrepancies may arise between evaluators, and estimates of SCC that correlate with CMT score vary greatly. Therefore the values listed in Table 8-4 are composites of several reported values of CMT scores versus SCC. Ample evidence demonstrates that loss of production correlates directly with CMT scores. This factor may be useful when convincing owners to use mastitis detection aids. Production losses from quarters with CMT trace values may be 5% or more, and losses from quarters having CMT +3 values may be 25% to 50%.

pH Indicator Papers. These test strips, which are widely used in Europe, detect the more alkaline pH in quarters with mastitis. Normal milk has a pH of approximately 6.5 to 6.7, whereas mastitic milk often approaches plasma pH of 7.4.

Palpation of the Udder. Perhaps becoming a lost art, udder palpation once formed the heart of mastitis control programs. Careful udder palpation is helpful for detection of fibrosis caused by chronic subclinical contagious *S. aureus* infection. Palpation also is useful for differentiation of high mastitis-related CMT results from false-positive CMT scores as a result of acute dry off or systemic illness. The palpation of a swollen udder and serum-like appearance of mastitic milk are both findings that suggest the cow will need to be treated for several days. Palpation also is valuable following resolution of

TABLE 8-4	Relationship of Linear Scores to Actual Somatic Cell Counts
CMT Score	**Approximate Somatic Cell Count**
Negative	0-200,000
Trace	150,000-500,000
+1	400,000-1 million
+2	800,000-5 million
+3	>5 million
Linear Score	**Somatic Cell Count Midpoint**
0	12,500
1	25,000
2	50,000
3	100,000
4	200,000
5	400,000
6	800,000
7	1.6 million
8	3.2 million
9	6.4 million

acute clinical mastitis to detect glandular changes that may be associated with infarction, abscessation, or chronic infection.

Somatic Cell Counts

The SCC has become the most widely used indicator of infection within individual cows and herds. Monitoring of somatic cell numbers has been simplified by automated cell counters that allow large numbers of milk samples to be evaluated quickly. Monitoring individual quarters or composite samples from all four quarters allows specific information helpful in decisions regarding treatment or culling. Monitoring bulk tank samples for SCC gives the owner and veterinarian a frequent reminder of the overall level of mastitis control in the herd.

Mastitis increases the relative proportion of neutrophils in mammary secretions to 95%. Other cell types in mastitic milk include mononuclear and sloughed alveolar epithelial cells. Economic losses are caused by reduced productivity that begins whenever the SCC reaches 50,000 and increases with each doubling of the SCC from 50,000 up to 400,000. Above 400,000 cells/ml of milk, production losses continue to increase but not as dramatically as below this level. A bulk tank sample showing an SCC of 500,000 or greater indicates a greater than 50% infection rate.

As regards bulk tank SCC, just a few cows with acute *S. agalactiae* mastitis may elevate the total tank SCC greatly because large numbers of neutrophils tend to be

produced in acute *S. agalactiae* infection. Perhaps more dangerous is that contagious *S. aureus* may be present in 50% or more of the herd before the bulk tank SCC reaches a level causing alarm (500,000 cells/ml).

SCCs, as discussed with CMT, tend to be higher for individual cows during the first 2 weeks and last 2 weeks of lactation and lower during peak lactation. A decrease in daily milk production of 20 lb for example increases the SCC because of nonspecific concentration of cells. Somatic cells tend to be higher in afternoon milkings, which undoubtedly occurs because of the shorter milking interval and less fluid milk dilution of the sloughed cells. Therefore increased frequency of milking (3 to 4 times/day) may elevate SCC but may benefit the herd because with increased milking frequency there is less time for new intramammary infections to develop. Therefore the tendency for increased SCC caused by shorter milking intervals may be offset by a lesser incidence of mastitis in well-managed dairies. Other factors such as season, age of cows, and relative numbers of cows at various stages of lactation may influence SCC from bulk tanks or individual cows. Debate continues concerning the effect, if any, of aging on the SCC. Some experts state that SCC increases with age, whereas others argue that this just reflects increased probability of infection or the results of previous infection in older cattle. Older cattle with two consecutive monthly SCCs greater than 600,000 (or heifers having >400,000) probably are infected.

Because of the variation in SCC as a result of multiple factors, a linear score method has been devised and is used by many dairy herd improvement cooperatives and mastitis control services. The relationship of linear scores to SCCs is listed in Table 8-4. Linear scores less than 4 indicate less than a 10% probability of infection, whereas a linear score greater than 5 indicates a greater than 90% probability of infection with causes of contagious mastitis. Accuracy of correlation is not as great with environmental pathogens, however. Reported linear score values can be averaged and are reported as current, average, and last year's on dairy herd improvement (DHI) records. When examined concurrently with culture results, linear score values are very helpful to decision making for treatment of infection, dry cow therapy, and culling. Heifers may lose an average of 200 pounds of production with each linear score value of 3 or more during the first lactation. Multiparous cows may lose an average of 400 pounds of production per lactation with each increase in linear score starting at 3. Goals for herds include linear scores of less than 4, and concern is amplified by a linear score of greater than 5.

SCCs from all individual cows are more valuable than only bulk tank SCCs because a treated cow's milk does not enter the tank. Because of this, a high incidence of clinical mastitis could exist despite a normal bulk tank SCC. Combining the tank SCC with bacterial plate counts and cultures from the bulk tank may add more information, especially revealing milking and storage problems, but information from individual cows may be essential when mastitis problems exist.

As regards bulk tank samples, goals include an SCC less than 300,000, and this figure should be no more than 200,000 in well-managed dairies. Many herds that practice good milking techniques and hygiene, as well as control of contagious mastitis problems, have bulk tank SCCs of less than 100,000, and this level should be sought by all dairies striving for excellent milk quality. Milk with low SCCs yields cheese with superior flavor and greater quantity. The National Conference of Interstate Milk Shipments recently lowered the allowable bulk tank SCC standard in the Grade "A" Pasteurized Milk Ordinance to 750,000 cells/ml from the previous level of 1 million cells/ml. Dairies are monitored by at least four bulk tank SCC tests every 6 months. If the SCC exceeds limits in three of five samples, the producer permit for grade A milk will be suspended. In some states, sanctions will be imposed if two of the four samples have SCCs greater than 750,000. Individual states may further restrict SCC limits, and the trend for the future will be continued reduction in allowable SCC limits.

Culturing

Bulk tank cultures may be used as an indication of specific contagious mastitis organisms such as *S. agalactiae* and *Mycoplasma* sp. or as an indicator of milking hygiene. Filthy environments, poor udder preparation, milking wet udders, and other milking procedural problems may increase the numbers of coliforms and other environmental bacterial numbers on plate counts. Other causes of increased bacterial numbers in bulk tank samples are inadequate cooling of milk as a result of mixing or refrigeration problems and poorly sanitized equipment or pipelines. If the sample is taken with the intent of identifying mastitis problems in the herd, the sample should be taken 1 or 2 hours after a milking is added to the tank.

Many different culture methods have been recommended for bulk milk, but probably the most important are the SPC, laboratory pasteurized count (LPC), *Mycoplasma* culture, coliform count, and cultures for other contagious forms of mastitis. The milk should be agitated before collecting the sample, and it should be collected by a sterile dipper into the tank rather than from the outlet valve, which might have a high concentration of environmental bacteria.

Public health concerns may dictate special culture procedures. Bulk tank milk can be contaminated by zoonotic organisms such as *Salmonella* sp. or *Listeria monocytogenes* that may be concurrently causing other health problems in the herd (see Table 8-3).

Bulk tank cultures may identify high numbers of specific contagious organisms *(S. agalactiae)* and indicate a herd problem that requires individual cow cultures. *Mycoplasma* and *S. aureus* may be shed intermittently in

milk by a small percentage of the herd and may be detectable only after repeated cultures.

Except for cases of *S. agalactiae* mastitis, SPCs are general indicators of milking and management problems. The SPCs do not reflect cases of *E. coli* mastitis because the affected milk would most likely be discarded or affected animals would be agalactic because of the systemic effects of the condition. Therefore high bulk tank milk coliform counts usually reflect a combination of poor hygiene, bad milking technique, refrigeration failures, or unsanitary milking equipment. Coliform counts should be well <50 CFU/ml. Excellent total plate counts should record fewer than 1000 colonies/ml milk, whereas counts greater than 100,000 cause milk to be rejected by processing plants. Plate counts should be less than 5000 in well-managed herds, and counts of 10,000 or more warrant a complete evaluation of milking and mammary health in the herd.

The LPC, which measures heat-resistant bacterial numbers in postpasteurized milk, is run by the processing dairy and may give helpful information. The postpasteurization count is performed on milk that has left and consequently is an indicator of hygiene in the tank truck or the milk-processing equipment. The LPC measures heat-resistant bacteria in the bulk tank milk at the farm. Bacteria that survive pasteurization are environmental contaminants from udder skin or from contaminated, milking equipment, including pipelines. Biofilms on the surfaces of milking equipment make excellent incubators for pasteurization-resistant bacteria. LPCs of >200 CFU/ml are most often caused by equipment cleaning problems. The preliminary incubation count (PIC), performed by holding the tank milk at 55° F for 18 hours before culturing, gives an indication of on-farm sanitation. If the PIC is three times the SPC, and the SCC is <250,000, this would indicate a problem with milking and storage sanitation.

Individual cow (composite) or quarter samples provide the most in-depth means of monitoring herd mastitis status and provide the only clear-cut method to monitor new intramammary infections. Debate exists as to whether milk samples for culture should be collected before or after milking. Currently the New York State Mastitis Program recommends postmilking samples because fewer contaminants occur in them. The teats should be clean and *dry*. Alcohol swabs should be used to wipe the teat end carefully before and after sampling. Collection tubes should be sterile and held horizontally with the cap downward to minimize contamination by the teat end or material falling off the udder. After collection, milk should be stored at 4.0 to 5.0° C until cultures are instituted. On farm cultures of mastitis cases may be accomplished by Petrifilm culture system.

Well-managed herds free of contagious organisms with excellent bulk tank and individual cow SCC monitoring may not need to culture as often or as many cows to stay abreast of current pathogens and new intramammary infections. Whenever contagious organisms are identified or high SCCs are the rule, every cow should be cultured to establish the causative organism(s), and the potential for successful lactation or dry cow therapy should be factored into all cull decisions.

Veterinarians should encourage clients to enlist the services of mastitis control programs to aid them in interpreting results and institute programs to improve udder health in each herd.

Prevention and Control of Mastitis

Milking Hygiene

Premilking hygiene can be accomplished by washing the teats with clean, uncontaminated water with or without sanitizers or by predipping teats in an approved teat dip. Excessive wetting of the udder should be avoided because the flowing water can carry bacteria down the teat and into the milk, increasing the risk for new infection and contaminating raw milk with excessive amounts of environmental bacteria. Washing should be done with individual towels, and milkers should wear latex or nitrile gloves. Gloved hands should be rinsed and sanitized often during milking, especially when milkers' hands become contaminated with milk. Iodine at 25 to 75 ppm can be added to the wash solution. Large dairies with automated group sprinklers or washers should allow the udder and teat skin to dry for 10 to 15 minutes before milking. Under no circumstances should milking units be applied to wet teats. Environmental bacteria are suspended in the water droplets and increase the risk for infection to individual cows. Common washing solutions, sponges, or rags should not be used because of the high risk for bacterial contamination. Use of a common washcloth is a well-established cause of cow-to-cow transmission of contagious forms of mastitis including *S. aureus* and *S. agalactiae*. Forestripping should be completed before or during the premilking cleansing. This procedure removes bacteria from the teat end and streak canal and allows surveillance for abnormal milk.

Predipping teats with a teat dip approved for premilking teat sanitation has become a common practice throughout North America. This procedure may be especially effective at reducing new coliform and *S. uberis* infections. When properly used, this technique reduces the number of environmental bacteria on the teat end but is not necessary on dairies that have effective mastitis and hygiene control programs. Predipping with 1% iodophor after washing the udder is most effective when used on cows in their first and second lactations. The predip should be allowed to stay in contact with the teat for 20 to 30 seconds before being wiped away with a single-use towel before milking. Proper contact time and removal of the predip to avoid residual iodine contamination of milk are essential.

Backflushing of the teat cups and claw is another disinfection technique that is effective in minimizing the spread of contagious bacteria and mycoplasma on some farms. Usually acid-iodophor sanitizers diluted to a final concentration of 30 to 40 ppm iodophor and phosphoric acid are used. Iodine concentrations of >50 ppm have been used but may cause ocular irritation to milkers. Alkaline water and hard water decrease the effectiveness of iodophor sanitizers. Backflushing sanitizers are effective for killing both staphylococci and mycoplasma. The use of backflushing increases the amount of time that is required for milking, and therefore some farms are reluctant to use this procedure. However, the effectiveness of backflushing for minimizing spread of contagious pathogens has varied from farm to farm. The considerable cost of backflushing technology has also contributed to its limited adoption.

Postmilking teat dips are important for reducing new intramammary infections from contagious organisms and, to a lesser degree, from environmental pathogens. Teat dips can only help prevent new intramammary infections and will not affect the duration of existing infections. Both dips and sprays are available. Sprays do not become contaminated after successive uses but must be carefully applied to completely contact the teat end. Cup application of teat dips will provide more effective and uniform coverage of teat skin. Teat dips provide superior contact with the sphincter, but the contents must be replaced frequently to prevent contamination by environmental pathogens. Iodophors are combinations of iodine and complexing agents that establish equilibrium but do not bind I_2 molecules. The free I_2 molecules are the active form and continue to be released from the complexing agent as the solution is used. Iodophors are very effective against contagious pathogens when used as a 1% or 0.5% solution. Lower strength iodophor dilutions also may be effective and are less irritating to tissue but are rapidly inactivated by organic debris. Teat dips with alternative sanitizers, including quaternary ammonia, chlorhexidine, hydrogen peroxide, chlorous acid, chlorine dioxide, and sodium hypochlorite, that are approved by the U.S. FDA for postmilking teat dips are also available. The National Mastitis Council (NMC) maintains a bibliography of premilking and postmilking teat dips evaluated under NMC guidelines. Although the NMC does not endorse any particular teat dip product, this bibliography provides information concerning specific products evaluated scientifically in accordance with NMC protocols and published in peer-reviewed scientific journals. Some germicides may harbor pathogenic bacteria in contaminated applicators or initiate teat-end irritation and decrease resistance in the cow. It is critical that teat dippers be cleaned and sanitized daily.

Physical barrier dips made of latex and acrylics are among the other products marketed to reduce the risk for new infection of the mammary gland. Barrier dips were designed to provide prolonged protection against environmental pathogens. Barrier dips must be carefully removed before the next milking to avoid contamination of milking equipment, lines, and claws with latex when these products are used. Teat dip should be stored carefully to avoid either freezing or exposure to high temperatures. Freezing of dips has caused separation of the contents or layering that rendered the solution ineffective or irritating.

Iodine concentrations in milk are a public health concern; however, iodophors used properly in udder wash, backflushing, and dipping results in less than 500 μg/L iodine residue in milk.

Selection of a teat dip should be based on the identity of a herd's pathogens, knowledge of the environment, milking procedures, hygiene, and mastitis prevalence. Teat dip programs that have been effective should not be changed. When used in accordance with the label instructions, most teat dip programs decrease new intramammary infections caused by contagious pathogens by more than 50%. When environmental pathogens are the major mastitis problem, barrier dips and predipping may be considered. When extremely low environmental temperatures or wind chill predispose to frostbite, teat dipping with aqueous solutions may be suspended. Suspending postmilking teat dipping may place the herd at greater risk for new infections particularly if contagious pathogens (*S. agalactiae*, *S. aureus*, or *Mycoplasma* mastitis) are present in the herd. In these situations, rapid drying dips are best to avoid damage to the teat end. If cows experience teat-skin or teat-end irritation, teat dip ingredients should be evaluated carefully, and a change should be considered. Addition of emollients such as glycerin, lanolin, and polypropylene glycol to teat dips prevents excessive drying of teat skin. High concentrations of some emollients, especially glycerin, however, may decrease the germicidal activity of teat dips. Cows should have access to feed following milking to keep them standing until the teat end dries and the streak canal closes completely. This technique helps to avoid environmental contamination of the teat ends immediately after milking.

Milking Procedures and Equipment

Recent investigations on the influence of milking procedures on milk harvest efficiency and udder health have demonstrated the importance of adequate stimulation of milk let down and time spacing of milking procedures (prep-lag time). Studies have shown that premilking stimulation provided by forestripping, washing, and wiping of teats, and the time interval required to take full advantage of oxytocin release and milk let down leads to greater peak milk flows and shorter unit on time. Milk is stored as two distinct fractions in the udder. Cisternal milk is stored in the gland and teat cistern. It accounts for approximately 20% of stored milk and is immediately harvestable. Alveolar milk accounts for the remaining 80% of milk in the udder and requires the action of oxytocin release to make this fraction harvestable in a timely manner.

Ten to 20 seconds of vigorous stimulation of teats is required to stimulate the release of oxytocin from the pituitary gland. The time period from the initiation of stimulation of milk let down is referred to as the prep-lag time. Optimal prep-lag time can be influenced by a number of factors, including parity, stage of lactation, presence of a calf, and other stimuli that may startle or induce a flight reaction in the cow. Forestripping three squirts of milk from each teat provides the best opportunity to visually evaluate milk from each quarter and provides the necessary stimulation to induce milk let down. It is believed that a time of 60 to 90 seconds is the optimal prep-lag time. Adequate prep-lag time is created by organizing other premilking procedures including predipping, cleaning, and drying teats in a manner that creates the optimal prep-lag time.

The dynamics of milk flow are important and can influence the development of teat-end hyperkeratosis, which is a recognized risk for new infections if teat-end lesions are severe. Characteristics of milk flow from a properly prepared cow include a rapid increase to peak flow and maintenance of a relatively uniform peak flow until the cow is milked out. The initial increase in the milk flow rate and peak flow is strongly influenced by the level of teat stimulation and prep-lag time. The decline phase of milk flow is largely an individual cow characteristic and not influenced by milking procedures.

Milk flow rate can be assessed simply by observing the flow of milk from the cow into the claw of the milking unit. The first milk to be harvested immediately after the milking unit is attached is cisternal milk. If adequate stimulation and prep-lag times have been provided, milk flow will be uninterrupted until all milk is harvested from the cow. If stimulation of let down is inadequate or prep lag time is short, milk flow into the claw will decrease substantially or cease for a period after cisternal milk is harvested (often a minute or more), and let down of alveolar milk then occurs. A more precise means of measuring milk flow from individual cows is with a LactoCorder (WMB AG, Balgach, Switzerland). Milk flow graphs below were generated with the LactoCorder. These graphs can be a valuable diagnostic tool and teaching aid for milker training (Figures 8-50 and 8-51).

A basic understanding of the milking machine and equipment is essential when evaluating mastitis or milk quality problems on a dairy. Improperly functioning machines may contribute to the spread of contagious pathogens, create new infections by environmental organisms, may damage teat ends, or may create reverse flow of milk at the teat end, thereby predisposing to mastitis. The following information is condensed and summarized from three basic references pertaining to

Foam   Amount of milk: 10.94 kg   Date: 02.08.06   Time:13:22:07

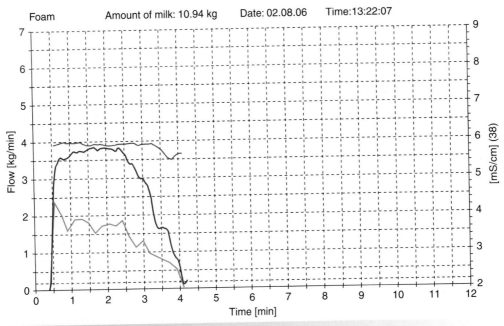

Figure 8-50

Milk flow graph generated by the LactoCorder (WMP AG, Wegenstrasse 6, CH-9436, Balgach, Switzerland. Internet: www.lactocorder.ch.). This graph demonstrates a desirable milk flow curve. Peak milk flow is achieved within 15 to 30 seconds and is sustained uninterrupted. Milk is completely harvested in less than 4 minutes.

Amount of milk: 11.59 kg   Date: 25.03.03   Time: 15:09:46

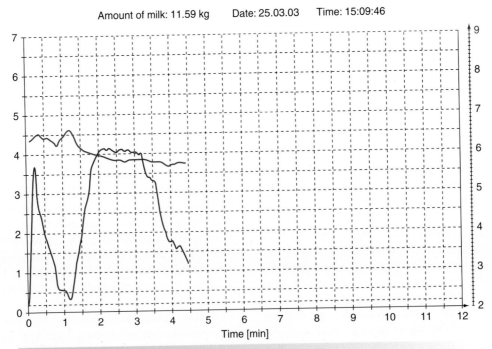

Figure 8-51

This graph demonstrates "bimodal milk flow." Bimodal flow is a consequence of inadequate stimulation of milk let down, inadequate prep-lag time, or a combination of both issues. Bimodal milk flow results in inefficient milk harvesting by extending machine-on time. The extended machine-on time results in overmilking and excessive trauma to teat ends, which may increase teat end hyperkeratosis and the risk for new mastitis infections.

milking machines. Although slight differences exist, the major principles and techniques are very similar. Poorly functioning or poorly maintained milking systems and machines may contribute to teat-end injuries, the spread of contagious organisms, and low milk quality. Poorly cleaned equipment may contribute to high bulk tank bacterial counts and postpasteurization counts.

Schematic illustrations of the milking and massage phases of the two-chamber teat cup milking machine are illustrated in Figure 8-52. Most current liners are narrow bore to maintain a snug fit along the entire length of the teat and lessen the chances of liner slips, air leaks, or teat cups that ride too high on the teat. These latter problems may occur more commonly with wide-bore liners. The inside of the liner is under constant vacuum from the short milk tube from the claw. During the milking phase, the vacuum is also applied between the outside of the liner and the shell. This space is also known as the pulsation chamber. During milking, the liner maintains its normal shape. The opening of the streak canal that allows milk to flow into the liner is primarily caused by the vacuum that is applied at the teat end. Pulsation creates differential pressures between the teat end and the cavity between liner and shell. This differential pressure is created by the action of the pulsators. When the cavity is vented to atmospheric pressure, negative pressure at the teat end collapses the liner, which massages the teat end. If pulsations did not occur, application of a constant vacuum on the teat end would produce edema and blood engorgement of the walls. Massage of the teat wall purges the congestion and increases the milk flow during the next milking cycle. As milking progresses and the gland cistern empties, gradual reduction in the slight positive pressure of the gland cistern and teat cistern occurs. Thus milk flow is reduced, and milkout is less efficient during the latter phase of milking.

Reduced milk flow toward the end of milking may be caused by obstruction of flow from the gland cistern to the teat cistern as the vacuum inside the liner pulls the teat deeper into the liner. Excessive or prolonged milking results in teat-end injury because massage is less effective at counteracting the congestion and trauma to the teat end and wall. Several points regarding vacuum at the teat and within lines are important as regards teat injury and mastitis:

1. *Vacuum fluctuations*—cyclical vacuum fluctuations may occur in the claws or liner and often correlate with improper pulsator function or inadvertent admission of air into the teat cup (liner squawk). Decreased vacuum during the massage phase may result in teat end trauma, and subsequent reduction in the natural defense mechanisms of the teat end. Vacuum fluctuations may also cause liner slips or teat cup drop off. Vacuum fluctuations during the milking phase may initiate reverse milk flows and droplet jets that spray against the teat ends. Milk flow reversal may force pathogens into or through the streak canal.
2. Rules of thumb:
   a. Line vacuum should not exceed 13.5 in Hg for systems with low milk lines and should not exceed 15 in Hg for high milk lines. No system should exceed 15 in Hg.
   b. The volume of air displaced at a given vacuum level is expressed in cubic feet per minute (CFM). Current recommendations for reserve air flow for a pipeline system (around the barn and parlor systems) are a basic level of 35 CFM and an additional CFM per milking unit. This may vary slightly with various milking systems.

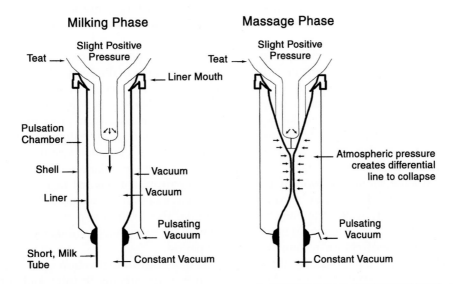

Figure 8-52

Schematic illustration of the milking and massage phases of the two-chamber teat cup milking machine.

c. Pulsator line sizes:
  1 to 2 in for up to 6 units
  2 to 3 in for 7 to 15 units
  Lines should be sloped toward pump with drains at risers and no dead ends
d. Vacuum levels:
  14 to 15 in Hg for high lines
  12.5 to 13.5 in Hg for low lines and buckets
e. Milk lines
  Sloped 1 to 2 in/10 ft
  Milk inlet at top third of line
  Looped with no dead ends
  1 in size = 2 units per slope
  2 in size = 4 units per slope
  2 in size = 5 to 6 units per slope
  3 in size = 7 to 9 units per slope
f. Milk hoses should be 9/16-in or 5/8-in inside diameter and not excessively long (maximum length 7 ft)
g. Vacuum to the teats should be shut off before removal from the cow. Either the claw or each individual inflation should be vented. This is an extremely important part of milking procedure to prevent droplet jets to the teat end and exposure to, or inoculation of, pathogens.

Pulsation rate is normally from 45 to 60/min, and most units approximate 60/min. The higher rates milk faster but must be maintained carefully to provide adequate time for the rest phase. Very slow rates may cause pain to the teat, increase the risk for teat-end damage (hyperkeratosis), and slow milking.

The pulsation ratio is the amount of time a pulsator creates vacuum to open the lines compared with the amount of time it admits air to collapse the liner. The pulsation ratio of various types of units may vary from 50:50 (milk/massage times) to 70:30, with 60:40 or 65:35 as common compromises. Ratios of 70:30 have been used in an attempt to milk faster but require excellent machine performance and maintenance, lest inadequate time for massage is allowed. Because 0.3 seconds are essential for massage phase, a machine set at 60 pulsations/min with a 70:30 ratio leaves little room for error. Teat-end injuries or chronic damage is propagated by inadequate massage phase. The rate of milking is not greatly different for pulsation ratios of 60:40 versus 70:30, thus 60:40 may provide more room for slight imperfections or deficiencies in the system while still providing adequate massage.

Excessive machine stripping should be avoided because it contributes to liner squawks and claw vacuum fluctuations and mechanical injury to the teat end and wall, which predisposes to mastitis. Liners should be replaced regularly according to manufacturers' recommendations. Recent research indicates that molded synthetic rubber liners should be replaced every 800 individual cow milkings (ICM), and natural rubber should be replaced every 500 ICM.

Cracked or damaged liners are difficult to clean and disinfect. They act as reservoirs for pathogens and do not function properly during milking. When worn or overused liners stretch, their performance changes. Average milking time increases, the frequency of liner slips grows, and teat condition and cow behavior worsen. The amount of milk left in the quarters when the milking units are removed increases. These changes in teat condition and liner slips will lead to a higher rate of new infections. Special continuing education programs and regular consultation with mastitis control professionals are the best means to evaluate a milking system during routine or troubleshooting analysis.

Teat Sealants

The use of teat sealants (i.e., bismuth subnitrite) as a component of dry cow therapy or as an "organic" alternative to intramammary infusion of antibiotics at the beginning of the dry period has become more commonplace. There is currently evidence to support a combination of teat sealant and intramammary antibiotic infusion at dry off, particularly in cattle that have experienced late lactation mastitis in the previous lactation. Furthermore teat sealant usage on its own at dry off has been shown to reduce the prevalence of new intramammary infections in the subsequent lactation compared with non–dry-treated, unsealed controls. This offers considerable promise for those producers who elect not to use antibiotic therapy at dry off for reasons of residue avoidance.

Natural Resistance Mechanisms of the Udder

Physical Mechanisms. The streak canal (teat canal) provides the most important physical deterrent to the entry of pathogens. Keratin in the streak canal not only serves as a physical barrier that tends to trap bacteria but also inhibits pathogens through a chemical defense system composed of antimicrobial lipids and proteins. Bacteria attached to keratin in the teat canal may be sealed in this location by tight closure of the sphincter muscle or extruded during milking as keratin desquamates. Thinning of the keratin layer predisposes to mastitis, as does any relative dysfunction of tight sphincter muscle tone. Because milking opens the teat canal for up to 2 hours, management procedures such as feeding cows after milking to keep them standing may lessen the chances of environmental mastitis.

Fear of excessive dilatation of the streak canal during dry cow treatment has led to research concerning the advantages of partial insertion of the dry cow infusion cannula. This technique may significantly decrease the number of new intramammary infections during the dry period.

As discussed in the section on staphylococcal mastitis, dirty environments, fly bites, and nursing by a group of poorly weaned calves fed mastitic milk may all play a role in teat-end colonization by staphylococci. Infection of the teat canal may lead to overt staphylococcal mastitis before or at the onset of lactation.

The udder is most susceptible to new intramammary infections during the early dry period before the teat canal has formed a thick keratin plug but is most resistant to new infections during the middle of the dry period.

Cellular Mechanisms. Macrophages and neutrophils along with sloughed alveolar epithelial cells compose the majority of somatic cells in milk. Lymphocytes compose a small fraction of these cells as well. Macrophages may be the most populous in noninflamed glands, but neutrophils predominate (90% or more) in inflamed glands. Following infection, neutrophils home toward the distal teat end and may migrate through the parenchyma rather than the cistern of the gland. Neutrophils work in conjunction with the keratinized teat canal defense mechanism to trap and kill bacteria before they can infect the glandular tissue. Because neutrophils have a relative impairment in milk as compared with blood, large numbers of neutrophils are necessary for an effective response to bacterial infection. This altered performance of neutrophils in milk is thought to be because of lack of opsonins, lack of energy source, and interference with phagocytosis by casein and fat. Experimental attempts to stimulate neutrophil numbers in the mammary gland, and consequently the teat end, have utilized indwelling intramammary devices of various types. Plastic and polyethylene coils, either smooth or braided, and chains of small glass beads are some of the types of intramammary devices that have been used. The desired result is to produce enough neutrophils or somatic cells to prevent bacterial colonization in the milk. This is an offshoot of the reduced coliform incidence in herds or cows with high SCC because of subclinical mastitis. Controversy continues regarding the usefulness and success of these devices in preventing new intramammary infections, but one large field study in Israel using abraded devices showed decreased clinical mastitis and increased milk yield. Other studies have shown less dramatic results and a slightly negative production response. Research with intramammary devices will be ongoing. Although a high SCC is likely with such devices, the neutrophils tend to be near the teat end, and forestripping may remove large numbers of cells.

Cellular defense mechanisms are altered at various stages of lactation. The SCC increases dramatically in noninfected quarters during the dry period and decreases dramatically in the peripartum period because of dilution. Macrophages predominate followed by lymphocytes and then neutrophils in noninfected dry quarters. Lymphocytes may be increased in dry cow secretions and colostrum in conjunction with increased IgA concentrations compared with those found in normal milk.

Secretory Antibodies. Passively transferred IgG is the major antibody class in milk, whereas IgA and IgM are in lower concentrations and are locally synthesized and transferred through the mammary epithelium. Immunoglobulins are selectively transported to the udder in the 3 weeks before freshening to concentrate in colostrum. Despite this high concentration of colostral antibodies at this time, the udder remains susceptible to infection. As regards defense of the udder versus pathogens, antibodies aid opsonization of bacteria. Subclinical mastitis with various pathogens does not seem to generate sufficient immune response to eliminate most infections. Attempts at systemic and local immunization have been attempted for *S. aureus* for many years, and the results have been variable (see staphylococcal mastitis).

Promising research and field trials support the use of the J-5 *E. coli* vaccine, a molecularly engineered vaccine that stimulates protection against lipopolysaccharide (LPS) endotoxin and therefore coliform mastitis. In well-managed herds that have minimal incidence of contagious pathogens, coliform mastitis may be the predominant cause of acute mastitis. Vaccination of large numbers of dairy cattle in California during controlled studies shows that bacterins significantly reduce the prevalence of coliform mastitis.

Lactoferrin and Other Soluble Factors. Lactoferrin, a whey protein, chelates iron in the presence of bicarbonate and therefore reduces iron availability for some pathogenic bacteria, particularly coliforms and most staphylococci. Conversely, streptococci require very little iron for optimal growth. Lactoferrin increases greatly in the well-involuted dry cow gland and helps prevent new intramammary infections caused by coliform organisms during this time. Citrate is low and bicarbonate is high in the involuted gland. As parturition approaches and colostrum is secreted into the udder, lactoferrin is reduced, and citrate, which competes with lactoferrin for iron, is increased. Therefore more iron becomes available for bacterial growth during this period.

Lysozyme and lactoperoxidase are other soluble components of the defense mechanism of the mammary gland. Cattle with low concentrations of lysozyme in milk are more prone to mastitis than cows whose milk has normal levels. Lactoperoxidase, an enzyme that is produced by mammary epithelial cells, oxidizes thiocyanate to hypothiocyanate, in the presence of H_2O_2. The oxidation reaction liberates free radicals that induce bactericidal cell membrane damage.

Pharmacology of Mammary Gland Therapy

Obtaining effective levels of antibiotics in milk by either systemic or intramammary routes is difficult. The following discussion will highlight the major points regarding antibiotic therapy for mastitis.

Systemically administered antibiotics must reach the udder and be able to effect inhibitory concentrations in milk and, for many pathogens, the udder parenchyma. Appropriate systemic antibiotics must be used at effective dosages and frequency and for sufficient duration to successfully eliminate bacteria. Unfortunately compromises often are made by veterinarians because of drug costs and expense of discarded milk, as well as fear of contaminating food products by antimicrobial residues. Intramammary antibiotics must diffuse well into the gland and must work in the presence of milk and inflammatory debris. Clinical and bacteriologic cures are not always coincident. This is especially true with organisms such as *S. aureus* when intracellular bacteria or L-forms produced by beta-lactam antibiotic therapy may not grow in standard media, yet may remain alive in the mammary tissues. The effectiveness of blood to milk transfer of systemic drugs depends on three factors:

1. *Lipid solubility*—more lipid solubility equates with better passage across biological membranes
2. *Degree of ionization*—poorly ionized drugs enter milk better
3. *Degree of protein binding*—less protein bound means better transfer into milk

In addition, the concentration gradient, which serves as a driving force for drugs into various tissues and secretion, is a function of a drug's total dose, frequency of administration, and rate of absorption from the site. The higher the dose or frequency of administration, the greater the concentration gradient pushing the drug to areas of the body. Without question, failure to establish effective concentration gradients may be one of the most routine pitfalls in dairy cattle treated with systemic antimicrobials. As is well known to clinicians, antibiotic dosages, frequencies of administration, and duration of treatment are less than optimal to satisfy regulatory agencies with respect to voluntary withholding period.

Milk has a pH of ≈6.5 versus a plasma pH of 7.4. Therefore after systemic administration, weak bases such as erythromycin and other macrolides diffuse into milk at higher concentrations than in plasma at corresponding times. However, when mastitis develops, the pH of milk increases and may approximate that of plasma. The higher pH reduces the concentration of erythromycin that diffuses into the gland. Similarly penicillin, amoxicillin, and ampicillin are weak acids that normally do not diffuse into the milk very well following systemic administration. Serum levels of penicillin following systemic administration may be 37 times higher than milk levels in healthy quarters but may only be 15 times higher than those in mastitic milk because of the higher pH of mastitic milk. Ampicillin may achieve serum levels eight times greater than in normal milk and six times greater in mastitic milk. Ceftiofur levels in mastitic milk were approximately 0.28 μg/ml compared with 1.0 μg/ml in the serum. Therefore high doses of relatively nontoxic drugs may improve concentrations of these drugs in mastitic milk. Tetracycline,

which is amphoteric, is distributed equally into healthy and mastitic quarters.

Partitioning and ionization of alkaline drugs in fluid with pH less than the pKa and greater than the pKa of acidic drugs lead to ion trapping and enhancement of antimicrobial efficacy within the udder. Site of injection into the cow may affect drug absorption and distribution as well. Sick or dehydrated cattle will not absorb non-IV administered drugs at normal rates—and will have prolonged tissue and milk levels because of reduced circulation and elimination of drugs.

In acute or peracute mastitis with severe edema and swelling, frequent stripping out may not only be therapeutic but may also greatly enhance the passage of systemically administered antibiotics such as gentamicin, ticarcillin, and polymyxin B. This could be especially important because many drugs, especially the aminoglycoside antibiotics, tend to be poorly distributed to the udder.

As regards systemic antibiotics, the following examples of distribution are for information purposes rather than specific recommendations. Because regulations controlling antibiotic usage in dairy cattle are changing constantly, these drugs may or may not be available for label or extra-label use in the future. In all instances, it is the veterinarian's responsibility to know what can be used and to know appropriate withdrawal times for milk and meat.

Macrolides, florfenicol, oxytetracycline, some fluoroquinolones, and rifampin have good distribution to the udder following systemic administration. Trimethoprim has good distribution into the mammary glands but is rapidly inactivated by rumen microflora, even when given IV to adult cattle. Sulfa drugs, penicillin G, ampicillin, ticarcillin, and cephalosporins have intermediate or limited distribution following systemic administration. Ceftiofur, the aminoglycosides, spectinomycin, and polymyxin B have poor distribution to the udder following systemic use. The dosage of beta-lactam drugs may be greatly increased without fear of toxicity to force a higher blood/mammary concentration gradient, but this principle would be extremely dangerous for aminoglycosides because of the potential for nephrotoxicity.

Intramammary (local) therapy also has pharmacologic principles that should be considered. As with systemically administered drugs, intramammary antibiotics may diffuse back into plasma depending on pKa of the drug, pH of the milk, degree of inflammation in the gland, and other factors. Oils added to mastitis preparations reduce the rate of distribution and inhibit drug diffusion from the udder. Mixing of drugs with an oil vehicle is particularly effective in dry cow preparations in which aluminum monostearate or benzathine is used to delay absorption of an antibiotic from the udder.

Distribution and the effects of inflammatory debris on the active antibiotic are also concerns when intramammary treatment is used. Increased dosages of antibiotics may be necessary and helpful to some cows, especially those with large udders. A double or triple dose of commercially approved mastitis treatments may be advantageous as the initial treatment of mastitis for cows with large udders but would prolong milk withdrawal times. Antibiotics in the milk may also affect neutrophil function, with most drugs diminishing neutrophil activity, whereas enrofloxacin increases neutrophil activity.

A limited number of products are approved for lactation and dry cow therapy (see Table 8-1). These are likely to change over time. Effective use of intramammary products requires extensive background information concerning mastitis status in each herd. Periodic reevaluation of treatment strategies is aided by complete culture surveys and mastitis control programs. As with systemically administered drugs, intramammary antibiotics are differentially distributed in the udder. Intramammary erythromycin, macrolides (except spectinomycin), pirlimycin, ampicillin, hetacillin, amoxicillin, novobiocin, rifampin, and fluoroquinolones have good distribution. Intramammary penicillin G, cloxacillin, cephalosporin, ceftiofur, and oxytetracycline have intermediate distribution, and the aminoglycosides and polymyxin B have poor distribution. This may be affected by the pH of the milk.

Clinical improvement following treatment should dictate continuation rather than discontinuation of therapy. The fact that bacteriologic cure rates are lower than "clinical" cure (cow and quarter improve but bacteria still can be cultured intermittently from gland, and quarter may suffer flareups) is partly because of premature cessation of treatment. It should also be noted that there is some evidence that cure rates with drugs with in vitro sensitivity to the mastitic agent are no different than cure rates when a drug having in vitro resistance is used. This may indicate a large number of "self-cures," inflammation from the drug/vehicle providing a beneficial effect, or sensitivity in vivo despite in vitro resistance.

Veterinarians are responsible for all drugs used in food-producing animals when a valid doctor-client-patient relationship exists. Although legislative and regulatory guidelines are available for approved and extra-label usage of drugs, the ultimate decision rests with the veterinarian. Recently the American Veterinary Medical Association has supported the 10-Point Quality Assurance Program to help maintain safety of milk and meat. Practicing veterinarians must remain informed on approved drugs and extra-label drug restrictions. Many milk residue antibiotic detection screening tests are available. Newer tests have greatly increased the sensitivity of detection of drug residues. Testing to detect infinitesimally low levels of antibiotics is illogical to rational people but not to zealots such as extreme animal rights groups or others who look for reasons to condemn milk and meat.

Perhaps more worrying is that many of the newer tests used to detect antibiotics in milk may yield false-positive results. Plasma or serum leaking into inflamed quarters because of coliform mastitis (untreated) seems to be commonly responsible for a false-positive antibiotic residue test. Therefore cows with mastitis that have not been treated with antibiotics could show a false-positive test, necessitating milk discard and causing significant economic and professional losses. An inherent problem with the use of tests such as the Penzyme Milk Test, Delvo-SP and Snap β-lactam assays is that they are intended, and have been validated, for use on commingled milk from tankers before processing for food. In field situations, these same tests are often employed using milk from individual cows, and recent studies have shown that although they may demonstrate high sensitivity and specificity, they have modest positive predictive values when assaying milk from mastitic cows that have undergone antibiotic treatment.

Stray Voltage

Stray voltage consisting of as little as 10-V potential difference has been suggested as a cause of milk let down failure and mastitis. The relationship between the mastitis and the stray voltage was thought to result from cow discomfort, poor let down because of apprehension, and incomplete milkout. Decreased production is explained by both incomplete milkout and a decreased appetite or water consumption associated with the stray voltage. Cows apparently react to recurrent flow or amperage, although voltage may be the measured assessment.

Experimental attempts to create stray voltage and then monitor productivity and appetite have yielded varying results. When there is stray voltage, cows can be subjected to voltage potential differences between electrified water cups or milking machines and their milking platform. There are numerous causes of stray voltage, including short-circuiting of electrical wiring through the milking machines, induction currents in ground through power lines, and direct voltage leaks from distant high intensity electrical sources. Cows that are subjected to stray voltage may be reluctant to enter milking areas, may kick at milking units, or may show decreased appetite and water consumption. The economic importance of stray voltage in individual cases is controversial, however, because at least one study has not detected lowered production in dairy cattle exposed to low levels of stray voltage, but others have shown significant improvements in productivity after correction of stray voltage in the dairy barn.

A study that exposed cows to 1.8 V for prolonged periods found no detrimental effects on the cows.

Given the controversy about the economic effects of stray voltage, obvious management deficiencies contributing to mastitis or other bottlenecks of productivity should not be overlooked on problem farms. Unless the cow's behavior suggests stray voltage problems, low-level stray voltage may not be as important as other management components when mastitis problems exist in a herd.

Milk Allergy

Milk allergy is the result of an immediate autoallergic reaction in cattle that are sensitized to their own casein. Milk allergy occurs within hours of dry off. Although observed in all major dairy breeds, the condition has the highest incidence in Jersey and Guernsey cattle. Retention of milk for any reason can stimulate the immediate hypersensitivity. The mediator release results in variable degrees of urticaria and dyspnea. The condition may be life-threatening when dyspnea caused by pulmonary or laryngeal edema develops. The condition is characterized by urticarial swellings of the eyelids, lips, vulva, and skin. Other instigating causes of milk allergy include delayed milking or "bagging" a cow for a show, sale, or photography session. The physiologic mechanisms that initiate the attack are unknown because these same cows that developed allergic disease after several hours of dry off seem to tolerate routine 12-hour milking intervals without problems. A cow may have only one episode or may develop repeated episodes so that drying off is impossible. A genetic basis for milk allergy is suspected.

Treatment includes immediate milkout, NSAIDs, antihistamines, and epinephrine. Corticosteroids may only be used in nonpregnant cows; any pregnant animals being dried off routinely should not be treated with corticosteroids.

Teat Amputation

Teat amputation is indicated when the teat presents a barrier to effective drainage of a severely infected mammary gland that threatens the cow's life. Typically, severe toxic or necrotizing mastitis has caused thick clots or toothpaste-like secretions that cannot be milked out of the teat in an efficient manner. Gangrenous mastitis is another indication for teat amputation. Clostridial mastitis may necessitate amputation as well. Badly mangled teats that have suffered repeated trauma and allowed secondary mastitis sometimes are amputated to allow salvage of the cow.

A decision on teat amputation is based on the potential value of the affected cow. If better drainage from a quarter seems essential and milkout is incomplete because of the character of the secretion, amputation may be elected. Teat amputation is only considered when the future productivity of the affected gland is likely to be lost or the gland threatens the cow's life.

Teat amputation is performed following anesthesia of the teat (unless it is gangrenous) by first clamping a Burdizzo at the base of the teat. The proximal udder should not be damaged because of the large venous plexus present in that location. After clamping with the Burdizzo, the teat is excised with heavy serrated scissors below the emasculatome. It is recommended that the excision be performed before releasing the emasculatome. If the teat and quarter are gangrenous, anesthesia and Burdizzo clamping before excision are not necessary.

KILLING A QUARTER (CHEMICAL DESTRUCTION) OR MASTECTOMY

A quarter that continues to produce grossly abnormal milk, has frequent clinical flareups that require treatment, or has a chronic active necrotizing inflammation may be a candidate for chemical destruction.

Chemical destruction or "killing" of a quarter obviously requires the teat to be functional to hold in whatever chemical is used. Therefore amputation of the teat cannot be performed in conjunction with chemical destruction. Chemical destruction of a quarter tends to be used for chronic problems that are not life-threatening to the patient but require treatment, make the cow slightly ill, or risk spread to other cows by contagion. Glands chronically infected with A. pyogenes or S. aureus probably constitute the majority of cases that undergo chemical destruction. Teat amputation, on the other hand, is indicated in life-threatening inflammations of the gland that are acute or chronic. Chemical destruction should not be considered in peracute or acute mastitis because it tends to worsen toxemia and illness associated with the primary inflammation. Chemical destruction can be performed with a variety of preparations. All are injected into the quarter in sufficient volume to penetrate the entire gland—thus a sizeable volume of chemical or chemical plus diluent may be necessary. The solution is left in the udder and, if possible, never milked out. All solutions cause inflammatory swelling, edema, and discomfort within 24 to 48 hours. However, unless the patient acts ill (inappetence, fever), the solution should not be milked out. If the cow acts ill, the quarter may be stripped out at 24 to 48 hours following instillation of the chemical. Successful destruction of a gland will be indicated by progressive atrophy of the gland following the initial acute inflammatory reaction. Chemicals that have been used include:

1. 100 ml of 10% formalin diluted to 500 ml with sterile saline and 30 ml of lidocaine. Infuse as much as the quarter will hold by gravity flow.
2. 50 to 100 cc of 3% silver nitrate solutions
3. 20 ml of 5% $CuSO_4$
4. Acriflavine 1 g/500 ml in sterile water: administer 250 ml by gravity infusion
5. Chlorhexidine, 60 ml. There is no transference of chlorhexidine into nontreated quarters; however, the disinfectant is present in infused quarter samples for as long as 42 days. Chlorhexidine is not very effective in killing the gland and may require multiple infusions to be effective.

6. 120 ml of 5% povidone iodine solution after milk-out has also been used stop lactation in chronically infected *S. aureus* quarters. In one study, this was a preferable method to chlorhexidine infusion.

Intramammary administration of any of the listed compounds does not conform to the existing Food and Drug Act regulations regarding approved drug use in food-producing animals. The systemic absorption of these compounds is unknown, and several of the chemicals are proved carcinogens. For chemicals that are noncarcinogenic, valid voluntary waiting periods are unknown; consequently the use of any drying off agent to a food-producing animal cannot be recommended.

Mastectomy has been performed in some cows with chronic mammary gland disease. This procedure must be performed by an experienced surgeon.

ABNORMAL MILK FLAVOR

Although not a "disease," a rancid flavor to milk can have a serious impact on consumers. Milk with a rancid flavor is soapy or bitter. Lipase activity that forms free fatty acids from milk fat continues to occur until milk is pasteurized. Intact protein membranes normally encapsulate milk fat molecules and protect the fat from enzyme activity. Conditions that interfere with or destroy protein membranes accelerate milk fat breakdown and should be avoided. S. E. Barnard of Pennsylvania State University states that rancidity may be found in as much as 70% of regular milk bought by consumers. He lists the following potential causes of milk rancidity:

1. Lack of adequate protein in the cows' diet
2. Milking cows greater than 305 days
3. Air leaks in pipeline milkers
4. Foaming or flooding of pipelines and receivers
5. Holding raw milk more than 48 hours after collection
6. Partial or less than every-other-day collection of milk from farms
7. Failure to empty and wash raw milk storage tanks on every processing day
8. Exposure of milk to copper or oxidizing metals
9. Contamination by chlorine sanitizers, acid water, and chlorine sanitizers
10. Exposure of milk to fluorescent lights
11. Ingestion of onions and *Helenium* (sneezeweed) or *Hymenoxys* by lactating cows
12. Excessive agitation of milk in bulk tank
13. Low dietary vitamin E, feeding high levels of vegetable fats, soybeans, and cottonseed meals
14. High iron or copper content in the drinking water
15. Diets that have strong odors, such as butyrous feed stuffs
16. Diets that are low in green forage or that depress milk fat

Rancidity of milk fats may cause more than 50% of the objectionable flavors detected in retail milk. Rancidity is produced by hydrolysis of the fatty acids from the glycerol backbone of the triglyceride. The release of the fatty acids produces a "goat acid" or rancid taste to the consumer. Rancidity can be detected using the acid degree value (ADV), in which the short chain fatty acids are measured. The test is recommended for use on individual farm samples rather than in tanker truck or composited creamery samples. The ADV of nonrancid, sweet-tasting milk is <0.8. Rancid milk usually has an ADV of 0.8 or greater.

SUGGESTED READINGS

Anderson KL, Smith AR, Gustafsson BK, et al: Diagnosis and treatment of acute mastitis in a large dairy herd, *J Am Vet Med Assoc* 181:690-693, 1982.

Anderson KL, Walker RL: Sources of *Prototheca* spp in a dairy herd environment, *J Am Vet Med Assoc* 193:553-556, 1988.

Arighi M, Ducharme NG, Honey FD, et al: Invasive teat surgery in dairy cattle. Part II. Long-term follow-up and complications, *Can Vet J* 28:763-737, 1987.

Barkema HW, Schukken YH, Zadoks RN: Invited review: the role of cow, pathogen, and treatment regimen in the therapeutic success of bovine *Staphylococcus aureus* mastitis, *J Dairy Sci* 89:1877-1895, 2006.

Bayoumi FA, Farver TB, Bushnell B, et al: Enzootic mycoplasmal mastitis in a large dairy during an eight-year period, *J Am Vet Med Assoc* 192:905-909, 1988.

Berry EA, Johnston WT, Hillerton JE: Prophylactic effects of two selective dry cow strategies accounting for interdependence of Quarter, *J Dairy Sci* 86:3812-3919, 2003.

Bleul UT, Schwantag SC, Bachofner C, et al: Milk flow and udder health in cows after treatment of covered teat injuries via theloresectoscopy: 52 cases (2000-2002), *J Am Vet Med Assoc* 226:1119-1123, 2005.

Bloomquist C, Davidson JN: Zearalenone toxicosis in prepubertal dairy heifers, *J Am Vet Med Assoc* 180:164-165, 1982.

Bowman GL, Hueston WD, Boner GJ, et al: *Serratia liquefaciens* mastitis in a dairy herd, *J Am Vet Med Assoc* 189:913-915, 1986.

Brka M, Reinsch N, Kalm E: Frequency and heritability of supernumerary teats in German Simmental and German Brown Swiss cows, *J Dairy Sci* 85:1881-1886, 2002.

Burvenich C, Van Merris V, Mehrzad J, et al: Severity of E.coli mastitis is mainly determined by cow factors, *Vet Res* 34, 521-564, 2003.

Bushnell RB: *Mycoplasma* mastitis, *Vet Clin North Am (Large Anim Pract)* 6:301-312, 1984.

Bushnell RB: The importance of hygienic procedures in controlling mastitis, *Vet Clin North Am (Large Anim Pract)* 6:361-370, 1984.

Butler JA, Sickles SA, Johanns CJ, et al: Pasteurization of discard Mycoplasma mastitis milk used to feed calves: thermal effects on various Mycoplasma, *J Dairy Sci* 83:2285-2288, 2000.

Chester ST, Moseley WM: Extended ceftiofur therapy for treatment of experimentally-induced *Streptococcus uberis* mastitis in lactating dairy cattle, *J Dairy Sci* 87:3322-3329, 2004.

Constable PD, Morin DE: Treatment of clinical mastitis using antimicrobial susceptibility profiles for treatment decisions, *Vet Clin North Am Food Anim Pract* 19:139-155, 2003.

Couture Y, Mulon PY: Procedures and surgeries of the teat, *Vet Clin North Am Food Anim Pract* 21:173-204, 2005.

Cullor JS: The *Escherichia coli* J5 vaccine: investigating a new tool to combat coliform mastitis, *Vet Med* August:836-844, 1991.

Deluyker HA, VanOye SN, Boucher JF: Factors affecting cure and somatic cell count after pirlimycin treatment of subclinical mastitis in lactating cows, *J Dairy Sci* 88:604-614, 2005.

Denamiel G, Llorente P, Carabella M, et al: Anti-microbial susceptibility of *Streptococcus* spp. isolated from bovine mastitis in Argentina, *J Vet Med B Infect Dis Vet Public Health* 52:125-128, 2005.

Ducharme NG, Horney FD, Baird JD, et al: Invasive teat surgery in dairy cattle. Part I. Surgical procedures and classification of lesions, *Can Vet J* 28:757-762, 1987.

Erskine RJ, Bartlett PC, Johnson GL 2nd, et al: Intramuscular administration of ceftiofur sodium versus intramammary infusion of penicillin/novobiocin for treatment of *Streptococcus agalactiae* mastitis in dairy cows, *J Am Vet Med Assoc* 205:258-260, 1996.

Erskine RJ, Bartlett PC, VanLente JL, et al: Efficacy of systemic ceftiofur as a therapy for severe clinical mastitis in dairy cattle, *J Dairy Sci* 85:2571-2575, 2002.

Erskine RJ, Eberhart RJ, Hutchinson LJ, et al: Incidence and types of clinical mastitis in dairy herds with high and low somatic cell counts, *J Am Vet Med Assoc* 192:761-765, 1988.

Erskine RJ, Tyler JW, Riddell MG Jr, et al: Theory, use, and realities of efficacy and food safety of antimicrobial treatment of acute coliform mastitis, *J Am Vet Med Assoc* 198:980-984, 1991.

Erskine RJ, Unflat JG, Eberhart RJ, et al: *Pseudomonas* mastitis: difficulties in detection and elimination from contaminated wash-water systems, *J Am Vet Med Assoc* 191:811-815, 1987.

Erskine RJ, Wilson RC, Tyler JW, et al: Ceftiofur distribution in serum and milk from clinically normal cows and cows with experimental *Escherichia coli*-induced mastitis, *Am J Vet Res* 56:481-485, 1995.

Foret CJ, Corbellini C, Young S, et al: Efficacy of two iodine teat dips based on reduction of naturally occurring new intramammary infections, *J Dairy Sci* 88:426-432, 2005.

Fox LK, Kirk JH, Britten A: Mycoplasma mastitis: a review of transmission and control, *J Vet Med B Infect Dis Vet Public Health* 52:153-160, 2005.

Galton DM, Petersson LG, Erb HN: Milk iodine residues in herds practicing iodophor premilking teat disinfection, *J Dairy Sci* 69:267-271, 1986.

Galton DM, Peterson LG, Merrill WG: Evaluation of udder preparations on intramammary infections, *J Dairy Sci* 71:1417-1421, 1988.

Gibbons-Burgener S, Kaneene JB, Lloyd JW, et al: Reliability of three bulk tank antimicrobial residue detection assays used to test individual milk samples from cows with mild clinical mastitis, *Am J Vet Res* 62:1716-1720, 2001.

Godden S, Rapnicki P, Stewart S, et al: Effectiveness of an internal teat seal in the prevention of new intramammary infections during the dry and early-lactation periods in dairy cows when used with a dry cow intramammary antibiotic, *J Dairy Sci* 86:3899-3911, 2003.

Goff JP: Major advances in our understanding of nutritional influences on bovine health, *J Dairy Sci* 89:1292-1301, 2006.

González RN, Cullor JS, Jasper DE, et al: Prevention of clinical coliform mastitis in dairy cows by a mutant *Escherichia coli* vaccine, *Can J Vet Res* 53:301-305, 1989.

González RN, Sears PM, Merrill RA, et al: Mastitis due to *Mycoplasma* in the state of New York during the period 1972–1990, *Cornell Vet* 82:29-40, 1992.

Green MJ, Green LE, Bradley AJ, et al: Prevalence and associations between bacterial isolates from dry mammary glands of dairy cows, *Vet Rec* 156:71-77, 2005.

Grohn YT, Gonzalez RN, Wilson DJ, et al: Effect of pathogen-specific clinical mastitis on herd life in two New York State Dairy herds, *Prev Vet Med* 71:105-125, 2005.

Hallberg JW, Wachowski M, Moseley WM, et al: Efficacy of intramammary infusion of ceftiofur hydrochloride at drying off for treatment and prevention of bovine mastitis during the nonlactating period, *Vet Ther* 7:35-42, 2006.

Hemmatzadeh F, Fatemi A, Amini F: Therapeutic effects of fig tree latex on bovine papillomatosis, *J Vet Med B Infect Dis Vet Public Health* 50:473-476, 2003.

Hill AW, Shears AL, Hibbitt KG: The pathogenesis of experimental *Escherichia coli* mastitis in newly calved dairy cows, *Res Vet Sci* 26:97-101, 1979.

Hillerton JE, Berry EA: The management and treatment of environmental streptococcal mastitis, *Vet Clin North Am Food Anim Pract* 19:157-169, 2003.

Hillerton JE, Bramley AJ, Staker RT, et al: Patterns of intramammary infection and clinical mastitis over a 5 year period in a closely monitored herd applying mastitic control measures, *J Dairy Res* 62:39-50, 1995.

Hillerton JE, Kliem KE: Effective treatment of *Streptococcus uberis* clinical mastitis to minimize the use of antibiotics, *J Dairy Sci* 85:1009-1014, 2002.

Hoe FG, Ruegg PL: Relationship between antimicrobial susceptibility of clinical mastitis pathogens and treatment outcome in cows, *J Am Vet Med Assoc* 227:1461-1468, 2005.

Hoeben D, Burvenich C, Heyneman R: Influence of antimicrobial agents on bactericidal activity of bovine milk polymorphonuclear leukocytes, *Vet Immunol Immunopathol* 56:271-282, 1997.

Hogan J, Smith KL: Coliform mastitis, *Vet Res* 34:507-519, 2003.

Hortet P, Seegers H: Calculated milk production loss associated with elevated somatic cell counts in dairy cows: review and critical discussion, *Vet Res* 29:497-510, 1998.

Janett F, Stauber N, Schraner E, et al: Bovine herpes mammillitis: clinical symptoms and serologic course, *Schweiz Arch Tierheilkd* 142:375-380, 2000.

Jarp J, Bugge HP, Larsen S: Clinical trial of three therapeutic regimens for bovine mastitis, *Vet Rec* 124:630-634, 1989.

Jones GF, Ward GE: Evaluation of systemic administration of gentamicin for treatment of coliform mastitis in cows, *J Am Vet Med Assoc* 197:731-735, 1990.

Jones TO: Correct use of intramammary treatments at drying off, *Vet Rec* 154:799, 2004.

Kang JH, Jin JH, Kondo F: False-positive outcome and drug residue in milk samples over withdrawal times, *J Dairy Sci* 88:908-913, 2005.

Knight AP: *Plants affecting the mammary gland. A guide to plant poisoning in North America*, Ithaca, NY, 2004, Teton NewMedia, IVIS.

Kristula MA, Rogers W, Hogan JS, et al: Comparison of bacteria populations in clean and recycled sand used for bedding in dairy facilities, *J Dairy Sci* 88:4317-4325, 2005.

LeBlanc SJ, Lissemore KD, Kelton DF, et al: Major advances in disease prevention in dairy cattle, *J Dairy Sci* 89:1267-1271, 2006.

Leininger DJ, Roberson JR, Elvinger F, et al: Evaluation of frequent milkout for treatment of cows with experimentally induced *Escherichia coli* mastitis, *J Am Vet Med Assoc* 222:63-66, 2003.

Letchworth GJ, Carmichael LE: Local tissue temperature: a critical factor in the pathogenesis of bovid herpesvirus 2, *Infect Immun* 43:1072-1079, 1984.

Makovec JA, Ruegg PL: Characteristics of milk samples submitted for microbiological examination in Wisconsin from 1994 to 2001, *J Dairy Sci* 86:3466-3472, 2003.

McDermott MP, Erb HN, Natzke RP: Predictability by somatic cell counts related to prevalence of intramammary infection within herds, *J Dairy Sci* 65:1535-1539, 1982.

McDonald JS, Anderson AJ: Experimental intramammary infection of the dairy cow with *Escherichia coli* during the nonlactating period, *Am J Vet Res* 42:229-331, 1981.

McDougall S: Efficacy of two antibiotic treatments in curing clinical and subclinical mastitis in lactating dairy cows, *N Z Vet J* 46:226-232, 1998.

McDougall S: Intramammary treatment of clinical mastitis of dairy cows with a combination of lincomycin and neomycin, or penicillin and dihydrostreptomycin, *N A Vet J* 51:111-116, 2003.

McLennan MW, Kelly WR, O'Boyle D: Pseudomonas mastitis in a dairy herd, *Aust Vet J* 75:790-792, 1997.

Middleton JR, Hebert VR, Fox LK, et al: Elimination kinetics of chlorhexidine in milk following intramammary infusion to stop lactation in mastitic mammary gland quarters of cows, *J Am Vet Med Assoc* 222:1746-1749, 2003.

Middleton JR, Timms LL, Bader GR, et al: Effect of prepartum intra-mammary treatment with pirlimycin hydrochloride on prevalence of early first-lactation mastitis in dairy heifers, *J Am Vet Med Assoc* 227:1969-1974, 2005.

Milne MH, Biggs AM, Barrett DC, et al: Treatment of persistent intra-mammary infections with *Streptococcus uberis* in dairy cows, *Vet Rec* 157:245-250, 2005.

Morin DE, Shanks RD, McCoy GC: Comparison of antibiotic admin-istration in conjunction with supportive measures versus support-ive measures alone for treatment of dairy cows with clinical mas-titis, *J Am Vet Med Assoc* 213:676-684, 1998.

Nickerson SC: Immune mechanisms of the bovine udder: an over-view, *J Am Vet Med Assoc* 187:41-45, 1985.

Nickerson SC: Resistance mechanisms of the bovine udder: new im-plications for mastitis control at the teat end, *J Am Vet Med Assoc* 191:1484-1488, 1987.

Nickerson SC, Owens WE: *Staphylococcus aureus* mastitis: reasons for treatment failures and therapeutic approaches for control, *Agri-Practice* 14:18-23, 1993.

Nickerson SC, Pankey JW: Cytologic observations of the bovine teat end, *Am J Vet Res* 44:1433-1441, 1983.

Ogawa T, Tomita Y, Okada M, et al: Broad-spectrum detection of pap-illomaviruses in bovine teat papillomas and healthy teat skin, *J Gen Virol* 85:2191-2197, 2004.

Oliver SP, Almeida RA, Gillespie BE, et al: Efficacy of extended pirli-mycin therapy for treatment of experimentally induced *Streptococ-cus uberis* intramammary infections in lactating dairy cows, *Vet Ther* 4:299-308, 2003.

Oliver SP, Almeida RA, Gillespie BE, et al: Efficacy of extended ceftio-fur intramammary therapy for treatment of subclinical mastitis in lactating dairy cows, *J Dairy Sci* 87:2393-2400.

Oliver SP, Gillespie BE, Ivey SJ, et al: Influence of prepartum pirlimy-cin hydrochloride or penicillin-novobiocin therapy on mastitis in heifers during early lactation, *J Dairy Sci* 87:1727-1731, 2004.

Oliver SP, Matthews KR: Analytical review of new teat dip efficacy claims, *Bov Proc* 26:79-83, 1994.

Owens WE: Evaluation of antibiotics for induction of L-forms from *Staphylococcus aureus* strains isolated from bovine mastitis, *J Clin Microbiol* 26:2187-2190, 1988.

Owens WE, Ray CH, Watts JL, et al: Comparison of success of antibi-otic therapy during lactation and results of antimicrobial suscepti-bility tests for bovine mastitis, *J Dairy Sci* 80:313-317, 1997.

Owens WE, Watts JL, Boddie RL, et al: Antibiotic treatment of mastitis: comparison of intramammary and intramammary plus intramus-cular therapies, *J Dairy Sci* 71:3143-3147, 1988.

Parkinson TJ, Vermunt JJ, Merrall M: Comparative efficacy of three dry-cow antibiotic formulations in spring-calving New Zealand dairy cows, *N Z Vet J* 48:129-135, 2000.

Polk C: Cows, ground surface potentials and earth resistance, *Bioelec-tromagnetics* 22:7-18:2001.

Povey RC, Osborne A: Mammary gland neoplasia in the cow, *Pathol Vet* 6:502-512, 1969.

Power E: Gangrenous mastitis in dairy herds, *Vet Rec* 153:791-792, 2003.

Querengasser J, Geishauser K, Querengasser K, et al: Comparative evaluation of SIMPL silicone implants and NIT natural teat inserts to keep the teat canal patent after surgery, *J Dairy Sci* 85:1732-1737, 2002.

Reed DE, Langpap MS, Anson MS: Characterization of herpesviruses isolated from lactating dairy cows with mammary pustular derma-titis, *Am J Vet Res* 38:1631-1634, 1977.

Roberson JR, Warnick LD, Moore G: Mild to moderate clinical masti-tis: efficacy of intramammary amoxicillin, frequent milk-out, a combined intramammary amoxicillin, and frequent milk-out treatment versus no treatment, *J Dairy Sci* 87:583-392, 2004.

Robert A, Seegers H, Bareille N: Incidence of intramammary infections during the dry period without or with antibiotic treatment in dairy cows—a quantitative analysis of published data, *Vet Res* 37:25-48, 2006.

Ruegg PL: Investigation of mastitis problems on farms, *Vet Clin North Am Food Anim Pract* 19:47-74, 2003.

Sargeant JM, Scott HM, Leslie KE, et al: Clinical mastitis in dairy cattle in Ontario: frequency of occurrence and bacteriological isolates, *Can Vet J* 39:33-38, 1998.

Sears PM, Fettinger M, Marsh-Salin J: Isolation of L-form variants after antibiotic treatment in *Staphylococcus aureus* bovine mastitis, *J Am Vet Med Assoc* 191:681-684, 1987.

Sears PM, González RN, Wilson DJ, et al: Procedures for mastitis di-agnosis and control, *Vet Clin North Am (Food Anim Pract)* 9:445-468, 1993.

Sears PM, Smith BS, English PB, et al: Shedding pattern of *Staphylococ-cus aureus* from bovine intramammary infections, *J Dairy Sci* 73:2785-2789, 1990.

Serieys F, Raquet Y, Goby L, et al: Comparative efficacy of local and systemic antibiotic treatment in lactating cows with clinical masti-tis, *J Dairy Sci* 88:93-99, 2005.

Shim EH, Shanks RD, Morin DE, et al: Milk loss and treatment costs associated with two treatment protocols for clinical mastitis in dairy cows, *J Dairy Sci* 87:2702-2708, 2004.

Smith GW, Gehring R, Craigmill AL, et al: Extralabel intramammary use of drugs in dairy cattle, *J Am Vet Med Assoc* 226:1994-1996, 2005.

Smith GW, Lyman RL, Anderson KL: Efficacy of vaccination and anti-microbial treatment to eliminate chronic intramammary *Staphylo-coccus aureus* infections in dairy cattle, *J Am Vet Med Assoc* 228:422-425, 2006.

Sol J, Sampimon OC, Snoep JJ, et al: Factors associated with bacterio-logical cure during lactation after therapy for subclinical mastitis caused by *Staphylococcus aureus*, *J Dairy Sci* 80:2803-2808, 1997.

Taponen S, Simojoki H, Haveri M, et al: Clinical characteristics and persistence of bovine mastitis caused by different species of coagu-lase-negative staphylococci identified with API or AFLP, *Vet Micro-biol* 115:199-207, 2006.

Thornsberry C, Marler JK, Watts JL, et al: Activity of pirlimycin against pathogens from cows with mastitis and recommendations for disk diffusion tests, *Antimicrob Agents Chemother* 37:1122-1126, 1993.

Tyler JW, Wilson RC, Dowling P: Treatment of subclinical mastitis, *Vet Clin North Am (Food Anim Pract)* 8:17-28, 1992.

Waage S, Mork T, Roros A, et al: Bacteria associated with clinical mas-titis in dairy heifers, *J Dairy Sci* 82:712-719, 1999.

Waage S, Odegaard SA, Lund A, et al: Case-control study of risk factors for clinical mastitis in postpartum dairy heifers, *J Dairy Sci* 84:392-399, 2001.

Warnick LD, Nydam D, Maciel A, et al: Udder cleft dermatitis and sar-coptic mange in a dairy herd, *J Am Vet Med Assoc* 221:273-276, 2002.

Wenz JR, Barrington GM, Garry FB, et al: Bacteremia associated with naturally occurring acute coliform mastitis in dairy cows, *J Am Vet Med Assoc* 219:976-981, 2001.

Wenz JR, Garry FB, Lombard JE, et al: Short communication: efficacy of paternal ceftiofur for treatment of systemically mild clinical mastitis in dairy cattle, *J Dairy Sci* 88:3496-3499, 2005.

Wilson DJ, Gonzalez RN, Case KL, et al: Comparison of seven antibi-otic treatments with no treatment for bacteriological efficacy against bovine mastitis pathogens, *J Dairy Sci* 82:1664-1670, 1999.

Wilson DJ, Kirk JH, Walker RD, et al: *Serratia marcescens* mastitis in a dairy herd, *J Am Vet Med Assoc* 196:1102-1105, 1990.

Woolford MW, Williamson JH, Day AM, et al: The prophylactic effect of a teat sealer on bovine mastitis during the dry period and the following lactation, *N Z Vet J* 46:12-19, 1998.

Wraight MD: A comparative efficacy trial between cefuroxime and cloxacillin as intramammary treatments for clinical mastitis in lactating cows on commercial dairy farms, *N Z Vet J* 51:26-32, 2003.

Wraight MD: A comparative field trial of cephalonium and cloxacillin for dry cow therapy for mastitis in Australian dairy cows, *Aust Vet J* 83:103-104, 2005.

Yamagata M, Goodger WJ, Weaver L, et al: The economic benefit of treating subclinical *Streptococcus agalactiae* mastitis in lactating cows, *J Am Vet Med Assoc* 191:1556-1561, 1987.

Younis A, Krifucks O, Fleminger G, et al: *Staphylococcus aures* leucocidin, a virulence factor in bovine mastitis, *J Dairy Res* 72:188-194, 2005.

Zadoks RN, Allore HG, Barkema HW, et al: Cow and quarter level risk factors for Streptococcus uberis and Staphylococcus aureus mastitis, *J Dairy Sci* 84:2649-2663, 2001.

Zdanowicz M, Shelford JA, Tucker CB, et al: Bacterial populations on teat ends of dairy cows housed in free stalls and bedded with either sand or sawdust, *J Dairy Sci* 87:1694-1701, 2004.

Ziv G: Treatment of peracute and acute mastitis, *Vet Clin North Am (Food Anim Pract)* 8:1-15, 1992.

CHAPTER 9

Reproductive Diseases

Robert Hillman and Robert O. Gilbert

The scope of theriogenology is beyond simple summation within a single chapter of a general textbook. Therefore no effort will be made to cover all gynecologic and reproductive topics. Emphasis in this chapter will be directed toward diseases of the reproductive tract that cause signs of illness or disease and require medical attention in dairy cattle. Standard theriogenology textbooks should be consulted for more in-depth reading and discussions of infertility, endocrinology, dystocia, and abortion.

DISEASES OF THE UTERUS

Hydrops

Etiology

Uterine dropsy or hydrops is a sporadic condition usually occurring during the last trimester of pregnancy. Hydrops of the amnion results from fetal anomalies that prevent fetal swallowing or intestinal transport of amniotic fluid and is responsible for approximately 10% of the cases of hydrops. Hydrops of the allantois is the more common condition and is usually accompanied by abnormal placentation characterized by reduced numbers of placentomes and adventitious placentation (multiple areas of adhesion between the endometrium and allantochorion, appearing as miniature placentomes). Therefore hydrallantois usually is considered a maternal abnormality of placentation, whereas hydramnios is considered more likely a fetal problem. Hydrallantois tends to cause rapid (days to weeks) abdominal distention that results in a rounded abdominal appearance as the patient is viewed from the rear, whereas hydramnios usually results in a slow progressive enlargement with eventual pear-shaped appearance. Twinning or multiple fetuses are more likely associated with hydrallantois. Fetal anomalies are common with hydramnios. Pregnancies that are the result of modern in vitro reproductive technologies such as those producing cloned or transgenic fetuses are more commonly beset by abnormal placentation and subsequently represent a greater risk for hydrops allantois. It is possible for nutritional deficiencies to cause hydrops allantois. Fetal hydrops

may occur due to accumulation of cerebrospinal fluid (hydrocephalus) or from ascites (usually in Ayrshire calves). These calves, if delivered alive, can survive, but should not be used for breeding.

Signs

The major outward sign of hydrops is progressive abdominal distention during the last trimester that worsens to such a degree as to decrease appetite and cause difficulty in moving or rising (Figure 9-1). Although abnormal fetuses causing hydramnios rarely can cause abdominal distention as early as the midtrimester, this is much less common than hydrops that appears during the last 4 to 6 weeks of pregnancy. The distended uterus

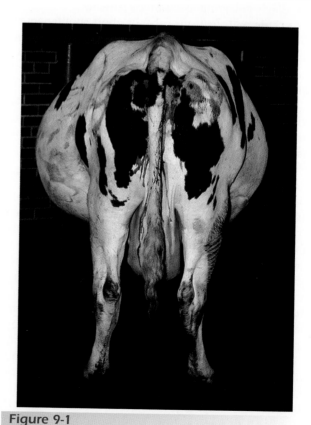

Figure 9-1

Hydrops allantois in a Holstein cow that was 8 months pregnant.

takes up so much room in the abdomen that affected cows have reduced appetites because of visceral compression. Weakness results both from reduced feed consumption and from the increased weight of uterine fluids. Secondary ketosis and other metabolic conditions are possible complications as a result of decreased feed intake and fetal nutritional needs—especially if twins are present in cows with hydrallantois. Rectal examination may help to differentiate hydramnios and hydrallantois. In hydramnios, the fetus and placentomes are palpable, but the uterine horns are more difficult to palpate. In hydrallantois, the distended uterine horns appear to fill the abdomen, but palpation of the fetus and placentomes may not be possible because the uterus is stretched tightly by the increased fluid content. Rectal or transabdominal ultrasound examination is helpful in making a diagnosis. Unless the conditions are diagnosed promptly, musculoskeletal complications such as exertional myopathy, hip injuries, hip luxations, and femoral fractures can occur because of struggling to rise or slipping brought on by the tremendous abdominal weight. (As much as 200 liters, or 440 pounds, of additional fluid may accumulate in the case of hydrops allantois.) Rupture of the prepubic tendon and ventral hernias also may occur. Because hydrallantois tends to cause more rapid fluid accumulation, musculoskeletal injuries appear to be more common with this condition than in the slowly enlarging hydramnios patients.

If cattle with hydrops calve or abort spontaneously, the thick viscid amniotic fluid present in hydramnios also can help differentiate this condition from the watery transudative excessive fluid discharged from cattle with hydrallantois.

Cattle with hydrops have normal temperatures but will show progressive tachycardia, anxiety, reduced appetite, and dehydration associated with severe abdominal distention. Fetal hydrops may cause dystocia.

Treatment

Treatment decisions must be tempered by the potential immediate and delayed complications anticipated. Prognosis usually is worse for hydrallantois because abnormal maternal placentation may be expected to cause severe and intractable problems with retained placenta and metritis, making future fertility extremely unlikely. If neglected or allowed to "run their course," most cattle with hydrallantois will progress to recumbency, cardiovascular collapse, and overwhelming myopathy. Hydramnios may have fewer severe immediate complications with retained placenta and metritis, but in these cases survival of the fetus is unlikely. Perhaps the most important consideration is the overall systemic state. Most hydrops cattle are in a negative energy balance, are 4 to 6 weeks from parturition, have slack udders, and may or may not come into lactation—at least to productive lactation levels. Therefore salvage should be considered unless the cow is particularly valuable or is within 2 weeks of term. Cattle that are recumbent and unable to rise or that already have severe musculoskeletal injuries should be euthanized.

When treatment is elected, several options exist. Induction of parturition is preferable if the uterus has not already been stretched beyond physiological limits, which is unfortunately usually the case. If surgery is elected, uterine fluid should be released over a period of 30 minutes to 2 hours, via a Foley catheter, while intravenous fluids are administered rapidly. This prevents the rapid onset of shock, which may result from venous fluid shifting into the splanchnic pool with abdominal decompression. Although some authors have not found hydrops patients to be markedly dehydrated, our experience differs and supports the comments of Roberts that those patients usually are dehydrated. Dehydration further increases the risk of compartmental pressure changes, subsequent splanchnic pooling, and shock for hydrops patients treated by cesarean section.

Dr. Rebhun's preference was to induce parturition with IM injections of 30 to 40 mg prostaglandin $F_{2\alpha}$ ($PGF_{2\alpha}$) and 20 mg of dexamethasone. Cervical relaxation may also be attempted by the manual application of synthetic prostaglandin E in the external os and cervical canal. Specific human gynecologic preparations of prostaglandin E are very expensive, but I have had success using misoprostol (1000 µg mixed in sterile obstetrical gel applied thrice daily) as an aid to cervical ripening in some cattle. Pregnant women should not handle this product! Most cattle treated with this combination calve within 24 to 48 hours and should be monitored closely. IV fluids—hypertonic saline is especially useful—are administered to cattle showing any degree of dehydration or inappetence. Supportive glucose or calcium may be indicated when ketosis or hypocalcemia is present. Treated cows are kept in well-bedded box stalls with good footing and are monitored closely because they may require assistance in calving. Milking is started as soon as the fetus is delivered, even when little milk is present in the udder. Most fetuses or calves delivered are abnormal, small, or nonviable. If the calf is more valuable than the cow and ultrasound examination indicates a viable fetus, treatment of the cow with dexamethasone and cesarean section 24 hours later would provide the best chance of having a live calf. In the case of an apparently viable calf, colostrum should be provided from another cow because the patient seldom has normal colostrum. Prognosis is better for those cows near term. Metritis and retained fetal membranes (RFM) should be anticipated and prophylactic antibiotic therapy instituted. Clinicians should anticipate that the cow will have a large, potentially enormous, atonic uterus after calving and will experience highly protracted and challenging involution. Although fetal kidney anomalies are more likely to be associated with hydrallantois, Dr. Rebhun once treated a hydramnios cow that subsequently delivered a calf having poly-cystic kidneys. Cattle with hydrallantois that survive delivery and avoid life-threatening postpartum metritis should not be bred again. If fetal hydrops causes dystocia, the excessive fluid can be drained to allow fetal extraction.

Because of the common complications of intractable retention of fetal membranes and associated metritis and infertility, and the poor prognosis for survival of the fetus, culling of the cow with hydrops allantois may represent the most economical option. Survival and subsequent fertility are much more likely in cows with hydrops amnios but they should not be bred again to the same sire.

Rupture of the Prepubic Tendon and Ventral Hernia

Etiology
Rupture of the prepubic tendon and ventral abdominal hernias usually occur during the last month of pregnancy. Contributing causes include the weight of a gravid uterus and periparturient edema of the ventrum. Further predisposition occurs in cattle with twin or multiple pregnancies and those with hydrops. Although more common in pluriparous cattle with a pendulous abdomen, the condition may occur in primiparous cattle. Injuries from direct trauma (especially from animals with horns), being cast or trapped on inanimate objects, or slipping on treacherous footing may be contributing or initiating factors. Factors that increase the uterine mass remain the major cause in cattle. Rarely, rupture of the body wall in the flank area with hematoma formation and obvious swelling occurs at parturition.

Clinical Signs and Diagnosis
Rupture of the prepubic tendon causes a bilateral and complete loss of fore udder definition, and the fore udder points ventrally in continuum with the pendulous ventrally directed abdominal wall (Figure 9-2). The cow assumes a sawhorse stance because of exquisite pain in the abdomen and is reluctant to lie down (Figure 9-3).

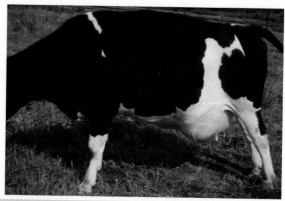

Figure 9-3

Rupture of the prepubic tendon in a first-calf heifer that was confirmed to have twins. The heifer has a sawhorse stance and would not lie down because of severe abdominal pain.

When the cow does lie down, she tries to assume lateral recumbency to avoid putting pressure on the ventrum. Abdominal distention usually is obvious. The owner usually observes overt or atypical extensive abdominal distention before rupture of the tendon, and cows (like mares) may have the rupture preceded by both extreme abdominal distention and a large plaque of ventral edema. These characteristics have been referred to as "impending rupture of the prepubic tendon" and are a grave sign.

Cattle with ventral hernias have the same predisposing causes as for rupture of the prepubic tendon but may have unilateral abdominal sagging coupled with an abnormal relationship of the fore udder to the affected side of the abdomen. Ventral hernias have been reported to be more common on the right side in cattle but can occur on either side.

Cattle with either condition become acutely painful at the moment that an "impending" situation becomes a hernia. Tachycardia, tachypnea, an anxious expression, reluctance to move or lie down, and a sawhorse stance are typical findings. Prepubic tendon rupture usually results in more overt pain than ventral hernia, but this is far from absolute.

Rectal examination may help to differentiate the conditions as a purely didactic measure. When true rupture of the prepubic tendon has occurred, the cranial brim of the pelvis may be tipped slightly upward, and the hand may be cupped under the brim because of loss of the prepubic tendon. In ventral hernias, the hernia may or may not be palpable, but the prepubic tendon can be palpated in the caudal abdomen as it attaches to the pelvic brim.

Cattle with either condition may require assistance in calving because pain and inability to generate normal abdominal press may lead to dystocia. In addition, twins or hydrops may be apparent and further the chances of

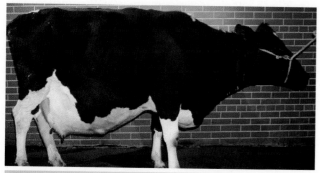

Figure 9-2

Rupture of the prepubic tendon in a 6-year-old Holstein cow.

dystocia. Cows with rupture of the prepubic tendon should be salvaged or euthanized because they are in extreme pain. Cows with ventral hernias that do not appear to be in severe pain may be kept for the current lactation but should not be bred back. Cattle thought to be showing signs of "impending rupture" or those suspected to have hydrops should be induced to calve immediately or undergo elective cesarean section in an effort to prevent herniation or rupture of the prepubic tendon. Cattle with either condition that are recumbent and unable to stand or those already having secondary musculoskeletal complications should be euthanized.

When parturition is induced in these cases, it should always be attended. Inserting a nasotracheal or orotracheal tube helps prevent abdominal press with further exacerbation of the abdominal wall rupture, while the calf may still be delivered by traction.

Rupture of the prepubic tendon and ventral hernias are specifically diagnosed based on clinical signs alone but should be differentiated from large hematomas or abscesses cranial to or dorsal to the udder, severe preparturient ventral edema, and inflammatory ventral edema or edema secondary to thrombosis of the mammary vein. The anatomic relationship of the udder to the ventral abdomen usually suffices to differentiate these conditions. Ultrasound examination will help in making a more definitive diagnosis. Anemia would be present with large udder hematomas, and fever might be present with abscesses. Ultrasonography could be very useful whenever the diagnosis is in doubt.

Uterine Torsion

Etiology

Bovine practitioners are familiar with uterine torsion as a cause of dystocia in dairy cattle. Although the exact cause of torsion seldom is discovered in an individual case, prolonged confinement, sudden falls or slipping, a pendulous abdomen, strong fetal movements, and poor uterine muscle tone may predispose. Unicornual pregnancy (where the conceptus fails to occupy both uterine horns) and especially unicornual twin pregnancy may cause instability of the uterus and predispose to torsion. Torsion is less common in Bos indicus breeds, where the uterine broad ligament is attached over a greater length of the uterine horns than in Bos taurus cows. Many parturient torsions occur during the latter part of the first stage of labor or early in the second stage. Other partial torsions of 45 degrees or more may be maintained in this position for weeks or months during late gestation but do not result in signs unless further rotation occurs that interferes with fetal or uterine blood supply.

In addition to these parturient problems, however, uterine torsion can result in clinical signs during the second or third trimester well before term. Such cattle have torsions greater than 180 degrees, and colic signs similar to intestinal obstruction may occur. Roberts states that uterine torsions in the cow have been observed as early as 70 days of gestation. Most cases occurring during the mid-trimester of gestation are characterized by colic and abdominal pain.

Clinical Signs and Diagnosis

Although an uncommon cause of colic, uterine torsion should be considered in the differential diagnosis of any cow showing colic and more than 4 months pregnant. The early signs shown by these cows are similar to those observed in the more common term uterine torsions and include restlessness, treading, anxiety, tachycardia, reduced appetite, and swishing of the tail. The cow may be reluctant to lie down or may get up and down frequently or may perhaps act irritable. As the condition progresses, complete anorexia, progressive tachycardia, and true colic with kicking at the abdomen may appear. Because the condition is seldom suspected in cattle in mid-gestation, further delay in diagnosis may occur if the signs are interpreted as intestinal in origin and treated symptomatically. Rectal examination allows definitive diagnosis because a clockwise or counterclockwise torsion will be identified. Most mid-pregnancy torsions are greater than 180 degrees, thereby causing the right broad ligament to be pulled downward under the torsed organ while the left broad ligament is pulled over the top of the reproductive tract (clockwise or right torsion). The opposite arrangement occurs in counterclockwise or left torsions. The viability of the calf should be determined by palpation and/or ultrasound examination. Counterclockwise torsions are slightly more common, since the uterus rolls toward and over the non-gravid horn.

Treatment

Unlike treatment methods available for term uterine torsions (e.g., manual detorsion, mechanical detorsion, "plank in the flank," and rolling), mid-trimester uterine torsions are best managed by manual correction following laparotomy. Attempts to roll the cow or use the plank-in-the-flank technique are usually unsuccessful because of lack of fetal mass and tend to further damage the already compromised uterus while risking hemorrhage or further transudative or exudative peritoneal effusion. When rolling was attempted in some early cases, the technique failed and subsequent laparotomy revealed severe serosanguineous peritoneal effusion and some frank hemorrhage. When diagnosed early and corrected by laparotomy, cattle with mid-trimester uterine torsions have a better chance of delivering a live calf. Fetal death and eventual abortion are likely following correction in neglected cases, severe torsions, or those with obvious vascular compromise. Prolonged cases can have uterine necrosis and die from septic shock.

Uterine Rupture

Etiology

Uterine rupture is an unfortunate consequence of dystocia in cattle. Although the condition rarely is observed following unassisted delivery, most cases occur following forced traction, uterine torsions, fetotomy, or delivery of emphysematous fetuses. Iatrogenic ruptures can also result from frustrated manipulations as the veterinarian becomes exhausted following prolonged attempts to relieve dystocia. Prolonged dystocias, emphysematous fetuses, and failure to lubricate sufficiently during extraction can increase the resistance and "drag" between fetus and maternal reproductive tract and predispose to rupture of the uterus. Abdominal pressure of the uterus against the pelvic brim can cause pressure necrosis and spontaneous uterine rupture.

Clinical Signs

When a veterinarian is present for the dystocia, manual examination of the cervix and uterus through the vagina should be performed following delivery of the calf. Full-thickness uterine tears usually can be diagnosed at this time unless the injury occurs in the uterine horns distal to the reach of the veterinarian.

When the condition is undetected initially or a veterinarian has not been present for the dystocia, clinical signs usually appear within 1 to 5 days postpartum. Depression, inappetence, fever, tachycardia, rumen stasis, and abdominal guarding because of peritonitis appear as the major signs. Some cattle progress rapidly to a condition of septic shock because of massive peritoneal contamination. This is especially common when prolonged dystocia, RFM, or a dead or emphysematous fetus allows bacterial inoculation of the uterus that quickly spreads to the abdomen. The fetal membranes may enter the abdominal cavity through the uterine tear and cause severe, potentially fatal peritonitis. Cattle with large uterine tears and tenesmus associated with dystocia may prolapse intestine through the reproductive tract and have these organs appear at the vulva. Spontaneous rupture caused by unattended dystocia occasionally has resulted in the calf or fetus being extrauterine in the abdomen. Signs of overt peritonitis greatly worsen the prognosis because fibrinous adhesions spread quickly through the abdomen and lessen the chances for uterine repair. When the condition is suspected, a manual vaginal examination following careful preparation of the perineum and vulva is indicated. If the cow is fresh less than 48 hours, a hand may enter the uterus easily, but it may be difficult for the hand to pass through the cervix in cows greater than 48 hours postpartum. A speculum may be helpful, but manual palpation of the tear remains the best means of absolute diagnosis. Most tears are dorsal and just cranial to the cervix. When uterine rupture is detected immediately following delivery, options should be discussed with the owner. Salvage is the best option for cows of average value. Conservative treatment may be attempted when the uterine tear is dorsal and small. Broad-spectrum systemic antibiotics and repeated administration of oxytocin have been used for conservative therapy. The success of conservative therapy is often poor because of the primary problems of dystocia allowing heavy bacterial contamination of the uterus and abdomen. Cows that experience small dorsal uterine tears following manipulation/delivery of a live calf and in which fetal membranes do not contaminate the abdomen have the best prognosis.

When the cow is judged to be extremely valuable direct aggressive therapy including repair of the uterine tear may be necessary.

Treatment

Specific therapy includes surgical correction of the laceration, intensive antibiotic therapy to treat or prevent peritonitis, and supportive measures that may vary in each case. Surgical repair has been accomplished through the birth canal, but obviously this is difficult, is often done blindly, and is frequently unsuccessful. Epidural anesthesia and special extra-long surgical instruments facilitate this technique, but it remains, at best, difficult. This technique is possible only when the condition is recognized immediately and the cervix is wide open to allow two-handed manipulation.

Surgical repair following laparotomy is a better choice but also has inherent difficulties because the site of the tear often is dorsal and close to the cervix—consequently it is difficult to reach and to suture effectively from a flank approach once uterine involution has commenced. Incisions for this type of repair need to be made as far caudal in the paralumbar fossa as possible to facilitate visualization and repair of the rupture. It may be helpful to have an assistant direct the reproductive tract toward the operator by placing an arm through the birth canal. Flank laparotomy also is necessary for those rare cases having the fetus or fetal membranes free in the abdomen.

Recently we have attempted repair of uterine tears in dairy cattle after medical prolapse of the uterus by inversion through the caudal birth canal. This technique requires pharmacologic relaxation of the organ to allow manual prolapse. A slow IV infusion of 10 ml of 1:1000 epinephrine is administered by an assistant while the veterinarian holds the uterus after passing a gloved arm through the cervix. As uterine relaxation occurs, the uterus is retracted through the vagina and a surgical repair of the uterine tear completed. The uterus then is returned to normal position similar to replacing a spontaneous uterine prolapse. Despite the epinephrine-induced relaxation of the organ, retraction still may be difficult. In addition, the cardiovascular consequences of IV epinephrine constitute a risk to the patient but may be the lesser of two evils when contrasted with the disadvantages of other repair methods.

Bactericidal antibiotics are indicated preoperatively and for at least 2 weeks postoperatively if repair has been successful. Intraperitoneal lavage with saline and antibiotics or very dilute Betadine is indicated and facilitated when the uterine tear is repaired through a flank approach. Further supportive therapy such as IV fluids, NSAIDs, or short-acting corticosteroids for cattle showing early signs of shock may be indicated. Prognosis is poor to guarded for cattle with uterine rupture.

Uterine Prolapse

Etiology

Prolapse of the uterus is a condition well-known to bovine practitioners. In dairy cattle, the condition is not thought to be inherited and seldom recurs in subsequent parturitions. Although the exact cause for an individual patient may be difficult to determine, predisposing causes include dystocia, tenesmus, and hypocalcemia. Primiparous cows can be affected, but pluriparous ones are probably at greater risk. Prolapse of the uterus also is fostered by confinement, lack of exercise, and gravitational effects when cattle are allowed to calve with their hindquarters lower than their forequarters, as happens when confined cows calve into the drop of conventional barns. Uterine atony is the common inciting cause and is frequently associated with hypocalcemia in multiparous dairy cattle.

Prolapse usually occurs within hours of calving and almost always within 24 hours of calving. Instances of uterine prolapse occurring several days following calving are cited by many practitioners but are extremely rare.

Clinical Signs and Diagnosis

The clinical signs are dramatic and suffice for definitive diagnosis (Figure 9-4). Occasionally neophyte handlers or those privileged to have never seen the condition will confuse uterine prolapse with vaginal prolapse, but the sight of a fully prolapsed uterus is difficult to confuse with other conditions. Conspicuous placentomes on the exposed endometrium make the prolapsed uterus impossible to confuse with any other organ. The cow may appear healthy otherwise; this is often the case in primiparous cattle. Pluriparous cows with uterine prolapse often show varying degrees of hypocalcemia such as weakness, depression, subnormal temperature, anxiety, struggling or prostration, and coma. Tenesmus is common to most cases. Signs of shock should be differentiated from those of hypocalcemia because a small percentage of prolapse patients may develop hypovolemic shock secondary to blood loss (internal or external), laceration of the prolapsed organ, or intestinal incarceration within the prolapsed organ. Extreme pallor, a high heart rate, and prostration are grave signs in such cattle. Rarely the cow is found dead, especially when an unobserved calving has occurred. The prolapsed uterus often is heavily contaminated with bedding, feces, dirt, and placenta. Some bleeding is common from exposure injuries to the placentomes or endometrium. If the affected cow is able to stand and walk, the massive organ hangs near the hocks and can be stretched, traumatized, or lacerated as it flops back and forth against the rear quarters.

Treatment

Uterine prolapse is one of the true emergencies in bovine practice, and rapid owner recognition followed by prompt veterinary treatment greatly improves the prognosis. When notified of the condition, the veterinarian should instruct the owner to keep the cow quiet and to cleanse the exposed organ and keep it moist. Warm water containing dilute (1%) iodine and a clean towel or sheet work well for this purpose. If possible, the owner also may be instructed to elevate the organ to the level of the ischium or higher to relieve vascular compromise and subsequent edema, as well as lessen the chance of injury. When the veterinarian arrives at the scene, overall assessment of the situation is in order before proceeding with specific treatment. The cow's position, overall physical status, and the environment should be assessed. Specifically:

1. Can the cow's position be altered easily given the available help and environment to provide a mechanical advantage for replacement?
2. Is the cow hypocalcemic? Would correction of the hypocalcemia be beneficial immediately, or can it wait until after replacement of the organ? Would the cow be more likely to stand if treated with calcium? Some practitioners prefer replacement with the animal standing; others do not. Calcium treatment increases uterine tone and makes it substantially more difficult to replace; deferment until after uterine replacement is preferred if the cow can withstand the delay.

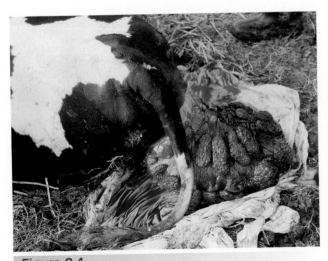

Figure 9-4

Uterine prolapse.

3. Is the cow in shock? If so, the owner should be made aware of the poor prognosis, lest veterinary treatment be blamed for her death during or after treatment.

4. Is footing adequate to allow the cow to stand, or should moving the cow to better footing be considered?

This overall assessment and a very quick history and cursory physical examination can be completed within minutes and may improve the end results greatly.

Specific treatment is subject to great individual variation as regards when to administer calcium, whether to perform the repair with the patient recumbent or standing, when to give certain drugs, and aftercare. The basic premises are, however, agreed on by most practitioners.

1. An epidural anesthetic is administered to relieve tenesmus and avoid fighting with the cow during replacement.

2. The cow is positioned to the veterinarian's advantage. The cow already may be able to stand, or the veterinarian may choose to treat the cow for hypocalcemia and allow her a short time such that she may stand for the procedure. Recumbent cows on a flat surface that have the hind legs pulled behind them so they are in sternal recumbency and the hind legs pulled caudally so the animal lies on the cranial stifle areas are easier to correct (Figure 9-5), but this position may predispose to coxofemoral injury if the cow struggles to get up. This tips the pelvis forward and allows a mechanical and gravitational advantage. If the cow is in an uneven posture, it also may be possible simply to angle her front end downhill to give significant mechanical advantage. In difficult situations where labor is unavailable or the environment is not conducive to gaining a mechanical or gravitational advantage, hip slings can be used to elevate the cow's rear quarters to hasten replacement. In some cases it

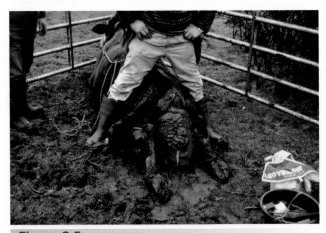

Figure 9-5

Adult cow positioned in sternal recumbency for replacement of uterine prolapse *(Courtesy Dr. Nigel Cook.)*

may be possible to hoist the hindquarters of the cow using farm equipment such as a skid steer. While this does facilitate replacement of the uterus, care must be taken to support the uterus as the cow's hindquarters are raised. Excessive tension on the prolapsed uterus may result in rupture of the uterine artery, already compromised by stretching in the prolapsed organs.

3. The uterus should be elevated to at least the level of the ischium to relieve vascular compromise and edema. One or two assistants can do this by suspending the organ in a towel, sheet, or prolapse tray when the cow is standing. In recumbent cows, the assistant can sit on the cow's sacral region facing backward and elevate the organ by holding it in his or her lap or suspended by a towel.

4. The uterine surface should be gently and thoroughly cleaned of debris and dirt and the placenta removed carefully. Usually the edematous placentomes allow easy separation of cotyledons from caruncles. Dilute antiseptics can be added to the water used for this purpose and the organ protected from further contamination. During this cleansing, gentle pressure and kneading of the organ are helpful to start restoration of uterine tone and relieve edema.

5. Systemic injection of oxytocin or ergonovine before replacement is controversial. Some practitioners will administer these tonic drugs before replacement—especially when the uterus is completely flaccid, atonic, or edematous, and the risk of iatrogenic perforation during replacement is deemed a considerable risk. Others (probably most practitioners, including these authors) prefer to administer tonic drugs following replacement for fear that the contracting organ will become more difficult to replace and cause greater resistance.

6. After the cow is positioned and the organ cleansed, replacement begins by slowly kneading and pushing the organ starting at the cervical end nearest the vulva. Lubrication with mild soaps and water or obstetrical lubricants is essential to facilitate these manipulations. Glycerol, if available, makes a useful lubricant because it is also hydroscopic and reduces uterine edema. The veterinarian must be careful not to push fingers through the friable endometrium or uterine wall; cupped hands work best. If iatrogenic uterine tears occur, they should be sutured with an inverting pattern. Candid discussion with the client regarding salvage should be undertaken when significant abdominal contamination is deemed to have occurred through uterine tears acquired following prolapse. Individual caruncles must be eased through the vulva, and rest periods during extreme tenesmus may be necessary. A slow, gradual replacement usually ensues

until only a portion of the gravid horn remains exposed. At this time, the tip of the horn is identified, and hand and arm pressure is exerted to evert the horn and uterus completely back into the abdomen. Once everted, the organ should be rocked gently and shaken to ensure complete eversion of the horns and minimize the chances of reprolapse. Some practitioners also use a bottle as an "arm extension" to aid in complete eversion of the horns. It is very important to completely evert both gravid and nongravid horns to prevent tenesmus from causing reprolapse after the epidural wears off.

7. Oxytocin or ergonovine is administered systemically and the organ palpated further to assess the response (e.g., increased tone). Intrauterine antibiotic therapy may be administered, and systemic antibiotics such as penicillin or ceftiofur should be used for 3 to 4 days to counteract the anticipated metritis. The cow should not be allowed to lie with her hind end "downhill" or in a gutter. Hypocalcemic cows not treated before replacement should be given appropriate calcium.

Retention sutures placed in the vulva following replacement of uterine prolapses are also controversial. They are ineffective for prevention of reprolapse and may rarely mask the condition by allowing the uterus to become trapped in the vagina. Since the common predisposition for uterine prolapse is uterine atony, complete restoration of the uterus to its normal position and treatment to enhance uterine tone are sufficient to prevent recurrence of the condition.

Prognosis

The prognosis for uncomplicated uterine prolapse is good, and most cows that respond promptly will breed back following routine monitoring and treatment of their metritis. Furthermore, dairy cows that have had prolapses do not have a higher incidence of the problem at future calvings. Of cows with uterine prolapses, 75% or more should do well.

Of cows that do not do well, a low percentage will reprolapse within 1 to 3 days, some cannot be replaced at all, some die as a result of intestinal incarceration in the prolapse or bleed out, some develop severe peritonitis or perimetritis from uterine tears, and some do irreparable damage to the prolapsed organ. The owner should be made aware that the cow could die at any time during or following replacement when shock is obvious. Reprolapse is an extremely bad sign, and cows that repeatedly prolapse after initial correction seldom do well. It is wise to reexamine all prolapse patients 3 days after repair to assess the overall systemic state and make specific recommendations regarding metritis or uterine injury. Decisions on further antibiotic and other therapy can be discussed with the owner at this time.

Retained Fetal Membranes

Etiology

RFM or retained placenta is a very common condition in dairy cattle. Fetal membranes should be expelled in less than 8 hours following normal parturition; therefore retention for longer than 8 to 12 hours is considered abnormal. Abortion, either infectious or sporadic, occurring during the last half of pregnancy frequently results in RFM. Hydrops, uterine torsion, twinning, and dystocia in general result in increased incidence of RFM when compared with normal parturitions. Heat stress and periparturient hypocalcemia also predispose to the condition. Cows induced to calve by pharmacologic means such as exogenous corticosteroid administration should be anticipated to have RFM. Nutritional causes such as overconditioning of dry cows and carotene and selenium deficiencies also have been incriminated. Low levels of vitamin A as occur in hyperkeratosis and polybrominated biphenyls toxicity are associated with RFM, metritis, and abortion. In selenium-deficient areas, cattle that have low selenium values may have an increased incidence of RFM, metritis, and cystic ovaries. Vitamin E, which has been shown to enhance neutrophil function, also may be involved. Cattle fed stored feeds from areas that are selenium deficient should be monitored for selenium status and supplemented routinely. Selenium and vitamin E could be related to RFM either as a result of pure deficiency or altered neutrophil function.

Cattle that have RFM following parturition may be at greater risk of the condition in subsequent years. Perhaps more importantly, epidemiologic studies show that cows with RFM have a higher incidence of metabolic diseases, mastitis, metritis, and subsequent abortion. Therefore despite the fact that many cows with RFM remain asymptomatic as regards immediate uterine health, associated diseases are a definite risk. Decreased resistance to uterine and other infections in cattle with RFM is partially explained by proven neutrophil dysfunction associated with the condition in periparturient cows. In addition to reduced neutrophil function, cattle with acute metritis associated with RFM could have a depletion of neutrophils in the peripheral blood as a result of acute recruitment of neutrophils to the infected uterus as evidenced by the degenerative left shift in the leukogram observed in some septic metritis patients. Although septic metritis or chronic endometritis does not occur in most cattle with RFM, the urge to treat RFM is based primarily on the inability to predict which cows will develop clinically significant sequelae.

Recent evidence strengthens the hypothesis that RFM is mediated by impaired neutrophil function beginning in the late dry period. Reduced neutrophil migration toward tissue extracts of placentomes can be detected as long as 2 weeks before calving in cows that go on to develop RFM. Other neutrophil functions, such as oxidative burst (a component of neutrophil bacterial killing action) are also impaired in these cows. Impaired neutrophil function has also been recorded in hypocalcemic cows. Indeed, many of the etiological factors associated with RFM have also been correlated to impairment of neutrophil function, including vitamin and mineral deficiencies, heat stress, or exogenous corticosteroid administration. The poor neutrophil function in affected cows extends into the postpartum period and probably mediates most of the complications usually associated with RFM.

Clinical Signs and Diagnosis

Clinical signs are obvious when the fetal membranes protrude from the vulva or hang ventral from the vulva to the escutcheon, rear udder, or hocks (Figure 9-6). The condition is less apparent when the membranes are retained within the uterus or only project into the cervix or vagina and require a vaginal examination to be detected. Other clinical signs are completely dependent on evolution of associated diseases. Metritis is the most common secondary complication, and clinical signs of metritis or endometritis are identical to those discussed in the metritis section. Secondary metabolic conditions may be linked directly to RFM when metritis exists or merely concurrent when the metritis is insignificant. As previously mentioned, mastitis, metabolic diseases, ascending urinary tract infections, and displaced abomasum may be associated with RFM complicated by metritis or, in the case of infections, because of less than optimal neutrophil function.

Tenesmus may appear in some cattle because of constant tension and irritation of the caudal reproductive tract by the protruding membranes. Eventually a fetid odor emanates from the RFM, especially when metritis develops, and this may be the initial prompt for producers to seek veterinary attention or instigate treatment themselves.

Untreated, most RFMs separate and fall away 3 to 12 days following calving. Unfortunately some cattle with RFM completely confined to the uterus may retain the membranes for a longer time because of cervical closure or antibiotic treatments, and only pass the RFM after the first estrus. These cows may become quite ill because of secondary metritis and retention of fetid fluid but go undetected initially because of a minimum of discharge and odor.

Clinical debate is sparked when the significance of RFM in dairy cattle is discussed. Because only a small percentage of cattle with RFM become ill and because numerous studies show that the subsequent fertility of cattle allowed to discharge RFM spontaneously is largely unaffected, why should veterinarians ever consider treating a cow with RFM? A frequently quoted reference from 1932 that details the subsequent fertility of 44 cows with untreated RFM compared with 44 herdmates without RFM showed no difference in subsequent fertility. Many other studies have since proven that manual removal of RFM is not only unnecessary but may be harmful. Although accepting these data as regards the simple issue of RFM, the studies tend to ignore the effects of the condition on the overall well-being of the cows with RFM. For example, in Palmer's 1932 article, only 31.8% of cattle with RFM had normal appetites for the 7 weeks following calving and only 29.5% had "good" milk production. It seems that these data support the observations of owners of cattle with RFM who believe that complete therapeutic disregard for cattle with RFM can lead to disaster. This is particularly true for obese cows with RFM. Reduced appetites leading to metabolic diseases or abomasal displacement are a definite problem in many cows with RFM that develop moderate or severe metritis. Even though the primary problem of RFM can clearly resolve itself naturally given time, the potential for associated and secondary problems exists, and "doing nothing" is often perceived as a potential economic gamble by owners of the modern high-producing dairy cow.

Treatment

A fascinating historical summation of treatment for RFM in cattle involving thousands of patients treated over several decades by the Ambulatory Clinic of the New York State Veterinary College is detailed in Roberts' text.

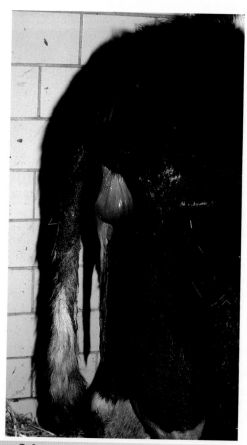

Figure 9-6

Retained fetal membranes.

A summary of these data would suggest that less invasive, less manipulative treatments in association with intrauterine or systemic antibiotics (as indicated by the individual patient's need and degree of metritis) progressively lessened the mortality rate for cattle with RFM. Cattle that resolve RFM and cycle normally should have fertility rates comparable with unaffected herdmates when breeding is begun at 90 days but may require adjunctive therapy in herds that begin breeding at 50 to 60 days as is common today.

Decisions to treat RFM may be based on medical need when metritis or other illnesses coexist or for the purpose of prophylaxis against metritis and associated problems. Some practitioners and owners take a "wait and see" attitude to avoid antibiotic concerns or unnecessary treatment whenever possible. Others who have herds that historically have a high incidence of metritis, ketosis, or abomasal displacement secondary to RFM tend to intervene prophylactically and therapeutically. Cattle that had dystocia, twinning, induced parturition, obesity, hepatic lipidosis, and RFM should be considered at high risk for metritis and probably justify prophylactic therapy. It is likely that the greatest benefits will accrue when measures are taken to improve management of cows in late gestation, rather than focus attention on cows actually suffering from RFM.

Treatment options include:

1. Do nothing—this course of action can be used when the affected cow appears completely healthy otherwise. Routine prebreeding reproductive exams can dictate the need for hormonal or antibiotic therapy following discharge of the membranes.
2. Administer systemic antibiotics prophylactically— usually ceftiofur (2.2 mg/kg once daily) is chosen to lessen milk withholding concerns. Treatment is started as soon as the RFM are judged pathologic (12 or 24 hours) and continued daily for 3 to 7 days or until the membranes separate. Systemic antibiotics immediately postpartum have a lesser economic impact because milk often is discarded during this time and penicillin could be used, but continued or long-term therapy can have significant economic impact because of drug costs and lost milk. Cows with high risk for metritis, e.g., overweight cows with RFM and suspected hepatic lipidosis, should be treated prophylactically with antibiotics and oxytocin in the immediate postpartum period. Although oxytocin does not promote release of membranes (indeed, cows with RFM have increased uterine tone relative to unaffected herd mates), evacuation of the uterus is a desirable consequence of treatment.
3. Administer intrauterine antibiotics prophylactically—usually tetracycline, ceftiofur, or penicillin is administered once daily or once every other day until the placenta falls away. In each case this represents extra-label drug use and the treatment has not been found to improve subsequent fertility. Tetracyclines may delay release of the placenta by inhibiting local metalloproteinases that play an important role in placental release. Catheter infusion of recently postpartum (<1 week) cattle is contraindicated—especially when performed by laypeople—because perforation of the cranial vagina or uterine body is an all-too-common sequela when the reproductive tract is too heavy to retract.
4. Combination of techniques 2 and 3.
5. Manual removal of RFM—this technique is no longer favored. More harm than good may come from manual attempts to remove RFM that are still firmly adhered to maternal caruncles, and further injury or irritation to the uterine endometrium can occur in badly infected or traumatized uteri. If the placenta is not easily removed with minimal tension, any further attempt to remove it manually should be abandoned. Some owners still request removal of RFM, and veterinarians must be emphatic that the procedure is not wise in most instances, lest the removal cause more subsequent damage than the existing condition.
6. Treatment of RFM complicated by metritis—see the section discussing metritis because all therapeutic decisions are based on resolution of that disease.
7. Hormonal treatment of retained placenta—oxytocin, prostaglandins, and estrogens have been proposed in varying dosages and times of administration to prevent or cause more rapid expulsion of RFM. There is little, if any, evidence that these treatments have any effect. In our hospital, oxytocin (5 U IM every 2 to 4 hours) is given for metritis and/or RFM <5 days duration in an attempt to decrease the volume of septic fluid in the uterus.
8. RFM protruding outside the vulva should be placed in a clean plastic bag (rectal sleeve) so gross contamination of the udder does not occur from the RFM. Although many practitioners prefer not to trim the protruding membranes in the belief that the weight of the dependent membranes speeds detachment, there is little supporting evidence for this view. Indeed, fetal membranes left intact at cesarean surgery are usually expelled spontaneously within a few days.

Acute Puerperal Metritis

Etiology

Postparturient metritis is extremely common in dairy cattle and is best thought of as a spectrum of diseases depicted as a biologic bell-shaped curve. The most severe manifestation of metritis, perimetritis, implies full-thickness infection of the uterus with subsequent serosal leakage resulting in pelvic and peritoneal complications.

Perimetritis is rare, potentially fatal, and most often follows severe dystocia. Septic metritis (acute puerperal or postpartum metritis, toxic metritis) refers to a severe puerperal uterine infection of the endometrium and deeper layers that results in systemic signs of toxemia. Puerperal metritis usually occurs from 1 to 10 days postpartum. "Metritis" is sometimes used as a general term for postpartum uterine infections of the endometrium or endometrium and deeper layers that may or may not cause systemic signs but may have implications for future reproductive performance. Infectious causes of reproductive failure such as brucellosis, leptospirosis, trichomoniasis, and campylobacteriosis may also cause varying degrees of metritis, but this discussion will be limited to conventional postpartum metritis.

Bacterial contamination of the uterus following parturition is extremely common during the first 2 weeks postpartum. As many as 93% of dairy cattle may have some bacterial contamination during this early postpartum period, but most infections appear to clear spontaneously because the infection rate decreases to 9% by days 46 to 60. Dystocia, RFM, dirty calving facilities, hepatic lipidosis, uterine atony, and iatrogenic vaginal contamination increase the occurrence of metritis.

The most common bacterium involved in early postpartum (<10 days) metritis is *Arcanobacterium pyogenes*. *Fusobacterium necrophorum*, *Prevotella melaninogenica*, and other anaerobes frequently complicate *A. pyogenes* infection, and these anaerobes act synergistically with *A. pyogenes* so the collective pathogenicity of each is increased. During the early postpartum period infection with *Escherichia coli*, hemolytic streptococci, *Pseudomonas* sp., *Proteus* sp., and *Clostridium* sp. may also be found. *E. coli* infections during the first 2 weeks postpartum seem to predispose to *A. pyogenes* infection and clinical or subclinical endometritis later in lactation. Persistent *A. pyogenes* infection after about 3 weeks postpartum is characterized by white or white-yellow purulent discharge. Although mild infections frequently resolve spontaneously, persistent or severe infections cause endometrial pathology and threaten future fertility. In many cases mild endometrial inflammation persists in the absence of frank uterine discharge, in a condition known as subclinical endometritis, which is common in North American dairy cows and has a severely detrimental effect on subsequent fertility. Involution of the uterus, host defense mechanisms, and regular reproductive cycling postpartum aid resolution of infection.

Mechanical influences such as severe uterine stretching as occurs in hydrops and twinning, physical injury to the reproductive tract resulting from dystocia, and uterine atony caused by hypocalcemia definitely predispose to infection as well. Dirty calving environments created by repeated use of maternity pens, calving in gutters or free stalls, and calving during periods of prolonged confinement act to increase environmental contamination

and increase the prevalence of metritis in dairy cattle. Field observations frequently imply an association between increased prevalence of metritis during periods of extreme heat or extreme cold and during the last months of confinement in conventionally housed cattle in northern climates. Management influences, although hard to define scientifically, are intuitively obvious because clinical metritis is rare in some herds and exceedingly common in others.

The consequences of postpartum metritis are not limited to reproductive matters, and many bovine practitioners believe that clinically significant metritis is *the* most common primary predisposing cause to displacement of the abomasum for cows in many herds. Affected cows are also predisposed to mastitis and clinical or subclinical endometritis.

Bovine practitioners should be familiar with variation in normal uterine involution and lochia. Normal postpartum uterine discharges tend to be mixtures of mucus and blood, with more mucus the better finding. Blood associated with uterine involution will often color uterine discharges red, orange, or "tomato soup." The consistency and odor of postpartum uterine discharges are important clues to the presence and severity of metritis in dairy cattle. Highly mucoid discharges in the early postpartum period (<10 days) usually indicate healthy uterine involution and minimal, if any, endometritis.

Although normal cattle have the greatest amount of lochia (several liters) within the first 48 hours postpartum, the amount subsequently discharged from the vulva varies from less than 100 ml (primipara) to 1 L or more (pluripara), and some may be absorbed via the uterus. Lochia consists of mucus, sloughing maternal placental tissue, and blood. Discharge of lochia usually begins at 3 days postpartum and continues through day 10. Around day 9 or 10 postpartum, the yellow-brown to red discharge may show increasing amounts of pink, brown, or red blood coinciding with sloughing of the maternal caruncles and their stalks, which leaves a denuded vascular surface. Such bloodstained mucoid discharge may be apparent as late as day 15 to 18. Cows with excellent postpartum health generally have their first postpartum ovulation around day 15, the second around day 32 or 33, and subsequent ones at regular 21-day cycles. Most of the first postpartum ovulations do not result in observable behavioral signs of estrus.

$PGF_{2\alpha}$ and its metabolites maintain high levels for 1 to 3 weeks postpartum and tend to remain elevated longer in cattle with metritis or delayed involution. In conjunction with elevated $PGF_{2\alpha}$ levels, progesterone levels remain at baseline until prostaglandin levels decrease. Administration of exogenous $PGF_{2\alpha}$ in the first weeks postpartum is unlikely to promote clinically relevant uterine motility or tone.

On rectal palpation, early postpartum uteri have good muscular tone and may have palpable longitudinal ridges associated with muscular contraction. Pluriparous cows usually have uteri too large to retract manually or to palpate fully before day 10 to 14. Some primiparous cows may have sufficient involution to allow full definition of the uterus per rectum by days 10 to 14. Rectal palpation may not, however, be the best means to detect abnormalities in uterine involution during the first 14 days following parturition, and veterinarians should not hesitate to perform clean vaginal examinations and a vaginal speculum examination as adjuncts. The onset of estrus causes a remarkable difference in the size of the organ in most cattle, and slightly cloudy or clear mucus may be massaged from the uterus and cervix at this time. Most grossly detectable uterine involution is completed by 25 to 30 days postpartum, although the uterine horns still may feel thicker or more doughy than normal until days 35 to 40. The process of involution is completed more quickly in primiparous cattle than older cattle, in cattle free of metritis, cattle without RFM, cattle without metabolic disease, and cattle that have not had dystocia. Normally during a vaginal examination at 2 days postpartum, a hand cannot be passed through the cervix, and by day 4, only two fingers can be passed into the cervix. Cervical involution may be delayed by dystocia, cervical trauma, or RFM.

Perimetritis is the most severe manifestation of metritis in cattle. Infection progresses through the entire uterine wall to cause serosal inflammation, exudation, and fibrinous adhesions. Almost invariably this condition is a consequence of dystocia because physical compromise and trauma to the uterus and caudal reproductive tract promote dissemination of bacteria from the uterine lumen and endometrium to the deeper layers. Vascular compromise as occurs in severe uterine torsions and subsequent manipulations to deliver the calf also predispose to perimetritis. True perimetritis results in peritonitis because this condition is not limited to retroperitoneal tissues. Extensive peritoneal exudates, fibrin deposition and adhesions to other viscera, and localization of septic exudates are common in perimetritis patients.

Clinical Signs and Diagnosis

Cattle with septic or toxic metritis become ill within the first 10 days—usually the first 7 days—postpartum. Signs of toxemia such as fever (103.0 to 106.5° F/39.5 to 41.39° C), tachycardia, inappetence, decreased production, rumen stasis, depression, dehydration, and diarrhea are common. Note that fever may be absent in a significant number of cows with acute puerperal metritis. Extremely severe infection may cause recumbency secondary to toxemia, weakness, and metabolic disorders, and death may ensue. A fetid watery uterine discharge may be obvious at the vulva, may stain the tail, or may require a vaginal examination to be detected. Such uterine discharges vary in color from brown to

amber to gray or red but always are fluid, low in mucus content, purulent, and have an extremely fetid odor that permeates one's clothes, hair, and arm even when guarded by an obstetrical sleeve. Although most cows with acute puerperal metritis have a history of dystocia, giving birth to twins, or RFM, not all do. Because these patients are very early postpartum, uterine infection and resultant appetite and gastrointestinal consequences predispose to metabolic diseases such as hypocalcemia and ketosis. The general term toxemia is used because (depending on the exact mix of causative organisms) endotoxins, exotoxins, and other mediators may be involved in the pathophysiology of the systemic signs.

Rectal examination usually reveals a hypotonic or atonic uterus with fluid distention. Physometra also may be present and cause the gas-fluid filled uterine horn to be confused with other viscera such as a distended cecum. Although attempts to retract the uterus should not be forced, gentle massage of the uterine body, cervix, and anterior vagina quickly causes fetid uterine discharges to be expelled from the vulva. A vaginal examination following cleaning of the perineal area is imperative to complete the diagnosis because this procedure allows differentiation of necrotic vaginitis or cervicitis and also allows detection of RFM and other pathology. Transabdominal ultrasound examination can be useful in determining size of the uterus, thickness of the wall, and the presence of fetal membranes or intrauterine gas. Cattle with septic metritis are at increased risk of abomasal displacement as a result of toxemia-induced gastrointestinal stasis and secondary metabolic conditions. A complete physical examination should be completed to rule out concurrent abomasal displacement and other conditions such as septic mastitis.

Clinical signs usually suffice for definitive diagnosis of septic metritis. Ancillary data support an overwhelming infection as evidenced by a degenerative left shift in the leukogram and elevated fibrinogen values. Acute recruitment of neutrophils to the uterus out of the bloodstream weakens the patient's cellular defenses against other infections—especially mastitis. A mild metabolic alkalosis is anticipated in cattle with gastrointestinal stasis. Differential diagnosis includes consideration of septic mastitis, peritonitis of any source, and acute pyelonephritis. Cultures of the uterine fluid never are contraindicated but, frankly, seldom are performed in dairy cattle. It is assumed that *A. pyogenes*, anaerobes such as *F. necrophorum* and *Prevotella melaninogenica*, and other organisms are present. Coliforms are common following dystocia or RFM and could cause additional endotoxin production. Clostridial organisms also have been identified in some septic metritis patients, and *Clostridium tetani* has been identified rarely in the uterine flora from cattle that develop tetanus secondary to septic metritis. If cultures are elected, both aerobic and anaerobic testing should be performed.

Because of the wide spectrum of severity observed in postpartum endometritis-metritis, some recently post-partum (<14 days) cattle are neither toxemic nor perfectly healthy. This intermediate group of cattle has signs of reduced appetite and depression and frequently has metabolic diseases such as ketosis and hypocalcemia. These cows may or may not be febrile and, if febrile, only mildly so (103.5 to 104.5° F/39.72 to 40.28° C). If rectal examination reveals a poorly involuting hypotonic uterus containing excessive fetid fluid, these animals should be treated for puerperal metritis. These patients also are at risk for abomasal displacement caused by decreased fiber intake and intermittent or constant gastrointestinal dysfunction.

Signs of peritonitis predominate and become apparent 1 to 5 days following parturition. Fever, tachycardia, gastrointestinal stasis, depression, anorexia, and dehydration are present. The patient may assume an arched stance, be reluctant to move or rise from recumbency, have a guarded abdomen, and groan during expiration. Tenesmus is present in some patients. Rectal examination reveals the profound consequences of perimetritis—fibrinous adhesions and inflammation of all pelvic viscera are present such that the rectum cannot be moved and the examiner's arm is locked in a constant position. If the uterine body can be palpated, crepitus caused by extensive fibrin deposition, adhesions, and abscesses may be palpable. Rectal examination findings coupled with the other signs usually suffice for diagnosis. Once the characteristic circumferential inflammation in the pelvis is palpated, however, it is best to discontinue the rectal examination for fear of worsening the situation, rupturing the uterus, causing the patient severe pain, or increasing the risk of severe tenesmus.

Ancillary data also may be helpful when the condition must be differentiated from retroperitoneal inflammation caused by vaginal perforations or extensive pelvic hematoma or inflammation secondary to dystocia. Abdominal paracentesis will indicate peritonitis based on increased protein and white blood cell counts in perimetritis patients but may be normal or have only moderately increased protein in retroperitoneal conditions. A complete blood count usually shows a degenerative left shift when perimetritis is peracute or acute. Neutrophilia is possible in subacute or chronic cases. Serum albumin tends to be decreased because of extensive protein loss into the uterus and peritoneal cavity in severe perimetritis cases (Figure 9-7). Vaginal examination may be indicated to rule out purely vaginal conditions and should be performed very gently following epidural anesthesia to avoid "malignant tenesmus," which is a constant straining fueled by movement of air into the rectum.

The prognosis is extremely poor for perimetritis, and most cows with this condition die within 1 to 7 days after diagnosis. If the cow's value allows intensive treatment,

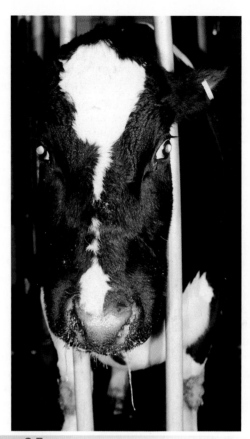

Figure 9-7

Severe facial edema caused by hypoproteinemia secondary to perimetritis.

systemic broad-spectrum antibiotics should be started immediately. IV fluid therapy is necessary because the extensive peritonitis usually results in complete anorexia. Penicillin, tetracycline, and ceftiofur are the most common antibiotics used for systemic therapy. Local or intra-uterine therapy is contraindicated in most cases because extensive compromise of the uterine wall increases the risk of perforation. Prostaglandins may be used to encourage evacuation of the uterus but probably are of limited value because the uterus adheres to adjacent visceral and parietal peritoneum. Epidural anesthesia may be necessary if tenesmus exists. NSAIDs may be helpful during the first few days of treatment to counteract endotoxemia and provide a degree of analgesia. Dosage and duration of therapy using these drugs must be limited to minimize the potential for abomasal or renal toxicity.

Cattle that survive show slow but continual improvement as evidenced by a gradual return to normal temperature, normal heart rate, and return of appetite. Long-term (3 to 4 weeks) antibiotic therapy is indicated, and attempts to palpate the reproductive tract should be avoided for 3 to 4 weeks so as not to disturb adhesions. Surviving cows will always have extensive adhesions of the reproductive tract in the caudal abdomen and pelvis. It is best to allow complete sexual rest; prostaglandins should be administered at 14-day intervals to encourage uterine evacuation. Evacuation obviously is hampered by uterine adhesions. The cow should be assessed by rectal palpation once monthly. Despite the presence of extensive adhesions, surviving cattle eventually may resolve many of the adhesions over a 5- to 6-month period and conceive. Frequently these cows only "work on one side"—meaning that one uterine horn, uterine tube, or ovary (or all these) continues to be confined by adhesions. Therefore such a cow may conceive only when an ovulation occurs on the healthy or nonadhered ovary. Careful evaluation of the caudal reproductive tract and the presence of mature fibrous adhesions within the pelvic canal are critical before a decision as to breeding the cow back is made. Some cattle with persistent adhesions may be able to conceive and carry a pregnancy to term but should undergo elective cesarean section rather than attempting a natural or assisted vaginal delivery.

Cattle that do not improve following initial intensive therapy may either die as a result of diffuse peritonitis within the first few days following parturition or else linger as chronic peritonitis patients with persistent low-grade fever, partial anorexia, abdominal distention, hypoproteinemia resulting from albumin loss into the peritoneal space, and wasting.

Clinical Endometritis

Much of the veterinary professional literature on bovine endometritis suffers from lack of a universally accepted definition of the disease and associated uniformity in diagnostic criteria. The lactation incidence of endometritis has been estimated at 7.5% to 8.9% based on visible mucopurulent vaginal discharge to over 40%. Interpretation of these data is difficult in view of the known high incidence of a transient inflammatory response in the postpartum bovine uterus.

Diagnosis of endometritis by rectal palpation (and fortuitous observation of a vaginal discharge, if present in adequate quantities) is probably the basis for treatment of most cows in the field in North America. Repeated observations that this is an insensitive and nonspecific method of diagnosis have generally passed unheeded. Of 157 cows suspected of having endometritis based on rectal palpation alone, 22% were culture positive, but 59% of positive uterine cultures were obtained from 59 cows in which a diagnosis of endometritis was based on vaginal speculum examination. The nature of cervical discharge determined by vaginoscopic examination is well-correlated to both the overall rate of positive bacterial cultures and to the rate of recovery of *A. pyogenes*.

Although endometrial biopsy and histopathology may constitute the ideal method of diagnosis of endometritis, the procedure is invasive, expensive, and time consuming. Furthermore, the procedure itself may be associated with delayed conception.

A 2002 publication by LeBlanc et al has done much to dispel confusion and provide a rational basis for diagnosis of clinical endometritis in dairy cows. They used survival analysis to derive a case definition of endometritis based on factors associated with an increased time to pregnancy. (Although this approach ignores the fact that "endometritis" is a term with a pathological definition—namely inflammation of the endometrium—it does yield a set of criteria that are clinically valuable.) LeBlanc et al examined 1865 cows in 27 herds between 20 and 33 days after parturition. This group concluded that the reproductive consequence of clinical signs depended on the time of their observation. The presence of a purulent uterine discharge or cervical diameter greater than 7.5 cm after 20 days postpartum or a mucopurulent discharge after 26 days postpartum defined clinically relevant endometritis in their study. Using this definition, prevalence was 17%. Vaginoscopy was an important component of the examination; failure to perform vaginoscopy would have resulted in failure to identify 44% of cases of clinically relevant endometritis. However, if vaginoscopy is not feasible, consideration of uterine horn diameter greater than 8 cm is an acceptable alternative. Cows with endometritis were 27% less likely to conceive in a given period, and 1.7 times more likely to be culled than cows without endometritis. Using pregnancy by 120 or 150 days as the main outcome measure, these diagnostic criteria were nearly 90% specific and had a sensitivity of about 20% (reflecting a multitude of other causes of reproductive failure).

Clinically relevant endometritis was more prevalent in mature cows. Cows in the third or higher lactation had a prevalence of 21%, compared with 13% for second lactation animals and 12% for first lactation cows. Cows with endometritis were more likely to have no palpable ovarian structures at the time of examination. The risk of clinically relevant endometritis was increased by retention of fetal membranes, birth of twins, or toxic puerperal metritis. Season of calving had no influence on prevalence of the condition.

Overall, the median time to pregnancy for cows with endometritis was 32 days longer than in normal cows. There was a slight (3 day) delay in days to first insemination, and a pronounced (30%) reduction in first service pregnancy risk.

Evaluation of treatment options has been limited by lack of a widely accepted definition of clinical endometritis and a failure to concentrate on reproductive outcomes. Thus intrauterine infusion was the mainstay of treatment of bovine endometritis for decades. In spite of this, there was no convincing evidence that this mode of therapy had any beneficial effect on future reproductive performance of affected cows. In the face of mounting public concern about medicinal remedies in edible animal products, it is hard to justify antimicrobial treatment of dubious efficacy. It is interesting to note that the first words of skepticism regarding intrauterine infusions were raised in 1956 by Roberts. The primary alternative to intrauterine therapy has been systemic administration of PGF$_{2\alpha}$. Unfortunately, evidence for this approach is not entirely convincing either.

Recently, however, a new product has emerged for which some positive evidence has accumulated. Administration of cephapirin, a first-generation cephalosporin antibiotic, specifically formulated for intrauterine administration, has been found effective in improving reproductive performance of dairy cows with risk factors for uterine disease and of those with clinical endometritis. In conjunction with the study in which they developed a definition of clinically significant endometritis, LeBlanc et al examined treatment with cephapirin or prostaglandin and found both to be superior to no treatment in terms of reproductive performance. LeBlanc et al found no benefit to treatment before 4 weeks postpartum. Cephapirin-treated cows had a significantly shorter time to pregnancy than control animals. Interestingly, they found a detrimental effect of PG administered to cows without a palpable corpus luteum.

The lack of convincing experimental data and variable availability of products from country to country make it impossible to promote a single approach to therapy of clinical endometritis with confidence. All intrauterine infusions, with the exception of cephapirin, seem to be contraindicated. Given current sensitivity to antimicrobial use in food-producing cows, more trials are necessary before cephapirin can be endorsed in all cases. Although the evidence in favor of PGF$_{2\alpha}$ is weak, this product is inexpensive in most markets, and not harmful. It is useful in reproductive management programs and may be beneficial independent of the presence of endometritis.

Subclinical Endometritis

Subclinical endometritis can be defined as endometrial inflammation of the uterus usually determined by cytology, in the absence of purulent material in the vagina. It is only of significance at the stage at which normal involution is complete (i.e. after about 5 weeks postpartum). In animals without signs of clinical endometritis, subclinical disease can be diagnosed by measuring the proportion of neutrophils present in a sample collected by flushing the uterine lumen with a low volume (20 ml) of sterile saline solution, or using a cytobrush. Although investigation of subclinical endometritis is at an early stage, presence of greater than 5% neutrophils after about 40 days postpartum constitutes a level of inflammation related to significantly impaired reproductive performance in affected cows. Alarmingly, several studies in different parts of the United States have indicated that as many as 50% of cows meet this definition.

Use of endometrial cytology in individual cows is not economically feasible, and attention should be devoted to preventing this disease, which has been associated with depressed dry matter intake beginning 2 weeks before parturition, negative energy balance, and impaired immune function.

Treatment with intrauterine infusion of cephapirin or PGF$_{2\alpha}$ has been associated with improved conception to first service and fewer days open.

Treatment Options

Review of the literature regarding the treatment of metritis and endometritis in cattle quickly reveals that few treatments have scientific merit. This lack of scientific data seems at odds with the empiric success enjoyed by most practicing bovine practitioners. Do we give too much credit to our treatment of endometritis patients when, in fact, spontaneous cures are responsible for most success? How then does the veterinarian decide intelligently which cows require treatment and what, if any, drugs to use? Is the veterinarian willing to assume the risk of benign neglect? The consequences of unresolved endometritis such as failure to cycle, failure to conceive, and early embryonic death or abortions are well known and accepted. Therefore when and how should we intervene? This decision is easier when cattle with metritis have associated systemic illness. In cattle without systemic signs, endometritis may resolve spontaneously if normal estrus activity, normal phagocytic cell function, and adequate nutrition all exist.

Perhaps the best decisions regarding therapy are made in light of an accurate diagnosis. Cattle with minimal delays in involution, minimal uterine fluid or discharge, and normal estrus activity are likely to cure themselves. However, cattle with systemic signs resulting from metritis, with large amounts of uterine fluid or discharges, ovarian inactivity or cysts, or failure of estrus should be considered abnormal and treatment should ensue. Most studies of treatment, or lack thereof, for cattle with metritis do not detail the severity of the problem and are subject to some criticism for this fact, as well as their failure to define the time postpartum when the diagnosis was reached and whether control populations were maintained.

Intrauterine Therapy

Intrauterine antibiotics have fallen largely into disfavor despite having been used for decades in the treatment of metritis in cattle. Intrauterine antibiotics also are often absorbed from the uterus to establish blood and milk levels that cause concern for milk residues and discard, resulting in significant economic losses. Absorption is more likely from healthy uteri, at the time of estrus, and following uterine involution. Certain antibiotics may interfere with phagocytic cell function, may be made inactive by beta-lactamase-producing bacteria, may irritate the endometrium, or may not work well in the relative anaerobic state thought to exist in the uterus. Perhaps the greatest impediment to using intrauterine antibiotics lies in the fact that large amounts of uterine fluid may simply overwhelm or inactivate small doses of locally administered antibiotics. Many intrauterine treatments may be compared to a "drop in the ocean" when used in severe metritis cases. Cephapirin, a first-generation cephalosporin, is available in some countries in a formulation designed specifically for intrauterine administration (Metricure, InterVet). It is not available in the United States. In several trials it has been found to be beneficial for treatment of clinical and subclinical endometritis. Its use in acute puerperal metritis has not been reported.

Despite these scientific reservations, intrauterine therapy may be helpful and is frequently used as a component of therapy. Why does it seem to help? Antibiotics may kill a proportion of the total bacterial populace when administered as intrauterine therapy even when pharmacokinetics and pharmacology are imperfect. Much of the referenced "pharmacology" is extrapolated from data collected in other species rather than specifically documented scientifically for cattle. Intrauterine oxytetracycline (5.5 mg/kg) administered to early postpartum cows did establish high luminal, caruncular, and endometrial levels for at least 24 hours. Another study showed that 3 g of oxytetracycline daily for 3 days (intrauterine) was more successful at sterilizing *A. pyogenes* metritis than either 3 consecutive days of $PGF_{2\alpha}$ or no treatment. The numbers of cows in this study were small, however. A more recent study demonstrated that 0.5 g of cephapirin (available in Europe) given within 24 hours of calving improved reproductive performance in cows with RMF or a dead calf. Similarly a recent study using intrauterine ceftiofur (1 g) demonstrated a positive effect in cows with either RFM or twins.

As previously mentioned the early postpartum uterus—especially when infected—does not absorb drugs into the deeper uterine wall or systemic circulation as effectively as an involuted, noninfected uterus. This may be beneficial to intrauterine antibiotics in early postpartum cattle because the major drug levels appear in the lumen and superficial endometrial tissue. Penicillin has been used as an intrauterine therapy. Either 10 million units of procaine penicillin or 10 million units of sodium penicillin have been used to establish effective luminal and endometrial concentrations for 24 hours.

In summation, regarding intrauterine antibiotic therapy as a treatment for endometritis, few drugs have been evaluated thoroughly, the magnitude of infection in treated cattle is difficult to evaluate, the dosage and duration of reported therapies vary tremendously, and many pharmacologic reasons exist as to why intrauterine therapy may not work. Based on literature review and common sense, the disadvantages of intrauterine therapy include:

1. In severe metritis or in cases having copious amounts of uterine fluid, a simple intrauterine treatment cannot possibly cure the problem because of dilution of the drug.
2. Drugs may be inactivated by purulent debris, beta-lactamase-producing microbes, or other factors such as an anaerobic environment.
3. Intrauterine antibiotics result in detectable blood and milk levels of antibiotic residues that require milk discard. Even though absorption may be less efficient in noninvoluted infected uteri, it has been demonstrated that daily intrauterine therapy with 5 g of oxytetracycline in early postpartum cattle with RFM resulted in elevated residues in milk for more than 2 days and, in other cases, 4 days, after the last treatment.

Despite these disadvantages, veterinarians may choose to use intrauterine therapy in certain circumstances. Based on the previous discussion, it means that rational use of intrauterine therapy requires several considerations.

1. Milk must be discarded and should be checked individually for residues following the use of antibiotics because extra-label use is the rule.
2. Treatment should be repeated daily.
3. Treatment should use appropriate dosages of drugs and consider the "volume" of the uterus and fluid or pus to be treated. Uterine lavage to remove large volumes of purulent material before administration of intrauterine antibiotics increases effectiveness of treatment.
4. Intrauterine therapy probably would be much more successful if the exact cause were identified by cultures in each patient.
5. In my opinion, intrauterine therapy for metritis is helpful in early postpartum infections (often in conjunction with systemic antibiotics) with watery purulent material and in later postpartum *A. pyogenes* infections with small amounts of residual pus. Intrauterine therapy is not as helpful in cattle 10 to 30 days postpartum that have large accumulations (>200 ml) of thick *A. pyogenes* pus.
6. Some antibiotics such as undiluted tetracycline are irritating to the endometrium. Nitrofurazone was also an irritant but is now illegal. Antiseptics such as diluted Lugol's iodine (1% to 2%) and chlorhexidine also are irritating and cause chemical necrosis and sloughing of the endometrium. However, tetracycline can be used safely in cattle as a powder in gelatin boluses or by direct infusion in early postpartum metritis cases. In addition, Lugol's iodine and oxytetracycline have been used successfully by many practitioners for selected chronic endometritis patients that conform to the following criteria: a fully or almost completely involuted uterus, poor uterine

tone, minimal purulent discharge, rectal palpations performed 2 to 3 weeks apart that have confirmed ovarian inactivity or ovarian cysts, in addition to evidence of abnormal discharge on more than one occasion. In these selected patients, judicious infusion of irritants may cause release of endogenous prostaglandins from the uterus that may cause the cow to cycle and thereby promote natural resistance mechanisms and a return to estrus.

Systemic Antibiotics

Systemic antibiotics have become the "in vogue" treatment for metritis in dairy cattle over the past decade. The use of systemic antibiotics is justified and often required for metritis that causes systemic illness. However, systemic therapy is definitely overused in cattle with metritis or RFM that do not have a fever or are not systemically ill. This overuse results in significant economic loss for owners because of antibiotic costs and loss of income resulting from discarded milk, although ceftiofur can be used without discarding milk. Veterinarians inexperienced with other treatment options do not discriminate or differentiate metritis based on severity, duration, or association with systemic signs and may be too quick to suggest systemic antibiotic therapy.

Systemic antibiotics are indicated when metritis causes systemic illness in recently postpartum cattle. Knowing that most recently (<10 days) postpartum cattle have mixed (*A. pyogenes*, anaerobes, coliforms, or others) infections and that chronic endometritis patients are more likely to be mainly *A. pyogenes* influences the choice of antibiotic. For example, penicillin would be effective against *A. pyogenes* and most opportunistic anaerobes such as *F. necrophorum* and *Bacteroides* sp. It is, however, unlikely that penicillin would eliminate concurrent coliform infection. Procaine penicillin (22,000 U/kg once daily) would likely maintain effective concentration in the uterus. Ceftiofur may be more effective against coliforms and was found to have lower mean inhibitory concentration (MIC) against *A. pyogenes* and anaerobic bacteria cultured from the uterus than did oxytetracycline. Ceftiofur derivatives have been shown to reach concentrations in both uterine tissue and uterine fluid of healthy postpartum cows that exceeds the MICs for *E. coli*, *F. necrophorum*, *Bacteroides* spp., and *A. pyogenes*. Ceftiofur is currently the most commonly used antibiotic for treating metritis in our hospital. Valuable cows are sometimes treated with ceftiofur at a dosage higher than the label dose of 2.2 mg/kg once daily. Oxytetracycline dosed at 11 mg/kg twice daily may only establish uterine tissue concentrations of 5 µg/kg—a level thought to be less than that required to kill *A. pyogenes*. This is interesting and somewhat difficult to fathom in light of the apparent widespread success experienced by veterinarians treating septic metritis patients with once-daily systemic oxytetracycline. The apparent contradiction

may be explained partially by dosage because many veterinarians administer 13.2 to 15.4 mg/kg oxytetracycline, which can be nephrotoxic. It could also be theorized that oxytetracycline somehow manages to control or reduce populations of organisms other than *A. pyogenes* that produce endotoxins or exotoxins that result in the majority of systemic signs. A combination of a systemic sulfa drug (sulfadimethoxine) and oxytetracycline also has been used successfully by many practitioners as systemic therapy for metritis associated with illness in recently postpartum cattle. Unfortunately few scientific data are available regarding antibiotics such as ampicillin and sulfonamides as regards systemic therapy of metritis.

Hormonal Therapy

Historically estrogenic compounds have been administered systemically to cows with metritis or endometritis—usually subacute to chronic cases. At present, estrogen therapy is seldom used. Some practitioners believed that estrogenic drugs enhanced the sensitivity of the uterus to oxytocin during natural oxytocin release or following exogenous administration, thereby promoting uterine tone and evacuation. It also was thought that such therapy might duplicate the inherent resistance of the uterus that occurs naturally during estrus and that is reduced by the influence of progesterone as previously mentioned. However, double-blind, prospective clinical trials have established convincingly that estradiol treatment of postpartum cows has no merit for improving health, survival, or later reproductive success. Because of withdrawal of estrogenic compounds from the market, public health fears regarding estrogenic compounds in food products, and lack of efficacy, estrogens are not indicated for use.

The commercial availability of $PGF_{2\alpha}$ and prostaglandin analogues has been a significant development in the treatment of metritis and endometritis in cattle. The use of prostaglandins largely has replaced antibiotic therapy and intrauterine antibiotics for endometritis patients without systemic signs and provides useful adjunctive therapy in some patients with systemic illness resulting from severe metritis. It is known and accepted that $PGF_{2\alpha}$ and other analogues such as cloprostenol, fenprostalene, and prostalene induce luteolysis. Therefore cattle with endometritis that also have a functional corpus luteum can be expected to return to estrus when given these products. Return to estrus stimulates uterine tone, enhances evacuation of uterine fluid, and causes endogenous estrogen levels to increase, whereas progesterone levels decrease. All of these effects are desirable. Less is known regarding the effects of these drugs in cattle that do not have a "functional" corpus luteum, including cows with puerperal metritis in the first 2 weeks postpartum. It has been suggested that $PGF_{2\alpha}$ and other analogues affect uterine evacuation by producing uterine contraction and may enhance phagocytic activity. However, these latter two mechanisms have not been demonstrated in cows. Further confusion is created by the fact that, as previously mentioned, recently postpartum cattle having metritis maintain higher than normal prostaglandin levels without exogenous help. Although the exact mechanisms of action for these drugs are only partially understood, $PGF_{2\alpha}$ and its analogues have replaced intrauterine therapy in most instances of subacute or chronic endometritis in dairy cattle (after 3 weeks postpartum).

Treatment of Cattle with Acute Puerperal Metritis

This requires therapy for systemic manifestations and control of local infection in the uterus. Systemic antibiotics should be administered once or twice daily. Oxytetracycline (13.2 to 15.4 mg/kg) administered intravenously (IV) once or twice daily (renal injury from the tetracycline must be considered at the high dosage and/or in dehydrated cows), procaine penicillin G (22,000 U/kg) given intramuscularly (IM) once or twice daily, ceftiofur (2.2 mg/kg) once daily, ampicillin (11.0 to 22.0 mg/kg) once or twice daily, and sulfadimethoxine have all been used for systemic treatment. Most practitioners now use ceftiofur. Supportive treatment includes parenteral dextrose, calcium, oral or IV fluids, and nonsteroidal antiinflammatory drugs (NSAIDs). Because most cows with septic metritis are fresh less than 10 days, associated or secondary hypocalcemia and ketosis are common problems. Cows that are completely off feed benefit from IV fluids, whereas those with functional rumen activity can be economically rehydrated and provided with an energy substrate with fluids and alfalfa meal administered through a stomach tube. NSAIDs such as flunixin meglumine (0.25 mg/kg thrice daily, 0.5 mg/kg twice daily, or 1.0 mg/kg once daily) are used by many practitioners for antiendotoxic, antipyretic, and antiinflammatory activity. Although commonly used in our hospital at 0.25 mg/kg thrice daily, Dr. Rebhun preferred to reserve flunixin for the most severely ill cattle because the drugs artificially decrease temperature, thereby interfering with effective monitoring of the effects of antibiotic therapy on the infection. In addition, these drugs may increase the potential for abomasal ulceration. Local therapy of the uterine infection also is important. A vaginal examination should be performed after proper cleaning of the perineum and uterine discharges evacuated by gentle manipulation whenever possible. Uterine siphoning and saline or dilute Betadine (Purdue Pharma, Cranbury, NJ) lavage is used by some practitioners and is common practice in our hospital. If siphoning and lavage are used, it is imperative they be performed gently by gravitational lavage only and with respect for the already compromised uterine wall, lest perforation occur. Lavage has rarely been associated with apparent worsening of clinical signs in some cattle. This subjective finding may be the result of uterine irritation and increased absorption of endotoxins or exotoxins through the inflamed uterine tissue. An epidural anesthetic (lidocaine) may be helpful in lessening the discomfort of the cow during and after the lavage and may prevent repeated straining both during and following the procedure. Cattle that are more than 3 days postpartum and found to have easily removable RFM can have these membranes removed to lessen the "plug" effect that they may create to effective uterine drainage. Forced physical removal of RFM is no longer performed in our hospital. If the clinician elects to administer intrauterine antibiotics, then the same antibiotic should be used systemically. Intrauterine therapy can be used once daily during the lavage until improvement is obvious. Oxytetracycline powder or solution may be administered intrauterinely as 2 to 4 oz of powder or 4 to 6 g of solution. Penicillin (10 million U of sodium penicillin in 250 ml of saline solution), ceftiofur, or ampicillin may be used in the same manner. Polymyxin (1.6 million units) has also been used to bind endotoxin in some valuable cows, but proper milk (at least 5 days) and meat withdrawal guidelines must be provided. Irritant chemical (concentrated iodine, chlorhexidine) infusions should be avoided. Obvious dilution and loss of intrauterine antibiotics occur because of the large volume of fluid present in the uterus of cows with septic metritis, dictating daily repetition of treatment. When uterine atony accompanies septic metritis, parental calcium solutions and oxytocin 10 units every 2 to 4 hours for up to 5 days postpartum may be used as adjunctive therapy, but their inclusion is empiric rather than scientific unless hypocalcemia is confirmed. $PGF_{2\alpha}$ and analogues have been used to improve uterine tone, but their effectiveness in the early postpartum cow is debatable. It may be preferable to wait until at least 8 days postpartum before using these products.

A return to normal temperature, heart rate, hydration, and appetite are the hallmarks of successful therapy. Systemic and local therapy should be continued a minimum of 3 days and the patient monitored for metabolic disease and abomasal displacement. Observance of withdrawal times for meat and milk should be established by milk or urine testing of individual patients. There is considerable individual variation in drug metabolism according to drug dosage, severity of systemic disease, and the route of administration chosen such that clients should be made aware that nonparenteral administration of antibiotics can still result in violative residues.

Cattle with severe early postpartum metritis that are not "toxic" but mildly to moderately ill may or may not require systemic antibiotics. However, they will frequently benefit from intensive local and supportive therapy as outlined above. In addition, these cows should receive two doses of $PGF_{2\alpha}$ 8 hours apart at 8 days postpartum and repeated when a functional corpus luteum has been palpated.

Cattle that are not systemically ill but have an obvious large volume of purulent discharge associated with endometritis generally are more than 10 days into lactation, have *A. pyogenes* as the major pathogen, and are treated by systemic $PGF_{2\alpha}$ or analogues with or without local antibiotic therapy. This treatment should again be repeated at least once when a functional corpus luteum is palpated. Although some of these cattle may recover spontaneously without treatment, assuming that normal estrus occurs, it often is impossible to predict which cows will cure themselves. Potential consequences of persistent endometritis and owner concern usually make the veterinarian err on the side of treatment rather than benign neglect. Intrauterine antibiotic therapy may be considered so long as the reservations listed above are recognized. Intrauterine therapy in those subacute to chronic endometritis patients is best performed after most or all uterine fluid has been evacuated. It also would seem wise to administer intrauterine therapy for several consecutive days to improve the chances of sterilizing the uterus.

The most difficult decision for therapy arises in the last category—*chronic, low grade endometritis with intermittent or small amounts of purulent discharge.* Such patients may or may not be cycling, and repeated rectal examinations are necessary to confirm or deny effective cycling. As mentioned previously, chronic endometritis may be the cause or effect when ovarian inactivity, ineffective ovulation, or cystic ovaries coexist with it. Rectal palpation may be helpful in some cows with detectable uterine fluid, thick-walled uteri, consistently poor uterine tone, or consistently increased uterine tone. Pus flecks or pus mixed with normal mucus may be observed or massaged from the reproductive tract in such cows. Cervicitis and vaginitis must be ruled out by vaginal speculum examination. Ideally treatment would be preceded by uterine cultures in these patients. *A. pyogenes* is assumed to be the causative organism, but this may not be true in all patients. Intrauterine antibiotic therapy is best performed daily for several consecutive days using either a ram's horn indwelling uterine catheter or Foley catheter. Cysts should be treated with gonadotropin-releasing hormone (GnRH) or chorionic gonadotrophin, and those cattle with a functional corpus luteum could be treated with prostaglandins to cause a return to estrus. Unfortunately these patients frequently have a vicious cycle of low grade infection and ovarian dysfunction that is extremely frustrating. When infection persists, use of prostaglandins frequently results in formation of follicles that fail to ovulate, and cysts result. Uterine biopsies for prognosis and/or culture of the uterus followed by intensive antibiotic therapy may be indicated in such cases.

Treatment of Cows with Clinical and Subclinical Endometritis

Most authors concur that treatment with $PGF_{2\alpha}$ or its analogues improves subsequent fertility in cows with clinical or subclinical endometritis, whether it does so by facilitating remission of the inflammation or by other mechanisms. Infusion of cephapirin in a formulation designed specifically for intrauterine infusion has consistently been beneficial. No other intrauterine infusion can be supported by the available evidence. Systemic administration of antibiotics has not been tested as a treatment for endometritis.

Uterine Abscesses and Adhesions

Etiology

Uterine abscesses and adhesions may originate from spontaneous compromise of the uterine wall during calving, small uterine perforations, or extension of endometrial infection through the uterine wall or uterine tube. Such causes result in focal or diffuse inflammation and infection. The pathology represents a mild version of uterine rupture or perimetritis, and affected cows usually are asymptomatic. A history of dystocia is usually but not always reported. The major iatrogenic cause is pipette injuries to the uterine body. Attempts to infuse cows less than 14 days postpartum are the usual cause of pipette injuries to the dorsal uterine body just distal to the cervix. These injuries are generally created by laypeople who fail to consider that the weight of the involuting uterus frequently precludes adequate retraction of the cervix and uterine body to safely administer infusions. Partial-thickness or full-thickness uterine tears created in this way allow seeding with bacteria that result in abscesses or adhesions, especially when postpartum endometritis has existed. Pipette injuries can also occur during conventional reproductive procedures involving the uterus, such as insemination or embryo transfer manipulations.

Clinical Signs and Diagnosis

There are usually no systemic signs, and the conditions are not recognized until routine rectal palpation is performed for reproductive purposes. A history of dystocia, endometritis, retained placenta, and treatment for these conditions is typical but not necessary. On palpation, uterine wall abscesses are firm, round or oval masses intimately attached to the uterine body or horn. Abscesses vary from the size of an egg to that of a basketball and may or may not have a network of fibrinous or fibrous adhesions associated with their juncture at the uterus. Such masses require differentiation from tumors, hematomas, and cysts. Differentiation may be difficult by palpation alone, but ultrasonography or aspiration provides definitive proof. In some cattle with uterine wall abscesses, intermittent or persistent purulent discharge from the vulva is noticed by the owner. These abscesses have a communicating tract into the uterine lumen. Other affected cattle have no evidence of purulent discharge. Blood work seldom is helpful because the leukogram and hemogram usually are normal and serum globulin is elevated only when the uterine wall abscess is large and of chronic duration. *A. pyogenes* is the usual isolate identified in these abscesses.

Uterine adhesions generally are found as sporadic problems in cattle without systemic signs but with possible historical evidence of parturient or immediate postparturient uterine problems. The owner should be questioned about the possibility of pipette injuries or vaginally administered medications. A network of adhesions may involve part of or the entire reproductive tract, and it usually is impossible to fully retract the uterus as adhesions hold the organ in the cranial pelvis, at the pelvic brim, or along the caudal prepubic tendon region. Some adhesions may be friable, thin, or fibrinous and can be broken down manually. However, it is best to leave these undisturbed so as not to tear the uterine tubes or horns. Cattle with extensive adhesions may have residual endometritis because the dependent arrangement of the uterus interferes with effective discharge of luminal contents. The patient may or may not have been noticed in estrus depending on the magnitude of ovarian involvement and health of the uterine endometrium. Rectal palpation often suffices for diagnosis but can be significantly and helpfully augmented by transrectal ultrasound.

Treatment

Conservative therapy for uterine abscesses consists of systemic antibiotics. Penicillin (22,000 U/kg once daily) or ceftiofur (2.2 mg/kg once daily) is administered for 2 to 4 weeks. Twenty percent sodium-iodide administered IV at 30 g/450 kg once followed by 1 oz of organic iodide orally, once daily until signs of iodism appear can be an additive treatment. Conservative therapy is not very successful, however. Valuable cattle with uterine abscesses usually require surgical drainage or amputation of the affected horn through a caudal flank or inguinal incision. When the uterine body is involved, surgical drainage coupled with the aforementioned medical therapy usually is attempted. Cattle with uterine wall abscesses confined to one horn may be candidates for removal of the affected horn, abscess, and ipsilateral ovary. Such surgery is very difficult because of problems gaining adequate exposure to the abscess and the fact that coexisting adhesions may further limit delivery of the mass into a flank incision. Rarely a uterine abscess will drain into the uterine lumen and resolve spontaneously. Subsequent endometritis can be managed by repeated prostaglandin injections and antibiotic therapy.

Uterine adhesions are best managed conservatively. My experience has been that many of these cows can conceive eventually if given sufficient time for natural resolution of the adhesions. Usually 4 to 6 months of sexual rest is necessary, so the cow must be deemed valuable enough to allow a prolonged lactation. Cattle with uterine and reproductive tract adhesions should be palpated gently once monthly by the same examiner to monitor progress. Those with associated endometritis can have intermittent injections of prostaglandin (PGF$_{2\alpha}$ or analogues) to encourage evacuation of purulent material—especially if palpation confirms the presence of a functional corpus luteum. Attempts at intrauterine therapy are contraindicated because further damage may result. Systemic antibiotics and iodide can be administered as outlined previously for treatment of uterine abscesses but seem less important than time. During the past 20 years, I have managed an average of two to three patients with extensive uterine adhesions per year. Given sufficient time, these cows have had a 50% to 66% chance of subsequent conception and successful pregnancy. Interestingly, the slow and steady stretching of the pregnant uterus and passing time frequently cause the majority of the adhesions to resolve by the time of next calving. Some cows are left as "one-sided" breeders because severe inflammation and adhesions permanently destroy function of one ovary, one uterine tube, or one horn. Breedings in these animals can be adjusted for ovulation from the functional ovary by prostaglandin therapy following palpation, or the ovary on the affected side can be removed via colpotomy or celiotomy. Those cattle with bilateral ovarian or uterine tube involvement and those with persistent endometritis have a poor prognosis.

Pyometra

Etiology

Pyometra is defined as an intrauterine accumulation of pus accompanied by a persistent corpus luteum and failure of estrus. Apparent failure of the endometrial luteolytic factor or endogenous prostaglandin to cause luteolysis makes pyometra cows "think they are pregnant" and fail to cycle. The same conditions that result in endometritis can result in pyometra. Roberts reports that the retained corpus luteum usually is the corpus luteum that develops following one of the first few ovulations following parturition. This definition of pyometra implies a failure to discharge material from the uterus or cycle as is the usual case with endometritis patients having similar uterine fluid. Pyometra also may occur following conception and embryonic death associated with infection. *A. pyogenes* is the usual predominant organism, but trichomoniasis always should be considered, especially if more than one case occurs on the premises or in a bull-bred herd. Routine prebreeding and postbreeding rectal examinations tend to detect pyometra earlier and result in less confusion when differentiating the disorder from pregnancy.

Clinical Signs and Diagnosis

Clinical signs are limited to failure to show heats, persistence of a corpus luteum, and fluid accumulation in the uterus. Many cases have intermittent or frequent mucopurulent discharge from the reproductive tract that has been noticed by the owner. Prebreeding checks of cattle not observed to have heat and not having been bred simplify the diagnosis. More confusion exists when prebreeding examinations are not routinely performed or the cow develops pyometra following breeding. In these latter instances, pyometra must be differentiated from pregnancy. Because the amount of fluid in pyometra cases varies from several ounces to several gallons, the amount of fluid may or may not correlate with an appropriate amount of fluid associated with pregnancy depending on days postbreeding. Such cases may be more difficult to differentiate than one would assume. Palpation of uteri with pyometra may find the uterus as thick-walled, atonic, or alternatively thin-walled. Usually thick pus and a lack of fetal membranes are detected. However, some cases have so much distention and thick pus that the examiner mistakenly suspects "membrane slip." In pyometra of longer than 90 days' duration, cotyledons are not present and uterine arteries are not enlarged, as in pregnancy. If the cow has been bred and confusion exists, the veterinarian should either recheck the cow in 30 days to evaluate evolution of a normal pregnancy or perform ultrasound to differentiate the conditions.

Treatment

Currently $PGF_{2\alpha}$, cloprostenol, and other analogues are the most satisfactory treatment. Most pyometra cases can be successfully evacuated by one or more injections of prostaglandin drugs. Treatments may be repeated at 14-day intervals. $PGF_{2\alpha}$ (35 mg) or 500 µg of cloprostenol has given excellent results. This treatment also works well for most cases of mummified fetus, although in some cows even repeat injections are not successful. On occasions fetal mummification/maceration will be refractory to exogenous hormonal attempts at abortion. The remaining fetal tissues in such circumstances may be removed by hysterotomy via a caudal flank or inguinal incision, but this may be technically challenging (Figure 9-8, *A* and *B*).

Duration of pyometra is inversely related to subsequent fertility. Cattle with pyometra for longer than 2 months and those with large amounts of pus have lesser chances of subsequent fertility. Recurrence of pyometra, ovarian cysts, and adhesions also are observed in a small percentage of treated pyometra cases. Early detection through routine rectal palpation and prompt treatment improve the prognosis.

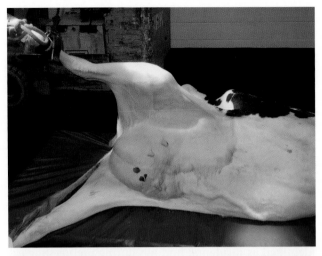

A

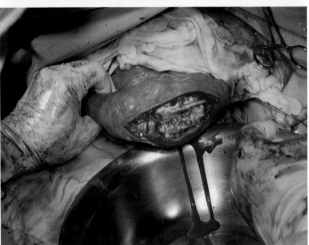

B

Figure 9-8

A, Cow positioned for inguinal approach for removal of macerated fetal remnants by hysterotomy. **B,** Bony fetal remnants being removed at surgery. *(Courtesy Dr. Mike Pritchard.)*

Uterine Tumors

Etiology

The most common neoplasm to affect the uterus of dairy cattle is lymphosarcoma. Adenocarcinomas, leiomyomas, fibromyomas, fibromas, and others are rarely reported.

Clinical Signs and Diagnosis

Cattle with lymphosarcoma of the uterus usually have detectable tumors of lymph nodes or other target organs in addition to lesions in the reproductive tract. Because of routine rectal palpation for reproductive examination, the uterine masses may be discovered either before the cow shows systemic signs or at the onset of illness associated with multifocal lymphosarcoma (see the section on lymphosarcoma in Chapter 15). Lymphosarcoma can appear in several forms in the reproductive tract such that focal, multifocal, or diffuse neoplastic infiltration is possible. The uterus is the most common portion of the reproductive tract to be affected, but ovaries, uterine tubes, the cervix, and the caudal reproductive tract can be affected. The typical uterine form of lymphosarcoma consists of multiple firm umbilicated masses in the uterine wall that feel similar to residual maternal caruncles (Figure 9-9). Diffuse firm thickening of the uterine horns, body, or both are found in other cows. Occasionally only a single smooth- or rough-surfaced uterine wall mass is palpated. A complete physical examination will usually allow identification of other lymphosarcoma tumors in these cattle.

Cattle with uterine tumors other than lymphosarcoma usually are asymptomatic, and the tumors are identified as incidental findings during prebreeding examinations. Some affected cattle are examined because of repeat breeding or failure to conceive. Pulmonary metastases and subsequent respiratory signs have been described in association with uterine adenocarcinomas, and may become clinically evident long before the primary tumor. Adenocarcinomas tend to be hard, rough surfaced, and involve one uterine horn. Leiomyomas are firm, rounded, and have distinct borders. Other tumors vary in gross appearance, shape, and consistency. Depending on the tumor type, metastases may or may not constitute a risk. Ultrasound and biopsy are helpful ancillary procedures.

Treatment

Cattle with lymphosarcoma of the uterus usually will be dead in less than 6 months as a result of multicentric disease. Pregnant cattle with lymphosarcoma of the uterus usually deliver small or nonviable calves if several weeks or months remain until term. Pregnant cattle that are less than 6 months pregnant seldom produce viable calves. Therefore treatment for this tumor is usually not indicated.

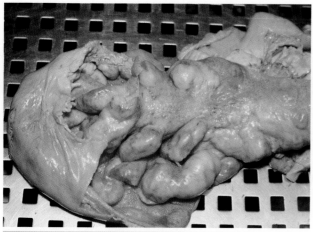

Figure 9-9

Lymphosarcoma of the uterus.

Unilateral horn neoplasia resulting from other tumors may be treatable by partial hysterectomy if the condition is detected early and the cow is deemed valuable enough to warrant surgical approach through a caudal flank incision.

DISEASES OF THE UTERINE TUBES OR OVIDUCTS

Etiology

The uterine tubes (oviducts, fallopian tubes) constitute a critical anatomic link between the ovary and uterus. Congenital or acquired abnormalities of the uterine tubes directly interfere with effective transport of ova or spermatozoa, depending on the anatomic region involved. The uterine tube is divided into an infundibulum, which possesses fimbria that aid collection of oocytes; an ampulla, which is long and thin walled; and an isthmus, which is thick, tortuous, and terminates at the uterotubal junction. Uterine tubes are lined with mucosa, have active cilia that tend to move material toward the uterus, have secretory activity, and are regulated by hormonal influences on muscle and blood supply.

Uterine tube disease occurs much more commonly than one would suspect and likely explains many cases of infertility characterized by repeat services without other overt signs or palpable abnormalities of the reproductive tract. Palpation detects some obvious uterine tube adhesions and enlargements but is a poor means of detection for subtle yet significant tubal adhesion, injury, or inflammation. Studies of slaughtered cattle suggest that 10% or more of cattle may have pathology in one or both uterine tubes.

Uterine tube congenital anomalies do exist but are less common than acquired pathology. Infections of the reproductive tract during the postpartum period, persistent endometritis, perimetritis, and other infections may involve the uterine tubes (salpingitis). Similarly, less spectacular but damaging salpingitis may be associated with *Tritrichomonas foetus*, *Campylobacter fetus* var *venerealis*, *Ureaplasma diversum*, *Mycoplasma* sp. and other organisms that infect the caudal reproductive tract and are discussed elsewhere in this chapter.

Traumatic injuries to the uterine tubes may accompany severe dystocia and were more common when manual removal of corpus luteum was practiced to instigate cycling in dairy cattle. Manual rupture of ovarian cysts also presents risk of trauma to the uterine tubes.

Clinical Signs and Diagnosis

Clinical signs of uterine tube disease are usually limited to infertility unless other portions of the reproductive tract are obviously infected or damaged. Diagnosis generally has relied on palpation but can be aided greatly by ancillary techniques such as ultrasonography, laparoscopy, laparotomy, dye studies, or cannulization.

Palpation is most likely to detect adhesions or enlargement of the uterine tubes and is unlikely to identify subtle changes. Palpation of the uterine tubes can best be performed by inserting one's fingers into the ovarian bursa. If the fingers are spread apart within the bursa, the uterine tube comes to lie along the fingertips. Although the normal uterine tube can not be identified, swelling or nodules indicative of pathologic change can be detected if present.

Treatment

Treatment is of limited value unless infections such as endometritis or other infections of the reproductive tract coexist and can be treated with antibiotics, prostaglandins, and other specific therapy. Sexual rest is indicated for adhesions, and the time required varies in each case. Usually 1 to 6 months is necessary. Lesions limited to one uterine tube allow the cow to be bred when ovulation occurs from the opposite ovary, and the opposite oviduct is thought to be normal.

DISEASES OF THE CERVIX

Etiology

Abnormalities of the cervix may be congenital or acquired. Congenital cervical malformations and anomalies may represent individual lesions or be a component of multiple congenital anomalies of the reproductive tract. Segmental aplasias, double external os, short or convoluted cervix, and other anomalies have been described, may interfere with breeding, may be hereditary, and seldom lead to clinical signs other than infertility.

Acquired cervical infections or injuries may result in overt clinical signs, including purulent discharges and severe tenesmus, or merely result in infertility. Injuries to the cervix commonly follow dystocia and may cause immediate signs such as hemorrhage or delayed signs of cervical infection, cervical abscesses, or cicatricial fibrosis that interfere with future breeding (Figure 9-10). Cervicitis also may develop secondary to chronic endometritis or vaginitis. Chronic vaginitis resulting from windsucking or urine pooling following vaginal or vulvar injuries predisposes to cervicitis. This especially affects the external cervical rings. Prolapse of the external cervical rings in older cows or cows that have had severe dystocias also predisposes to external cervical infection. Rough use of insemination pipettes, and especially insemination rods commonly used today, can puncture or damage the cervix, allowing chronic infection or abscessation. Most chronic infections of the cervix are caused by *A. pyogenes*, although mixed infections are encountered occasionally.

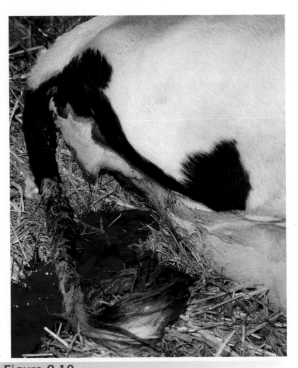

Figure 9-10

Hemorrhage from the cervix that recurred at each of the first three postpartum heats following dystocia. The exact site of the origin in the cervix could not been seen, and the condition resolved.

Clinical Signs and Diagnosis

Cervical abnormalities may be detected or suspected during routine rectal examination but are best diagnosed by vaginal speculum examination. Ultrasound currently provides an additional diagnostic tool when cervical masses, abscesses, or internal cervical lesions are suspected. A mucopurulent discharge is frequently observed by the owner, and repeated breeding, infertility, or difficulty passing an insemination pipette may be reasons veterinary attention is sought. Because cervical infections are much less common than endometritis or vaginitis, the condition can be missed easily unless palpation and speculum examinations are performed.

Speculum examination usually allows viewing of an edematous, dark red, and swollen external cervix with purulent discharge. Because of the high probability of endometritis or vaginitis associated with the cervical infection, therapy may need to be directed against the primary uterine or vaginal infection. This is necessary because infections limited to the external cervical region seldom occur as single lesions and are seldom a cause of infertility by themselves.

Cervical abscesses most commonly follow dystocia or pipette and insemination gun injuries. These lesions usually can be palpated during rectal examinations and may be confirmed with the aid of ultrasonography.

Cervical stenosis may be either congenital or acquired. Injuries subsequent to dystocia or fibrosis secondary to chronic endometritis and cervicitis are the usual causes of acquired lesions. Failure to conceive or inability to pass insemination pipettes or guns through the cervix brings attention to the problem.

Treatment

Cervicitis associated with vaginitis or endometritis requires treatment of the primary problem and the cervix. Treatment of chronic endometritis has been discussed and includes evacuation via luteolysis with $PGF_{2\alpha}$ or analogues coupled with antibiotic therapy. Cultures and antibiotic susceptibility testing may provide useful ancillary data when the condition is chronic. Local therapy of vaginitis includes therapeutic douching to cleanse the caudal reproductive tract and appropriate antibiotic therapy. Specific treatment for primary cervicitis using antiseptic swabbing of the affected rings (especially if these are the external rings and therefore accessible) has been practiced with iodines, iodine and glycerol combinations, 1% acriflavine, and other drugs. Cervical forceps are used to retract the cervix and allow local treatment, which may need to be repeated several times over a 2-week period. Cervicitis secondary to endometritis or vaginitis usually resolves if the primary condition is corrected. If straining becomes persistent, frequent administration of lidocaine via needle or epidural catheter may be needed to "break" the straining cycle.

Cervical abscesses are treated by sexual rest and systemic iodide therapy. If drainage into the cervical lumen from the abscess is present, cultures may be obtained to guide selection of an appropriate systemic antibiotic as well. Systemic iodide therapy includes treatment with 20% sodium iodide (30 g/450 kg IV) once or twice at 72-hour intervals or the use of 1 oz of organic iodide orally each day until iodism occurs. For abscesses smaller than 5.0 cm in diameter, prognosis is fair to good. Larger abscesses may require specific surgical drainage and long-term antibiotic therapy and have a poor prognosis. Dr. Rebhun reported treatment of two cows in the same herd that had cranial cervical abscesses probably associated with a newly trained inseminator. Following 2 months of rest and iodides, the abscesses shrank to small palpable fibrotic masses, and both cattle later conceived. One of these patients subsequently aborted a 3-month fetus. It could be argued that sexual rest and spontaneous healing may have been as important as iodide therapy, but treatment at least helped focus the owner on the need for gentler insemination techniques.

Acquired cervical stenosis interferes with effective insemination. Because many inseminators merely drop semen in the cervix rather than the uterine body, the only complaint may be repeat service. Alternatively, a few cows with cervical stenosis do not cycle, and although they do not have associated pyometra, they have a persistent corpus luteum. Palpation of the cervix may be suggestive of stenosis but frequently is inconclusive because of the great variation in the palpable size and conformation in normal cervices. A Chamber's or Woelffer's catheter is most useful for exploring the cervical lumen and attempting to "open" the stenosis. In particularly difficult cases, an epidural anesthetic may improve patient comfort during the procedure. Usually the slight bend and stiff metal consistency of a Chamber's catheter or Woelffer's catheter allow careful and gradual entry through the stenosed or narrowed region of cervix. If the stenosis is bypassed, an infusion of saline or saline-antibiotic fluid is administered and the catheter withdrawn. The cow can then be cycled with prostaglandin and bred on observed heat. Surprisingly this technique is highly successful in most instances and does not necessarily present a problem during the next lactation. Extremely scarred cervices that are stenosed or those that have both stenosis and chronic cervicitis have a very poor prognosis.

VAGINAL, VESTIBULAR, AND VULVAR DISEASES

Parturient Injuries

Etiology

The vagina and caudal reproductive tract may suffer multiple insults associated with parturition. These insults are much more common in conjunction with first calvings but can occur secondary to dystocia even in multiparous cows. Lacerations, hemorrhage, pressure necrosis, and other injuries frequently occur during difficult births. In first-calf heifers, these injuries may occur without apparent dystocia. Vaginal trauma may be obvious immediately following dystocia when hemorrhage or prolapse of perivaginal fat occurs. Distortion of the normal vaginal-vulvar anatomy also may be apparent as external lacerations in the vulva or perineum. Delayed evidence of vaginal trauma such as necrotic vaginitis is most common in first-calf heifers and tends to cause signs 2 to 10 days following calving or dystocia. Perivaginal hematomas in the pelvic inlet usually are subclinical but manifested as multiple palpable firm masses in the pelvic inlet on routine postpartum palpations of cows less than 30 days fresh. Rarely, extensive perivaginal hemorrhage may lead to a large hematoma that fills the retroperitoneal space and/or perineal area, causes blood loss anemia, and constricts the rectum and vagina. Perivaginal abscesses are another delayed consequence of vaginal trauma.

The integral relationship between conditions of the vagina, vestibule, and vulva allow discussion of these diseases as a group. For example, distortion or laceration of the normal vestibule-vulva conformation may result in an abnormal anatomic positioning that allows windsucking and secondary vaginitis.

Clinical Signs and Diagnosis

Acute clinical signs of hemorrhage, prolapse of perivaginal fat, or lacerations may require specific therapy or merely recording such that healing may be monitored. Subacute consequences of caudal reproductive tract birth trauma such as necrotic vaginitis-vulvitis cause clinical signs of tenderness or tenesmus accompanied by a foul necrotic odor. A gentle vaginal examination is necessary to differentiate the condition from metritis and to determine the extent of the condition. Perineal lacerations represent a problem that may be noticed immediately or not recognized until routine prebreeding examination. Perivaginal hematomas and abscesses usually are not recognized until routine prebreeding examination. Hematomas are firm, may be smooth or rough surfaced, usually are moveable, and often are multiple. Abscesses tend to be fluctuant to firm, rounded, and tense. The rare diffuse pelvic hematoma occurring from perivaginal hemorrhage can be compared with perimetritis because the rectum is tightly constricted and held in one position. Firm swelling throughout the pelvic inlet prevents meaningful rectal palpation. Overt anemia may be present in these cattle, and the condition is differentiated from perimetritis by absence of fever coupled with anemia.

Delayed or chronic consequences of birth trauma include windsucking (pneumovagina), chronic vaginitis, "tipped vulva" that assumes a horizontal position rather than a vertical one, vaginal stenosis, vaginal mucosal adhesions, and urovagina. All of these conditions predispose to chronic vaginitis through irritation, inflammation, and allowing opportunistic infection. Therefore fertility may be affected.

Treatment

Acute injuries to the caudal reproductive tract may require immediate attention when hemorrhage is severe or persistent and when lacerations that may have future impact on reproduction are present. Severe vaginal bleeding occurring immediately after delivery of a calf may require isolation and ligation of the bleeding vessel. This can be accomplished in a variety of ways depending on anatomic location and how easily the site may be visualized or reached. Retraction of the vulva by sutures, instruments, or retractors may allow viewing of the site. Ligatures of absorbable suture material or clamping with a hemostat that is subsequently removed in 24 to 48 hours suffices for hemostasis in most cases. When hemorrhage is associated with vaginal or vulvar mucosal lacerations, hemostasis and repair of the mucosal defect both may be accomplished with absorbable suture material. Prolapse of perivaginal fat may or may not require treatment. Débridement of prolapsed fat and closure of mucosal defects are indicated for large lacerations.

Conservative therapy with or without systemic antibiotics may suffice for smaller prolapses. Fat necrosis and scarring are anticipated consequences of conservative therapy, and perivaginal fat necrosis may subsequently be palpated per rectum as perivaginal masses similar in consistency to perivaginal hematomas.

Perineal and vulvar lacerations occurring during dystocia may be repaired immediately, but periparturient edema, inflammation, and contamination often result in failure of acute repair and make delayed repairs slightly more successful.

Subacute conditions such as necrotic vaginitis-vulvitis usually require treatment during the first postparturient week. A fetid odor and vaginal discharge are present and may be accompanied by tenesmus, pelvic tenderness, and soft tissue swelling. The offensive odor may cause the owner to suspect metritis or RFM as the cause of the cow's problem. Treatment starts with careful cleansing of the perineum and vulva followed by gentle manual vaginal examination or speculum examination. Regions of mucosal pressure necrosis are obvious, and opportunistic infection with *A. pyogenes*, anaerobes, and coliform organisms is common. Careful douching of the vagina with mild disinfectants should be followed by application of oily antiseptic or antibiotic ointments that have antimicrobial and lubricant properties to deter side-to-side mucosal adhesions in the vagina or vulva. Fibrinous adhesions of mucosa to mucosa may need to be gently broken down. If metritis is present, this should be treated as well. When perivaginal pelvic inflammation or fever accompanies necrotic vaginitis, systemic antibiotics such as penicillin or ceftiofur may be helpful. Anesthetic epidurals and NSAID treatment often causes dramatic improvement in the affected cow's appetite and demeanor.

Perivaginal hematomas usually are incidental findings during routine physical or reproductive examinations in cows fresh less than 30 days. These lesions are most common in first-calf heifers, do not require specific therapy, and usually resolve by 40 to 60 days postpartum. Rare instances of large perivaginal hematomas or pelvic hematomas that result in massive pelvic swelling and blood loss anemia may require blood transfusion to save the animal's life and may have a negative impact on future breeding potential because of diffuse adhesions in the pelvis. Such large hematomas may also eventually lead to pelvic abscessation, a condition with a grave prognosis. Perivaginal or pelvic abscesses represent delayed manifestations of vaginal injury, laceration, or necrosis. Affected cows may be asymptomatic or have chronic vaginitis with discharge. Diagnosis is suspected on routine rectal palpation and may be confirmed by ultrasonography or aspirates obtained through the vaginal wall. Perivaginal abscesses adherent to the vaginal wall may be surgically drained into the vagina. This drainage usually is curative unless multiple abscesses or multiloculated abscesses exist. Systemic antibiotics (best based on culture) or iodides may be used following drainage to hasten resolution of the condition. When palpation or ultrasound fails to confirm a distinct attachment of the abscess to the vaginal wall, treatment becomes much more complex and less successful. Because such abscesses usually are retroperitoneal, the cow shows no signs of peritonitis, but attempts at drainage are anatomically difficult. Drainage sometimes has been tried through the area lateral to the vulva and anus or using laparotomy. Complications and recurrence are common. Conservative therapy likewise has poor success, but long-term systemic antibiotic therapy, iodide therapy, or both may be tried.

Other delayed consequences of birth trauma such as "tipped vulva," urovagina, and chronic vaginitis will be discussed in the treatment of vaginitis.

Other Vaginal Injuries

Etiology
Although parturient injuries are the most common cause of vaginal trauma, rare cases of vaginal laceration or irritation can follow natural breeding, injuries caused by insemination pipette or rod, and sadism. Natural breeding of small heifers to adult bulls occasionally can lead to cranial vaginal perforations or laceration at intromission. Punctures of the cranial vagina by insemination instruments can occur when inexperienced or rough neophyte inseminators attempt breeding cows or heifers. Unfortunately sadism also must be considered—especially when more than one animal on a given premises is affected.

Clinical Signs and Diagnosis
Small punctures caused by insemination instruments may go completely undetected, although pelvic abscesses, peritoneal abscesses, or peritonitis can develop, depending on the location and severity of the puncture. Natural breeding injuries with full-thickness laceration of the cranial vagina result in typical signs of peritonitis with loss of appetite, tachycardia, an arched stance, reluctance to move, and fever. Tenesmus may be present. Rectal examination may allow detection of pelvic tenderness and fibrinous adhesions of varying degree. Similar signs are present when sadism has caused vaginal lacerations. Vaginal speculum examination is necessary to identify the site and extent of the vaginal injury. Retroperitoneal or localized infection can lead to perivaginal adhesions, abscesses, or tenesmus. Peritoneal cavity contamination causes distinct signs of peritonitis and caudal abdominal or reproductive tract adhesions.

Treatment
Treatment includes sexual rest for 30 to 60 days and systemic antibiotics to control retroperitoneal or peritoneal infection. Antibiotic therapy may need to be continued for 1 to 2 weeks, and analgesics may be helpful during the acute phase. Local therapy usually is contraindicated unless perivaginal abscesses are identified and require drainage.

Vaginitis

Etiology
Vaginitis may appear as an acute or chronic condition. As previously discussed, birth trauma is a common cause of acute, necrotic, and chronic vaginitis that is either a primary condition or secondary to chronic endometritis and cervicitis. Cloudy or mucopurulent discharge is the hallmark of vaginitis but does not specifically differentiate the condition from cervicitis or endometritis. Necrotic vaginitis has a fetid odor that accompanies discharge and is more easily diagnosed.

Conditions that result from dystocia and alter the normal caudal reproductive tract anatomy predispose to vaginitis. Windsucking, perineal lacerations, and urine pooling are the major primary conditions. Alteration of the normal perineal anatomy encourages vaginal contamination. This is true for cattle with tipped vulvas or perineal lacerations. Chronic "windsucking" that allows air to be trapped in the vagina causes irritation that promotes opportunistic infection by organisms normally present in the vaginal flora or by organisms present in feces or on the skin. Urine pooling or urovagina may result from birth trauma, partial bladder paralysis from birth trauma, or chronic tension on the cranial vagina by a heavy uterus and cervix. Urine pooling in the cranial vagina may bathe or enter the cervix and predisposes to cervicitis and endometritis. Urea is irritating to the tissue and may allow secondary opportunistic infection. Urine also is toxic to spermatozoa, and urovagina frequently leads to conception failure for this reason or because of interference with implantation when endometrial irritation results. Extreme pelvic laxity as observed in chronic cystic ovaries tends to worsen both pneumovagina and urovagina.

In addition to physical conditions that result in vaginitis, specific infectious diseases can cause vaginitis. These organisms include *Mycoplasma* sp., *Ureaplasma* sp., *Histophilus somni*, infectious b ovine rhinotracheitis virus (Figure 9-11), and others. Such organisms can cause endemic or epidemic vaginitis in dairy cattle and will be discussed separately. More recently an outbreak of vulvovaginitis caused by *Porphyromonas levii* was reported, but I have no first-hand experience with this disease.

Clinical Signs and Diagnosis
Subacute or chronic vaginitis without anatomic distortion of the caudal reproductive tract is most likely residual from traumatic consequences of dystocia or infection following parturition. Coexisting endometritis or cervicitis is common in these conditions. Cloudy mucopurulent or purulent discharge may be the only

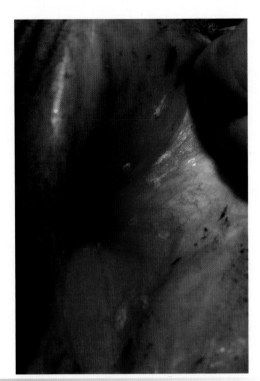

Figure 9-11

Vulvar plaques caused by bovine herpesvirus.

sign or may be accompanied by occasional tenesmus. Tenesmus and severe infections are more common in acute vaginal injury and necrotic vaginitis. Rectal palpation and vaginal speculum examination usually suffice for diagnosis. Ultrasonography and uterine biopsy may be useful to further evaluate the uterus when palpation or speculum examination is inconclusive about primary uterine pathology. A reddened, edematous vaginal mucosa with purulent discharge is usually observed when speculum examination is performed.

Signs of vaginitis in cows with tipped vulvas that predispose to intermittent contamination of the caudal reproductive tract make the tipped vulva the likely primary cause. Similarly cattle having vulvar malformations, cicatricial separation of the vulvar lips, or other conditions that allow pneumovagina are prone to secondary vaginitis. Rectal examination confirms pneumovagina, and the air can be expressed by firm pressure on the cranial vagina and retraction of the reproductive tract.

Vaginitis secondary to urine pooling is very common and usually follows anatomic distortion of the vagina and vestibule from injuries during parturition. It may also follow calving injuries that mechanically or neurologically interfere with bladder emptying. Chronic persistent or intermittent mucopurulent vaginal discharge is observed, and rectal palpation results in discharge of clear or cloudy urine when backward pressure on the vagina, back-raking of manure, or retraction of the uterus is performed. Rectal palpation should eliminate cystic ovaries as a

complicating factor whenever pneumovagina or urovagina is diagnosed.

Treatment

Therapy of subacute or chronic vaginitis unassociated with anatomic disorders necessitates local therapy including douching of the vagina with dilute antiseptic solutions and treatment of concurrent metritis or cervicitis. Chronic cases may benefit from local antibiotic infusion of the vagina and uterus following cleansing douches. Antibiotic therapy is best used when a culture has identified a specific organism and susceptibility testing has been completed. Vaginitis may be primary or secondary to endometritis and cervicitis; it may be difficult to determine an absolute primary origin in chronic cases. Therefore treatment of the entire reproductive tract is indicated. Treatment should be repeated daily or as often as possible for best results.

Treatment of vaginitis associated with tipped vulva, perineal laceration, or other vulvar anatomic abnormalities requires treatment of vaginitis and correction of the anatomic primary cause. For tipped vulvas, pneumovagina, and simple vulvar abnormalities, a simple closure of the dorsal portion of the vulvar cleft (Caslick's procedure) usually prevents further vaginal contamination and pneumovagina. This procedure is performed with epidural anesthesia, careful removal of approximately 2.0 mm of skin at the mucocutaneous junction of the entire dorsal portion of the vulvar cleft, and closure with a continuous fine suture. Depending on the length of the vulvar cleft, usually 3.0 to 5.0 cm is left open ventrally. Correction of these problems by surgical closure is coupled with antiseptic or antibiotic treatment of the vaginitis, as well as treatment of any endometritis present. Spontaneous resolution of vaginitis also may occur after the primary anatomic defect is corrected and probably is caused by normal defense mechanisms associated with effective cycling and prevention of further exogenous contamination of the caudal reproductive tract.

Treatment of urovagina may be conservative or surgical. Decisions about conservative versus surgical treatment are made based on the cow's value, severity of the problem, success of previous treatments, the cow's stage of lactation, and the number of failed inseminations. Urovagina identified before breeding may be associated with ventral traction on the vagina and urethra by a heavy uterus and cervix. If endometritis is present, it should be corrected by evacuation with prostaglandin or other treatment and the uterus allowed to involute. If following involution urovagina persists, then the condition must be treated specifically. Similarly if ovarian cysts are detected and the entire reproductive tract and pelvic ligaments are relaxed and sloppy, the cystic condition should first be treated and the urovagina reassessed.

Conservative treatment of urovagina consists of evacuation of pooled urine by ventral and caudal pressure through the rectum before insemination. Insemination is performed by a double-sheathing technique. Some practitioners also recommend another evacuation 24 hours postbreeding followed by an intrauterine antibiotic infusion. Many cows with mild to moderate urovagina can be bred successfully in this manner, although two to three repeat services are not unusual.

Invasive surgical correction of urovagina may be necessary when the cow is extremely valuable or when conservative efforts have failed to allow conception. Urethral extension is the procedure generally recommended in cattle with urovagina. The patient may be sedated, and epidural anesthesia is administered. A single- or double-layer mucosal canal is structured following a vaginal mucosal incision starting at the transverse fold at the cranial urethral opening into the vagina. The incision is then continued as a U-shaped mucosal incision to a point 2.0 to 2.5 cm from the vulvar lips. The mucosa then is undermined both dorsally and ventrally from the incision line to loosen and relax tension on the mucosa, which is then apposed over a Foley catheter placed in the bladder and exiting the urethra. A continuous Lembert suture is used for closure of the ventral and then dorsal layers. This repair is derived from a surgical technique developed by Brown and colleagues for mares. The surgery can be completed successfully in a single layer, using only the ventral tissue flap. The exposed submucosa usually granulates and reepithelializes without any complication. Closure in a single layer has the advantage of preserving a larger vestibular lumen, with less likelihood of reinjury at subsequent calving. Systemic antibiotics and NSAIDs are administered preoperatively and postoperatively. It is preferable to leave a Foley catheter in place for 48 to 72 hours after surgery because some cattle initially fail to urinate spontaneously following the procedure. It is wise to continue systemic antibiotics and place a Heimlich valve on the exposed end of the Foley catheter to minimize the chance of ascending urinary tract infections. An alternative surgical technique involves a buried purse-string suture at the level of the vestibule-vaginal junction, taking care not to penetrate the urethra, which should be catheterized so that its location is clear. The suture is tightened to allow a lumen of only 2 to 3 cm. The surgery is simple, is rapid, and has resulted in a high success rate in a small number of cows to date.

Prevention

Prevention of vaginal, cervical, and vulvar injury is superior to treatment. Veterinarians should be alerted to a potential need for management changes when multiple cases of caudal reproductive tract injury are observed, particularly in first-calf heifers on an individual farm. Modern dairy management practices often utilize laypeople for assistance of calf delivery and relief of dystocia. Dystocia may be real or perceived in such circumstances, and despite good intentions, calving assistance may be prematurely instigated by lay staff, resulting in an increased prevalence of reproductive tract trauma. Inadequate lubrication, brutal technique, and impatience for complete cervical dilation can also contribute to the problem. Inappropriate sire selection for smaller body frame heifers may also contribute, as can overconditioning in the dry period and an increased prevalence of periparturient metabolic disease resulting from poor transition cow management.

Vaginal Prolapse

Etiology

In dairy cattle, vaginal prolapse occurs primarily in dry cows that are overconditioned or that have had anatomic injuries at previous parturitions that resulted in excessive pelvic or perineal laxity. Increasing estrogenic influence during late gestation further contributes to laxity of the caudal reproductive tract. The condition is observed when the cow is lying down and especially if the cow lies with her rear parts lower than the foreparts, as occurs in confined cattle that lie over or in a gutter. Apparently the abdominal mass helps push the cervix and vagina caudally. Laxity, deformity of the vulvar lips, and obesity predispose to vaginal prolapse as well.

When vaginal prolapse is observed in cows that are not in advanced gestation, excessive estrogen levels should be suspected. Cystic ovaries and highly estrogenic feeds may be responsible for some cases. Zearalenone, a mycotoxin, can cause vaginal prolapse in addition to other problems such as swollen vulva, cystic ovaries, and premature udder development when moldy corn or other feed containing the mycotoxin is fed. Rarely a cow that suffered extreme dystocia with severe physical stretching and perhaps damage to pelvic innervation may develop recurrent or persistent vaginal prolapse that does not respond to simple corrective measures. This specific form of vaginal prolapse has the most devastating impact on productivity and future fertility.

Clinical Signs and Diagnosis

Diagnosis is obvious based on clinical signs of a round pink or reddened mucosal prolapse that protrudes from the vulva (Figure 9-12). Usually the ventral vagina protrudes, since the prolapse invariably begins with the ventral floor of the caudal vaginal rolling over the vestibule-vaginal junction, and the cervix and lateral vaginal walls only appear in more severe cases. In many dry cows, the condition is benign, only appears when the cow lies down, and returns to normal position when the cow rises. If the cow is close to term and the condition is mild, it may be neglected. Cattle that are weeks or months from term usually require treatment, lest a vicious cycle of vaginal prolapse, vaginal irritation and exposure damage, vaginitis, and tenesmus develops. Such cows suffer vaginal irritation simply from drying of

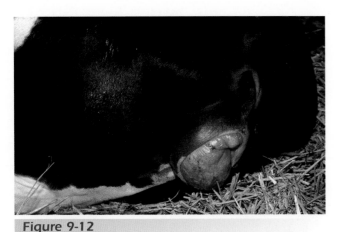

Figure 9-12

Vaginal prolapse in a dry cow.

the mucosa and abrasions created by their own tails. Exposure damage may result in edema, inflammation, superficial necrosis, or the formation of diphtheritic membranes as the vaginal mucosa continues to be exposed during recumbency. Eventually tenesmus and vaginitis make the cow uncomfortable and disturb appetite. In severe cases that expose the cervix and a large part of the vagina, cervicitis and abortion are possible. Hematoma of the vagina, cystic vestibular glands, and tumors may be mistaken for vaginal prolapse.

Cattle that are not pregnant should be examined for the presence of ovarian cysts. Mycotoxins such as zearalenone should be considered especially when more than one animal in the herd or group of heifers has signs of vaginal prolapse. Cattle that develop persistent or recurrent vaginal prolapse following dystocia usually have had a "big calf," and physical examination will detect extreme laxity of the perineum, vulva, pelvic ligaments, and ischial region. These cattle may also have partial loss of innervation to the caudal reproductive region, perineum, and bladder. Vaginal prolapse is also encountered in cows repeatedly superovulated for embryo recovery because of the chronically high estrogen level to which they are exposed.

Treatment

Mild vaginal prolapse in dry cows that are near term may not require any therapy. These cows may be helped by removal from confinement and placement in a well-bedded box stall, clean maternity area, or pasture when their rear quarters are less likely to be dependent or over a gutter.

Pregnant cows with mild to moderate vaginal prolapse that have weeks or months until term can be treated by the aforementioned management changes or may be helped by aluminum or rope trusses that are held in place by rope surcingles around the neck and chest. Pessaries have also been used in the past but are seldom used today. Moderate to severe vaginal prolapse in heavy dry cows not close to term usually can be managed best

by a Caslick's procedure to close the dorsal vulvar cleft. This procedure is performed easily under epidural anesthesia and is described in the treatment of vaginitis caused by windsucking. Only a thin portion of mucocutaneous junction is apposed, so that the incisional area may be slit just before calving such that vulvar tears do not occur.

Many other surgical procedures have been suggested. Those that depend on closure of the vulvar lips are not suitable because they do not prevent the prolapse. Neither do they contain it effectively in any but the mildest cases.

Severe vaginal prolapses, especially those that are postpartum, may require more drastic measures. Buhner's method consists of a buried suture that constricts the vestibule region. In this method, incisions are made below the lower commissure of the vulvar lips and above the dorsal (close to the anus but not in the anal sphincter) commissure. A Buhner's needle, which is a 12-in-long needle with the eye in the point, is passed through, and the procedure is repeated on the opposite side of the vulva. This "purse-string" suture then is tied tightly. The well-placed suture will migrate cranially and come to lie close to the vestibule-vaginal junction, the area where the prolapse begins. Correctly performed, this suture prevents recurrence. If this procedure is performed in prepartum cattle, the suture should be tightened to a point where three or four fingers can enter the vulva. The suture should then be knotted, leaving long ends that will ease removal when calving is imminent. When postpartum cattle are treated, the sutures may need to be even tighter and left in place until fibrosis occurs in the vestibular caudal vagina— thereby reducing the chances of recurrence.

Minchev's method passes heavy suture from the cranial vagina through the gluteal region, where the suture is anchored by buttons or other devices. Abscessation and damage to sciatic nerve branches have developed occasionally following this technique; it is thus not recommended. Similarly radical techniques such as cervopexy rarely are indicated in dairy cattle. Reefing procedures that resect large areas of affected vaginal mucosa could be considered only for extremely severe cases when the cow's value justifies the surgery.

Early intervention is perhaps the best means of ensuring successful management of vaginal prolapse in dairy cattle and preventing the vicious cycle of events that result in vaginal injury and tenesmus. Simple techniques work most effectively when used before severe vaginal exposure damage, edema, necrosis, and diphtheritic membrane formation have resulted.

All of the aforementioned surgical techniques require epidural anesthesia, careful cleansing of the exposed area of vagina, replacement of the organ, and then surgical repair. Rarely the bladder is prolapsed, preventing easy replacement of the vagina; aspiration of the urine will decrease the size of the prolapse and allow replacement.

Antibiotics and other supportive measures are seldom necessary except in neglected cattle. Cows having severe exposure damage and vaginitis that result in tenesmus may require repeated epidural anesthesia for a day or longer until vaginal irritation subsides.

Nonpregnant cattle with vaginal prolapse secondary to cystic ovaries should be treated for the primary condition.

Vaginal and Vulvar Tumors

Etiology

Fibropapillomas are occasionally observed in the vulva or vagina of young cattle and heifers (Figure 9-13). These tumors are caused by a bovine papillomavirus and are also common on the penises of young bulls (Figure 9-14, A and B). Venereal transmission is possible when natural service is practiced. Fibropapillomas of the vulva and vagina are probably more common than we realize because only large warts that protrude from the vulva or bleed cause detectable signs. These tumors are benign and usually regress spontaneously but may require treatment when large enough to protrude through the vulva because they then result in bleeding and tenesmus.

In adult cattle, many tumor types are possible. Squamous cell carcinoma of the vulva (Figure 9-15) in older cattle with lightly pigmented vulvas can be an aggressive tumor that spreads by both local infiltration and metastases unless diagnosed early. Lymphosarcoma can involve the vagina, especially when diffuse neoplasia of the reproductive tract occurs. Other tumor types are exceedingly rare in cattle.

Signs and Diagnosis

Unexplained bleeding from the vulva, vaginal discharge, tenesmus, or an obvious mass protruding from the vulva may signal a vaginal or vulvar tumor. Vaginal examination by speculum determines the extent of the lesion and

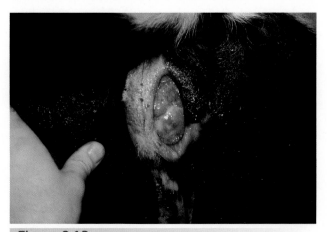

Figure 9-13

Large vaginal fibropapilloma protruding from the vulva of a bred Holstein heifer.

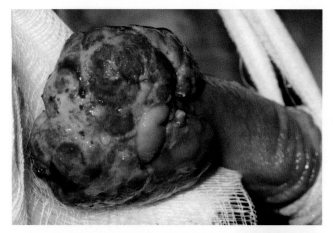

A

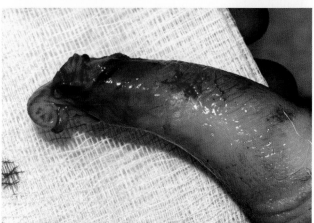

B

Figure 9-14

A, Fibropapilloma on the penis of a 2-year-old Holstein bull. **B,** The same tumor as shown in *A* following debulking and before cryosurgical treatment of the base of the mass.

allows biopsy or excisional biopsy. Fibropapillomas may be left untreated unless they disturb the heifer or are large enough to protrude from the vulva.

Squamous cell carcinoma causes raised or ulcerative (or both) pink cobblestone-like tissue proliferation on the vulva. The tumor is more common in cows with nonpigmented vulvas and more frequent in geographic areas where cows receive a great deal of exposure to sunlight. The lesion may be singular or multifocal and causes progressive erosion of the affected tissue. Neglected cases have a characteristic necrotic odor, purulent or crusted discharge, and may invade deeper structures or metastasize to regional lymph nodes and other visceral locations. Sometimes precursor plaquelike lesions or warty epitheliomas precede carcinomas similar to lesions observed in ocular squamous cell carcinoma.

Other tumors are extremely rare, and biopsy is indicated to identify the tumor type and offer treatment or prognostic aid. Although lymphosarcoma can involve the caudal reproductive tract, tumor masses in other target organs are more likely to be responsible for clinical

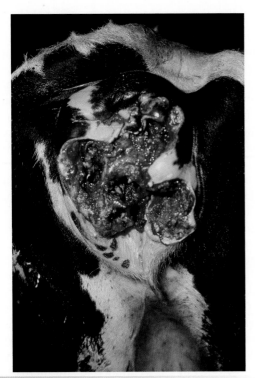

Figure 9-15

Squamous cell carcinoma on the vulva of a 12-year-old Holstein.

signs, and therefore lymphosarcoma in this region usually is an incidental finding.

Treatment

Removal of large fibropapillomas, and those that protrude from the vulva or penis, may be necessary. Surgical debulking or removal should be followed by cryosurgical destruction of the tumor base to prevent recurrence. Vaginal fibropapillomas occasionally have a very thick and vascular base that bleeds profusely if the tumor is simply excised. Hemostasis may be difficult in such cases, and the surgeon should anticipate this problem. Bulls with penile warts may spread the problem to many heifers. The efficacy of wart vaccines as preventive medicine for such fibropapillomas is debatable, and wart vaccines are not an effective form of treatment.

Treatment of squamous cell carcinoma of the vulva is most successful when the condition is diagnosed early. Affected areas should be treated with cryosurgery, radio-frequency hyperthermia, or other means. Radiofrequency hyperthermia is best used for small, superficial lesions. Cryosurgical destruction of early vulvar squamous cell carcinoma is often successful. Serial injections of Bacillus Calmette Guérin are usually avoided as a treatment option in dairy cattle because these injections could sensitize the cow to tuberculin and cause a false-positive result on a tuberculin test. Intralesional chemotherapy with cisplatin and 5-fluorouracil or topical imiquimod as used in horses may become useful in the future, but as yet suf-

ficient experimental data and legality of use are lacking in cattle. Advanced cases that have invaded the pelvic region or regional lymph nodes usually are hopeless.

Cystic Bartholin's Glands

Cystic Bartholin's (or vestibular) glands occasionally are noticed by owners when an affected cow lies down and the pink or red cystic structure protrudes through the vulvar cleft (Figure 9-16). It may be confused with mild vaginal prolapse. One gland exists on each lateral vestibular wall, and cyst formation is thought to represent obstruction or atresia of the emptying duct. Most are unilateral, and the condition is sporadic—perhaps seen once a year in bovine practice. Some cattle with lesser degrees of the condition may escape detection because the cystic structure does not protrude from the vulva. Usually the condition goes unobserved until the cyst is greater than 5.0 cm in diameter. The cyst is soft, smooth, and fluid filled. Chronic exposure damage may change the appearance and also predispose to contamination of the caudal reproductive tract as the cyst repeatedly prolapses and then returns to the vaginal region.

Treatment merely involves scalpel incision of the cyst, which will usually drain a thick, slightly cloudy, mucoid fluid. Occasionally the condition coexists with cystic ovaries, but the two generally are considered unrelated. It simply may be that increased laxity of the caudal reproductive tract associated with cystic ovaries allows the cyst to protrude more easily.

Infectious Causes of Vaginitis

Infectious Bovine Rhinotracheitis (IBR)/Infectious Pustular Vulvovaginitis (IPV)

The bovine herpesvirus I type 2 causes IPV. This form of IBR manifests as typical plaques (see Figure 9-11), erosions, ulcers, and inflammation of the vaginal and vulvar

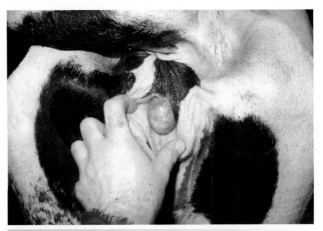

Figure 9-16

Cystic Bartholin's gland in a mature Holstein.

mucous membranes. Swelling and discharge are apparent at the vulva, and affected animals may be uncomfortable. Although not as common as the respiratory or conjunctival forms of IBR, IPV is observed occasionally. The condition may be spread by coitus from infected bulls with lesions on the prepuce or penis and through use of infected semen. As with other forms of IBR, a septicemic spread of the virus does occur despite localization of signs to the caudal reproductive tract. Therefore systemic signs of fever, depression, and inappetence may accompany the lesions. Lactating cattle or those under stress for other reasons are more likely to show systemic signs than heifers. The condition may appear as the only sign of IBR in a group or may appear in conjunction with the respiratory form. Abortion is a possible sequela as a result of septicemia and is more common when severe systemic signs appear. Abortions are not as common with IPV as with the other forms of IBR but always are a risk when the disease appears. Abortions may occur at any stage of pregnancy but are more common in cattle in the last half of pregnancy.

Diagnosis. Clinical signs in acute cases are pathognomonic and include white plaques, erosions, and ulcers in the vulvar and vaginal mucous membranes. Diagnosis may be confirmed by smears subjected to fluorescent antibody (FA) testing or viral cultures. If lesions are older than 7 to 10 days, virus may no longer be present in the lesions, and serologic (paired) testing is indicated. It has been reported, however, that neutralizing antibody response may occur very slowly following IPV in females or similar lesions in bulls. Therefore FA and isolation procedures may be indicated even after the acute phase if serology does not yield definitive information. Abortions may occur during the recuperative period or be delayed for weeks following clinical signs of IPV and other forms of IBR. Therefore cattle that subsequently abort are usually seropositive and may not show an increase in titer with paired samples. Recrudescence of the virus is always possible once an animal has been infected.

Treatment and Prevention. No specific treatment exists. Prevention includes using semen from IBR-negative bulls and ensuring adequate immunization against IBR in all cattle (see IBR in Chapter 4). Young stock should be vaccinated after maternal antibodies subside; good primary immunity is established by two vaccinations at 2- to 4-week intervals when killed or inactivated products are used. Cattle should be boostered against IBR every 6 to 12 months for life.

Granular Vulvitis Complex

A condition of controversial significance and etiology, granular vulvitis is diagnosed when signs of vaginitis, including a cloudy or mucopurulent discharge, appear chronically or intermittently; infertility or repeat services recur as an epidemic or endemic problem; and typical vulvar lesions that are raised nodules, granules,

or lymphoid follicles are found on the vulvar mucous membrane—especially near the clitoris. It is not known whether these lesions are specific, semispecific, or simply nonspecific lymphoid hyperplasia tissue responses to any of the opportunistic or pathogenic organisms inhabiting the caudal reproductive tract. Lesions are more common in heifers and younger cows but can be seen at any age. Mild lesions also can be observed in normal cows with no known reproductive problems. Moderate to severe lesions occurring with a high prevalence in a herd experiencing reproductive problems and vaginal or vulvar discharges should be considered abnormal and suggestive of contagious infection.

Many causes have been suggested for the condition, but currently *Mycoplasma* sp., *U. diversum*, and *H. somni* have received the most attention and will be discussed here. That these organisms may be isolated from the caudal reproductive tracts of both healthy and diseased cattle further frustrates a clear-cut definition of disease.

Ureaplasma diversum. *U. diversum* has been associated with granular vulvitis and caudal reproductive tract infection. The organism resides primarily in the vagina and vulva but can gain entrance to the uterus during insemination. Although *U. diversum* usually does not cause chronic endometritis, experimental inoculation of the organism into the uterus of susceptible cows produced endometritis and salpingitis. Experimental infection of pregnant cows has resulted in abortion. Natural infections of the uterus are thought to be cleared relatively quickly but may create an unhealthy environment for implantation or toxicity to embryos if present at the time of insemination. Early embryonic deaths also have been observed in field outbreaks of this disease. Experimental infection of the vulva causes red or tan granular vulvitis lesions and may in severe cases produce heavy purulent discharge, swelling of the vulva, and pus-filled white nodules several millimeters in diameter on the vulvar mucous membrane. These lesions may be confused with those seen with IBR-IPV. However, IPV tends to be erosive and/or ulcerative.

Bulls commonly have *U. diversum* as a commensal (or pathogen) in their urethra or prepuce and can spread the organism to cows through natural service or via fresh or frozen semen. Although *U. diversum* has been shown to establish infection in the vesicular glands of bulls when inoculated there experimentally, infection of accessory sex glands in bulls is thought to occur less often than urethral contamination of semen.

Field infections with *U. diversum* may be sporadic and tend to go undiagnosed unless an endemic or epidemic condition involving multiple cows within a herd appears. Cloudy or mucopurulent discharges on the vulva, tail, and perineum signal the condition. Many of the affected cows have not been observed to have endometritis during the early postpartum period and may have had "clean" early postpartum reproductive examinations.

Discharge may be found in cows at any stage of lactation but is most common in those cows due to be bred and cows that have been bred but returned to service. Some cows may not show obvious discharge until a few days following breeding. Examination of affected cattle usually reveals typical lesions of granular vulvitis or atypical, more purulent, focal vulvar lesions. Repeat services at regular or irregular (suggestive of early embryonic death) intervals and early abortions frequently accompany clinical signs of vulvar discharges in these infected herds. Sporadic cases in herds not considered to be having reproductive problems usually are dismissed as cases of chronic endometritis or chronic vaginitis. Crowding, dirty environments, and other stressors may contribute to herd infections, and selenium deficiency has been identified as a coexisting problem in a few dairy herds investigated. It is not known how the organism spreads. Crowding and spread by tails has been theorized, as has "sniffing" by cows during heat activity that might spread the organism by respiratory secretions. Dogs licking discharges from infected cattle and transmitting the pathogen to other cows also has been theorized but seems unlikely on most farms. Once *U. diversum* establishes infection, it persists for a prolonged period and apparently fails to cause any effective immune response.

Positive diagnosis requires isolation of *U. diversum* from multiple cows that have had signs of disease. Ideally these signs include discharges, granular vulvitis lesions, and reproductive failure. A single isolate is less than conclusive because the organism has often been found as an apparent commensal in the reproductive tract of cows and bulls. Treatment and control measures include:

1. Improve management to minimize crowding, clean dirty facilities, and improve sanitation.
2. Avoid natural service if it is currently practiced in the herd. Most artificial insemination (AI) stud services add antibiotics to semen to control *Mycoplasma* spp. and *Ureaplasma* spp. in processed semen.
3. Inseminate cows using "double-sheathing" techniques to avoid contamination of the uterus with vaginal organisms.
4. Consider use of systemic antibiotics in specific animals.
5. Assess the herd for concurrent diseases and nutritional status. Assess selenium levels in feed and blood when the disease occurs in unsupplemented herds that reside in selenium-deficient areas.

Mycoplasma **spp.** Although *Mycoplasma* spp. are linked less specifically to granular vulvitis than *U. diversum*, they have been isolated from cows with the condition, and *Mycoplasma* can infect the reproductive tract to cause infertility. Similar to *U. diversum*, *Mycoplasma* also can be isolated from the caudal reproductive tract of healthy cattle without overt reproductive disorders. Therefore cause and effect relationships, data on experimental infections, and significance of individual isolates often are questioned.

Mycoplasma bovigenitalium can be cultured from the vagina or cervix of many cattle. Some of these cows may have histories of reproductive failure or granular vulvitis lesions. Uterine infection appears much less commonly than caudal reproductive tract infection, and some strains of *M. bovigenitalium* may be more pathogenic than others. One study found that heifers bred to an infected bull developed purulent infections and had biopsy-confirmed evidence of endometritis. *M. bovigenitalium* (at least some strains) definitely can infect the prepuce, urethra, and vesicular glands of bulls. Because of this, antibiotic mixtures of gentamicin, tylosin, and lincocin-spectinomycin commonly are added to collected semen to be used in AI. Natural service use of infected bulls would likely constitute a major risk.

Mycoplasma bovis does not appear to infect the reproductive tract of cows or bulls very commonly, but when experimental infections have been produced, severe uterine, oviduct, and vaginal pathology may occur.

Based on current understanding, *M. bovigenitalium* appears to be a more common isolate from the caudal reproductive tract of cows. This organism tends to remain in the caudal reproductive tract but, similar to *U. diversum*, could be introduced to the uterus by insemination and cause transient endometritis, interfere with implantation, or kill embryos. It should be considered a pathogen only when signs of granular vulvitis, discharge, and reproductive failure in multiple cattle are found in conjunction with isolation of the organism. Control measures may be similar to those for *U. diversum* but also include antibiotic additives to semen for bulls in AI use. In addition, *systemic* treatment of infected cattle with tetracycline appears effective.

Histophilus somni. *H. (Haemophilus) somni* can be isolated with great regularity from the cervicovaginal area of cows with and without signs of reproductive tract infections. Similar to *Mycoplasma* sp. and *U. diversum*, the significance of an isolate may be difficult to determine. This gram-negative pleomorphic coccobacillus has been discussed in Chapter 4 and Chapter 12. It is capable of causing infections in many systems of the cow. Neurologic disease including thrombotic meningoencephalitis in growing cattle, meningitis in adult dairy cattle, polyarthritis, pneumonia, myocarditis, upper respiratory tract infections, septicemia, and reproductive conditions have been attributed to the organism. Although microbiologists disagree regarding the existence of strain differences between isolates as regards organ trophism and pathogenicity, field outbreaks suggest that strain variation is real. Some strains may cause neurologic disease but not reproductive disease and vice versa. The pathophysiology and route of infection sometimes are difficult to determine, but the respiratory tract appears the most likely entry point. Septicemia is thought to follow infection regardless of entry site. Because of the frequent isolation of *H. somni* from the reproductive tract, some have theorized that this may be a site of entry. Isolation of the organism from the reproductive tract of healthy, fertile cattle raises questions as to pathogenicity of the organism, but perhaps again this reflects strain differences.

Klavano worked with field outbreaks of infertility associated with *H. somni* isolates and then experimental infections, which confirmed that the *H. somni* in these animals was capable of causing vaginitis with acute mucopurulent discharge and persistent isolation of the organism for almost 2 months. Therefore vaginitis certainly is a possible consequence of *H. somni* infection.

Uterine infections also have been attributed to *H. somni*. Such infections may represent postpartum ascending infections from the caudal reproductive tract or be a result of septicemia. Abortion and early embryonic death also have been attributed to *H. somni* in some field studies and experimental infections.

In addition to the frequent isolation of *H. somni* from the caudal reproductive tract of cows, the organism is often isolated from the sheath and semen of bulls. Infection of the reproductive tract or accessory glands is possible, but the organism frequently is isolated from bulls with no evidence of macroscopic or histologic lesions. Infected bulls can have reduced semen quality and certainly could transmit the disease through natural breeding or semen. Semen usually is treated with antibiotics to minimize this possibility, as discussed already.

A diagnosis of *H. somni* infertility should be based on isolation of the organism from several animals, aborted fetuses, or other samples. Treatment recommendations or indications are nebulous, but it appears that systemic treatment with tetracycline is preferable to local intrauterine or intravaginal therapy.

Control is best attempted by immunization using *H. somni* bacterins even though proof of vaccine efficacy in preventing or controlling reproductive infections is sparse. Animals should be vaccinated twice within 2 to 4 weeks or according to manufacturer's recommendations and then given booster shots annually or semiannually depending on risk. Little is known regarding immunity to the organism, but vaccines generally are considered helpful—regardless of the system infected. Vaccines may be improved significantly in the future if distinct strains of *H. somni* are identified and strains having specific system tropism confirmed. Some manufacturers currently attempt to address this issue by formulating bacterins from isolates from various systems.

OTHER CAUSES OF INFERTILITY

Campylobacteriosis (Vibriosis)

C. fetus var *venerealis* is the cause of campylobacteriosis—formerly called vibriosis in cattle. Although the disease seldom occurs in dairy herds using only AI with semen

from commercial production, it still is common in beef cattle and could be introduced to dairy cows or dairy heifers if infected bulls or heifers are purchased. *C. fetus* var *venerealis* is an obligate parasite of the reproductive tract of cattle and prepuce of bulls. Following infection of the vagina, the organism quickly establishes an endometritis that persists for weeks to months. Salpingitis also may occur. The major consequences of the disease are early embryonic death, fetal death, and infertility. Immunity slowly develops following infection, and most cows subsequently conceive after two or more repeat services even when the organism continues to persist in the caudal reproductive tract. Young bulls are reported to be difficult to infect but act as mechanical carriers of the infection from infected to susceptible heifers and cattle during natural service. Older bulls (>5 years) more commonly are found to be chronically infected, harbor the organism in their prepuce, and contaminate semen with the organism.

Endometritis associated with *C. fetus* var *venerealis* usually is subclinical and seldom causes detectable evidence of infection on rectal examination. Evidence of purulent discharge is unusual. Immunoglobulins of the IgG type eventually are produced and found in the uterus in recovered animals, whereas IgA antibodies are found in the vagina. Infertility in infected cows may be apparent as repeat services at regular or irregular intervals. Irregular intervals are associated with embryonic death. Abortion can also occur, and although most observed abortions occur at 4 to 7 months gestation, probably a greater incidence occurs at less than 4 months, thereby going undetected or only suspected following a return to heat.

Diagnosis of the disease requires culture of the organism from vaginal mucus or reproductive discharges of infected cattle, aborted fetuses (lung and stomach contents), or sheath aspirates from bulls. Material can be collected with sterile insemination pipettes passed through a straw or speculum for cranial vaginal mucus or sheath samples. Diagnostic laboratories should be contacted before sample collection to determine appropriate handling, transport media, and temperature for shipment. Tampons to collect vaginal mucus also have been used to assess antibody levels in the mucus via agglutination tests. When such agglutination tests are chosen, sampled cows should be suspected to have infection for more than 30 days, and samples should be avoided from cows in estrus or that are recently fresh because antibody levels may be diluted by large quantities of mucus at those times. Samples from several animals should be collected. Cultures are more likely to be diagnostic in early infection, and agglutinating antibody tests are more useful in late infections or recovered animals.

Control of the disease includes using only commercial antibiotic-treated semen from AI companies and avoiding natural service. Vaccination also is effective as both a control and treatment method because it evokes IgG production that results in elimination of infection in the uterus of cows and sheaths of bulls. Vaccination should be performed according to manufacturer's instructions and repeated yearly. If natural service is continued, it must be emphasized that noninfected vaccinated bulls may transmit the disease mechanically even though they themselves are immune.

Trichomoniasis

Etiology

T. foetus, a flagellate protozoan, is the cause of trichomoniasis—a venereal disease of bull-bred cattle. Although herds using semen from commercial AI stud services as the exclusive source of semen are not at risk, herds that use custom collected and frozen semen or natural service are at risk. The disease is much more prevalent in beef cattle but deserves mention to remind us that dairy cattle are susceptible.

Trichomoniasis is spread by carrier and infected bulls. Older bulls are more likely to be infected chronically because *T. foetus* establishes infection on the epithelium and in the epithelial crypts of the prepuce and glans. These crypts become more numerous as bulls age, thereby causing greater risk for older bulls. Although young bulls are infected less commonly, they certainly can be, and they also may be chronic carriers.

Infected bulls have no outward signs of infection and may shed large numbers of *T. foetus* when mated to only a few cows. Heavy breeding, as occurs during seasonal breeding in beef animals, tends to dilute or reduce the number of organisms shed during coitus, thereby somewhat reducing infectivity. Infected bulls kept on dairy farms and bred year-round would likely be more infective at all breedings. Even noninfected bulls and bulls that develop immunity or resistance to *T. foetus* (rare) may act as mechanical carriers of infection from infected to noninfected cattle.

Cows infected with *T. foetus* usually clear the infection spontaneously within a few months. The mechanisms of immunity involved in the self-limiting infection are unclear, but few cattle remain persistently infected or carriers. Cattle that have been infected, resolve the infection, conceive, and calve but then are reinfected seem to clear the infection more rapidly, which suggests some immune responsiveness. Infected cows suffer from infertility thought to be the result of early embryonic death. Such embryonic death is related to uterine and oviduct inflammation. Infected cows either become repeat breeders or return to estrus at irregular intervals that suggest early embryonic death. Most infected cattle resolve the infection spontaneously within 3 to 4 months and then are able to conceive and maintain a normal pregnancy. A small percentage of infected cows develop pyometra or suffer abortion. The occurrence of multiple pyometra cows in a bull-bred herd may be a major indicator of trichomoniasis. Abortions usually occur before the fifth month of gestation, and those that occur before 90 days seldom are observed. When abortion is observed, the fetus is autolyzed and may be macerated.

Following inoculation of the organism into the reproductive tract of susceptible cows, infection is established in the vagina, cervix, endometrium, and tubules. Some cattle show postcoital discharge several days following breeding, and mild vulvovaginitis and cervicitis are possible. However, most cows have little observable discharge. The vaginal infection usually resolves within 1 to 2 months because of vaginal antibody production, but the uterine infection lingers for 3 to 4 months, after which time immunity or resistance is established.

Clinical Signs and Diagnosis

Clinical signs other than infertility may be minimal. Therefore a careful history and examination of breeding records may be required before the disease is suspected. Postcoital discharges, pyometra, and abortion are helpful signs but are far less common than simple return to service at regular or irregular intervals.

Diagnosis requires identification and isolation of *T. foetus*. It is recommended that bulls be sampled by preputial scrapings and aspirates. These are collected using a dry pipette inserted into the preputial fornix, simultaneously scraping and while aspirating any available smegma. Because the organism lives in the mucosal crypts, the procedure must be done vigorously, and it is desirable to induce mild irritation or even bleeding while collecting the sample. The pipette also may be introduced through a dry straw, and preparation of the prepuce should include clipping preputial hair. Cows may be sampled by collection of cranial vaginal mucus but are not as likely to yield organisms from this technique unless infected recently. Pyometra cases may yield the organism if fluid is aspirated directly from the uterus, and the abomasal fluid of aborted fetuses also is worth sampling. Sampling of bulls is considered the prime means of diagnosis and surveillance in infected herds.

Field samples may be transferred to sterile physiologic saline solution or lactated Ringer's solution and quickly transported to a qualified diagnostic laboratory for identification. Alternatively, and perhaps preferably, the collected samples may be inoculated immediately into appropriate isolation media. Diamond's medium is time tested for isolation of *T. foetus*. Some authorities do not recommend field inoculation of Diamond's medium. More recently it has been recommended that screw-top culture tubes containing Diamond's medium or In-Pouch TF medium chambers (Biomed Diagnostics, Santa Clara CA) be inoculated in the field to reduce loss of viable organisms in transport diluents. In this study, the In-Pouch TF medium allowed more rapid detection of *T. foetus* and superior detection of infection when smaller inoculums were collected.

Treatment and Control

Elimination of infected and carrier animals coupled with prevention of reintroduction of the disease are the hallmarks of control programs. In dairy herds, this can be simplified by stopping all natural breeding, getting rid of all bulls, and using only reputable commercially prepared semen. If bulls must be retained, they should be cultured and treated if positive. Treatment currently consists of three injections of 15 to 30 g (deeply IM) of ipronidazole at 24-hour intervals. Because this imidazole ring compound (ipronidazole) may be inactivated by the normal preputial flora that includes micrococcus organisms, systemic antibiotics should be administered for several days before starting ipronidazole. One injection of long-acting tetracycline or daily injections of penicillin for 2 to 3 days have been used for this purpose. Ipronidazole is very acidic and irritating to tissue, so that injection site abscesses are common. Other imidazoles including metronidazole and dimetridazole also have been used but have disadvantages (IV use for metronidazole and the unpalatability and gastrointestinal tract dysfunction associated with dimetridazole) when compared with ipronidazole. Practitioners should familiarize themselves with the legality of administering antibiotics belonging to the azole family in their respective geographic region before use. For example, use of the substituted azoles (metronidazole, dimetridazole, and ipronidazole) in food producing animals is currently forbidden by the Food and Drug Administration in the United States.

Infected cows may be segregated, allowed several months of sexual rest, or repeatedly cycled with prostaglandin or analogues to hasten elimination of the infection from the reproductive tract. There are currently very few vaccines available worldwide against *T. foetus*; the one product that is available in the United States is a whole cell product with no efficacy claim regarding protection in bulls.

The best treatment is to eliminate natural service and use only commercially prepared semen by AI.

Neospora sp.

Neospora caninum has been identified as a cause of abortion in cattle. Similarities to other carnivore-borne protozoans suggest that carnivores, specifically the domestic dog, are the primary host and shed oocysts in their feces that are infectious to cattle. *N. caninum* has been confirmed as a major cause of abortion in cattle in the United States and other countries. Abortions may occur between 3 and 9 months, with the majority occurring at 4 to 6 months gestation. Following transplacental infection, the central nervous system of the fetus is the major target area, and protozoan encephalomyelitis ensues. In addition to abortions, calves may be born weak or with obvious neurologic deficits. Some cattle that have aborted once because of *Neospora* sp. infection may subsequently deliver calves with neurologic lesions and concurrent paresis as a result of congenital *Neospora* infection. On-farm studies of precolostral antibody levels in calves on endemic premises suggest that the risk of endogenous vertical transmission by a chronically infected dam may be as high as 95%, but the vast majority of congenitally infected calves will be normal.

Vertical transmission is the primary mode of transmission once the infection has been introduced into a herd. Experimental confirmation of vertical transmission in cattle is well documented. Nonsuppurative myocarditis has also been reported in fetuses or calves with congenital focal necrotizing encephalomyelitis.

Neospora parasites have been isolated from aborted fetuses. In addition, other workers have found protozoan abortion in one herd of cattle that was concurrently infected with *Hammondia pardalis* thought to be related to a large feral cat population.

In most affected herds, protozoan abortion has seemed to be associated with close confinement of cattle. Abortions may be sporadic, endemic, or epidemic, and the prevalence varies greatly.

Clinical signs are limited to abortion and the birth of calves with neurologic signs secondary to congenital infections of the central nervous system. Infected cows are asymptomatic. Diagnosis is based on immunohistochemical staining of fetal or calf tissues and an enzyme-linked immunosorbent assay (ELISA) test on serum. The current immunohistochemical procedure performed on tissue samples is an immunoperoxidase test using antisera against *N. caninum* or the bovine *Neospora* (BPA1) isolate on paraffin-embedded sections. All tissues should be examined, but the brain and heart are most likely to show lesions. The ELISA test currently is recommended for screening of cattle and precolostral calves showing signs or considered at risk of congenital infections. Serology may be a helpful screening procedure to detect the presence of the *Neospora*-like organism in a herd or suspect calf. If all tested animals are negative, the disease is not likely to exist on that farm, and immunohistochemical staining may not be indicated. Milk ELISA test may be useful to assess herd status. Diagnostic laboratories studying aborted fetuses will need to use immunohistochemical stains to detect the organism in fetal tissues, however. Practitioners should inquire regarding the availability of these tests before sending samples to specific laboratories. A vaccine has recently become available in many parts of the world. Although efficacious in reducing incidence of abortion, it does not eliminate it.

Epizootic Bovine Abortion

Etiology

Epizootic bovine abortion is a disease of uncertain etiology that occurs in the foothill regions of the Sierra Nevada Mountains, including parts of Nevada, Oregon,

California, and northern New Mexico. Although the specific etiologic agent is unknown, the disease occurs only in areas harboring *Ornithodoros coriaceus*, so the disease is thought to be tick-borne. Cattle and deer are the primary hosts of this tick. Chlamydia was long considered to be the cause, but this assumption appears to be erroneous. Spirochetes and more recently a novel delta protobacterium have also been incriminated in the etiopathogenesis of the disease.

Abortions occur 3 months or more following tick exposure and tend to be correlated with seasonal implementation of grazing. Resistance to the disease appears to occur and is important for prevention and control. Susceptible cows and heifers moved to tick-infested areas for the first time are at greatest risk. Abortion generally occurs during the last trimester of pregnancy. Following initial exposure, cattle develop resistance, and therefore cattle sometimes are moved to tick-infested areas several months before first breeding in an effort to allow immunity to develop. The duration of immunity is unknown but appears adequate for one or two seasons.

Clinical Signs and Diagnosis

Infected cattle show no signs other than abortion—or delivery of weak calves—and diagnosis requires laboratory confirmation of compatible histopathology in aborted fetuses or calves. Gross lesions include lymphadenopathy, splenomegaly, and hepatomegaly. Ascites is present in some fetuses. Histopathology identifies lymphohistiocytic infiltration of many tissues. This infiltration suggests chronic inflammatory disease that may have a proliferative component. Lymphoreticular tissues and other organs may be involved, and thymic lesions are extensive. The disease can be experimentally reproduced in susceptible animals by innoculation of thymic tissue from aborted fetuses.

Control measures other than avoiding endemic areas or preimmunizing cattle by exposure to tick-infested areas several months before breeding await further elucidation of the specific etiology.

Prolonged Gestation

Etiology

Prolonged gestation in dairy cattle results from fetal anomalies and requires differentiation from fetal loss or fetal mummification because affected cattle fail to show signs of impending parturition at their due date. Adrenal abnormalities of the fetus are a major cause of prolonged gestation because parturition normally is triggered by fetal cortisol release. Prolonged gestation may occur in calves produced by cloning, in vitro fertilization, or embryo transfer as part of the "large newborn calf" syndrome. It also is possible that adenohypophyseal and pituitary abnormalities coexist or contribute to adrenal insufficiency in such fetuses. The condition is reported in Holsteins and

Ayrshires, and I have observed it in Brown Swiss cattle; it is thought to represent a recessive trait. Cattle with this form of prolonged gestation appear normal but do not show signs of udder edema or pelvic laxity at the predicted calving date. Gestation may be prolonged 1 to 3 months or more. Palpation of the cow reveals a large fetus; errors in breeding dates or records must be ruled out before confirming the condition. Fetuses with adrenal insufficiency may be normally formed, are very large (up to 150 to 200 lb in Holsteins and Brown Swiss), and often require delivery via cesarean section. Spontaneous parturition seldom occurs in true prolonged gestation unless the fetus dies in utero. If induction of parturition is elected, dystocia should be anticipated. If the fetus is alive, it will be nonviable because of adrenal insufficiency, and most calves with this condition die shortly before, during, or within 48 hours of birth.

Another form of prolonged gestation occurs in fetal anomalies involving the skull and brain. Calves are miniature rather than giant and may have a cyclopian-like head deformity with accompanying adenohypophyseal hypoplasia or pituitary abnormalities. A recessive trait is suspected as the cause of this condition in Guernseys, Ayrshires, and Swedish Red and White cattle. Roberts also has observed another anomaly of the skull and brain that includes cerebral hernia as a cause of prolonged gestation. Adrenal, hypophyseal, and pituitary anomalies are likely, and calves are large—often requiring cesarean section.

Prognosis is guarded for cattle with prolonged gestation because:

1. They usually are not prepared to produce milk.
2. They usually experience dystocia or require cesarean section.
3. Inheritance is suspected as the cause.

REPRODUCTIVE MONITORING OF DAIRY CATTLE

Although this section cannot, and will not try to, address the subject of reproduction in dairy cattle fully, a brief synopsis, review, and summary based on my experience will follow. Bovine practitioners should consult standard theriogenology and reproductive textbooks for more in-depth reading.

Reproductive programs have been, and will continue to be, devised and revised based on herd management styles, owner preferences, veterinary preferences, available labor, and pharmacologic manipulations. Veterinarians tend to be products of their education and experience when it comes to recommending or devising reproductive monitoring programs for their clients. It is idealistic for veterinarians to assume that clients always will accept a set protocol. In fact, veterinarians will suffer less damage to their egos and gain better client compliance when a reproductive monitoring program evolves from collective bargaining between client and doctor. Such collective bargaining minimizes client reservations, allows consideration of time-tested successful components on each farm, and allows the veterinarian to suggest and implement new or corrective measures to address unsuccessful components. Therefore the program should be tailored to the individual farm. Monthly herd checks may be acceptable for cow herds of 40 but obviously are unacceptable for herds with a population of 400 or more. Decisions as to which open cows should be monitored also will vary. Some herds have all postpartum cows evaluated, whereas others check only those 30 days or more postpartum and those with known postpartum problems. Ideally all cows not observed in heat by 30 to 40 days should be checked; however, the intensity and effort put into estrus detection is extremely herd variable, and many larger herds now prefer to arbitrarily schedule reproductive examinations for all cows beyond a certain number of days in milk before first breeding. Regardless of the program chosen, it is imperative that a program exists that allows a regular, timely, and interactive relationship between veterinarian and client that forces both to concentrate on the herd reproductive performance.

Postpartum cows should be evaluated regularly by routine rectal examinations to monitor involution and to allow detection of postpartum abnormalities such as endometritis, cervicitis, vaginitis, and cystic ovarian disease. In some herds, all postpartum cattle are included on the check list, whereas in others only those fresh 2 weeks or more are palpated. Rectal palpation of recently fresh cows (<14 days) is limited somewhat because uterine retraction is not always possible. However, evaluation of the uterine tone, degree of muscular contraction, and palpation of obvious abnormalities may still be helpful. In addition, repeated pressure directed downward and backward on the cervix and anterior vagina allows the examiner to propel discharges to the vulva and thereby evaluate reproductive tract discharges that might be missed otherwise. Vaginal examinations and speculum examinations are indicated for cows less than 14 days postpartum suspected to have endometritis, RFM, necrotic vaginitis, and other caudal reproductive tract pathology.

Estrus Cycle

Cattle undergoing normal involution usually ovulate for the first time 13 to 15 days following calving. This ovulation usually does not result in detectable signs of heat but will cause a detectable follicle, increased uterine tone, and increased amounts of mucus discharge. The mucus discharge may be mixed with purulent material, bloody lochia, or appear fairly clear. The second ovulation follows another shorter than 21-day cycle and generally occurs 30 to 35 days following parturition.

This ovulation is more likely to result in observable signs of heat than the first ovulation but still may go undetected in approximately 50% of cows. Following this second ovulation, dairy cows usually assume a regular estrus interval of 20 to 23 days. A small percentage of cows will have cycles that are regular but shorter or longer than the average 20- to 21-day cycle.

Veterinarians monitoring reproductive programs try to determine whether cows are cycling normally and to anticipate heat dates (based on rectal palpation findings). History, including observed heats, reproductive tract discharges, treatments for postpartum conditions, and notes recorded at the time of earlier examinations are essential when palpating cows during prebreeding examinations. Veterinarians must palpate thousands of cows before being comfortable with predicting stage of cycle, anticipated heat date, and the variations in normal findings that are encountered. Uterine tone, the cervix, the oviducts, reproductive tract discharges, and ovarian structures constitute the major palpable entities during routine rectal palpation of the nonpregnant cow.

Follicular development during the estrus cycle in cattle is characterized by two or more waves of follicular growth that produce 5 to 10 follicles on each ovary. Of these follicles, one usually becomes dominant and larger than the others within 1 to 2 days of the start of the wave, and the others undergo atresia. In cattle that have two follicular waves during their cycle—one may start on the day of ovulation and the second wave starts around day 10 of the cycle. The dominant follicle from the first wave enlarges for 5 to 6 days, becomes stationary for 5 to 6 more days, and then regresses. The dominant follicle from the second wave is the eventual ovulatory follicle. It follows that a palpable follicle may be present from about day 4 or 5 until ovulation because regression of the first wave-dominant follicle overlaps with the production of the second wave-dominant follicle. Ovulatory follicles usually are 12 to 16 mm in diameter. Nonovulatory dominant follicles reach a similar size. Therefore the presence of a follicle should not be interpreted mistakenly always to mean a cow is near heat. Some research suggests that many cows have three waves of follicular activity, and some may even have four.

Cows that have three follicular waves have the waves start at about days 0, 9, and 16 of the cycle. Cows with three wave cycles tend to have longer luteal phases and longer cycles of 22 to 24 days.

The last wave-dominant follicle is the ovulatory follicle. Luteolysis is associated with increased concentrations of $PGF_{2\alpha}$ in the uterine endometrium that eventually reach the corpus luteum following transport into the uteroovarian veins and then into the ovarian artery. Regression of the corpus luteum causes reduced progesterone levels and triggers a large secretion of luteinizing hormone (LH) from the anterior pituitary gland after hypothalamic release of GnRH. At the same time that LH is peaking, estradiol levels are increasing and will result in estrus behavior. The dominant follicle is being acted on by both LH and follicle-stimulating hormone (FSH) as follicular maturation occurs in the preovulatory period. LH acts on theca interna cells and increases androgen synthesis, which eventually causes effects on granulosa cells, whereas FSH enhances estradiol production.

The preovulatory LH peak is associated with complex and poorly understood effects on the follicle, but the result is follicular rupture, ovulation, and corpus luteum production. The estradiol peak associated with follicular maturation is thought to be responsible for the physical and behavioral signs of heat or estrus. Increased uterine tone, clear mucus discharge, hyperemia of the reproductive tract, and a palpable follicle 12 to 18 mm in diameter occur as the cow approaches "standing heat." Cows in heat should have a small or barely detectable regressing corpus luteum.

Estrus and Heat Detection

Estrus is usually regarded as lasting 10 to 18 hours, but there is evidence that estrus in modern high-yielding dairy cows is much shorter—about 8 hours. Ovulation generally occurs about 12 hours after estrus ends or 24 to 30 hours following the onset of estrus. Heat detection is the traditional heart of all reproductive programs and cannot be overemphasized. Observed duration of heat may be less than 10 hours and can be split in some cows such that physiologic duration of heat may be longer than apparent based solely on observation. Despite urging by lay publications, heat detection techniques and aids, and veterinary encouragement, many farms continue to do a poor job of heat detection. A study from the 1970s revealed that at that time approximately 50% of estrus periods went undetected on the average dairy farm in the United States; current biology and management of high-yielding cows mean that far fewer estrus periods are detected now. Owners who insist that cows do not show heats are reluctant to accept rectal palpation findings that suggest normal cyclic activity in their cows. Veterinarians who have grown up or worked on dairy farms know all too well the reasons for poor heat detection. When the labor force is spread too thin, assigned to field or mechanical chores, or fails to turn out confined cows, heat detection will be compromised. Some dairy farm workers and owners simply are poor observers, are impatient, or only check cows for a 5- to 10-minute period each day. Veterinarians must understand owner limitations but must not reinforce bad habits by agreeing that all cows have had "silent heats." Owners should be encouraged to observe cows several times daily. Bonuses may be paid to workers who detect heats, and this may encourage workers to observe the cattle more closely. Owners who refuse to turn cows out or only do so once a day for a short time

are at an automatic disadvantage. Free stall housing is not limited by turnout time but can suffer heat detection problems for other reasons. Because estrus occurs over a limited time of 12 to 18 hours, cows showing estrus at night frequently go undetected. Owners should check tails and perineums for clear mucus discharges that suggest proximity to, or recent, estrus; metestrus bleeding can be detected in the same manner. Cows suspected to be in or near heat because of previous heat charting, prostaglandin treatment, or rectal predictions should be observed closely and perhaps have a rectal examination performed by the person responsible for insemination. Increased uterine tone or clear mucus discharge can be detected by this examination. Behavioral or physical signs of standing for other cows to mount, decreased milk production, increased activity, frequent mounting of other cows, roughed up topline or foot stains along the flank region from allowing other cows to mount are things to look for in cows showing heat. Mechanical aids include heat detector strips attached to the tail head, progesterone levels, pedometers, teaser bulls of various types, instruments to measure vaginal mucus electrical resistance (lower resistance or increased conductivity during estrus because of increased chloride levels), an organized highly visible heat expectation chart, and easily observed means of animal identification. When video monitoring of cattle to detect heat is compared with observed visual detection of heats, the pattern of heat detection is brought into perspective. For the first three postpartum heats, approximately 20%, 44%, and 64% were observed by visual observation, whereas the video camera recorded approximately 50%, 94%, and 100%.

Not all blame for failure to detect estrus accrues to labor, however. High-producing cows consume more dry matter to sustain the high yield. High dry matter intake, in turn, stimulates increased liver blood flow and liver size, both of which result in increased metabolism of steroid hormones. These cows have lower circulating concentrations of progesterone and estrogens, which undoubtedly contributes to reduced intensity of estrus expression, and potentially to pregnancy recognition and failure.

Time of Insemination

Once heat is detected, the next problem is deciding when to breed the cow. Ovulation generally occurs 24 to 30 hours after the onset of estrus or 12 hours after the end of estrus. Much debate exists regarding the appropriate time for insemination. Some farms breed in the afternoon for morning-observed heats and breed the following morning for afternoon-observed heats. Others breed once daily. If breeding is in the afternoon, cows in heat that morning are bred, and cows in heat that afternoon are bred the next day. Although recommendations vary greatly, it appears clear that conception rate is improved if insemination occurs before ovulation, and insemination probably should be performed within 12 to 20 hours following the onset of heat.

Concerns regarding timing of ovulation versus timing of insemination frequently are raised for repeat breeder cows or cows that seem to have heats that are prolonged or persist for 2 consecutive days. Some benefit may exist in the use of 100 μg of GnRH administered at the time of breeding for repeat breeder cows that have had at least two previous services, but this same treatment does not appear to be helpful to first service heifers. Individual cows that are determined to have delayed ovulation based on rectal examination also may benefit from GnRH treatment in conjunction with the next breeding if they repeat. Cattle having multiple ovulations may ovulate those follicles at different times, and this is not necessarily abnormal as long as the ovulations occur within 30 hours of the onset of estrus. Roberts reports that 55% to 60% of ovulations and subsequent pregnancies occur in the right ovary and uterine horn.

A small percentage of pregnant cows will show heat despite being pregnant. Although this is more commonly observed in the early months of pregnancy, some cows show heats at regular intervals throughout pregnancy.

Following ovulation, a corpus luteum forms from the theca and granulosa cells of the follicle under the influence of the LH surge and begins to secrete progesterone. The postovulatory ovary and uterus usually have characteristic palpable changes that are present for the first few days of the cycle. The early corpora hemorrhagica (CH) is friable, crepitant, or spongy and generally smaller than the mature corpus luteum. In addition, the uterus feels edematous, thickened, has progressively decreasing tone, and may be flaccid. These changes occur more quickly in some cows than others, and persisting uterine tonus accompanying a small corpus luteum can cause confusion between a preheat and postheat palpation—especially in the 48 hours before or after heat. Usually other determinants such as a dominant preovulatory follicle, a small, firm, regressing corpus luteum, a clear mucus discharge, or metestrus bleeding will assist in accurate determination of the cycle stage, but this may not always be easy. Metestrus bleeding commonly occurs 1 to 3 days following heat and usually is expected to signal a heat that occurred 2 days previously. Although suggestive that ovulation has successfully occurred, this bleeding has nothing to do with conception or lack thereof—despite lay opinions to the contrary.

Rectal palpation following recent ovulation may reveal uterine edema and reducing tone for up to 7 days, after which time a mature corpus luteum and "normal" mid-cycle tone return to the uterus. Increased uterine tone returns as the next heat approaches and is more obvious in young cows than in older ones. As mentioned previously,

it is common and expected to palpate dominant follicles throughout the estrous cycle of cattle. Therefore palpation of uterine tone, corpus luteum size, consistency, shape, and other factors must be evaluated jointly when predicting stage of cycle and anticipated time of heat. It always is useful to attempt to "back-rake" cervical and vaginal discharges forcefully per rectum during routine evaluations—especially in older cows in which uterine tone can be misleading because the appearance of clear mucus discharge may signal an impending heat, and cloudy or purulent discharge may allow diagnosis of inflammatory conditions.

Reproductive Goals and Programs

Each farm must have an established set of goals for reproductive performance. Criteria to be considered include heat detection efficiency, average day to first service, average days open, services per conception, and the voluntary waiting period (VWP). Each farm will have strengths, weaknesses, and different goals. Currently the use of bovine somatotropin (BST) is having significant impact on some time-tested rules of thumb for reproduction efficiency. Before BST, a calving interval of 12.0 to 13.0 months was considered ideal for cows to complete a 305-day record and have an adequate dry period between calvings. Financial manipulation can formulate many theories regarding appropriate calving intervals, but it still is more likely that small to moderate cow-number farms will profit more from the cow that completes four lactations in 48 months than a cow that completes three lactations in 48 months. Large cow-number farms with greater than 40% annual cull rates and concurrent use of BST may not care as much about cow longevity as smaller family farms. Therefore a more prolonged calving interval of 15 to 18 months may be acceptable—especially if the cow will be culled at the end of profitable production levels in that lactation.

Most farms using BST will try to get cows bred back early and then institute BST use. Although the topic is controversial, it is the opinion of many veterinarians that cows on BST and not bred by 150 to 180 days of lactation are very difficult to get bred. Most farms use a VWP of 50 to 60 days before first insemination. Farms that push the VWP to 45 days or less must anticipate a higher services per conception rate because many cows have not fully involuted or have residual problems such as low grade endometritis at the time of first service. Regardless of goals, the reproductive program should emphasize routine diagnosis and treatment of postpartum conditions that may have a negative impact on conception. Regular reproductive checks, treatment of problem cows, and the use of prostaglandin to force cyclicity and aid uterine evacuation and involution all are essential.

Prostaglandin or prostaglandin analogues are the most common therapeutic drugs used in the dairy industry today. In addition to treatment of endometritis and pyometra, these drugs are used to force cows into heats through luteolysis. Many management programs have been and will continue to be devised for wholesale use of prostaglandin treatment of open cows to improve reproductive efficiency. Herd veterinarians must involve themselves in recommendations for, and evaluation of, prostaglandin-dependent breeding programs. It is best that cows at or beyond the VWP be evaluated by rectal palpation to rule out obvious problems such as endometritis, cystic ovarian disease, ovarian inactivity, and to confirm that the corpus luteum and uterus are at an appropriate stage for prostaglandin therapy to be successful. The body condition of the cow, as well as concurrent diseases, stresses, or lameness, may negate the use of prostaglandin for certain individual cows. Programs have been devised that direct prostaglandin treatment of all open cows beyond the VWP regardless of rectal status. These programs suffer from some obvious disadvantages, ignore veterinary advice, and often are a crutch for deficient management, poor heat detection, and inadequate labor efforts as regards reproductive health. Programs have been suggested wherein cows to be bred are given prostaglandin every 10 days, every 14 days, or every 7 days (Monday morning program). Large herds may be forced to implement these programs, but it takes little critical analysis to realize that, without concurrent rectal palpation, the economic justification for these programs often does not consider failures caused by cystic ovarian disease, noncycling cows, caudal reproductive tract infections, and many other conditions that increase days open for some members of the herd. Furthermore, prostaglandin-induced heats are only an aid to conception when adequate heat detection exists on that farm. Managers who do a poor job of heat detection will often miss heats—regardless of whether the heats are spontaneous or induced by prostaglandin. Timed breeding, for example, at 80 hours after prostaglandin dosing is not highly efficient in adult dairy cattle. Dairy cattle at appropriate stages of the estrus cycle that are treated with $PGF_{2\alpha}$ or analogues are expected to show heat 2 to 5 days following the injection. However, in reality, some cows do not respond during this interval. This variability may be related to the effects of follicular wave development rather than simply because of age of the corpus luteum. Recent work shows that cows treated on day 10 of the cycle may have a more variable and longer interval from treatment to estrus than those treated before or after this midpoint. It appears from these studies that the presence of a dominant follicle available to become the ovulatory follicle is important to ensure a normal treatment-to-estrus interval following $PGF_{2\alpha}$ administration.

The major advantage to prostaglandin use for inducing heats is that it usually forces owners to observe the cows more closely during the window of time that heat is anticipated. A further advantage is provided by producing estrus, thereby enhancing uterine defense mechanisms as discussed in the section on endometritis. Targeting breeding strategies involving repeated administration of prostaglandin alone followed by either timed insemination or insemination to observed estrus have been largely superceded by modified targeted breeding protocols, the Ovsynch and Ovsynch/Presynch programs. The modified targeted breeding system involves the administration of prostaglandins to eligible cows followed by GnRH 14 days later, and a second prostaglandin injection 7 days after that. Breeding to observed estrus or 72 to 80 hours after the second $PGF_{2\alpha}$ should be performed.

Ovsynch is an ovulation synchronization protocol that allows timed insemination of cattle without the need for heat detection. This technique involves administration of GnRH at random stages of the estrous cycle followed by $PGF_{2\alpha}$ 7 days later. Forty-eight hours after the $PGF_{2\alpha}$, a second shot of GnRH is administered, and the cow is inseminated 16 to 20 hours later. Several studies have demonstrated that fertility in dairy cows is further improved when cows on the Ovsynch program are presynchronized by administering $PGF_{2\alpha}$ one or two times before initiating Ovsynch. The second (or only) presynchronizing prostaglandin injection is administered 12 days before Ovsynch is begun. Optimally insemination should be timed alongside GnRH administration 72 hours after the final prostaglandin injection of the Presynch/Ovsynch program.

The ability to deemphasize estrus detection has been one of the main selling points for the Ovsynch and Ovsynch/Presynch programs, but it is sobering to realize that in multiple studies, 5 to 8 week pregnancy rates rarely exceed 35% to 40% with these programs. (Of course, this is offset by the 100% submission rate.) Furthermore, field experience suggests that many farms only achieve more modest numbers. These facts should be discussed openly with clients, alongside the economic implications of increased hormone usage. With these programs should come a commitment to excellent record keeping, timing, and semen handling and insemination technique.

Although GnRH and human chorionic gonadotropin (hCG) have also been used in experimental and field cases as a one-time treatment to enhance ovarian function in early lactation cattle (usually around day 14 postpartum), the results of these studies have been variable. Although available and popular for many years overseas, intravaginal progesterone-releasing controlled internal drug release (CIDR) devices have only recently become available in the United States. At this time it is unclear whether these devices confer much of a benefit on pregnancy rates when combined with the aforementioned Ovsynch and Ovsynch/Presynch programs.

CONDITIONS THAT RESULT IN REDUCED FERTILITY

The preceding section discussed reproductive monitoring and briefly reviewed current practices for cycling cattle. A complete listing and discussion of causes of infertility or reduced reproductive performance is beyond the scope of this textbook, but several major causes of reduced herd fertility deserve mention. Readers also are directed to discussions in this chapter of specific infectious conditions and infectious diseases that affect reproduction.

Cystic Ovaries

Cystic ovaries (cystic ovarian disease, "cysts") are one of the most common causes of infertility in dairy cattle. Classically cystic ovaries are defined as anovulatory follicles larger than 25 mm diameter that persist for 10 days or more in the absence of a corpus luteum. This definition no longer holds for all cases of cystic ovaries currently identified in dairy cattle. During the past 10 years, it has been increasingly obvious to many veterinarians that a percentage of cystic ovary cows have anovulatory follicles much smaller than 25 mm and that anestrus is far more common than nymphomania. Cysts may also coexist with a corpus luteum in some cows. Contemporary ultrasound studies have shown that in many cases cysts are dynamic, with a new cyst replacing a receding one with each succeeding follicular cohort. Compared with 20 years ago, routine rectal palpation performed on high-producing herds currently identifies more cystic ovaries, more cysts less than 25-mm diameter, and more cystic ovary patients with owner complaints of anestrus rather than nymphomania. Cows with cystic ovaries that show nymphomania or appear "to be in heat every day" represent danger to themselves and herdmates. Although these cows may aid heat detection by being "bullers," they also may cause injuries to themselves and herdmates, and they spend a great deal of time and effort in chasing other cows in the herd. Chronic cystic ovaries cause estrogen-induced physical alterations in conformation and behavioral changes. Relaxation of the pelvic ligaments, swelling of the vulva and perineum, mucometra, a raised tail head ("sterility hump"), thick neck, and overcondition or steerlike appearance may eventually be seen in cattle affected by chronic (months) cystic ovaries.

Pathologic ovarian cysts may be follicular or luteal and may be single or multiple on one or both ovaries. Follicular cysts are thin-walled, fluid-filled structures associated with low plasma progesterone levels. Luteal cysts are partially luteinized fluid-filled structures that result in higher plasma progesterone levels. Both types are thought to represent the same disease, may persist, be replaced by other cysts without a distinct ovarian cycle, and can change from follicular to luteal. Follicular cysts are more common and can occur in the early postpartum period or any time thereafter. For practical purposes there is little value in distinguishing between these. In contrast to follicular and luteal cysts, cystic corpora lutea are normal structures that do not alter either cyclicity or pregnancy. Cystic corpora lutea have fluid cavities, usually 7 to 10 mm in diameter, surrounded by normal luteal tissue and are nonpathologic. They will not be discussed further in this chapter.

It is not always easy to diagnose cystic ovarian structures accurately by rectal palpation alone. Despite a palpator's confidence or experience, it appears that rectal palpation is a poor means of differentiating follicular and luteal cysts. Ultrasonography and plasma progesterone levels are much more accurate except in those cases of very large follicular cysts for which palpation is sufficient. It is more difficult to identify luteal cysts than follicular cysts accurately by palpation. However, palpator experience seems to be directly proportional to accuracy of differentiation of the two types. Because of the extreme variability in progesterone levels and sensitivities of many milk progesterone tests, it appears that ultrasonography is the most accurate means of clinically differentiating luteal and follicular cysts.

The causes of cystic ovaries are likely multifactorial and frequently difficult to determine. However, several factors require consideration and have been reviewed recently. Nutritional and hormonal influences have been suggested, but absolute cause and effect relationships are scarce or largely theoretical. Highly estrogenic feeds or estrogenic drugs may contribute to ovarian cysts. Interactions and responsiveness to estrogen levels as regards LH release may be involved, but pituitary release of LH following GnRH stimulation appears normal in cattle with cystic ovaries. Stress that causes cortisol elevations may contribute to cystic ovaries because adrenocorticotropic hormone (ACTH) appears to block preovulatory LH surges. If this theory holds, it helps explain cysts in early lactation but is less tenable in cows in mid-lactation or stale cows. Cystic ovarian disease in high-producing cows may also be associated with hypoinsulinemia. Occasionally herds experience an increased incidence of cystic ovaries because of selenium deficiency or excessive soluble protein levels in the diet. Further questions are raised because high milk production has been blamed for increased incidence of cystic ovaries, but epidemiologic studies tend to deny this as a significant cause. The interaction between a healthy uterine endometrium and ovarian function seems very important in the field, and evidence supporting endometritis as a contributing cause for ovarian cysts has been published. Field work often identifies problem cows greater than 90 days into lactation that have poor fertility as a result of both recurrent cystic ovaries and low grade endometritis. Genetics are also most likely involved, and certain cow families have notoriously high incidence of cystic ovaries. Current selection of cows and sires for production may propagate this problem even though heritability of cysts is considered to be low. Cysts are more common in multiparous cows but are not rare in primiparous heifers. Cows overconditioned at dry off also are more prone to development of cystic ovaries in the next lactation.

It is most likely that cystic ovaries occur because of both environmental and genetic reasons. Poor uterine health, nutritional or mineral imbalances, chronic reproductive tract infections, stresses, hormonal interactions, and other factors may be involved.

Treatment of cystic ovaries is indicated in most cases. Early lactation cysts (<30 days postpartum) may resolve spontaneously, but it is impossible to know which ones will not. Therefore treatment at the time of diagnosis has been shown to be the best decision. Although many follicular cysts are fluctuant and can be ruptured manually during rectal palpation, manual rupture is usually contraindicated because the success of this treatment is limited (probably one third of cases or less), and direct or indirect damage to the ovary or uterine tube is a potential risk. Fibrosis, adhesions, and hemorrhage associated with manual rupture of cysts are specific possibilities.

Treatment of cystic ovaries involves the use of GnRH, hCG, and $PGF_{2\alpha}$. GnRH is a decapeptide that, when injected into cattle, causes release of LH from the anterior pituitary gland. Although the standard dose used in the United States is 100 μg (Cystorelin, CEVA Labs, Overland Park, KS), a dose-related response has been shown to exist for this drug, and European doses are often larger than 100 μg. Although 100 μg is the usual recommended dose, better response in repeat cystic ovary patients may be expected with larger doses when the additional expense can be justified. Approximately two thirds to three quarters of cystic ovary patients respond to 100 μg of GnRH with a good estrus 18 to 23 days following treatment. In an effort to speed return to estrus in treated cows, rectal examination may be performed 9 to 12 days later, and if an obvious corpus luteum has formed, $PGF_{2\alpha}$ may be administered to induce heat. Other GnRH analogues are available, and more may be forthcoming. More potent analogues including nonapeptides should be used according to manufacturer's recommendations. Insemination of a cow with cystic ovarian disease subsequent to GnRH treatment, even when behavioral signs of estrus are seen, has historically been discouraged because of perceived lesser fertility. In practice, it is most convenient to treat cows with cystic ovaries by submitting them to the routine OvSynch protocol. Because there is evidence that some cystic cows are unable to mount a normal ovulatory LH surge until after exposure to progesterone, inclusion of progesterone, in the form of a CIDR, is probably beneficial.

hCG is another time-tested treatment for cystic ovarian disease, is comparable to LH, and is used by IV or IM injection. Generally 10,000 IU are injected IM or 5000 to 10,000 IU IV. Treatment success is comparable with GnRH, but some negative consequences exist for hCG. First, hCG is more expensive than GnRH. Second, because the product contains foreign proteins (from another species), repeat injections may lead to either sensitivity or increased refractoriness to treatment as cows treated repeatedly with hCG develop antibodies against the foreign protein. Third, the drug has recently been classified as a controlled substance. However, hCG remains a valuable drug for one-time use or as an alternative therapy for cystic cows that appear refractory to GnRH.

$PGF_{2\alpha}$ may be used as the only treatment for luteal cysts because the luteinized tissue in the cyst, albeit less than in a normal corpus luteum, usually responds to $PGF_{2\alpha}$ and estrus will be induced. Obviously treatment with $PGF_{2\alpha}$ alone is based on assumption or knowledge that the cyst is luteal. Because clinical differentiation of follicular versus luteal cysts is difficult by palpation alone, ultrasonography or progesterone levels may be necessary for absolute diagnosis of a luteal cyst. These ancillary aids add further expense to therapy and are often neglected for this reason. Milk progesterone tests may be helpful in this regard because cystic cows with low milk progesterone levels treated with GnRH and cystic cows with high milk progesterone treated with $PGF_{2\alpha}$ had a higher cure rate than those receiving a form treatment of both types with GnRH. Other authors suggest concurrent treatment of all cystic cows with GnRH and $PGF_{2\alpha}$ to cover all contingencies. This approach may not, however, be as successful as progesterone determined treatments. The obvious advantage to specific treatment of luteal cysts with $PGF_{2\alpha}$ is a quick return to estrus. Therefore some additional expense (as in milk progesterone test) may be justified. In addition to specific treatment of cystic ovarian disease, concurrent reproductive tract abnormalities such as endometritis should be treated. When a higher than expected incidence of cystic ovaries exists in a herd, nutritional and other management factors should be evaluated.

Variable success has been encountered when GnRH has been used as a preventive by administration to all cows approximately 2 weeks following parturition; this technique requires further study. Culling of problem cystic cows probably is not practiced enough—often because the cows are thought to have desirable production or genetic traits.

Ovarian Tumors

Ovarian tumors of many types have been described, but all are rare. Granulosa cell tumors occasionally are identified on one or both ovaries as cystic or lobulated masses that may be quite firm. Some cows having granulosa cell tumors exhibit nymphomania apparently associated with elevated estrogen levels. Although granulosa cell tumors are rarely diagnosed clinically, they are not uncommon in slaughterhouse surveys, suggesting that some cases dismissed as intractable cystic ovaries are actually granulosa cell tumors. Rarely lymphosarcoma may affect the ovary of cattle, and the lesion usually represents just one of many anatomic areas affected by multicentric lymphosarcoma.

Nutritional Causes

Poor nutrition and poor body condition have drastic negative influences on fertility. Field observations and many scientific references implicate poor body condition and inadequate energy balance as causes of reduced fertility. Cows that calve in poor condition because of deficiencies in dry cow management are more likely to have prolonged anestrus postpartum. In addition, those cows with the greatest decline in body condition postpartum have more problems reproductively. Negative energy balance in early lactation may depress luteal function, lower progesterone levels, and lower fertility because corpus luteum production of progesterone can suffer a lag-phase depression from depressed metabolic condition 40 to 70 days before ovulation. Therefore regardless of specific pathophysiology, cows that freshen in less than desirable body condition or those that lose more condition than desirable during the first 5 to 8 weeks of lactation are likely to have reduced fertility. Although it is expected that early lactation is a time of negative energy balance because of peak production preceding peak dry matter intake, those cows that suffer the most severe losses will be likely to have altered fertility and metabolic diseases that could further compromise fertility. Cows with severe energy imbalances do not cycle and have a persistent corpus luteum, have inactive ovaries, or cycle but fail to show heat. Repeat services are common even in those cows showing heat. Although some studies do not support similar problems in nulliparous heifers in negative energy balance, I find this difficult to believe based on field experience that has often confirmed inactive ovaries associated with poor body condition and growth in heifers that are maintained in a negative energy balance.

Cattle with extreme energy imbalances have a reduced tendency to cycle normally, reduced conception rates, and may suffer early fetal losses. These cows should not be bred until they are in a positive energy balance. Negative energy balance increases hypothalamic sensitivity to estradiol, resulting in negative feedback of GnRH and gonadotrophins. Dominant follicles in affected animals regress before they reach ovulatory size or estradiol production. (This mimics the endocrinology of prepubertal heifers.)

Dietary protein is another nutritional factor that affects fertility. Inadequate protein significantly lowers conception rates and too much protein with resultant increases in urea nitrogen levels may do the same. Excessive urea or ammonia levels resulting from excessive dietary protein may affect spermatozoa or early embryos, but the exact mechanism of infertility is unknown. Discrepancies in the results of various studies on excessive protein levels in the diet of dairy cows may be explained somewhat by the variations in protein sources. Experimental studies and field work support the theory that excessive rumen-degradable protein is harmful to reproduction. Diets that result in serum urea nitrogen levels greater than 20 mg/dl have been associated with infertility. This work is supported by field observations that confirm a high incidence of repeat breedings, early embryonic death, and cystic ovarian disease in herds feeding excessive rumen-degradable protein. It has been recommended that 35% of dietary protein be present as rumen bypass protein and that excessive protein may not only be harmful to reproduction but also expensive. In addition, certain protein supplements derived from cotton sources may contain excessive gossypol, which has negative implications for both reproductive performance and cow health.

In selenium-deficient areas, low selenium levels in dairy cattle can have a significant negative effect on reproduction. In addition to an increased incidence of RFM, selenium-deficient herds have a higher incidence of endometritis, cystic ovarian disease, failure to show estrus, and embryonic death. Supplementation with selenium to correct blood-selenium deficiencies results in dramatic improvement in the herd reproductive status within 60 days. Selenium supplementation is best performed by adding the mineral to the ration at approved rates rather than administering selenium in slow-release boluses or by injection. Herds confirmed as selenium deficient should have periodic assessment of selenium status provided by analysis of blood samples from cows in various stages of lactation and from heifers. Practitioners in selenium-deficient areas that have identified selenium-deficient herds and observed response following dietary supplementation remain perplexed by the logic behind recent regulatory efforts that limit selenium supplementation to livestock. The supposition that dairy cattle in selenium-deficient areas somehow release excessive selenium into the environment seems unlikely to say the least.

Heat Stress

High ambient temperature and humidity can create heat stress in dairy cattle, especially when management deficiencies in ventilation or cooling exacerbate the problem. Cows experiencing heat stress may secrete higher levels of progesterone to a degree that interferes with the LH surge of estrus. Alteration in the steroidogenic function of ovarian tissue and the resultant negative implications for folliculogenesis are likely primary physiologic forces behind the diminished reproductive performance observed during periods of severe heat stress in dairy cattle. Anestrus and reduced evidence of estrus behavior may be observed. Thyroxine and triiodothyronine levels decrease to effect lower heat production to help the cow accommodate, but these same reductions lower feed intake. Reduced feed intake can contribute to decreased production and energy imbalances. The combined effects of high temperature and humidity result in heat stress. Conception rates plummet in cows under severe heat stress, and some farms discontinue breeding during periods of high temperature and humidity because of frustration with poor heat detection and poor conception. Heat stress has been associated with increased numbers of abnormal embryos and unfertilized ova. Conception failure, early embryonic death, and even abortion can be observed in herds suffering heat stress. Late gestation cows may calve early with resultant RFM and have metabolic problems that are amplified by decreased feed intake. Cows tend to be inactive, do not want to move about to feed bunks or demonstrate heat activity, and tend to congregate in areas of better ventilation or around water troughs. Severe heat stress will cause some cows to show open-mouth breathing and all cows to show tachypnea. Heat stroke is a possible sequela.

Management must anticipate the possibility of heat stress caused by weather extremes during warm months and ensure adequate ventilation by proper barn construction that includes escape of hot humid air through the roof, increased use of powerful fans, water misters, open or screened sides, and other measures to ameliorate cow comfort and performance during hot weather. Decreased dry-matter intake and electrolyte losses through panting, sweating, and salivation may contribute to a decrease in rumen pH. Supplemental buffers such as bicarbonate and additional potassium may aid appetite and increase rumen pH value. Cattle that have not fully shed out winter hair coats should be clipped to help avoid heat stress.

Cold Stress

Cold stress during periods of inclement weather is largely a problem for free stall-housed dairy cattle that must increase energy intake to maintain body heat. In this instance, thyroid hormones may increase to enhance dry-matter intake. However, regardless of exact pathophysiology, reproductive performance is diminished. Cows are reluctant to interact, tend to lose weight, may suffer production losses as more energy is directed toward body heat, and do not like to move about on icy floors and hard irregular surfaces created by frozen manure on floors. Roughened hair coats and losses in body condition are observed in many animals in cold-stressed herds. Heat detection and conception suffer. A more energy-dense ration may need to be formulated when herds suffer from cold stress-induced fertility problems, metabolic problems, or production losses.

Slippery Surfaces

Slippery surfaces may exist in free stall barns without grooved floors, frozen icy surfaces of free stalls during cold extremes, poorly cleaned free stalls, muddy areas, and frozen barn yards. Cattle that fall on slippery surfaces are reluctant to stand for or mount other cows and therefore show reduced estrus activity or shortened evidence of behavioral estrus.

Lameness and Other Stresses

One of the most common causes of sporadic infertility and an occasional cause of reduced herd fertility in dairy cattle is lameness. Lame cows do not want to stand, move about, or interact with other cows. The obvious consequences are less time spent eating, less movement to bunks, subsequent weight and production losses, and failure to show heat. Extreme lameness with weight loss causes a negative energy balance and can cause anestrus. Special consideration for lame cows must be made. Treatment must be the foremost consideration, and the cow should be placed in a well-bedded box stall with good footing. If this is not possible, the cow is likely to suffer other musculoskeletal injuries, be battered by herdmates, and develop secondary conditions in addition to having infertility. Lame cows in negative energy balance are unlikely to conceive, and breeding is best attempted after correction of the lameness and evidence of a positive energy balance. Even when lame cows are in estrus, they do not interact for fear of injury or pain and therefore are reluctant to stand to be mounted. Herd epidemics of lameness caused by laminitis, foot rot, hairy heel warts, or interdigital fibropapillomas can have a drastic effect on herd fertility for all of the previous reasons.

Nonspecific stress associated with infectious, metabolic, musculoskeletal, environmental, and nutritional conditions also can have a negative impact on fertility. It is impossible to quantify or scientifically explain "stress," but veterinarians recognize the importance of this poorly defined condition. Most explanations theorize that cortisol levels are increased. Studies wherein heifers were given exogenous ACTH during proestrus resulted in delayed LH surges, delayed onset of estrus, and shortened behavioral estrus. Progesterone and cortisol levels both may be elevated in cattle receiving ACTH. Progesterone alone may prevent estrus, or other hormonal interactions may contribute to the problem. In any event, estrus may be shortened or nonexistent, and fertility suffers. Recognition and treatment of conditions that cause cow stress are essential to restoration of fertility in affected cattle.

Semen Quality and Delivery

Many dairy farms own their own semen tanks to store commercial semen from a variety of bull stud services regardless of whether insemination is performed by professional representatives of AI studs or a farm employee. Errors in semen handling can have profound effects on conception rates and frequently are overlooked as a cause of reduced fertility. A well-maintained semen tank is critical to preservation of quality semen. Temperature must remain at $-196.0°$ C in liquid nitrogen tanks and even brief periods of exposure to ambient temperatures can be disastrous. Temperatures above $-130.0°$ C can lead to recrystallization that allows water molecules to leave ice crystals, attach to other crystals, and create some larger crystals that can damage cellular structures. Straws of semen are much more subject to damaging thermal variations than the older semen ampules because of volume differentials. Recrystallization damage may be cumulative. Tanks must be monitored closely, and a repeated need to add liquid nitrogen to a tank may signal a vacuum leak that eventually could cause severe problems. If vacuum is lost completely, all liquid nitrogen may be gone within 24 hours.

American Breeders Service has produced a monitoring device composed of ampules with color detectors that can signal inappropriate temperature increases in semen tanks. These devices are available from Minitube of America Inc. (Madison, WI).

Expertise of the inseminator is another concern—especially when a recently trained or neophyte farm employee assumes the role of inseminator. The uterine body is the best site for semen deposition, and personnel involved in insemination must be trained properly to deliver semen to this location. There is a great deal of variation in the skill of individual inseminators, and profound conception rate decreases associated with a new inseminator warrant investigation of technique. Veterinarians involved in herd reproductive programs often are placed in the middle of disputes when owners perceive inseminator errors. A more difficult situation, however, is created when the owner or a family member of the owner becomes inseminator following a 1- or 2-day short course. Criticism by the veterinarian may not be well accepted in these instances. Neophyte inseminators also can cause cervical or uterine injuries, abscesses, or perforations of the reproductive tract and even rectal lacerations. I have worked with many owners and farm personnel who generate exceptional conception rates over many years and have been fortunate to work with many talented professional inseminators. Unfortunately I also have worked on many farms where owners persist in performing inseminations on cattle despite a poor conception rate because of economic reasons or because of personal vendettas against professional inseminators.

In such instances, the result is economic loss because of repeat service and poor conception rates.

PREGNANCY DIAGNOSIS

Accurate and safe diagnosis of early pregnancy in dairy cattle is a required skill for bovine practitioners. Economics dictate that cows be checked for pregnancy as early as possible so that open cows not observed in heat following breeding be identified promptly. Practitioners must be confident and comfortable with whatever limit of detection is established for each herd. Most practitioners choose to diagnose pregnancy any time after 30 days, but some only feel confident at 40 days or more. Heifers and young cows can be diagnosed as early as 28 days in most instances, and previous recommendations to wait until 60 days of pregnancy no longer are tenable because of the potential for economic loss if cows are found open after this length of time.

Fears regarding palpation during early pregnancy (28 to 40 days) centered around embryonic losses associated with palpation. These concerns appear unfounded when skilled and experienced palpators perform the examinations. Furthermore, owners should be made aware of the fact that as many as 20% to 25% of pregnancies existing at 28 days suffer spontaneous embryonic or fetal death before 90 days gestation whether cows are palpated per rectum or not. Therefore although owners often blame veterinarians for "knocking a calf out of a cow" when a cow previously diagnosed pregnant returns to heat, this seldom is the case, assuming the examining veterinarian is well-trained and practiced in pregnancy diagnosis.

Five techniques are available to diagnose early pregnancies. The first is palpation of the uterus for fluctuation of fluids. The second is palpation of the amniotic vesicle, and the third consists of slipping the fetal membranes (chorioallantois). The fourth is rectal ultrasound examination. The fifth is hormonal assays for pregnancy, which are still in the developmental stage, but promise earlier pregnancy detection than other methods.

Slipping of fetal membranes is best performed between days 35 and 90. Membrane slip must be performed gently to avoid injury to the fetus or membranes. This technique is most helpful when differentiating pregnancy from other causes of uterine fluid accumulation, such as pyometra and mucometra. It also is helpful when diagnosing pregnancy in bull-bred herds or herds that do not practice prebreeding examinations that would tend to rule out previous uterine pathology. Slipping membranes may, in the hands of some examiners, result in increased fetal loss over those observed with other techniques.

Diagnosis of pregnancy by palpation of the amniotic vesicle can be used for pregnancy diagnosis as early as 30 days but must be performed very gently to avoid embryonic injury, which may result in fetal death or atresia coli. As with membrane slipping, palpation of the amniotic vesicle is most valuable when prebreeding examinations have not been performed to rule out pathologic fluid distention of the uterus.

The first technique, palpation of the uterus for fluid distention and fluctuation, is what I prefer. The pregnant horn develops "live" fluid distention that can be detected as early as 28 days postbreeding. The nongravid horn usually is not distended until approximately 40 days or more and thereafter varies greatly as to the degree of fluid distention and placentation present. Retraction of the uterus, as performed with all three techniques, is followed by a gentle palpation of each horn by allowing the horn to slide through the thumb and index or middle finger of the palpating hand. No pressure is directed against the fluid distention, and the membranes are not slipped. The area of the amniotic vesicle frequently is apparent but is not palpated specifically. This technique is most appropriate when cows being tested for pregnancy have had prebreeding examinations that have confirmed a normal uterus without pathologic fluid retention, pyometra, or mucometra.

Regardless of the technique used for early pregnancy diagnosis, the uterus must be retracted to facilitate examination of both uterine horns. In addition to assessment of the uterine horns, a tight, firm, and narrow cervix usually is associated with pregnancy, and a palpable corpus luteum usually is present in the ovary on the same side as the pregnant horn. The advantages of early pregnancy diagnosis before 40 days include more easy retraction and palpation of the uterus, diagnosis of obviously open cows that then allows treatment or intensified observation for next heat, economic gain in identifying open cows as early as possible, and detection of abnormal pregnancies.

The safety of early pregnancy diagnosis (28 to 42 days) was studied recently. Results indicated that a significantly low probability of fetal injury existed early in this period and that the risk increased slightly as the fetal age approximated 42 days. Thereafter, no association was made between palpation and abortion. It was theorized that manipulation during the period of placental attachment (complete at 45 days) may be involved, and it is also possible that variations in examiners' techniques for pregnancy diagnosis closer to 42 days may be involved. This study was of particular interest because my personal experience has been that cows around 40 to 42 days pregnant often have increased uterine tone and more tightly coiled uterine horns that may be slightly more difficult to uncoil and palpate. This increased tone is associated with physiologic increases in tone that occur in many cows at regular 21-day (or regular heat interval for that cow) intervals even during pregnancy.

Abnormal pregnancies are usually characterized by lesser amounts of fluid in the gravid horn than would be expected based on experience and normal variation for cows bred a specific number of days. When pregnancy determinations are made before 40 to 45 days, less fluid than normal usually equates to embryonic death that has not yet resulted in expulsion or absorption of the uterine contents. Any cow suspected to have an abnormal pregnancy based on decreased amounts of fluid in the gravid horn should be rechecked in 1 to 2 weeks unless she returns to heat before this. Some of these cows also will have decreased uterine tone or edematous-feeling gravid horns that further raise suspicion that embryonic death already has occurred. Because some biologic variation exists in the volume of fluid present at any specific day, however, discretion is called for, and a recheck in 1 to 2 weeks is a safer alternative than immediate PGF$_{2\alpha}$ treatment. Experimental induction of embryonic or fetal death has demonstrated that expulsion or resorption of dead embryos and fetal fluids, as well as return to estrus, can be delayed beyond the time of death.

It is not rare for pregnant cattle to demonstrate behavioral evidence of estrus at regular intervals. This is most common during the first half of pregnancy, but some cows show behavioral signs of heat at regular intervals throughout a normal pregnancy. Many cows have palpable increased uterine tone when palpated on days 21, 42, and 63 following breeding, despite having had a normal pregnancy; therefore some evidence of a tendency for cyclicity seems likely based only on clinical observations.

Cows diagnosed pregnant that subsequently develop purulent or bloody discharges or have behavioral signs of estrus should be rechecked by rectal palpation; they are excellent candidates for ancillary examination using ultrasound. Ultrasound examination for pregnancy is being routinely used by many bovine practitioners today, which enables diagnosis of pregnancy as early as 20 days and allows earlier detection of open cows in need of rebreeding. The technique has numerous applications for bovine reproduction and could be used in problem breeders, cattle suspected to have abnormal pregnancies, and cattle suspected to have uterine fluid accumulations that require differentiation from pregnancy. Utilization of ultrasound, uterine cultures, and uterine biopsies should be practiced more when individual valuable cattle have fertility problems. Ultrasound is also used in select circumstances for fetal sexing, typically around the eighth and ninth week of gestation. Determination of fetal sex may be of greater economic benefit to the beef rather than dairy industries, although clients may believe that pregnant, genetically superior dairy cattle may economically justify the expense of fetal sexing before contract sale of a calf. Semen sorting into sex-specific spermatozoa may also become a common service offered by the commercial AI industry in the near future, allowing clients to choose the likely sex of the fetus at the time of breeding.

An excellent discussion by Roberts regarding pregnancy diagnosis, variables, and normal fetal development is recommended for all veterinarians interested in bovine reproduction.

PREPUTIAL AND PENILE INJURY

Penile Hematoma

Most dairy practitioners now have little or no contact with dairy bulls, but a few practitioners may have a "bull raising" or bull study in their practice area and be asked to look at reproductive injuries to a bull. Although this is rare compared with incidences in beef bulls, both penile hematomas and preputial lacerations occur in dairy bulls. Penile hematoma may be seen in a dairy bull used for natural breeding as a "clean up" bull or young sire program. The clinical signs are a classical swelling just in front of the scrotum (Figure 9-17). The hematoma is dorsal to the penis and caused by a rupture of the tunica albuginea. Treatment could be either surgical repair for large (>15 cm) or recent (<3 days) hematomas or medical treatment, which would consist of hydrotherapy of the hematoma and once-daily injection of penicillin. Regardless of the treatment, there should be sexual rest for at least 2 months. Mild prolapses of the prepuce may occur with penile hematomas and should be prophylactically treated with moisturizing/antibiotic creams. The prognosis for recovery from penile hematomas is good.

Prolapse of Prepuce

Although rare in dairy bulls, prolapse of the prepuce may occur following injury to the prepuce. Medical treatment may be attempted with hydrotherapy, antibiotic creams, and preputial slings to decrease edema formation. If the lesions are severe and/or chronic, surgical repair (posthioplasty) would be the preferred treatment. If adhesions have developed and the penis cannot be extended, the prognosis is guarded to poor.

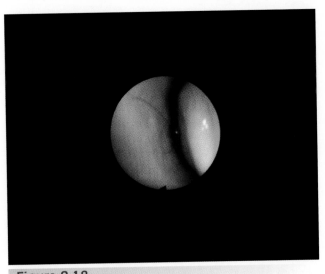

Figure 9-18

Hair ring seen around the penis during endoscopic examination.

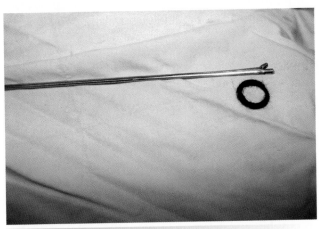

Figure 9-19

Hair ring after removal from the bull with uterine biopsy.

Hair Rings

Young bulls may occasionally rub hair onto the glands penis, and the accumulation of hair may form a ring around the penis, causing pain and inability to breed. A diagnosis can be made by observing the hair ring around the penis. An endoscope can be used to aid in the diagnosis (Figure 9-18). A uterine biopsy probe can be used to cut and remove the hair ring (Figure 9-19).

VESICULITIS/SEMINAL VESICULITIS/ VESICULAR ADENITIS

Etiology

Inflammation of the vesicular gland, referred to as vesiculitis, vesicular adenitis or seminal vesiculitis, in bulls will be discussed because the condition occasionally

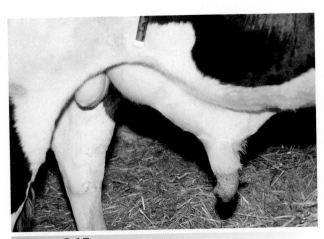

Figure 9-17

Penile hematoma (swelling just in front of the scrotum) in a 3-year-old Holstein.

results in systemic signs that can be confused with peritonitis of other origins. Independently its negative effect on semen quality makes it an economically important disease in the AI industry.

Individually housed bulls appear to be at lesser risk of seminal vesiculitis than group-housed bulls kept at bull stud services. Bulls of any age may develop the condition, and it is thought that the incidence of infection increases in young group-housed bulls because of repeated homosexual mounting activity that allows contamination of the penis and sheath with subsequent ascending infection. *A. pyogenes* has been the most common bacterial cause of seminal vesiculitis in the United States. Ascending, descending, and systemic infections have been identified as causes of *A. pyogenes* vesiculitis. *Brucella abortus* is a common cause of the disease when brucellosis is endemic and natural service is used. Other bacteria, such as *H. somni* and *Mycobacterium* sp., have been incriminated sporadically but are much less common than *A. pyogenes*.

Mycoplasma and *Ureaplasma* organisms currently are a common cause of vesiculitis in bulls. These organisms may be the sole isolate or compose a part of mixed infections that also include bacteria. *M. bovigenitalium* has been shown to cause vesiculitis experimentally and naturally. *M. bovis* also has been shown to be capable of causing vesiculitis when introduced experimentally. It is not known whether *M. bovigenitalium* seminal vesiculitis originates from ascending infection from the prepuce or from systemic spread of the organism.

U. diversum, as discussed in the section on vaginitis, may cause reproductive failure in cattle yet can be isolated from the caudal reproductive tract of cattle with normal reproductive function. The organism also may be isolated from the sheath of bulls and is thought to occasionally result in ascending infection and subsequent vesiculitis.

Clinical Signs and Diagnosis

Most bulls affected with vesiculitis have no outward signs of infection. In such latent cases, abnormalities in semen quality and reduced fertility constitute the only evidence of infection. Semen abnormalities range from gross findings of purulence, clots, increased viscosity, ropiness, lowered motility, decreased fructose content, and other abnormalities in bacterial infections to simple reduced motility in the case of *Mycoplasma* sp. or *U. diversum* infections.

Physical findings in latent infections may include palpable abnormalities of the vesicular glands during rectal examinations. The glands may be firm, swollen, and nodular in some instances or grossly abnormal with irregularity, abscesses, fibrosis, and adhesions when chronic *A. pyogenes* or mixed infections exist. Palpation cannot identify all cases, however, and the lesions may

be unilateral or bilateral. Ultrasonography may be a valuable adjunct to rectal palpation.

Severely affected bulls may show systemic signs that mimic peritonitis caused by hardware disease, perforating abomasal ulcers, and other conditions. Such bulls may have an arched stance, pain on defecation, urination, or rectal examination, and be reluctant to mount or thrust. Fever may or may not be present. Rectal examination of such bulls is likely to identify abnormal seminal vesicles.

Diagnosis requires a combination of physical examination, rectal findings, ultrasonography, semen evaluation, and culture of urethral fluid in such a manner as to avoid preputial contamination. Culturing of semen alone is not recommended because of possible contamination of the sample.

Treatment

Treatment is based on the severity and etiology. Mild cases in young bulls sometimes spontaneously resolve. Specific antibiotic therapy may be used for bacterial infections and consists of long-term (>2 weeks) treatment with appropriate systemic antibiotics. The therapy of *Mycoplasma* sp. and *U. diversum* infection is often empiric and consists of systemic tetracycline or macrolide-type antibiotics. Chronic infections with *A. pyogenes* may be treated with long-term penicillin (22,000 U/kg IM, twice daily) or penicillin and oral rifampin (2 to 5 mg/kg orally, twice weekly) for several weeks. Unfortunately in many chronic cases, medical therapy is unsuccessful, prompting consideration of surgical excision. Surgical removal of severely infected seminal vesicles has been historically performed through the ischiorectal fossa when conservative therapy has failed to resolve the problem and the affected bull is of significant economic value. An alternative technique described by Dr. Bruce Hull of an approach in the floor of the rectum allows the surgeon to better visualize the diseased gland.

Prognosis should remain guarded in all cases.

SUGGESTED READINGS

Abbitt B, Ball L, Kitto GP, et al: Effect of three methods of palpation for pregnancy diagnosis per rectum on embryonic and fetal attrition in cows, *J Am Vet Med Assoc* 173:973-977, 1978.

Abbitt B, Craig TM, Jones LP, et al: Protozoal abortion in a herd of cattle concurrently infectecl with *Hammondia-pardalis*, *J Am Vet Med Assoc* 203:444-448, 1993.

Allrich RD: Estrous behavior and detection in cattle, *Vet Clin North Am (Food Anim Pract)* 9:249-262, 1993.

Anderson ML, Blanchard PC, Barr BC, et al: *Neospora*-like protozoan infection as a major cause of abortion in California dairy cattle, *J Am Vet Med Assoc* 198:241-244, 1991.

Antony A, Williamson NB: Recent advances in understanding the epidemiology of Neospora caninum in cattle, *N Z Vet J* 49:42-47, 2001.

Ball HJ, McCaughey WJ: Distribution of mycoplasmas within the urogenital tract of the cow, *Vet Rec* 104:482-483, 1979.

Ball L, Dargatz DA, Cheney JM, et al: Control of venereal disease in infected herds, *Vet Clin North Am (Food Anim. Pract)* 3:561-574, 1987.

Barr BC, Anderson ML: Infectious diseases causing bovine abortion and fetal loss, *Vet Clin North Am (Food Anim Practice)* 9:343-388, 1993.

Barr BC, Conrad PA, Breitmeyer R, et al: Congenital *Neospora* infection in calves born from cows that had previously aborted *Neospora*-infected fetuses: four cases 1990–1992, *J Am Vet Med Assoc* 202:113-117, 1993.

Barth AD: Factors affecting fertility with artificial insemination, *Vet Clin North Am (Food Anim Pract)* 9:275-290, 1993.

BonDurant RH: Diagnosis, treatment, and control of bovine trichomoniasis, *Compend Contin Educ Pract Vet* 7:S179-S184, 1985.

Borchardt KA, Norman BB, Thomas MW, et al: Evaluation of a new culture method for diagnosing *Trichomonas foetus* infection, *Vet Med* February:104-112, 1992.

Bosu WTK, Peter AT: Evidence for a role of intrauterine infections in the pathogenesis of cystic ovaries in postpartum dairy cows, *Theriogenology* 28:725-736, 1987.

Bretzlaff KN: Rationale for treatment of endometritis in the dairy cow, *Vet Clin North Am (Food Anim Pract)* 3:593-607, 1987.

Bretzlaff KN, Ott RS, Kortiz GD, et al: Distribution of oxytetracycline in genital tract tissues of postpartum cows given the drug by intravenous and intrauterine routes, *Am J Vet Res* 44:764-769, 1983.

Brown MP, Colahan PT, Hawkins DM: Urethral extension for treatment of urine pooling in mares, *J Am Vet Med Assoc* 173:1005-1007, 1978.

Butler WR, Smith RD: Interrelationships between energy balance and postpartum reproductive function in dairy cattle, *J Dairy Sci* 72:767-783, 1989.

Callahan CJ, Horstman LA: Treatment of postpartum metritis in dairy cows caused by *Actinomyces pyogenes*, *Bov Pract* 27:162-165, 1993.

Chenault JR, McAllister JF, Chester ST Jr, et al: Efficacy of ceftiofur hydrochloride sterile suspension administered parenterally for the treatment of acute postpartum metritis in dairy cows, *J Am Vet Med Assoc* 224:1634-1639, 2004.

Curtis CR, Erb HN, Sniffen CJ, et al: Path analysis of dry period nutrition, postpartum metabolic and reproductive disorders, and mastitis in Holstein cows, *J Dairy Sci* 68:2347-2360, 1985.

Datgatz DA, Mortimer RG, Cheney JM: Bovine trichomoniasis, *Bov Clin* Fall:3-5, 1985.

Day N: The diagnosis, differentiation, and pathogenesis of cystic ovarian disease, *Vet Med* July:753-760, 1991.

Day N: The treatment and prevention of cystic ovarian disease, *Vet Med* July:761-766, 1991.

Dinsmore RP, White ME, English PB: An evaluation of simultaneous GnRH and cloprostenol treatment of dairy cattle with cystic ovaries, *Can Vet J* 31:280-284, 1990.

Dinsmore RP, et al: Oxytetracycline residues in milk intrauterine infusion of dairy cows, *Bov Proc* 26:186-187, 1994.

Doig PA, Ruhnke HL, Palmer NC: Experimental bovine genital ureaplasmosis: I. granular vulvitis following vulvar inoculation, *Can J Comp Med* 44:252-258, 1980.

Doig PA, Ruhnke HL, Palmer NC: Experimental bovine genital ureaplasmosis: II. granular vulvitis, endometritis, and salpingitis following uterine inoculation, *Can J Comp Med* 44:259-266, 1980.

Dubey JP, Lindsay DS, Anderson ML, et al: Induced transplacental transmission of *Neospora caninum* in cattle, *J Am Vet Med Assoc* 201:709-713, 1992.

Elad D, Friedgut O, Alpert N, et al: Bovine necrotic vulvovaginitis associated with Porphyromonas levii, *Emerg Infect Dis* 10:505-507, 2004.

Ellington JE, Schlafer DH: Uterine tube disease it cattle, *J Am Vet Med Assoc* 202:450-454, 1993.

Elliott L, McMahon KJ, Gier HT, et al: Uterus of the cow after parturition: bacterial content, *Am J Vet Res* 29:77-81, 1968.

Elmore RG: Focus on bovine reproductive disorders: managing cases of placental hydrops, *Vet Med* January:73-77, 1992.

Erb HN: High milk production as a cause of cystic ovaries in dairy cows: evidence to the contrary, *Compend Contin Educ Pract Vet* 6:S215-S216, 1984.

Erb HN, Martin SW, Ison N, et al: Interrelationships between production and reproductive diseases in Holstein cows. Path analysis, *J Dairy Sci* 64:282-289, 1981.

Erb RE, Hinze PE, Gildow EM, et al: Retained fetal membranes: the effect of prolificacy of dairy cattle, *J Am Vet Med Assoc* 133:489, 1958.

Farin PW, Estill CT: Infertility due to abnormalities of the ovaries in cattle, *Vet Clin North Am (Food Anim Pract)* 9:291-308, 1993.

Farin PW, Youngquist RS, Parfet JR, et al: Diagnosis of luteal and follicular ovarian cysts by palpation per rectum and linear-array ultrasonography in dairy cows, *J Am Vet Med Assoc* 200:1085-1089, 1992.

Farin PW, Youngquist RS, Parfet JR, et al: Diagnosis of luteal and follicular ovarian cysts in dairy cows by sector scan ultrasonography, *Theriogenology* 34:633-642, 1990.

Ferguson J: The effects of protein level and type on reproduction in the dairy cow. In *Proceedings: Annual Meeting Society of Theriogenologists*, 1986, pp. 164-185.

Fortune JE, Quirk SM: Regulation of steroidogenesis in bovine preovulatory follicles, *J Anim Sci* 66:1-4, 1988.

Frazer GS: A rational basis for therapy in the sick postpartum cow, *Vet Clin North Am (Food Anim Pract)* 21:523-568, 2005.

Garverick HA, Smith MF: Female reproductive physiology and endocrinology of cattle, *Vet Clin North Am (Food Anim Pract)* 9:223-247, 1993.

Gearhart MA, Curtis CR, Erb HN, et al: Relationship of changes in condition score to cow health in Holsteins, *J Dairy Sci* 73:3132-3140, 1990.

Gilbert RO, Grohn YT, Guard CL, et al: Impaired post partum neutrophil function in cows which retain fetal membranes, *Res Vet Sci* 55:15-19, 1993.

Gilbert RO, Oettle EE: An outbreak of granulomatous vulvitis in feedlot heifers, *J S Afr Vet Assoc* 61:41-43, 1990.

Gilbert RO, Shin ST, Guard CL, et al: Prevalence of endometritis and its effects on reproductive performance of dairy cows, *Theriogenology* 64:1879-1888, 2005.

Gilbert RO, Schwark WS: Pharmacologic considerations in the management of peripartum conditions in the cow, *Vet Clin North Am (Food Anim Pract)* 8:29-56, 1992.

Gilbert RO, Wilson DG, Levine SA, et al: Surgical management of urovagina and associated infertility in a cow, *J Am Vet Med Assoc* 194:931-932, 1989.

Ginther OJ, Kastelic JP, Knopf L: Composition and characteristics of follicular waves during the bovine estrous cycle, *Anim Reprod Sci* 20:187-200, 1989.

Gröhn YT, Erb HN, McCulloch CE, et al: Epidemiology of reproductive disorders in dairy cattle associations among host characteristics disease and production, *Prev Vet Med* 8:25-40, 1990.

Grooms DL: Reproductive consequences of infection with bovine viral diarrhea virus, *Vet Clin North Am Food Anim Pract* 20:5-19, 2004.

Guitian J, Thurmond MC, Hietala SK: Infertility and abortion among first-lactation dairy cows seropositive or seronegative for Leptospira interrogans serovar hardjo, *J Am Vet Med Assoc* 215:515-518, 1999.

Gustafsson BK: Therapeutic strategies involving antimicrobial treatment of the uterus in large animals, *J Am Vet Med Assoc* 185:1194-1198, 1984.

Habel RE: Prevention of vaginal prolapse in the cow, *J Am Vet Med Assoc* 130:344, 1957.

Haddad JP, Dohoo IR, Van Leewen JA: A review of Neopsora caninum in dairy and beef cattle—a Canadian perspective, *Can Vet J* 46:2302-2343, 2005.

Hall CA, Reichel MP, Ellis JT: Neospora abortions in dairy cattle: diagnosis, mode of transmission and control, *Vet Parasitol* 128:231-241, 2005.

Hammon DS, Evjen IM, Dhiman TR, et al: Neutrophil function and energy status in Holstein cows with uterine health disorders, *Vet Immunol Immunopathol* 15(113):21-29, 2006.

Hjerpe CA: Bovine vaccines and herd vaccination programs, *Vet Clin North Am Food Anim Pract* 6:171-260, 1990.

Hoeben D, Mijten P, de Kruif A: Factors influencing complications during caesarean section on the standing cow, *Vet Q* 19:88-92, 1997.

Jubb KVF, Kennedy PC, Palmer N: *Pathology of domestic animals,* ed 4, vol 2, New York, 1993, Academic Press, Inc.

Kassam A, BonDurant RH, Basu S, et al: Clinical and endocrine responses to embryonic and fetal death induced by manual rupture of the amniotic vesicle during early pregnancy in cows, *J Am Vet Med Assoc* 191:417-420, 1987.

Kastelic JP: Understanding ovarian follicular development in cattle, *Vet Med* January:61-71, 1994.

Kastelic JP, Knopf L, Ginther OJ: Effect of day of prostaglandin f-2-alpha treatment on selection and development of the ovulatory follicle in heifers, *Anim Reprod Sci* 23:169-180, 1990.

Kennedy PC: Epizootic bovine abortion. In Kirkbride CA, editor: *Laboratory diagnosis of livestock abortion,* ed 3, Ames, IA, 1990, Iowa State University Press.

Kesler DJ, Garverick HA: Ovarian cysts in dairy cattle: a review, *J Anim Sci* 55:1147-1159, 1982.

Kimura K, Goff JP, Kehrli ME Jr, et al: Decreased neutrophil function as a cause of retained placenta in dairy cattle, *J Dairy Sci* 85:544-550, 2002.

King GJ, Hurnik JF, Robertson HA: Ovarian function and estrus in dairy cows during early lactation, *J Anim Sci* 42:688-692, 1976.

Kirkbride CA: *Mycoplasma, ureaplasma* and *Acholeplas* infections of bovine genitalia, *Vet Clin North Am (Food Anim Pract)* 3:575-591, 1987.

Klavano GG: Observations of *Haemophilus somnus* infection as an agent producing reproductive diseases: infertility and abortion. In *Proceedings: Annual Meeting Society of Theriogenologists,* 1980, pp. 139-149.

Konigsson K, Gustafsson H, Gunnarsson A, et al: Clinical and bacteriological aspects on the use of oxytetracycline and flunixin in primiparous cows with induced retained placenta and postpartal endometritis, *Reprod Domest Anim* 36:247-256, 2001.

LaFaunce NA, McEntee K: Experimental *Mycoplasma bovis* seminal vesiculitis in the bull, *Cornell Vet* 72:150-167, 1982

LeBlanc SJ, Duffield TF, Leslie KE, et al: The effect of treatment of clinical endometritis on reproductive performance in dairy cows. *J Dairy Sci* 85:2237-2249, 2002.

Lee CN, Maurice E, Ax RL, et al: Efficacy of gonadotropin-releasing hormone administered at the time of artificial insemination of heifers and postpartum and repeat breeder dairy cows, *Am J Vet Res* 44:2160-2166, 1983.

Lein DH: The current role of ureaplasma, mycoplasma, and *Haemophilus somnus* in bovine reproductive disorders. In *Proceedings: 11th Technical Conference on Artificial Insemination and Reproduction,* 1986, pp. 27-32.

Lindell JO, Kindahl H, Jansson L, et al: Postpartum release of prostaglandin$_2$ and uterine involution in the cow, *Theriogenology* 17:237-245, 1982.

Lucy MC: Reproductive loss in high-producing dairy cattle: where will it end? *J Dairy Sci.*84:1277-1293, 2001.

Magdub A, Johnson HD, Belyea RL: Effect of environmental heat and dietary fiber on thyroid physiology of lactating cows, *J Dairy Sci* 65:2323-2331, 1982.

Miller HV, et al: Endometritis of dairy cattle: diagnosis, treatment and fertility, *Bov Pract* 15:13-23, 1989.

Miller RB, Lein DH, McEntee KE, et al: *Haemophilus somnus* infection of the reproductive tract of cattle: a review, *J Am Vet Med Assoc* 182:1390-1391, 1983.

Morrow DA: *Current therapy in theriogenology,* ed 2, Philadelphia, 1986, WB Saunders.

Murray RD, Allison JD, Gard RP: Bovine endometritis: comparative efficacy of alfaprostol and intrauterine therapies, and other factors influencing clinical success, *Vet Rec* 127:86-90, 1990.

Newman KD, Anderson DE: Ceasarean section in cows, *Vet Clin North Am Food Anim Pract* 21:73-100, 2005.

Olson JD, Ball L, Mortimer RG: Therapy of postpartum uterine infections, *Bov Proc*17:85-88, 1985.

Palmer CC: Clinical studies on retained placenta in the cow, *J Am Vet Med Assoc* 80:59-68, 1932.

Parish SM, Maag-Miller, Besser TE, et al: Myelitis associated with protozoal infection in newborn calves, *J Am Vet Med Assoc* 191:1599-1600, 1987.

Parsonson LM, Hall CE, Settergren I: A method for the collection of bovine seminal vesicle secretions for microbiologic examination, *J Am Vet Med Assoc* 158:175-177, 1971.

Peter AT, Bosu WTK: Relationship of uterine infections and folliculogenesis in dairy cows during early puerperium, *Theriogenology* 30:1045-1052, 1988.

Pursley JR, Mee MO, Wiltbank MC: Synchronization of ovulation in dairy cows using PGF2 and GnRH, *Theriogenology* 44:915-923, 1995.

Randel RD: Nutrition and postpartum rebreeding in cattle, *J Anim Sci* 68:853-862, 1990.

Refsal KR, Jarrin-Maldonado JH, Nachreiner RF: Endocrine profiles in cows with ovarian cysts experimentally induced by treatment with exogenous estradiol or adrenocorticotropic hormone, *Theriogenology* 28:871-889, 1987.

Rhoads ML, Rhoads RP, Gilbert RO, et al: Detrimental effects of high plasma urea nitrogen levels on viability of embryos from lactating dairy cows, *Anim Reprod Sci* 91:1-10 2006.

Risco CA, Donovan GA, Hernandez J: Clinical mastitis associated with abortion in dairy cows, *J Dairy Sci* 82:1684-1689, 1999.

Risco CA, Hernandez J: Comparison of ceftiofur hydrochloride and estradiol cypionate for metritis prevention and reproductive performance in dairy cows affected with retained fetal membranes, *Theriogenology* 60:47-58, 2003.

Risco CA, Reynolds JP: Uterine prolapse in dairy cattle, *Compend Contin Educ Pract Vet* 10:1135-1143, 1988.

Roberts SJ: *Veterinary obstetrics and genital diseases (theriogenology),* ed 3, Woodstock, VT, 1986, published by the author.

Ruegg PL, Marteniuk JV, Kaneene JB: Reproductive difficulties in cattle with antibody titers to *Haemophilus-somnus, J Am Vet Med Assoc* 193:941-942, 1988.

St. Jean G, Hull BL, Robertson JT, et al: Urethral extension for correction of urovagina in cattle: a review of 14 cases, *Vet Surg* 17:258-262, 1988.

Saint-Jean G, Rings DM, Hoffsis GF, et al: Adenocarcinoma of the uterus with pulmonary metastasis in two cows, *Compend Contin Educ Pract Vet* 10:864-867, 1988.

Samuelson JD, Winter AJ: Bovine vibriosis: the nature of the carrier state in the bull, *J Infect Dis* 16:581-592, 1966.

Schonfelder A, Sobiraj A: Etiology of torsio uteri in bovines: a review [article in German], *Schweiz Arch Tierheilkd* 147:397-402, 2005.

Scott HM, Schouten MJ, Gaiser JC, et al: Effect of intrauterine administration of ceftiofur on fertility and risk of culling in postparturient cows with retained fetal membranes, twins, or both, *J Am Vet Med Assoc* 226:2044-2052, 2005.

Sheldon IM, Bushnell M, Montgomery J, et al: Minimum inhibitory concentrations of some antimicrobial drugs against bacteria causing uterine infections in cattle, *Vet Rec* 155:383-387, 2004.

Sheldon IM, Lewis GS, LeBlanc S, et al: Defining postpartum uterine disease in cattle, *Theriogenology* 65:1516-1530, 2006.

Sirois J, Fortune JE: Ovarian follicular dynamics during the estrous cycle in heifers monitored by real-time ultrasonography, *Biol Reprod* 39:308-317, 1988.

Sprecher DJ, Nebel RJ, Whittier WD: Predictive value of palpation per rectum vs milk and serum progesterone levels for the diagnosis of bovine follicular and luteal cysts, *Theriogenology* 30:701-710, 1988.

Sprecher DJ, Strelow LW, Nebel RL: The response of cows with cystic ovarian degeneration to luteotropic or luteolytic therapy as assigned by latex agglutination milk progesterone assay, *Theriogenology* 34:1149-1158, 1990.

Stoebel DP, Moberg GP: Effect of adrenocorticotropin and cortisol on luteinizing hormone surge and estrous behavior of cows, *J Dairy Sci* 65:1016-1024, 1982.

Théon AP, Pascoe JR, Carlson GP, et al: Intratumoral chemotherapy with cisplatin in oily emulsion in horses, *J Am Vet Med Assoc* 202:261-267, 1993.

Thurmond MC, Picanso JP: Fetal loss associated with palpation per rectum to diagnose pregnancy in cows, *J Am Vet Med Assoc* 203:432-435, 1993.

Trimberger GW: Breeding efficiency in dairy cattle from artificial insemination at various intervals before and after ovulation, *Nebraska Agricultural Experimental Station Research Bulletin* 153, 1948.

Vaillancourt D, Bierschwal CJ, Ogwu D, et al: Correlation between pregnancy diagnosis by membrane slip and embryonic mortality, *J Am Vet Med Assoc* 175:466-468, 1979.

Villa-Godoy A, Hughes TL, Emery RS, et al: Association between energy balance and luteal function in lactating dairy cows, *J Dairy Sci* 71:1063-1072, 1988.

Weaver LD: Effects of nutrition on reproduction in dairy cows, *Vet Clin North Am Food Anim Pract* 3:513-532, 1987.

Wehrend A, Reinle T, Herfen K, et al: Fetotomy in cattle with special reference to postoperative complications—an evaluation of 131 cases [article in German], *Dtsch Tierarztl Wochenschr* 109:56-61, 2002.

Weiss B, Hogan J, Smith L: Vitamin E and selenium: key nutrients for health, *Hoard's Dairyman* April 10:288-289, 1994.

West JW, Mullinix BG, Sandifer TG: Changing dietary electrolyte balance for dairy cows in cool and hot environments, *J Dairy Sci* 74:1662-1674, 1991.

White ME, Erb H: Treatment of ovarian cysts in dairy cattle—a decision analysis, *Cornell Vet* 70:247-257, 1980.

Wiltbank MC, Gumen A, Sartori R: Physiological classification of anovulatory conditions in cattle, *Theriogenology* 57:21-52, 2002.

Wolfe DF, Baird AN: Female urogenital surgery in cattle, *Vet Clin North Am (Food Anim Pract)* 9:369-388, 1993.

Younquist RS, Braun WF Jr: Abnormalities of the tubular genital organs, *Vet Clin North Am (Food Anim Pract)* 9:309-322, 1993.

CHAPTER 10

Urinary Tract Diseases

Thomas J. Divers

ABNORMAL URINARY CONSTITUENTS AND CONDITIONS

Urinary tract diseases are less common in dairy cattle than disorders of the gastrointestinal, respiratory, musculoskeletal, and other systems. For this reason and because signs of renal disease may be subtle, the urinary tract often is overlooked as a cause of illness. Evaluation of urine for abnormal constituents, urinalysis, and serum chemistry may be necessary to confirm urinary tract disease. Additionally, ultrasound examination of the kidneys and/or cystoscopic examination may be warranted in some cases. Percutaneous examination of both kidneys can be achieved easily in adult dairy cows and calves through the paralumbar fossae with a 2.5- to 5-mHz probe, and excellent images of the left kidney, ureter, and bladder can often be obtained during rectal examination using a conventional 5- or 10-mHz reproductive probe. Geographic differences in the incidence of diseases also may affect the relative frequency of urinary tract disease in cattle. Most practitioners utilize the gross appearance of urine, evaluation of abnormal urine constituents based on multiple reagent test strips, and signs found on physical examination as indicators of urinary tract disease. Vague illnesses that originate from the urinary system may require more ancillary data in the form of complete urinalysis, serum electrolytes and chemistry, and complete blood counts (CBCs) for diagnosis. Fortunately urine is obtained routinely during completion of physical examination for evaluation of urinary ketones, and this provides a sample for other routine screening processes when indicated. Abnormal urinary constituents identified by multiple reagent strips seldom are specific but give direction as to other ancillary tests to be performed. The following discussion of abnormal urinary constituents will give examples of diseases to be considered in a differential diagnosis. Although midstream samples are usually sufficient for cultures, on rare occasion it may be necessary to collect a catheterized sample. Catheterization is difficult in the cow because of the urethral diverticulum, and the technique is shown in Figure 10-1.

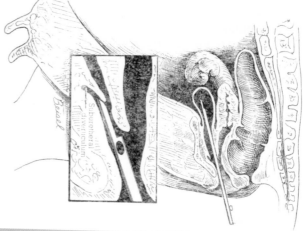

Figure 10-1

Drawing of the urinary system of the cow and proper urinary catheterization technique. The urethral diverticulum makes catheterization difficult.

Proteinuria

Because positive values for proteinuria obtained using multiple reagent test strips are relative rather than absolute, a urinalysis including sulfosalicylic acid test (SSA) or urine protein/creatinine ratio evaluation of protein is indicated before attributing much significance to these levels. For example, highly alkaline urine in ruminants may cause a false-positive protein reaction on reagent test strips (tetrabromphenol blue). An even more specific test would be to perform simultaneous protein and creatinine measurements and to calculate the urinary protein/creatinine ratio.

Proteinuria may be normal in ruminants less than 2 days of age that have ingested adequate or large amounts of colostrum. This physiologic phenomenon should correct quickly after this time, and the urine should then be negative for protein. Any insult to the renal glomeruli or tubules could lead to mild or moderate proteinuria. For example, renal infarcts secondary to severe dehydration and reduced renal perfusion could cause mild proteinuria, whereas glomerulonephritis, tubular nephrosis, amyloidosis, pyelonephritis, and other severe renal diseases would lead to more significant proteinuria with eventual hypoalbuminemia. Nonspecific inflammation or irritation of the postrenal urinary tract as found in cystitis, urolithiasis, trauma, or neoplasia also may result in proteinuria. Finally, false-positive proteinuria may occur from admixture of urine with vaginal discharges, preputial discharges, uterine discharges, or fecal material and is therefore particularly common in free-catch samples obtained from normal, healthy postparturient cattle.

Glycosuria

In cattle, exogenous sources of glucose such as intravenous (IV) glucose solutions, exogenous cortisone, and stress-induced glycosuria account for most positive reactions on multiple reagent test strips. False-positive reactions also may result from other reducing agents present in the urine, such as penicillin, tetracycline, some other antibiotics, and aspirin. Therefore, except for use in monitoring parenteral nutrition, this constituent seldom is helpful in dairy cattle.

Ketonuria

Ketone segments contained in multiple test reagent strips (Multistix, Bayer, Elkhart, Ind.) are specific for diacetic (acetoacetic) acid and do not react with acetone in urine. The urine strip test is approximately 90% sensitive and 75% to 85% specific for ketosis when the lower detection level of 5 μmol/L is used as a positive test. A Ketostix (Bayer, Elkhart, Ind.) that measures acetone and acetoacetate has a high sensitivity and specificity for diagnosing ketosis if interpreted within 5 to 10 seconds. A complete physical examination, anamnesis, and additional chemistry testing may be required to separate secondary from primary ketosis.

Hematuria

Gross hematuria is apparent by inspection, whereas occult or microscopic hematuria is detected by a positive reaction on the orthotoluidine test strip of multiple reagent test strips. This orthotoluidine reagent cannot differentiate among hematuria, hemoglobinuria, or myoglobinuria, and all three must be considered unless urine color, precipitation of red blood cells (RBCs), or complete urinalysis indicates the exact component.

Microscopic hematuria could originate in the kidney (e.g., infarct, tubular nephrosis, pyelonephritis, or other causes), ureter (e.g., calculi, tumor, or pyelonephritis), bladder (e.g., cystitis, calculi), urethra, or falsely through blood contamination of urine in the vagina. Gross hematuria usually is associated with pyelonephritis, urinary calculi, urolithiasis, or cystitis in dairy cattle.

Cattle affected with malignant catarrhal fever (MCF) often have hematuria caused by renal vasculitis or hemorrhage from the bladder due to hemorrhagic cystitis.

Hemoglobinuria

Gross hemoglobinuria may be apparent as reddish urine when marked intravascular hemolysis has occurred and subsequently exceeded the renal threshold for hemoglobin. Such conditions as water intoxication in calves, hypotonic IV fluids, onion and rye grass toxicity, bacillary hemoglobinuria caused by *Clostridium hemolyticum*, leptospirosis in calves, babesiosis, and postparturient hemoglobinuria may cause obvious hemoglobinuria during acute hemolysis. Early or late stages of these diseases may only yield occult or microscopic hemoglobinuria causing a positive reaction on the blood (orthotoluidine) component of multiple strips. Many plant and heavy metal toxicities also cause hemoglobinuria.

Myoglobinuria

Gross evidence of myoglobinuria in the form of brown or brownish-red urine may be apparent in severe myopathies such as exertional myopathy in downer cows, coffee weed poisoning, and diffuse nutritional myopathy involving the heavy muscle groups in vitamin E/selenium deficiency (white muscle disease). Frequently, however, occult myoglobinuria is detected in such cases as a positive reaction in the orthotoluidine component in multiple reagent test strips and positive protein reaction.

Bilirubin and Urobilinogen

Urinary bilirubin may be increased in a rare case of obstructive jaundice in cattle such as biliary stones, abscess, or neoplasia. Urobilinogen evaluation has not been of any diagnostic value in cattle.

Specific Gravity

Assessment of urine specific gravity is an essential test when renal pathology is suspected or if serum chemistry confirms azotemia. Isosthenuria may be indicated by specific gravity values between 1.006 and 1.014 in cattle that are dehydrated because normal renal function concentrates urine in a dehydrated patient. Unilateral renal ischemia usually will not result in isosthenuric specific gravity of urine. With acute renal failure the specific gravity will not always be in the isosthenuric range, but the specific gravity is no higher than 1.022, even in the face of dehydration.

White Blood Cells

Microscopic evidence of white blood cells (WBCs) merely provides evidence of urinary tract inflammation or degeneration. The most common causes include renal inflammation or degeneration, ureteral infection or obstruction, and cystitis. Contamination of free-catch samples by normal lochia or abnormal uterine/vaginal discharges is common in postpartum cows. The finding of 1 to 5 WBCs per high power field should be considered normal in urine samples obtained from cattle. Tubular degeneration caused by nephrosis or nephritis must be differentiated from lower urinary tract infection or inflammation. Gross pyuria is observed most commonly in pyelonephritis or cystitis in cattle. Urine samples demonstrated to have gross or microscopic pyuria should be submitted for bacterial culture; ideally such samples should be obtained following aseptic preparation and bladder catheterization.

Casts

Hyaline casts usually are composed of protein and are most common in severe nephrosis. Granular casts usually originate from damaged tubular epithelium.

RENAL DISEASES

Embolic Nephritis

This condition occurs in septicemic calves and cows or occasionally in endocarditis patients with left-sided valvular disease (Figure 10-2). Fever, other signs of septicemia, and specific organ dysfunction (e.g., mastitis, joint infections) also may be present. Urine multiple reagent test strips may be positive for blood and protein, whereas microscopic examination of the urine will reveal increased numbers of WBCs, RBCs, and bacteria in some cases. Nephritis is seldom the most significant component of disease in these animals but is another sign of septicemia. Therapy must be directed against the primary disease.

Renal Ischemia

A common but often undetected problem, renal ischemia results from decreased renal perfusion with subsequent reduced glomerular filtration in dehydrated patients. Renal failure is more common when both sepsis and dehydration are concurrent. Another possible cause of ischemic renal failure is severe ruminal distention. Cattle with severe dehydration resulting from gastrointestinal obstruction or diarrhea frequently develop renal infarcts that result in some RBCs, WBCs, and protein in the urine.

Finding these abnormal constituents in urine from dehydrated patients should arouse suspicion of renal failure and alert the clinician to the need for rehydration and avoidance of nephrotoxic drugs. If renal failure is present, urine concentration is <1.022; therefore evaluation of specific gravity is imperative to rule out renal failure. This is especially true when serum chemistry indicates azotemia in dehydrated patients. Further laboratory tests that help distinguish between

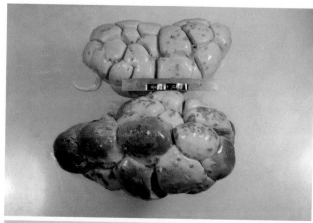
Figure 10-2

Kidneys of a 5-year-old Holstein that died from septic metritis. Numerous large infarcts can be seen.

prerenal and true renal azotemia should be utilized including fractional excretion of electrolytes, particularly sodium. There is considerable variation in urinary fractional excretion of sodium in normal dairy cattle according to diet, stage of lactation, and gestational status, but values for pregnant and periparturient dairy cattle rarely exceed 1%, whereas normal cows in early and peak lactation may occasionally reach 2% to 3%. Neonatal calves typically have urinary fractional sodium excretion values of <1%. Prerenal azotemia is properly diagnosed only when a dehydrated, azotemic cow possesses the ability to concentrate urine. As in other species, renal prostaglandin levels are cytoprotective to the kidney during reduced perfusion. Therefore prostaglandin inhibitors such as nonsteroidal antiinflammatory drugs (NSAIDs) should be used in reduced dosages or not at all in severely dehydrated cattle, lest further ischemic damage with increased infarction or papillary necrosis occurs. If sepsis is present, the benefits of the NSAID would likely outweigh the negative effects on the kidneys, such as might be the case in individuals with severe gram-negative mastitis or severe metritis.

Treatment should be directed toward the primary disease and the patient rehydrated with IV fluids to improve renal perfusion, urine production, and to correct existing prerenal azotemia. Nephrotoxic drugs such as aminoglycosides, oxytetracycline, and NSAIDs should be avoided if possible. If potentially nephrotoxic drugs must be used, repeated serum creatinine values, serial urinalyses, and fractional excretion ratios should be considered to monitor renal function.

Toxic Nephrosis

Damage to the renal tubules by toxins, certain drugs, and physiologic events linked to hemoconcentration, endotoxemia, and ischemic changes may cause tubular degeneration, inflammation, and in some instances interstitial nephritis. Usually both kidneys are affected equally.

Etiology

Antibiotics such as aminoglycosides, tetracycline, and sulfa drugs are known to be nephrotoxic. Neomycin, gentamicin, amikacin, and other aminoglycosides can cause renal tubular damage in cattle and other species. Tetracycline, and perhaps the vehicles used in certain injectable forms of tetracycline, may contribute to renal tubular nephrosis. Propylene glycol and polyvinylpyrrolidone vehicles are used in many oxytetracycline hydrochloride preparations, and these vehicles may cause hemodynamically mediated reduced renal perfusion, thereby accentuating any basic nephrotoxicity of the antibiotic itself. Sulfa preparations possess the ability to damage kidney tubules and precipitate in the renal tubules. Most antibiotic nephrotoxicity occurs as a result of two factors that deserve emphasis:

1. Overdosage
2. Proper dosage but administered to calves or cattle that are dehydrated, hypovolemic, and have reduced renal perfusion, thereby increasing the potential for renal damage

Overuse of calcium salts has also, on rare occasions, caused renal tubular nephrosis. In some instances, recumbent cattle received inordinate amounts of calcium solutions as therapy for suspected hypocalcemia.

Nephrosis also may result from physiologic progression of minor renal ischemia associated with septic conditions, gastrointestinal diseases, and other problems that reduce renal perfusion and glomerular filtration rate (GFR). Early manifestations of renal ischemia include renal infarcts and papillary necrosis. These conditions are much more common in dehydrated cattle than most veterinarians realize but are relatively benign if the cow's primary disease and dehydration status are treated. When severe renal ischemia occurs, widespread reduction in renal perfusion results in further organic necrosis of tubulointerstitial renal tissue. Acute renal failure is possible in this instance and would be indicated by azotemia and isosthenuria, despite severe dehydration in the patient.

Reduced renal perfusion also is a possible result of overuse of NSAIDs in cattle. Drugs such as phenylbutazone and flunixin meglumine are potent inhibitors of prostaglandin synthesis within many tissues, including the kidney. Renal prostaglandins are "cytoprotective" because they help maintain renal perfusion through small vessels during times of hypotension or dehydration. Loss of this protective effect occurs when NSAIDs have reduced the production of renal prostaglandins. Therefore the kidneys are more susceptible to ischemic damage. Although renal papillary necrosis frequently is associated with the use of NSAIDs, minor (infarction)

or major (tubular nephrosis) renal organic disease also may occur. Once again, the use of NSAIDs in dehydrated patients increases the risk of nephrotoxicity. The risk of toxicity can be further exacerbated by hypoalbuminemia such as occurs with acute gastrointestinal diseases because more of the NSAID being administered will be non–protein bound and therefore pharmacologically active drug. Therefore reduction of the dosage or total avoidance of these drugs, unless concomitant fluid therapy restores renal perfusion, should be practiced when devising therapy for a dehydrated patient.

Other nephrotoxins include the heavy metals (i.e., lead, mercury, and arsenic) and plant toxicities, such as oxalates, oak, and pigweed, that occur in some parts of the United States. Toxicities may involve several animals within a group, thus raising an index of suspicion regarding a toxic etiology. Oak poisoning most commonly affects heifers at pasture, with acorns being ingested in the fall and oak buds in the spring.

Clinical Signs

Cattle affected with toxic nephrosis usually have nonspecific signs, including depression, anorexia that varies from mild to absolute, dehydration, and potentially recumbency. Cattle with drug-related nephropathies usually have more blatant lesions in other body systems, such as septic mastitis, septic metritis, abomasal disorders, diarrhea, pneumonia, and so forth. Therefore coexisting or primary diseases may mask the existence of nephrosis. Polyuria may be present in some, but certainly not all, calves and cattle with nephrosis. When present, this sign is helpful because an obviously dehydrated animal is observed to void grossly dilute urine frequently. Rectal palpation may suggest enlargement of the left kidney.

In nephrosis associated with ingestion of heavy metals, neurologic signs (lead, arsenic) or gastrointestinal signs (lead, arsenic, and mercury) may be present and raises suspicion of intoxication. In plant toxicities, an absence of historical evidence of previous antibiotic or NSAID use, as well as absence of obvious infectious diseases, may lead to suspicion of plant poisoning. In many such plant toxicities, however, diagnosis must be assisted by clinical pathology and necropsy.

Clinical Pathology and Diagnosis

The diagnosis is linked primarily to clinical pathology data and history. Renal failure will be documented by a urine specific gravity in the isosthenuric range (<1.022) despite obvious dehydration. RBCs, WBCs, granular casts, and proteinuria usually are confirmed by urinalysis in acute nephrosis. Azotemia is present and characterized by elevations of serum urea nitrogen and creatinine. Specific causes may be suggested by the history (i.e., previous use of aminoglycosides, NSAIDs) or merely suspected (severe dehydration in a patient with salmonellosis). Serum chemistry often confirms hypochloremia, which may be more severe than that seen with intestinal obstruction, hypokalemia, hyponatremia, hypocalcemia, hyperphosphatemia, and hypermagnesemia.

Renal biopsy is the most definitive means of diagnosis and can be accomplished by percutaneous biopsy of the left kidney, which is pushed during rectal examination into the right paralumbar fossa, or either kidney can be biopsied from the right with ultrasound guidance. A Tru-Cut biopsy needle (Baxter Health Care, Deerfield, Il.) is used for this procedure. Evaluation of a coagulation panel may be indicated before biopsy because some renal diseases of cattle have been associated with a bleeding diathesis.

Ultrasound study of the kidney may be a helpful ancillary procedure if available.

Treatment

Therapy must attempt to reestablish renal function and to correct primary disorders that may have contributed to nephrosis. Previous use of nephrotoxic drugs should be discontinued and other potentially nephrotoxic drugs avoided in the therapy.

Aggressive fluid therapy to ensure adequate renal perfusion and accomplish diuresis is the primary therapeutic goal. IV fluids that are balanced to address associated electrolyte or acid-base abnormalities must be tailored to the individual patient. Because hypochloremia, hypokalemia, and hyponatremia usually are present, physiologic sodium chloride with supplemental KCl added at 20 to 40 mEq/L is frequently used. Unless the patient is anuric, large volumes of IV fluids are required to address existing dehydration, allow for anticipated fluid losses, and establish diuresis. If an adult patient is anuric or oliguric following an initial 20 to 40 L of IV fluids, 250 to 500 mg of furosemide may be administered IV one or more times at 15- to 30-minute intervals in an effort to initiate diuresis. Failure to produce urine in the face of high volume fluid therapy alongside diuretic administration should be taken as a negative prognostic sign. Repeated bladder evaluation by rectal palpation or ultrasonography to confirm urine production and accumulation may be a useful monitoring technique. Patients that are severely hypoproteinemic, produce inadequate urine despite large volume fluid administration, or show evidence of dependent edema may need additional monitoring for an increasing central venous pressure. A 500-kg cow that is azotemic, isosthenuric, and 10% dehydrated requires 50 L of fluids simply to counteract her existing dehydration. Therefore she may require a total of 80 to 100 L during the first 24 hours of therapy to establish adequate diuresis.

Judicious IV calcium or subcutaneous (SQ) calcium borogluconate should be utilized in those patients that are hypocalcemic. A low percentage of dextrose may be added to the basic fluids by adding 1 L of 50% dextrose to each 20 L of saline/KCl if desired.

Although adult cows with renal failure resulting from nephrosis seldom become hyperkalemic, calves that have acute diarrhea and metabolic acidosis may be hyperkalemic. Therefore initial fluid therapy should be formulated based on the individual patient's acid-base and electrolyte status. Acidotic, hyperkalemic patients should receive IV saline, dextrose (half-strength physiologic saline solution [PSS] mixed equally with 2.5% dextrose), and supplemental $NaHCO_3$. Salmonellosis patients (either calves or cows) with secondary tubular nephrosis may be acidotic and require bicarbonate therapy if balanced crystalloid administration does not correct the acidosis. Oliguric or anuric patients also may require 20 L of 10% dextrose solution in addition to furosemide to instigate osmotic diuresis. Anuria that is unresponsive to fluid diuresis and furosemide therapy may also necessitate dopamine (3 to 5 μg/kg/min) and/or dobutamine (2 to 5 μg/kg/min) in 5% dextrose if all other therapy fails. Other potential treatments include mannitol, norepinephrine, vasopressin, and aminophylline.

Once diuresis is established, fluid therapy is adjusted to maintain diuresis and assist renal excretion of wastes. Serum urea nitrogen and creatinine initially should be monitored each day to establish a trend. The length of treatment varies from a few days to 2 weeks in most cases. The prognosis is guarded until normal renal function is reestablished. The more prolonged the azotemia, the more likely the patient is to develop chronic renal failure. Initially the clinician must proceed with therapy in the hope that nephrosis is acute and reversible. The exact degree of renal damage is impossible to assess initially. Response to therapy and the results of renal biopsies, once available, afford the best means of prognosis.

If a potential nephrotoxic drug must be used to treat a primary condition, reduced dosages and monitoring of blood levels, if available, are essential to continued usage.

Pyelonephritis

Infectious nephritis caused by bacterial infection of the kidney is usually an ascending infection from the lower urinary tract. Pyelonephritis is the most commonly diagnosed disease of the kidney in dairy cattle. Reported incidence in practice settings seems to far outnumber other renal diseases such as nephrosis and glomerulonephritis. This may be a true representation or merely supposed because of the relative ease of diagnosis of pyelonephritis as opposed to other conditions that require more ancillary laboratory data for diagnosis.

Etiology

In cattle, bacterial pyelonephritis has been attributed to ascending infection of the urinary tract by *Escherichia coli* or *Corynebacterium renale* (Figure 10-3). At least three *C. renale* serotypes exist as normal flora of the caudal

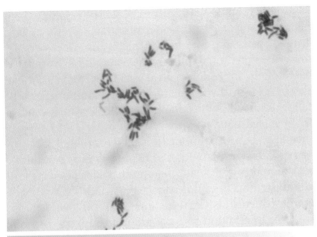

Figure 10-3

Gram stain of the urine from a cow with *C. renale* pyelonephritis.

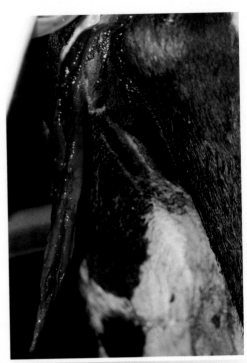

Figure 10-4

Large blood clot protruding from the vulva of a 3-year-old Holstein with acute pyelonephritis. The visible clot was part of a larger clot occluding the urethra, causing the animal to show signs of colic.

portion of the reproductive tract of female cattle and the sheath of male cattle. Unlike most gram-positive organisms, *C. renale* possesses pili that promote attachment to and colonization of the urinary tract mucosa. Conditions that provide physical or chemical damage to the mucosa in the lower portion of the urinary tract such as dystocia, bladder paralysis, or catheterization may predispose the cow to pyelonephritis as a result of *C. renale* ascending infection from the urinary bladder to the ureters and kidneys. *C. renale* causes a humoral antibody response when renal infection develops but not when infection is limited to the bladder. Because routine catheterization of cattle to assess urinary ketones has been abandoned, pyelonephritis caused by *C. renale* is seen less frequently, whereas pyelonephritis caused by gram-negative organisms is seen more frequently. Pyelonephritis as a result of *E. coli* infection has a similar pathogenesis to pyelonephritis caused by *C. renale* in that ascending infection from the lower urinary tract occurs following damage to the caudal portion of the reproductive tract.

Clinical Signs

Acute primary pyelonephritis causes fever of 103.5 to 105.5° F (39.72 to 40.83° C), anorexia, and a precipitous decrease in milk production. Some cows with acute pyelonephritis have colic manifested by kicking at the abdomen, restlessness, and treading. Signs of colic usually are associated with renal or ureteral inflammation and pain, but urinary obstruction caused by blood clots blocking urine outflow from a kidney (ureter) or bladder (urethral) also may contribute to colic (Figure 10-4). Further agitation, such as swishing of the tail, may be observed if the affected cow also has cystitis as a precursor lesion of pyelonephritis. Stranguria, polyuria, an arched stance, gross hematuria (Figures 10-4 and 10-5), blood clots, fibrin, or pyuria also are observed in some patients with *C. renale*

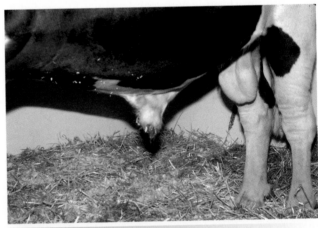

Figure 10-5

Hematuria and pyuria in a bull with *C. renale* pyelonephritis.

infection. Acute pyelonephritis should be considered as a differential for acute colic in postparturient cattle. Consequently left kidney and ureter palpation per rectum should be mandatory components of the physical examination of any sick cow with signs of colic.

Chronic pyelonephritis is associated with weight loss, poor hair coat, anorexia, poor production, diarrhea, polyuria, anemia, stranguria and gross urine abnormalities. Lordosis and stretching out may be apparent in some cows affected with chronic pyelonephritis because of renal pain.

Latent or subclinical pyelonephritis may exist in cattle with multiple medical problems, especially during the first few months of lactation. Cattle with concurrent abomasal displacement, metritis, mastitis, or cattle that had dystocia may develop pyelonephritis that is "masked" by more obvious signs in other systems. Only through screening urine and subsequent urinalysis will the condition be confirmed. Specific physical signs of pyelonephritis in these instances are minimal unless, on rectal palpation, the left kidney is large, painful, and has indistinct lobulations, thereby increasing the possibility of pyelonephritis.

Diagnosis

Diagnosis of pyelonephritis is made by combining the clinical signs, rectal palpation findings, vaginal palpation findings, and urinalysis. Fever usually is present in acute pyelonephritis but may be absent in chronic pyelonephritis. Urinalysis abnormalities such as RBCs, WBCs, protein, and bacteria may be present in both cystitis and pyelonephritis. However, cystitis does not usually lead to systemic illness, and the ureters would not be enlarged (as one or both are in pyelonephritis) as determined by palpation per vagina or per rectum. Vaginal palpation remains an essential aid to diagnosis because it allows detection of unilateral or bilateral ureteral enlargement that is too subtle to be detected per rectum.

Rectal palpation may reveal enlargement of the left kidney in unilateral left kidney infection or bilateral infections. Normal lobations of the kidney may be lost; the kidney may feel "mushy"; and there may be a pronounced arterial pulsation. Rectal palpation is not helpful to diagnosis in right kidney infections unless the infection is very chronic with massive enlargement of the right kidney. Ultrasonography is another helpful ancillary aid to diagnosis and may reveal valuable prognostic information (see video clips 20 and 21).

Other laboratory tests may be performed in valuable cattle or when a diagnosis is not definitive. Hypoalbuminemia is present in most pyelonephritis patients and is more severe in chronic pyelonephritis. Proteinuria appears to be very significant in pyelonephritis and occurs in most cases. Serum globulin values may be higher (>5.0 g/dl) if infection has been chronic. Generally a period of 10 to 14 days of renal infection is necessary to elevate globulin values, and adult cattle tend to have higher globulin levels than calves with chronic infection.

Gross examination of the urine may be diagnostic in acute cases in which fibrin, blood clots, and pus are apparent in voided urine. Some cows with acute pyelonephritis will suffer severe renal hemorrhage that may obstruct the ureter or urethra, thus leading to intermittent or continuous urinary blockage. On occasion

blood clots may be so substantial as to fill and occlude the bladder and urethra. Cattle with less obvious urinary abnormalities will have positive blood and protein reactions on reagent test strips, and urinalysis will confirm the presence of RBCs, WBCs, protein, and bacteria. Routine use of multiple test reagent strips to screen urine during the routine physical examination is an excellent means to detect pyelonephritis and other urinary tract diseases.

Urine culture is the most important laboratory aid because it allows identification of the causative organisms and more importantly the sensitivity of the causative organism to antibiotics. Previous treatment with antibiotics by the owner may interfere with in vitro growth. Therefore antibiotics should be discontinued for 24 to 48 hours before culture of the urine. Urine for culture should be obtained using catheterization or a midstream voided sample to avoid contamination, and a colony count should be requested. Colony counts ($>10^3$/ml on a catheterized sample or $>10^4$/ml on a midstream voided sample) are often necessary to determine the infectious organism(s).

Azotemia is cause for prognostic concern and may indicate prerenal conditions such as dehydration, bilateral pyelonephritis with subsequent renal failure, or postrenal urinary obstruction. Postrenal obstruction usually is obvious following the physical examination and rectal examination. Prerenal azotemia should be suspected if the animal is very dehydrated but is capable of concentrating urine to a specific gravity >1.022. Prerenal azotemia also should respond to rehydration using oral or IV fluids. Most cattle with pyelonephritis that also are azotemic have bilateral disease and renal failure (Figure 10-6). These usually are chronic infections and also have elevated globulin levels, hypoalbuminemia, inability to concentrate urine, and may have electrolyte abnormalities such as hypochloremia, hyponatremia, hypokalemia, and hypocalcemia. Therefore cattle with bilateral pyelonephritis and azotemia have a guarded prognosis.

Anemia may be suspected based on physical examination or confirmed by a CBC. Anemia may develop from blood loss alone in acute cases or more commonly by blood loss from the urinary tract coupled with reduced erythropoiesis subsequent to renal parenchymal damage in chronic cases.

Treatment

The causative organisms and their susceptibility to antimicrobial agents constitute the major economic decision involved in case management. After the organism is identified and antimicrobial susceptibility determined, an antimicrobial agent should be selected that maintains high concentrations in urine, is not nephrotoxic, and is approved for use in cattle. These guidelines may need to be compromised in occasional patients. For example,

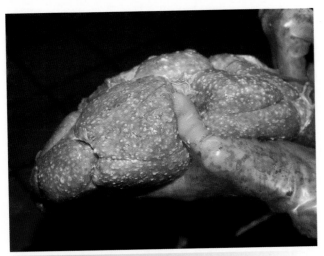

Figure 10-6

Necropsy view of kidney with severe pyelonephritis caused by *C. renale* in a Holstein cow that died from the disease. Both kidneys appeared similar. *(Photo courtesy Dr. John M. King.)*

aminoglycosides may be indicated based on sensitivity results, but these agents possess the potential for nephrotoxicity. Penicillin, because of its urinary route of excretion, has an exponential concentration in urine versus plasma that may make the drug effective in vivo against some *E. coli*, which are resistant to penicillin in vitro. After a catheterized urine sample has been collected for culture, standard therapy in our clinic consists of penicillin (22,000 U/kg, intramuscularly [IM] every 12 hours), which is given until culture and susceptibility results are returned in 72 to 96 hours. When *C. renale* is identified, penicillin is continued for 3 weeks because the organism is uniformly susceptible to penicillin. If the disease is severe and peracute, IV penicillin may be administered for the initial treatment. When *E. coli* is identified, penicillin is continued if objective data (e.g., serial urinalyses, temperature) and subjective data (e.g., appetite, attitude) are returning to normal. If no improvement has occurred during the initial 72 to 96 hours of penicillin therapy in *E. coli* pyelonephritis patients, another agent must be chosen based on antimicrobial susceptibility.

Recommended therapy for bovine pyelonephritis, as with any urinary tract infection, is long term—at least 3 weeks. Short-term antimicrobial therapy has been ineffective.

The prognosis for cows with acute pyelonephritis and treated with long-term antimicrobial therapy is good unless functional or mechanical urogenital abnormalities persist. Pyelonephritis secondary to bladder paralysis or rectovaginal fistula after dystocia would have a poorer prognosis because recurrence of urinary tract infection would be likely.

The prognosis for chronic pyelonephritis is guarded because abscesses of the kidney or total loss of the kidney parenchyma may occur (Figure 10-7). Cows affected with chronic pyelonephritis also have a greater risk of developing a bilateral infection, leading to azotemia and renal failure. Chronically affected cattle also have increased incidence of renal stone formation.

Surgical therapy to remove a massively enlarged and infected kidney occasionally is indicated for treatment of chronic unilateral pyelonephritis (Figure 10-8). The abnormal kidney usually is palpable per rectum, even if the right kidney is involved. The kidney simply feels like a mass the size of a football or basketball and has suffered chronic pyelonephritis, abscessation, and hydronephrosis.

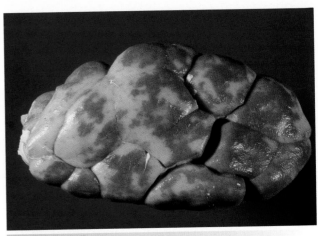

Figure 10-7

Necropsy specimen from a cow with bilateral chronic pyelonephritis, showing pale, fibrosed, chronically infected zones of renal cortex. *(Photo courtesy Dr. John M. King.)*

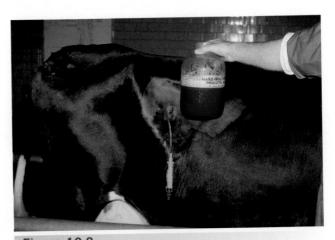

Figure 10-8

Nephrectomy of the right kidney that had ruptured because of chronic pyelonephritis. The red fluid is urine and blood and debris collected from the retroperitoneal space.

Glomerulonephritis

Glomerulonephritis, a rare clinical condition in cattle, causes progressive renal failure and severe proteinuria, hypoalbuminemia, weight loss, and ventral edema.

Etiology

Glomerulonephritis is thought to develop either as a result of antigen-antibody complexes deposited in the glomeruli or specific antibodies produced by the affected animal that attack glomerular basement membranes. In either event, damage to the glomeruli interferes with normal filtration such that protein loss from the kidney occurs and renal failure follows. In the cow, glomerulonephritis usually is associated with infections in body cavities, udder, or uterus and is thought to be caused by circulating antigen antibody complexes. Walled-off infections, such as abscesses that continue to promote antibody production against the somewhat protected antigen, may result in large amounts of antibody, thereby predisposing to glomerulonephritis.

Dr. Rebhun observed one family of dairy cows in which three full siblings (two heifers and one bull) developed glomerulonephritis and nephrotic syndrome and subsequently died. These animals appeared healthy until 18 to 30 months of age and then developed signs that resulted in death within several months of onset (Figure 10-9). This familial problem was most likely a genetic disorder with an antibasement membrane antibody responsible for the glomerular lesions. Unfortunately, only one of the three animals was presented for workup and subsequent necropsy. We have also confirmed renal failure caused by glomerulonephritis in a group of 5- to 8-week-old heifers. The heifers had a rather acute onset of diarrhea and edema caused by the marked proteinuria leading to hypoproteinemia

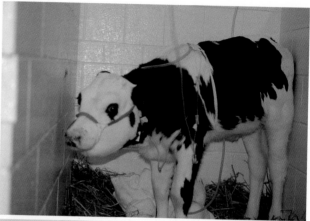

Figure 10-10

A 6-week-old calf with severe edema caused by glomerulonephritis. The calf had marked hypoproteinemia and hypertension.

(Figures 10-10 and 10-11). The heifers were also severely hypertensive. The heifers were from two unrelated farms. Cause of the glomerulonephritis was undetermined, although a common antiserum had been administered to the calves within the first days of life.

Clinical Signs

Weight loss, decreased appetite and production, poor hair coat, and ventral edema are typical signs in cattle affected with glomerulonephritis. Some patients have diarrhea. Because these signs are nonspecific and concurrent or chronic infections may be present in these patients, the possibility of renal disease may be overlooked.

Rectal palpation of an enlarged left kidney may be the only specific physical abnormality detected. Proteinuria will be detected by a positive protein reaction on the multiple test reagent strips and can be confirmed by SSA protein or finding a urine protein/urine creatinine ratio >3.

Diagnosis

Because the clinical signs are similar for glomerulonephritis and amyloidosis, renal biopsy is essential to confirm the diagnosis. If the nephrotic syndrome (i.e., ventral edema, hypoalbuminemia, and proteinuria) is present, the condition probably is advanced and renal failure is present.

Ventral edema, an enlarged left kidney (the right kidney cannot be reached) (Figure 10-12), absence of urinary constituent abnormalities other than proteinuria, and azotemia with isosthenuria should allow a tentative diagnosis of glomerulonephritis or amyloidosis. Renal biopsy will confirm the diagnosis. Ultrasonography generally is not helpful to the diagnosis but may be useful during biopsy. Laboratory data as regards serum urea nitrogen, and creatinine and electrolyte levels may show mild abnormalities in early cases or dramatic

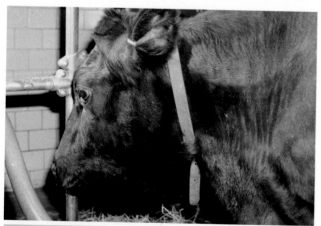

Figure 10-9

Intermandibular edema associated with severe hypoproteinemia and hypoalbuminemia in a 2-year-old Holstein having glomerulonephritis of possible genetic origin.

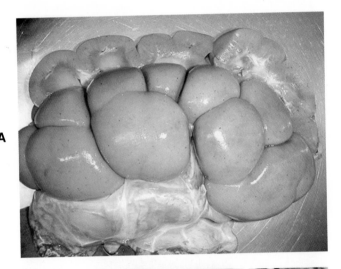

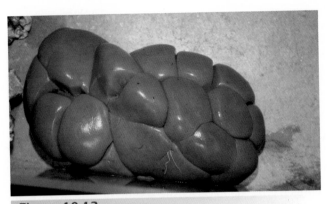

Figure 10-12

Gross specimen of kidney having glomerulonephritis from a cow that had chronic cellulitis in one hind limb. Both kidneys were enlarged and appeared similar.

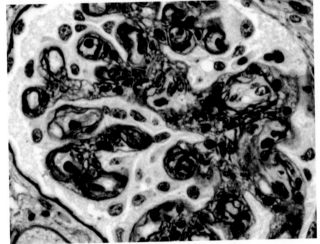

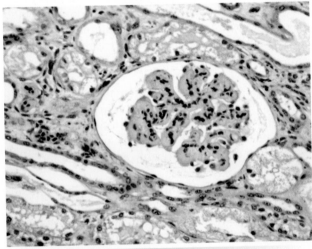

Figure 10-11

A, Kidney from the calf in Figure 10-10. Microscopic view of the glomeruli from the calf in Figure 10-10. **B,** Glomerular loops are expanded by eosinophilic material and increased mesangial cells and **(C)** marked diffuse thickening of glomerular basement syembrane.

abnormalities as renal failure ensues. Hypoproteinemia characterized by hypoalbuminemia is present in all cases. Anemia may develop in chronic cases. Diarrhea, although more typical of amyloidosis, may be present in some glomerulonephritis patients if hypoproteinemia is so severe as to lead to edema of the gut wall.

Unfortunately cattle with glomerulonephritis usually have progressed to renal failure by the time an accurate diagnosis is reached. Therefore attempts at treatment have been limited.

Treatment

Early or acute cases may be treated by supportive care for renal failure and specific therapy directed against any infections (e.g., mastitis, abscesses) thought to be primary to the glomerulonephritis. Once renal failure has developed, treatment usually is hopeless.

Amyloidosis

Amyloidosis is an infrequent systemic disease characterized by extracellular deposition of amyloid (abnormal deposits of glycoprotein) in the kidney, gut, liver, adrenal gland, spleen, and other tissues. Because the kidney appears to be a major site of deposition in the cow, proteinuria and a nephrotic syndrome develop in bovine amyloidosis patients. Affected cattle are 4 years of age or older.

Etiology

Both primary and secondary forms of amyloidosis exist. Primary amyloidosis is likely an immune-mediated or metabolic storage disease, whereas secondary amyloidosis (most commonly systemic AA type amyloid) has been associated with chronic infections in various organ systems. Approximately half of the reported cases in two case series had evidence of chronic infection that could be interpreted as contributory to the development of amyloidosis. Chronic infection currently is theorized to predispose to both secondary amyloidosis and glomerulonephritis. Inflammatory lesions of hardware disease, chronic pneumonia, mastitis, metritis, and abscesses have been associated with amyloidosis.

Signs

Weight loss, reduced production, diarrhea, and ventral edema characterize the early signs of amyloidosis in dairy cattle (Figure 10-13). As the disease progresses, nephrotic syndrome becomes more obvious with marked ventral edema, hypoalbuminemia, and proteinuria. Appetite may be fair to normal early in the course but tends to decrease as hypoproteinemia worsens and azotemia develops. Rectal palpation may allow detection of an enlarged, firm left kidney, and test reagent strips confirm marked proteinuria.

Diarrhea usually is present and may be profuse. Diarrhea is thought to originate from amyloid deposition in the gut. This deposition is not detectable grossly and so may require microscopic study. Diarrhea probably worsens the hypoalbuminemia because of protein loss from the intestine. Given the relative dearth of clinical signs other than diarrhea, weight loss resulting from Johne's disease or other primary gastrointestinal diseases need to be considered in the differential diagnosis. Although amyloidosis may be characterized by diarrhea, it should be emphasized that other causes of chronic renal failure or proteinuria also may be associated with diarrhea because of gut and mesenteric edema secondary to hypoalbuminemia.

Diagnosis

The diagnosis of amyloidosis requires renal biopsy or necropsy to differentiate the disease from glomerulonephritis. Diarrhea, an enlarged left kidney per rectum, weight loss, and other nonspecific signs of chronic illness will also be present. Other than hypoproteinemia caused by hypoalbuminemia and proteinuria, laboratory tests are not helpful. Degree of azotemia, electrolyte values, and urine specific gravity vary based on the duration and degree of renal involvement. Terminally, cattle with amyloidosis are azotemic, proteinuric, and isosthenuric.

Hypocalcemia is typical and associated with hypoalbuminemia and calcium-binding principles. At necropsy, affected kidneys are large, pale, and firm.

Kidney biopsy tissue or gross postmortem tissue may be stained with special stains to highlight amyloid depositions. Lugol's iodine has been used on gross renal tissue to detect the presence of amyloid (Figure 10-14). The iodine stains amyloid-infiltrated renal tissue mahogany brown, and further staining with sulfuric acid produces a blue color. Congo red stains highlight amyloid for light microscopy, whereas electron microscopy identifies a characteristic fibrillar appearance.

Treatment

No practical treatments exist, and the disease is fatal to affected cattle. As a result of the urinary losses of antithrombin III, which is similar in molecular weight to albumin, hypercoagulation may be present, causing an acute clinical demise associated with acute renal vein thrombosis (Figure 10-15).

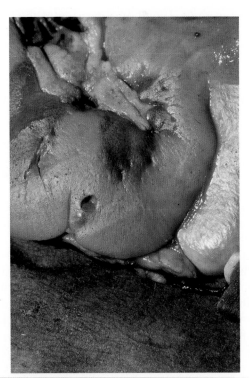

Figure 10-14

Kidney of a cow that died from amyloidosis. The kidneys were enlarged, tan colored, and firm. Lugol's solution has been poured on the cut surface, and brown dots can be seen in the glomeruli because of the Lugol's staining of the starch component of the amyloid.

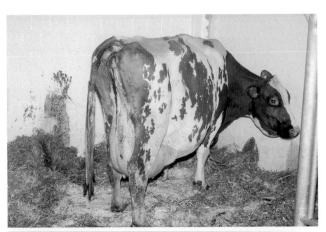

Figure 10-13

An 8-year-old Red and White Holstein with amyloidosis causing diarrhea, proteinuria, hypoproteinemia, azotemia, and edema. The kidneys were three or four times the normal size because of the amyloid deposition.

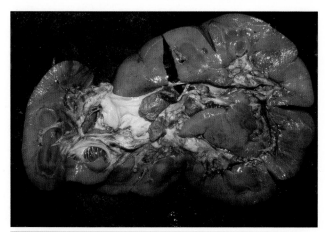

Figure 10-15

A large thrombus in the renal vein of a cow that had renal amyloidosis.

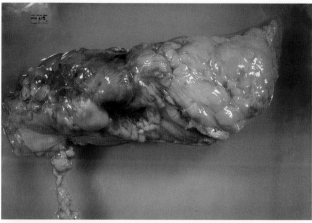

Figure 10-16

Lymphoma involvement of the kidney. The kidney was enlarged, had an abnormal shape, and had lost normal lobations.

Renal Tumors

Although primary renal adenomas, adenocarcinomas, and nephroblastomas are reported in cattle, these tumors are too rare to merit discussion. The neoplasm most commonly encountered involving the bovine kidney is lymphosarcoma (Figure 10-16). The kidney is one of many organs involved in multicentric lymphosarcoma in cattle. Lymphoma invasion of the left kidney may cause the kidney to develop an unusual shape when palpated per rectum.

Disorders of the Ureters

Few specific diseases of the ureters exist. Most conditions affecting ureters descend from the kidney or ascend from the bladder.

Ureteral inflammation and distention are seen commonly with pyelonephritis, and calculi in the ureter have been observed rarely in cattle. Either inflammation or calculi in the ureter may result in severe pain that is manifested as colic and requires differentiation from colic of gastrointestinal origin (Figure 10-17). When renal/ureteral stones are seen, they are usually bilateral, associated with chronic infection, and cause intermittent obstruction. Diagnosis can be confirmed by ultrasound examination (Figure 10-18). Antibiotic and fluid treatment will often result in clinical improvement (the ureteral stone likely moves back into the renal pelvis, temporarily relieving the obstruction). Congenital ureteral ectopia has been described in a dairy calf. Endoscopy and radiographs were not diagnostic for the case, but it was confirmed at surgery, and the calf recovered after nephrectomy of the affected side.

Lymphosarcoma may invade the ureters in cows with the adult form of lymphosarcoma and is the most common tumor of the ureter in my experience.

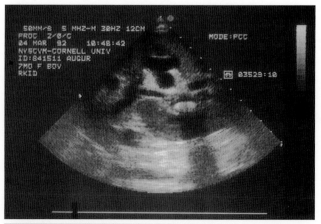

Figure 10-17

A calf demonstrating "colicky" signs (stretching out) because of ureteral obstruction.

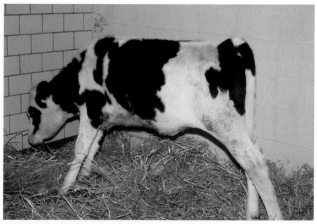

Figure 10-18

Ultrasound of the kidney of the calf in Figure 10-17 revealing a large nephrolith. *C. renale* was cultured from the urine of the calf and was likely the cause for the stones to form.

Palpation of the ureters is best accomplished per vagina as the ureters cross the pelvic brim. The ureters can be palpated by rolling them gently over the pubis.

Diseases of the urinary bladder include inflammatory, neurogenic, and neoplastic disorders, as well as formation of cystic calculi.

Cystitis

Etiology

Urinary bladder inflammation and infection occur secondary to bladder paralysis that allows urine stasis, dystocia with ascending contamination from the urethra, and chronic irritation from cystic calculi. Dystocia is a major cause of cystitis in dairy cattle because sacral innervation to the bladder may be damaged, thereby decreasing bladder tone, interfering with emptying, and predisposing to infection by either stasis or direct contamination through the urethra.

In calves, cystitis almost always is associated with urachal or umbilical remnants that act as a nidus of infection, or prevent complete bladder emptying by traction from fibrous adhesions.

Signs

Frequent attempts to urinate small volumes, strangury, tail swishing, treading on the hind limbs, and irritability are common signs of cystitis in adult cattle. Urethritis generally accompanies cystitis and may be responsible for some of these signs. Occasionally high-strung cows with cystitis may kick at the abdomen, but this sign is not as common as observed in pyelonephritis. Scalding of the perineum from urine dribbling is observed in some cattle if sacral nerve damage has caused relative bladder atony and subsequent urine dribbling. Sandlike particles may be present on the vulvar hair because of excessive crystalluria or uroliths (Figure 10-19, A and B). Umbilical infections in calves frequently produce a mild clinical or occult cystitis. Careful observation of calves with urachal or umbilical artery remnant infections may reveal polyuria, but stranguria is not common. Similarly, microscopic urinalysis may reveal pyuria and bacteruria, but the systemic signs are often mild or attributed to the presence of infection in the umbilical stalk. Pyelonephritis as a consequence of urachal remnant infection and cystitis in calves is extremely rare.

Rectal palpation may reveal a distended atonic bladder in cases with sacral nerve damage following dystocia or other neurologic diseases. In primary ascending cystitis without innervation defects, the bladder will be palpated as a firm, thick-walled structure the size of a baseball or softball. Cystic calculi, if present, also would be diagnosed on rectal palpation. Vaginal palpation of the ureters is normal.

Urine may show gross evidence of hematuria or pyuria (Figure 10-20). Multistix (Bayer, Medfield, MA) usually

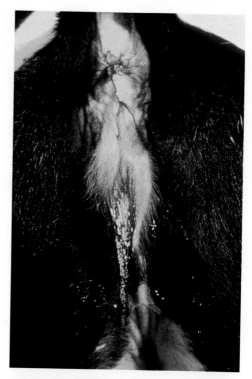

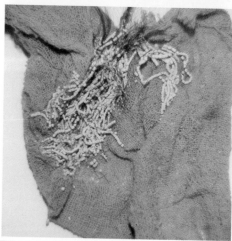

Figure 10-19

A, Crystals attached to the vulva hair of a heifer with chronic *C. renale* cystitis. **B,** Sandlike crystals and struvite precipitates removed from the vulvar hair of the heifer.

will show positive blood, positive protein, and a variable pH based on the organisms present and the diet. Fever is not common and is one means of differentiating cystitis from acute pyelonephritis. Affected cows do not act ill, but irritation from the infection may cause enough discomfort to affect appetite and thus production.

Diagnosis

The clinical signs, absence of systemic signs, normal ureters, and abnormal urine constituents contribute to the diagnosis. Ultrasonography of the bladder (per rectum)

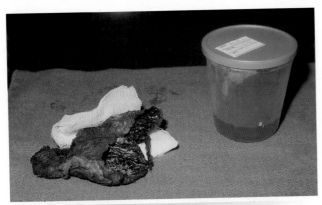

Figure 10-20

Large fibrin cast and urine with hematuria and pyuria from a cow with chronic cystitis. The fibrin cast was removed manually from the urethra where it had lodged.

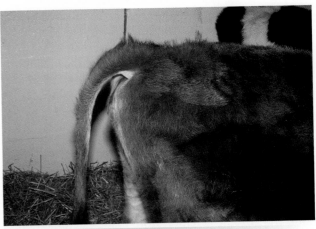

Figure 10-21

Elevated tail head and dysuria in a 6-month-old Brown Swiss with a chronic urachal abscess causing the bladder to be adhered to the ventral body wall. The urinalysis was normal. Surgical removal of the abscess and adhesion and part of the bladder alleviated the clinical signs.

and kidneys will confirm disease of the bladder and rule out pyelonephritis. Culture and sensitivity of urine for bacteria is helpful to confirm the bacteria responsible for infection and direct therapy. Bladder endoscopy can be used to determine the severity of mucosal lesions from cystitis (see video clip 22).

In calves with cystitis or recurrent cystitis, ultrasonography of the abdomen to detect urachal abscesses or umbilical remnants adherent to the bladder is imperative. On occasion calves with recurrent cystitis may have resolved the infection within the umbilicus and urachus but have been left with fibrous adhesions between the bladder and abdominal wall, resulting in incomplete voiding and repeated infections.

Treatment

Bacterial cystitis requires antibiotic therapy based on urine culture and antibiotic susceptibility tests. Therapy should be continued for at least 7 days. Antibiotics that obtain good inhibitory concentrations in urine should be selected when possible. While awaiting urine culture results, penicillin (22,000 U/kg) and ampicillin (11 mg/kg) are excellent choices for initial therapy. When bladder paresis or atony complicates cystitis, temporary placement of a Foley catheter may improve bladder emptying and decrease inflammatory sediment in the bladder. Bladder paresis decreases the prognosis and predisposes to relapse or reinfection following cessation of antibiotic therapy. Adequate salt and water should be available to encourage water consumption, and a high anionic salt diet may be used to both acidify the urine and promote diuresis in addition to antibiotics.

Bacterial cystitis associated with cystic calculi requires correction of the calculi problem and will be discussed in the section on urolithiasis.

Calves with dysuria secondary to umbilical or urachal adhesions and infection require abdominal surgery

through a ventral midline approach to free the bladder and resect septic lesions or adhesions (Figure 10-21).

Bladder Paralysis (Neurogenic Injury, Bladder Atony)

It is difficult to discuss bladder paralysis and cystitis separately because inadequate bladder emptying predisposes to cystitis by encouraging ascending infection.

Etiology

Sacral nerve injuries causing bladder dysfunction are most commonly caused by dystocia with intrapelvic injury to the nerves or by crushing injuries to the sacrum and tail head at the vertebral level from riding activity. Occasional cases of direct sacral trauma are observed in modern facilities with poorly designed free stall dividers or partitions. In either event, the bladder dysfunction seldom is diagnosed until cystitis develops or a large bladder is palpated during routine rectal palpation of the reproductive tract. If suspected in the acute phase following dystocia or crushing tail head sacral injuries, symptomatic therapy to reduce acute inflammation may be indicated. In some cases chronic infection may cause the paralysis rather than vice versa.

Signs and Diagnosis

Dribbling of urine and voiding of small amounts of urine despite efforts at complete urination are the major signs of bladder dysfunction. Urine scalding may be observed in cattle suffering crushed tail heads from riding injuries. Urine is normal unless secondary cystitis occurs. Cystitis is common following dystocia because of urethral compromise, trauma, and associated vaginitis. Crystalluria may result in sandy calculi formation on the vulvar hair ventral to the vulva.

Rectal palpation confirms an enlarged bladder, and the affected cow cannot empty the bladder when stimulated. Failure to conceive because of urine pooling in the vagina and chemical or bacterial vaginitis is a common reproductive complication to bladder paralysis in cows.

Treatment

In acute cases, placement of an indwelling Foley catheter coupled with prophylactic penicillin therapy may prevent urinary retention and cystitis. Systemic NSAIDs, dexamethasone (10 to 20 mg once daily for 3 days), or epidural administration of 5 mg of dexamethasone may be worthwhile to reduce edema and inflammation around the involved sacral nerves.

In chronic cases, the same therapy may be attempted but is less likely to be successful; use of antiinflammatory drugs probably is not justified.

When cystitis is present, therapy should be directed against the cystitis as outlined above. The prognosis is poor because recurrent cystitis and eventual pyelonephritis are probable.

Hemorrhagic Cystitis Associated with Malignant Catarrhal Fever

Etiology

In addition to the acute head and eye, chronic, enteric, and mild forms of MCF, acute hemorrhagic cystitis has been observed as a rare form of MCF. The disease is thought to be a variant of the more common forms resulting from infection by the causative herpesvirus of MCF. Instances are sporadic, as are most reports of MCF in dairy cattle, and affected cattle have been housed or pastured near sheep at some time within several months of disease onset.

Signs

Acute onset of high fever (106.0 to 108.0° F/41.11 to 42.22° C), depression, hematuria, strangury, and frequent attempts at urination constitute the major signs. Affected cattle progress rapidly to severe depression and inappetence with death occurring in 24 to 72 hours. Other grossly detectable signs of MCF (e.g., oral erosions, lymphadenopathy, and ocular lesions) may not be apparent.

Diagnosis

Necropsy reveals severe hemorrhagic cystitis with a thickened bladder wall and mucosal erosion. A retrospective diagnosis is made based on lesions of vasculitis in all major organs (e.g., kidney, brain, and lymph nodes) and exclusion of other causes of hemorrhagic cystitis.

Prevention

Because the disease is usually fatal, preventing exposure to sheep remains the best prevention of MCF in dairy cattle. Although other vectors of the virus have been theorized and are possible, most cases in dairy cattle result from environmental exposure to sheep.

Enzootic Hematuria

Etiology

A progressive noninfectious cystitis with tissue metaplasia of the bladder mucosa has been described in cattle allowed to graze bracken fern for extended periods. Sporadic cases also have been observed in cattle with no known exposure to bracken fern or, for that matter, any pasture. Although several toxic factors have been identified in bracken fern, the exact cause is unknown. There is also a putative role for bovine papilloma viruses (specifically BPV2) combined with bracken fern exposure in the etiopathogenesis of the disease in some parts of the world. Multiple types of neoplasms are possible in this syndrome, including both epithelial and mesenchymal origin tumors. Metastases are possible in some cases.

Signs

Severe hematuria, strangury, and anemia are found in affected cattle. Absence of fever suggests a noninfectious cause. Rectal examination in most cases allows palpation of multiple masses within the bladder wall. Early signs of hematuria may be the result of microscopic lesions in the urinary tract or associated with the pancytopenia typical of chronic bracken fern toxicity.

Diagnosis

Diagnosis is suggested if multiple animals are affected with similar signs following pasturing. In individual cases, necropsy findings of anemia, bladder masses, and hematuria, coupled with exclusion of infectious diseases, allow diagnosis.

Prevention

Removal from pasture is the best prevention but may not reverse the disease in severely affected cattle. Fortunately "pasture diseases," such as enzootic hematuria, are currently rare in dairy cattle in the United States because of reduced pasture availability.

Bladder Rupture

Etiology

Bladder rupture is rare in cattle but has been reported following parturition and in heifers with urachal adhesions or traction adhesions resulting from previous abdominal surgery. Urolithiasis is uncommon in dairy cattle, thereby decreasing the likelihood of urinary obstruction and secondary bladder rupture. Bladder rupture also has occurred secondary to urethral obstruction by large blood clots in severe cases of acute pyelonephritis in cattle. Although rare in cattle raised for milk production, urolithiasis may occur in dairy calves raised for veal or dairy steers and will be discussed below.

Signs

Abdominal distention, depression, inappetence, and a detectable fluid wave during ballottement of the abdomen are typical signs of bladder rupture in cattle. History may reveal previous signs of urinary abnormalities (e.g., pollakiuria, tenesmus, and colic), umbilical problems during calfhood, or previous surgery for umbilical or abdominal lesions. It will be impossible to palpate the bladder during rectal examination.

Diagnosis

Failure to palpate the urinary bladder and fluid abdominal distention arouse suspicion of bladder rupture. However, because this problem is rare in dairy cattle, laboratory aids are essential to diagnosis.

Abdominocentesis should result in copious fluid that may be analyzed for cytology, protein content, and creatinine levels. Comparison of serum creatinine with abdominal fluid creatinine should allow positive diagnosis of urinary bladder rupture because the abdominal fluid creatinine will be much higher than the serum value. Serum electrolytes usually show hyponatremia, hypochloremia, and variable values for potassium. In most species, uroperitoneum results in serum hyperkalemia, but reported cases in cattle (steers) have not done so.

Treatment

Treatment options include slaughter or surgical repair of the bladder defect. If repair is to be attempted, the patient benefits from preoperative IV fluids (PSS primarily) and slow drainage of urine from the abdomen via a peritoneal drain or Foley catheter (Figure 10-22). Antibiotics should be utilized preoperatively and postoperatively as well. Because the caudal ventral midline is the best surgical access to the urinary bladder, adult dairy cows are poor surgical candidates because the udder covers the ideal approach.

Eversion and Prolapse of the Urinary Bladder

Eversion of the bladder has been reported in dairy cattle following severe tenesmus associated with parturition or shortly thereafter. True eversion occurs through the urethral orifice, whereas bladder prolapse tends to follow a laceration in the floor of the vagina during parturition. A prolapsed bladder usually fills with urine, whereas an everted bladder obviously cannot contain urine. Both conditions are rare. Bladder eversion or prolapse may grossly mimic vaginal and uterine prolapse but can be

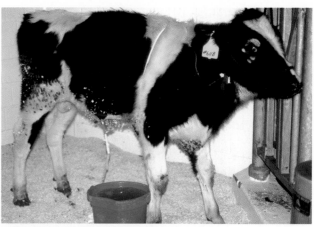

Figure 10-22

Urine being drained from the abdomen of a steer with ruptured bladder caused by urethral calculi.

differentiated easily following cleansing of the organ and vaginal examination. The bladder may rarely be involved in a vaginal prolapse and will prevent normal replacement of the vagina until the urine is drained.

Prognosis is guarded for these conditions. Repair of eversion is difficult because of rapid congestion and subsequent edema in the tissue. The narrow urethra of the cow makes replacement difficult. One case report describes a dorsal urethral incision to aid replacement. Necrosis of the everted bladder may lead to a fatal outcome even if repair has been apparently successful.

Similarly prolapse of the bladder requires emptying of the bladder, replacement through the lacerated vaginal floor, and repair of the vaginal wound. Peritonitis, bladder necrosis, and adhesions affecting urine outflow are possible complications.

Bladder Neoplasms

Most bladder neoplasms derive from enzootic hematuria and include hemangiomas, hemangiosarcomas, leiomyosarcomas, fibromas, fibrosarcomas, squamous cell carcinomas, transitional cell carcinomas, and papillomas. Experience with enzootic hematuria is limited in the northeastern United States, where the most common tumor found in an adult cow bladder is lymphosarcoma. Simply based on the incidence of lymphosarcoma and the potential for this neoplasm to attack any tissue, most neoplastic lesions involving the lower urinary tract (i.e., bladder, urethra, and ureter) prove to be lymphosarcoma. Biopsy can be obtained during endoscopy (see video clip 23).

Urolithiasis

Urolithiasis is the most important urinary tract disease in feed lot and range cattle but is seldom a problem in dairy cattle unless dairy veal and steers are included.

In modern management systems in the northeastern United States, few dairy calves, bulls, or cows have problems with urolithiasis, but a basic discussion of the condition is justified because the condition may exist in dairy cattle in other geographic regions.

Etiology
Many causes and contributing factors exist that predispose to urolithiasis in cattle:

1. High concentrate diets are thought to increase urinary mucoproteins and lead to "solidification" of urine solutes. These diets are a major cause of urolithiasis in feed lot beef animals.
2. High phosphorous diets or improper calcium-phosphorous balance in a ration, again usually associated with a high concentrate diet.
3. Pastures containing large amounts of silica or oxalate.
4. Vitamin A deficiency and excessive estrogens. Both conditions allow squamous metaplasia of mucosa creating solid nidus formation, narrowing of the urethral lumen, and excessive desquamation of epithelial cells. Estrogens may originate in pastures, feedstuffs, zearalenone, or from estrogenic tissue implants.
5. Hypervitaminosis D—perhaps because of increased urinary calcium levels.
6. Reduced water intake. Drought or extreme cold with subsequent freezing of water supplies causes severe concentration of urine solutes and encourages calculi formation. During the winter, animals are reluctant to drink normal amounts when water is extremely cold, even though it may not be frozen.
7. Early castration of male animals contributes to reduced diameter of the distal urinary tract and is an important contributing feature in beef steers and smaller ruminants.

Having reviewed most of the contributing causes of urolithiasis, it becomes obvious that dairy cows, calves, and bulls have few risks compared with beef cattle, sheep, and goats. Sporadic cases may occur in dairy calves or bulls. If endemic problems occur, the veterinarian must investigate all potential causes to rectify the problem as quickly as possible.

Signs
Obstruction of male cattle occurs most commonly at the distal sigmoid region of the urethra. Renal, ureteral, and cystic calculi also are possible, but urethral obstruction is the most common clinical situation. Signs of urinary obstruction include treading, tenesmus, pulsation of the urethra in the escutcheon proximal to the obstruction, colic characterized by kicking at the abdomen, sandy calculi or crystals on the preputial hair, and inappetence. If urine can be passed, it often appears blood-tinged. Rectal examination confirms the presence

of a greatly distended urinary bladder and pulsating pelvic urethra.

The signs are much different if rupture of the bladder has occurred as a result of prolonged urethral obstruction. Colic is replaced by depression, and tenesmus ceases. Abdominal distention follows. (This is discussed fully under the heading "Bladder Rupture.")

More commonly, rupture of the urethra in males allows the subcutaneous deposition of urine and appearance of diffuse pitting edema along the sheath and ventral abdomen referred to as "water belly" (Figure 10-23). This is a severe complication that often results in chemical necrosis and eventual sloughing of the affected tissue.

Diagnosis
Diagnosis is based on clinical signs. Rectal examination or abdominal ultrasonography is imperative to assess an intact bladder. In calves, as in small ruminants, radiography may be helpful to evaluate the number, location, and size of calculi within the urinary tract before surgery.

Treatment
Because of the sigmoid flexure, catheterization usually is impossible. Therefore therapy entails urethrostomy, and this may interfere with future breeding. Complete urethrostomy with penile amputation may be lifesaving but of course renders breeding animals worthless. Postpubic urethrostomy, catheterization, and medical therapy with smooth muscle relaxants and IV fluid therapy with saline solutions could be tried for bulls of valuable genetic base, but prognosis must be guarded. Aminopromazine has been used as a smooth muscle relaxant in feed lot cattle, but a paucity of controlled data exist regarding treatment of intact males.

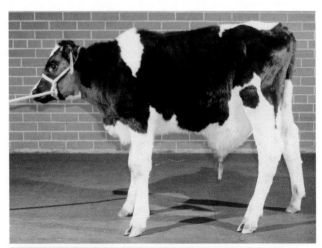

Figure 10-23

"Water belly" or urethral rupture in a Holstein steer with urolithiasis. Sandlike crystals form chains on the preputial hair.

Where geographic conditions or causes allow single calculus formation, dye studies or ultrasonography to localize the lesions and specific surgery to remove the calculus would theoretically be possible.

Prevention

In all instances, correction of the underlying causes or removal from offending pastures or feedstuffs should be used to prevent further cases. Providing free access to a source of nonfrozen water is very important, and adding NaCl to 4% to 5% of the ration will encourage water consumption and reduce precipitation or accumulation of urine solutes. This is especially helpful during extreme cold weather.

Patent Urachus in Calves

Persistence of a patent urachus in calves is less common than in foals but leads to similar predisposition to septicemia. Clinical signs consist of urine dribbling from the umbilical region or persistent moisture surrounding a small urachal opening at the umbilicus. Unless the urachus closes by 24 hours after birth, surgical resection is indicated to reduce the likelihood of septicemia. If economics disallow surgery, prophylactic broad-spectrum antibiotics systemically and cautery of the urachus with silver nitrate or Lugol's iodine are indicated.

Umbilical Infections

Etiology

Umbilical infections, hernias, and fetal vascular infections are common problems in calves. Some umbilical lesions (i.e., patent urachus) are evident at birth, whereas others, such as small hernias and abscesses, may not become obvious to the owner for 1 to 6 weeks.

Infection in the umbilical region may lead to a multitude of intraabdominal lesions and cellulitis or abscessation external to the body wall. Neonatal infections of the umbilical region result in painful swelling and palpable enlargement of the umbilical vessels. Septicemia resulting from bacteria ascending the umbilical vessels or urachus is always a threat. Infection through this route may cause acute septicemia or chronic septicemia with subsequent joint ill, meningitis, uveitis, and so on. In some instances, infection is low grade, and no clinical signs develop until the calf is several months old. Delayed problems often involve infected urachal remnants and bladder dysfunction or recurrent urinary tract infection.

Chronic infection of the umbilical vein may cause hepatic abscessation, whereas umbilical artery infection may cause chronic infection involving the urinary bladder. The plethora of pathology possible subsequent to umbilical infection requires that each calf be assessed as to its individual problems (Table 10-1).

Signs and Diagnosis

In acute neonatal umbilical infections, palpation and physical findings may suffice for diagnosis. Affected calves are febrile and have cellulitis in the region of the umbilicus with palpable enlargement of the umbilical vessels.

Signs of septicemia such as septic arthritis, uveitis, meningitis, or peritonitis may be present and would worsen the prognosis.

Subacute infections limited to the umbilicus may have purulent material that drains from the umbilical vessels or urachus after removal of a scab at the exterior umbilicus.

Latent infections of intraabdominal vascular remnants or the urachus are harder to diagnose. Affected calves may be several weeks old before signs of fever and depression occur. Depending on the pathology present, other signs may include signs of peritonitis, septic arthritis, or urinary tract infection. The umbilicus may appear normal on inspection, but deep palpation may detect thickened umbilical remnants intraabdominally.

Diagnosis is greatly aided by ultrasonography to detect the site and extent of infection (see video clip 24).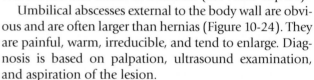

Umbilical abscesses external to the body wall are obvious and are often larger than hernias (Figure 10-24). They are painful, warm, irreducible, and tend to enlarge. Diagnosis is based on palpation, ultrasound examination, and aspiration of the lesion.

Umbilical Hernias

Etiology and Signs

Uncomplicated umbilical hernias in calves range from 1.0 to 10.0 cm in diameter, are soft and reducible, and not painful (Figure 10-25). Omentum and abomasum may be palpated in the hernia. Small hernias (diameter less than 4.0 cm) often close spontaneously by 3 to 4 months of age. Those that persist require therapy, as do larger hernias. Some hernias are thought to originate secondary to infected umbilical remnants; cordlike remnants of umbilical structures may be palpated in these hernias. Most hernias are of unknown origin. Although inheritance definitely is a possibility, heifer calves usually are not culled because of this problem unless an extremely large hernia exists. Most bull studs will not accept bull calves with hernias (or bulls that have had hernias repaired) for fear of perpetuation of the trait.

Treatment

Manual reduction of small hernias followed by snug taping around the midabdomen with an elastic adhesive tape has been a successful procedure for some practitioners for hernias less than 3 fingers width in diameter. The tape is left in place for several weeks, allowing the abdominal wall to close the defect. In healthy, rapidly growing calves postweaning, the tape may need to be changed at 1- to 2-week intervals to prevent it from

TABLE 10-1 Treatment of Umbilical Infections*

Physical Findings	Treatment

Neonatal calf, healthy other than palpable cellulitis or vascular thickening with possible fever.	1. Remove scab over umbilicus to allow drainage
	2. Broad-spectrum antibiotic therapy to counteract probable *Arcanobacterium pyogenes* or mixed infection
	   a. Penicillin 22,000 U/kg once or twice daily
	   or
	   b. Ceftiofur 2.2 mg/kg twice daily
	   or
	   c. Trimethoprim-sulfa 22 mg/kg once daily (7 days)

Neonatal calf with fever, palpable umbilical lesions, and evidence of septicemia	1. Assess adequacy of passive transfer of immunoglobulins
	2. Remove umbilical scab, and culture any discharge
	3. Consider blood culture if valuable calf
	4. Intensive broad-spectrum antibiotic therapy for gram-negative organisms
	   a. Penicillin and gentamicin, 22,000 U/kg once daily and 2.2 mg/kg twice daily, respectively
	   or
	   b. Trimethoprim-sulfa 22 mg/kg twice daily
	   or
	   c. Ceftiofur (Naxcel) 2.2 mg/kg twice daily
	5. Attend localized infections such as septic joints via lavage, etc.
	6. Surgical resection of umbilicus once calf is stabilized (1-3 days)

Calf 2 wk or older with fever and evidence of urinary tract infection	1. Urine culture and sensitivity 2. Ultrasonography of umbilicus 3. Surgical resection of umbilicus and urachus or umbilical artery infection 4. Appropriate systemic antibiotics for 7-14 days. *A. pyogenes* and gram-negative organisms most common
Calf 2 wk or older with fever and septic arthritis in one or more joints. Umbilicus may appear normal or thickened; vascular remnants may be palpable through the abdominal wall	1. Blood culture and culture of infected joints 2. Resection of umbilicus and infected remnants. This may be complicated by hepatic abscessation or require dissection of multiple adhesions 3. Lavage of infected joints 4. Appropriate systemic antibiotics for 7-21 days. *A. pyogenes* almost always present but may be complicated by anaerobes or gram-negative organisms
Apparently healthy calf 1-8 mo of age with umbilical abscess external to body wall	1. Aspirate to confirm presence of pus 2. Liberal drainage of abscess followed by daily flushing 3. If concerned about possible intraabdominal lesions, ultrasound after resolution of external abscess

Specific therapeutic recommendations must address the pathology present in each patient.

becoming too tight. Some owners report successful resolution with repeated manual reduction of small hernias, but these cases may have resolved spontaneously. In larger hernias, or when physical therapy fails, surgery is the only option.

Surgery for uncomplicated hernias is performed under local anesthesia with the calf sedated with xylazine (up to 0.22 mg/kg IV). The hernia sac is opened and examined for problematic remnants, and the abdominal wall closed with mattress sutures. Surgical preference dictates the exact suture pattern, but our clinic has been pleased with far-near-near-far suture patterns for large hernias.

Complicated hernias with intraabdominal adhesions or infected umbilical remnants are difficult surgical procedures requiring larger incisions, advanced knowledge of abdominal anatomy, and superior surgical skills. Surgical referral should be considered for these patients.

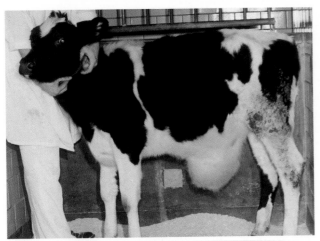

Figure 10-24

Large umbilical abscess in a Holstein heifer.

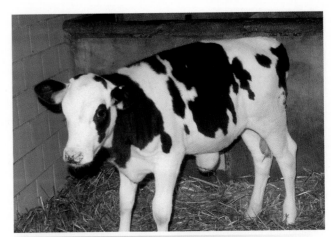

Figure 10-25

Large but reducible umbilical hernia in a Holstein heifer.

SUGGESTED READINGS

Bertone AL, Smith DF: Ruptured bladder in a yearling heifer, *J Am Vet Med Assoc* 184:981-982, 1984.

Braun U, Nuss K, Wapf P, et al: Clinical and ultrasonographic findings in five cows with a ruptured urachal remnant, *Vet Rec* 159(23):780-782, 2006.

Carrier J, Stewart S, Godden S, et al: Evaluation and use of three cow-side tests for detection of subclinical ketosis in early postpartum cows, *J Dairy Sci* 87:3725-3735, 2004.

Chandler KJ, O'Brien K, Huxley JN, et al: Hydronephrosis and renal failure in two Friesian cows, *Vet Rec* 146:646-648, 2000.

Divers TJ: Diagnosis and therapy of renal disease in dairy cattle. In *Proceedings: Annual Convention American Association of Bovine Practitioners*, 15:74-78, 1983.

Divers TJ: Assessment of the urinary system in physical examination, *Vet Clin North Am* 8:373-382, 1992.

Divers TJ, Crowell WA, Duncan JR, et al: Acute renal disorders in cattle: a retrospective study of 22 cases, *J Am Vet Med Assoc* 181:694-699, 1982.

Divers TJ, Reef VB, Roby KA: Nephrolithiasis resulting in intermittent ureteral obstruction in a cow, *Cornell Vet* 79:143-149, 1989.

Donecker JM, Bellamy JE: C. Blood chemical abnormalities in cattle with ruptured bladders and ruptured ureters, *Can Vet J* 23:355-357, 1982.

Ducharme NG, Stein ES III: Eversion of the urinary bladder in a cow, *J Am Vet Med Assoc* 179:996-998, 1981.

Flock M: Ultrasonic diagnosis of inflammation of the umbilical cord structures, persistent urachus and umbilical hernia in calves [article in German], *Berl Munch Tierarztl Wochenschr* 116:2-11, 2003.

Flock M: Sonographic application in the diagnosis of pyelonephritis in cattle, *Vet Radiol Ultrasound* 48(1):74-77, 2007.

Franz S, Winter P, Baumgartner W: Cystoscopy in cattle a valuable additional tool for clinical examination, *Acta Vet Hung* 52:423-438, 2004.

Hammer EJ, Divers TJ, Tulleners EP: Nephrectomy for treatment of ectopic ureter in a Holstein calf, *Bov Pract* 34:101-103, 2000.

Johnson R, Jamison K: Amyloidosis in six dairy cows, *J Am Vet Med Assoc* 185:1538-1543, 1984.

Morse EV: *A study of Corynebacterium renale and penicillin therapy in the treatment of specific pyelonephritis of cattle*, MS Thesis, Ithaca, NY, 1948, Cornell University.

Mueller PO, Hay WP, Allen D, et al: Removal of an actopic left kidney through a ventral midline celiotomy in a calf, *J Am Vet Med Assoc* 214:532-534, 496, 1999.

Rebhun WC, Dill SG, Perdrizet JA, et al: Pyelonephritis in cattle: 15 cases (1982-1986), *J Am Vet Med Assoc* 194:953-955, 1989.

Trent AM, Smith DF: Pollakiuria due to urachal abscesses in two heifers, *J Am Vet Med Assoc* 184:984-986, 1984.

Tulleners EP, Deem DA, Donawick WJ, et al: Indications for unilateral bovine nephrectomy: a report of four cases, *J Am Vet Med Assoc* 179:696-700, 1981.

Vaala WE, Ehnen SJ, Divers TJ: Acute renal failure associated with administration of excessive amounts of tetracycline in a cow, *J Am Vet Med Assoc* 191:1601-1603, 1987.

Wiseman A, Spencer A, Petrie L: The nephrotic syndrome in a heifer due to glomerulonephritis, *Res Vet Sci* 28:325-329, 1980.

Yamada M, Kotani Y, Nakamura K, et al: Immunohistochemical distribution of amyloid deposits in 25 cows diagnosed with systemic AA amyloidosis, *J Vet Med Sci* 68:725-729, 2006.

Yeruham I, Elad D, Avidar Y, et al: A herd level analysis of urinary tract infection in dairy cattle. *Vet J*, 171:172-176, 2006.

CHAPTER 11

Musculoskeletal Disorders

Charles Guard

DIGITAL LAMENESS—LESIONS AND TREATMENTS

Throughout this section on therapy of hoof diseases, reference will be made to functional hoof trimming. This refers to the method developed and promoted by the Dutch veterinarian Toussaint Raven and described fully in his excellent book *Cattle Hoof Care and Claw Trimming*. Toes are cut to 75 mm or 3 in as measured along the dorsal wall from the point near the coronet where the wall becomes hard (this measurement may be increased 3 mm for each 75 kg over 750 kg, or $^1/_8$ in for every 150 lb over 1600 lb). Following this cut, a wedge of sole and wall are removed that is thickest at the toe and tapers toward the heel. The toe thickness is maintained at 5 mm or $^1/_4$ in at the tip where the first cut was made. These dimensions preserve adequate sole thickness (5 mm) at the toe tip to prevent bruising. The heel of the taller claw is trimmed to balance the weight bearing between the two digits. To complete the job, the sole is dished along the axial border of both digits from the heel-sole junction to the point where the axial wall and white line are evident. This is usually between one third and one half the length of the sole.

General principles of therapy for digital diseases are to eliminate the pain first and foremost and then to correct the underlying problem if possible. Hoof horn that is detached from underlying layers of hoof or corium should be removed. Around areas of exposed corium the wall or sole should be thinned to make the existing hoof capsule more flexible along the border of newly developing cornified epithelium. Bandages do not promote healing but may be used to control hemorrhage or to maintain some antibiotic or antiseptic in contact with a wound. Regardless of original intent, most bandages should be removed in a few days and the lesion left uncovered. Hoof blocks are an essential tool for managing painful conditions, and their use should be routine (Figure 11-1). Nonsteroidal antiinflammatory drugs (NSAIDs) such as flunixin and ketoprofen (although the latter is not approved for use in dairy cattle in the United States) should be considered to reduce the pain of some severe claw horn diseases and following surgery of the digit. Their use is not encouraged enough by most veterinary practitioners.

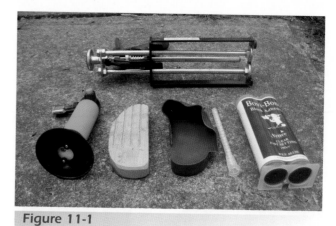

Figure 11-1

Polyurethane hoof block adhesive, two types of blocks, and a heat gun for drying the hoof surface.

Basic tools for lame cow therapy include left and right hoof knives and small hoof nippers. Additional tools that are in wide use are long-handled hoof nippers and electric angle grinders with carbide-toothed chipper wheels. There is a wide variety of restraint devices present on farms, and still some farms have nothing. Practitioners should encourage every client to have a safe and efficient place or device for lameness work because every herd will have lame cows, and most practitioners, at least in the United States, do not travel with a trimming chute to every call. Because most lameness occurs in the rear feet, simple devices for small herds should be made available to make rear limb lifting and examination easy. Examples are illustrated in Figure 11-2, *A* to *C*.

Simple Overgrowth

Although not a painful condition itself, overgrowth is considered a predisposing cause of hoof horn lesions and is often present in lame cows with painful lesions. The practitioner should trim such hooves to normal conformation when treating lameness. The practitioner should also be aware of the general condition of hoof overgrowth in a herd to advise on the need for maintenance trimming.

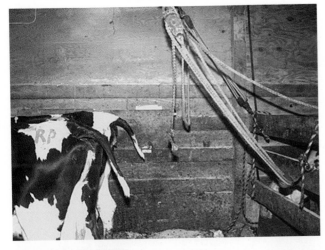

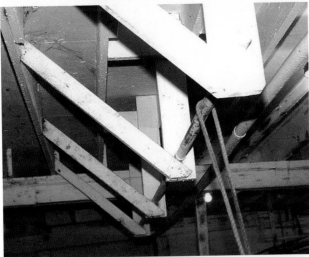

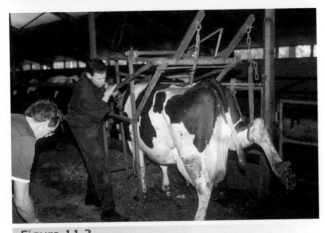

Figure 11-2

A to C, Simple devices that can provide adequate restraint and support for hoof work on rear limbs.

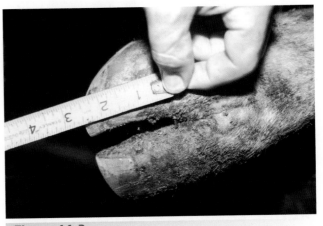

Figure 11-3

Toe length of 2.5 in, in a herd with severe overwear as a result of abrasive sand used as bedding combined with steeply sloped travel lanes. Normal length after trimming is 3 in.

(Figure 11-3). There may be no other hoof diseases, but the lameness caused by subsolar bruising or exposure of the corium at the white line can be very painful. Individual animal treatment is to apply hoof blocks to allow regrowth of the overworn sole. Some hoof trimmers have suggested placing a layer of hoof block adhesive on the sole to increase its thickness and to reduce wear of the horny tissue. As a herd problem, environmental modification is indicated, which usually means installing rubber in the holding pen and travel lanes to and from the free stall pens.

White Line Abscess

The most common location is in the posterior third of the white line of the rear lateral claw. The presence of this lesion may be detected with the response to finger pressure on the bulb of the heel of the affected digit. If the abscess is near the toe tip, it may be necessary to apply pressure with hoof testers to identify the location. In the forelimbs, the most common site is the posterior quarter of the medial claw. Usually white line abscesses are obvious after a thin layer of horn has been removed. There often is dark discoloration of a portion of the white line (Figure 11-4). Sometimes the white line is fissured with manure packed into the resulting crevice, which must be cleaned before the specific site of the abscess becomes visible. Relieving the pressure within the abscess provides some immediate pain relief. Abscesses near the heel may dissect between layers of sole horn to exit at the heel, resulting in a transverse flap of detached horn. Much less frequently than in the horse, abscesses under the wall may erupt at the coronary band. Treatment is to remove the detached horn and trim to allow walking without pressure on the inflamed corium. Large abscesses and those at the toe tip will benefit from the use of a hoof

Overwear, Thin Soles

Increasingly in large confinement dairies where cows walk long distances to and from the milking parlor and in some moderate-sized dairies using sand bedding, hooves wear away faster than new hoof is produced

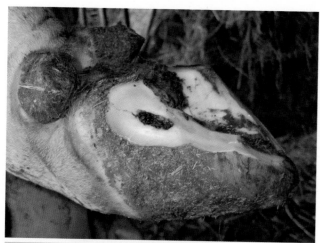

Figure 11-4

White line abscess near the heel of the lateral claw. The heel of this claw was further trimmed to remove weight bearing from this portion of the digit.

block on the healthy digit (Figures 11-5 and 11-6). Bandaging is discouraged. Most cows recover uneventfully, and reexamination is not necessary. Hoof blocks should be removed in about 4 weeks. Occasionally white line abscesses will extend into the soft tissue structures of the digital cushion and involve structures posterior to the distal interphalangeal joint. These conditions require surgical intervention that is described later.

Sole Ulcer

Ulceration of the sole may occur in any digit but is most common in the lateral claws of the rear feet and the medial claws of the forelimbs. Symmetrical ulcers occur

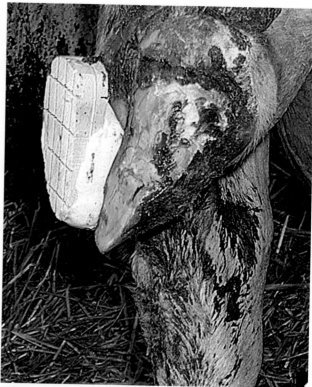

Figure 11-6

Same cow as Figure 11-5 after further trimming. No bandage was used in the therapy.

in both rear limbs or both forelimbs. The typical site for ulceration is in the corium that overlies the flexor process of the third phalanx (Figure 11-7). Ulceration at the toe tip is a less common lesion in housed cattle but the most common lesion in extensive grazing dairies of

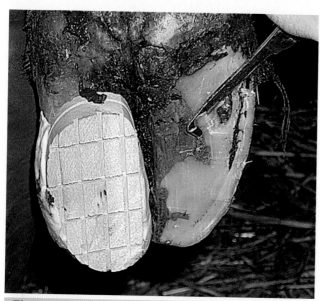

Figure 11-5

White line abscess in the lateral claw.

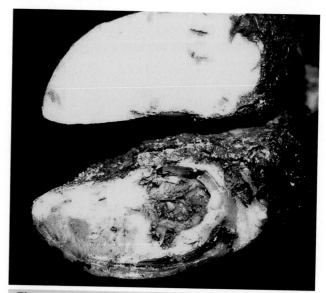

Figure 11-7

Sole ulcer in the typical site in the lateral claw superficial to the flexor tuberosity of P3.

the southern hemisphere. When it occurs in housed cattle, it is thought to be caused by either overtrimming at the toe or from wear that exceeds growth. A third location of ulceration is at the heel-sole junction. This may occur secondary to severe interdigital dermatitis or, as is usually seen in the medial claw of the rear foot, from unknown causes. The degree of damage to the sole and underlying corium varies from slight hemorrhage visible at trimming to complete absence of a portion of the sole to extensive necrosis of the underlying corium. The term complicated sole ulcer is used for those that have necrosis extending beyond the corium to include other tissues in the hoof.

Treatment for sole ulcer is to remove weight bearing from the affected portion of the digit. Depending on the location of the lesion and its severity, this may be accomplished by corrective trimming and lowering the heel horn of the affected claw. Most often a hoof block is applied to the healthy claw. If the ulcer is in the typical site or at the heel and there is sufficient heel depth of the healthy toe, a "heelless" trimming method may be used. This method, described by a Japanese hoof trimmer H. Manabe, is to remove all wall and sole from the posterior half of the digit to a depth that just preserves a thin layer of sole. When the cow stands, there should be space for a finger between the floor and the remaining portion of the affected area. The use of this technique eliminates the need for a block but is always dependent on the cow having sufficient heel depth on the healthy digit. Bandaging is discouraged. If the corium is intact, the swelling that is usually present throughout the posterior portion of the digit, including protrusion of the coronary corium, will usually subside within a few days. Reexamination in about 4 weeks is recommended to check the integrity of the hoof block and to trim the sole horn adjacent to the original lesion. Healing time for full-thickness sole ulcers is about 2 months. Reoccurrence in subsequent lactations is likely. Complicated sole ulcers require surgical intervention that is described later.

Toe Ulcer, Toe Necrosis

This condition results from overwear or overtrimming at the toe tip. The resulting thin sole at the tip is more susceptible to deformation from stepping on stones or irregular features of the flooring. If a hematoma results at the toe tip, it may lead to avascular necrosis of the soft tissues at the toe tip (Figure 11-8). If the lesion is open to the environment, miscellaneous bacteria may invade and produce osteomyelitis or pathologic fracture of the tip of the third phalanx (Figure 11-9). Conservative therapy with a hoof block and cleaning of the toe tip usually results in a chronic state of infection and mild pain. Our current approach to this problem is to place a hoof block on the sound digit and amputate the distal portion of the affected digit. Either obstetrical wire or hoof nippers may

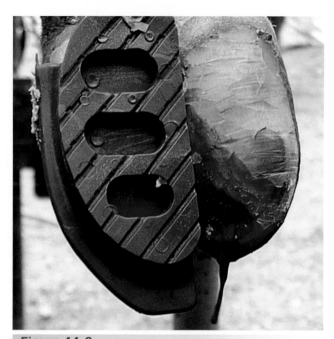

Figure 11-8

Toe ulcer in a heifer from an extensively grazed dairy in Uruguay.

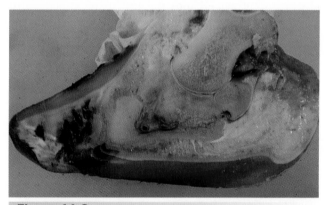

Figure 11-9

Sagittal section of amputated digit illustrating common changes at the apex of P3 and the remodeling of the associated hoof in chronic toe necrosis.

be used to remove slices of the affected digit until all tissue exposed appears healthy (Figure 11-10). A tight bandage is applied over some antibiotic powder to control hemorrhage. The bandage is removed in a few days. There is no need for parenteral antibiotics. Regrowth of functional cornified epithelium will cover the partial amputation in about 1 month. The prognosis is excellent.

Thimbling or Transverse Wall Separation

This condition results from an insult to the coronary corium that results in an interruption in growth and resulting break in continuity of the horn tubules of the hoof wall. It is not apparent until the hoof has grown

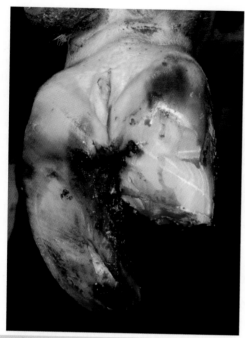

Figure 11-10

Partial toe amputation for toe necrosis. The hoof and all internal structures are resected until only healthy tissue remains.

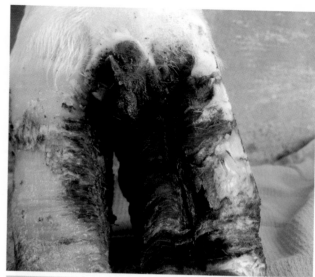

Figure 11-11

Vertical wall crack in a mature dairy cow.

sufficiently for the break point to be about 5 cm from the coronary band. It is always present in all eight digits but usually noticed because of pain in only one. The distal portion of the hoof capsule separates from the more proximal section along the entire axial, dorsal, and abaxial regions. The sole is normally attached to the younger healthy wall and the older detached wall. Pain occurs when movement of the distal portion relative to the rest of the hoof pinches the corium at the toe tip. The goals of trimming are to minimize weight bearing at the toe tip by shortening as much as possible and thinning the sole at the toe relative to the rest of the hoof. Pain may shift from one limb to another as successive thimbles become more detached from the younger hoof wall. Recovery is complete and without complications as the thimbles wear or are trimmed away.

Vertical Wall Cracks or Sand Cracks

Cracks in the dorsal or lateral hoof wall that extend from the coronary band distally are much more common in range cattle than in dairy cattle but do rarely occur (Figure 11-11). It is important to verify that the crack is the cause of lameness before proceeding. If the crack is causing pain, it should be carefully debrided of foreign material. There may be exposed corium or granulation tissue. Care must be taken to not extend the hoof wall defect during trimming. Removing granulation tissue may be necessary, followed by controlling hemorrhage and protecting the healing corium from

damage. Standard procedure is to stabilize the adjacent portions of the hoof wall with acrylic and to place a block on the sound claw.

Vertical cracks in the axial wall are more common in dairy cattle although far less frequently seen than ulcers and white line abscesses. The strategy of treatment is similar to that used in range cattle, although acrylic is less often used (Figure 11-12). The greatest challenge to treatment of the axial wall cracks is to visualize and trim affected tissues in the interdigital space. Separated or detached horn should be removed, granulation tissue resected, and a tight bandage with antibiotic powder, usually tetracycline, applied. The tight bandage is to help prevent the formation of granulation tissue. A hoof block is applied to the healthy digit. Several visits may be required at about 1-week intervals to achieve healing.

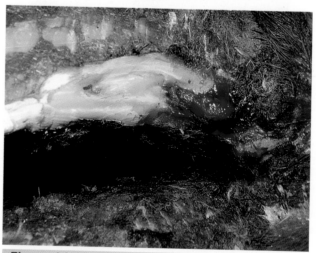

Figure 11-12

Axial wall crack in a yearling dairy heifer.

Corkscrew Claw, Splayed Toes— Inherited Defects

The appearance of corkscrew claws, although inherited, does not become evident until the cow reaches 3 or more years old. Both lateral rear digits, both medial fore digits, or all four may be affected. The entire configuration of the third phalanx, the soft tissues between the claw capsule and bone, and the claw capsule are abnormal. The external appearance is of a hoof that is rotating around an axis perpendicular to the articulation of the third phalanx. The abaxial wall develops a curvature that extends the wall into the normal location of the sole. The axial wall becomes dorsal, and the tip of the toe curls up from the ground (Figure 11-13). This conformation creates a mild predisposition to lameness but of more importance is the technique required for routine trimming to prevent exposure of the corium. The toe tip should be trimmed slightly longer than normal. Removal of the overgrowth of the abaxial wall can return weight bearing to the sole and wall in a flat plane. Care must be taken near the toe tip because the corium is abnormally close to the exterior, about one fourth of the distance from the toe tip to heel. Thus the toe tip should be left about 1 cm thick. Exaggerated dishing of the axial margin of the sole may prolong the time until the next trimming is needed.

Splayed toes is primarily a condition of beef cattle, which predisposes to interdigital fibroma and will not be further considered here.

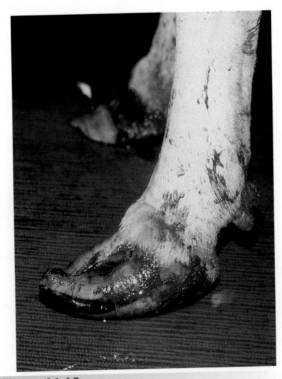

Figure 11-13

Corkscrew claw in a Holstein cow.

Traumatic Exungulation

Cows may get a toe caught in a manure grate or floor slot and detach the horny capsule of a claw while extricating themselves. If the corium is not badly damaged and the condition treated as an emergency, regrowth of a new, nearly normal claw capsule can occur. It is important to clean and disinfect the exposed tissues and bandage with a tissue-friendly antiseptic. A hoof block is necessary on the healthy digit, and parenteral antibiotics are recommended for 7 to 10 days. The limitations to recovery seem to depend on the degree of trauma to the soft tissues. If it is apparent that the corium or deeper structures are significantly damaged, then amputation or slaughter should be chosen.

Fracture of the Third Phalanx (P3)

This injury may occur in cattle of any age or size. In a hospital population, it is observed primarily in dairy bulls, but others report that young cattle and young milking cows are predisposed. Excessive dryness of the hoof, leading to reduced cushioning of routine weight bearing, or hoof trauma may predispose to P3 fracture. Trauma from a hoof becoming stuck in a floor slot may result in fracture (Figure 11-14). The incidence of P3 fractures may be increased when fluorine toxicity exists in a herd. Hoof trauma resulting from blunt injury or falling to the ground following mounting a cow also is a suspected cause of P3 fractures.

Acute severe lameness with no weight bearing in the affected limb is observed. Careful local examination frequently reveals warmth in the affected digit, and flexion of the hoof, hoof tester pressure, and percussion all elicit a painful response from the affected animal. If one digit is affected, the cow will attempt to touch the foot down only on the nonaffected digit, if at all, when forced to walk. Occasional bilateral fractures of the medial P3 in the forelimbs have been described wherein

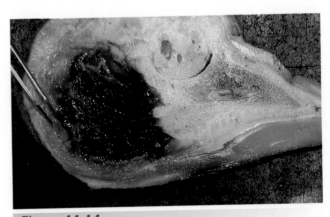

Figure 11-14

Fracture of the flexor process of P3 and hematoma in the heel region.

affected cattle stand with the forelimbs crossed in an effort to bear all weight on the nonaffected lateral claws. Bilaterally affected cattle may refuse to rise on their front feet and rest on their knees, similar to laminitis patients.

The diagnosis is confirmed by radiographs following elimination of more common causes of lameness through examination and paring of the affected claw. Acute laminitis is the most common differential diagnosis in the absence of obvious hoof lesions when considering a fracture of P3. Radiographs should be taken from at least two views. In addition, lateral radiographs are best obtained by placing the film in the interdigital area such that only the affected digit is evaluated.

Resting the affected digit by use of a standard hoof block applied to the normal claw is the treatment of choice. The affected animal should be placed in a comfortable box stall and the block renewed as necessary during the 4 to 8 weeks required for healing. Based on the size of the animal (e.g., an adult bull compared with a yearling heifer) and individual response to therapy, the exact recuperative time is difficult to predict. Response to therapy is usually good unless underlying nutritional deficiencies or fluorine toxicity exists. In the case of dairy bulls, the animal may require several additional weeks of sexual rest, lest the healing fracture be reinjured during dismounting a cow or an artificial insemination (AI) phantom.

Interdigital Fibroma

Redundant skin in the interdigital space is a hereditary condition associated with lax interdigital ligaments, resulting in a splay-toed conformation. It also occurs in cattle secondary to chronic interdigital dermatitis. By itself, it is not painful unless the fibroma becomes so large that the cow pinches it between the sole and floor when walking. However, fibromas predispose a risk of foot rot and are common sites of digital dermatitis in endemically infected herds. For most dairy cattle, fibromas occur secondary to interdigital dermatitis and should not be treated as a specific problem but as a reflection of the poor management of hygiene or foot bathing (Figure 11-15). There exists some pressure from farmers on veterinarians and hoof trimmers to remove fibromas as part of routine procedures, and this should be discouraged. Rather, the underlying causal factors should be addressed.

If the fibroma is a part of a significant painful process in a cow, then surgical removal is indicated. Anesthesia is discussed in the section on digit surgery. Sharp dissection of the skin around the base of the fibroma follows normal surgical site preparation. It is considered important for prompt healing to remove the interdigital fat and the protruding fibroma. Care must be taken to prevent surgical injury to the distal interphalangeal joint capsule and the cruciate ligaments when removing the

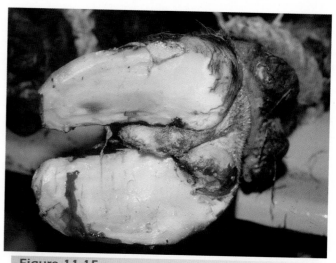

Figure 11-15

Interdigital fibroma in a bull.

fat. Some antibiotic powder may be placed in the wound, but no dressings or packings should be used before bandaging the foot to prevent splaying of the toes. The bandage may be removed in a few days because granulation tissue will fill the defect. Systemic antibiotics are optional.

Foot Rot or Interdigital Phlegmon

Recognition of this acute disease is straightforward. The bacterial causes are *Fusobacterium necrophorum* and *Bacteroides melaninogenicus,* with both required for disease to occur. There may be other important bacterial contributors from the genus *Prevotella.* The cow becomes lame over the course of a day or two with symmetrical swelling above the hoof. Pain may be severe with unwillingness to bear any weight on the affected limb. Rear limbs are more commonly affected. There is a fissure in the interdigital skin with necrosis of the underlying tissues (Figure 11-16). Usually this is a dry necrosis with no exudate, but some very virulent strains of *F. necrophorum* may produce tissue liquefaction. The odor of foot rot is strong and characteristic. Corrective claw trimming may be used along with some topical antiseptic to the interdigital space. Bandaging is strongly discouraged so that air may reach the interdigital tissues. Parenteral antibiotics are the most important part of therapy. For almost all cases of foot rot, many antibiotics are effective and the choice is unimportant. In the United States, as of this writing, ceftiofur is registered for foot rot and requires no milk discard. There are cases of foot rot caused by multiple drug-resistant *F. necrophorum.* Trial and error has determined that these cases respond to treatment with tylosin at label-recommended dosages. Recognition of the presence of drug-resistant strains in a herd comes after treatment failure with the usual choice of antibiotic. It is important to verify that

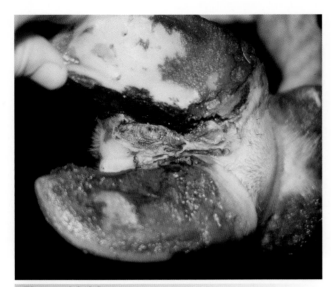

Figure 11-16

Necrosis of interdigital soft tissues in a cow with foot rot.

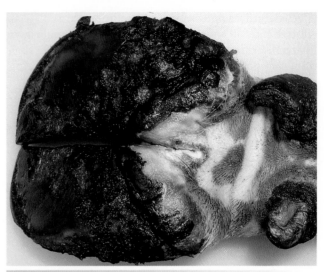

Figure 11-17

Eroded and roughened heels and slight hypertrophy around the interdigital cleft as a result of chronic interdigital dermatitis.

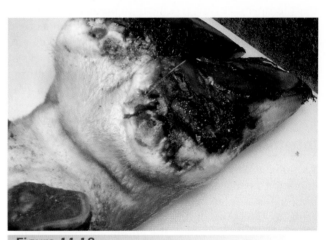

Figure 11-18

Scalloped layers of heel horn typical of heel horn erosion.

the disease problem is foot rot because many cases are diagnosed and treated by farmers or their employees. If the original problem was a sole ulcer, changing antibiotics will not help.

Interdigital Dermatitis, Heel Horn Erosion, and Heel Cracks

Chronic interdigital dermatitis caused by infection with *Dichelobacter nodosus* is very common in cattle that live in moist environments. The presence of infection may be detected in subclinically affected cattle by nonpainful erosion or ulceration of the interdigital skin (Figures 11-17 and 11-18). There is usually a moist, white exudate with a characteristic odor distinct from that of foot rot. The infection produces a mild irritation that results in underlying skin hypertrophy and may produce a faster growth rate of the adjacent axial hoof wall. Skin hypertrophy may result in an interdigital fibroma as discussed earlier or excessive horn accumulation along the axial wall. The axial wall may flare toward the interdigital space or cause an abnormally high region in the adjacent sole. Corrective trimming should remove all the excessive horn and open the interdigital space so that it is more self-cleaning and more accessible to air. If the infection spreads across the heels, it may erode the horny portion of the heel in irregular patterns or create a transverse crack at the heel-sole junction. *D. nodosus* produces proteases that are capable of digesting the keratin of hoof tissues.

Lameness results from interdigital dermatitis when the cracks in the heel combined with hypertrophy of heel bulb skin change the weight distribution to increase pressure on the heel. The discontinuity of tissues from sole to heel may also result in pinching of sensitive tissues beneath the crack. Cows are not usually severely lame but

may stand with their heel suspended over the manure gutter or off the rear of a free stall curb. Usually the problem is symmetrical in both limbs. Rarely a crack at the heel-sole junction penetrates to expose the corium. Treatment for these heel cracks is to remove the flaps of overlying horn and open the enclosed spaces to air. A hoof block is indicated in the rare cases of exposure of the corium. Topical disinfectants such as iodines or copper or zinc solutions are all effective in killing *D. nodosus*.

Digital Dermatitis, Mortellaro, or Heel Wart

The condition goes by the name of hairy heel warts, strawberry foot, verrucous dermatitis, digital warts, interdigital papillomatosis, and probably most correctly digital dermatitis (or papular digital dermatitis). Since

1994 the disease has developed to epidemic proportions in most of Europe and spread throughout the United States. One wonders why a disease that was reported originally in 1974 suddenly spread worldwide in dairy cattle in the past few years. Currently researchers are still trying to define the specific cause(s); several strains of spirochete bacteria of the genus *Treponema* are believed to be responsible for the disease. Histological specimens of lesions stained with silver that demonstrate spirochetes reveal their presence in great numbers throughout the stratum spinosum of the dermis.

The earliest lesion recognizable as digital dermatitis is a reddened circumscribed area typically just above the interdigital cleft on the plantar aspect of the pastern, the strawberry form of digital dermatitis. The most striking feature of the lesion is the degree of pain expressed by the cow (Figure 11-19). Hairs at the periphery of the lesion are often erect and matted in exudate to form a rim. As the lesion progresses, focal hypertrophy of the dermis and epidermis leads to raised conical projections appearing much like wet, grey terrycloth. In even later stages, papilliform projections of blackened keratin may extend 10 to 15 mm from the surface, the hairy wart stage. Typical lesions may be seen affecting any of the limbs, but rear limbs are more commonly involved. The location and extent of affected skin are variable and include interdigital skin, anterior and posterior margins of the interdigital cleft, and distinct lesions that do not touch the coronary band. Many cows have simultaneous infection with *D. nodosus*, leading to significant erosion of the horn of the heels in a hemispherical pattern surrounding the axial space (Figure 11-20). The hoof may be noticeably misshapen from abnormal wear caused by the altered use of the limb, resulting in short rounded toes and exaggerated heel depth. Interdigital fibromas, regardless of etiology, are commonly infected with digital dermatitis in endemic herds. In our experience, after digital dermatitis has been present in a herd for a year or so, most cases of

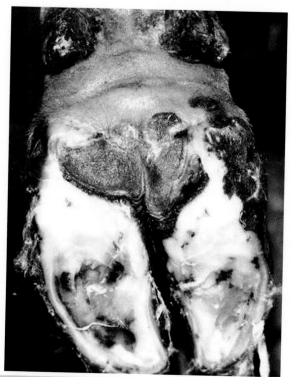

Figure 11-20

Digital dermatitis lesion at the skin-heel horn junction with erosion of heel horn and extension of the digital dermatitis into the solar region.

lameness are found in the first-lactation animals even though lesions may be seen on the digits of older cows during routine hoof trimming (Figure 11-21).

We recommend topical treatment of lame cows with oxytetracycline in the form of 5 to 15 cc of injectable 10% oxytetracycline applied on a cotton dressing with a flimsy wrap. Others use tetracycline powder under some form of bandage with or without a cotton pad. We have

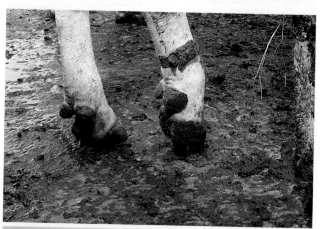

Figure 11-19

Typical posture of a cow with digital dermatitis affecting the plantar surface of the pastern region.

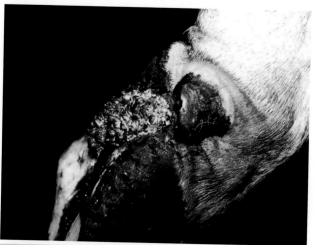

Figure 11-21

Chronic, proliferative lesion caused by digital dermatitis.

examined many of these cows after 2 to 5 days and have been amazed at the regression of the lesion and complete elimination of pain. Because the response is so rapid, we use less and less of a bandage so that the cotton will fall off in a few days. Reoccurrence in the same cow and even in the same location is common. Some cows in an endemic herd never develop lesions. However, all cows in endemic herds will have antibodies to at least two species of treponemes. Autogenous and commercial vaccines have come and gone with none proving efficacious in preventing the development of lesions. An apparently related skin disorder is udder cleft dermatitis on the ventral midline at the attachment of the fore udder. Histologically this lesion is undistinguishable from digital dermatitis, including the presence of spirochetes throughout the epidermis.

Deep Sepsis of the Digit

Untreated or late-treated foot rot, complicated sole ulcer, white line abscess that extends into retroarticular structures, and puncture wounds may all result in necrosis and/or infection of structures important for weight bearing. These problems have in common severe pain that is not relieved by hoof blocks or analgesic medication. Specific diagnosis of the problem may be aided by using a probe to explore fistulous tracts or by inserting a hypodermic needle (14 or 16 gauge) into joints or tendon sheaths but rarely requires radiography (Figure 11-22). Cows suffering from deep sepsis are truly suffering, and a decision should be made at the first recognition of this

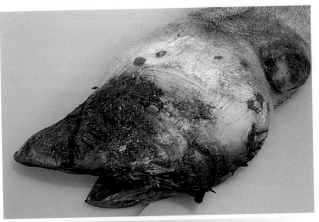

Figure 11-23

Chronic deep sepsis of the digit. Note several fistulous tracts and the upward tilt of the affected digit. Destruction of the deep flexor tendon or its attachment to P3 allows the toe to tip up. This slaughterhouse specimen showed no evidence of attempts at useful therapy.

problem to euthanize, slaughter, or perform surgery. Too many cases receive no treatment or systemic antibiotics in the hope that the problem will somehow resolve spontaneously (Figure 11-23). These cows deserve a more humane approach.

Surgery of the Digit

Anesthesia is most easily performed by intravenous infiltration of lidocaine distal to a tourniquet on the metatarsus or metacarpus. Lidocaine without epinephrine, 20 to 30 ml, is infused using a butterfly catheter (19 gauge, 15 to 25 cm) (Figure 11-24). Any accessible vein will result in complete anesthesia of both digits

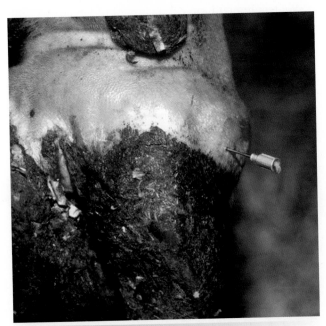

Figure 11-22

Demonstration of pus in the distal interphalangeal joint. The joint capsule enlarges and bulges proximal to the coronary band when the joint is septic.

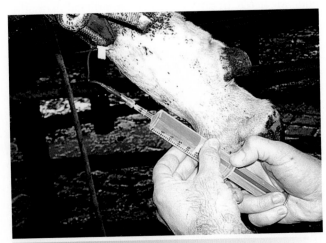

Figure 11-24

Intravenous regional anesthesia with lidocaine injected into the common dorsal digital vein. A butterfly catheter is easier to maintain in the vein than a needle and syringe alone.

after a few minutes. If no vein can be found, regional perfusion above the intended surgical site is an alternative. The distal limb is scrubbed and disinfected as for any surgery but usually not shaven because the hair is typically very short or absent. Surgical procedures are commonly done in the field and are considered "clean" procedures but not sterile. The goal is to debride necrotic tissues and provide drainage for pus and exudate. If a hoof block is to be used as part of the therapy, it should be attached before the surgery because adhesives require dry hoof to bond. Injecting the lidocaine followed by applying the block or scrubbing the area ensures adequate time for diffusion of the anesthetic to all tissues distal to the tourniquet.

Digit Amputation

Amputation of one digit at the proximal interphalangeal joint or just above is a common procedure in cattle practice. After preparation, a skin incision is made in the interdigital space and then beginning about 2 cm proximal to the interdigital cleft angling upward to a point on the lateral or medial side of the leg even with the distal margin of the accessory digit or dewclaw. All soft tissues can be sharply incised along the line of the skin incision. Obstetrical wire is then placed between the digits, and the distal end of the first phalanx is cut (Figure 11-25). If the cut misses this landmark and a portion of the second phalanx remains proximal to the cut, it should be

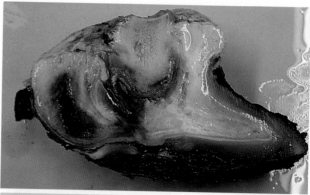

Figure 11-26

Digit amputated by disarticulation and cut sagittally illustrating sepsis of P2, P3, the navicular bone, and the deep flexor tendon.

removed. If the articular surface of the first phalanx is intact, it should be roughened with a knife. Alternatively, the digit may be amputated by sharp dissection to disarticulate the proximal interphalangeal joint (Figure 11-26). Some practitioners ligate one or two arteries, and others simply use a very tight bandage. The cut surface of the removed portion should be carefully examined for evidence of sepsis or necrosis. If damaged tissue extends above the amputation and it is not debrided, the outcome will be poor. After determining that all diseased tissue is removed, the surface of the wound is covered with an antiseptic or antibiotic dressing and a bandage applied to control hemorrhage. The bandage should be removed or changed in about 1 week if there was no need for maintaining drainage of septic regions proximal to the incision. If a tendon resection is performed, the bandage should be removed in 2 or 3 days. Depending on the environment in which the cow must live after surgery, either no bandage is placed after the first one is removed or a light wrap to minimize painful contact with environmental objects is used. Parenteral antibiotics are usually given for 5 days.

Flexor Tendon Resection

If, after amputation, it is evident that sepsis extends proximally along the deep flexor tendon, it should be resected. A 3-cm incision parallel to the path of the tendon is made over the affected branch of the flexor tendons beginning just proximal to the accessory digit. There is strong fascia surrounding the sheath of the combined superficial and deep flexor tendons. In fact, the superficial flexor tendon forms a tube around the deep at this level. Sharp dissection oriented along the skin incision through the superficial flexor tendon will reveal the deep flexor tendon. The deep flexor tendon is grasped with a strong instrument such as a dental extractor or exteriorized with the aid of curved hemostats (Figure 11-27). There may be adhesions of the deep

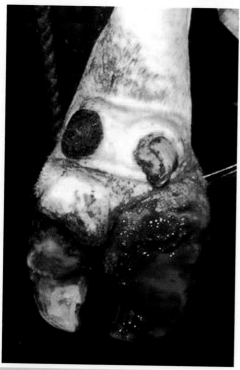

Figure 11-25

Amputation of a digit with a wire saw.

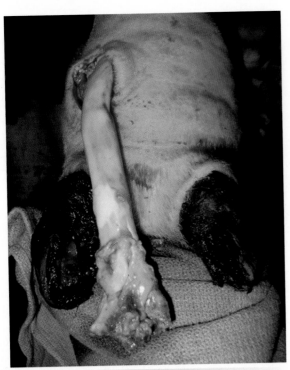

Figure 11-27

Deep flexor tendon with severe inflammation at the distal end resected through an incision above the corresponding accessory digit. A surgical drain was placed in the space left by removal of the tendon and the proximal incision closed with sutures.

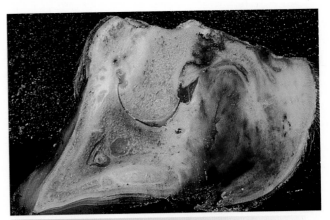

Figure 11-28

Retroarticular abscess in an amputated digit. Surgical debridement and drainage are alternatives to amputation.

flexor tendon to surrounding structures at the level of the distal transaction that require sharp dissection. In some cases, the tendon will simply be pulled to the outside from the proximal incision. The deep flexor tendon is transected at the most proximal exposed part, and surgical drainage tubing is placed through its original course to exit at the distal incision. It may be knotted into a loop or each end affixed by suture. One or two skin sutures are placed in the proximal incision. Systemic antibiotics are routinely given for 5 days. The drainage tubing is removed in 2 weeks.

Retroarticular Abscess

White line abscesses near the heel, penetrating foreign bodies, and deep flexor tendon avulsion or fracture of the flexor process of the P3 all may result in severe lameness with extensive painful swelling of the heel region of a single digit (Figure 11-28). Following anesthesia and standard surgical preparation, an incision is made into the heel bulb. The choices are a vertical incision extending into the sole (after paring away enough sole at the heel so that it is thin enough to make an incision with ordinary surgical instruments) or a transverse incision in the middle portion of the cornified heel. Exploration of the cavity encountered will dictate further steps. If the limits of the

abscess or hematoma do not involve the navicular bursa or deep flexor tendon, the prognosis is excellent and resolution should be prompt. The cavity is flushed with water and mild disinfectant such as povidone iodine. A surgical drain is inserted in the wound and affixed with sutures. Antibiotic powder is placed in the cavity, and the incision is closed with a few skin sutures. A hoof block should be placed on the healthy digit. If the condition resulted from mechanical disruption of the deep flexor tendon or an avulsion fracture of P3, there is risk of involvement of the navicular bone and bursa. If no sepsis is evident, the outcome should be satisfactory. The cow will probably need the hoof block renewed in 1 month, but no further treatment is necessary.

Septic Distal Interphalangeal Joint

When the distal interphalangeal joint is septic, there is enlargement of the joint space and distention of the joint capsule. This may be observed as painful swelling at the coronary band in the caudal third of the abaxial coronet. It is possible to insert a needle into the joint capsule through the coronary band to verify the nature of the joint contents. In those cases when there is no swelling of the heel or deep flexor tendon, a simple fenestration of the joint may result in a satisfactory cure following ankylosis of the joint. The most common means of this sepsis occurring are secondary to foot rot or to a complicated sole ulcer. In either case, after anesthesia and cleaning the sole, if it is intact, a 7- to 12-mm (³/₈ to ½ in) drill is used to fenestrate the joint. Beginning in the typical site for sole ulcer, the drill is directed in a sagittal plane to exit the digit just at the coronary band on the dorsal surface (Figure 11-29). This will satisfactorily provide drainage of the joint. Surgical tubing or braided nylon rope is passed through the drilled hole and tied around the abaxial side of the hoof (Figure 11-30). A block is placed on the healthy digit, and systemic antibiotics are given for

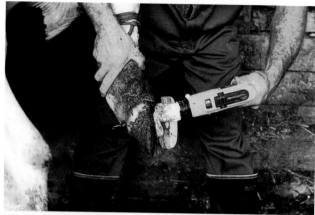

Figure 11-29

Fenestration of the distal interphalangeal joint with a drill to provide drainage and facilitate ankylosis of the joint.

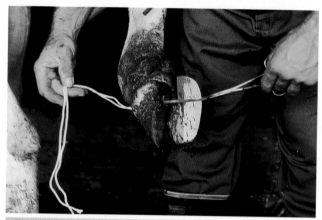

Figure 11-30

Nylon cord placed through the drilled hole to maintain drainage. The cord is removed in 2 weeks.

5 days. The drain is removed in 2 weeks. Full ankylosis requires several months, but the cow will usually be sound without a block in 1 month.

Extensive Deep Sepsis of the Digit

Amputation is an acceptable therapy for extensive deep sepsis of the digit. However, claw-sparing procedures have been adapted for field use and provide excellent results. We have combined the transverse heel incision (Figure 11-31) described above with drilling through the distal interphalangeal joint, navicular bone resection, and deep flexor tendon resection to resolve some extensive problems with deep sepsis. A hoof block should be applied before beginning surgery. The approach is as for retroarticular abscess but includes incising deeply just proximal to the navicular bone. This will transect the deep flexor tendon if it is still intact. Through the same skin incision, a more distally directed incision is made

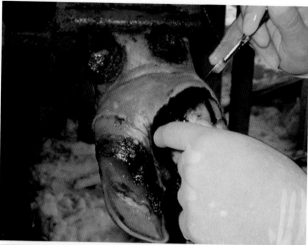

Figure 11-31

Initial incision across the heel bulb for exploration of a digit with deep sepsis.

to cut the distal attachments of the navicular bone and remove a wedge of tissue. In some cases, the navicular bone and its attachments are so necrotic that it has already disappeared or is easily removed through this incision, allowing visualization of the distal interphalangeal joint (Figure 11-32). If the collateral ligaments are intact and difficult to incise, use a 5-mm ($\frac{1}{4}$ in) drill to make a hole in the center of the navicular bone. Insert a stout metal rod or screwdriver into this hole to fracture the bone into two pieces. Each piece can then be grasped and twisted to rupture any remaining attachments. A useful inexpensive tool for this procedure is a canine dental extractor. If the flexor tendon is necrotic or septic, it should be resected as described above. Use a 7- to 12-mm ($\frac{3}{8}$ to $\frac{1}{2}$ in) drill to fenestrate the distal interphalangeal joint through the incision. To exit at the

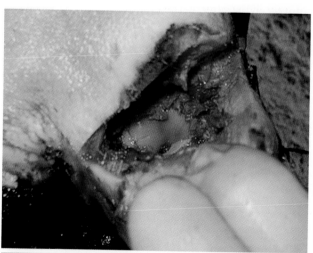

Figure 11-32

Visualization of the distal interphalangeal joint after removal of the navicular bone.

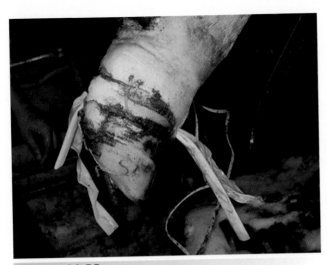

Figure 11-33

Drains placed through the distal interphalangeal joint after drilling through the incision made in Figure 11-31. Drains are removed in 2 weeks.

coronary band it will be necessary to overextend the distal interphalangeal joint. Surgery tubing should be placed through the joint and secured in a loop around the axial side (Figure 11-33). If tendon was resected a drain should be placed there as well. If there was an existing fistula that is not connected to the transverse heel incision, it should also have a surgical drain. Once all drains are in place, antibiotic powder is placed in the heel incision, and the incisions are closed with a few skin sutures. Parenteral antibiotics should be given for 5 days, and all drains should be removed in 2 weeks. We do not recommend wiring the toes of the two digits together as is done by others. The intended ankylosis of the distal interphalangeal joint will proceed more quickly if there is no motion in the joint. If the digits are fastened together, every step will cause motion of the joint receiving surgery. The block may need replacement at 1 month.

FUNCTIONAL ANATOMY OF CATTLE DIGITS: WHAT GOES WRONG THAT RESULTS IN LAMENESS

Introduction to Biomechanics

The structures of the bovine digit that support her body weight and work in normal locomotion can and do become diseased in predictable fashion. The bones, tendons, ligaments, corium, and hooves are all potentially involved when things go wrong. A better understanding of the biomechanical relationships in the digits of cattle can help with more rational therapeutics and appropriate preventive maintenance. The things that go wrong with the digits from a mechanical perspective are related

to the environmental influences of moisture, infection pressure, and standing surfaces. The distance walked and the characteristics of the substrate walked on also result in predictable problems. This section will describe the interplay between external forces and physiologic and pathologic events in the digits.

What we see as the current condition of the claws on any cow is a result of continuous growth, continuous wear, and intermittent trimming. The growth rate of hooves is relatively constant but subject to minor modifications. Nutrition can influence hoof growth rate. Hooves do not grow as fast during starvation as during adequate feeding. Because dairy cattle are never intentionally starved, this effect is unimportant. A small variation occurs during the lactation/gestation cycle and with season. The reports on this effect are difficult to interpret because the cattle described calved seasonally. In a study we conducted at Cornell on mid-lactation cows, growth rate was influenced by floor surface within the free stall pens. Cows grew hoof faster on concrete than rubber floors. The implication is that hoof growth can respond to environmental conditions by making more hoof when the standing or walking environment is more mechanically insulting. Typical growth rates are about 6 mm of hoof wall per month with variations caused by environment less than 10% of control rates. Wear rates are much more variable and depend on the abrasiveness of the walking surface and distance walked. Data are not available to compare the wear rates of dry versus wet hooves on the same walking surfaces.

Why do we see more disease in rear feet than fore? Why is there more disease in lateral rear claws than medial? The fore versus rear argument in dairy cattle has three components. The rear limbs of dairy cattle are forced to carry weight in excess of the original design criteria. The wild-type cow that gave us our modern dairy cows never had a large udder, even at calving. As geneticists have selected for more milk production, we do not think they have been able to simultaneously modify the musculoskeletal system to accommodate this extra weight at the rear of the cow. Second, the forelimbs are attached to the body by elastic components versus the direct bony connections in the rear limbs. Concussive forces created during locomotion must be absorbed by the digital cushion and the flexion of the hock and stifle. Third, rear feet are always more exposed to the bacteria and moisture of manure and urine. The skin near the hooves is more likely infected with bacteria as a result of maceration by this moisture, and the hoof capsule is softer because of greater hydration. The medial versus lateral argument is potentially more confusing. Lateral claws grow about 10% faster than medial claws and wear about 8% more in free stall-housed Holsteins. Thus lateral claws can progressively outgrow medial claws. They are larger even in fetal calves. Larger lateral claws are more heavily loaded than medial claws.

Larger loads result in more potential for mechanical insults. Cows may adopt a toed-out posture to help equilibrate the weight between the rear claws when overgrowth and some discomfort occur. This toed-out posture or being "cow hocked" can be used as an indicator of the need to trim an individual cow or by population evaluation to determine when a group or herd needs trimming.

Body weight is supported by the column of digital bones, resulting in the load being approximately evenly divided between the eight digits with normal claws and conformation. P3 is the end of these columns. The load on P3 is supported by several structures of importance in our concern for lameness. There are laminae in the mural corium that are tightly attached to lateral and cranial portions of P3 and that interdigitate with laminae in the hoof wall. These have less surface area of mutual contact per unit of supported weight than in the horse. Therefore the laminar region of the bovine digit, although very important, is not as significant as in the horse for support. There is also support of P3 by ligaments that suspend the caudal portion of the bone and blend with the interdigital cruciate ligaments axially and with the laminar corium abaxially. The tension of the deep flexor tendon on P3, in addition to fixing the bony column in a nearly vertical formation, pulls the distal tip of P3 ventrally and transfers some weight forward in the claw. Between P3 and the solar corium is a complex arrangement of fat deposits that cushion and distribute weight transferred to the sole. The fat pad is thickest at the heel and plays a dynamic role in cushioning during walking.

The structure of the horny capsule of the claw is different in different regions. Everyone who has trimmed a hoof knows this. The wall horn is the most rigid and hardest. It has the highest density of horn tubules that are arranged in parallel and develop from papillae in the coronary corium. The horn tubules are much less numerous in the sole, which makes it more flexible. The horn of the heel has the lowest density of horn tubules, and it is very pliable. The only nontubular horn of the claw is called cap horn and is produced at the distal ends of the laminae. It serves to cement the sole to the wall and is visually identified as the white line. This cap horn seems particularly vulnerable to the effects of laminitis. It may fail mechanically, allowing the wall and sole to separate, or fall out in portions of the white line, allowing entry of foreign matter. All of the horny tissue of the claw is able to absorb water. The higher the water content, the softer and more flexible is the horn. The most noticeable effect of continuous hydration of the claw is in the sole. The horn of the sole flakes away, leaving a concave surface and a relatively thin and consistent thickness of the sole when the hoof is dry most of the time. This occurs by slight contraction of the cells of the sole during desiccation and fracture along horizontal planes during walking. Under dry environmental conditions, the moisture within the sole is derived from the corium, which diffuses at a constant rate into the sole resulting in a constant thickness. In contrast, in free stall-housed cows, where slurry keeps the sole continuously moist, the sole does not flake away, and it must be worn or trimmed away.

When the events commonly known as laminitis occur, the vascular disturbance affects the corium of the laminae and the nonlaminar corium as well. The edema and resulting swelling reduce the ability of normal circulatory dynamics to oxygenate the corium. Some anoxic damage may occur. The mechanical properties of the corium that have suffered the distortion because of the edema and the biochemical changes as a result of anoxia can be altered with the result of lower tensile strength. As a consequence, P3 may move within the horny capsule beyond the limits occurring in healthy claws. With the exaggerated movement of P3, two specific lesions may develop. If P3 moves closer to the sole, abnormal pressure may cause further anoxic damage to the solar corium. If mild, this may appear as hemorrhage in the sole at a later trimming. If severe, the solar corium may die and result in a sole ulcer. In housed cattle, the ulcer is most common at the caudal portion of P3 in proximity to the flexor tuberosity where the subcorial fat pad is thin, and in extensively managed cattle it more often occurs under the distal portion of P3. The abnormal movement of P3 relative to the laminar corium may result in ruptured blood vessels that lead to hemorrhage. If the hemorrhage is very mild, it is later seen as a red line in the sole at the sole-wall junction or white line. If the hemorrhage is more extensive, it can result in a hematoma that later becomes either a sterile abscess or a septic abscess if the white line is separated and permits entry of environmental bacteria. Cattle that must make sharp turns on rough flooring may experience more white line lesions as a result of the lateral forces placed on the wall. During a turn, there may be claw deformation that can pull the wall from the corium or shear the corium if the structural integrity of the tissue is already compromised by edema.

It is important to note that the lesions of the corium that we recognize as and call laminitis require weight bearing during the period of primary damage to the corium. No one knows how long episodes of altered permeability and edema last following the chemical messengers from ruminal acidosis. However, if the cow did not stand during that period, there would be no mechanical damage to the corium. In the vast majority of cases, the lesions within the claw that we call laminitis are the consequence of standing or walking on damaged corium. Standing is perhaps a worse insult to the corium than walking. With each step there is normal movement of P3 within the horny capsule of the claw. This movement results in periodic perfusion of parts of the corium. When a cow stands without shifting her weight, these periodic changes in blood flow within the corium are probably interrupted. Thus standing motionless is potentially more damaging to an already insulted corium than walking. Only in the rarest cases do the lesions of laminitis develop while cows are lying. Thus the great stress in recent years on cow comfort and maximizing opportunities through time management and providing attractive lying surfaces are antilaminitis efforts.

Claws with abnormal shape, particularly of the ground contact surfaces, are more prone to mechanical insult to the corium. This is most commonly seen when excess horn production occurs at the axial border of the claws near the heel. The horn is probably being produced at an accelerated rate by this portion of the sole in response to stimulation by chronic dermatitis caused by *D. nodosus,* which is recognized to cause skin hypertrophy of the heels and interdigitally. Unfortunately this site on the sole where an excess rate of horn production is observed is also that of the common sole ulcer. During weight bearing, the corium deep to the horn buildup will be compressed in a fashion similar to when P3 movement within the claw is excessive.

Complications of the simpler lesions of the white line may occur when the pressure accumulating within the space between the hoof wall and the mural corium is not released to the exterior. The pressure within the abscess may be great enough to dissect along whatever path presents the least resistance. This may be proximally to the coronary band, axially across the sole, or caudally under the heel. Such abscesses result in greater disruption of the mechanical stability of the claw and the necessity of more horn removal.

Complications of sole ulcer are caused by extension of necrosis to the nearby structures around the coffin joint. The navicular bursa, deep flexor tendon, and coffin joint are all at risk of sepsis from free entry of bacteria through devitalized tissue. It is unclear whether necrosis of these connective tissue structures must precede invasion by bacteria or whether bacterial infection of a sole ulcer can proceed to extend into these other tissues if they are healthy.

Abnormally shaped claws may develop from genetic traits such as corkscrew claw or secondary to chronic or recurrent episodes of laminitis. The laminitic changes may manifest as concavity of the dorsal hoof wall as a result of displacement of the wall from the corium. Weakness of the capsule-corium attachment or corium-P3 attachment in conjunction with mechanical pressure on the hoof at the toe tip can result in turning up of the toe. Care must be taken in trimming of these claws because Dutch rules will not work unless the dorsal wall is first straightened. The thickening of the white line may be more widely distributed around its entirety, resulting in laterally flared claws. The claw capsule may also seem

to twist on its long axis because of laminitis resulting in so-called screw claw, although this is distinct from the genetically controlled condition. All of these claw shape abnormalities are likely at least uncomfortable for the cow to walk and stand on. In addition, they predispose to more severe lameness conditions as a result of abnormal loading of the corium. Thus trimming is of significant value in restoring normal weight bearing to already diseased claws.

Risk Factors for Lameness

Lameness appears to be an increasingly important problem for adult dairy cattle throughout the world. There are both economic and welfare concerns that motivate producers and their advisors to seek answers to the nature of the underlying causes. Specific causes of lameness can be divided into infectious agents that injure either the skin or underlying tissues of the digit with some effect on the horny claw capsule, internal injuries caused by metabolic and/or circulatory disturbances, and traumatic injuries. Any given cow can have all causes present in creating a painful condition recognized as lameness. This section will discuss what limited literature exists on the environmental risk factors contributing to herd problems of lameness and supplement this with anecdotal information gained in 25 years of examination of individual and herd problems throughout the Americas, Europe, and Australasia.

Environmental Risk Factors for Infectious Causes of Lameness

1. Foot rot is caused by specific pathogenic strains of *F. necrophorum* and *B. melaninogenicus* that gain entry through the interdigital skin. These bacteria can persist in wet soil or slurry for very long periods. They are also routinely present in the rumen and colon of cattle, although not necessarily pathogenic strains. Intact dry skin is resistant to penetration of these organisms. Thus conditions that produce breaks in the interdigital skin such as coarse sand or small stones becoming lodged in the interdigital space by walking through mud may predispose to foot rot. These conditions may prevail in cattle laneways, around water sources, or in riparian zones. Traditional control methods have been to fence cattle away from riparian zones and mudholes. A new approach for cattle laneways that is in use in the United Kingdom was recently described by Dr. Roger Blowey from Gloucester. A 40-in-wide roadway is constructed by excavating to a depth of 12 in. Eight inches of gravel or crushed stone is placed in the trench, covered with geotextile fabric, and the remainder of the excavation filled with shredded bark. The laneway remains dry on the

surface, stands up very well to traffic, and cows move comfortably along.

Foot rot in housed dairy cattle may be predisposed by the maceration of the interdigital skin, which is continuously moist. The severity of problems in housed dairy cattle is dependent on manure removal practices, which may influence both the infection pressure and the interdigital skin integrity. Footbathing with antibacterial compounds is a routine procedure to prevent new cases of foot rot.

2. Interdigital dermatitis is a chronic superficial infection of the interdigital skin caused by *D. nodosus*. It is very common in housed cattle with visible lesions present in the majority of cattle, whether housed in free stalls or tie stalls. One reference indicates a lower incidence of lameness as a result of interdigital dermatitis on slatted floors than solid floors. Pain and lameness are not present in most obviously infected cattle. Exposure to manure and urine predisposes to infection and influences the severity of problems. Most lameness caused by interdigital dermatitis is secondary either to skin (and possibly hoof sole) hypertrophy or to fissures in the heel horn caused by the bacterial elastases that are capable of cleaving the beta-pleated keratin of the hoof. The main environmental risk factors seem to be manure contact with the skin and anaerobic conditions between the manure layer and the skin. Control is as for foot rot.

3. Digital dermatitis is an infectious disease of the skin affecting cattle older than about 6 months of age anywhere from the vicinity of the dewclaws distally. The causal organism(s) have not been conclusively identified, but response to therapy with antibacterial drugs and the consistent observation of spirochetes in affected tissues supports a bacterial etiology. Environmental risk factors are the same as for interdigital dermatitis, and the two diseases often occur together with some synergy apparent. Infection with *D. nodosus* may facilitate establishment of the agents of digital dermatitis. Dry conditions as may occur in dry lot or some pasture conditions seem to prevent spread of the infection but do not influence the severity in already infected cattle. Control is with footbathing or spraying with the antibiotics (oxy) tetracycline or lincomycin. These plus some antiseptic solutions including formalin are used successfully in footbaths for control.

Environmental Risk Factors for Claw Horn Diseases

Most concern for the prevention of laminitis has been focused on the nutritional management of cattle to minimize the occurrence of ruminal acidosis. Ruminal acidosis is probably a necessary but not independently sufficient condition for the development of the most commonly observed lesions of subacute ruminal acidosis: sole and white line hemorrhages, white line abscesses, and sole ulceration. Environmental conditions and cow behavior appear to modify the final expression of the insult caused to the laminae and corium of the claws caused by ruminal acidosis. Subacute ruminal acidosis likely occurs in most dairy cattle in North America at some time during lactation. Despite this likely common occurrence, lameness is more variable and even severe in some herds. Experimental data are available on the ruminal effects of high concentrate diets. On the other hand, there are few data on the consequences within the claws of diet manipulations. The reports of Manson and Leaver, Livesey and Fleming, and Peterse et al describe the incidence of laminitis lesions in small groups of cattle in experimental herds with diet treatments that were either high or low concentrate feeding levels relative to forage. In each study there were more cases of lameness in the higher concentrate feeding groups. The groups fed low to moderate levels of concentrate were affected with some lesions of laminitis despite attempts to minimize the occurrence of ruminal acidosis. The author participated in a trial of rubber versus concrete flooring in free stall housing. The experiment was flawed by the cows available to populate the two barns; the groups were not well matched. Nevertheless, there were more lameness events in the cows living on concrete floors versus rubber floors. The consequences of standing on concrete are considered by many to be very important in the development of lesions of laminitis. Pressure exerted on specific portions of the claw may contribute to the observed vascular-derived lesions of either hemorrhage or necrosis. Cattle claws are commonly shaped in less than desirable forms. When these misshapen claws are supporting a cow on an unforgiving surface, the localized pressure can contribute greatly to damage of underlying structures. It is these consequences that have lead to our suggestion that barn floors be surfaced with something other than concrete and that routine trimming can prevent many of the more severe cases of lameness. It is of interest that the installation of rubber by feed alleys, in parlor holding areas, along alleys connecting pens to the milking parlor, and most recently complete alley covering with rubber mats has been increasing. Thus far there are no data on the effects of these changes on lameness, but our unquantified observations of cow behavior suggest that we are moving in the right direction.

Lameness incidence in bullocks housed on slatted floors, 4.75% of 12,010, in winter in Ireland was twice that of bullocks housed in straw yards, 2.43% of 2882, in 1984. Similarly a cross-sectional survey of Dutch dairy calves between 2.5 and 12 months of age observed more sole hemorrhages in heifers housed on slatted floors than in straw yards. Calves were examined on

117 farms. The prevalence of sole hemorrhage in straw yards was 5% compared with 45% on slatted floors. A comparison between 11 herds with chronic laminitis problems and 11 control herds was made during 2 years by Dr. Christer Bergsten in the vicinity of Skara, Sweden. There was a correlation between the stall surfaces, either concrete or with a rubber mat, and the occurrence of hemorrhages. Fewer sole hemorrhages occurred in stalls fitted with rubber mats. The cows were in tie stalls, and bedding use was not found to influence the prevalence of sole hemorrhages, although it was described as minimal in all stall types. The only publication suggesting an effect of environment on laminitis in free stall housing compared the problem in two herds with the same owner and stall design but managed differently because of the requirements of the manure removal system. The herd with a higher incidence of lameness used less bedding. Both the proportion of animals standing in the alleys and the proportion of animals standing half in the stalls were higher for the herd with more lameness. Increasing the bedding amount for the problem herd resulted in amelioration of the lameness.

Environmental circumstances for dairy cattle thus appear to have two possible avenues of influence on the development of laminitis. First are those environmental conditions that influence feeding behavior. Second are those conditions that predispose to excessive standing time, and standing on concrete in particular. Both feeding and lying behavior tend to be synchronized activities within a group of cows. Observations on the behavior of cattle in an experimental setting have shown that regardless of feed access, whether 100% can eat at once or 50% at once, most eating will occur in temporal clusters. When feed access is limited, the subordinate cattle will have less time available to eat and will slug-feed more often. Besides overcrowding the feeding space, heat stress probably influences feeding behavior the most adversely with regard to laminitis. Slug-feeding is predisposed by heat stress when the majority of feed consumed will be when the environment and the body temperature of the cow are comfortable. These two factors comprise the major influences of environment on feeding behavior with ultimate consequences mediated via ruminal acidosis on the development of laminitis.

Standing time on concrete is heavily influenced by the environmental design of dairy facilities and modified by overcrowding and management activities. Synchronization of behavioral activities again leads a group of cattle to mostly lie down at the same time. Overcrowding of free stall pens prevents some of the subordinate animals from access to a stall. When a stall becomes available, it may signal the pen is ready to collectively eat or be milked, thus preventing that timid animal from lying at all. Data from long-term observations of groups of cattle with known dominance structure showed that a very subordinate animal, usually a heifer, might stay in a stall

during some group eating times. Reasons for this are speculative, but regardless the result is slug-feeding for that animal when she does leave the stall. Subordinate animals are also more likely to stand in the alley altogether with the head placed in a stall or half in a stall. Interpretation of this behavior is that it provides a reduction in the danger posed by more dominant cattle. Housing first-lactation animals separately from older cows has resulted in a reduction of the negative effects of these social interactions on the heifers.

Standing in a free stall pen is heavily influenced by the design of the free stall itself. Great attention has justifiably been spent in the past 20 years on improving the design of free stall partitions, beds, and overall dimensions. Cow comfort has been a popular theme of the past decade with most of the emphasis placed on the stall. This emphasis has in great part been driven by the desire to improve lying time to reduce lameness. The goal of free stall facility design should be to provide a space for every cow. Cows should enter and exit freely including lying and rising without interference and ideally spend about 14 hours per 24 hours lying in the stall. Because mechanical loading of the claws contributes very importantly to the development of the serious lesions of laminitis, evidence of underutilization of stalls is a cause for alarm. Cows that have had an unpleasant experience in a stall are more reluctant to use a stall the next time it is appropriate. Those cows that stand half in and half out of stalls are often increasing the load on the rear digits and at an unnatural angle. Maintenance of the bedding in stalls is also critical for use and comfort. Hock lesions are a common complaint of many mattress stall designs because of the lack of adequate bedding at the rear of the stall. Plain concrete or hard rubber mat stalls with bedding appear to be the least desirable for overall comfort and utilization and hock lesions. Another notable study made comparison of two free stall designs utilizing 43 heifers through late pregnancy and early lactation. One stall type was the Dutch comfort with side openings and outfitted with rubber mats. The other was Newton Rigg, which prevented side lunging and had no rubber mat over the concrete base. Lying time was increased, and standing half in stalls was reduced in the Dutch comfort stalls. There were more sole hemorrhages and six cases of acute lameness in the Newton Rigg stalls versus one lame heifer in the Dutch comfort stalls.

For free stall–housed herds, the forced standing time imposed by management activities may contribute to laminitis problems. The milking parlor should be sized to limit holding period time to 3 hours out of every 24 hours, regardless of milking frequency. Other management activities such as bedding stalls or veterinary work should be organized to minimize the intrusion on potential lying time.

In many herds in North America, laminitis has a pronounced seasonal occurrence. Late summer through early fall is the peak of cases of white line abscess and sole ulcers. We believe that there are two primary environmental factors involved in this. First, cows experiencing heat stress will redistribute their meals to eat predominately in the morning. This slug-feeding increases the incidence of ruminal acidosis. Second, and of unknown importance relative to the increase in low rumen pH, is the increase in standing time. Cows stand huddled around waterers. They stand in the stalls, often concentrated where fans move the most air. Sometimes, apparently when stable flies (*Stomoxys calcitrans*) are bothersome, they stand in tight groups at one end of a pen. To avoid fly bites the goal of a cow is to be in the center of a group where the heat stress is likely maximal. Maybe they stand in the stalls because they perceive themselves to be cooler standing than lying down. For whatever constellation of reasons, the slug-feeding and excess standing lead to large increases in lame cows. Summer ventilation and strategies to cool cows have the possibility to significantly reduce this seasonal lameness problem.

Miscellaneous Environmental Considerations

Floor surfaces may contribute to lameness if they are uneven or have elevated protrusions as from small stones. The softness of moist hooves, as in most free stall–housed cattle, makes them more susceptible to traumatic lesions of the sole. Some floor grooving and some slatted floors have such large voids in the surface that the claws of cows can be injured as they push their claws into the grooves or holes. Small stones on solid floors may come from sand bedding that is not screened to exclude particles larger than about 5 mm or 0.25 in.

Many herds have experienced excessive lameness when cows were placed in facilities with new concrete. For the most part, these problems have been caused by excessive wear of the soles leading to exposure of the corium. Prevention of this problem of surfaces that are too abrasive at first can be done by dragging concrete blocks or scraping with a steel blade before cattle are introduced to the barn.

Conclusions

Environmental conditions play a significant role in the occurrence of lameness in dairy cattle. Manure and urine in constant contact with the hooves and digital skin may predispose to entry of infectious agents that produce lesions in the skin and hooves producing lameness. Control is enhanced when hooves and skin are clean and dry. Footbathing with antibacterial solutions in appropriately designed and located baths can reduce the incidence of lameness resulting from infectious causes. Laminitis is predisposed by ruminal acidosis and augmented by standing on concrete. Design strategies to

provide unimpeded access to feed for all members of a group will help minimize slug-feeding. Standing time is heavily influenced by facility design. Comfortable stalls and heat stress prevention will greatly minimize the development of lameness resulting from laminitis.

LAMENESS ABOVE THE DIGIT—SPORADIC DISEASES

Most upper limb lameness is caused by trauma, although degenerative arthritis does occur rarely in cattle. The outcome of any case will depend on the severity of the injury, what specific structures are damaged, and the enthusiasm the farm personnel have for nursing disabled or recumbent cows. Most upper limb injuries end in euthanasia or slaughter. It is valuable to determine a diagnosis and prognosis early for those cattle that have no chance of recovery. Most cattle do not warrant the expense of attempts at surgical correction of major tendon or ligament injuries, which, on the whole, are not very successful anyway. Good hospital pen circumstances with soft bedding and no competition for food and water are essential. Antiinflammatory medication with steroids such as dexamethasone or NSAIDs such as flunixin or ketoprofen is an important part of conservative therapy.

A second category of upper limb lameness is caused by infection either of muscles and tendons or joints. Septic arthritis or tendonitis may occur from wounds but more commonly occurs in neonates as a result of failure of adequate colostrum management and poor passive immunity. Arthritis and tendonitis caused by *M. bovis* appear to be a unique condition.

Stifle Injuries

Stifle injuries occur most commonly in adult cattle and bulls. Mounting injuries, falls, slipping on poor footing, and exertional activity in downer cows cause most stifle injuries in cattle. Degenerative joint disease also may contribute to stifle injuries in old cattle or bulls. Although many specific injuries have been reported for the bovine stifle, only the three most common injuries will be discussed in this section.

Cranial Cruciate Ligament Injury
Typical signs of acute stifle lameness characterized by flexion of the stifle and just touching the toe to the ground characterize cranial cruciate ligament rupture. Joint distention may be obvious, and the tibial crest may be more apparent than normal. When weight is forced onto the affected limb or the animal is forced to walk, palpation of the stifle will allow detection of an obvious "bone-on-bone" mobility within the joint and an audible clunking sound. The degree of pain varies but usually is moderate to severe, and the affected animal is reluctant

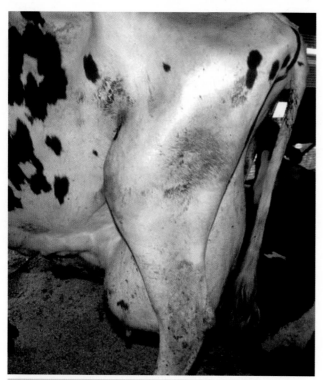

Figure 11-34

Localized swelling and rotation of the tibia in a cow with chronic rupture of the cranial cruciate ligament.

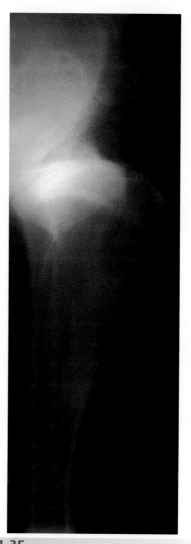

Figure 11-35

Stifle radiograph from cow with a chronic cranial cruciate ligament rupture. The femoral condyles appear caudal to the tibial spine, and the cranial joint space is wider than normal. Degenerative joint changes are present.

to bear weight on the limb. Chronically affected cows who tolerate the associated pain may have a severe limp but continue to be profitable members of the herd (Figure 11-34). A cranial drawer sign may be demonstrated if the animal will bear weight on the affected limb by standing behind the limb with the knees braced against the hock. A pull is exerted on the cranial proximal tibia, which will move into its normal position. In very large animals or animals that will not support weight, this test may not be helpful. Lateral radiographs may support the diagnosis because the femoral condyles appear caudal to the tibial spine and the cranial joint space seems wider than normal (Figure 11-35).

Treatment of cranial cruciate ligament injury may be conservative if lameness is only moderate, reflecting subtotal rupture. Conservative therapy consists of box stall rest, good footing, and antiinflammatory therapy. If the affected cow is able to maintain body weight and production, this may suffice. If lameness is severe and obvious pain causes weight loss, poor appetite, and poor production despite conservative measures, slaughter should be considered. The only alternative treatment is referral for surgical procedures that may reduce the abnormal mobility within the joint. These procedures include attempts at artificial replacement of the cranial cruciate ligament or imbrication procedures to tighten fascia around the joint but have a low proportion of success.

Prognosis is always guarded for cranial cruciate ligament rupture because a cow cannot be managed as an individual in most herds unless the animal is extremely valuable. In addition, risk of other musculoskeletal injuries increases, especially to the opposite hind limb. We have observed many cattle with cranial cruciate ligament rupture that develop the same lesion or other stifle injuries in the opposite limb within 1 to 2 years of the original injury. This may suggest a predisposition associated with degenerative joint disease or genetics in certain cattle.

Rupture of the Medial Collateral Ligament

Rupture or stretching of the medial collateral ligament results in an abducted limb and weight bearing on the medial claw. The injury is reported to be more common in heifers than adult cattle. Lameness is moderate to severe, and the animal prefers standing with the toe touching the ground and the limb held forward or behind the normal perpendicular weight-bearing position. Palpation of the medial aspect of the joint usually reveals local sensitivity when digital pressure is placed on the collateral ligament. Radiographs are usually not helpful.

Conservative treatment consisting of box stall rest, good footing, and antiinflammatory medication usually results in improvement within a few weeks. If no improvement is observed, referral for imbrication is the only treatment alternative. Prognosis is fair for valuable cows that can be individualized but poor for cattle that must interact with herdmates because continued pain and reinjury are more likely.

Meniscal Injury

Trauma or progressive deterioration secondary to degenerative arthritis may result in meniscal damage or rupture. Nonspecific signs of moderate stifle lameness including resting the toe on the ground with the stifle flexed and reluctance to bear full weight are observed. Flexion of the joint may cause pain, but distinct clunking, as in cranial cruciate ligament rupture, is not evident. A palpable click or crepitus is apparent in some acute cases, and joint effusion may be present. Synovial fluid suggests hemorrhage, trauma, or degenerative joint disease rather than sepsis. Treatment consists of conservative measures as previously mentioned or surgical referral if conservative therapy fails to alleviate the cow's pain. Prognosis is poor because degenerative arthritis either preexists or will likely follow meniscal injury or rupture.

Hip Injuries

The major hip injuries include coxofemoral luxation, fracture of the femoral head or neck, slipped capital femoral epiphysis, pelvic fractures involving the acetabulum, and rupture of the ligament of the head of the femur (round ligament). In heifers and adult animals, these injuries are caused by trauma, estrous mounting behavior, falls, slipping on poor footing, splitting the hind limbs by slipping or following obturator nerve paralysis, and struggling secondary to recumbency, myopathies, or neuropathies (Figure 11-36). In calves, some of these conditions follow forced traction during dystocia. Hip lameness resulting from inflammatory or degenerative arthritis (coxitis) also may result in similar signs but is less likely to be as acute as the aforementioned injuries.

The result of these hip conditions is severe lameness or recumbency. If the animal can stand, the stifle often will point outward. The animal is reluctant to bear weight, and the limb is advanced with a rolling outward motion

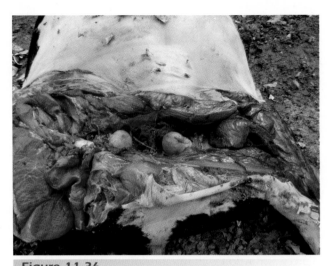

Figure 11-36

Bilateral ventral luxation of the hip joints in a heifer. She was injured by penmates during estrus.

and short stride that may cause the toe to drag. The history or posture of the patient may suggest diagnosis. This is especially true if the caretaker observed the animal as she slipped, split her hind legs, or if the cow tends to lie with the affected limb in forced extension. In newborn calves, a history of forced traction to relieve dystocia should arouse suspicion of hip injury or femoral nerve damage. If the affected animal can stand, the symmetry of the greater trochanter and pelvis (tuber ischii) should be assessed. In dorsal luxation of the hip, the affected limb may appear shorter, the greater trochanter may be palpated in a more cranial position than normal (farther away from the tuber ischii), and the limb may be rotated outward; the animal will try to avoid any weight bearing on the limb. In ventral luxation, the greater trochanter may be difficult to palpate, and the femoral head sometimes becomes trapped in the obturator foramen. In either dorsal or ventral luxation, excessive movement of the greater trochanter may be palpated when the limb is manipulated. In femoral neck fractures, slipped capital epiphysis, round ligament ruptures, and acetabular fractures, crepitus and a grinding sensation will be detected when the limb is manipulated and the greater trochanter is palpated simultaneously. Regardless of the exact diagnosis, manipulation of the limb to flex, extend, or swing causes the animal pain. In recumbent animals, palpation and manipulation are the keys to diagnosis. If the animal is supported by hip slings or other mechanical aids, the leg often is held extended, rotated outward, and is non–weight bearing. Flexion and manipulation of the standing animal (supported) may be done by an assistant while the clinician palpates the hip region and performs a rectal examination to check for acetabular fractures, ventral hip luxation into the obturator foramen, other pelvic fractures, or crepitus in femoral head or neck fractures.

Prognosis remains poor for most severe hip injuries and coxofemoral luxations. Therefore if a recumbent cow has obvious signs of hip luxation or fractures in this area and cannot stand, euthanasia should be performed. In valuable calves or cows that warrant further diagnostics, radiographs of the pelvis and hip are essential to accurately prognose the condition and offer treatment options, especially if the animal is able to rise and support weight on the three normal limbs, in which case nonsurgical or surgical replacement may be an option.

Femoral head and neck fractures, acetabular fractures, rupture of the round ligament, and slipped capital epiphysis carry a guarded to poor prognosis in large heifers or cows. In calves affected unilaterally, orthopedic surgery may be attempted with a guarded prognosis in some instances. Reduction with intramedullary pinning has been successful in some calves and young cattle with a slipped capital femoral epiphysis.

Coxofemoral luxation in calves and adult cows carries a fair prognosis, according to recent reports, but is best treated by open reduction (Figure 11-37). Prognosis is better for younger animals and cows that are able to get up and down using the normal opposite hind limb. Recumbent animals that are heavy or have bilateral hip lesions are not good candidates for surgical treatment.

Fractures

Although relatively uncommon, fractures require immediate attention and expertise in orthopedics for proper management. The bovine practitioner seldom gets enough experience with fractures to become an "expert" but may handle common fractures, especially those of the lower limbs, on the farm. Economics may

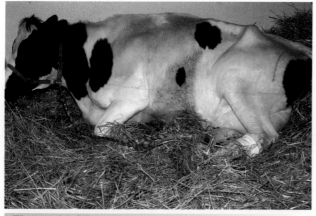

Figure 11-37

A 3-year-old cow that has had surgical repair of a coxofemoral luxation. The halter is loosely tied to the leg that has been repaired to force the cow to lie down on the opposite side. She is housed in a dirt stall with straw bedding.

preclude the referral of certain cattle or calves for internal or external fixation of fractures, but referral remains the best decision for upper limb fractures involving the tibia, humerus, femur, radius, and ulna. A full discussion of fractures is beyond the scope of this text, and the reader is referred to several excellent references concerning bovine fractures.

Diagnosis in closed fractures is based on non–weight bearing, limb deviation, and crepitus in the region of the limb deviation. In open or compound fractures, the bone may be grossly visible. Radiographs are required for prognosis in complicated fractures or luxation and are always helpful for decisions regarding initial management and follow-up assessment.

The most common bovine limb fracture involves the metacarpus of yearling heifers in free stall housing. Presumably the forelimb is extended laterally beneath a stall divider during rising, with the divider as the fulcrum under which the metacarpus fractures. The distal epiphysis is always involved. At the time of examination, there may be minimal displacement of the fracture but severe pain on manipulation. Sedation with xylazine and placing in lateral recumbency with the affected limb uppermost allow easy alignment of the distal limb and cast application. A fiberglass cast is placed from the hoof to about 10 cm above the distal end of the radius. The cast is removed in 4 to 6 weeks with an excellent prognosis for a normal lifespan.

Occasionally seen in newborn calves are fractures of the distal metacarpus or metatarsus resulting from the torque during forced extraction from the uterus. Usually the obstetrical chains have been malpositioned in the metacarpal area. These fractures may be associated with vascular compromise to the limb distal to the fracture site because of the "tourniquet effect" of the obstetrical chains that resulted in fracture or because of sharp bone fragments lacerating vessels supplying the digit. If the tissue distal to the fracture is cold, the prognosis is grave. Calves carry a much better prognosis than adult cattle, and noncontaminated closed fractures have a better prognosis than compound fractures. Standard treatment for metacarpal and metatarsal fractures uses either half-limb or full-limb casts, depending on the anatomic site of the fracture, size of the animal, and so forth. A fair to good prognosis is in order for promptly attended noncontaminated fractures.

Fractures above the carpus or tarsus (or involving these joints) require more assessment and planning for successful management. Referral is suggested if the value of the animal warrants this therapy. When economics are a concern but the owner wishes some treatment to be attempted, the clinician must use best judgment. Many humeral fractures in calves and heifers have healed with the only treatment being box stall rest. Femoral, tibial, and radius-ulnar fractures are not as likely to heal without internal or external fixation. Full-limb casting may suffice for hock and carpal fractures or luxations and also for distal radius-ulna fractures. Tibial and femoral fractures are difficult to manage in a field situation and are best managed by modified Thomas splints or internal fixation.

Owners must be made aware of the severity of the problem and informed that referral for treatment will be very expensive. Therefore only very valuable or potentially very valuable calves and cows are referred for repair of upper limb fractures. When referring fractures, the clinician should personally attend to a supportive bandage, splint, or cast, depending on the size of the animal and the bone involved. The support should extend dorsally beyond the joint above the site of the fracture. In this way, transport can be accomplished safely without worsening the injury. Long bone or vertebral fractures occurring as an epidemic problem in a group of growing animals signals metabolic disease, and nutritional consultation to assess calcium, phosphorus, and vitamin D concentrations in feed is imperative.

Rupture of the Gastrocnemius Muscle or Tendon

The gastrocnemius muscle and tendon in the cow are very critical structures for normal rising and weight bearing. Rupture of either prevents weight bearing in the affected limb and usually carries a hopeless prognosis. Cattle with hypocalcemia that make repeated efforts to rise or struggle to rise on a slippery floor are at risk for gastrocnemius rupture. Occasional younger animals may be affected if trapped in mud, deep manure, or have neurologic conditions that cause them to struggle excessively to rise. Tractor front-end loader accidents have also resulted in gastrocnemius rupture. However, the adult cow with hypocalcemia represents the typical patient.

Inability to rise is the typical complaint reported for adult cattle affected with this condition. Usually one limb is affected, but rare cases of bilateral rupture have been observed. The classic appearance of gastrocnemius rupture is the "rabbit leg" with the point of the hock resting on the ground such that a 90-degree angle exists between the tibia and metatarsus (Figure 11-38). Because many heavy cows with gastrocnemius rupture fail to rise even to a halfway point in the normal hind limb when attempting to rise, the clinician always should stand at the animal's rear to observe the condition when stimulating a recumbent cow to rise. The affected gastrocnemius muscle is firm and swollen because of hematoma formation around the ruptured muscle; the tendon proximal to the hock is relaxed. Less commonly, the gastrocnemius tendon has been ruptured, in which case the muscle will not be swollen.

Although most cases have complete rupture, partial rupture may occur, resulting in severe lameness in the

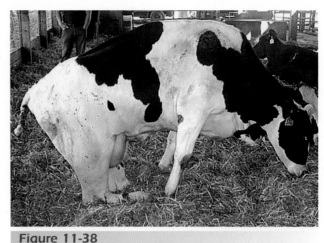

Figure 11-38

Bilateral rupture of the gastrocnemius muscles.

affected limb, a slightly dropped hock, and a tense, firm swelling in the affected gastrocnemius muscle. The animal can support some weight but prefers to rest the limb in a forward fashion by extending the stifle and flexing the fetlock.

Treatment for adult cattle with complete rupture of the gastrocnemius muscle or tendon is likely hopeless. Calves and younger animals with the problem that can rise to stand on three legs may be confined to a box stall with good bedding and footing for several months, but once again, the prognosis usually is hopeless for these animals as well.

Rupture of the Peroneus Tertius

Rupture of the peroneus tertius muscle results in inability to flex the hock, therefore preventing the reciprocal flexion of the hock when the stifle is flexed. Excessive struggling to rise on a slippery floor with or without concurrent hypocalcemia and slipping backward while trying to rise or mount another cow are the usual causes of rupture of the peroneus tertius.

An extended hock while the stifle flexes results in inability to advance the limb normally. The toes are dragged, and the dorsum of the pastern or fetlock may suffer abrasion. The gastrocnemius muscle and tendon appear relaxed. The stifle can be flexed with the hock fully extended (Figure 11-39). Although prognosis is guarded at best, some affected cattle may recover if placed in a box stall with good footing.

Flexor Tendon Lacerations

The most common cause of laceration to the superficial and deep flexor tendons of the hind limbs is sharp trauma from scraper blades on tractor-mounted manure scrapers in free stall barns. Alternatively, attendants cleaning stalls with sharp implements may startle a cow

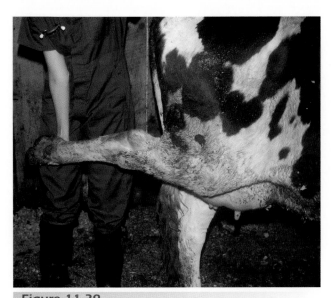

Figure 11-39

Rupture of the peroneus tertius in a recently fresh Holstein cow.

that then kicks out and contacts the sharp end of a shovel or other tool. Cattle may become entangled in miscellaneous circumstances and lacerate tendons in their struggles to escape.

Lacerations involving only the superficial flexor allow the limb to bear full weight but have a slight increased flexion of the digit if the superficial flexor is completely transected. In such cases, a thorough inspection of the wound is necessary to rule out partial laceration of the deep flexor, which may progress unless supported more intensively than normal therapy for superficial flexor injury. Lacerations that involve both the superficial and deep flexors result in inability to bear weight, the plantar aspect of the fetlock contacts the ground when the animal attempts to bear weight on the affected limb, and the toes point dorsally.

If only the superficial flexor tendon is lacerated, the wound should be cleaned, irrigated, and a sterile dressing applied with adequate support to prevent exuberant granulation tissue. The wound should be redressed at 3- to 7-day intervals. Antibiotics should be administered for 10 to 14 days.

If the superficial flexor tendon is lacerated and the deep flexor partially lacerated, a splint or cast should be considered because continued stress on the compromised deep flexor tendon could cause a complete rupture. If both the superficial and the deep flexor tendons are lacerated, a splint or cast is required following clipping, cleaning, and irrigation of the wound. For calves and heifers, splints work very well; for adult cattle, however, casts are necessary to withstand weight-bearing stress. Before splinting, the wound is protected by a sterile bandage, and heavy cotton rolls are applied from the ground to the top of the hock. Gauze wrap is used

to secure the cotton rolls, and the heel is raised 2.5 to 3.75 cm off the ground with a block or rubber wedge. A piece of polyvinyl chloride (PVC) pipe that has been measured for fit and split lengthwise is then applied to the plantar aspect of the limb from the ground to the top of the hock, and the entire apparatus then is pressure wrapped with strong self-adherent tape. It is important to incorporate the block or wedge pad under the tape to keep the heel raised, thus alleviating tension on the damaged tendons. A waterproof bag or piece of rubber may be applied to the portion of the splint contacting the ground to prolong its life. The animal should be confined to a box stall, and antibiotics should be administered for 1 to 2 weeks. The splint will need to be changed every few days for the first 1 to 2 weeks and then weekly until 6 to 8 weeks have elapsed. Xylazine is sufficient for sedation and restraint of calves and heifers during this procedure.

In casting, the wound is prepared as with splinting, but only a light sterile dressing is applied followed by stockinet and the cast. Cast changes are more time consuming than splint changes; therefore adequate sedation, anesthesia, and restraint are necessary during the procedures to prevent reinjury of the healing tendon. Adult cattle may require 6 to 12 weeks in a cast to allow complete healing.

Improper application of the cast or splint and infection of the tendon sheath constitute the major complications. Fracture of the limb proximal to the cast has also occurred rarely when the cast application has been improper or patients are housed on slippery floors. Prognosis is fair to good for calves and heifers but only fair for adult cattle because they have a higher complication rate.

Degenerative Arthritis

Degenerative arthritis may be secondary to poor conformation such as extremely straight hind limbs or abducted forelimbs. Previous septic arthritis or osteochondrosis lesions also may contribute to degenerative joint changes. Overnutrition of bulls and genetic factors also have been considered as potential causes of this condition.

Joint effusion, reduced range of motion in affected joints, a stiff gait, muscle atrophy, and a slow progressive course suggest the diagnosis. Radiographs confirm loss of articular cartilage and osteophyte production within the affected joints. The major joints of the hind limbs are most commonly affected, but occasional cases occur in the shoulder or carpal joints in the forelimbs.

Although no specific treatment is possible, analgesic antiinflammatory treatment with NSAIDs may relieve the animal's pain and allow continued production. In working bulls, these drugs may allow further semen collection with the use of electroejaculation. Intraarticular corticosteroids may provide transient improvement but contribute to further degeneration of the joint with time. Hyaluronic acid and other intraarticular medications used in horses also may be beneficial but seldom are used in cattle because of the expense. They may find use in valuable breeding cattle or bulls in AI facilities. Recently acupuncture and other nontraditional therapies have been used with some success in the treatment of valuable bulls.

Prognosis is poor because the condition is progressive. Some animals survive for 1 or more years if kept in comfortable surroundings and treated symptomatically. However, continued deterioration of the joints eventually causes so much pain that weight loss secondary to musculoskeletal injuries and loss of production are inevitable.

Septic Arthritis

Infectious arthritis is a common problem in dairy calves and a sporadic problem in older animals. A plethora of organisms have been isolated from septic joints in cattle and largely reflect a variety of primary endogenous and exogenous sources of infection. Fever and acute lameness are apparent in most cases. The causes, means of diagnosis, and treatment of septic tenosynovitis and osteomyelitis essentially are the same as for septic arthritis and will not be discussed separately.

In young calves, septic arthritis originates from umbilical infections or septicemia. Calves with failure of passive transfer of immunoglobulins are at great risk (Figure 11-40). Neonatal septicemic calves with septic arthritis or osteomyelitis frequently have other signs of

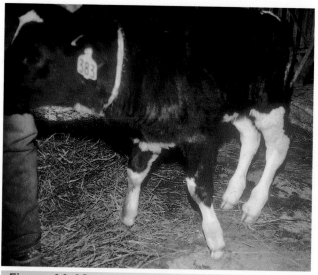

Figure 11-40

A colostrum-deprived calf with septic arthritis and osteomyelitis involving the distal limb, fetlocks, and pastern joints in all limbs.

gram-negative sepsis such as enteritis, meningitis, uveitis, or pneumonia. The prognosis for neonatal calves with arthritis—especially polyarthritis—secondary to failure of passive transfer of immunoglobulins is poor. Calves with umbilical infections also may develop septic arthritis in one or more joints resulting from a variety of gram-negative and gram-positive organisms. Calves also may develop septic synovitis, osteomyelitis, or arthritis from exogenous abrasions, wounds, and decubital sores that occur secondary to abrasive surfaces. Calves with other medical problems that result in prolonged recumbency are at greater risk. Although *Escherichia coli* may be identified as a cause of septic arthritis or osteomyelitis in neonatal calves, *Salmonella* sp. and *Arcanobacter pyogenes* are also frequently isolated.

Older calves (more than 3 weeks) and heifers may develop septic arthritis following exogenous wounds, periarticular cellulitis, punctures, or endogenous circulation of pathogens from the intestinal (*Salmonella* sp.) or respiratory tract (*Histophilus somni* and *Mycoplasma* sp.). *Mycoplasma* arthritis is common in growing calves 3 to 6 months of age, and affected calves frequently have concurrent pneumonia. Uncomplicated trauma to the carpus that results in bruising of the cranial surface may result in a reluctance to flex the carpus when recumbent. If the housing circumstances do not permit extension of the carpus when recumbent, further trauma to other extremities may result. This is not a problem of sepsis but from pain of nonseptic inflammation. Carpal trauma should be treated with antiinflammatory medication, bandaging when feasible, and appropriate housing. It should be distinguished from sepsis of the carpus, which is less common. Adult cattle may develop synovitis, arthritis, or osteomyelitis secondary to endogenous diseases such as endocarditis, septic mastitis, pneumonia, lung abscesses, liver abscesses, and chronic foot infections, as well as from exogenous infections secondary to traumatic wounds, decubital sores, and periarticular cellulitis or abscessation. *A. pyogenes* is the most common organism isolated from septic joints, osteomyelitis lesions, or tenosynovitis in older calves and adult cattle.

Although *Mycoplasma* arthritis is not thought to be as common in dairy animals as in beef, the disease probably is underdiagnosed and has been found in many herds in which *Mycoplasma* mastitis exists or *Mycoplasma* sp. are ubiquitous in the respiratory tract. Isolated cases of polytendonitis/arthritis affecting a single limb in weaning calves to aged cattle have been recognized in dairy animals caused by *M. bovis*. *Mycoplasma* arthritis may be associated with pneumonia (Figure 11-41), and the joint fluid typically has a very high protein and neutrophil count, but the neutrophils may be relatively well preserved.

Signs of septic arthritis include marked lameness with distention of the affected joint capsule, warmth over the joint, and a painful response when the joint is

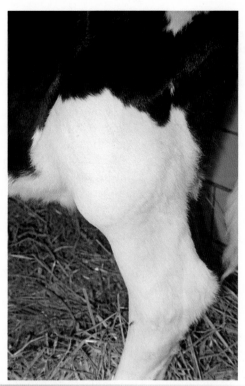

Figure 11-41

Distended left stifle of a 3-month-old calf with *M. bovis* arthritis and pneumonia. The tarsi and carpi are the most commonly affected joints in *Mycoplasma* infections.

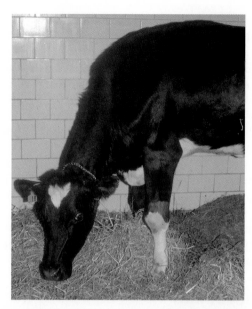

A

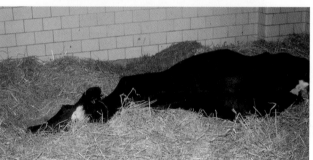

B

Figure 11-42

A first-calf heifer with a septic left carpus. **A,** Standing. **B,** When recumbent, the heifer would assume lateral recumbency so that the extremely painful joint need not be flexed.

manipulated, flexed, or extended. Fever usually is present and frequently is low grade (103.0 to 104.0° F/39.4 to 40.0° C). Cattle may assume an abnormal attitude in recumbency and lie with the affected limb extended or lie in lateral recumbency to extend the affected limb more easily (Figure 11-42, *A* and *B*). Calves or cattle with chronic polyarthritis tend to spend excessive time in recumbency and may develop secondary flexor tendon contracture that requires differentiation from primary flexor tendon contracture (Figure 11-43, *A* and *B*).

The definitive diagnosis of septic arthritis or tendonitis is made by examination of fluid aspirates from the affected structure. Arthrocentesis following aseptic preparation of the skin over the joint provides synovial fluid for cytology and culture. The diagnosis often is grossly apparent on inspection of abnormal synovial fluid, but laboratory analysis is helpful. Cytology usually reveals a white blood cell (WBC) count greater than 30,000 WBCs per μl and total solids greater than 3.0 g/dl. Bacteria may be apparent with Gram staining, or culture may be necessary for bacterial identification. In valuable calves or cattle, cytology and culture for aerobic and anaerobic bacteria and *Mycoplasma* are important diagnostic tools. Degenerative neutrophils are apparent in most bacterial arthritis cases but may be missing from acute *Mycoplasma* infections. In chronic septic arthritis, the synovial fluid may be grossly purulent. The purulent

material that accumulates in mycoplasmal tendonitis/ synovitis is always caseous in consistency and nonodorous in contrast to the characteristic odor of sepsis associated with *A. pyogenes*.

A history and thorough physical examination should be performed to determine the primary cause—umbilical infection, septicemia, or exogenous infection—and ancillary procedures such as ultrasonography of the umbilical region performed if a primary lesion is suspected in this area. Radiographs of acute joint infection show a widening of the affected joint space because of increased synovial fluid volume, whereas chronic infections may show a narrowing of the joint space as a result of loss of articular cartilage, erosion of the subchondral bone and bony proliferation, periostitis, and occasional osteomyelitis. Subtle lesions in acute cases make synovial fluid a better diagnostic test, but radiographs are extremely valuable for formulating a prognosis in chronic cases.

Treatment of septic arthritis must address the infected joint or joints, as well as any primary conditions

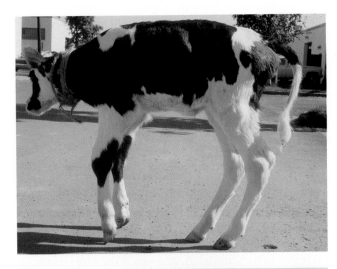

A

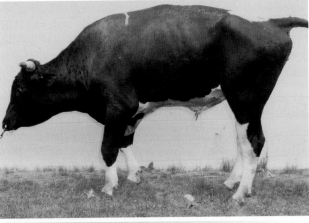

B

Figure 11-43

Polyarthritis causing a painful stiff gait, an arched stance, and secondary flexor tendon contracture as a result of excessive time spent in recumbency in a calf (A) and a Holstein bull (B).

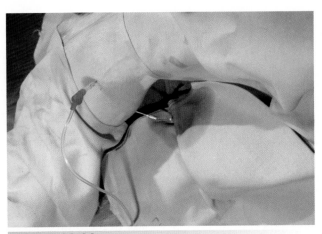

Figure 11-44

Joint lavage in a calf with a septic hock joint.

that have predisposed to septic arthritis/synovitis. Acutely infected joints have a much better prognosis than chronically infected joints that contain thick purulent debris. In acute infections, joint lavage is the key to successful management. The infected joint should be surgically prepared and lavaged by through-and-through flushing using two 14-gauge needles and buffered lactated Ringer's solution or normal saline (Figure 11-44); 1 or 2 L per joint suffices. The technique involves arthrocentesis with a 14-gauge sterile needle followed by distention of the joint capsule and subsequent joint puncture by a second 14-gauge needle at the opposite side of the joint. The lavage solution is then pumped through the joint to flush out causative organisms, fibrin, WBCs, and mediators of inflammation. A light sterile dressing is placed over the joint after squeezing as much fluid out of the needles as possible. Systemic antibiotics are more effective than antibiotics injected into the joint or added to the lavage solution

and should be started as soon as possible. Antibiotic selection is based on cytology (Gram stain evaluation) initially and culture results eventually. Alternatively, a broad-spectrum antibiotic such as florfenicol or ceftiofur may be empirically selected without culture results.

Joint lavage is repeated daily or as needed (1 to 3 days) to continue flushing the joint of products of inflammation and debris. The degree of lameness and joint distention dictates the need for additional lavage procedures. Most cases require three to seven lavage procedures over a 1- to 2-week course. Appropriate systemic antibiotics are continued for a minimum of 2 weeks, and the animal should be kept in a dry, well-bedded stall.

An alternative to joint lavage is becoming more popular with surgeons in our clinic. An arthrotomy is performed on the affected joint, the joint is flushed with saline, and surgical drains are placed that permit continuous drainage of joint contents. Flushing of the joint may or may not be utilized after the initial procedure. We have had success with septic tarsal joints in adult cattle by simply inserting a surgical drain with the use of a Buhner needle after ensuring that the entry and exit points are sufficiently large for drainage around the tubing.

Primary problems must be addressed. In septicemic calves, passive transfer of immunoglobulins and the umbilicus must be assessed. Blood or plasma transfusions and umbilical resection may be required to prevent further joint seeding. Exogenous wounds and other sites of sepsis must be treated if they are thought to be primary to the septic arthritis.

Chronic septic arthritis carries a guarded prognosis because sterile ankylosis of the joint becomes the only acceptable result. Repeated joint lavage or arthrotomy for drainage of thick purulent joint fluid may be necessary. In calves, chronic infections, usually caused by *A. pyogenes*, require arthrotomy to drain thick pus from the joints. Open lavage of the joint coupled with systemic antibiotics and physical therapy to prevent tendon contracture follow arthrotomy. Physical therapy may be as simple as manipulation or may necessitate splints or casts for support and immobilization in the most serious cases. Calves are more likely to recover from a single chronic septic joint than an adult animal because calves can more easily support weight on three limbs during the time necessary for treatment and recovery. Treatment of *Mycoplasma* arthritis in cattle is empiric because little documentation of effective resolution of *Mycoplasma* infection in cattle is available. In districts where fluoroquinolones are registered for cattle, they appear to be the first choice. In the United States, newer macrolides such as tulathromycin are probably the best choice for nonlactating cattle. There are no highly effective, approved antibiotics available for lactating adult cattle in the United States.

Prognosis always should be guarded but is better for acute than chronic cases, better for single joints than multiple ones, and better when the primary etiology may be corrected.

Osteomyelitis and Bone Sequestra

Both of these conditions usually result in chronic or recurrent purulent drainage from the skin overlying a bony swelling (Figure 11-45). In some instances, soft tissue swelling precedes drainage of pus and formation of a fistula originating at the necrotic or infected bone.

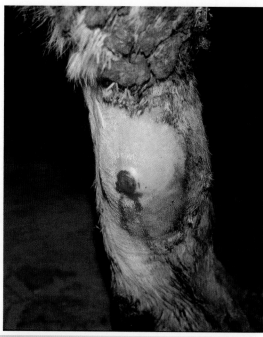

Figure 11-45

Osteomyelitis in a springing heifer's metacarpal region. Recurrent swelling, lameness, and subsequent drainage had been observed for 3 months.

The history may suggest improvement while on antibiotics, but recurrence of the lesion follows cessation of therapy. Affected animals may be slightly lame and resist palpation of the affected area of bone. Most lesions involve the metatarsus or metacarpus.

Diagnosis is confirmed by radiographs of the area. Bone sequestrum must be differentiated from osteomyelitis because a sequestrum necessitates surgical intervention, whereas osteomyelitis may only require medical therapy. Field removal of a sequestrum is not difficult with the aid of radiographs and a bone-cutting chisel. There is frequently significant cancellous bone surrounding the sequestrum, which must be removed before the sequestrum can be extricated. In addition to radiographs, culture and sensitivity of the purulent discharge should be performed. Although *A. pyogenes* is the most common organism identified, other organisms requiring broad-spectrum antibiotic therapy occasionally are isolated. Long-term antibiotic therapy (4 to 6 weeks) is usually required for osteomyelitis. Therefore the animal's value must be sufficient to warrant the costs of therapy.

Spastic Paresis, Spastic Syndrome

Spastic paresis is a rare, progressive muscular disorder that causes overextension of the hind limbs secondary to spastic contraction of the gastrocnemius muscle. One or both hind limbs may be involved, and affected cattle have very straight hind limbs with overextension of the hock. In Holstein calves, spastic paresis has been called Elso heel because the condition tends to appear in animals whose genealogy dates back to a bull called Elso. Calves usually begin showing signs between 2 and 10 months of age. Calves with the disease have extremely straight hind limbs, and the affected limb or limbs often is held in extension behind the body with only the toes contacting the ground (Figure 11-46; see video clip 46). In the early stages, the leg may relax or intermittently relax following the gastrocnemius contraction that occurs after the animal rises. The calf also may raise its head and neck upward when showing overextension of the limb. Because of the progressive nature of the problem, if both hind limbs are affected, the calf is in extreme pain because of gastrocnemius cramping or spasticity and eventually will lose weight and prefer lying down to standing. When forced to stand, the affected limbs are held back rigidly in extension caudal to the body, and the gait is stiff because of difficulty advancing the limb. At rest, the limb may be flexed easily. Palpation of the gastrocnemius in standing animals confirms a tense, contracted muscle in the affected limb. The condition appears in many beef and dairy breeds, but of the dairy breeds, Holsteins and Guernseys are the most commonly affected.

Spastic syndrome in adult animals is distinct from Elso heel, has been called "crampiness," and becomes progressively more severe with age. Confined bulls at

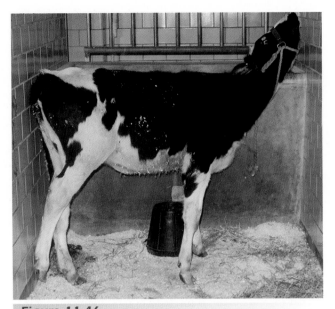

Figure 11-46

Elso heel in a Holstein calf. The right hind limb is held in spastic extension as the calf dorsoflexes the neck.

bull-studs and older cows confined to a box stall are most commonly affected. The first signs usually appear between 2 and 6 years of age. Holsteins and Guernseys are the most frequently affected dairy breeds. Initially affected cattle show crampiness as they attempt to rise and subsequently extend the affected hind limb behind their bodies in an effort to relax the gastrocnemius contractions. In confined cattle, this results in the animals standing off the curb or placing the hind feet in the manure drop. Lowering of the loin and raising the head and neck appear to provide relief from a bout of spasticity. Within minutes, the muscles relax, and the cow may assume a more normal stance. As the condition progresses, affected cattle become more spastic as they attempt to rise and, after rising, may extend the hind limbs behind the body and shake them. Intermittent cramping while standing may occur, causing the cow to extend the limbs backward, shake them, or stand with the hind limb placed caudal to the normal position. If severely affected cows are confined without exercise for several days, they may experience such severe muscle cramping as to be unable to rise.

Diagnosis is based on the physical signs and palpation of the affected gastrocnemius muscles.

Treatment of calves with Elso heel is popular in Europe, where the animals may be raised only for meat production. Treatment using tenotomy of the gastrocnemius tendon or gastrocnemius tendon plus a portion of the superficial digital flexor tendon has yielded improvement in most but not all cases. Neurectomy of branches of the tibial nerve supplying the gastrocnemius muscle has also been successful. In the United States, at least in

dairy cattle, probable inheritability of the condition makes it unwise to treat affected animals, and slaughter should be recommended.

Treatment of adult cows and bulls with spastic paresis is not practiced except for occasional suggestions for the use of muscle relaxants or analgesics to help make an individual cow or bull comfortable. Unfortunately it is a commonly observed condition in bull studs, and affected animals have been used extensively for AI, thereby propagating the condition within the affected breeds. It also is unfortunate that some valuable show cows are treated to mask signs of spastic paresis before being shown.

Contracted Tendons

Contracted flexor tendons in calves and young cattle are either congenital or acquired. Congenital flexor contracture generally occurs in the forelimbs of calves. If no other congenital defects are present, treatment is indicated for valuable calves. It is important to rule out arthrogryposis as a potential cause.

Affected calves knuckle at the fetlock and may either support weight on the toe or, in severe cases, stand on the dorsum of the fetlock (Figure 11-47). The carpus also may be slightly flexed in severe cases. When present at birth, the diagnosis is obvious. Acquired flexor tendon contracture occurs when young calves remain recumbent for prolonged periods because of various conditions, including septicemia, white muscle disease resulting in recumbency, polyarthritis, laminitis, malnutrition, and neurologic diseases. In growing heifers and bulls, recumbency following injury or laminitis

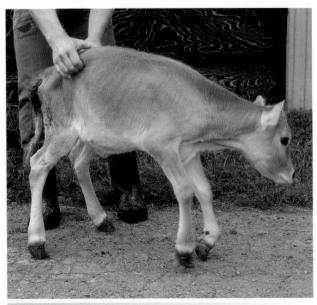

Figure 11-47

Congenital contracted tendons in a Jersey calf.

predisposes them to forelimb flexor tendon contracture, although polyarthritis and other causes are identified occasionally.

Treatment of flexor tendon contracture requires only physical therapy in the simplest congenital cases. Frequent extension of the digit to stretch the tendons gently and encouraging the calf to stand on the limbs for exercise may be all the treatment required. In severe congenital cases, splints or surgical transection of the superficial, deep, or both flexor tendons followed by application of a cast may be necessary. Splints are elected for those individuals that do not appear to respond to physical therapy but are still able to bear weight on the toes. The calf is sedated, and PVC splints are applied over cotton wraps to prevent further knuckling. The splints are changed every week, and the tendons are stretched manually in an effort to gain a degree of extension each time the splints are applied. The calf is made to stand and exercise several times daily. In valuable calves in which the aforementioned conservative measures fail, surgical referral for tendon section of the superficial digital flexor or deep digital flexor tendon or both may be required. This is best done by surgeons who have experience with equine tendon contracture. Casts are required for several weeks following surgery until the sectioned tendons heal; the prognosis must be poor for calves that require tendon section of both the superficial digital and deep digital tendons. High doses of oxytetracycline, as used in foals for contracted tendons, do not appear to be as effective in cattle, and high-dosage administration is a significant risk for acute renal failure in cattle.

In calves or growing animals that develop flexor tendon contracture secondary to other diseases, conservative physical therapy coupled with correction of the underlying condition constitute the grounds for therapy. The longer that these young animals remain recumbent as a result of their primary disease, the less likely they are to respond to conservative physical therapy for flexor tendon contracture.

OTHER MUSCULOSKELETAL PROBLEMS

Ventral Fracture of the Coccyx

Crushed tail head is the common term for compression-type fractures or luxations of the sacral and proximal coccygeal vertebrae (Figure 11-48). This condition is very common in dairy cattle as a result of mounting activity during estrus. Usually spinal nerves are injured in the process with resulting tail paresis or paralysis in most cases. In intermediate cases, the tail is paralyzed, and the bladder never empties but rather trickles urine into the vagina continuously; however, the cow has normal control of the hind limbs. In more serious cases involving the sacrum, proximal sacral nerves may be

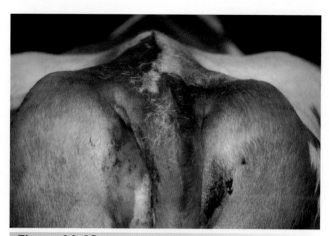

Figure 11-48

Fractured fourth sacral vertebrae causing ventral depression of the tail head and diminished ability to move the tail in a Guernsey show cow. The fracture was surgically repaired, and the cow recovered a normal appearance of the tail head and improved function of the tail.

damaged, leading to sciatic nerve deficits with bilateral knuckling of the hind limbs.

Diagnosis is made by inspection. The normal alignment of the sacrum and proximal coccygeal vertebrae is disturbed, and abrasions may be apparent over the tail head from mounting activity by other cows. Manipulation of the tail and tail head may be painful to the cow. In chronic cases, atrophy of the musculature at the tail head and coccygeal muscles may be apparent. The major complication of tail-head injuries resulting in tail paralysis is soiling of the perineum and tail with feces and urine. The affected cow is unable to raise her tail to defecate or urinate; subsequently manure and urine become smeared on the vulva, perineum, and tail. In some instances, this condition promotes vaginal contamination, which may interfere with conception because of ascending reproductive tract infection. Severe sacral fractures also may injure the pudendal nerve with consequential loss of caudal reproductive tract sensation.

Conservative treatment is unlikely to change the clinical signs, but cattle with severe injuries resulting in apparent sciatic nerve damage should be treated with antiinflammatory drugs during the acute course in an effort to reduce edema and inflammation around the sacral nerves. After healing of the luxation, the pelvic canal may be too small for passage of a normal calf; if the cow is pregnant, a surgical delivery should be planned.

Sacroiliac Luxation

Although rather uncommon, sacroiliac luxation occurs during the periparturient period, generally 1 week before to 1 week after parturition. The physiologic laxity of

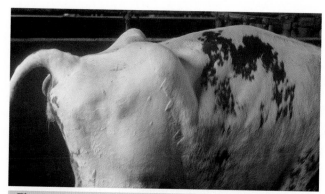

Figure 11-49

Sacroiliac luxation in a mature Ayrshire cow. The tuber coxae project dorsally far above the level of the vertebral column.

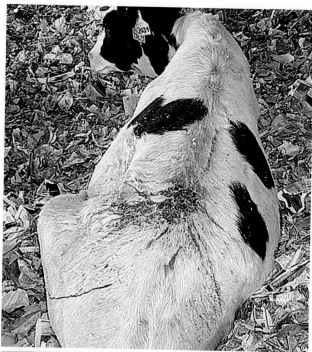

Figure 11-50

Back injury in a cow that became entrapped in a stall. She was unwilling to rise for several days but did recover.

ligamentous structures that occurs during the estrogen peak associated with parturition apparently predisposes to sacroiliac luxation or subluxation.

The signs of luxation are apparent by inspection, as the tuber coxae appear raised above the plane of the vertebral column, and they rock back and forth when the cow walks because the hind limbs and pelvis now move independently of the vertebral column (Figure 11-49). In subluxation, the tuber coxae may be slightly raised above the vertebral column or there is small but painful motion between the sacrum and ilium. Some cattle with complete luxation experience severe pain and refuse to move or eat, whereas others seem to experience less pain, move about with a stiff gait, and continue to eat. If luxation occurs before calving, the cow should be assisted during delivery or may require a cesarean section because of the dorsoventral compression of the pelvic inlet.

Prognosis is guarded to poor in all instances of sacroiliac luxation and favorable for sacroiliac subluxation because scarring of the joint will likely occur. Cattle obviously in extreme pain should be slaughtered. Those cattle that continue to eat, give milk, and move about may finish the current lactation. Knowledge on reoccurrence does not exist because of the rarity of the condition. Cattle with complete luxation should not be bred back because dystocia will be inevitable.

Back Injuries

Efforts to rise while accidentally positioned or trapped under stall partitions cause most back injuries in cattle. Cattle in free stalls or tie stalls may become positioned under divider bars if stalls are improperly designed or maintained. Adult cows with lameness or metabolic diseases may inadvertently become malpositioned. Other causes of back injuries include being ridden by larger cows or falling while being ridden by another cow.

Often cows with an injured back are able but unwilling to stand. Thus the examination is often conducted on a recumbent cow. An arched stance with the hind limbs placed further caudal than normal typifies the posture of a cow with a back injury (Figure 11-50). Inspection of the top line may allow rapid diagnosis if multiple abrasions or hematoma formation is observed. The gait is stiff and shuffling, and the cow may get up and down in a very awkward fashion. Rectal temperature is normal, but heart and respiratory rates may be elevated because of pain. The appetite may be normal or slightly reduced. Palpation of the back and dorsal spinous processes of the cow's vertebrae may elicit a painful response. History may suggest the diagnosis if back trauma has been observed by the caretaker.

Diagnosis is reached by history, observation, palpation, and the patient's characteristic posture. Other causes of an arched stance, such as localized peritonitis, are ruled out by the physical findings of normal gastrointestinal tract, normal temperature, and fair to normal appetite. Spastic syndrome may cause the hind limbs to be held caudal to the perpendicular, but spastic cattle tend to lower the loin rather than being arched. In laminitis, cattle stand with the hind limbs under the body and show sensitivity to hoof testers and warmth in the claws.

Rest and analgesics are the therapy for back injuries in cattle. A clumsy animal should be moved to a box stall until healing occurs. Keeping the cow isolated from others will prevent further injury from riding behavior.

Dexamethasone or NSAID therapy greatly aids the affected animals and should be used for 3 days to 2 weeks, depending on severity. Improvement is suggested when stance becomes less arched and gait more normal.

Downer Cows—Myopathy

Exertional myopathy is caused by struggling; uncoordinated efforts to rise; being entangled in mud, manure, wires, or equipment; or repeated attempts to rise on treacherous footing such as ice or wet concrete. Repeated muscular exertion results in microscopic or gross muscle injury with breakdown of cells, edema, hemorrhage, release of lactic acid, and eventual necrosis or fibrosis. Various muscle groups may be involved, depending on the patient's position, weight, or environment, but the hind limb musculature is most commonly affected. Adductor musculature may be involved if cattle have split their hind limbs secondary to obturator paralysis or splaying their legs by splitting on slippery flooring. The quadriceps may be involved in "creeper cows" that struggle to move or rise with their hind limbs extended behind the body. The gastrocnemius or semimembranosus-semitendinosus musculature in the caudal thigh may be involved when the patient repeatedly struggles to rise but is too weak to do so. In most instances, a primary disease (e.g., hypocalcemia, nerve dysfunction following dystocia or injury, hypokalemia) has caused recumbency, and myopathy follows in those patients that struggle excessively or are left on slippery footing.

Compartmental syndrome is another secondary complication of primary metabolic, neurologic, or musculoskeletal diseases that results in prolonged recumbency. Compartmental syndrome results in ischemia to the down-side limbs—usually the hind limb in a recumbent cow. This ischemia will result in swelling of the limb distal to the stifle and combined neurologic-muscular damage because of edema and pressure necrosis of muscle bundles and nerves confined within fascial borders. In addition, the sciatic nerve may experience pressure damage at the caudal aspect of the upper portion of the femur, and the peroneal nerve is subject to direct pressure at the proximal fibula below the stifle. Those conditions are discussed in Chapter 12. The peroneal nerve frequently is involved in compartmental syndrome or pressure myopathy-neuropathy in the region between stifle and hock of the down-side limb in recumbent cattle.

The clinical result of exertional myopathy or compartmental syndrome is limb dysfunction characterized by inability to rise or bear weight normally on affected limbs. Signs may include limb swelling, muscular swelling, rigid extension of the limb, inability to rise, and flexion of the limb with knuckling, among others. Obviously the exact posture and signs will vary based on the muscle groups involved and other skeletal injuries or neuropathies. Muscle swelling in acute myopathy may be associated with firm swelling, but in most cases the muscle will be relatively flaccid or soft such that physical diagnosis relies on detection of muscular swelling, asymmetry, and characteristic signs when the patient is standing, lying in recumbency, or attempting to rise. Simple ancillary data confirmation may be obtained by using test reagent strips on the patient's urine. In the most severe myopathies, frank myoglobinuria will be apparent as distinctly brown or deep red urine that is also cloudy. In less severe cases, the urine may be clear and brown, or clear and yellowish but show a strong positive to the hemoglobin and protein reagents on the multiple test strips. Because the m-orthotoluidine reagent composing the hemoglobin test also responds to myoglobin, it is useful in detecting myoglobin in a field setting. In valuable cattle or questionable cases, serum creatine kinase (CK) and aspartate aminotransferase (AST) should be assessed as a prognostic aid. Most recumbent cattle have some degree of elevated CK and AST values, so slight elevation may not be diagnostic of severe myopathy. The relative level of CK and AST elevation is the important diagnostic-prognostic indicator. It also is important to realize that CK peaks very quickly following muscular injury and has a short (4 to 8 hours) serum half-life, whereas AST peaks more slowly but remains elevated or steady for several days. Therefore CK would be a better diagnostic test for the cow recumbent only 24 to 48 hours, whereas a cow that has been recumbent for 7 days might be better assessed by AST, assuming muscle damage occurred early in her recumbent course. CK values greater than 5000 to 10,000 IU/L are typical in acute exertional myopathies and frequently exceed 20,000 IU/L if severe heavy muscle damage has occurred. Severe myopathies may cause AST elevations of 3000 or greater that persist for several days after reaching peak levels. In general, CK values exceeding 100,000 IU/L or AST levels exceeding 10,000 IU/L carry an extremely poor prognosis. These cattle may have elevated serum potassium in the acute phase as a result of muscle cell breakdown and are at risk for myoglobin nephrosis. Metabolic acidosis may be present because of profound lactic acid release from muscle cells and/or poor perfusion. In cattle with drastic exertional myopathy (e.g., having been trapped in mud) that destroys many heavy muscle groups, a shock-like state and neurologic signs may be seen secondary to release of lactic acid, potassium, and probably many other products from damaged muscle.

Following diagnosis of myopathy, the clinician must decide whether the primary cause of recumbency has been resolved or requires further treatment and whether the animal can survive the degree of myopathy present. In many instances, the primary problem has been corrected (e.g., hypocalcemia), and only myopathy remains as a cause of recumbency. In other instances (such as septic mastitis or obturator paralysis), primary conditions remain that, along with secondary myopathy, contribute additionally to a poor prognosis. Frank myoglobinuria suggests the possibility of myoglobin nephrosis with subsequent renal failure and worsens the prognosis. If myopathy is confirmed, clinical judgment dictates the likely success of therapy. Cattle that are bright, alert, willing to attempt to rise, and have resolved the primary problem that resulted in recumbency are the best patients with which to work. If treatment is deemed practical, the following therapeutic principles should be followed:

1. Nursing care: Be sure to have the recumbent animal on good footing with a nonslip surface. This may be a manure pack, dirt box stall, well-bedded box stall, or solid ground outside. Cows lunge forward when rising, and straw bales can be placed around the inside of the stall to prevent the cow from lying down with her head near the wall. The cow also should be fed and watered where she lies; preventing other cows sharing the same pen from eating the downer cow's feed seems a regular challenge in larger dairies. Cows with a tendency to abduct the hind limbs because of calving paralysis should be hobbled to prevent splitting. Recumbent cattle should be rolled from one side to the other several times daily to reduce the possibility of compartment syndrome.

2. Analgesics: Exertional myopathy is an extremely painful condition, and either flunixin or ketoprofen or dexamethasone is indicated.

3. Fluid therapy: Indicated when frank myoglobinuria is present and renal damage is possible or present. Balanced electrolytes are indicated unless laboratory data show hyperkalemia and metabolic acidosis that require specific fluid and electrolyte replacement.

4. Vitamin E and selenium: Most adult cattle have sufficient levels of blood selenium, but empirically it does no harm to administer a therapeutic dose of vitamin E and selenium to ensure that the cow has an adequate rebuilding capacity for muscle repair. Empiric treatment is utilized because laboratory evaluation of selenium or glutathione peroxidase values may have a rather long turnaround time, and it may be best to provide these supplements rather than wait for laboratory confirmation or denial of low selenium levels.

5. Manual or mechanical assistance in rising: This portion of supportive care is the most controversial and is subject to individual clinical experience. The simplest means is to provide manual assistance by lifting the cow by her tail when she attempts to rise. Other mechanical means include the use of hip slings, cattle walkers, inflatable air bags, or slings. All mechanical aids must be used judiciously, lest they do more harm than good. It usually is best not to rush into the use of mechanical devices if good nursing care is available, but cattle in compromised environments may require mechanical aids within 48 hours of initial recumbency to determine whether they can support weight once raised. Raising the recumbent cow also allows a more thorough physical examination, including an easier rectal examination and evaluation of weight-bearing abilities in each limb. This can be an extremely helpful aid to prognosis.

The newest tool available for physical therapy of the downer cow is the flotation tank. There are commercial units available, including those with the capacity to heat the large volume of water required to about 36° C or 95° F. There is probably more therapeutic benefit than diagnostic value in supporting a cow with water. After 24 to 36 hours in the tank, the cow can be released onto good footing such as deep sand, which will give her confidence in her ability to remain upright and control her posture. It is best, although not always possible, to fill the tank quickly to minimize panic on the cow's part. Most tanks are equipped with large-diameter drain spigots so that the water can be removed quickly. When used in cold ambient temperatures, either periodic heating of the water or replacement of some of the water with hot water is needed. In hot ambient temperatures, a shade may be important to protect the cow from hyperthermia. In our clinic, some cows have failed to stand after three or four sessions yet eventually recovered fully. Cows that have stood squarely in the tank have generally had a better prognosis than those that constantly shift weight (Figure 11-51, *A* and *B*).

Although maligned by many clinicians, we prefer well-padded hip slings as mechanical aids (Figure 11-52) because they are relatively inexpensive, can be used indoors (beam hooks) or outdoors (hydraulic tractor lift), and they require fewer people for their use. The best patient-candidates for mechanical aids are those that want to stand, will try to stand, and can stand once they are assisted to their feet. These cattle usually only require mechanical assistance twice daily for 1 to 5 days before being able to rise by themselves. Some recumbent cattle are apprehensive and frightened when raised for the first time and will refuse to bear weight. Therefore the initial attempt should not be overinterpreted but rather thought of as a "training session." The individual value of the animal and the manpower available for nursing care will dictate the length of time devoted to care of the recumbent myopathy patient. No absolute rules exist regarding length of time a cow may remain down before the prognosis becomes hopeless. However, each additional day spent in recumbency obviously worsens prognosis because further musculoskeletal and neurologic damage is made more likely. Subtle signs of improvement such as progressively bearing more weight on the affected limbs when raised day by day are the keys to prognosis and the decision as to whether to treat for a longer time. If hip slings or other slings are used, they should be well-padded and removed within 1 to 5 minutes after the animal is standing to reduce the possibility of pressure necrosis over the skin on the tuber

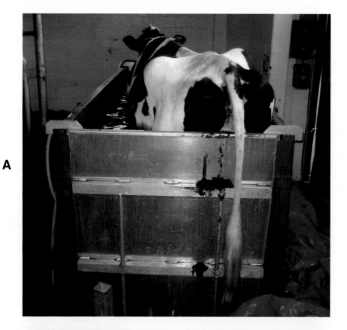

A

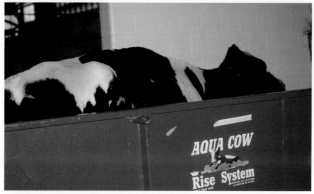

B

Figure 11-51

Stance of two cows placed in float tanks because of inability to stand. **A,** The cow was recumbent because of a metabolic disease and when placed in the tank stood squarely and recovered. **B,** The cow did not stand squarely, was euthanized after 3 days of treatment, and was found to have a pelvic fracture on necropsy examination.

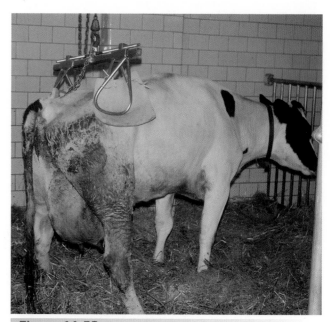

Figure 11-52

Hip slings being used to raise the rear quarters of a cow suffering from exertional myopathy.

coxae region. If the cow cannot support weight within 1 to 5 minutes after being lifted, she should be milked out promptly and allowed to lie down again. Hip slings never should be left in place for longer than 5 to 10 minutes during any lifting episode, and they always should be heavily padded. Properly managed, some patients with mild to moderate myopathies can be saved. Cattle with severe myopathies or cattle with lesser myopathies that are improperly managed have poor prognoses.

White Muscle Disease

Nutritional myodegeneration characterized by Zenker's degeneration was once common in dairy calves in selenium-deficient geographic areas. The disease can occur in growing animals, and although most common in

calves less than 6 months of age, it can be observed in animals up to 2 years of age. All commercial diets in the United States are now supplemented with the allowable levels of selenium. Herds that formulate their own mineral/vitamin mixtures or have them custom-made may be feeding more than allowable levels (which may be necessary to meet requirements because they are based on an allowable concentration and not on milligrams of selenium consumed per day). As a consequence of this widespread use of selenium supplementation, clinical cases of white muscle disease are now mostly seen in calves from hobby farms where commercial diets are not fed.

Deficiency of selenium, vitamin E, or both may play a role in predisposing to the disease. Selenium is an important precursor for enzymes such as glutathione peroxidase that protect tissues against oxidation. Vitamin E also protects against superoxide damage resulting from the normal oxidation of unsaturated lipids in the diet. Forages and grain should contain at least 0.1 to 0.3 ppm selenium (on a dry matter basis) to be considered adequate. Aging, fermentation, and other factors may have a negative impact on vitamin E content of stored feeds such that levels of this vitamin are much lower when fed than when originally harvested. Studies in other species suggest that certain dietary minerals may interact with selenium to increase or decrease bioavailability, but this work has not been repeated in cattle.

Signs of white muscle disease may involve any striated muscles, including those in the pharynx, larynx, tongue, respiratory muscles, heart, neck musculature, or limb musculature. In newborn calves, the tongue may be the only tissue affected, and the animal will be unable to nurse. The tongue feels slightly flaccid, and the calf wants to eat but the tongue merely lolls when a finger is inserted into the calf's mouth to evaluate the sucking reflex. Inhalation pneumonia may develop in several calves within a group, or obvious dyspnea may appear when pharyngeal, laryngeal, and respiratory muscles such as the intercostals and diaphragm are affected.

Classic signs of a stiff gait may be observed early in the course, especially in calves that have just moved from close confinement to a large area where more exercise occurs. A stilted gait may be apparent in just the hind limbs, just the forelimbs, or all limbs. When present, this sign requires differentiation from laminitis, polyarthritis, and tetanus. Diffuse muscle degeneration leads to weakness, and this is a common sign in young calves (Figure 11-53). When lifted to a standing position, these calves will have muscular tremors within seconds after trying to support weight, and then within a short time, the head will drop as a result of cervical musculature weakness. If made to stand longer, the limbs may collapse or the animal may show obvious dyspnea. Severe diffuse muscular degeneration leads to complete collapse, and the calves or yearlings appear paralyzed at first glance. The worst cases are depressed, dyspneic, and may show apparent neurologic signs secondary to metabolic acidosis associated with high levels of lactic acid released from damaged musculature. Gross myoglobinuria usually is present in these severely affected animals.

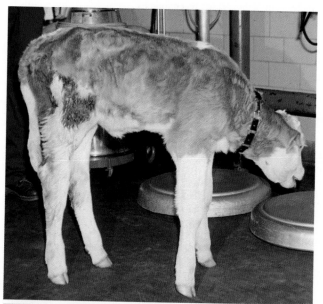

Figure 11-53

A 1-week-old calf with diffuse white muscle disease. After being raised, the calf could only support itself for a few seconds before collapsing. The calf is unable to raise its head because of neck musculature weakness. Open-mouth breathing is apparent as a result of myopathy involving the muscles of respiration.

When the myocardium is affected, arrhythmias, heart murmurs, dyspnea associated with pulmonary edema, or sudden death with no premonitory signs may be observed. Exercise accentuates the signs in affected animals, and exercise or handling may precipitate the signs in apparently normal but deficient animals.

In acute cases with localized Zenker's degeneration in heavy muscle groups, the muscle may be firm and swollen when palpated. In most instances, however, and certainly in those with severe diffuse Zenker's degeneration, the affected muscles are soft when palpated. Chronic cases that have been recumbent for days may show obvious muscle atrophy and fibrosis.

Clinical signs, especially if more than one animal is affected, coupled with myoglobin in the urine suffice for clinical diagnosis. Gross myoglobinuria is more common in diffuse degeneration or in older calves that have heavy musculature affected. Less obvious myoglobinuria will be suspected when urine dipstick evaluation confirms a positive blood (hemoglobin [Hb], red blood cell [RBC], and myoglobin) and protein reaction. Laboratory findings of very elevated CK and AST values help confirm the diagnosis. Values for CK increase quickly and, because of the short half-life of this enzyme, may decrease within 2 to 4 days unless continued muscle destruction occurs. Values for AST tend to increase slowly over 1 to 2 days and then reach a plateau for nearly 1 week. Therefore the history coupled with these values can be helpful in interpretation. CK values will be greater than 1000 IU/L and frequently exceed 10,000 IU/L. Values for AST usually exceed 500 IU/L. These values tend to be much higher in older animals in which the sheer volume of affected musculature tends to elevate the enzymes far more than in a young calf, for example, that has only myocardial or muscles of deglutition affected. Final confirmation of the diagnosis rests on laboratory assessment of whole blood selenium (heparinized sample) or glutathione peroxidase (ethylenediaminetetraacetic acid sample). Selenium is incorporated in glutathione peroxidase in erythrocytes, and this enzyme facilitates cellular breakdown of peroxides. Because selenium must be incorporated into RBC glutathione peroxidase during erythrogenesis, an increase in measured glutathione peroxidase requires 4 to 6 weeks. Therefore glutathione peroxidase can be evaluated even if an affected or suspected calf has recently received supplemental selenium, although selenium values from the same calf may not be as valuable. In untreated calves, whole blood selenium usually is assessed. Ranges for selenium and glutathione peroxidase are listed below, although individual laboratories may establish slightly different normal ranges:

	Whole Blood Selenium, µg/dl	Glutathione Peroxidase U/g Hb
Normal	>12.0	>30
Marginal	8.0-12.0	20-30
Deficient	<8.0	<20

White muscle disease is a "selenium-responsive" disease so that, regardless of the exact etiology (selenium, vitamin E, or binding of selenium by other minerals), treatment and prevention require supplementation with selenium products through injection or feeding.

Affected calves require injection of selenium and vitamin E at manufacturers' recommended dosages, and these injections may be repeated three to four times at 3-day intervals.

Overtreatment with selenium/vitamin E preparations by injection is dangerous because selenium toxicity may develop with subsequent death of the patient. Therefore it is important to adhere strictly to label dosage recommendations when treating with commercial vitamin E/selenium preparations.

SUGGESTED READINGS

Adams SB: The role of external fixation and emergency fracture management in bovine orthopedics, *Vet Clin North Am (Food Anim Pract)* 1:109-129, 1985.

Anderson DE, St-Jean G, Morin DE, et al: Traumatic flexor tendon injuries in 27 cattle, *Vet Surg* 25:320-326, 1996.

Bentley VA, Edwards RB III, Santschi EM, et al: Repair of femoral capital physeal fractures with 7.0 mm cannulated screws in cattle: 20 cases (1988-2002), *J Am Vet Med Assoc* 227:964-969, 2005.

Berg JN, Loan RW: Fusobacterium necrophorum and Bacteroids melaninogenicus as etiological agents in foot rot in cattle, *Am J Vet Res* 36:115, 1975.

Bergsten C: Haemorrhages of the sole horn of dairy cows as a retrospective indicator of laminitis: an epidemiological study, *Acta Vet Scand* 35:55-66, 1994.

Bicalho RC, Cheong SH, Warnick LD, et al: The effect of digit amputation or arthrodesis on surgery culling and milk production in Holstein dairy cows, *J Dairy Sci* 89:2596-2602, 2006.

Blood DC: Arthrogryposis and hydrancephaly, *Aust Vet J* 32:125-131, 1956.

Bouckaert JH, DeMoor A: Treatment of spastic paralysis in cattle: improved denervation technique of the gastrocnemius muscle and postoperative course, *Vet Rec* 79:226, 1966.

Colam-Ainsworth P, Lunn GA, Thomas RC, et al: Behaviour of cows in cubicles and its possible relationship with laminitis in replacement dairy heifers, *Vet Rec* 125:573-575, 1989.

Cox VS: Understanding the downer cow syndrome, *Compend Contin Educ Pract Vet* 3:S472-S478, 1981.

Cox VS, McGrath CJ, Jorgensen SE: The role of pressure damage in pathogenesis of the downer cow syndrome, *Am J Vet Res* 43:26-31, 1982.

Crawford WH: Intra-articular replacement of bovine cranial cruciate ligaments with an autogenous fascial graft, *Vet Surg* 19:380-388, 1990.

Dermirkan I, Walker RL, Murray RD, et al: Serological evidence of spirochaetal infections associated with digital dermatitis in dairy cattle, *Vet J* 157:69-77, 1999.

Desrochers A, Anderson DE, St.-Jean G: Lameness examination in cattle, *Vet Clin North Am (Food Anim Pract)* 17:39-51, 2001.

Ewoldt JM, Hull BL, Ayars WH: Repair of femoral capital physeal fractures in 12 cattle, *Vet Surg* 32:30-36, 2003.

Ferguson JG: Management and repair of bovine fractures, *Compend Contin Educ Pract Vet* 4:S128-S136, 1982.

Ferguson JG: Principles of application of internal fixation in cattle, *Vet Clin North Am (Food Anim Pract)* 1:139-152, 1985.

Ferguson JG: Special considerations in bovine orthopedics and lameness, *Vet Clin North Am (Food Anim Pract)* 1:131-138, 1985.

Firth EC, Kersjes AW, Kik KJ, et al: Haematogenous osteomyelitis in cattle, *Vet Rec* 120:148-152, 1987.

Francoz D, Desrochers A, Fecteau G, et al: Synovial fluid changes in induced infectious arthritis in calves, *J Vet Intern Med* 19:336-343, 2005.

Frankena K, van Keulen KAS, Noordhuizen JP, et al: A cross-sectional study in prevalence and risk indicators of digital haemorrhages in female dairy calves, *Prev Vet Med* 14:1-12, 1992.

Gangl M, Grukle S, Serteyn D, et al: Retrospective study of 99 cases of bone fractures in cattle treated by external coaptation or confinement, *Vet Rec* 158:264-268, 2006.

Garrett EF, Nordlund KV, Goodger WJ, et al: A cross-sectional field study investigating the effect of periparturient dietary management on ruminal pH in early lactation dairy cows, *J Dairy Sci* 80(suppl 1):169, 1997 (abstract).

Greenough PR, MacCallum FJ, Weaver AD: *Lameness in cattle*, ed 3, St. Louis, 1997, WB Saunders.

Grubelnik M, Kofler J, Martinek B, et al: Ultrasonographic examination of the hip joint region and bony pelvis in cattle, *Berl Munch Tierarztl Wochenschr* 115:209-220, 2002.

Gütze R: Spastic paresis of the hindquarters of calves and young cattle, *Dtsch Tierärztl Wochenschr* 40:197, 1932.

Hull BL, Koenig GJ, Monke DR: Treatment of slipped capital femoral epiphysis in cattle: 11 cases (1974-1988), *J Am Vet Med Assoc* 197:1509-1512, 1990.

Hum S, Kessell A, Djordjevic S, et al: Mastitis, polyarthritis and abortion caused by Mycoplasma species bovine group 7 in dairy cattle, *Aust Vet J* 78:744-750, 2000.

Leonard FC, O'Connell J, O'Farrell K: Effect of different housing conditions on behaviour and foot lesions in Friesian heifers, *Vet Rec* 134:490-494, 1994.

Livesey CT, Fleming FL: Nutritional influences on laminitis, sole ulcer and bruised sole in Friesian cows, *Vet Rec* 14:510-512, 1984.

Logue DN, Offer JE, McGovern RE: The housing effects of first calving Holstein Friesian heifers separately or with the adult herd on claw conformation and lesion development. In Lischer CJ, Ossent P, editors: 10th International Symposium on Lameness in Ruminants, Lucerne, September 1998, pp. 60-62, Department of Veterinary Surgery, University of Zurich.

Maas JP: Diagnosis and management of selenium-responsive diseases in cattle, *Compend Contin Educ Pract Vet* 5:S393-S399, 1983.

Madison JB, Tulleners EP, Ducharme NG, et al: Idiopathic gonitis in heifers: 34 cases (1976-1986), *J Am Vet Med Assoc* 194:273-277, 1989.

Manson FJ, Leaver JD: The influence of concentrate amount on locomotion and clinical lameness in dairy cattle, *Anim Prod* 47:185-190, 1988.

Martens A, Steenhaut M, Gasthuys F, et al: Conservative and surgical treatment of tibial fractures in cattle, *Vet Rec* 143:12-16, 1998.

Maton A: The influence of the housing system on claw disorders with dairy cows. In Wierenga HK, Peterse DJ, editors: *Cattle housing systems, lameness, and behaviour: Proceedings of Commission of European Communities*, Brussels, June 1986, Dordrecht, 1987, Martinus Nijhoff Publishers, pp. 151-158.

McDuffee LA, Ducharme NG, Ward JL: Repair of sacral fracture in two dairy cattle, *J Am Vet Med Assoc* 202:1126-1128, 1993.

Metz JHM, Wierenga HK, Behavioural criteria for the design of housing systems for cattle. In Wierenga HK, Peterse DJ, editors: *Cattle housing systems, lameness, and behaviour: Proceedings of Commission of European Communities*, Brussels, June 1986, Dordrecht, 1987, Martinus Nijhoff Publishers, pp. 14-25.

Murphy PA, Hannan J, Monaghan M: A survey of lameness in beef cattle housed on slats and on straw. In Wierenga HK, Peterse DJ, editors: *Cattle housing systems, lameness, and behaviour: Proceedings of Commission of European Communities*, Brussels, June 1986, Dordrecht, 1987, Martinus Nijhoff Publishers, pp. 67-72.

Nelson DR: Surgery of the stifle joint in cattle, *Compend Contin Educ Pract Vet* 5:S300-S306, 1983.

Nelson DR, Kneller SK: Treatment of proximal hind-limb lameness in cattle, *Vet Clin North Am (Food Anim Pract)* 1:153-173, 1985.

Nuss K, Weaver MP: Resection of the distal interphalangeal joint in cattle: an alternative to amputation, *Vet Rec* 128: 540-543, 1991.

Pejsa TG, St. Jean G, Hoffsis GF, et al: Digit amputation in cattle: 85 cases (1971-1990), *J Am Vet Med Assoc* 202:981-984, 1993.

Peterse DJ, Korver S, Oldenbroek JK, et al: Relationship between levels of concentrate feeding and incidence of sole ulcers in dairy cattle, *Vet Rec* 115:629-630, 1984.

Potter MJ, Broom DM: The behaviour and welfare of cows in relation to cubicle house design. In Wierenga HK, Peterse DJ, editors: *Cattle housing systems, lameness, and behaviour: Proceedings of Commission of European Communities*, Brussels, June 1986, Dordrecht, 1987, Martinus Nijhoff Publishers, pp. 129-147.

Rajkondawar PG, Liu M, Dyer RM, et al: Comparison of models to identify lame cows based on gait and lesion scores, and limb movement variables, *J Dairy Sci* 89:4267-4275, 2006.

Read DH, Walker RL, Castro AE, et al: An invasive spirochete associated with interdigital papillomatosis of dairy cattle, *Vet Rec* 130:59-60, 1992.

Rebhun WC, Payne RM, King JM, et al: Interdigital papillomatosis in dairy cattle, *J Am Vet Med Assoc* 177:437-440, 1980.

Rebhun WC, de Lahunta A, Baum KH, et al: Compressive neoplasms affecting the bovine spinal cord, *Compend Contin Educ Pract Vet* 6:S396-S400, 1984.

Reiland S, Stromberg P, Olsson SE, et al: Osteochondrosis in growing bulls, *Acta Radiol* 358:179-196, 1978.

Scholz RW, Hutchinson LJ: Distribution of glutathione peroxidase activity and selenium in the blood of dairy cows, *Am J Vet Res* 40:245-249, 1979.

Studder E, Nelson JR: Nutrition related degenerative joint disease in young bulls, *Vet Med* 66:1007-1010, 1971.

Thyssen I: Foot and leg disorders in dairy cattle in different housing systems. In Wierenga HK, Peterse DJ, editors: *Cattle housing systems, lameness, and behaviour: Proceedings of Commission of European Communities*, Brussels, June 1986, Dordrecht, 1987, Martinus Nijhoff Publishers, pp. 166-178.

Toussaint-Raven E: *Cattle footcare and claw trimming*, Ipswich, UK, 1989, Farming Press.

Toussaint-Raven E: The principles of claw trimming, *Vet Clin North Am (Food Anim Pract)* 1:93-107, 1985.

Trent AM, Plumb D: Treatment of infectious arthritis and osteomyelitis, *Vet Clin North Am (Food Anim Pract)* 7:747-778, 1991.

Trott DJ, Moeller MR, Zuerner RL, et al: Characterization of Treponema phagedenis-like spirochetes isolated from papillomatous digital dermatitis lesions in dairy cattle, *J Clin Microbiol* 41:2522-2529, 2003.

Tulleners E, Divers TJ, Evans L: Bilateral bicipital bursitis in a cow, *J Am Vet Med Assoc* 186:604, 1985.

Tulleners EP: Metacarpal and metatarsal fractures in dairy cattle: 33 cases (1979–1985), *J Am Vet Med Assoc* 189:463-468, 1986.

Tulleners EP, Nunamaker DM, Richardson DW: Coxofemoral luxation in cattle: 22 cases (1980–1985), *J Am Vet Med Assoc* 191:569-574, 1987.

van Amstel SR, Shearer JK: Review of Pododermatitis circumscripta (ulceration of the sole) in dairy cows, *J Vet Intern Med* 20:805-811, 2006.

Van Pelt RXVW: Idiopathic septic arthritis in dairy cattle, *J Am Vet Med Assoc* 161:278-284, 1972.

Van Vleet JF: Amounts of eight combined elements required to induce selenium-vitamin E deficiency and protection by supplements of selenium and vitamin E, *Am J Vet Res* 43:1049-1055, 1982.

Verschooten F, Vermeiren D, Devriese L: Bone infection in the bovine appendicular skeleton: a clinical, radiographic, and experimental study, *Vet Radiol Ultrasound* 41:250-260, 2000.

Walker RL, Read DH, Loretz KJ, et al: Spirochetes isolated from dairy cattle with papillomatous digital dermatitis and interdigital dermatitis, *Vet Microbiol* 47:343-355, 1995.

White SL, Rowland GN, Whitlock RH: Radiographic, macroscopic, and microscopic changes in growth plates of calves raised on hard flooring, *Am J Vet Res* 45:633-639, 1984.

CHAPTER 12

Neurologic Diseases

Alexander de Lahunta and Thomas J. Divers

BOVINE NEUROLOGIC EXAMINATION

There are five components of a neurologic examination: sensorium, gait, postural reactions, spinal reflexes, and cranial nerves (CNs). The order and degree to which these can be performed will depend on the clinician's choice and the size and attitude of the patient.

Sensorium

This is best assessed by observing the patient before it is handled. Abnormalities that reflect intracranial interference with the ascending reticular activating system (ARAS) include (in increasing severity): depression, lethargy, obtundation, semicoma (stupor), and coma. Behavioral changes occur with prosencephalic disorders, especially those that affect the limbic system and include propulsive pacing and circling, head pressing, agitation, excessive licking, charging, and mania.

Gait

If the patient is ambulatory, its gait should be observed in a closed area, ideally while being led. Observation from the side is the most informative and while being walked in small circles in each direction. The quality of the deficits observed with the various anatomical sites of lesions will be described at the beginning of each anatomical area that is covered in this chapter. For difficult cases, it helps to video the gait abnormality so that it can be studied repeatedly and with slow motion. With recumbent animals, it is essential to try to sling the animal to determine which limbs are affected, how much voluntary limb movement is present, and the quality of the paresis or paralysis. Be aware that compression of a large muscle mass in heavy animals that are recumbent can reduce the accuracy of your assessment.

Postural Reactions

In calves and young stock that are cooperative, you can assess their ability to hop on each limb by holding up the opposite limb and pushing the patient laterally on the limb being tested. Difficulty in supporting weight with rapid attempts to do so suggests neuromuscular disease. Brainstem or spinal cord disorders that interfere with descending upper motor neuron (UMN) and ascending general proprioceptive (GP) pathways will mean a delay in the hopping response or none at all. (Despite what has been written about neurologic examinations, there is NO test that is specific for conscious proprioception, and that misconception should be discarded.)

Spinal Reflexes—Muscle Tone and Size

Denervation atrophy is best observed in the standing animal. Realistically, spinal reflex testing is only of value in the recumbent patient and that will be influenced by the extent of muscle compression secondary to the recumbency. Limbs can be manipulated to assess muscle tone, but in adult animals hypotonia can be difficult to determine. The only reliable tendon reflex is the patellar reflex (femoral nerve: L4, L5 spinal cord segments, roots, and nerves). Withdrawal (flexor) reflexes can be done in each limb to assess the integrity of the respective spinal cord intumescence and the peripheral nerves that arise from each.

The spinal reflexes will be influenced by how much nociception and voluntary movements are still present in the patient. Tail and anal tone and reflexes are readily assessed in the standing or recumbent animal. In animals with severe peripheral nerve or spinal cord disease, the determination of nociception has prognostic importance. Using forceps to produce a noxious stimulus may not be adequate in the recumbent patient, and it may be necessary to use an electric (hot shot) stimulus. This is NOT a pain stimulus. Pain is not a sensory modality. Pain is the subjective response of the patient to a noxious stimulus and varies considerably between individual animals.

Differentiating "superficial and deep pain" as is often described is not only a misnomer but also superfluous and of no practical value in localizing lesions even if one thought he or she could determine the difference.

Cranial Nerves

In most animals and especially young calves, this part of the examination is best done initially without handling the patient, and consists of the following:

Assess the menace response with your hand (eye – II – central visual pathway – VII)

Assess the symmetry of the pupils and the pupillary light reflex (eye – II – rostral brainstem – III – ciliary ganglion – iris)

Look for strabismus (III, IV, and VI – vestibular)

Look for resting nystagmus – jerk nystagmus (vestibular VIII), pendular nystagmus – ocular tremor (idiopathic)

Look for the size of the palpebral fissure (VII, III, sympathetic), ear position, and movement (VII)

All of the above can be done without handling the animal.

Move the head side to side for normal physiologic nystagmus (vestibular VIII – brainstem– III, VI)

Hold the head to each side and in extension, and look for development of a positional nystagmus (vestibular VIII)

Evaluate the palpebral reflex (V-brainstem-VII), lip tone (VII), and the response to stimulating the nasal mucosa with your finger (V – brainstem – prosencephalon). Palpate the size of the muscles of mastication, and assess for jaw tone and movement (motor V). Assess the tongue for its strength and size (XII). The ability to swallow is the only way to realistically check the function of the pharyngeal branches of IX and X.

BRAIN

Clinical Signs of Brain Dysfunction

Prosencephalic signs include all forms of seizure disorders and behavioral changes that range from mild alterations in the animal's relationship with its environment to changes in its habits, propulsive pacing and circling, head pressing, and extreme aggression and mania. Changes in the animal's sensorium range from depression to lethargy to obtundation to semicoma (stupor) and to coma. The most profound of these (obtundation to coma) most often reflect disorders involving the ARAS in the diencephalon (i.e., pituitary abscess). Cerebral disorders cause blindness with normal pupillary light reflexes. Lesions of the eyeballs, optic nerves or chiasm will cause blindness with abnormal pupillary light reflexes.

There are three features of the neurologic examination that localize lesions in the prosencephalon. All three would be contralateral to a unilateral prosencephalic lesion. (1) A normal gait with postural reaction deficits: In animals too large to hop, this may be reflected by observing limbs on one side slide out on a slippery surface or seeing hooves scuff or drag when going over rough ground or a curb; (2) loss of the menace response; and (3) cutaneous or nasal mucosa hypalgesia.

CN deficits help localize brainstem lesions: II, diencephalon; III, IV, mesencephalon; V, pons; and VI-XII, medulla.

Gait abnormalities usually occur with lesions caudal to the diencephalon from involvement of the UMN and GP pathways. With unilateral lesions, these deficits are usually ipsilateral.

Vestibular system signs (e.g., balance loss, head tilt, and abnormal nystagmus) occur with lesions in the pons, medulla, and cerebellum. Involvement of the brainstem ARAS results in depression, lethargy, or obtundation. Severe mesencephalic or pontine lesions may cause semicoma or coma.

Cerebellar lesions usually cause a dysmetric gait with a delay in the onset of protraction, followed by an overresponse creating a sudden burst flexor action that is poorly directed. Balance loss often accompanies this gait, as well as an abnormal nystagmus and a head tilt if the lesion is asymmetric. Severe rostral cerebellar lesions may cause opisthotonos.

Malformation of the Brain

Cerebellar Hypoplasia/Atrophy

This is the most common brain malformation observed in the northeastern United States and is the result of an in utero infection with the bovine virus diarrhea virus (BVDV) agent, usually between 100 and 200 days of gestation. The inflammation peaks about 14 days after infection and resolves before birth. The small malformed cerebellum seen at birth reflects atrophy of the already differentiated cerebellar parenchyma at the time of the infection and hypoplasia from the destruction of the embryonic precursor cells primarily in the external germinal layer (Figure 12-1). In most affected calves, the cerebellum is largely absent with only a few remnants of cerebellar folia remaining (see video clips 25 to 27). Clinical signs vary. Some calves are unable to stand and often thrash around in their attempts to get up, and they exhibit periods of opisthotonos and sometimes abnormal nystagmus. Others can stand and walk but have a base wide posture, stagger, and weave from side to side with a hypermetric gait and balance loss (Figure 12-2).

In some calves, the retina and optic nerves are affected, resulting in blindness. In these calves, the optic nerves, chiasm, and tracts are less than one half their normal size. Cataracts can also occur. Occasionally there are cavities in the cerebrum (porencephaly), which do not contribute to recognizable signs.

It is important to obtain a necropsy diagnosis for these calves because their clinical signs do not differ

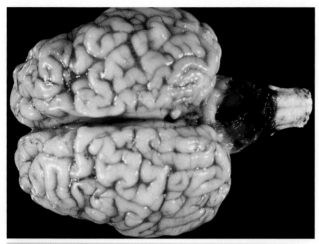

Figure 12-1

Brain from a 3-week-old calf with cerebellar hypoplasia and atrophy caused by in utero BVD infection. Amazingly the calf was able to stand.

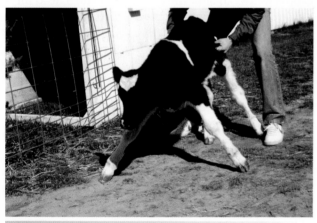

Figure 12-2

A 3-week-old calf with severe cerebellar hypoplasia and atrophy (see Figure 12-1) that was able to stand; notice the base-wide stance and lowered head position.

from a possible genetically induced cerebellar malformation. The latter has been observed in Angus and Scottish Highland calves with a symmetrically reduced cerebellar size but no gross or microscopic evidence of any destructive process. In addition, there is no trapezoid body on the ventral surface of the rostral medulla, but there is an abnormal band of parenchyma passing across the fourth ventricle just caudal to the cerebellar peduncles with a nucleus at each end. This may be the trapezoid body and the cochlear nuclei in an abnormal position that cannot be explained by an in utero viral infection. The fourth ventricle is remarkably reduced in size.

Congenital Cerebellar Function Disorder

On a few occasions, we have seen Holstein calves unable to get up at birth that exhibit opisthotonos and extensor rigidity on attempts to rise. If assisted, voluntary movements are delayed and overreactive. These calves are unable to balance and have abnormal nystagmus but are alert, responsive, and visual. Their anatomical dysfunction is primarily cerebellar. At necropsy, there are no gross or microscopic lesions anywhere in the nervous system. This is presumed to be a functional cerebellar disorder that may be inherited, but the latter remains unproven.

Hydranencephaly

This is primarily a cerebral abnormality in which the neopallium is reduced to a thin transparent membrane of pia and glial tissue as a result of complete destruction of the cerebral parenchyma. The lateral ventricle, containing a huge volume of cerebrospinal fluid (CSF), expands to take up the space vacated by the parenchymal loss. This is compensatory hydrocephalus. The hippocampus and olfactory bulb and peduncle and the basal nuclei are usually spared. The skull has a normal shape because CSF circulation is not obstructed in these calves. Akabane or bluetongue virus in utero infection at around 125 days of gestation is a recognized cause of this lesion. BVDV has also been reported as a cause, but this has not been seen in the northeastern United States where the BVDV-induced cerebellar lesion is common. The Aino and Chuzan viruses have also been implicated. The lesion is probably the result of the destruction of mitotically active progenitor germinal cells, as well as a vasculitis of the branches of the arterial circle that compromises the blood supply to the developing cerebrum. If the lesion is limited to cerebral hydranencephaly, the clinical signs are prosencephalic, and the animal will be able to ambulate but will be obtunded and blind.

Congenital Obstructive Hydrocephalus (Hypertensive)

Inherited forms are described in numerous breeds: Hereford, Charolais, Dexter, Ayrshires, and Holstein. The obstructive hydrocephalus is often accompanied by other brain malformations, which will influence the character of the clinical signs. A common cause of the obstruction is a failure of the mesencephalic aqueduct to develop normally. The latter may be associated with the presence of a single structure representing the rostral colliculi. The cause of this mesencephalic malformation is unknown in cattle but is inherited in laboratory rodents. Clinical signs will be prosencephalic, but brainstem and cerebellar signs may be present if there is significantly increased intracranial pressure.

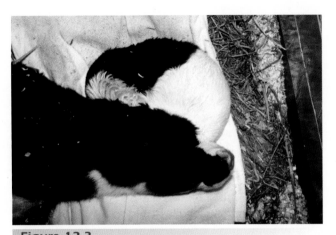

Figure 12-3

A newborn calf with a large fluctuant swelling of the head (meningoencephalocele).

Meningoencephalocele

This malformation occurs along the midline of the calvaria through an opening referred to as cranioschisis or cranium bifidum. The size of the extracranial accumulation of CSF may be extensive, producing a soft fluctuant pendular skin-covered structure (Figure 12-3). Although it is possible that some of these malformations may just be meningoceles, microscopic study of the tissues containing the CSF usually reveals a thin layer of brain parenchyma associated with the meninges beneath the skin, and therefore these are meningoencephaloceles.

Lipomeningocele

These also can occur along the midline of the calvaria or vertebral column through a cranioschisis or spina bifida, respectively. They consist of fat-filled meningeal tissue continuous with the falx cerebri in the head or the dural surface in the vertebral canal. With no associated neural tube malformation, there are no neurologic signs in these animals. The cause is unknown.

Complex Nervous System Malformation

A unique multifocal bone and neural tube malformation described in calves has been called an Arnold-Chiari malformation, presumably because of an assumed similarity to a human malformation given this eponym. Although there are some similarities, the distinct differences in the bovine disorder make use of this eponym incorrect. These calves are usually born recumbent and unable to coordinate their limb and trunk function to stand. They often exhibit opisthotonos and abnormal nystagmus. There is a sacrocaudal spina bifida with a meningomyelocele, a malformed tail, and associated loss of tone and reflexes in the anus and tail. At necropsy, the meningomyelocele consists of sacrocaudal nerves connecting from their spinal cord segments in the exposed vertebral canal into the skin-covered swelling over the spina bifida. The ganglia for these nerves are located in this skin. Myelodysplasia is present in the sacrocaudal segments. In the head, the cerebellum is flattened and elongated into a cone-shaped structure, and it is displaced into the foramen of the atlas and cranial axis along with the medulla. The associated CNs are elongated to extend back into the cranial cavity to exit through their respective foramina. There is a bilateral abnormal extension of each occipital lobe into the caudal cranial fossa space vacated by the cerebellum. These abnormal extensions of the otherwise normal occipital lobes pass ventral to the tentorium, which results in a groove on the lateral side of each of these extensions. These are not herniations of the normal occipital lobes. This malformation has been sporadically recognized in calves since the early 1900s.

Partial Diprosopus/Dicephalus

Occasionally calves are born with partial duplication of the face (diprosopus). This usually consists of varying degrees of two separate nasal regions; therefore four nares, parts of two lower jaws, and three orbits with the central one enlarged to accommodate two separate or fused eyeballs. The cranial region is broad, but there are two normal ears and a single normal atlantooccipital joint. These calves have four cerebral hemispheres (one for each naris formed from the embryonic olfactory placode, which gave rise to the olfactory nerves). Each cerebral hemisphere has a normal olfactory bulb, which resides in the cribriform plate related to each nasal cavity. There are four ethmoid bones. Two diencephalons are present (one for each set of eyes, two pairs of optic nerves, and two optic chiasms). The brainstem usually becomes single somewhere in the mesencephalon. The pons, medulla, and cerebellum are single structures. This is a partial dicephalus. These calves are usually born alive but are recumbent and unable to stand.

Prosencephalic Hypoplasia-Telencephalic Aplasia

Calves with this sporadic unique malformation are alive at birth and unable to stand. Their cranium is flattened between two normal orbits with normal eyeballs. A dorsal midline skin defect is present at the level of the caudal aspect of the orbits. There usually is a slight bloody discharge from this opening, which probably contains CSF. The skin tissue surrounding the opening is continuous caudally with a malformed diencephalon at the rostral portion of the brainstem. There are no cerebral hemispheres, just a malformed brainstem and cerebellum. There are no recognizable geniculate nuclei, no mesencephalic colliculi, and the cerebellum is elongated. With the exception of the olfactory nerves, all the remaining CNs are present, including the optic nerves that extend to the two eyes. In humans, this defect is called anencephaly, which is inappropriate because there is a brainstem and cerebellum present. There is no adequate term for this combination of malformations, and we have chosen to call this prosencephalic hypoplasia with telencephalic aplasia. The cause is unknown in cattle but has been blamed on folic acid deficiency or hyperthermia in humans.

Congenital Tremors

Hypomyelinogenesis

Failure to develop normal central nervous system (CNS) myelin can be the result of an inherited defect in oligodendroglial function or an in utero infection of the fetus that interferes with this process. Some strains of the BVDV have been implicated. An inherited hypomyelinogenesis has been reported in Jersey calves. Calves are usually recumbent at birth, and any muscular activity elicits diffuse whole body tremors. The more excited the calf becomes and struggles to move, the worse the tremor. It disappears when the calf is completely relaxed. These calves are usually alert, responsive, and visual. Occasionally calves affected by an in utero BVDV infection will improve over a few weeks, suggesting they became able to develop CNS myelination (see video clips 28 to 30).

Axonopathy

We recently studied a group of related Holstein calves that at birth were usually able to stand and walk but had a constant coarse tremor primarily of the trunk and pelvic limbs. At necropsy, they all had a diffuse primary axonopathy throughout the spinal cord with secondary demyelination.

INFLAMMATION OF THE BRAIN

Meningitis

Etiology

Gram-negative septicemia in neonates is the most common cause of meningitis in dairy cattle. Calves given inadequate amounts of high quality colostrum have insufficient levels of passively acquired immunoglobulins to fend off opportunistic organisms. Septicemia may originate in umbilical infections or more commonly by oral inoculation of pathogens. Gram-negative organisms such as *Escherichia coli*, *Klebsiella* sp., and *Salmonella* sp. predominate, with *E. coli* being the most common organism to infect neonatal calves. In colostrum-deficient calves, *Streptococcus* spp. may also cause bacteremia with meningitis, endophthalmitis, and peritonitis. Although any opportunistic or environmental organism may infect a calf with inadequate amounts of passively acquired immunoglobulins, only extremely pathogenic organisms will cause meningitis in a calf having adequate immunoglobulin supplies.

Although meningitis is a sporadic disease on well-managed farms, endemic problems may develop when calf husbandry is poor. Certain strains of causative gram-negative or less commonly gram-positive bacteria seem to result in meningitis in a high percentage of calves that develop septicemia. The owner may report similar signs in other calves that have subsequently died. An unusual strain of *E. coli* was identified as the cause of endemic meningitis in a "baby beef" Holstein calf operation. Affected calves were 2 to 5 months of age. This outbreak represents the first time that we have seen *E. coli* meningitis in calves of this age that are immunocompetent.

Acute bacterial meningitis in adult dairy cattle is not as common, and most cases are sporadic. Confirmed sporadic cases of meningitis in adult cows have been caused by septicemic spread of bacterial organisms from acutely infected organs such as the mammary gland or uterus, or foci of chronic infection such as traumatic reticuloperitonitis abscesses. Coliform mastitis may be the most common predisposing cause of sporadic bacterial meningitis in adult cattle in our practice area. Mycotic encephalitis has been observed as a sequela to mycotic mastitis and mycotic rumenitis with subsequent embolic septicemia. Direct extension of chronic infections such as pituitary abscesses and chronic frontal sinusitis may also result in meningitis in adult dairy cattle. When multiple cases of acute meningitis occur within a herd of adult cattle, *Histophilus (Haemophilus) somni* infection should be suspected. It must be emphasized that *H. somni* may cause meningitis rather than thrombotic meningoencephalitis (TME) in adult dairy cattle. Rarely, TME is observed in dairy heifers between 6 and 24 months of age.

Signs

Signs of meningitis in neonatal calves may be overt, with classical fever, somnolence, intermittent seizures, head pressing, and blindness, or be masked by hypovolemic shock and collapse in overwhelming septicemias. When meningitis precedes other major organ infection, signs of fever, depression, head pressing or "headache" appearance, seizures, and cerebral blindness signal the diagnosis (Figure 12-4). The gait is stiff, and the head is often held straight, with the muzzle extended. The condition is painful, and the animal may appear to have a "headache" with the eyelids partially closed and the head and neck extended. However, when meningitis coexists with other organ infection such as uveitis, septic arthritis, and omphalophlebitis, it may be difficult to recognize specific signs of meningitis. Overwhelming septicemia results in rapid deterioration of the neonate such that shock may mask clinical signs of meningitis (see video clip 31). Some calves affected with meningitis have opisthotonos—perhaps caused by cerebral inflammation and edema exerting pressure on the cerebellum and caudal brainstem (Figure 12-5). Affected calves are generally between 2 and 14 days of age with the mean being 6 days of age.

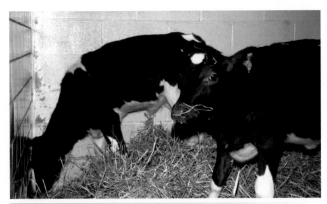

Figure 12-4

Two calves with meningitis. The calf on the left is head pressing into the wall. The calf on the right is unaware of its surroundings and has hay in its mouth but is not chewing. Both calves are blind.

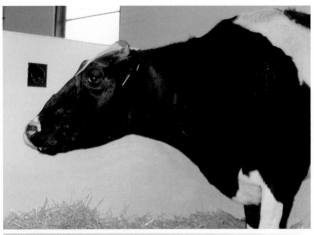

Figure 12-6

An adult cow exhibiting depression with a rather rigid "stargazing" appearance. The cow had a fractured skull, bacterial sinusitis, and meningitis.

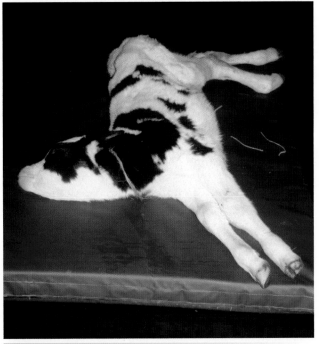

Figure 12-5

A 10-day-old Holstein calf with bacterial meningitis causing severe opisthotonos. The CSF was grossly abnormal.

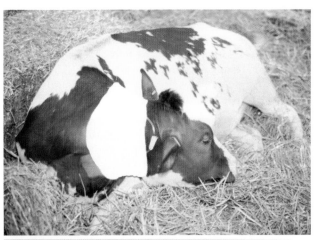

Figure 12-7

A 13-month-old recumbent red and white Holstein with *H. somni* meningoencephalitis. The heifer was treated with ampicillin and supportive treatment and recovered in 1 month. This favorable outcome is unusual in such a severely affected animal.

Adult cattle affected with meningitis usually have fever and profound depression. A stiff, stilted gait and "headache" appearance (stargazing or continually pressing head or muzzle against an object) are common (Figure 12-6), but seizures are less common than in calves. Inflammation of the visual cortex can result in blindness with normal pupillary function.

Meningitis caused by *H. somni* is acute, with affected cows becoming extremely depressed within a few hours. Fever usually is present and may be as high as 106.0° F/ 41.11° C. The depression progresses over 12 to 24 hours

to total inappetence and somnolence, and the affected cow may be unable to rise (Figure 12-7). Depression is so severe that presence or absence of vision may be difficult to determine, and occasional seizures are observed in some patients. Affected cows die within 24 to 48 hours of onset unless treated specifically for *H. somni*. Herds experiencing *H. somni* meningitis often have multiple cases over a period of several months, until appropriate diagnostics and preventive measures are used. TME caused by *H. somni*, although rare, does occur in growing dairy heifers and causes acute severe neurologic disease that may be accompanied by retinal lesions (Figure 12-8).

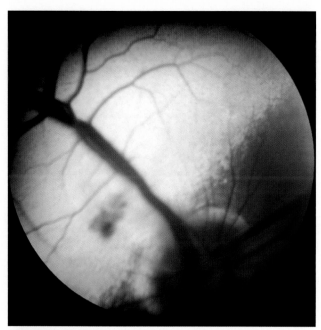

Figure 12-8

Focal chorioretinitis with hemorrhage dorsal to the optic disc in a Holstein yearling with thrombotic meningoencephalitis. *H. somni* was isolated from a cerebrospinal fluid (CSF) tap obtained from this patient.

Diagnosis

Clinical signs coupled with a CSF analysis confirm the diagnosis. Increased values for protein (normal = ≤40 mg/dl) and white blood cells (WBCs) (normal = ≤6 nucleated cells/μl) are present in the CSF, and the WBCs are mostly neutrophils in acute cases. In subacute cases, macrophages may predominate. The fluid can appear normal on visual examination, or it can be grossly discolored (red to orange). Neonatal calves showing neurologic signs that also have omphalophlebitis, uveitis, or septic arthritis should be suspected of having meningitis.

Bacterial cultures of the CSF and blood are indicated to determine the exact causative organism. Serum protein and immunoglobulin levels should be evaluated in neonatal calves to assess adequacy of passive transfer of immunoglobulins and thereby assess calf management procedures.

Diagnosis may be more difficult in adult cattle with meningitis secondary to acute or chronic infections elsewhere in the body. These cattle have been ill for variable lengths of time, and the developing signs of meningitis may be mistakenly assumed to be progressive systemic illness associated with failure to respond to therapy for the primary condition. Depression, an extended head and neck, head pressing, blindness with intact pupillary light responses, and seizures are all possible signs that may exist in individual patients. To repeat, CSF evaluation is necessary for diagnosis and will yield increased protein and WBCs—primarily

neutrophils in acute cases and macrophages in more chronic cases.

Treatment

Broad-spectrum antibiotics constitute the primary treatment for meningitis in calves and adult cattle. Although the blood-brain barrier normally interferes with effective CSF levels for most antibiotics, the barrier is compromised by inflammation in meningitis patients. Therefore most antibiotics will enter the CSF in higher levels than would be possible in the healthy state. Antibiotics should be chosen based on the likely causative organism. For example, in neonatal calves, the anticipated cause would be a gram-negative organism such as *E. coli*, and appropriate antibiotics would include an aminoglycoside or other antibiotic effective against *E. coli* (e.g., ceftiofur 2 to 4 mg/kg twice daily or amikacin 20 mg/kg once daily plus ampicillin 10 mg/kg twice daily, or florfenicol 20 mg/kg twice daily). If amikacin is used, fluids should be given and proper meat withdrawal time advised. Although not permitted in North America, enrofloxacin would be an excellent antimicrobial selection for gram-negative meningitis. In adult cattle with secondary meningitis, the likely cause of the primary disease (e.g., mastitis, metritis) should be addressed when choosing a systemic antibiotic. Gram stain evaluation of CSF may be rewarding in some cases and thereby guide antibiotic selection. When *H. somni* is suspected, ampicillin (11.0 to 22.0 mg/kg twice daily) and florfenicol (20 mg/kg twice daily in replacement heifers) are reasonable antibiotic choices. Without early treatment, the prognosis for recovery is grave. Some calves that are aggressively treated too late with proper antibiotics may live for several days but never regain reasonable mentation and have necrotic lesions in the brain at necropsy.

Supportive treatment with a single dose of corticosteroids (5 to 10 mg of dexamethasone and/or mannitol 0.5 mg/kg slowly intravenously [IV]) may help decrease life-threatening inflammation and cerebral edema associated with meningitis. Some practitioners administer nonsteroidal antiinflammatory drugs (NSAIDs) instead of corticosteroids. If the inflammation cannot be immediately controlled, the calf will probably die despite proper antimicrobial therapy. Seizures may be controlled with 5 to 10 mg of diazepam in neonatal meningitis patients.

Prevention

Adequate passive transfer of immunoglobulins through well-managed colostrum feeding of each newborn calf is the most important method of prevention. Dipping navels and providing a clean, dry environment will minimize opportunities for navel infection, septicemia, and meningitis. Herd vaccination against *H. somni* is indicated whenever meningitis or TME is found to be caused by this organism.

Brain Abscesses and Pituitary Abscesses

Etiology

Brain abscesses, similar to abscesses affecting the spinal cord, usually arise from embolic spread of bacteria from distant sites of infection or during septicemic episodes. Calves develop brain abscesses most commonly from umbilical sepsis and extensions from otitis media/interna, whereas those in adult cattle have been associated with chronic infections, such as abscesses resulting from hardware disease, chronic musculoskeletal abscesses, or rumenitis. In addition, direct extension from chronic frontal sinusitis and bacterial seeding associated with nose rings in bulls are other potential causes of brain abscesses in adult cattle. Although the relationship with frontal sinusitis is obvious, the inferred higher risk of cattle or bulls with nose rings for brain or pituitary abscesses is very interesting. Theories to explain this phenomenon center around the complex rete mirabile circulation that encircles the pituitary region and is suspended in the cavernous sinuses, which drain the nasal cavity. *Arcanobacterium pyogenes* is the most common organism isolated from brain abscesses in cattle.

Signs

Signs vary tremendously, depending on neuroanatomic location of the brain abscess. Initial signs such as mild depression, dysphagia, hemiparesis, and hemianopsia may be subtle and will frequently go undetected by the owner. As the abscess enlarges, varying degrees of visual disturbance, paresis, ataxia, profound depression, and CN signs become apparent. Head pressing may be observed (see video clips 32 and 33). Calves tend to be affected between 2 and 8 months of age, thereby being past the typical age for neonatal meningitis. If the abscess becomes sufficiently large, it will interfere with venous return of blood from the orbital region and cause exophthalmos (Figure 12-9). Adult cattle can be of any age. Depression and a stargazing attitude have been observed in cattle with cerebral abscesses. Bradycardia coupled with depression and a stargazing attitude has been described to indicate a pituitary abscess (Fox FH, personal communication, 1985, Ithaca, NY), but other signs such as blindness, dysphagia, or CN signs are possible. A review of pituitary abscesses found that approximately 50% had bradycardia in addition to other neurologic signs. The bradycardia may result from involvement of hypothalamus or may be caused by the anorexia.

Abscesses localized to one cerebral hemisphere usually cause blindness with intact pupillary function in the contralateral eye (hemianopsia) as a result of optic radiation or cerebral cortical injury (Figures 12-10 and 12-11). Similarly, contralateral abnormal postural reactions would be anticipated with a normal gait in animals light enough to be hopped or a scuffing of the limbs

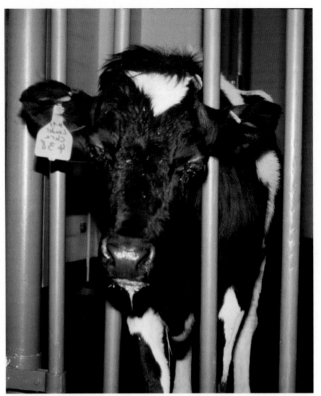

Figure 12-9

A heifer with exophthalmos, swollen conjunctiva, salivation, and depression caused by a brain abscess. Cerebrospinal fluid was normal.

when walked in a tight circle or over rough ground. Propulsive tendencies may appear also with large cerebral abscesses. Anorexia secondary to severe depression may be accentuated by specific CN dysfunction if the abscess directly or indirectly damages the brainstem. Some affected cattle continue to eat despite extensive space-occupying abscesses.

Neurologic signs worsen and become more numerous as the abscess (or abscesses) enlarges. Antiinflammatory or antibiotic therapy may stabilize or transiently improve the animal's signs, but regression coincides with stoppage of medications. Eventually locomotion is affected, and tetraparesis and ataxia followed by recumbency occur as the caudal brainstem becomes compromised. Occasionally a pituitary abscess will rupture, and the inflammation will spread caudally in the meninges, where it can involve and compromise numerous CNs.

Diagnosis

Antemortem confirmation of brain or pituitary abscesses may be difficult. The neurologic signs are the most helpful to diagnosis—especially in young animals in which inflammatory lesions are more common than other intracranial disorders. Serum globulin should be assessed because it frequently is elevated in adult cattle with brain abscesses but may be variable in calves and

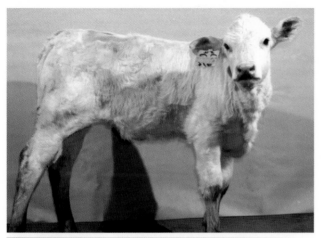

Figure 12-10

Calf with a brain abscess. The calf is profoundly depressed, unaware of its surroundings, has a "stargazing" head carriage with the head and neck turned to the right (pleurothotonos), and has right side hemianopsia and right hopping deficits. A left cerebral abscess was identified at necropsy.

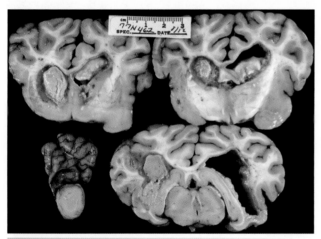

Figure 12-11

Sections of brain from calf shown in Figure 12-10. The left side of the photo illustrates the left side of the brain.

young cattle. A neutrophilic leukocytosis may be anticipated, but in fact the hemogram often is normal.

CSF may or may not be helpful. CSF may be normal in early cases but will be profoundly abnormal in advanced cases of abscessation with both protein and WBCs elevated. Generally a high percentage, but not all, of the WBCs are mononuclear because of macrophage activity instigated by the chronic infection. Erosion of the abscess to cause leptomeningitis incites a neutrophilic pleocytosis in the CSF.

Radiographs of the skull occasionally show fluid lines consistent with gas-fluid interfaces in large, advanced,

cerebral abscesses. CT and MR imaging procedures are the most reliable but are expensive and require general anesthesia.

Treatment

Other than long-term antibiotic therapy and potential drainage, therapy is limited and prognosis grave. We are unaware of successful surgery for brain abscesses in cattle, although this is occasionally possible in some other species. Symptomatic therapy with antibiotics and anti-inflammatories may cause a slight improvement in the animal's neurologic signs but is short-lived, and death is inevitable for most cattle affected with brain abscesses.

Listeriosis

Etiology

Listeria monocytogenes, a small gram-positive rod that is ubiquitous in soil, vegetable matter, and fecal material from humans and animals, is the cause of the most common meningoencephalitis of adult cattle. Although this facultative intracellular organism occasionally causes septicemia in young calves and abortion in adult cows, it is best known for the neurologic infection of the brainstem that is labeled listeriosis or "circling disease" in adult cattle and other ruminants. Use gloves when examining these animals because humans are susceptible to this infectious agent.

L. monocytogenes type 4b has been the most common serotype to cause meningoencephalitis in cattle. The organism is present in chopped forages such as corn silage and haylage owing to the presence of both soil and vegetable matter in these feedstuffs. Proper ensiling, wherein fermentation lowers the pH of the silage to <5.0, kills or prevents multiplication of *L. monocytogenes*. However, improper ensiling as a result of excess dryness of the forage, lack of fermentation caused by trench ensiling, silage inoculants, and other variables may prevent the silage from achieving a pH of <5.0, thereby allowing proliferation of *L. monocytogenes*. Corn silage is most incriminated as the forage source of organisms.

Infection is thought to occur following injury to mucous membranes of the oral cavity, nasal cavity, or conjunctiva with subsequent retrograde passage of the organisms via the sensory branches of the fifth CN (CN-V) to the brainstem. A possibility exists that cattle could become infected through the gastrointestinal tract with hematogenous spread to the brainstem as may occur in rodents and humans, but this route is thought less likely than following the peripheral nerve branches of CN-V.

Once established in the brainstem, the organism proliferates in the pons and medulla regions and may spread elsewhere. The trigeminal nerve and its neighboring CN nuclei are subject to injury as a result of neuritis, encephalitis, and meningitis. The classical histologic lesions of listeriosis consist of microabscesses subsequent to focal necrosis with abundant neutrophils and perivascular cuffing with mononuclear cells.

Fortunately, and rather inexplicably, given the common exposure of the whole herd to similar feedstuffs, the disease tends to be sporadic with only one animal in the herd affected. Endemics have been observed when two to six cattle become infected over a period of a few months, but this is much rarer in cattle than in sheep—where high flock morbidity is common. Calves are seldom affected, and the disease is seldom confirmed in cattle less than 12 months of age. This most likely coincides with less relative risk of exposure to feedstuffs containing *L. monocytogenes* in young animals but may be affected by increased dental eruption and therefore mucosal injury in young adult cattle.

Signs

Fever may be present, especially during the first few days of illness. The fever is not high (103.0 to 105.0° F/ 39.4 to 40.5° C), and absence of fever does not rule out listeriosis.

Depression coupled with a variable array of CN signs compose the major clinical signs of listeriosis in cattle. Classically the disease was known as circling disease because of the frequency of this clinical sign. The anatomic basis for this is unclear. Asymmetric involvement of vestibular nuclei with loss of balance and circling to that side is one explanation. However, the propulsive tendency to circle suggests involvement of extrapyramidal system nuclei such as the substantia nigra or the descending reticular formation. Although propulsion is a common prosencephalic sign, this portion of the brain is much less affected in listeriosis. Patients may circle until they collapse from exhaustion or eventually wander into solid objects. Stanchioned cattle constantly push or propel themselves into the stanchion in an effort to circle (Figure 12-12).

Anorexia, or perhaps an inability to eat, is present in most cattle affected with listeriosis and may be caused by specific CN deficits in CN-V, -VII, -IX, -X, and -XII, as well as depression. Inability to drink frequently accompanies the inability to eat but is not present in all cases. Individual or combinations of CN injuries unique to each patient may occur (Figure 12-13) (see video clips 34 and 35).

General signs of depression characterize brainstem disease but may be accentuated by dehydration and acid-base deficits in cattle affected with listeriosis.

Lesions of CN-V motor nucleus or mandibular nerve create weakness in the muscles of mastication. When severe and bilateral, a dropped jaw results (Figure 12-14). When mild, weakness may be appreciated during manual efforts to open the patient's mouth. Although this lesion may be unilateral, it is only obvious clinically when bilateral. Difficulty in prehension and mastication of food results.

Lesions of the abducent nucleus (CN-VI) are not common but, when present, cause a distinct medial strabismus.

Facial nerve deficits caused by lesions involving the facial nucleus or the intramedullary components of the facial nerve are a very common sign of listeriosis and often are unilateral, causing a drooped ear, ptosis, and

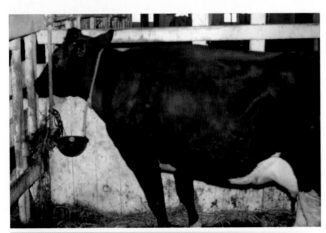

Figure 12-12

This cow with listeriosis would circle constantly to the left until finding respite by securing her muzzle between the water pipe and wall of the box stall.

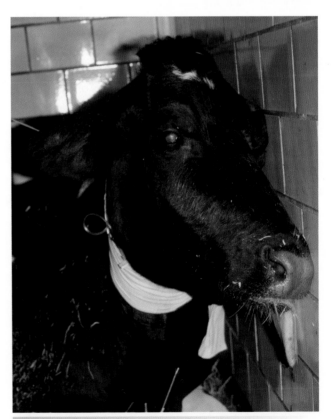

Figure 12-13

Listeriosis patient having multiple cranial nerve deficits including left side CN-VII and CN-VIII, as well as CN-V, -IX, -X, and -XII. The right ear is drooped here.

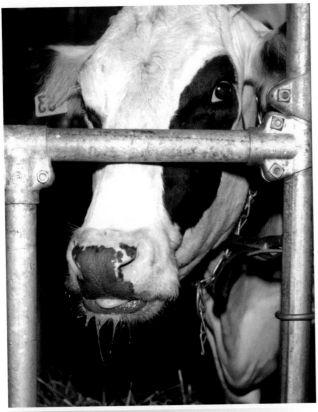

Figure 12-14

Listeriosis patient with major signs of depression and inability to close her jaw (CN-V) and swallow (CN-IX and -X). Tongue tone was normal.

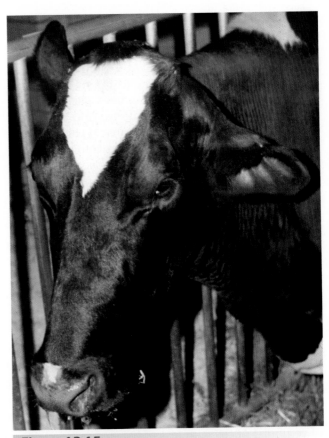

Figure 12-15

Listeriosis. Classical appearance of unilateral CN-VII paralysis with ear droop, ptosis, and flaccid lip.

flaccid lip (Figure 12-15). Very early cases or cases recovering from complete facial nerve paralysis occasionally have facial nerve irritability evidenced by eyelid or lip spasticity in response to noxious stimuli. Although unilateral deficits in CN-VII are classic for *Listeria* meningoencephalitis of cattle, the deficits may be subtle, incomplete, or bilateral and therefore require careful evaluation during the neurologic examination. Exposure keratitis is the major ophthalmic complication found in listeriosis patients and results from facial nerve dysfunction and subsequent failure of tear distribution to prevent corneal desiccation or injury. Additionally, involvement of the parasympathetic facial nucleus may cause a decrease in the aqueous phase of the tear secretion. Exposure keratitis can rapidly progress with resultant deep corneal ulceration, uveitis, corneal perforation, and endophthalmitis unless addressed promptly. Endogenous uveitis with hypopyon or endophthalmitis has been suggested as possible ophthalmic complications by some authors, but in our experience, exposure keratitis and exogenous infection of the eye are the most common ophthalmic complications of listeriosis in cattle (Figure 12-16).

Damage to vestibular nuclei affects central vestibular control, leading to head tilt, circling, and vestibular ataxia. Abnormal posture and truncal ataxia also are

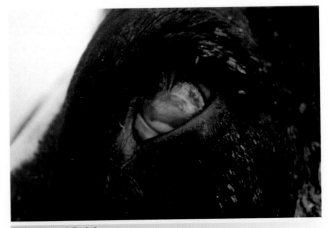

Figure 12-16

Exposure keratitis, hypopyon, and uveitis caused by listeriosis.

possible; when these signs are present, the cow's trunk leans toward the affected side and is flexed so a concavity toward the affected side is present. When abnormal nystagmus is observed, the direction (fast phase) is variable, as expected with a central vestibular deficit. Adjacent unilateral lesions affecting reticulospinal UMN and spinocerebellar GP pathways may cause ipsilateral paresis

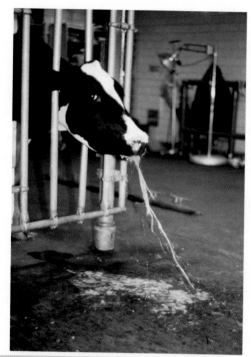

Figure 12-17

An adult Holstein cow with an acute onset of depression, bloat, and vomiting. The cow had listeriosis and recovered with treatment.

and ataxia. Bilateral lesions in this area resulting in spastic tetraparesis and GP ataxia may be severe enough to cause recumbency.

Lesions involving neuronal cell bodies of CN-IX and -X in the nucleus ambiguus cause dysphagia and salivation. Vomiting and/or bloat occasionally are observed (Figure 12-17) as an early sign of listeriosis in cattle and are thought to result from inflammatory irritation of the parasympathetic vagal neurons in the medulla.

Protrusion or weakness of the tongue is associated with lesions in the hypoglossal nuclei or the intramedullary components of CN-XII. Tongue protrusion caused by these lesions is accentuated if motor nuclei of CN-V lesions coexist, thereby allowing a dropped jaw.

Cerebellar signs also have been observed in listeriosis patients but are not common. Lesions caused by listeriosis are uncommon in the prosencephalon, and therefore blindness is very unusual. Spinal cord lesions are rare.

Diagnosis

Anorexia, depression, and possibly fever are the general signs that accompany specific CN signs in cattle having meningoencephalitis caused by *L. monocytogenes*. It is important to remember that "anorexia" may in fact be a result of inability to prehend or swallow food and water. A careful neurologic examination to confirm brainstem disease and specific CN deficits is essential when considering a diagnosis of listeriosis. In some cases, the deficits may only be detected on careful clinical examination.

In addition to the clinical signs, CSF analysis is the most valuable ancillary aid to support a diagnosis of listeriosis in cattle. With few exceptions, the CSF from listeriosis patients has elevated nucleated cells and protein levels. In one study 44 of 57 affected cattle had high leukocyte counts in the CSF. In addition, at least 50% of the nucleated cells are mononuclear cells, with macrophages being slightly more common than lymphocytes. CSF is usually obtained in the lumbosacral region unless the patient is recumbent and obtunded. The fluid is generally clear on visual inspection.

A complete blood count (CBC) may show mild leukocytosis and monocytosis, which is suggestive, but not absolute, of this disease. Unfortunately cattle affected with listeriosis do not frequently have the peripheral monocytosis that typically may be present in other species infected with this organism and that gave *L. monocytogenes* its name.

When salivation is obvious, an acid-base and electrolyte profile may be helpful for diagnosis and subsequent therapy because listeriosis patients can suffer profound salivary loss. Because the saliva of cattle is rich in buffer, patients so affected may have metabolic acidosis, low bicarbonate values, associated depression, and weakness.

Lactating cattle also may become ketotic because of continued (albeit reduced) milk production in the face of inappetence.

Many differential diagnoses exist for listeriosis, with rabies being the most important from a public health and medicolegal standpoint. Inner and middle ear infections may cause CN-VII and -VIII signs. Affected cattle are more alert and more able to eat and drink than are cows with listeriosis. In general, middle ear infections are common in calves up to yearling age, whereas listeriosis seldom occurs in cattle younger than 1 year of age.

Polioencephalomalacia (PEM), lead poisoning, and other diseases of the cerebral cortex can usually be differentiated from listeriosis unless the patient is recumbent or comatose, which limits the neurologic examination and a patient's responses. PEM causes profound depression, bilateral cortical blindness with intact pupillary function, and may cause a dorsomedial strabismus in calves (not necessarily present in adult cattle). Opisthotonos may develop in advanced cases. Similarly, lead poisoning manifests with bilateral cortical blindness, depression, seizures, and bellowing, but no CN signs as seen with listeriosis. In addition, listeriosis does not result in blindness unless a severe exposure ulceration from facial nerve paralysis leads to uveitis or endophthalmitis in the ipsilateral eye. The lack of a menace response in listeriosis is a result of the facial paralysis, which also causes a lack of a palpebral reflex. Listeriosis rarely causes blindness.

TME or pure meningitis caused by *H. somni* can lead to acute signs of brain disease in young cattle. Although

TME occurs mainly in beef cattle, we occasionally observe this problem in dairy heifers. Signs vary based on the multifocal nature of the septic thrombi within the brain, and CN signs are possible, as well as the typical cerebral signs and depression. Fever may be present in the acute phase, and blindness caused by chorioretinal hemorrhages and thrombosis is possible. The CSF, however, helps differentiate *H. somni* from listeriosis because, although protein values are elevated in both diseases, the nucleated cell count with *H. somni* usually is greatly elevated and consists primarily of neutrophils. The fluid may be grossly discolored on visual inspection.

Nervous ketosis can occasionally be confused with listeriosis in stanchioned cattle that become propulsive or constantly push forward into the stanchion, mimicking the propulsion seen in some listeriosis patients. However, a lack of CN signs, positive urinary ketones, history of early lactation, and, if necessary, a normal CSF would rule out listeriosis.

Subtle or mild cases of listeriosis have been confused with gastrointestinal disorders such as traumatic reticuloperitonitis. This can easily happen if the patient shows little or no evidence of CN dysfunction but cannot eat or drink. Subsequent dehydration or lack of water intake causes the rumen ingesta to become very firm and dry. Deep ventral abdominal pressure exerted on the rumen may lead to apparent painful responses that erroneously lead one to suspect peritonitis. In addition, occasional listeriosis patients show vomiting as one of their initial signs before other CN signs become apparent. Vomiting is more commonly associated with highly acidic diets, indigestion, irritation of reflex centers from ingested hardware, and other gastrointestinal disorders. Once again, a careful neurologic examination is essential, and a CSF analysis should be considered.

Space-occupying lesions in the cerebrum or brainstem (e.g., lymphosarcoma) or parasitic migration can rarely be confused for listeriosis.

Unfortunately rabies is the most difficult disease to differentiate from listeriosis when dysphagia or other CN signs are present. Because rabies can result in virtually any neurologic sign, it must be considered in the differential diagnosis of listeriosis in endemic areas. In general, CSF in rabies patients has fewer nucleated cells and protein than those found in listeriosis patients. In addition, the high percentage of mononuclear cells to neutrophils found in listeriosis patients is not typical in rabies, in which case small lymphocytes predominate. Because overlap may occur in these values, extreme caution is warranted for handling patients in rabies-endemic areas.

Treatment

Treatment usually consists of intensive antibiotic therapy with either penicillin or tetracycline, although other antibiotics are reported to be effective in vitro. Two major therapeutic obstacles exist to antibiotic therapy that

dictate higher dosages than normally used for other susceptible bacteria:

1. *L. monocytogenes* is a facultative intracellular organism that can survive and hide from drugs in macrophages.
2. The blood-brain barrier, although compromised by inflammation, may still impede antibiotic penetration of the brain to some degree.

Therefore we have chosen to use penicillin at 44,000 U/kg twice daily, either intramuscularly (IM) or subcutaneously (SQ), to treat listeriosis patients. This is used for at least 7 days before being reduced to either once daily or 22,000 U/kg twice daily, IM or SQ.

IV administered penicillin, 10 million units thrice daily, or ampicillin, 10 mg/kg thrice daily, would likely result in higher concentration in the CSF but is more expensive. Some clinicians prefer to use oxytetracycline HCl at 10 mg/kg twice daily, IV or SQ. Dosage reduction generally coincides with signs of obvious clinical improvement, such as a return to an ability to eat and drink. Although the exact duration of therapy will vary in each case based on severity of signs and many other factors, the treatment should continue for at least 1 week beyond apparent cure as based on appetite, attitude, and other factors. Most affected cows require 7 to 21 days of therapy. Premature reduction in dosage or discontinuation of treatment risks relapse in listeriosis patients. Some degree of facial neuronal signs may persist for a long time in recovered listeriosis patients, and neurologic signs tend to resolve in the opposite order of their original appearance. There may be no improvement in clinical signs for 7 to 9 days in some animals.

Fluid and electrolyte status may be very important to the well-being of listeriosis patients that lose the ability to drink. Cattle that cannot drink but are not salivating can be given water and balanced electrolytes through a stomach tube. This improves patient hydration and also softens the firm rumen contents and encourages rumen activity. Patients that are salivating should be monitored for buffer loss and will require bicarbonate replacement therapy and fluids. These may be given IV—although this is a more expensive route—or orally with substantial water to correct dehydration. Replacement therapy will be necessary daily until salivary losses stop. The depression and weakness that occur with severe metabolic acidosis may be confused with progression of the disease or lack of response to therapy for listeriosis. Depending on degree of salivary loss, 4 to 16 oz of sodium bicarbonate may be required daily to compensate. Cattle with facial paralysis also require frequent treatments of the affected eye with topical ointments to prevent keratitis and corneal ulcers.

Nursing care, including a well-bedded box stall with good footing, is essential to survival of cattle affected with listeriosis. Assuming intensive antibiotic therapy, fluid therapy, and supportive care are given, prognosis is fair to good for cattle infected with listeriosis that are ambulatory when the diagnosis is made. The prognosis for cattle that are recumbent and unable to rise at the time of diagnosis is very poor.

L. monocytogenes is capable of infecting humans and thus causing meningoencephalitis. This is especially true in the very young, the very old, and the immunocompromised person. Therefore public health concerns exist. Listeriosis patients may shed *L. monocytogenes* in their milk, and this fact requires veterinarians to warn owners and caretakers against the consumption of raw milk. Milk from these cattle should be discarded. Even pasteurized milk subjected only to low-temperature pasteurization may contain the organism. Pregnant cattle with the neurologic form of listeriosis may abort during the duration of their disease. The cause of the abortion is generally septicemic spread of *L. monocytogenes* to the uterus. Therefore handling of the fetus, placenta, and so forth should be done carefully.

Rabies

Etiology

Rabies virus is transmitted to cattle and other warm-blooded animals by bites from infected vectors such as foxes, raccoons, skunks, bats, and vampire bats. Cats and dogs are more routinely vaccinated against the disease, but unvaccinated cats and dogs also present a risk to cattle, humans, and other species. The rabies virus is a member of the genus *Lyssavirus* within the *Rhabdoviridae* family and is uniformly fatal to infected animals. Therein lies the tremendous fear of infection that the word "rabies" holds for humans. Public health and medicolegal implications are obvious.

Although aerosol transmission occurs in nature, mainly in bats within their caves, people and animals have been infected through aerosols in laboratory settings. Ingestion of infected tissues also may occasionally result in infection of carnivores. However, the primary means of transmission of this neurotrophic virus is through bites from an infected animal that inoculates virus-laden saliva into the tissue of a noninfected animal.

The virus replicates at the site of inoculation in an animal recently bitten. It then travels in retrograde fashion within the axons of peripheral nerves to spinal ganglia to the spinal cord and eventually the brain. The virus is then shed into the salivary and nasal secretions of the infected animal through centrifugal distribution following CN axons to these secretory glands. Therefore the virus is concentrated in saliva and nasal secretions—making these fluids the most feared source of exposure to uninfected animals or people.

Incubation periods vary widely. Most experts agree that 1 week is the minimum, but the range varies from 1 to 3 weeks, 10 to 60 days, or 3 weeks to 3 months; all authors agree that rare instances exist where the incubation may be as long as 6 months. Infection through bites closer to the brain (i.e., face and neck) may lead to shorter incubation periods than distal limb bites.

Clinical Signs

Clinical signs of rabies in cattle, as well as other species, are variable and may include spinal cord signs, brainstem signs including CN signs, cerebral signs, apparent lameness, genitourinary signs, gastrointestinal signs, and mixtures thereof.

Because of the variation in clinical signs of rabies, veterinarians practicing in endemic areas are more cautious of cattle with overt neurologic signs. Several points are important generalities when discussing signs of rabies in cattle.

1. The signs are progressive; this may mean, for example, that appetite continues to decline or neurologic signs observed on day 1 will be more pronounced on day 3. Most cattle will be recumbent in 4 to 5 days.
2. Death usually occurs by day 10 after the onset of signs with the average being around 5 days from onset of signs to death.
3. In endemic areas, rabies should be on the differential diagnosis for almost every sick cow with nervous system signs examined by the veterinarian.

The clinical signs at the onset relate to the area of the body that is bitten and where the virus first enters the nervous system. Spinal cord signs are seen frequently. These may include subtle hind limb lameness or shifting of weight in the hind limbs that progresses to knuckling of one or both fetlocks (see video clip 36). Ataxia and weakness may follow these signs and progress until the cow needs help getting up or becomes completely paralyzed in the pelvic limbs (Figure 12-18). In some cases, there is a spastic uncontrolled flexion of the limbs. Associated with these lumbar and sacral signs, constipation, tenesmus, paraphimosis (males), dribbling of urine from bladder paralysis, and a flaccid tail and anus may become apparent. Therefore progressive signs of spinal cord or spinal nerve dysfunction should raise concern for rabies. With head bites, CN signs may occur initially.

Cerebral signs include signs of progressive depression ("dumb form") or aggression ("furious form"). Few veterinarians would fail to identify quickly any newly aggressive cattle as rabies suspects, but certainly nervous ketosis and hypomagnesemia would need to be ruled out. Other accentuated cerebral responses observed in rabies patients are hypersexuality (e.g., frequent mounting), localized or generalized pruritus that can progress to self-mutilation, seizures, tremors, alert eyes and ears despite paresis or ataxia, head pressing, bellowing, and opisthotonos. Blindness can occur but is not common.

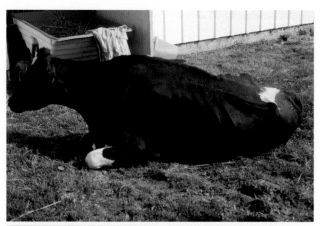

Figure 12-18

A 4-year-old Holstein that was first noticed to be abnormal when she buckled on both hind limbs coming into the parlor. Within 2 hours, she was recumbent, would not eat, and began bellowing. Cerebrospinal fluid had a lymphocytic pleocytosis. She tested positive for rabies.

Dysphagia, salivation, and a weak tongue are apparent in some cattle affected with rabies. An inability to drink usually accompanies these signs, which are reflective of pharyngeal paralysis. Bellowing is described as "peculiarly low pitched and hoarse and may progress to bubbly sounds prior to death." Laryngeal paralysis associated with pharyngeal dysfunction may contribute to these sounds.

Affected cattle may have all or none of the signs described above. These are signs reported and observed in past cases, but no sign is pathognomonic for rabies.

The differential diagnosis is exhausting, but several common diseases should be considered. In the paralytic form with spinal cord signs predominating, sacral injuries from estrus activities and vertebral canal lymphosarcoma or abscesses should be differentiated from rabies. As discussed above, a personality change to furious or aggressive behavior should be differentiated from nervous ketosis, hypomagnesemia, or the occasional cow recently transported to a new location that simply "goes crazy" but has neither rabies nor nervous ketosis. With brain signs, the differential list is too long to consider simply because the brain signs possible with rabies are unlimited. In our experience, atypical listeriosis that causes dysphagia with or without tongue paralysis but without facial or vestibular nuclear signs is the disease most confused with rabies. However, in an advanced rabies case that is approaching coma, many encephalitic and toxic CNS diseases would need to be considered.

Diagnosis
CSF from rabies patients may be normal, have only elevated protein values, or have both elevated nucleated cells and protein. Most nucleated cells in the CSF of

rabies patients are lymphocytes. No other premortem tests are helpful to the practicing veterinarian, and the brain from suspect animals must be submitted to the regional laboratory approved by the state health department for rabies testing. Currently fluorescent antibody (FA)-stained sections of brain offer the quickest and most accurate means of diagnosis. The FA test has replaced histologic examination of the brain for Negri bodies and the mouse inoculation tests. In addition, FA tests using monoclonal antibodies to epitopes of the virus can help distinguish the vector source of rabies (i.e., raccoon, fox, and bat) to aid epidemiologic studies.

No treatment is possible for rabies patients. However, cattle bitten by unknown assailants should have the wounds cleaned vigorously, as well as washed and disinfected, just as is done for people suffering bite wounds from animals of unknown rabies status.

When rabies is suspected in a cow or calf, gloves should be worn by the handlers and veterinarians during examination and treatment. A minimal number of people should be involved in treatment of the cow, and her milk should be discarded. If a cow is confirmed to have rabies, public health authorities should be consulted for advice on rabies prophylaxis therapy for any handlers that worked with the animal and had definite exposure to virus.

Rabies vaccination of cattle is now being practiced in many endemic areas and is a viable means to counteract the public and private anxiety regarding exposure to rabies while working with livestock. Vaccination also greatly reduces the likelihood of human exposure and subsequent expensive prophylaxis and treatment with globulin and human diploid vaccines. An entire herd (small size) of dairy cattle can be vaccinated for less than the cost of one human postexposure treatment. Therefore, vaccination of cattle in endemic areas is worthy of consideration. Veterinarians should be certain to use only vaccines approved for use in cattle because some modified vaccines are inappropriate for herbivores. At least two vaccines are currently available for use in cattle (RM Imrab3, Rhone Merieux Inc., Athens, GA and Rabguard TC, SmithKline Beecham Animal Health, West Chester, PA). Both vaccines can be given initially at 3 months of age for primary immunization and repeated annually.

Pseudorabies (Aujeszky's Disease, Mad Itch)

Etiology
This herpesvirus of swine is the cause of pseudorabies. Often a mild disease in swine, this disease is highly fatal in cattle and may cause signs similar to rabies—hence the name, pseudorabies. This is a rare disease in dairy cattle because pigs and dairy cows seldom are housed together. However, trends in agriculture change

constantly, and diversification that includes swine and dairy cattle operations located on the same premises could occur, thereby risking spread of this virus from swine to cattle.

The virus is shed in the nasal secretions and pharyngeal secretions of infected pigs. Contact with cattle may include contamination of feedstuffs, contamination of wounds (because intradermal and SQ routes of infections are possible), and nose-to-nose contact. Infected brown rats also have been incriminated in carrying pseudorabies virus from farm to farm. Following infection, the incubation period is between 2 and 7 days.

Signs

Intense pruritus that may be localized or generalized develops, with licking, rubbing, and mutilation possible. This pattern has led to the name "mad itch" in cattle. However, many other neurologic signs are possible—similar to rabies—and fever usually is present. Peracute cases may die suddenly or have primary brain signs, which vary from salivation, pharyngeal/laryngeal dysfunction, dyspnea, bloat, ataxia, paresis, abnormal nystagmus, depression or aggression, and seizures. The course of the disease is 2 to 3 days, and although rare instances of survival have been noted in cattle, most infected cows succumb. Differential diagnosis would include rabies and many other neurologic diseases, but historical proximity of swine would be a key point.

Diagnosis

Serology, viral isolation from CNS (especially from a spinal cord segment supplying localized pruritus lesions), or edematous fluid from a localized lesion, and FA tests are possible. Tests continue to change and improve for this disease, and if this diagnosis is suspected, it would be best to contact a regional diagnostic laboratory for advice on sample collection. Rabies may need to be ruled out as well. No treatment exists. We are unaware of published CSF values for cattle affected with pseudorabies virus.

Bovine Herpesvirus Encephalitis

Etiology

Both bovine herpes virus (BHV) 1 and 5 may cause encephalitis in cattle. BHV1, a cause of abortion, infectious bovine rhinotracheitis, and pustular vulvovaginitis, only sporadically causes meningitis in cattle. On the other hand, BHV5 has marked neurotrophism, and in some parts of the world, particularly South America, it is a common cause of meningoencephalitis in cattle. BHV5 encephalitis can cause single disease on a farm or herd outbreaks, mostly in young replacement heifers, but the incidence in North America appears much lower than in South America. BHV5 meningoencephalitis may result from initial exposure to the virus or

from a stress/corticosteroid reactivation at a later time. Clinical signs generally occur approximately 1 week after either initial exposure or reactivation of the virus. The virus invades the CNS via the olfactory mucosa following intranasal infection or reactivation. A trigeminal ganglionitis is found in infected calves, and this is an anatomical area of persistent infection in some calves.

Clinical Signs and Diagnosis

Clinical signs of respiratory disease may be concurrent with neurologic signs, especially with BHV1. Prosencephalic signs predominate and are usually accompanied by a fever. Most affected animals remain visual, which helps separate many of the infectious encephalitides from metabolic or toxic diseases affecting the cerebral cortex. I (TJD) have analyzed CSF on only one BHV encephalitic calf (Figure 12-19), and it had a lymphocytic pleocytosis. If BHV-infected cattle survive, they will seroconvert in 7 to 10 days. Animals that die with nonsuppurative encephalitis can be confirmed as having BHV by immunohistochemistry. Genomic analysis or polymerase chain reaction (PCR) can be used to differentiate between the two strains. The CNS lesion consists of a diffuse nonsuppurative meningoencephalomyelitis affecting both the gray and white matter.

Treatment and Prevention

Treatment is supportive and includes control of seizures when necessary, in addition to the use of NSAIDs. Corticosteroids would likely be contraindicated, although this is controversial. Although complete protection against either strain does not occur with vaccination, the modified live intranasal BHV1 vaccines have good efficacy against both strains.

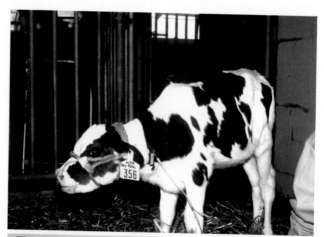

Figure 12-19

A 2-month-old calf with acute onset of fever and depression followed by seizures and respiratory distress. The CSF had a lymphocytic pleocytosis. BHV1 inclusion was present in the brain at autopsy.

Malignant Catarrhal Fever

Malignant catarrhal fever (MCF) is caused by a gamma herpes virus and sporadically causes fatal meningoencephalomyelitis in cattle. The virus that causes MCF in cattle in North America and Europe is sheep associated (ovine herpes virus 2). Most cases of MCF in cattle occur when affected cattle have had contact with sheep that are actively shedding the virus (especially weaned lambs). There have been some cases of MCF in cattle where a direct contact with sheep did not occur. The infection causes a vasculitis and lymphoproliferative reaction in many organs, including the CNS. The incubation period may be several weeks or more in cattle. We have recently identified the disease in pigs in contact with sheep.

Clinical Signs

Clinical signs are most common in cattle 1 to 2 years of age, and sporadic cases are the norm, although outbreaks can occur. There are basically two clinical forms: the head and eye or the intestinal form. Cattle with the head and eye form have a high fever, corneal opacity, nasal discharge, enlarged lymph nodes, hematuria, and diffuse neurologic signs. Similar to infectious bovine rhinotracheitis (IBR) keratitis, the corneal lesions often start at the limbus and spread centrally. Recovery with this form of the disease is rare. In the intestinal form, fever and diarrhea are the predominant clinical signs. Outbreaks are more common, as is recovery, compared with the head and eye form. We have collected CSF on only a few MCF/head and eye form cases. They had a remarkable mononuclear pleocytosis, and the exact type of some of the mononuclear cells was difficult to determine.

Diagnosis and Treatment

Diagnosis is based on signalment, clinical signs, history of sheep exposure (may be in distant past), and ruling out other diseases that may cause similar clinical signs (e.g., IBR). Hematuria, lymphadenopathy, and finding bizarre-appearing mononuclear cells in the CSF should help distinguish between the two diseases. An antemortem diagnosis can be made by performing PCR on whole blood (ethylenediaminetetraacetic acid [EDTA] anticoagulated sample). Postmortem diagnosis can be made by performing PCR on tissues. Lesions consist of a primary immune-mediated vasculitis with secondary parenchymal degeneration. Treatment is symptomatic.

Thrombotic Meningoencephalitis

TME is caused by *Histophilus somni*, formerly known as *Haemophilus somnus*. This small coccobacillus attacks vascular endothelium, causing a septic vasculitis with thrombosis. The parenchymal lesions of ischemic and hemorrhagic infarction are secondary to the primary vascular lesions that can occur anywhere in the CNS. In addition, similar vascular lesions can occur in the lung, heart, skeletal muscle, and joints. Death may occur acutely without evidence of neurologic signs. Pyrexia is present in clinically ill patients. This disease is more common in feedlot cattle than in pastured or dairy animals. In New York State pulmonary signs and lesions are the most common manifestation of this disease. Diagnosis and treatments for TME are discussed on p. 510.

Bovine Spongiform Encephalopathy

Although the purpose of this book is not to be all encompassing as regards exotic diseases but to concentrate on common problems in dairy cattle, bovine spongiform encephalopathy (BSE) deserves brief mention because of the threat of introduction into the United States, the possibility that at least one case has occurred in the United States, and the ensuing public health concerns. The abbreviation BSE should not be confused with sporadic bovine encephalitis (SBE or Buss disease), which is a chlamydial infection primarily seen in young beef cattle in the western United States. This is not an inflammatory disease but is caused by an unusual infectious agent.

Etiology

BSE is considered to be a form of scrapie in cattle. Scrapie is a disease of sheep and goats that is one of a group of diseases referred to as the transmissible spongiform encephalopathies (TSE). These include BSE, chronic wasting disease of deer, mink encephalopathy, and Creutzfeldt-Jakob disease of humans. The cattle disease first emerged in Great Britain in 1986 following the feeding of concentrates produced from slaughtered scrapie-infected sheep. Most investigators consider the infectious agent to be an altered host protein referred to as a prion.

One pathogenetic theory holds that BSE was most likely initially caused by scrapie-infected sheep-origin meat and bone meal products as part of calf starter rations or adult cattle concentrates. Another theory is that TSE developed in cattle and was exacerbated by feeding the tissues from infected cattle to other cattle. Public health concerns have focused on the similar features of the causative agent of Creutzfeldt-Jakob disease and kuru in humans to the prion-type causative agents found in scrapie and BSE. Because cattle were thought to have acquired this agent through ingestion, fears were raised relative to human consumption of meat products. Because the United States obviously has scrapie and chronic wasting disease as an endemic problem in sheep and deer, respectively, the threat of BSE in cattle raised in the United States seems to exist. However, great differences in amounts of sheep byproducts fed to cattle, as well as differences in rendering procedures, currently make the risk of BSE in U.S. cattle small. Additionally, there may be a species barrier, although not impermeable, to TSE transmission. There is also believed to be a genetic predisposition to the disease, and development of tests to determine resistant cows is being evaluated.

In addition to horizontal transmission, presumably from feeding contaminated ruminant tissue, there is vertical transmission of the TSE agent as well. BSE-infected cattle were three times more likely to have infected offspring than noninfected cows during the England outbreak. After banning the feeding of ruminant meat and bone meal to cattle in the United Kingdom, there has been a dramatic decrease in the incidence of BSE. In contrast, incidences in some other European and non-European countries have increased during the same period.

Signs

BSE occurs in adult dairy cattle 3 to 6 years of age or older. The disease is usually slowly progressive over 2 or more weeks. Hyperexcitability, an anxious expression, hypermetric ataxia, and hyperesthesia characterize the clinical signs. Affected cattle have facial and ear twitching, may kick repeatedly, and develop progressive ataxia and paresis that lead to stumbling, falling, and eventually recumbency. Only a small number of affected cattle display abnormal aggression (mad cow). Loss of weight is a significant sign in these cattle.

Diagnosis

Lesions consist of vacuoles in neuronal cell bodies or their processes in the neuropil sometimes associated with a mild gliosis but no inflammation. There is no serum antibody production, and the CSF is normal.

Immunodetection tests are available for detecting the prion in brainstem tissue. Currently in the United States, the disease has been confirmed in only a very few cows, which certainly justifies the many surveillance efforts that have been put into place.

DEGENERATIONS: METABOLIC AND TOXIC BRAIN DISEASES

Polioencephalomalacia

PEM describes a degenerative lesion of the gray matter of the cerebral cortex, a cerebrocortical necrosis for which there are many causes. These include thiamine deficiency, sulfur toxicity, lead poisoning, osmolality aberrations associated with salt and water imbalances, and hypoxia. Despite this, most clinicians equate PEM with thiamine deficiency, which is how it will be used in the following description.

Etiology

PEM or cerebrocortical necrosis is a thiamine-responsive disease that occurs in calves and adult cattle. In dairy calves, the disease usually is sporadic, but in grouped yearling heifers, the morbidity may reach 10% to 25%, similar to herd outbreaks in beef feeder calves or yearlings. The most common age for sporadic PEM in dairy

calves is 2 to 8 months of age; calves less than 3 weeks of age are seldom at risk for PEM. Adult dairy cattle are only rarely affected.

The cause of PEM has been the subject of much research regarding thiamine metabolism, thiaminase activity in the rumen, the effect of various feedstuffs on rumen microbial flora related to thiamine production or destruction, and chemicals that alter thiamine levels in ruminants. Thiamine must be present in adequate levels to allow production of the coenzyme thiamine diphosphate, which is the active form of thiamine and helps to form red blood cell transketolase, and pyruvate and alpha-ketoglutarate dehydrogenases. This transketolase is important to the pentose phosphate shunt pathway for glucose metabolism in the bovine brain. Thiamine also participates as a cofactor in the Krebs cycle production of ATP. The brain is at great risk when thiamine is inadequate because of the brain's dependence on aerobic metabolism where thiamine is a critical participant as a coenzyme. Within the CNS, specific groups of neurons are more susceptible to this interference with aerobic metabolism than others (i.e., neocortex, lateral geniculate nucleus, and caudal colliculus). It is important to appreciate that in severe cases the clinical signs represent a much more diffuse neuronal dysfunction than the distribution of histologic lesions seen at necropsy. This is a metabolic disorder that can disrupt neuronal function before causing ischemic-type degeneration or necrosis that is visible with the light microscope. The clinician's objective is to stop this process as soon as possible before the neuronal changes become permanent.

Cattle normally produce thiamine as a result of rumen microbial activity. However, thiamine deficiency or alteration of normal thiamine production can be induced by a variety of means. High grain/low fiber diets are one of the most commonly encountered problems associated with field outbreaks of PEM. Such diets may alter the rumen flora to allow production of thiaminase type 2 by various anaerobes or other organisms. Similarly feedstuffs that contain thiaminase activity, such as bracken fern ribozyme and horsetail, may alter thiamine levels via thiaminase type 1. Type 2 thiaminase appears to be most important in causing PEM in cattle. Worming with levamisole or thiabendazole and tranquilization with acepromazine have also been incriminated by field experience. Although the feeding of amprolium, a thiamine analogue, has been associated with PEM, experimental cases were fed extremely high levels to reproduce the disease.

The exact etiology in sporadic cases usually is impossible to determine, although herd outbreaks warrant close analysis of possible contributing factors—especially concentrate versus roughage ratios.

Clinical Signs

Cerebrocortical signs predominate in PEM. Depression and anorexia are present in both calves and adults, but these signs may only be present for a short time before more overt signs of cortical disease become apparent. Blindness with intact pupillary function is one of the first signs observed because of the sensitivity of the visual cortex to the ongoing pathology (see video clips 37 and 38). Pupillary response to light may be lost in some recumbent cases as the disease progresses and presumably the oculomotor nerve is compressed. Head pressing and odontoprisis may be observed or an extended head and neck typical of cattle with "headache"-type pain. A slow shuffling gait is usually apparent if the animal is able to walk. Vocalization, as observed in some early cases in goats, is usually not observed in calves or adult cattle with PEM. A dorsomedial strabismus thought to be caused by involvement of the CN-IV nucleus is common in calves and yearlings but observed less often in adult cattle. Muscle tremors and salivation also may occur.

If the disease has progressed enough to cause recumbency, opisthotonos frequently is observed, and abnormal nystagmus, seizures, or coma is likely to follow (Figure 12-20). Untreated cases may die within 24 to 96 hours, depending on the severity of the metabolic dysfunction. CN signs other than possible dorsomedial strabismus usually are not present (Figure 12-21). Although optic disc edema has been reported to occur, we have never observed this in any calf or cow affected with PEM. Therefore in our opinion, blindness is entirely of cortical origin (Figure 12-22). Associated with either cortical blindness or cerebral edema, cattle may have a stargazing appearance (Figure 12-23).

The major differential diagnoses are lead poisoning, sulfur toxicity, meningitis, encephalitides including rabies, salt poisoning, nervous ketosis (in adult lactating cows), hepatoencephalopathy, and clostridial enterotoxemia type D (calves only).

Diagnosis

In acute cases, the clinical signs and CSF evaluation usually allow a diagnosis. The CSF in acute PEM is usually clear, has no increase in nucleated cells, and may have a normal or slightly elevated protein. In chronic cases that have been affected 3 or more days, the CSF may show

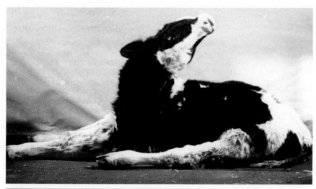

Figure 12-20

Profound opisthotonos in a calf with PEM.

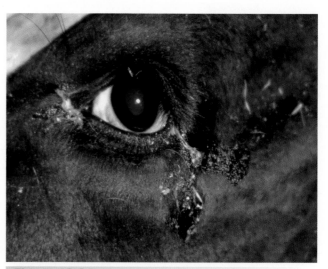

Figure 12-21

Dorsomedial strabismus in a yearling Holstein recumbent as a result of PEM. The strabismus was bilateral.

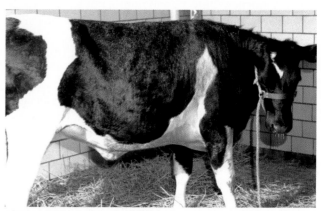

Figure 12-22

Two-year-old Holstein that was blind with intact pupillary light responses and profoundly depressed as a result of PEM.

increased protein and mild-to-moderate increases in nucleated cells—especially macrophages—as a result of advanced cerebrocortical necrosis. Therefore the CSF helps rule out most meningitis and encephalitides except rabies. Blood lead and tissue lead tests may be necessary to rule out lead poisoning if this disease cannot be completely eliminated by history. In addition, animals with lead poisoning tend to show more seizure activity than PEM patients, although this is a subjective statement. Blood ammonia can be measured to rule down a portosystemic shunt (see video clip 39). Urinary and blood ketones can be assessed in lactating cattle to rule down nervous ketosis. Comparative assessment of serum and CSF sodium levels would be necessary if salt toxicity/water deprivation was considered.

Many specific laboratory tests have been suggested to confirm PEM, but they all suffer from the disadvantages

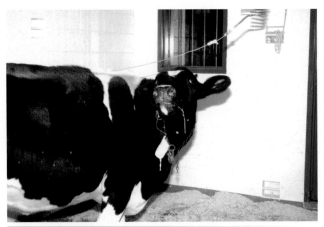

Figure 12-23

A 3-year-old Holstein cow with an acute onset of cerebrocortical blindness and stargazing appearance. The cow was treated with thiamine and IV crystalloids and appeared normal within 72 hours. The diagnosis was thiamine-responsive PEM, which is not common in adult cows.

of unavailability to the practicing veterinarian, expense, and the limited number of more research-oriented laboratories that offer the service. These tests include those measuring erythrocyte transketolase levels (should be decreased with PEM), blood pyruvate, blood lactate, pyruvate kinase, and fecal and ruminal thiaminase (all may be high with PEM). In herd outbreaks of PEM, the attending veterinarian may wish to contact regional laboratories as to the availability, practicality, turnaround time, and expense of these tests.

On a practical basis, necropsy becomes the most reliable means of diagnosis in those cattle that die or do not respond to therapy for PEM. Gross postmortem examination may reveal a slight yellow discoloration of neocortical gyri as a result of cortical edema. If brain edema is extensive, herniation of the caudal cerebellar vermis at the foramen magnum (cerebellar coning) may occur. An ultraviolet light may cause fluorescence of the cerebral cortex because of mitochondrial changes that occur in the affected cortex. Microscopic lesions vary from cytotoxic edema and ischemic-type degeneration to complete necrosis of the neocortex and selective brainstem nuclei. This depends on the severity and duration of the disorder. Response to specific therapy often is used as a clinical confirmation of PEM in the field. In many cases, these microscopic lesions are difficult to differentiate from those caused by lead poisoning and sulfur toxicity.

Treatment

Specific treatment for PEM requires thiamine hydrochloride administered at 10 to 20 mg/kg IV as an initial bolus and then repeated at 10 mg/kg IM twice daily for 3 to 10 days, depending on the severity of signs and response to treatment. Mannitol has been used in some valuable

calves, but its efficacy is unproven. This is administered as a 20% solution IV slowly over 20 to 30 minutes at 0.5 to 2.0 g/kg. This may be repeated once or twice at 3- to 4-hour intervals. Corticosteroids are generally not used.

In acute cases, improvement is apparent within hours, whereas subacute cases respond gradually over 24 to 96 hours. Blindness is usually the last sign to disappear, and we have observed one young animal that did not show evidence of vision until the ninth day of treatment. Blindness also may be permanent, despite resolution of all other neurologic signs.

Prevention

The diet should be assessed in all patients with PEM. This is especially true when multiple cattle or calves within a group have been affected. When all grain or mostly grain diets are identified, adding fiber in the form of long-stem hay at 5 to 10 lb/head/day will stop further incidence of PEM. Other possible nutritional factors discussed in the etiology section may be addressed where necessary. The addition of thiamine to the diet at a rate of 5 to 10 mg/kg of feed may help prevent further incidence. For group outbreaks in calves, injections of thiamine hydrochloride at 10 mg/kg IM may be given to unaffected animals and repeated weekly in the hope of deterring further cases.

Sulfur Toxicity

Diets or water high in sulfates may cause a similar PEM. Sulfur is metabolized to sulfide ion, which appears to be the toxic form. Sulfur, sulfates, and even sulfites (e.g., preservative in pretzels) may be found in feeds, water, or minerals. The clinical signs are the same as those that result from the PEM caused by thiamine deficiency. Elevated levels of hydrogen sulfide gas can be determined from trocarization of the ruminal gas cap. The treatment is the same as for PEM resulting from thiamine deficiency. Response to treatment is often poor and should emphasize the need to locate a possible source of sulfur to prevent other cattle from developing the same lesions.

Lead Poisoning

Etiology

Accidental or malicious exposure to materials containing lead predisposes cattle to lead poisoning or plumbism. Lack of discrimination in eating habits, coupled with the species' tendency for licking objects and ingesting odd-tasting foreign materials, also predisposes cattle to lead poisoning. Although modern housing tends to reduce the likelihood of lead toxicity in dairy cattle, ample opportunity still exists in many geographic areas where pasturing and other management techniques allow cattle to roam, escape from fences or enclosures, and thereby gain access to areas where lead-containing chemicals or materials may exist. Used motor oils, certain roofing materials, lead and aluminum-based paints, lead arsenate sprays, lead shot, linoleum, solder, used batteries, and weather-worn lead sheeting compose some of the more common sources of lead to which cattle may be exposed. Environmental contamination caused by industrial production of lead or lead wastes is possible in certain areas.

All animals are susceptible, but calves fed milk may be more susceptible than calves fed hay and grain. The dose of lead necessary to cause toxicity to cattle varies tremendously because one exposure to a massive quantity (1 g/kg body weight) could induce acute lethal signs, whereas exposure to 2 to 3 mg/kg body weight daily might require 1 month or longer before clinical signs appear. Other factors, such as age, diet, ruminal pH, previous or ongoing lead levels in diet before exposure, and many other details may influence the amount of lead required to cause clinical signs. It is simplest to remember that the incubation period is shortened, the clinical signs accentuated, and the mortality elevated by increasing dosages.

Signs
Neurologic signs predominate in cattle poisoned with lead, but gastrointestinal signs also may appear. Early signs induced by low levels of lead in the diet include excessive salivation (ptyalism) and teeth grinding (bruxism), muscle tremors, tongue wallowing, and hyperesthesia (see video clip 40b). More advanced cases or animals that ingested higher concentrations show classical signs of cerebrocortical disease with blindness with normal pupillary function, propulsive activity, seizures, abnormal posture, facial spasticity, head pressing, vocalization, bruxism creating foamy saliva at the mouth, or aggression as possible signs (Figure 12-24). Acute death without premonitory signs also is possible. Although various theories exist as to the cellular effect of lead on the CNS, the exact cellular pathophysiology is unknown.

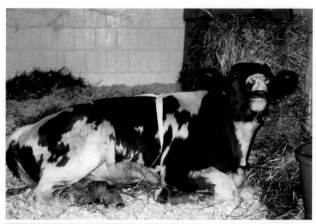

Figure 12-24

Lead poisoning causing recumbency, blindness, and bellowing. There also were uncontrolled jerking actions in this 16-month-old heifer.

Gastrointestinal signs including ruminal stasis, bloat, diarrhea, or constipation have been described. Abdominal pain characterized by colic also has been described and is thought to result from irritation of the bowel by the toxic material. Mild-to-moderate levels of exposure may result in both cerebrocortical and gastrointestinal signs. Such animals are noticed to be depressed, blind, sometimes wander aimlessly or head press, and have ruminal stasis. The clinical signs can look nearly identical to thiamine deficiency PEM. Occasionally during the clinical examination of the patient, the odor of used motor oil or some other chemical will be detected and can aid greatly in the diagnosis.

Normocytic, normochromic anemia, basophilic stippling, reticulocytosis, and mild elevation of blood urea nitrogen (BUN) and creatinine have been found in some chronic lead poisoning patients but are not common in bovine lead poisoning.

Diagnosis
The clinical signs coupled with a thorough search of the premises on which affected cattle have been housed or turned out constitute the principal means of diagnosis. Laboratory confirmation usually is essential.

Blood or tissue lead levels must be obtained to confirm the diagnosis of lead poisoning. Although references vary greatly, most laboratories use 0.05 to 0.25 ppm as reference ranges for blood lead (heparinized sample) and indicate that any values >0.30 ppm are abnormal. Kidney and liver lead values >10 ppm on a wet basis are considered toxic levels. Low-grade, chronic exposure may not generate greatly elevated blood lead levels.

Although blood and tissue lead values are the most practical means to confirm lead toxicity in cattle, other specific tests are available at some laboratories. These tests measure the effect of lead on porphyrin and heme metabolism. Specifically lead inhibits activity of delta-aminolevulinic acid dehydratase, which is essential to heme synthesis. Resultant low levels of delta-aminolevulinic acid dehydrase in blood and high levels of delta-aminolevulinic acid in urine may be measured to diagnose lead toxicity. These changes may occur before clinical signs are pronounced and thus may offer an early monitoring technique. These levels also offer a more sensitive means than blood lead analysis to monitor remaining tissue lead values following treatment. However, these tests are not widely available to veterinarians at present.

CSF analysis generally reveals normal protein and nucleated cell counts in acute cases. Subacute cases showing obvious neurologic signs may have mild protein and cellular elevations caused by cerebrocortical necrosis.

Gross necropsy offers little help unless oil, grease, or a particular suspect material such as paint is found in the rumen. Subacute cases may have enough cerebrocortical necrosis to be detectable as gross cortical swelling and yellow discoloration. Microscopic examination of the neocortex will reveal patches of cerebrocortical degeneration that vary with the severity and duration of the disorder. In the first 72 hours, these consist of cytotoxic edema, ischemic degeneration of neuronal cell bodies, and reactive blood vessels with increased and enlarged endothelial cells. In more prolonged lesions, necrosis is more extensive and macrophages will accumulate. These lesions are similar to those caused by thiamine deficiency. Mild liver and kidney changes also have been described in chronic cases. These include acid-fast intranuclear inclusion bodies in renal proximal tubular epithelium.

The major differential diagnosis to lead poisoning in dairy cattle is PEM resulting from thiamine deficiency, with salt poisoning, hepatic encephalopathy, vitamin A deficiency, rabies, and other causes of meningitis or meningoencephalitis, such as *H. somni,* also requiring consideration. In general, acute lead toxicity patients have more of a tendency to have seizures, vocalize, and appear irritable (e.g., facial twitching, hyperesthesia) than do cattle with thiamine deficiency PEM. Both diseases cause cortical blindness with intact pupil function, and both may lead to depression, head pressing, bruxism, and other signs. Dorsomedial strabismus may be more common in PEM. It may be difficult in a single patient to appreciate these differences, but in herd outbreaks, the pattern of clinical signs may be more obvious. Also in PEM, ruminal activity may be unaltered, whereas lead poisoning tends to depress ruminal activity.

Meningitis or meningoencephalitis is characterized by inflammatory CSF, fever, or other signs indicative of inflammation. Rabies must be considered in all differential diagnoses, but blindness is not as common with rabies as with lead poisoning.

Treatment

Unless history confirms the source of lead, prevention of further exposure must be the primary concern of the veterinarian. This may require removal of all suspect feedstuffs, confinement of cattle heretofore pastured, or other measures. When the history confirms that the only affected cow is the one who "got loose and was found in the machinery shed," then the mystery of exposure is usually solved. Much more difficult are herd outbreaks with multiple cattle affected and no known means of exposure. Much detective work must be completed to find the source in feed, water, or on the premises. Suspect feed material should be sent to toxicology laboratories for confirmation.

Specific treatment requires disodium calcium EDTA (Na$_2$,Ca-EDTA) given systemically—but not orally. Suggested doses for IV Na$_2$,Ca-EDTA vary between 62 and 110 mg/kg body weight given once or twice daily. Some clinicians recommend dividing the dose and giving half of the total daily dose twice daily. SQ administration also

is acceptable. During IV administration, Na$_2$,Ca-EDTA should be given very slowly because reactions (e.g., increased heart and respiratory rates, trembling, hair elevation) are common if the drug is administered rapidly. The mechanism of action of Na$_2$,Ca-EDTA is chelation of lead held in bone, thereby allowing solubilization and urinary excretion. It does not chelate lead in soft tissue, and continued treatment depends on soft tissue lead equilibrating with the decreasing bone levels. Therefore treatment with Na$_2$,Ca-EDTA is designed to be intermittent. One well-controlled study used 62.0 mg/kg body weight Na$_2$,Ca-EDTA IV twice daily for 4 days, skipped 4 days, and then treated again for 4 days. In summary, a twice-daily IV treatment with 60 to 110 mg/kg Na$_2$,Ca-EDTA should be used to treat lead poisoning in cattle. The exact number of days is not likely to be important, but a period of 3 to 5 days seems reasonable. This initial therapy should then be repeated after a lag time of 3 to 5 days, during which time soft tissue accumulation of lead may be shifted to bone and thus, once again, subjected to chelation by Na$_2$,Ca-EDTA.

Thiamine should be administered as well at a dosage of 2 mg/kg body weight or higher. Thiamine does not protect against or remove lead accumulation in tissue but does seem to improve clinical signs in lead-poisoned cattle. In fact, treatment with Na$_2$,Ca-EDTA alone may worsen the clinical signs, whereas treatment with thiamine or thiamine and Na$_2$,Ca-EDTA in combination improves the clinical signs in lead-poisoned cattle. Thiamine's exact mechanism is unknown. However, because the cerebrocortical lesions of PEM and lead toxicity are so similar, it has been theorized that lead interferes with thiamine levels or metabolism to some degree and that some of the cerebrocortical lesions are in fact the result of relative thiamine deficiency. IV mannitol as described for PEM resulting from thiamine deficiency is the treatment of choice for cytotoxic edema.

When recent ingestion of a known lead-containing material has occurred, a rumenotomy offers the best opportunity to remove the material, wash out the rumen, and institute supportive therapy. Magnesium sulfate laxatives are indicated to cause formation of insoluble lead sulfides that can be passed in the feces.

Prognosis is best for those cattle with mild neurologic signs or gastrointestinal signs. Cattle that are having seizures or showing opisthotonos, blindness, and dementia have a poorer prognosis. Anticonvulsants are not of great use in adult cattle, but diazepam (5 to 10 mg IV) has been used in calves.

Salt Intoxication

Etiology

Salt intoxication (water deprivation) or hypernatremia is an occasional cause of neurologic signs in calves or adult cattle. Feeding errors that allow excessive sodium chloride in the diet are the usual cause, but occasional cases have resulted from dilutional errors when compounding large quantities of IV fluids for cattle. Failure to dilute electrolyte solution or milk replacers for calves may result in hypernatremia because calves seem willing to drink solutions containing excessive sodium chloride. Failure to provide access to water for milk replacer–fed calves is a common cause of salt intoxication.

Adult cattle have suffered salt intoxication primarily as a result of water deprivation that was accidental or brought on by natural disasters or droughts. We have observed an outbreak of salt poisoning in replacement heifers during freezing weather when both their water source and walkways were covered with ice; salt was sprinkled on the walkways to melt the ice, resulting in the cattle drinking the surface water, which contained very high amounts of salt. Consumption of salt water also has caused the disease in beef cattle. We have observed one instance of salt poisoning in heifers fed liquid whey that contained excessive amounts of sodium chloride. Excessive salt in the ration generally is not a problem as long as plenty of fresh water is available to cattle. However, excessive salt in the water (>0.25%) may decrease milk production in dairy cattle.

Although both sodium and chloride levels are greatly elevated in the serum and CSF, sodium is of more concern because hypernatremia apparently inhibits glycolysis in cerebral neurons. Beware that the signs of cerebrocortical degeneration may follow the consumption of excessive quantities of water after a period of hypernatremia. The sudden effect of the hypo-osmolar serum can result in cytotoxic brain edema. This can occur when water is suddenly restored to cattle deprived of it during a period of frozen water pipes.

Clinical Signs

In calves, depression, diarrhea, and weakness are the major signs, but seizures may occur in advanced cases. Serum and CSF sodium levels usually are >160 mEq/L, and neurologic signs tend to be directly proportional to serum sodium levels. Diarrhea caused by saline catharsis and enteric pathogens in calves contributes to dehydration, which worsens the electrolyte problems. Seizures may occur spontaneously or following administration of IV fluid intended to correct dehydration. Rapid administration of isotonic IV fluids or excessive intake of water orally to hypernatremic patients decreases extracellular fluid osmolarity faster than intracellular osmolarity in the brain cells; the net result is imbibition of water into brain cells, subsequent edema, and neurologic signs such as seizures.

Adult cattle that are water deprived tend to show gastrointestinal signs, including anorexia, diarrhea, and vomiting. Polyuria is common. Neurologic signs initially reflect the prosencephalic cerebrocortical lesion—depression, blindness, and seizures. More severe lesions will involve the brainstem and cerebellum, causing cerebellar ataxia and UMN/GP locomotor deficits.

Ancillary Aids and Diagnosis

Definitive diagnosis requires laboratory confirmation of hypernatremia in the serum and CSF of patients showing typical clinical signs. Most cases in calves go undiagnosed in the field because of lack of laboratory data. Groups of calves or cows that are affected usually stimulate greater diagnostic efforts. Most calves with salt poisoning have a severe azotemia.

Rations and water should be analyzed for salt content when adult dairy cattle or heifers are affected with hypernatremia. When calves are affected, investigation into feeding protocols, dilution rates of fed milk replacer or oral electrolyte solutions, and the availability of ad libitum access to fresh water is required.

The differential diagnosis in calves may include acid-base electrolyte abnormalities associated with neonatal infectious enteritis, meningitis, and PEM. In adult cattle, PEM, lead poisoning, and rabies may be considered.

Treatment

Treatment should be designed to produce a slow, gradual decrease in serum and CSF osmolarity. For adult animals, this means allowing access to small amounts of fresh water at regular intervals. Free-choice water would likely create cerebral edema as previously discussed because extracellular fluid osmolarity decreases much more rapidly than brain intracellular osmolarity. In addition, a too rapid recovery of normal osmolality may result in brain stem myelinolysis. The use of diuretics such as furosemide (0.50 mg/kg) may be indicated if the patient's hydration status is adequate.

Calves having hypernatremia should be placed on slow drip IV therapy with low percentage dextrose solutions containing half-strength to normal saline until serum sodium values return to normal. Some clinicians have enjoyed success using gradually diminishing concentrations of hypertonic saline in the treatment of hypernatremic neonates. Ideally correction of hypernatremia should be <2 mEq/hr. Therapy is complicated if severe dehydration exists because the patient needs intensive fluid therapy for dehydration but will likely suffer neurologic complications if administered fluids too rapidly. Generally the azotemia resolves, and calves with sodium concentration as great as 201 mEq/L have completely recovered. Supportive therapy with thiamine may be of benefit and is unlikely to be harmful. If the sodium has returned to normal but the calf has not responded appropriately, a dose of mannitol (0.5 mg/kg) can be given.

Nervous Ketosis

Etiology

Nervous ketosis is simply an encephalopathic form of metabolic ketosis and may occur at any time during the first 8 weeks of lactation. The pathophysiology of ketosis is discussed in Chapter 14. Resultant ketoacidosis and hypoglycemia cause the clinical signs associated with the wasting and neurologic forms of the condition. In severe ketosis, the relative energy imbalance causes extreme ketonemia. The reason for the neurological signs in nervous ketosis are not known but may be caused simply by hypoglycemia, acetoacetic acid levels that are toxic to the brain, or through the production of isopropyl alcohol from acetoacetic acid breakdown in the rumen. A degree of hepatic encephalopathy could contribute to neurologic signs in these cattle, but we are unaware of studies to confirm or deny this theory.

Signs

Signs observed in cattle affected with nervous ketosis vary from recumbency to aggression. Many cows having nervous ketosis act demented, constantly licking one or more spots on their own body or on inanimate objects. Some cows bite objects such as drinking cups and have been known to break cups off water pipes (Figure 12-25) (see video clip 40a). Other cows, if confined, show propulsive tendencies by constantly leaning into a stanchion or tie stall. Cattle not confined to tie stalls may wander about, appear ataxic, blind, and will head press. Sometimes hyperesthesia is observed. Some severely affected cattle become recumbent as their degree of hypoglycemia worsens. Once recumbent, the patient may appear similar to hypocalcemic or hypomagnesemic patients. Signs of constant licking or depraved appetite in recumbent cattle suggest nervous ketosis (Figure 12-26). Overly fat periparturient cows may develop severe ketosis and signs of nervous ketosis within days following calving. Therefore if recumbent, these cows are often assumed to be hypocalcemic or hypomagnesemic but may have nervous ketosis or combined metabolic problems. In conventional housing, cattle with severe ketosis may walk short distances following release for exercise and then collapse because of hypoglycemia.

Cattle showing irritation or aggression are obviously more dramatic and can be dangerous to handlers, veterinarians, and themselves. Irritability resulting from hypoglycemia, just as in people, can worsen if the patient is stressed. Therefore uncontrolled activity including aggression, wild running, bellowing, and a wild-eyed appearance may be seen by the clinician. Usually this form is observed following attempts to capture or restrain the patient.

Blindness is observed occasionally in cattle having nervous ketosis. Most cattle regain vision following treatment, which has caused many authors to describe this blindness as "transient" or "apparent." However, blindness may persist and be permanent in some nervous ketosis patients, even though all other signs have resolved with treatment. This bilateral blindness, first described by Fox, is a cerebrocortical blindness with intact pupillary function and is most likely caused by permanent damage to the visual cortex. The visual cortex is extremely sensitive to

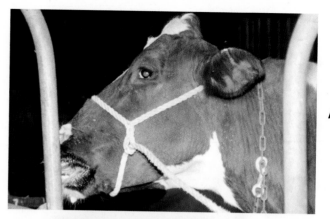

A

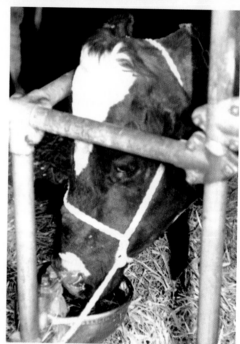

B

Figures 12-25

A and B, Nervous ketosis. This cow appeared demented and repeatedly licked her side and stall pipes, and bit the water cup.

metabolic derangements, such as severe hypoglycemia, making this the most likely cause. The retinas and optic nerves are normal in appearance in such patients.

Diagnosis

Diagnosis depends on identification of ketonuria in cattle showing bizarre neurologic signs. Ketonemia and ketonuria are usually dramatic, and test tablets quickly turn purple. However, not all patients have strongly positive urine ketones. This may be a dilutional effect if the cow has been drinking large quantities of water or chewing on a salt block because of a depraved appetite. Therefore some variation in the degree of ketonuria exists in nervous ketosis patients. Reagents to detect ketones in urine, blood, or milk also vary. Many of the tests detect

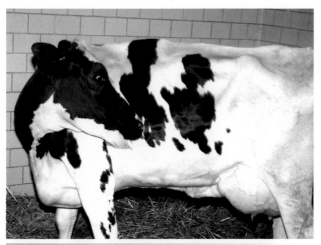

Figure 12-26

A cow with nervous ketosis propulsively licking on only one side of the thorax.

only acetoacetate and do not detect acetone or beta-hydroxybutyric acid.

Clinical signs of constant licking, chewing, or biting objects make this diagnosis likely. More bizarre signs cause the clinician to consider a wider differential diagnosis, including other metabolic diseases (e.g., hypocalcemia, hypomagnesemia) when recumbency, hyperesthesia, and tetany are apparent. Aggression brings the fear of rabies into consideration. Blindness, if present, requires a wide-ranging differential diagnosis, including PEM and lead poisoning, among others. Leaning into a stanchion or propulsive activity by the patient requires consideration of listeriosis. Despite the broad differential diagnosis, the triad of early lactation, positive (usually strongly) urine or milk ketones, and nervous signs generally allow accurate diagnosis.

Occasionally cows with other neurologic diseases such as listeriosis, and especially those with dysphagia, may become ketotic secondary to continued milk losses. However, in these instances, neurologic signs have usually preceded ketosis by several days.

Overly fat periparturient cows with nervous ketosis require further workup, including acid-base electrolyte status, serum calcium, serum magnesium, and serum biochemistry to evaluate liver function.

Treatment

IV dextrose (300 to 500 ml of 50% dextrose) is the initial therapy for nervous ketosis patients. In aggressive or demented patients, it may be necessary to sedate the animal with xylazine (20 mg IM or IV) before IV dextrose. Dextrose should be repeated in 6 to 12 hours in field settings. If possible, slow constant administration of 20 L of 5% dextrose over a 24-hour period is superior followup to initial concentrated dextrose. If this is not practical, repeat treatments with dextrose should be suggested at 12-hour intervals for at least three treatments. A single

treatment is never sufficient to correct the underlying metabolic rearrangement. In addition to dextrose, low-dose corticosteroids usually are used as therapy for ketosis. An initial dose of 10 to 20 mg of dexamethasone is followed by 10 mg daily for 3 to 4 additional days. Dexamethasone treatment is contingent on the fact that the patient has no contraindications to use of this drug.

Other supportive measures are controversial and vary greatly. Most clinicians use propylene glycol or glycerol at 6 to 8 oz, usually twice daily, as a supplemental energy source. It is important not to use these products in excessive doses because they may contribute to decreased ruminal activity and diarrhea. Therefore they are most useful in patients that have good ruminal activity. On some farms, propylene glycol may be the only treatment required for ketosis, whereas on others, owners refuse to use the product because of lack of perceived benefit.

Chloral hydrate (30 g orally in gelatin capsules) may be extremely helpful as initial therapy in very agitated patients because of the sedative properties of the drug. It may also contribute to starch metabolism in the rumen and aid glucose production in some unknown ways.

Periparturient patients with nervous ketosis have a guarded prognosis. These patients usually require many other treatments. Prognosis for nervous ketosis patients, other than those that are periparturient, is good with therapy as directed. With the exception of the rare permanent blindness observed in some patients, most cattle fully resolve the neurologic signs within hours and only relapse if maintenance therapy is neglected.

Vitamin A Deficiency

Etiology and Signs

An absolute or relative deficiency of vitamin A may cause a multitude of abnormalities in growing cattle. Poor growth, blindness, inappetence, seizures and other neurologic signs, dermatitis, diarrhea, xerophthalmia, and pneumonia have been observed in young dairy cattle experimentally deprived of vitamin A. Mature cattle may show blindness and gastrointestinal, neurologic, and reproductive abnormalities.

Most natural outbreaks of vitamin A deficiency involve growing or feedlot beef cattle, but much experimental work has been completed with dairy animals. Because natural occurrence in dairy animals is rare, discussion of this deficiency will be brief and primarily useful as a differential diagnosis to PEM and lead poisoning.

Clinical signs are the result of (1) increased intracranial pressure secondary to meningeal thickening and altered arachnoid villi that interfere with CSF absorption, and (2) abnormal bone growth with deficient bone resorption contributing to optic nerve compression. The meningeal fibroplasia and a narrowing of the caudal cranial fossa and foramen magnum result in caudal cerebellar vermal herniation.

Neurologic signs, in both experimental and natural outbreaks, include blindness, seizures, circling, disorientation, opisthotonos, depression, and elevated head carriage. Blindness is a classic finding and is primarily caused by progressive optic disc edema from increased CSF pressure in adult cattle. Optic disc edema must be severe to result in blindness because many deficient cattle will remain visual despite mild-to-moderate edema. In growing cattle, optic disc edema and blindness are caused by both elevated CSF pressure and dural fibroplasias in the optic canals with resultant optic nerve compression. In severe cases, this causes dilated pupils with deficient pupillary responses to light. These pupillary abnormalities help to differentiate this form of blindness from that which occurs in PEM, in which case they are normal. Nyctalopia or night blindness also is associated with vitamin A deficiency and, although it is one of the earliest signs, may be difficult to assess in field settings. Vitamin A is essential for rhodopsin regeneration required for photoreceptor activity during dark adaptation. Rod photoreceptors may be more affected than cones, thus contributing to nyctalopia.

Diets consisting of aged feed material, all grain diets that have not been supplemented with vitamin A, diets in which vitamin A may have been destroyed by heat, or diets completely devoid of green forage can lead to natural outbreaks of vitamin A deficiency. Similarly animals pastured during extreme drought conditions or only offered coarse roughage in addition to pasture may become deficient.

Diagnosis

Optic disc edema with associated retinal edema and hemorrhages will be present in vitamin A–deficient animals (Figure 12-27). The finding of optic disc edema in a group of animals showing signs of blindness with abnormal pupillary light responses and other neurologic signs is pathognomonic for vitamin A deficiency. Although optic disc edema has been reported in lead toxicity and PEM in cattle, it rarely, if ever, occurs in these diseases. Therefore optic disc edema, especially in multiple animals, should make vitamin A deficiency the most likely diagnosis.

Rations and blood from affected animals should be assessed for vitamin A or carotene levels. Normal values for vitamin A in serum range from 25 to 60 μg/dl. The severity of clinical signs is inversely proportional to the level of vitamin A when serum levels decrease to <20 μg/dl.

Histopathology in active cases in growing animals reveals optic nerve degeneration resulting from dural fibrosis within the optic canal, squamous metaplasia of parotid salivary ducts, and many other changes.

Treatment

Normally vitamin A deficiency is prevented by feeding green forage or a diet supplemented with vitamin A. However, if the disease occurs, all animals in the group

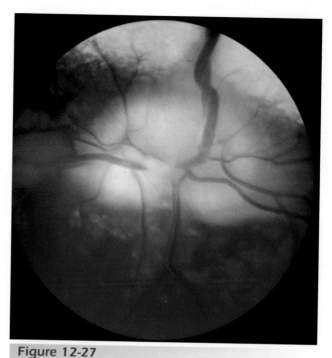

Figure 12-27

Optic disc edema, peridiscal retinal edema, and hemorrhage in a vitamin A–deficient heifer.

should receive 440 IU/kg body weight of vitamin A by injection. This may be repeated, and dietary supplementation should begin immediately with sufficient levels of vitamin A in the diet to provide 40 IU/kg body weight/day for the cattle.

Hepatic Encephalopathy

Hepatic encephalopathy (HE) is a metabolic disorder that results from a diffuse liver deficiency that causes a hyperammonemia along with other circulating toxic factors that interfere with neuronal function. In calves, this is usually caused by a portosystemic shunt (PSS). In older cattle, HE is usually secondary to diffuse liver disease caused by the consumption of pasture grasses that contain large quantities of plant species that produce a pyrrolizidine alkaloid. Species of *Crotalaria* and *Senecio* are most commonly implicated. The chronic consumption of this alkaloid causes liver degeneration that can result in HE. Most clinical signs are prosencephalic in origin with changes in behavior and seizures. Calves with PSSs may seem normal for the first couple of weeks of life until the rumen becomes functional; then the increase in blood ammonia causes waxing and waning signs of both cerebral and spinal cord disease (Figure 12-28). Diagnosis can be made by serum chemistry changes that reflect liver failure including hyperammonemia. PSS can be diagnosed by ultrasound and contrast radiography. One calf has been surgically corrected, but the surgery is difficult even when there is a single extrahepatic shunt. If surgery is being contemplated,

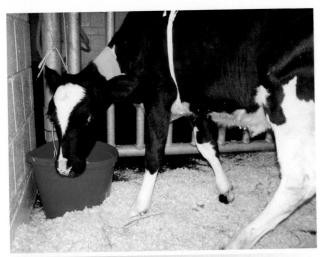

Figure 12-28

A 3-month-old calf with intermittent depression, falling, shuffling gait (which can be seen by the tracks in the shaving) caused by a portosystemic shunt.

medical management would include thiamine and fluids administered IV and vinegar given per os to lower the ruminal pH. If the calf is eating, it should continue to be fed a low protein feed because removing all feed will increase ruminal pH and may increase blood ammonia. Pyrrolizidine toxicity can be diagnosed by liver biopsy that shows a triad of fibrosis, megalocytosis, and bile duct proliferation. The CNS lesions of astrocyte proliferation and alteration and dilated myelin sheaths are reversible. Pyrrolizidine toxicosis is usually fatal but can be prevented by avoiding pastures containing these plant species.

Nervous Coccidiosis

Neurologic signs in calves infected with intestinal coccidia are rare in the northeastern United States and most common in the northwest states and western Canada. Coccidiosis in calves is discussed in detail in Chapter 6. Neurologic signs are more common in heavily infected feedlot beef cattle in severe winter weather. The pathophysiology of these neurologic signs is unknown and assumed to be neurotoxic in nature because there are no brain lesions. Signs include partial or generalized seizures, tremors, and recumbency with opisthotonos and abnormal nystagmus. The mortality rate is high.

Toxins

Mycotoxicosis is rare in cattle in the northeastern United States. The toxins are produced by fungal agents that contaminate various grass species consumed by the cattle. A list of these tremorgenic neurotoxins, along with other miscellaneous toxins that can cause neurologic signs, can be found in table form in Chapter 16.

INJURY

Intracranial injury from external causes is uncommon. Newborn calves are most susceptible because of their less dense calvaria and less resistant brain at this age. Most injuries relate to falls and striking their heads on the concrete in their environment. Brain swelling from hemorrhage and edema leads to herniations.

NEOPLASIA

Brain neoplasms are uncommon in cattle, which may relate to their short life span. Intracranial lymphosarcoma is the most common (Figure 12-29). Intracranial lymphoma is usually not caused by bovine leukemia virus (BLV). Gliomas have also been reported. One of us (TD) has seen two calves (both approximately 2 months of age) with medulloblastomas causing opisthotonos (Figure 12-30) (Table 12-1).

SPINAL CORD

Clinical Signs

Based on clinical signs, the spinal cord can be divided into four regions: C1-C5, C6-T2, T3-L3, and L4-Cd. Lesions that interfere with the gray matter of the intumescences (C6-T2, L4-S2) will cause a gait quality that reflects lower motor neuron (LMN) paresis accompanied by loss of tone, spinal reflexes, and denervation atrophy. The posture and gait will reflect degrees of inability to support weight, and if the patient is ambulatory, there will be short strides sometimes accompanied by trembling. Lesions that spare the intumescence gray matter but affect the white matter

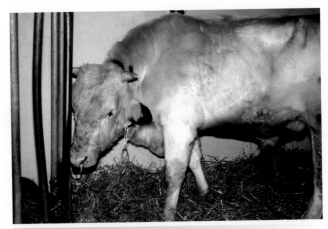

Figure 12-29

A 3-year-old Holstein bull depressed and propulsively circling to the left. The bull was blind in the right eye but had normal pupillary response to light. A large mass (lymphosarcoma) was found in the left cerebral hemisphere.

A

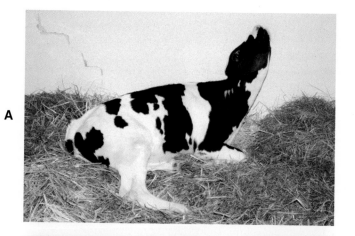

B

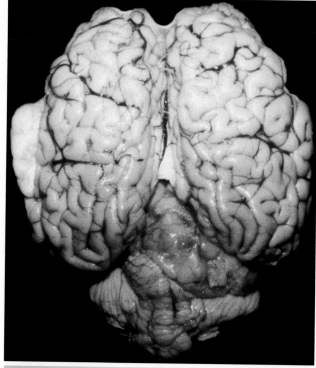

Figure 12-30

A, A 2-month-old calf with severe opisthotonos caused by a medulloblastoma. The clinical signs of opisthotonos often suggest brainstem or cerebellar dysfunction and can look identical to other diseases such as the calf in Figure 12-31 with cerebellar abiotrophy. **B,** Gross appearance of the medulloblastoma.

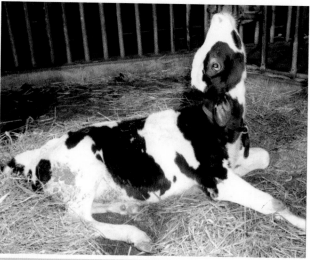

Figure 12-31

Inherited cerebellar abiotrophy in a 6-month-old Holstein heifer. When standing, the heifer had a base-wide stance and a hypermetric gait. Searching head movements and tremor were observed.

tracts that connect with the gray matter will result in a gait quality that reflects interference with the UMN and GP systems. The UMN tracts are descending from nuclei in the caudal brainstem and function to maintain normal muscle tone and to influence the central pattern generators in the intumescences to generate the limb movements for the gait. Interference with these pathways will result in UMN quality paresis. The ascending GP pathways function to provide the sensory information necessary to result in smooth coordinated limb movements. Interference with this pathway results in a GP quality ataxia. The resultant gait abnormality is a reflection of the loss of function of the pathways of both of these two systems, which are adjacent to each other at every level of the spinal cord. It is not possible, nor necessary, to distinguish between the signs because of the interference with these two systems. The clinician's goal is to recognize the signs and locate the region of the spinal cord involved.

Sacrocaudal lesions cause a loss of tail and anal tone, reflexes, and nociception. S1 and S2 contribute primarily to the tibial nerve component of the sciatic nerve. Loss of their function will result in an overflexed tarsus, "dropped hock," and a unique dorsal buckling of the fetlock. Incontinence with dribbling of urine and rectal impaction or pneumorectum may occur. L4-L6 lesions cause varying degrees of difficulty in supporting weight in the pelvic limbs and very short strides if the patient is ambulatory. There will be a tendency to collapse when weight is placed on the limb. L6 primarily contributes to the peroneal component of the sciatic nerve. Loss of its function will cause the animal to stand on the dorsal surface of the digits. Depending on the severity of the lesion, there will be varying degrees of loss of tone, spinal reflexes, and nociception.

T3-L3 lesions cause a delay in the onset of protraction of the pelvic limbs, a longer stride with inaccurate placement of the hooves, a swaying of the trunk and limbs, an excessive adduction or abduction of the limb as it is protracted, and a scuffing of the hooves at the onset of protraction or landing on their dorsal surface at placement. Severe lesions can cause complete pelvic limb paralysis. With caudal thoracic and cranial lumbar lesions, the recumbent patient may use its thoracic limbs and cranial trunk muscles to sit up like a dog (dog-sitter posture). In all situations, the pelvic limb

TABLE 12-1   Uncommon Causes of Brain Signs

Disease	Etiology	Clinical Signs
Bovine "hysteria" or "Bonkers"	Anhydrous ammonia	Intermittent wildness, aimless wandering, bellowing, seizures, recumbency, aggression
Sporadic bovine encephalomyelitis (Buss disease)	Chlamydial organisms have been incriminated, as have paramyxovirus	Fever, depression, respiratory signs, ataxia, weakness, mostly adult cattle with a subacute to chronic course
Hypomagnesemia	Magnesium deficiency	Tremors, seizure-like activity, recumbency
Hypoglycemia	Low blood glucose; most common in young calves, although occasionally seen in cows with overwhelming sepsis or ketosis	Mostly depression and weakness, rarely seizure
Nervous coccidiosis	High levels of Coccidia–often complicated by inclement weather	Convulsions, recumbency, hyperesthesia, diarrhea, high mortality
Neosporosis	*Neospora caninum*	Mostly abortion with early fetal infection but a few clinically affected calves will be born. Most calves infected after 30 weeks gestation will be normal. Both brain and spinal cord signs may exist
Sarcocystis infection	Ingestion of *Sarcocystis* sp. from carnivore feces in contaminated feeds	Poor growth, fever, "rat tail," weakness, gastrointestinal signs, many possible neurologic signs depending on site and severity of lesion in central nervous systems
Pyrrolizidine alkaloid poisoning	Hepatic encephalopathy	Depression, head pressing, aggression, seizures, tenesmus, rarely detected jaundice
Portosystemic shunt; patent ductus venosus	Hepatic encephalopathy	2- to 3-month-old calf, poor growth, intermittent neurologic signs such as ataxia, weakness, depression, bruxism, and tenesmus also noted
Enterotoxemia	Epsilon toxin of *Clostridium perfringens* type D	Acute death or convulsions, mania, and coma in well-grown and well-fed calves
Grass staggers	Rye grass, Dallis grass (*Claviceps paspali*)	Mostly tremors, hypermetria, ataxia, and change in behavior
Cerebellar hypoplasia	Bovine virus diarrhea virus (BVDV) infection of fetus during midtrimester of pregnancy	Strong but uncoordinated calf with intention head tremor. If stands has base wide stance and hypermetric gait. May have ocular or visual signs such as cataracts, retinal scarring, optic nerve lesions, microphthalmia
Cerebellar abiotrophy	Inherited in Holstein breed	Acute onset of cerebellar signs at 3 to 8 months of age. Intention head tremor, base-wide stance, hypermetric, ataxia (Figure 12-31)
Blue-green algae toxicosis	Ponds contaminated with blue-green algae (microcystin toxin)	Multiple cattle with muscle tremors, ataxia, over-response to stimuli, bloody diarrhea, profuse salivation

Differential Diagnosis	Diagnosis	Treatment
Rabies Lead poisoning	History of feeding with good quality forage treated with anhydrous ammonia	Stop feeding ammoniated forage: toxic agent not known—may be substituted imidazole
Malignant catarrhal fever	Rare, nonsuppurative encephalomyelitis, culture of organisms, serology	Oxytetracycline
Toxicities Vitamin A deficiency Rabies	Low serum magnesium and CSF magnesium and absence of magnesium in the urine	Magnesium and calcium, which is also low in most cases
Metabolic diseases	History and very low blood glucose from a sample measured within 2 hours of collection	50% glucose initially followed by continual administration of glucose
Toxicities PEM	Usually beef calves Not blind; usually associated with high levels of Coccidia in feces but direct cause:effect relationship not established	Check serum electrolytes, Mg^{++}, Ca^{++}, glucose, treat if necessary Coccidiostats and supportive therapy
Cerebellar hypoplasia and other congenital anomalies	Necropsy and histopathology	No proven treatment
Many	Serology or histopathology	Prevent contamination of cattle feeds by carnivore feces
Encephalopathies Rabies	Elevated serum liver enzymes and blood ammonia values Gross and microscopic pathology Multiple animals affected	Supportive—usually fatal
Encephalitis	Rare Elevated blood ammonia Normal liver enzymes	Surgical repair if valuable
Polioencephalomalacia Lead poisoning Rabies	Culture of organism or toxin assay on fresh postmortem gut specimen	Prevent by vaccination
Other toxicities (e.g., organophosphates) Hypomagnesemia	History, detection of fungi on plants.	Remove from suspect pastures, diazepam may calm excitable cattle
Congenital cerebellar disease Trauma	Grossly small cerebellum at necropsy Pre-colostral blood samples for BVDV isolation and serology If virus isolated = calf persistently infected; if no virus but positive pre-colostral antibodies, calf formed antibodies to virus due to infection after fetal immune system competent	None—some actually adapt to ataxia and compensate
Brain abscess PEM	Acute onset of cerebellar signs that progress Cerebellum may be grossly normal size at necropsy but histopathology shows distinct loss of Purkinje cell layer	No
Other toxicities	Culture of blue-green algae from pond	Supportive Activated charcoal Copper sulphate to pond water (0.0001% concentrate in pond water desired)

Continued

TABLE 12-1	Uncommon Causes of Brain Signs—cont'd	
Disease	Etiology	Clinical Signs
Hydrocephalus	Congenital accidents	Newborn calf with gross abnormality of skull or profound neurologic deficits
Hydranencephaly	Viral insults in utero	
Encephalocele	Toxic insults in utero	
Hypomyelinogenesis	Inherited in Jersey breed	Neonatal calf head and body tremors that worsen when the calf tries to move; spastic gait—possible cerebellar signs

tone and spinal reflexes will vary from normal to hyperactive. Severe transverse lesions will cause complete paralysis and analgesia caudal to the lesion.

· C6-T2 lesions cause the same signs in the pelvic limbs as a T3-L3 lesion but LMN quality paresis in the thoracic limbs with difficulty supporting weight and short strides if ambulatory. Muscle tone and spinal reflexes will be diminished in the thoracic limbs and normal to increased in the pelvic limbs.

C1-C5 lesions cause the same signs in all four limbs that were described for the pelvic limbs with a T3-L3 lesion. The longer strides seen in the thoracic limbs will appear like an overreaching movement with the limb in extension, sometimes referred to as a floating movement.

MALFORMATION

Malformations of the spinal cord are common in calves and are almost confined to the thoracolumbar and sacrocaudal segments. In most of these myelodysplasias, the gray matter of the lumbosacral intumescence is normal or not depleted of neurons, and usually considerable voluntary movement can be generated. However, there may not be enough interaction of the long tracts (UMN-GP) and the ventral gray columns to permit the animal to stand. Most of these calves will exhibit some limb movement when supported in a standing position. A few can walk unaided. However, characteristic of nearly all myelodysplasias, the flexor responses to advance the limb or in response to a noxious stimulus in the recumbent calf occur simultaneously in both pelvic limbs. The common description of these simultaneous voluntary movements is "bunny hopping." Nociception is usually normal unless an aplasia has occurred. These are very consistent clinical signs regardless of the nature of the myelodysplasia in most instances. In all cases, the clinical signs are present at birth and do not get progressively worse.

Severe myelodysplasias in which there is a failure of the lumbosacral intumescence to develop will cause a severe pelvic limb deformity. Joint and muscle development are dependent on the muscle being innervated. If this does not occur, the muscle remains undeveloped, and the joints are abnormal in their development and position and cannot be moved. This joint fixation is often referred to as "contractures or arthrogryposis."

A common clinical finding in calves with myelodysplasia is the presence of a vertebral column malformation such as kyphosis, scoliosis, spina bifida, absence of one or more vertebra or their arches, and shortened and/or crooked caudal vertebrae in the tail. Simultaneous malformation of the spinal cord and vertebral column is common because of the close relationship of the development of the somitic sclerotomes and the neural tube. Both are influenced by the growth factors elaborated from the adjacent notochord.

Although a great variety of myelodysplasias can affect the T3 to caudal spinal cord segments, the neurological signs are usually the same. Examples include segmental hypoplasia of one or more segments; syringomyelia, which often consists of numerous cavities with no specific gray or white matter location; abnormal gray matter formation without apparent dorsal or ventral gray column differentiation; diplomyelia, which is a duplication of the spinal cord all within one meningeal sheath; and diastematomyelia, which is a duplication of the spinal cord with each spinal cord in its own meningeal sheath and the two spinal cords are usually separated by a bony partition. The latter two can both occur in the same calf at different levels of the spinal cord. Diplomyelia is the most common myelodysplasia seen in our experience (see video clips 41 to 43).

Segmental aplasia is uncommon. One Simmenthal calf was presented recumbent with remarkable rigidity of the pelvic limbs. Neurologic function was normal in the head, neck, and thoracic limbs. Pelvic limbs were held in rigid extension, but any stimulus caused a rapid simultaneous flexion of both limbs. Nociception was absent caudal to the midlumbar level. When supported by the tail, any contact of the hooves with the floor elicited flexion movements at the hips and a short limb advancement. Forceps stimulation of the tail, anus, or pelvic limbs elicited the same response. The cranial lumbar region was depressed where no vertebral spines could be palpated.

Differential Diagnosis	Diagnosis	Treatment
	Consider pre-colostral blood for viral isolation and serology (BVDV, bluetongue, akabane)	None—congenital
	Consider pre-colostral blood for viral isolation and serology (BVDV, bluetongue, akabane)	None—congenital
Hereditary neuraxial edema (Herefords) BVDV infection	Pre-colostral blood for viral isolation and titers	None—congenital

At necropsy there was no spinal cord (segmental aplasia) from the T13 segment through the L3 segment and no vertebral arches over T13 through L2. All the pelvic limb "hopping movements" represented the uninhibited activity of the lumbosacral intumescence and would classify as an example of spinal reflex walking. This case exemplifies the major role of the UMN in the inhibition of motor neuron activity, especially that of extensor motor neurons to the antigravity muscles.

Alternate limb movements are dependent on a subset of commissural interneurons in the intumescences. Because the lack of these alternate movements is so common in these myelodysplasias, a lack or abnormality of development of these commissural interneurons may be the basis for this unique clinical sign.

In contrast to the above description, a severe myelodysplasia with diplomyelia and large syrinx formation in the lumbosacral segments was observed in a 2-year-old Holstein bull with just a very slight ataxic gait and no loss of alternate limb movements. Observations like this tend to keep the clinician humble!

INFLAMMATION

Myelitis is uncommon in cattle as a primary lesion. Occasionally a vertebral column-epidural abscess will invade the meninges causing a suppurative leptomeningitis and myelitis. Newborn calves infected in utero with *Neospora caninum* may be born with a diffuse myelitis caused by this protozoal agent.

Abscesses

Etiology

Although most common in calves, epidural abscesses occasionally occur in adult cattle. These abscesses may originate either within vertebrae as areas of osteomyelitis or adjacent to the vertebrae in the epidural space. Calves with acute or chronic septicemia secondary to umbilical infections are at risk for vertebral abscesses. These same calves may have polyarthritis, meningitis, uveitis,

pneumonia, or other sites of infection as well. Pneumonia and coughing may predispose to the bacteremic organism localizing in the vertebral vessels because there are significant pressure changes and bidirectional flow of blood in those blood vessels associated with the coughing. Adult cattle with vertebral abscesses generally have suffered septicemic spread of bacterial organisms from areas of acute or chronic infection such as lung abscesses. *A. pyogenes* remains the most common organism isolated from vertebral abscesses, but gram-negative organisms, such as *Pasteurella* sp., *Fusobacterium necrophorum*, *Streptococcus* sp., and Strain 19 *Brucella abortus*, also have been isolated. Although bacteria reach the vertebrae or epidural location through embolic spread (endogenous) in most cases, we have observed several cows that developed exogenous origin abscess from external trauma to the lumbosacral region and subsequent large subcutaneous abscesses. Cauda equine neuritis and abscessation can occur from tail docking, and *Clostridial* organisms are often the infective agent. This problem has become more common since the first edition of this book because of the widespread practice of tail docking dairy cattle.

Signs

Fever, a painful stance, and stiff gait compose the initial signs observed in cattle with epidural abscesses. Fever may be low grade and does not occur in all cases but is very helpful to the diagnosis when present. When cervical vertebrae are involved, the discomfort causes the animal to have a "weather vane" neck, resists attempts at neck movement or flexion, and tends to hold the head and neck extended (Figure 12-32). If the abscess is in the caudal cervical or cranial thoracic vertebrae, the animal may refuse to lower its head and eat from the ground. When thoracic or lumbar vertebrae are involved, the animal assumes an arched stance. A more remarkable arched stance and contracted flexor tendons may be present if polyarthritis coexists or if prolonged recumbency has been observed. Palpation of the vertebrae may cause a painful response when pressure is exerted on the affected bone. Neurologic signs consistent with spinal cord disease are present as the vertebral abscess or epidural abscess

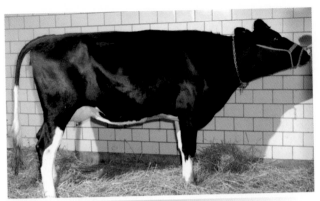

Figure 12-32

Cervical vertebral abscess that was in the vertebral body of C4. Note the anxious expression and the stiff "weather vane" neck

progressively exerts pressure on the spinal cord. Paresis, ataxia, and paralysis occur as the lesions progressively damage the spinal cord. Occasionally the infection invades the meninges and spinal cord causing a focal meningitis and myelitis. Paraparesis and "dog sitting" would be expected with severe thoracolumbar lesions (Figure 12-33) and tetraparesis with cervical abscesses. Abscesses located in the lumbosacral region, which seems to be the most common location in calves, or sacrum may cause difficulty in urination, defecation, tail paresis, and progressive sciatic nerve dysfunction that usually is bilateral. Therefore a neurologic examination is essential to identify the neuroanatomic location of the lesion. Peracute spinal cord signs may occur associated with a fracture of the infected vertebral body (see video clip 44). Cauda equina neuritis following tail docking often results in a rapidly progressive ascending disease. Initially tail, anal, and bladder function become hypotonic, but there can be rapid progression to pelvic limb LMN paresis and recumbency in addition to marked swelling of the gluteal area.

Radiography is the most definitive means of confirming a diagnosis of vertebral abscessation (Figure 12-34). Radiographic studies are more easily accomplished in calves than adult cattle because of their size difference. CSF may be normal or have slight elevation in protein values unless the abscess has extended into the subarachnoid space, resulting in both increased numbers of WBCs (neutrophils and macrophages) and protein. A case series of five vertebral body abscesses reported that only one of the five had abnormal CSF values, whereas another recent report found six of six vertebral body or spinal abscess patients had grossly elevated nucleated cell (macrophage and neutrophil) counts and protein values.

Epidural and vertebral body abscesses must be differentiated from congenital vertebral malformations, degenerative spinal conditions, white muscle disease, spinal cord trauma, tumors, and vertebral fractures. Radiographs, CSF analysis, serum biochemistry to assess creatinine kinase and aspartate aminotransferase, and blood selenium values provide ancillary data when necessary. Adult cattle with abscesses frequently have elevated serum globulin levels that support the diagnosis, but calves with this disease may not. Rectal examination rarely identifies the site of the lesion when the abscess has created detectable swelling ventral to an affected vertebral body. This is most likely to be helpful if the neurologic examination suggests a lumbosacral lesion.

Clinical signs coupled with radiographic study and CSF analysis remain the most reliable diagnostic tools.

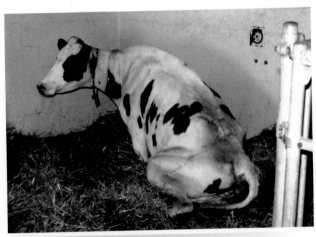

Figure 12-33

Vertebral body abscess of T12 in an adult Holstein causing severe pelvic limb paresis and a dog-sitting position.

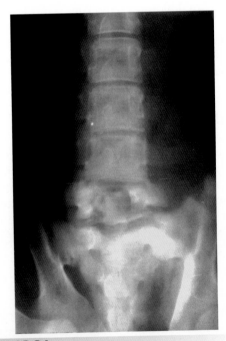

Figure 12-34

Radiograph of a calf with lumbar 6 vertebral body abscess. The calf had no tail tone, dribbled urine, and was paretic in the hind limbs.

Treatment

The causative organism is usually unknown unless a culture from a suspected primary focus of infection, blood culture, or other secondary areas of infection has been obtained. *A. pyogenes* is the most commonly isolated organism. Appropriate antibiotics and analgesics constitute the therapy for vertebral abscesses. Penicillin, tetracycline, and cephalosporins have been used. Tetracycline (11 mg/kg twice daily) is a good choice because this antibiotic maintains good tissue penetration in bony tissues. Treatment needs to be long term (minimum of 2 to 4 weeks) and should be directed by cultures where possible. Analgesics such as flunixin or other nonsteroidal antiinflammatories in standard dosages encourage patient mobility and appetite. Recently, surgical curettage of a cervical abscess was successful. Clinical signs of improvement include resolution of fever, improved appetite, and increased range of mobility (cervical lesions) or lessening of the arched stance (thoracolumbar lesions).

Prognosis is poor, but cattle without detectable septicemia, severe spinal cord signs, or other sites of infection have the best chance for recovery. Acute lesions obviously carry a better prognosis that chronic ones.

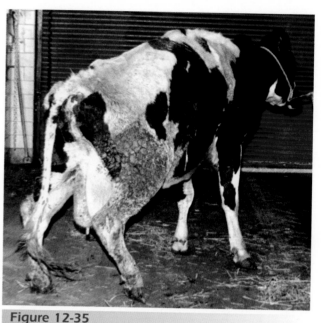

Figure 12-35

Pelvic limb ataxia and weakness in a cow with thoracolumbar spinal cord compression caused by lymphosarcoma.

COMPRESSIVE NEOPLASMS

Etiology

Extradural compression of the spinal cord by neoplasms is one cause of focal or multifocal spinal cord injury that may result in spinal cord signs in the pelvic limbs or all four limbs. Lymphosarcoma is the most common neoplasm identified, but nerve sheath neoplasms occasionally cause similar spinal cord compression. Lymphosarcoma is usually located in the epidural space at any level of the vertebral canal, although involvement of the lumbosacrocaudal spinal cord and spinal nerves seems most common. Lymphosarcoma lesions usually, but not always, can be identified in other target organs in cattle affected with spinal cord compressive lymphosarcoma.

Clinical Signs

Progressive spinal cord signs in a cow that is bright, alert, responsive, and eating are the major clinical signs of extradural tumor compression of the spinal cord. The history may be acute, subacute (5 to 14 days), or chronic (longer than 2 weeks) and indicate progression from mild paresis and ataxia to recumbency. Signs usually are bilaterally symmetric. Neurologic examination frequently allows neuroanatomic location of the mass or masses (see introductory description of spinal cord signs). Lesions from T3 to L3 cause spastic paresis and ataxia in the pelvic limbs because of white matter compression (Figure 12-35). These patients tend not to "dog sit" with the forelimbs bearing weight as observed in distal lumbar and sacral lesions. Pelvic limb reflexes and tone are judged normal or exaggerated.

Lesions from C6 to T2 lead to greater paresis in the forelimbs, and the forelimbs may lose tone and reflexes, whereas the pelvic limbs remain normal or exaggerated as regards reflexes. Recently a Holstein cow with subacute to chronic bloat and bilateral forelimb weakness and muscle atrophy that was progressive was found to have massive neurofibromatosis of the brachial plexuses, heart, and other spinal nerves. A large lesion in the thoracic inlet interfered with effective eructation. Lesions from C1 to C5 cause spastic paresis and ataxia in all four limbs. Rarely lymphosarcoma may occur diffusely in the subarachnoid space.

As mentioned, the history may indicate great variation in the duration of clinical signs. Owners often notice the cow developing progressive weakness or difficulty in rising; she may require manual assistance to rise. Overt ataxia and paresis usually ensue within days or weeks (Figures 12-36 and 12-37). Treatment with corticosteroids by the owner or veterinarian may temporarily alleviate the signs, but the effect is short lived, and obvious paresis returns within days of discontinuing corticosteroids. Cattle with compressive neoplasms affecting the spinal cord that have acute histories must be differentiated from cattle with injuries from bulling or riding activities, metabolic diseases such as hypocalcemia, *Hypoderma* larvae migration, and chute injuries. Those with subacute or chronic histories must be differentiated from patients with vertebral or epidural abscesses, ascending

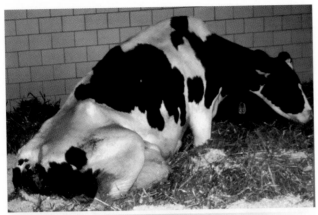

Figure 12-36

Pelvic limb paralysis in a cow still able to rise with the thoracic limbs but affected with compressive lymphosarcoma tumors subsequently identified in the lumbar and sacral epidural region.

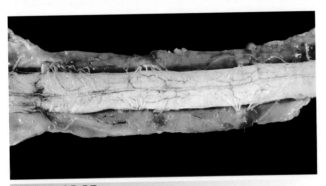

Figure 12-37

Cranial lumbar spinal cord from the cow in Figure 12-36 showing lymphosarcoma infiltrates in the meninges surrounding the cord.

meningitis from tail injuries or epidural injections, rabies, musculoskeletal injuries, and other conditions.

Diagnosis

Physical examination must be thorough both to rule out other causes of paresis and to seek out other evidence of neoplasia in the patient. Limbs and joints must be manipulated to rule out musculoskeletal causes of paresis or recumbency. Peripheral nerve injuries must be ruled out. Peripheral and abdominal lymph nodes palpable per rectum should be assessed for enlargement consistent with lymphosarcoma. Cardiac arrhythmias occasionally are present if the heart is affected with either lymphosarcoma or neurofibromatosis lesions. Muffling of heart sounds caused by myocardial, epicardial, or pericardial lymphosarcoma masses also may occur. Melena may indicate abomasal infiltration with subsequent ulceration. Palpation of the uterus may reveal masses consistent with lymphosarcoma, and unilateral or bilateral exophthalmus may indicate retrobulbar infiltration with this neoplasm.

Because cattle affected with extradural neoplasms usually are bright and appetent, many diseases that include anorexia as a sign can be ruled down. If no other target organ infiltration is identified during the physical examination, ancillary data will be helpful. CSF should be evaluated. In one review of 14 cattle with spinal cord compression caused by neoplasia, 10 cattle had CSF evaluations. Elevated protein levels (>40 mg/dl) were found in 5 of 10, whereas only 1 of 10 had elevated nucleated cells. In another study involving cattle with lymphosarcoma, CSF values were abnormal in three of four patients. Therefore as with epidural abscesses, the CSF may not be specifically diagnostic but tends to rule out some diseases. On several occasions, we have attempted lumbosacral puncture to obtain CSF from recumbent cattle suspected to have extradural lymphosarcoma only to be unable to obtain any fluid after feeling the characteristic "pop" associated with needle entrance into the lumbosacral subarachnoid space. On these occasions, aspiration with a syringe attached to the spinal needle allowed neoplastic cells to be recovered that were made into smears on microscopic slides, stained, and confirmed a diagnosis of lymphosarcoma.

Serum globulin values are usually normal in cattle affected with tumors, as opposed to cattle with epidural or vertebral abscesses in which serum globulin may be elevated. Similarly fever and neutrophilia in the peripheral blood usually are absent in tumor patients. Metabolic diseases may be ruled out by serum evaluation of major organ function, as well as magnesium, calcium, and potassium values.

Rectal examination helps to rule out recent sacral or caudal injury and allows the reproductive tract to be examined to determine whether the cow is in heat or just past heat—this is useful primarily in acute pelvic limb paresis where bulling or injuries from being ridden by other cows must be ruled out. The iliac lymph nodes should be carefully palpated because these are frequently enlarged if the lymphoma involves the caudal spinal cord.

A CBC will not confirm a diagnosis of lymphosarcoma but may raise the index of suspicion if lymphocytosis is present. Similarly assessment of the patient's serum for antibodies against the BLV does not confirm the diagnosis (because many cows are positive but never do develop clinical tumors), but a positive result raises the index of suspicion. Most cows with lymphosarcoma masses causing extradural compression will test positive for BLV unless they have the juvenile form of lymphosarcoma, as did a single 5-month-old calf in the case series. Calves with the juvenile, thymic, or skin form usually test negative for BLV antibodies.

Treatment

No effective treatment exists for these patients, and necropsy frequently reveals multifocal masses in the epidural region of the vertebral canal. Symptomatic improvement that is temporary and short lived has been observed in some cattle treated with dexamethasone, or other corticosteroids. This treatment is usually reserved for nonpregnant cattle, and the owner has a short-term goal such as embryo transfer from an extremely valuable patient. We have used isoflupredone in late pregnant cows to improve the clinical signs long enough to allow delivery of the calf. However, the calf may be infected with BLV. L-asparaginase has also been used successfully as short-term therapy but is expensive.

INJURY

Spinal cord injury can be external in origin from trauma or internal from compressive lesions such as a tumor or abscess causing a compressive myelopathy, as just described.

Traumatic (External) Injury— Vertebral Fractures

Etiology

Trauma is the most common cause of vertebral fractures in adult cattle. Nutritional factors must be considered in calves and growing heifers when vertebral fractures or multiple instances of long-bone and vertebral fractures occur within a group of calves. Riding injuries either caused by great weight discrepancy between mounted and mounting cows or the mounted cow slipping on a slippery surface may predispose to thoracolumbar vertebral fractures. Cattle traumatized by automatic chutes or that fall while caught in chutes or even stanchions may fracture cervical vertebrae. The latter is more likely if the head is restrained in the chute or stanchion when the animal falls. Cattle trapped under divider bars in tie stalls or free stall barns may struggle excessively and fracture thoracolumbar vertebrae. Mature bulls with ankylosing spondylosis eventually may fracture a vertebral body if forced to mount after showing early signs of spondylosis.

Vertebral fractures or displacements of the sacral and caudal vertebrae are usually caused by cows being mounted during estrus activity or because of cystic ovaries. Dystocia also may be a cause of sacral and caudal vertebral injury or fracture. Self-induced trauma from being caught under pipe partitions also may injure the sacral-caudal vertebrae. Malicious or sadistic handlers often fracture caudal vertebrae by excessive force applied to the tail during tail restraint. Excessive traction, especially rotational traction, during dystocias can fracture the thoracolumbar vertebrae of the calf.

Calves or heifers with metabolic bone disease such as vitamin D deficiency or calcium-deficient diets may experience vertebral compression fractures. With nutritional causes, frequently more than one animal in the group will suffer either long bone or vertebral fractures within a

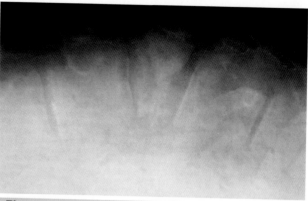

Figure 12-38

Compression fracture of L1 in an 8-month-old Holstein calf that had been fed a calcium-deficient diet. Several other calves in this group suffered long bone or vertebral fractures over a period of 4 weeks.

period of a few weeks or month. A nutritional secondary hyperparathyroidism occurs in calves or heifers fed a diet extremely low in calcium, such as poor quality or aged grass hay, Sudan grass, or high phosphorous/low calcium diets (Figure 12-38). As mentioned above, cattle with a vertebral body abscess may develop acute spinal cord signs if the diseased bone acutely fractures.

Clinical Signs

Clinical signs are sudden in onset and not obviously progressive unless the patient struggles excessively or is handled too vigorously (i.e., a nondisplaced fracture becomes displaced). The clinical signs will reflect the fracture site and the neuroanatomic diagnosis (see introductory section on spinal cord signs) (see video clip 45). Cattle with cervical fractures may lie in lateral recumbency, have an anxious expression, and be unable to right themselves into sternal recumbency. Physical examination may raise suspicion of the fracture location based on observation and palpation of dorsoventral or lateral deviation of the vertebral spines. This is most helpful in calves and heifers but more difficult in heavily muscled or fat adult animals. In severe cases, nociception and the cutaneous trunci reflex may be reduced caudal to the site of the fracture and these are easily performed tests during the neurologic examination. A cow with severe thoracolumbar spinal cord injury seldom demonstrates the Schiff-Sherrington syndrome with thoracic limb extension and hypertonia coupled with paraplegia and hypotonia in the pelvic limbs.

Cattle with sacrocaudal or caudal vertebral fractures usually have obvious swelling at the site, demonstrate extreme pain when the affected area is palpated or the tail moved, and may show a crushed tail head if the injury was caused by being mounted. Affected cattle may have reduced tail mobility and varying degrees of perineal anesthesia. Cattle having sacral fractures may show evidence of sciatic nerve dysfunction, as well as bladder atony; tail paresis; hypalgesia or analgesia of the anus, perineum, or vulva; and an atonic anus allowing pneumorectum (Figures 12-39 and 12-40).

The acute onset and nonprogressive course helps differentiate fractures from vertebral abscesses and neoplasms, both of which tend to have progressive courses that begin as paresis but progress to paralysis.

Pain is a pronounced feature of most vertebral fractures, and cattle with fractures may show anorexia and increased heart and respiratory rates. Certainly vertebral or epidural abscess patients also show pain, but cattle with compressive neoplasms usually do not.

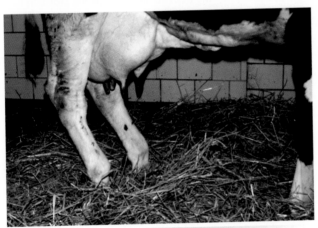

Figure 12-39
Sacrocaudal injury with crushed tail head and associated bilateral overflexed hocks and fetlock dorsal buckling and weakness in the hind limbs caused by injury of the spinal nerve roots that contribute to the tibial nerves. The cow was in heat on the day the injury occurred.

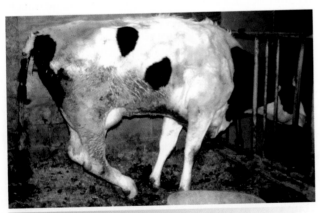

Figure 12-40
Sacrocaudal spinal injury with partial sciatic (tibial) nerve paralysis in a first-calf Holstein heifer that had forced extraction of a large calf 1 month earlier. Initially the heifer could not stand with her pelvic limbs. Now, with assistance, she can support weight. Tail paralysis and bladder paralysis also are present. The sacrocaudal vertebrae are elevated dorsally from the lumbosacral junction caudally.

Diagnosis

The history, neurologic examination, and radiographs are key features for diagnosing vertebral fractures. The CSF usually is normal unless spinal cord injury from a displaced fracture is severe enough to cause bleeding, in which case the CSF may be xanthochromic and have increased numbers of red blood cells and protein. Radiographs, if available, are diagnostic. Special equipment may be necessary to perform diagnostic radiography of adult animals, but calves and younger cattle may be radiographed easily. Particular attention should be directed to bone density if nutritional causes are considered in young cattle.

Treatment

Treatment is symptomatic and may include corticosteroids (0.10 mg/kg body weight) and supportive care. The use of large doses of corticosteroids is no longer considered to be efficacious and should not be used in pregnant cows or cattle thought to be at high risk of infection. Neck braces may be indicated for nondisplaced cervical fractures. Prognosis is guarded-to-poor for all cattle with vertebral fractures, but younger animals with nondisplaced fractures have the best chance of recovery. Extremely valuable calves may be candidates for referral to orthopedic specialists. It may also be possible to surgically repair crushed tail heads having sacral and caudal vertebral injuries or displacements. If orthopedic repair is performed promptly, neurologic deficits may be minimized and cosmetic appearance improved.

Assessment and correction of dietary inadequacies must be performed whenever multiple animals are involved.

Vertebral Malformation

Vertebral malformations without a spinal cord malformation are uncommon. They usually involve thoracic vertebrae and slowly compress the spinal cord secondary to a progressive kyphosis that develops at the site of the malformation as the calf grows. Progressive T3-L3 signs occur at a few months of age. Diagnosis can be made by observation and palpation of the kyphosis and radiographs. Surgical repair has not been attempted (Figure 12-41).

DEGENERATION

Degenerative Myeloencephalopathy of Brown Swiss Cattle (Weaver Syndrome)

Etiology

Degenerative myeloencephalopathy is an inherited disorder in Brown Swiss cattle that causes progressive neurologic signs. It is commonly called Weaver syndrome because of the layperson's impression of a weaving gait that some affected animals show.

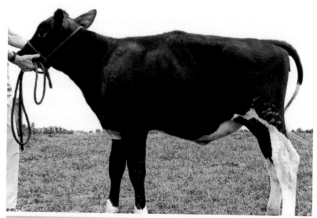

Figure 12-41

Vertebral malformation causing a kyphosis visible as a focal arch in the topline of an 8-month-old Holstein heifer. Although the vertebral malformation was present since birth, overt signs of ataxia and paresis did not become obvious to the owner until the heifer was 6 months old and the kyphosis was observed.

Signs

The disease becomes apparent at 5 to 8 months, and signs continue to worsen until the animals become unable to rise—usually between 18 and 36 months of age. The earliest signs reflect a T3-L3 spinal cord lesion with UMN/GP signs of spastic paraparesis and ataxia. As the degeneration progresses, thoracic limbs will be similarly affected, and these cattle will fall if turned quickly or if they attempt to run. There are no signs of brain involvement.

Diagnosis

The progression of neurologic signs with no evidence of associated discomfort tends to rule out trauma or vertebral fracture. Vertebral or epidural abscesses would likewise cause pain, perhaps fever, and might lead to evidence of chronic inflammation (e.g., neutrophilia, monocytosis) in the hemogram or an elevated globulin. In contrast, animals with Weaver syndrome would not be expected to have abnormal hemogram or globulin values. In addition, the CSF should be normal in those with Weaver syndrome, whereas it may or may not be in cattle with an abscess. Spinal cord compression from neoplasia such as lymphosarcoma also may be a differential for cattle with Weaver syndrome, but generally neoplasms progress quickly to cause recumbency, whereas those with Weaver syndrome are more slowly progressive.

Ruling out other diseases and histopathology are the only means to confirm a diagnosis. Histopathology of the spinal cord from cattle with Weaver syndrome has shown a primary axonal degeneration and secondary demyelination. Lesions appeared more severe in the thoracic region.

Weaver syndrome is thought to be an inherited recessive trait, and bulls that may carry this trait have been identified.

Motor Neuron Disease

A congenital motor neuron disease occurs in Brown Swiss calves that is inherited as an autosomal recessive gene. These calves exhibit a progressive neuromuscular disorder at birth or within the first few weeks of life. When ambulatory, their gait is very short-strided, and they fatigue rapidly and collapse. They progress in a short period to recumbency with loss of tone and reflexes and develop severe muscle atrophy. At necropsy, the spinal cord ventral gray columns contain neuronal cell bodies in various stages of degeneration or glial scars where neurons have been lost. Secondary Wallerian degeneration occurs in their intramedullary axons and throughout their distribution in the peripheral nerves. Both North American and European bulls have been identified as carriers.

Delayed Organophosphate Toxicity

Cattle that have access to some forms of organophosphate may develop a diffuse primary axonopathy of the spinal cord and exhibit a slowly progressive UMN/GP gait abnormality. This will begin with a spastic paresis and ataxia in the pelvic limbs and progress to the thoracic limbs. The form of organophosphate is one of the many triorthocresyl phosphates, which are often a component of machinery lubricants. There is usually a delay of a few weeks between the period of consumption and neurologic signs. The toxicity affects the ability of neurons to maintain their axons, which results in a dying back axonopathy. This pattern is observed in the spinal cord funiculi at necropsy.

Postanesthetic Poliomyelomalacia

A rare spinal cord ischemic disorder has been observed in a calf that was anesthetized for surgery to evacuate the contents of the abomasum. Postsurgically this calf was unable to stand in the pelvic limbs and exhibited a mixture of LMN signs with some loss of nociception along with UMN/GP signs that were asymmetric. After 2 weeks, there was no change in the neurologic signs. At necropsy there was an asymmetric severe ischemic degeneration in the lumbosacral segments centered in the ventral gray column with varying degrees of extension into the adjacent dorsal gray column and white matter. This lesion is similar to what has been described in horses that have been anesthetized for various surgical procedures that require a period of dorsal recumbency. It is hypothesized that during surgery some organ position compresses the blood supply in the lumbar spinal arteries that are distributed to the area of ischemic spinal cord.

FUNCTIONAL DISORDERS

Spastic Paresis

Spastic paresis is a progressive, presumably spinal cord, disorder that causes overextension of the pelvic limbs secondary to severe contraction of the gastrocnemius muscles. One or both pelvic limbs can be involved, and affected cattle have very straight pelvic limbs with overextension of the hock. In Holstein calves, spastic paresis has also been called Elso heel because the condition tends to appear in animals whose genealogy dates back to a bull in Europe called Elso.

Calves usually begin showing signs between 2 and 10 months of age. Affected calves have extremely straight pelvic limbs and a stiff gait. When forced to stand, the affected limb (or limbs) is often held extended caudally with only the tips of the hooves contacting the ground (Figure 12-42). The gait is awkward and stiff because of the difficulty advancing the limb. In the early stages, the limb may relax or intermittently relax following the gastrocnemius contraction that occurs after the calf rises (see video clip 46). The calf may also raise its head and neck dorsally when showing overextension of the limb. Because of the progressive nature of the problem, the calf will be in extreme discomfort if both pelvic limbs are affected because of the excessive prolonged gastrocnemius contraction, "cramping." The calf will prefer lying down to standing and will eventually lose weight. When the calf is lying down, the affected limb can be readily flexed. Palpation of the gastrocnemius muscle in the standing calf confirms a tense contracted muscle in

the affected limb. The condition occurs in many beef and dairy herds, but Holsteins and Guernseys are the most commonly affected of the dairy breeds.

A similar syndrome that occurs in adult cattle, especially confined bulls at sire centers or older cows that are kept in box stalls, has been called spastic syndrome or "crampiness" with the first signs appearing between 2 and 6 years of age. Holsteins and Guernseys are the most frequently affected dairy breeds. Preexisting "post-leggedness" (straight pelvic limbs) may be observed as a conformational defect in most animals before the onset of signs. Signs in adult animals are slowly progressive over a period of years. Initially affected cattle show crampiness as they attempt to rise and subsequently extend the affected pelvic limb caudal to their body. In confined cattle, this results in the animal standing off the curb or placing the hooves in the manure drop. The pelvis is lowered, and the head and neck may be raised. Within minutes, the muscles relax, and the animal may assume a more normal stance except for the conformational straight pelvic limbs. As the condition progresses, the affected cattle become more spastic when they attempt to rise and after rising may extend their pelvic limbs caudally and shake them as if attempting to relieve the gastrocnemius muscle contraction. The same pelvic limb caudal extension and shaking may occur intermittently in the standing animal. If severely affected cattle are confined without exercise for several days, they may experience such severe muscle cramping as to be unable to rise.

No microscopic lesions have been observed in the spinal cord or peripheral nerves that are involved in the innervation of the caudal crural muscles of affected calves or adults with this disorder. In calves, experimental studies have determined that the clinical signs are caused by uninhibited ventral gray column gamma neuron activity. The cause of the hyperactive gamma neurons is unknown and presumed to be at a neurochemical or membrane channel level.

Diagnosis is based on the physical signs and palpation of the affected gastrocnemius muscles. A tibial nerve block may improve hock flexion and the gait.

Treatment of calves with spastic paresis is popular in Europe, where the animals may be raised only for meat production. Treatment using tenotomy of the gastrocnemius tendon or gastrocnemius tendon plus a portion of the superficial digital flexor tendon has yielded improvement in most but not all cases. Neurectomy of branches of the tibial nerve supplying the gastrocnemius muscle has also been successful. In the United States, at least in dairy cattle, the probable inheritability of the condition makes it unwise to treat affected calves, and slaughter should be recommended.

Treatment of adult cows and bulls with spastic syndrome is not practiced except for occasional suggestions for the use of muscle relaxants or analgesics such as

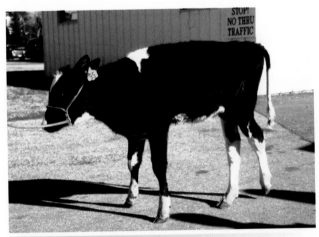

Fig 12-42
A Holstein calf with spastic paresis. Notice that although the calf is standing still she keeps the left pelvic limb extended caudally, only touching the hooves to the ground.

flunixin to help make an individual cow or bull more comfortable. Unfortunately this is a commonly observed condition in bull studs, and affected bulls have been used extensively for artificial insemination, thereby possibly propagating the condition within the affected breeds. See Table 12-2 for uncommon causes of spinal cord disease.

PERIPHERAL NERVES

Injury

Peripheral nerve injuries are very common in dairy cattle. Frequently peripheral nerve injuries accompany myopathy in recumbent cattle and cattle that develop exertional myopathy from metabolic weakness or slippery surfaces. Peripheral nerve injuries may be confused with musculoskeletal lameness in dairy cattle, so it behooves the veterinary practitioner to be well versed in the variable gaits and stances that accompany peripheral nerve injuries.

Spinal cord root and nerve injuries from vertebral injury may create peripheral nerve dysfunction in the limbs—especially the hind limbs in cattle. Therefore it is best to consider the entire course and origin of peripheral nerves when attempting to localize the neuroanatomic site of injury.

THORACIC LIMB

Suprascapular Nerve Injury

Etiology

The suprascapular nerve is a motor nerve to the supraspinatus and infraspinatus muscles. Because of its location and origin (C6-C7), it is subject to occasional injuries caused by chutes or other objects cattle run into forcefully and are abruptly stopped as pressure is placed against the caudal cervical or shoulder area. The suprascapular nerve winds around the neck of the scapula and could be injured at this site. Inadvertent injections of irritating material into the caudal neck or cellulitis secondary to SQ injections may inflame the nerve. Working oxen of dairy breeds occasionally may be at risk, depending on the type of yoke or collar used for pulling.

Signs

Cattle with suprascapular nerve paralysis abduct the shoulder when placing weight on the affected side and may circumduct when advancing the limb. The stride is shortened. The affected limb tends to jut out at the shoulder joint when bearing weight, and this appearance becomes more prominent if permanent nerve injury has occurred because of neurogenic atrophy involving the supraspinatus and infraspinatus. In working draft horses this has been called "Sweeney" when the collar is too tight and compresses the suprascapular nerve at the neck of the scapula. (Sweeney was a brand of horse collar.)

In severe cases, loss of the lateral rotatory function of the infraspinatus muscle at the shoulder may cause the elbow to rotate laterally on weight bearing. In acute cases, a reluctance to bear weight on the affected limb may be apparent and will require differentiation of suprascapular nerve injuries from radial paralysis, scapulohumeral fractures, or bicipital bursitis.

Treatment

Treatment of suprascapular nerve injuries is symptomatic. Acute injuries may be treated with hydrotherapy if possible. Antiinflammatory drugs such as dexamethasone (10 to 40 mg IM) and appropriate dosages of NSAIDs (see the section on the peroneal nerve that follows) are indicated. Best results are found in cases treated immediately following injury such as a suprascapular nerve injury resulting from a cattle chute injury. Chronic or neglected cases have obvious signs of muscle atrophy and excessive shoulder laxity as seen in horses with sweeney.

Radial Nerve Injury

Etiology

Complete or partial injury to the radial nerve may result from direct trauma, humeral fractures, or chute injuries but most commonly occurs secondary to recumbency on tilt tables for surgery or foot trimming. The latter cause may result in direct pressure on the nerve or, more likely, a compartmental syndrome that involves the radial nerve as it courses laterally over the distal humerus proximal to the elbow joint.

Signs

Signs of radial nerve injury proximal to the innervation of the triceps brachii involve loss of extensor muscle function of the entire forelimb. Collapsing on the limb due to the inability to extend the elbow to bear weight is the most obvious sign of paralysis. In addition there is inability to advance the lower forelimb and digit by extending the carpus, fetlock, and digits (Figure 12-43). The hooves may be dragged, thus leading to abrasions on the dorsum of the digit, or the limb may be carried off the ground. The elbow may be "dropped" or carried lower than in the normal opposite limb but does not become as dramatic or severe as when brachial plexus paralysis exists. Analgesia of the dorsum of the digits and metacarpus may be present. With partial lesions proximal to the innervation of the triceps muscle, the patient will walk "lame"—short-strided—because of the partial loss of weight support, and occasionally the hooves will drag from partial inability to extend the fetlocks and

Table 12-2   Uncommon Causes of Spinal Cord Disease

Disease	Clinical Signs	Differential Diagnosis	Diagnosis	Treatment
Hemivertebrae	Spinal cord signs usually pelvic limb paresis and ataxia. May progress or be more obvious after calf is several months of age (see Figure 12-41)	Trauma, abscess, tumor, white muscle disease	Obvious deviation of vertebral column. Radiographs	None—congenital
Myelodysplasia	Spinal cord signs at birth: ataxia, paresis, or paralysis	Trauma, myelitis, white muscle disease	Radiographs	None—congenital
Fibrocartilaginous emboli	Rare in cattle but may cause acute nonprogressive spinal cord dysfunction	Iliac thrombosis, fracture	Histopathology	Might improve with time and supportive care
Protozoan myelitis	Spinal cord signs at birth with paresis or tetraparesis and ataxia. Maybe more than one involved	Trauma, white muscle disease	Histopathology (toxoplasmosis, sarcocystosis, *Neospora caninum*), serology of dam	None
Degenerative myelopathy	Holstein or Holstein X Gir crossbred calves, both sexes with progressive gait disturbances beginning by 3 months of age	Abscess, trauma, rarely copper deficiency, delayed organophosphate toxicity	Histopathology	None
Delayed organophosphate toxicity	Tetraparesis–may be progressive	Abscess, tumor	Histopathology (diffuse axonal degeneration)	None
Hypoderma bovis larvae–induced spinal cord disease	Pelvic limb paresis and ataxia within 2 to 3 days of administration of larvicidal anthelmintics. More than one animal may show signs	Trauma, abscess, tumor	History—usually normal or slightly abnormal cerebrospinal fluid. Eosinophils *not* typical. (Signs may be from toxins. Larvae are extradural and do not usually cause direct spinal cord injury.)	Antiinflammatories such as steroids, nonsteroidals. Do not use grub treatments or other larvicidal anthelmintics after October in Northern climates and August/September in Southern climates.
Motor neuron disease (spinal muscular atrophy)	Holstein calves with progressive paraparesis or tetraparesis within first 1-2 months of life	Trauma, abscess, rarely copper deficiency	Age, breed, genetics and histopathology demonstrating degeneration and loss of motor neurons in the spinal cord. Electromyography will be consistent with denervation atrophy	None

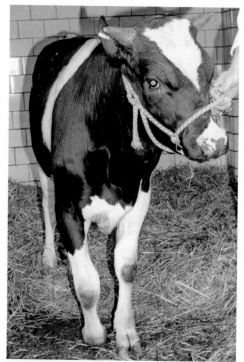

Figure 12-43

Radial nerve paralysis following tabling of yearling Holstein bull.

digits. Partial injuries at the level of the elbow joint may be associated with the ability to support weight and no elbow drop but less ability to readily extend the carpus, fetlock, and digits causing the digits to be dragged. This reflects an injury distal to the nerve supply to the triceps brachii muscle where the radial nerve courses over the lateral surface of the brachialis muscle.

Most radial nerve injuries respond to therapy or improve spontaneously but should be attended promptly for best results.

Treatment

When acute radial paralysis is detected as a cow recovers from surgery or comes off a tilt table, the cow should be encouraged to stand and walk a few steps on good footing. Many mild cases spontaneously recover function within minutes. If the paralysis is still present after 5 minutes, it is better to overtreat than to neglect the injury. If there are no contraindications (e.g., pregnancy) for corticosteroids, dexamethasone (20 to 50 mg IV or IM) and an NSAID (aspirin 240 to 480 grains orally twice daily) or flunixin meglumine (0.5 to 1.1 mg/kg every 24 hours) are given. Hydrotherapy by hosing is especially helpful when a concurrent myopathy or compartmental syndrome exists. If the affected animal has great difficulty standing and/or rising, which may be the case in some adult cows, they can be placed in a float tank for as many days as necessary to give the nerve a

chance to return to better function. The float tanks are generally better for muscle diseases but have saved the life of some cows with nerve paresis that could not stand otherwise. If the cow cannot place the limb in the proper position in the tank, which is sometimes the case with severe radial paralysis, the tank flotation is not very successful. Following these initial treatments, antiinflammatory drugs are continued for 2 to 3 days and then discontinued or tapered. Prognosis is good in most cases when therapy can be instituted quickly following the onset of signs. However, prognosis worsens in direct proportion to the length of time the cow was recumbent or tabled. Humeral fractures causing radial nerve paralysis have a guarded to poor prognosis for return of nerve function.

Neglected or chronic cases have no specific therapy, but hydrotherapy and NSAIDs for analgesia may help slightly. Spontaneous healing may take 3 to 6 months in some severe cases. The prognosis in chronic cases is better for younger or light animals. Multiparous cows or adult bulls do poorly because of the stress placed in the opposite forelimb and secondary injuries.

Prevention

Prevention of radial paralysis requires using adequate padding for the shoulder and elbow region of recumbent cattle. It is best if extra padding is built into or added to existing tilt tables. If tables are not supplied with extra padding, each animal tabled should have a shoulder pad inserted to protect the area from the scapula distal to the carpus on the down side. At least an 8- and 12-in-thick pad should be used for cows and bulls, respectively. Similarly cattle in lateral recumbency for surgery should have the down forelimbs padded heavily. The down forelimb should be pulled forward as well.

Brachial Plexus

Etiology

Injury to the brachial plexus is rare in dairy cattle, but it has been associated with severe lacerations of the axilla, excessive traction on the forelimbs of a calf during dystocia, and severe abduction of a forelimb.

Signs

Signs of brachial plexus injury are profound with complete inability to advance the forelimb or support weight. The limb is dragged on the dorsum of the digit and fetlock and is dramatically limp. The elbow is "dropped" below the level of the sternum, and the affected animal may assume a stance with the hind limbs more cranial than normal and the opposite forelimb extended forward to support weight. Severe lesions will be associated with extensive loss of nociception in the affected limb distal to the elbow.

The prognosis for brachial plexus injury is guarded and depends on the cause and extent of injury as regards permanence of paralysis.

Treatment

Medical treatment for brachial plexus injury is identical to that described for radial nerve injury. Wounds in the axilla, if present, should be treated as indicated. Prognosis is guarded, and the condition must be differentiated from fractures of the olecranon and humerus.

PELVIC LIMB

Femoral Paralysis

Etiology

Unilateral or bilateral femoral nerve paralysis is most commonly observed in calves following dystocia—especially those requiring forced traction—and is thought to occur because of overextension of the hip and tearing of the femoral nerve where it emerges from the iliopsoas muscle and enters the proximal portion of the quadriceps femoris. In a necropsy of a 3-month-old Hereford calf with femoral paralysis since birth, the L4 and L5 spinal nerve roots were torn from the spinal cord. Traction trauma to the quadriceps femoris muscle may contribute to the inability to support weight. Severe lesions will cause analgesia in the autonomous zone of the saphenous nerve when tested on the medial side of the crus. Loss of nociception suggests a poor prognosis for recovery. Femoral nerve injury or paralysis in adult dairy cattle is most common in cattle that struggle to rise when their hind limbs are retracted caudally. Cattle that are positioned on slippery footing and have metabolic diseases such as hypocalcemia or are trapped may struggle excessively and repeatedly until direct femoral nerve injury or quadriceps femoris muscle damage and compartmental damage to the femoral nerve occurs. Frequently the femoral nerve injury is bilateral in adult cattle. In dairy cattle, "creeper" cows that have had hypocalcemia are most at risk for femoral nerve injury. Slippery concrete surfaces in some free stalls also contribute to possible femoral nerve injury because it is not at all rare to see cows fall in free stall alleys with their hind limbs extended caudally. Such cows are lying on the ventral abdomen, udder, and cranial surface of the stifles. Occasionally these animals have difficulty getting their hind limbs back under them and risk femoral nerve injury.

Signs

The femoral nerve supplies motor innervation to the quadriceps femoris to extend the stifle and a portion of the iliopsoas muscle to help flex the hip. The femoral nerve also gives rise to the saphenous nerve, which supplies skin sensation to the medial aspect of the limb from the mid-thigh to the tarsus. The major clinical sign of femoral nerve paralysis is inability to support weight on the affected hind limb. Loss of extensor and reciprocal apparatus function causes the stifle and all joints distal to the stifle to be flexed (Figure 12-44). However, there is no loss of muscle function distal to the stifle. With complete paralysis, attempts to bear weight will lead to collapse. The limb can be advanced by hip flexion with the iliopsoas muscle that is also innervated by the ventral branches of all the lumbar spinal nerves. With partial paralysis, the limb will be flexed, be lowered, and struggle to bear weight. The stride will be shortened, creating a "lame" gait. Trembling is obvious in the quadriceps femoris muscles (see video clips 47 and 48). In bilateral partial paralysis, affected cows struggle to rise with all joints in the hind limbs flexed and bearing weight on the dorsal surface of the digits, and they assume a "squatting" posture. The forelimbs are placed caudal to normal position to assume greater weight bearing.

Calves with femoral nerve paralysis have been studied extensively. Complete bilateral paralysis results in recumbency, and unilateral paralysis still carries a guarded prognosis in calves. Neurogenic muscle atrophy involving the quadriceps femoris appears within 10 days and worsens dramatically over the next several weeks. Associated with this muscle atrophy, the patella becomes freely

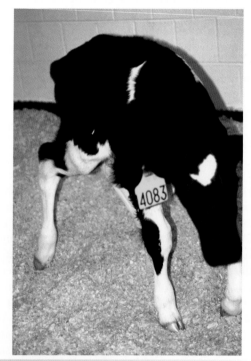

Figure 12-44

A calf with femoral nerve paresis of the right pelvic limb. This was believed to be caused by a difficult delivery and "hip lock" while passing through the maternal pelvis.

moveable, and the cause of limb dysfunction may be misdiagnosed as patellar luxation.

Treatment

Medical therapy of femoral nerve paralysis should be instituted immediately on recognition of the problem. Dexamethasone and NSAIDs (see the earlier section on the radial nerve injury) should be administered. The cow should be moved to a well-bedded box stall or an area where good footing is available. Slippery floors must be avoided, lest the condition be worsened or the cow experience further musculoskeletal injury. Placing the cow's hind limbs in proper position and rolling her onto her opposite side helps. Warm compresses applied to the quadriceps femoris may be helpful, as may massage. Appropriate dosages of vitamin E and selenium are recommended empirically. Assistance in rising should be given. The cow may only need manual assistance by tail lifting or judicious use of mechanical aids, such as well-padded hip slings. When mechanical aids are used, it is important not to further damage the quadriceps femoris muscles. If the cow is affected unilaterally, prognosis is fair. If bilateral femoral nerve paralysis has occurred in a cow, the prognosis is guarded to poor, but some cows so affected can be slowly nursed back over a 2- to 3-week convalescence with assistance in rising. Cattle that are improving gradually return to a full-standing position in the hind limbs rather than a flexed, squatting trembling posture in the affected hind limbs.

Analgesic therapy is continued as long as necessary. Corticosteroids usually are a one-time treatment but may be tapered over 3 to 4 days in severely affected cattle.

Calves with femoral nerve paralysis following forced traction have a poor prognosis. Symptomatic therapy should be intense as outlined for adult cattle, and vitamin E/selenium should be given at recommended dosages. Good bedding and footing are especially important to avoid decubital sores in calves. If muscle atrophy and patellar laxity develop, the prognosis is very poor.

Sciatic Nerve Paralysis

Etiology

Injury to the sciatic nerve and its branches are the most common peripheral nerve injuries affecting limb function in dairy cattle. When the characteristic clinical signs are observed, the neuroanatomic diagnosis includes the origin of the sciatic nerve from spinal cord segments L6, S1, and S2, their nerve roots and spinal nerve ventral branches and their distribution to the caudal thigh, and distal to the stifle through the peroneal (L6, S1) and tibial (S1, S2) nerve branches.

Damage to the sciatic nerve proper most commonly results from iatrogenic injury from injections of irritating

drugs in the gluteal region or too close to the course of the nerve near the hip joint between the greater trochanter and the tuber ischium. These reactions or injuries seldom cause complete or permanent loss of sciatic function in adult cattle but may do so in calves. Calves are particularly at risk for sciatic nerve injury from injections made in the gluteal or caudal thigh regions. Although irritating injectables are most risky, direct injury through needle puncture is possible because of the paucity of gluteal and caudal thigh musculature in dairy calves.

Pelvic fractures involving the ilium or femoral fractures may do severe damage to the sciatic nerve as well. In a prolonged dystocia, compression of the ventral branch of the L6 spinal nerve where it courses caudally over the ventral surface of the sacrum will cause a peroneal nerve dysfunction in the cow.

Signs

Complete sciatic nerve paralysis results in slight lowering or "dropping" of the hip and hock with overflexion of the fetlock (Figure 12-45). The animal can advance the limb by hip flexion and support weight, but the digit may drag as the limb is advanced, and the animal usually stands on the dorsum of the digit and fetlock with the hock overflexed, or "dropped." Analgesia of the limb is present distal to the stifle with the exception of the medial surface. When incomplete or partial sciatic nerve paralysis exists, the cow can support weight but has overflexion (dorsal buckling) of the fetlock and a slightly dropped hock compared with the unaffected hind limb. Tell-tale swelling or "blood tracks" in the gluteal region of the affected limb allow diagnosis of iatrogenic injury from injections and should be looked

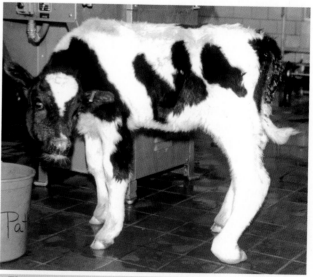

Figure 12-45

Complete sciatic paralysis secondary to IM injection of irritating drug in a calf.

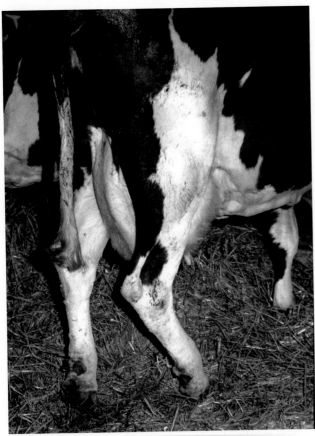

Figure 12-46

Partial sciatic nerve injury in an adult Holstein that received repeated IM injections in the gluteal region. Note the dropped hock and dorsal buckling of the fetlock.

for because laypeople may not always volunteer such information in the history (Figure 12-46). Sciatic nerve injuries must be differentiated from tibial nerve injury, peroneal nerve injury, partial rupture of the gastrocnemius tendon or muscle, and sacral root and sacral nerve injuries associated with vertebral and spinal cord diseases.

Treatment

Treatment for acute sciatic nerve injury is symptomatic. Fortunately most peripheral sciatic nerve injuries are partial rather than complete. Educating clients to avoid giving injections in the gluteal region of adult dairy cattle is imperative. There is a distinct difference between dairy and beef cattle in that beef cattle have more gluteal mass, are moved through chutes where gluteal injection is safer and easier, and injections in the hamstrings of beef cattle are contraindicated, lest meat quality be compromised at slaughter. Dairy cattle, on the other hand, have a "dished out" gluteal area with little muscle protection for sciatic nerve branches. If an abscess has formed at the site of a gluteal injection,

drainage is indicated to relieve pressure on the sciatic branches. Direct injury through needle laceration or indirect injury through an irritating drug placed adjacent to nerve branches is possible.

In dairy calves, the giving of gluteal injections constitutes malpractice. Even well-placed injections into the caudal thigh muscles occasionally cause sciatic or tibial nerve injury in calves.

Acute injuries may be treated symptomatically with antiinflammatory drugs and hydrotherapy. A support wrap or gutter-pipe splint may need to be applied to the lower limb if buckling and walking on the dorsum of the fetlocks occurs. Further injections into the affected limb should be avoided, and the animal should be placed on the best footing available to minimize further complications.

Tibial Nerve Injury

Etiology

Injury to the tibial nerve in dairy cattle and calves may result from injection of an irritant drug or a large volume of drugs distally in the caudal thigh muscles. This is more of a risk in calves than adult cattle. Abscesses, hematomas, and seromas in this region also may compress the nerve. "Downer" cows may develop compartmental syndromes involving this nerve and associated musculature. Be aware of sacral fractures that injure the ventral branches of S1 and S2 that contribute to the tibial nerve and cause a tibial nerve paralysis.

Signs

The tibial nerve supplies motor innervation to the gastrocnemius, popliteus, superficial digital flexor, and deep digital flexor muscles. Therefore tibial nerve paralysis or partial injury will affect function of these muscles, causing a dorsal buckling of the fetlock and reduced extension or increased flexion of the hock (Figure 12-47). The hock does not appear as "dropped" or lowered as with sciatic nerve paralysis, but this is often difficult to assess because of fetlock buckling (see video clips 49 and 50). The cow is not observed to stand on the dorsum of the digit nor does she drag the digit when walking, as in peroneal or complete sciatic paralysis. The limb bears full weight during walking but may be favored slightly at rest.

The skin of the plantar metatarsal area and digits may be analgesic because the tibial nerve supplies sensation to this region.

Tibial nerve injury or paralysis must be differentiated from partial sciatic nerve injury (and doing so may be difficult), partial rupture of the gastrocnemius and/or superficial digital flexor tendon or muscle, and peroneal paralysis.

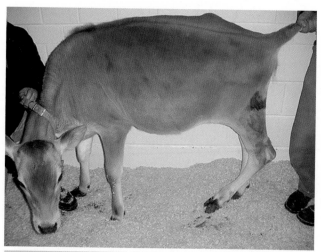

Figure 12-47

Tibial nerve paresis, as part of partial sciatic nerve injury, of a heifer caused by an injection abscess in the hind limb.

Treatment

Treatment of tibial nerve paralysis is symptomatic and similar to sciatic nerve injury. Tibial nerve injury may, in some instances, be a manifestation of a partial sciatic nerve injury. If present, abscesses, hematomas, or seromas in the distal thigh area should be treated accordingly.

Peroneal Nerve Injury

Etiology

Peroneal nerve injury is common in downer cows, including milk fever patients, because of the superficial location of this nerve where it crosses the lateral surface of the lateral head of the gastrocnemius muscle and fibular head to enter the craniolateral crural muscles. Prolonged recumbency with the hind limbs in normal position allows pressure injury to the nerve at this site. The anatomic location of this injury is often highlighted by abrasions or decubital sores just distal to the stifle on the lateral surface of the limb in cows suffering from prolonged recumbency. Even relatively short periods of recumbency on hard surfaces or when the cow is recumbent with the stifle region resting on the edge of a concrete platform may produce peroneal injury.

Signs

The peroneal nerve supplies motor function to flexor muscles of the hock and extensor muscles of the digit. Therefore paralysis of the peroneal nerve results in straightening or overextension of the hock, and the affected limb may bear weight on the dorsum of the

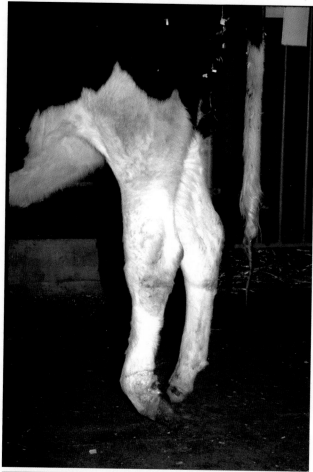

Figure 12-48

Peroneal nerve paralysis caused by trauma in a heifer.

flexed fetlock and digits (Figure 12-48). Because the hock cannot flex normally, the limb is advanced with the hock extended and the limb stiff. The dorsum of the metatarsus fetlock and digits may show analgesia because of loss of sensory function of the peroneal nerve.

Treatment

Recumbent cattle should be bedded heavily and kept on good footing to minimize direct pressure to the peroneal nerve or compartment syndrome affecting this nerve. These nursing recommendations suffice for prevention and treatment. In addition, recumbent cattle should be rolled to the opposite side every hour to minimize pressure damage to muscles and nerves on the down limb. Physical therapy, including warm compresses, massage, and vigorous manipulation of the limb, may be helpful to cattle suffering from peroneal paralysis.

Systemic therapy with corticosteroids (10 to 30 mg of dexamethasone) and NSAIDs (aspirin 240 to 480 grains orally, twice daily) or flunixin meglumine (0.5 to 1.1 mg/kg every 24 hours for lactating dairy cows) may be helpful—especially in acute cases, assuming there are no contraindications for the use of these drugs.

Encouraging the cow to stand and assisting her in rising by manually lifting the tail promotes circulation in the limb if the cow can support weight on the opposite limb and can stand for short periods.

Prognosis is fair to good for acute unilateral cases diagnosed promptly because owner education is very important. Each cow should be managed individually, preferably in a well-bedded box stall or one with a dirt or sand surface and nursed accordingly. Prognosis is guarded when recumbency persists or in bilateral peroneal paralysis because cattle so affected are extremely prone to other musculoskeletal injuries. Hip luxations, fractures of the femoral head or neck, and exertional myopathy are all possible complications if the cow falls or struggles to rise in an awkward fashion.

Obturator Nerve Injury (Calving Paralysis)

Etiology

The classical description of obturator nerve paralysis causing unilateral or bilateral inability to adduct the hind limbs following calving may or may not be explained simply by obturator nerve dysfunction. Experimental studies in calves and cows have shown that both the obturator nerve and the L6 lumbar nerve root of the sciatic nerve are probably involved in the clinical signs previously associated with calving paralysis. These studies showed that bilateral obturator neurectomy did not produce lasting recumbency and total adductor failure but did predispose the animal to slipping and abduction on slippery footing. Dystocia, especially in first-calf heifers or dams with an oversized fetus, may compress the obturator nerve as it courses down the medial shaft of the ilium. In addition, the sixth lumbar spinal nerve passes ventral to the prominent ridge of the sacrum and is vulnerable to compression and injury during dystocia. The obturator nerve supplies motor function to several adductor muscles of the hind limb, whereas the sixth lumbar spinal nerve contributes to the sciatic nerve branches to the semitendinous and semimembranosus muscles, as well as contributing to the peroneal nerve, which innervates the cranial crural muscles.

A syndrome similar to calving paralysis may occur in cattle that "split" on slippery floors or ice and tear adductor musculature in the hind limbs.

Signs

Cattle with unilateral or bilateral damage only to the obturator nerves will be able to rise and support weight, assuming they have good footing. They may show a tendency for abduction when standing, and this tendency is accentuated on slippery surfaces.

Cattle with true calving paralysis caused by simultaneous damage to the sixth lumbar nerve component of the sciatic nerve and the obturator nerve may have unilateral or bilateral signs. Unilateral signs include inability to adduct the affected hind limb and standing on the dorsum of the fetlocks and digits. These latter two signs correlate well with sciatic nerve damage, especially involving fibers supplying the peroneal nerve. Depending on the cow's weight and agility, unilateral cases may be able to rise with assistance and support weight. Cattle with bilateral damage to both the sciatic nerve and obturator nerve are unable to rise, frequently lie in a frog-like position on the ventral abdomen with the hind limbs flexed but abducted, and may, in the worst cases, have the hind limbs split and extended perpendicular to the body's long axis.

Adductor muscle myopathy frequently accompanies calving paralysis in a limb and complicates the condition. Cattle with calving paralysis are also at extremely high risk of developing hip and femoral complications, including hip luxation, femoral head or neck fractures, and femoral shaft fractures.

Cattle recumbent because of calving paralysis must be differentiated from those suffering pure adductor muscle myopathy, pelvic fractures, femoral fractures, hip luxations, metabolic disorders, and severe septicemia/endotoxemia. Prognosis is fair for unilateral cases and poor to guarded for bilateral calving paralysis associated with recumbency. First-calf heifers generally have a better prognosis than multiparous cows because of their size, their smaller abdominal visceral mass, and their overall agility.

Treatment

Therapy is most successful when started immediately on recognition of signs indicating calving paralysis following dystocia. Otherwise, muscular damage is likely to complicate the already serious neuropathy. Initially dexamethasone (20 to 40 mg) parenterally and a NSAID at the discretion of the veterinarian (see the previous discussion in the section on the peroneal nerve) should be administered. The hind limbs should be hobbled together in the metatarsal region with 24 to 30 in (60.96 to 76.20 cm) allowed between the hobbles, depending on the size of the cow. A soft connecting rope can be connected to nylon or rope straps applied to the metatarsal region when formulating the hobbles. The hobbles should be fashioned to minimize trauma and so as not to compromise circulation at their attachments to the metatarsal areas. The cow must be placed on the best footing available, such as a well-bedded, dirt-based, or manure-packed box stall or outside on grass with a quickly constructed fence to prevent excessive room for movement.

It should be determined whether the cow can rise with assistance provided by one or two people lifting the tail as she attempts to rise. If she can stand, albeit briefly, the cow should be milked out; standing also promotes circulation to the hind limbs. A rectal examination should be done to rule out pelvic fractures or separation of the pelvic symphysis.

Any associated metabolic or infectious diseases should be treated, and analgesic therapy with NSAIDs should be continued for at least several days; dexamethasone may be continued for 1 to 2 days.

Cattle unable to rise with manual assistance should be assessed daily as to the benefits of slings, cattle walkers, or hip slings that might be mechanical aids used to assist the animal in standing. Well-padded hip slings can be used judiciously to lift the cow to a standing position to assess her ability to support weight once standing. If the cow can support weight, the slings can be removed quickly with the cow allowed to stand as long as she is comfortable. Because many cows are frightened or "give up" when initially lifted by slings or other mechanical aids, the devices should not be ruled out until at least a second or third attempt is made at 8- to 12-hour intervals.

Recumbent cattle should be rolled to the opposite side as often as practical and kept in well-bedded areas. Other symptomatic therapy may include vitamin E/selenium injections IM according to manufacturer's recommendations. Recumbent cattle require daily reassessment to detect complications that may alter the prognosis. Adductor muscle damage usually appears as obvious muscular swelling between the medial thigh and rear udder attachment (Figure 12-49). Hip and femoral complications are possible, as well as gastrocnemius injuries (Figure 12-50). Neglected cases or cattle with previous severe adductor myopathy have a poor prognosis.

Animals that regain the ability to rise require at least 10 to 14 days or longer before they can be safely moved to milking facilities. Decisions regarding removal time for hobbles and allowable exercise must be made on an individual case basis.

CRANIAL NERVES (NERVES VII AND VIII)

Otitis Media/Interna

Etiology

Middle ear infections are common in dairy calves from 1 to 6 months of age. Although exogenous infections from otitis externa are possible, most cases arise from endogenous ascending infections from the nasopharynx. Exogenous infections from filthy surroundings, manure contamination, and ear sucking by penmates cause malodorous, purulent otitis. Endogenous infections, unless very chronic, seldom show signs of otitis externa. *Mycoplasma* sp. is the cause of most acute

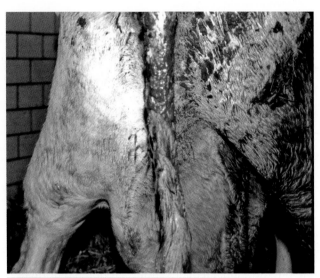

Figure 12-49

Left adductor muscle myopathy causing filling of the normal space between udder and medial thigh in a cow with calving paralysis. The cow cannot stand and is being supported by hip slings.

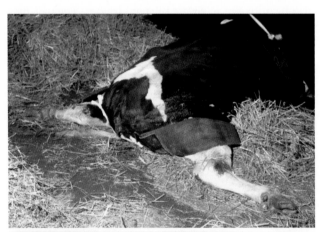

Figure 12-50

Severe complications of calving paralysis. Despite suffering calving paralysis, this cow was allowed on a slippery floor. Bilateral femoral neck fractures and massive adductor myopathy are present.

otitis media/interna of endogenous origin. This organism is a common inhabitant of the upper respiratory tract and therefore is capable of ascending infections. Herds that have *Mycoplasma* mastitis appear to have a high incidence of otitis media/interna. *Pasteurella multocida* and *H. somni* occasionally have been isolated from acute otitis media/interna cases as well. In chronic cases, *Mycoplasma* sp. may be joined by or replaced by *A. pyogenes* or *Corynebacterium pseudotuberculosis*. Exogenous infection generally results in a mixed infection with *A. pyogenes* eventually predominating.

Signs

Acute unilateral or bilateral signs of dysfunction in CN-VII and -VIII occur with acute otitis media-interna. If the clinical signs are unilateral, the syndrome is easily diagnosed because there is often a head tilt toward the affected side with ipsilateral dropped ear, reduced palpebral reflex, and hypotonic lip present (Figure 12-51) (see video clips 51 and 52). Low-grade fever (103.0 to 105.0° F/39.44 to 40.56° C) may occur, but the calf remains fairly bright and does not show signs of brainstem disease. In some cases, dysphagia and depression are present. The dysphagia presumably is associated with inflammation extending beyond the boundaries of the tympanic bulla to involve CN-IX and X as they course near the tympanic bulla (Figure 12-52, *A* and *B*). Mild balance loss with drifting to the affected side and circling may accompany the head tilt, but the animal remains strong. Hopping is normal. If abnormal nystagmus is present, the fast phase is away from the side of the lesion. Acute bilateral otitis media/interna is difficult to diagnose because an observable head tilt is absent. With bilateral vestibular lesions, wide head excursions to both sides may be exhibited, especially when the calf is blindfolded (Figure 12-53). Deafness may also be apparent in severe bilateral lesions. The gait may be awkward, and the head may be carried low. Partial or complete facial nerve paralysis may be present bilaterally in this instance and may only be determined by a careful clinical examination. Pneumonia and chronic cough often accompany otitis interna/media.

Chronic or neglected cases may have pronounced head tilt, other vestibular signs, complete facial paralysis, and exposure keratitis. These same patients may have purulent otitis externa from rupture of the tympanic membrane. Purulent otitis externa may be observed in the affected

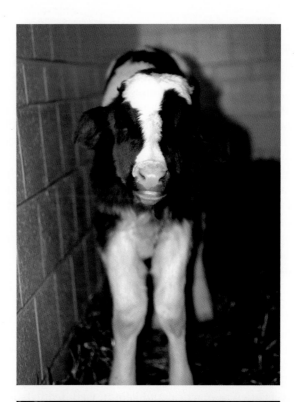

A

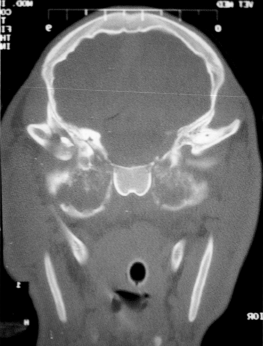

B

Figure 12-52

A, Bilateral purulent otitis interna/media in a red and white Holstein. This calf had dysphagia and was depressed. **B,** CT of the calf showed distention of the bony areas surrounding the bulla and exudates in the bulla. Antibiotics were not effective in this calf, but surgical drainage was.

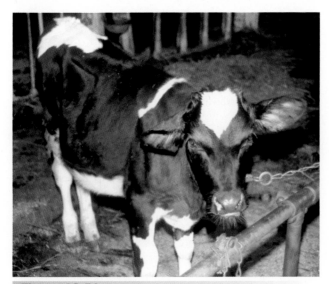

Figure 12-51

Facial paralysis and drooped ear as a result of middle/inner ear infection in a 3-month-old Holstein calf.

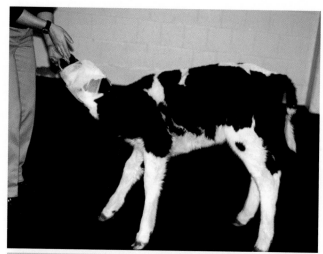

Figure 12-53

Blindfolding a calf with otitis interna/media, which exacerbates the abnormal head carriage of the affected calves.

side when exogenous infection has caused the disease but generally is absent in endogenous infections.

Diagnosis

Clinical signs and farm history suffice for diagnosis in most cases. Oblique or dorsoventral skull radiographs of the tympanic bullae would be helpful but are seldom necessary. Radiographs sometimes and CT will always demonstrate the fluid-filled tympanic bulla and bony destruction, if present (see Figure 12-52, *B*). A CSF analysis will be normal unless, as in many chronic cases, there is intracranial extension of the inflammation.

Treatment

Rigorous therapy is required to prevent this infection from extending into the cranial cavity and causing a meningitis and a brain abscess. Response to appropriate antibiotic therapy is commonly thought to confirm a diagnosis of acute otitis. Because *Mycoplasma* sp. is the usual causative organism for acute endogenous infections, tetracycline (11 to 17.6 mg/kg) IV or IM, once or twice daily, is a good initial therapeutic choice. Unfortunately a significant number of *Mycoplasma* organisms are resistant to tetracycline and most other approved antibiotics for dairy cattle. Almost all strains remain sensitive to enrofloxacin, but this drug is not approved for use in dairy animals in the United States. Most opportunistic *P. multocida* and *A. pyogenes* are sensitive to tetracycline, cephalosporins, and even penicillin (22,000 U/kg twice daily). Acute infections respond within 5 to 7 days. If facial paralysis is obvious, antibiotic or protective ophthalmic ointments should be applied to the ipsilateral cornea to prevent exposure keratitis, although calves seem much more resistant to this than horses.

Chronic or neglected cases require longer-term therapy, and the possibility of *A. pyogenes* infection should

be considered. Therefore long-term penicillin, cephalosporin, or penicillin may be considered. Surgical drainage may be required in cases that are not responsive to antibiotics. The prognosis is good for acute cases and fair to poor in chronic disease.

Facial Nerve Injuries

Etiology

Peripheral injuries to the facial nerve usually are caused by halters or collars that become excessively tight over facial nerve branches. Animals that struggle in lateral recumbency or are tightly held with ringed halters on tilt tables may also develop signs of facial nerve paralysis. Mass lesions such as an abscess, granuloma, or rarely tumors in the area of the stylomastoid foramen may injure the facial nerve.

Frightened or nervous cattle held in stanchions often pull back violently to escape the stanchion if approached from the front. This occasionally results in a cow trapped caudal to the orbital rim along the zygomatic arch. If the cow remains trapped this way in the stanchion for a period of time, bilateral traumatic injury to the auriculopalpebral nerve occurs as the cow tries to move back or forward or tilts her head to escape "stanchion paralysis." The resultant bilateral auriculopalpebral nerve injury causes loss of palpebral response and occasionally is severe enough to also show a bilateral ear droop.

Signs

Signs of ptosis, loss of palpebral response, and flaccid ipsilateral lip are most apparent with traumatic facial nerve injuries. Deeper injuries or massive lesions may injure the nerve where it emerges from the stylomastoid foramen, resulting in a dropped ear as well. Exposure keratitis may be present in chronic cases and should be anticipated in acute cases.

The auriculopalpebral nerve, a branch of the facial nerve, carries motor function to the orbicularis oculi muscle and muscles of the ear. The palpebral branch is more commonly injured by stanchion trauma than the auricular branch, but both may be. The key to diagnosis is observation of bilateral ptosis, tearing, loss of palpebral response (Figure 12-54), and possible bilateral drooped ears. Exposure keratitis evidenced by bilateral central corneal ulcers may be apparent in subacute or chronic cases. Close examination of the head may reveal obvious swelling along the zygomatic arch caudal to the orbits and may aid diagnosis. Cattle may be slightly off feed as a result of pain associated with temporomandibular joint movement; the owner's complaint is that the cow looks "droopy" and may be tearing bilaterally. Stanchion paralysis must be differentiated from bilateral middle ear infections and brainstem disease. Lack of vestibular signs, normal gait and strength, and

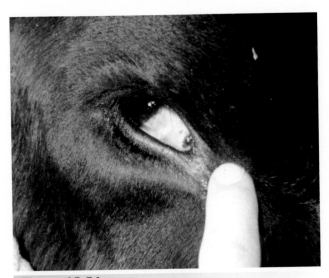

Figure 12-54
Inability to close the eyelids in response to stimulation of the palpebral reflex in a Holstein cow with "stanchion paralysis." The condition was bilateral.

usually the ability to eat help rule out other causes. The same signs could occasionally occur in animals run through a chute, but this is less common because the aberrant catch location is apparent immediately, unlike a stanchion in which a trapped cow may go unobserved for hours.

Treatment

Symptomatic therapy with topical and systemic antiinflammatories is indicated for traumatic lesions. Topical application of warm compresses may help reduce soft tissue edema at the site of injury. The cornea must be treated prophylactically with lubricant or broad-spectrum antibiotic ointments to prevent exposure keratitis until nerve function returns. The prognosis is good for injuries and poor for other causes (i.e., neoplasia).

For auriculopalpebral nerve injury caused by a stanchion, warm compresses and topical antiinflammatory drugs may suffice for therapy. The corneas need to be protected with ophthalmic lubricants or broad-spectrum antibiotic ointments three to four times per day. If there are no contraindications to the use of dexamethasone, one IM injection of 20 to 30 mg in an adult cow may quicken resolution of the problem.

Cranial Nerves IX, X

Retropharyngeal abscesses or cellulitis may involve the pharyngeal branches of CN-IX and CN-X, resulting in varying degrees of dysphagia. One cause of such infection is the trauma secondary to excessively vigorous use of a balling gun pilling device. Treatment of the infection may resolve the dysphagia.

Sympathetic Nerves

Although not a CN, the function of the sympathetic nerves that innervate the head will be examined during the CN examination. The preganglionic sympathetic axons in the cervical portion of the sympathetic trunk are at risk of injury when needles are placed in the external jugular vein for drug injection or for obtaining blood samples. The sympathetic trunk is in the carotid sheath associated with the vagus nerve (vagosympathetic trunk) and the common carotid artery. Although this sheath is deep to the sternomastoideus muscle, which separates it from the external jugular vein, occasionally it is injured during a difficult venipuncture. This results in a unique paralysis referred to as Horner's syndrome. The most obvious clinical signs are the ipsilateral ptosis and the dry muzzle only on the paralyzed side. There will be slight miosis and a very slight elevation of the third eyelid on the paralyzed side (see video clip 53). The skin will be slightly warmer on that side of the face, which is best felt in the ear. This is because of the cutaneous vasodilation that occurs, which also causes a nasal mucosal congestion and a decreased airway through that nasal cavity. On a cold wintry day, the astute observer will see less mist at this nostril during expiration. Usually this sympathetic paralysis will resolve spontaneously over a few days if it is only because of some local hemorrhage at the needle puncture site. Some drugs and calcium solutions that are injected inadvertently into the perivascular connective tissues at this site will result in an inflammation that can involve the components of this carotid sheath and produce a sympathetic paralysis, which may be more difficult to treat and resolve.

NEUROMUSCULAR JUNCTION

Botulism

Etiology

Signs of botulism in cattle usually follow the ingestion of toxin produced by various strains of *Clostridium botulinum*. This organism is a gram-positive spore-forming rod that is an obligate anaerobe and has been subdivided into types based on antigenic variation of the potent exotoxin produced. These neurotoxins that result in the clinical disease of botulism are extremely potent blockers of acetylcholine release at neuromuscular junctions and other cholinergic nerve endings. Currently at least eight toxin types are recognized: A, B, Ca, Cb, D, E, F, and G. *C. botulinum* is ubiquitous in soil and decaying plant and vegetable material. In general, type B is the most common cause of botulism in the eastern United States, whereas type A is much more common west of the Rocky Mountains. Types C and D are found in the intestinal tract of animals and birds. Therefore contamination of feedstuffs or water supplies with carrion or dead animals may increase the risk of botulism in cattle ingesting this feed or water. Similarly phosphorous deficiency may create pica in cattle, so decaying carcasses are attractive food sources for these cattle. This scenario has led to botulism in South African cattle, and the disease has been called "lamziekte." Types other than C and D usually are saprophytes of soil and water that proliferate in stagnant or decaying vegetable matter.

Ingestion of preformed toxin followed by intestinal absorption is the most common route of entry, but occasional cases of toxicoinfectious botulism and wound botulism may be encountered. Toxicoinfectious botulism implies vegetative growth of *C. botulinum* spores in an anaerobic or necrotic region of gastrointestinal tract of the patient with subsequent absorption of the toxin. Wound botulism—similar to tetanus—implies that a necrotic wound that provides an anaerobic environment may allow the vegetative growth of *C. botulinum* spores and subsequent absorption of the toxin into the bloodstream of the patient. However, ingestion of preformed toxin in feedstuffs such as silages and brewer's grains contaminated with *C. botulinum* and, more importantly, its toxin has caused most outbreaks of this disease in cattle. Improperly ensiled forages that never reach a pH less than 4.5 may be of much greater risk of harboring live *C. botulinum* and toxin. Cattle may be slightly less sensitive to botulinum toxin than horses.

Clinical Signs

Clinical signs occur within 1 to 7 days of ingestion of the toxin. Anorexia and weakness predominate as clinical signs of botulism. Affected cattle that can still stand may tremble, stumble, or hang their heads because of weakness in the neck musculature. Salivation, pharyngeal paralysis, and mild tongue weakness are the major signs that indicate inability or reduced ability to prehend and swallow food or water. Affected animals may continually chew the same bite of food without swallowing it. Animals that retain the ability to drink and eat—albeit reduced transiently—may have a better chance for survival. A recumbent cow may lie with the head tucked in the flank and muzzle resting on the ground (Figure 12-55). Although tongue tone seems preserved better in cattle than horses, the tongue may protrude from the mouth in severe cases, and salivation is common.

Ruminal contractions are weak or absent, and feces may vary from excessively dry (lack of water intake, hypocalcemia) to diarrhea (perhaps associated with feed materials that contained toxin). Reported heart rates in affected cattle usually are normal or elevated, although Fox has taught that bradycardia is typical (Fox FH, personal communication, 1985, Ithaca, NY).

Urine dribbling may be observed, resulting from atonic distention of the urinary bladder and loss of tone in the

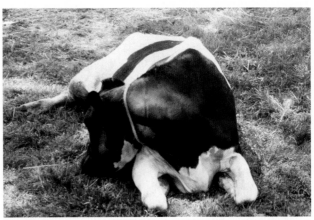

Figure 12-55

An adult cow with generalized weakness from botulism. She was one of several that became affected when a new grass silage that had not been properly fermented was fed. The cow was recumbent for nearly 30 days but recovered with supportive care.

urethralis muscle. Tail tone is also lost. Ptosis and a mild mydriasis with slower than normal pupillary response to direct light have been detected in some patients.

Severity of disease is directly proportional to the amount of toxin ingested. Unfortunately this amount is impossible to assess clinically. In general, recumbency and inability to rise are bad prognostic signs. Severely affected cattle may die within 1 to 3 days. Cattle that show signs of botulism but can still rise from recumbency, eat, and drink have a much better chance of survival.

Diagnosis

Other than clinical signs, identification of toxin in the ruminal contents, feces, or suspected feed or water is the only means possible to diagnose botulism. Unfortunately the amount of toxin necessary to cause toxicosis in animals is often very small and may be difficult to detect. Mouse inoculation with extracts of feed or intestinal contents is the standard laboratory test. Both susceptible mice and mice passively immunized with antitoxin are used in these methods. Few laboratories provide this service, and the attending veterinarian will need to contact diagnostic laboratories if confirmation is essential. Necropsy reveals no diagnostic lesions.

Treatment and Prevention

Treatment is largely supportive because toxin already fixed to neuromuscular receptors is irreversibly bound until natural deterioration occurs. Antitoxin may be indicated, as in tetanus, as an immediate treatment to counteract circulating toxin not yet bound to receptors. Polyvalent antitoxins for *C. botulinum* are available and have been used occasionally in the treatment of botulism patients. Although certainly indicated, polyvalent antitoxins may not be readily available, are expensive, and do not ensure efficacy because the exact type (e.g., B, C, D, and so on) of *C. botulinum* toxin affecting the patient may not be known. If available and indicated based on geographic probability of toxin type (type B in the eastern United States), they may be of use as initial treatment.

If ingestion of feedstuffs containing toxin is the suspected source, cathartics and oral medication to prevent further absorption are indicated. Mineral oil and high volume saline cathartics administered through a stomach tube may be helpful in this regard. Magnesium products should be avoided because they may further neuromuscular weakness. Similarly antibiotics such as procaine penicillin, tetracycline, and aminoglycosides should be avoided. Cholinergic drugs have been used but are of little clinical use, may serve to excite the animal, and subsequently contribute to respiratory failure. Obviously, feeding of forage or water suspected to be the source of toxin should be stopped.

In individuals suspected of having wound origin botulism or toxicoinfectious botulism, crystalline penicillin, drainage and aeration of wounds, and supportive therapy are indicated.

Dehydrated patients or those that cannot eat or drink may be given water, alfalfa pellet gruels, or rumen transfaunates through a stomach tube.

Toxoid may be administered when the type of botulinum toxin is known. This should be repeated two to three times at 2-week intervals. Yearly boosters are then recommended. In one type B outbreak, this allowed the contaminated forage to be fed rather than destroyed after cattle had been fully immunized. These authors also recommended not using the manure from affected or recovering cattle for fertilization of gardens or fields that will contain forage crops for at least 8 weeks.

Vaccination of affected animals with toxoid is indicated, regardless of apparent recovery, because the dose of toxin required to cause disease is so minute that it may not induce lasting humoral antibody production against *C. botulinum*.

Myasthenia Gravis

Myasthenia gravis is rare in cattle. There is no description of the acquired immune-mediated form. A congenital form occurs in Brahman calves, and the gene defect responsible for the inability to form functional acetylcholine receptors on the muscle cell membrane has been determined. This is an autosomal recessive inherited disorder (see video clip 54). Affected calves have difficulty standing, prefer to lie in sternal recumbency, walk with very short strides, and quickly fatigue, tremble, and collapse. They show immediate brief improvement after IV anticholinesterase treatment using Tensilon (edrophonium). The defect is permanent.

MUSCLE DISORDERS

Myotonia

A form of inherited congenital myotonia has been recognized in a breed of buffalo cattle in Brazil that is similar to what has been seen since the late 1800s in goats. This is a disorder of the muscle cell membrane that permits episodes of continuous contraction of muscle cells without relaxation. The limb extensor muscles are primarily affected. The myotonic episodes can be elicited by sudden exciting events. Affected cattle will suddenly develop extensor rigidity of their limbs and often fall onto their sides. If left alone, they will relax in a few minutes, stand and walk with a mild stiffness, and then be normal for a short period in which they are refractory to further episodes. Diagnosis can be supported by electromyographic studies. In goats a chloride channel defect in the muscle cell membrane has been described. This remains to be determined in these cattle.

Metabolic Disorders

Diffuse neuromuscular signs will occur acutely in hypokalemic, hypocalcemic, and/or hypomagnesemic cattle.

Hypokalemia leading to severe paresis and recumbency may occur because of overzealous treatment with mineralocorticoid drugs used for treating ketosis or mastitis. The clinical signs of severe neuromuscular paresis mimic those seen with hypocalcemia. Occasionally cattle are found dead. Affected cattle generally have plasma potassium levels <2.2 mg/dl and are recumbent. Treatment is generally unsuccessful in larger cattle because of secondary muscle damage from being down. Potassium chloride (½ to 1 lb) given via oral-rumen tube is the best treatment. Sporadic cases of hypomagnesemia occur in dairy cattle, and the reason for these is rarely proven. Clinical signs are generally hyperexcitability leading to recumbency and constant flashing of the third eyelid and seizure-like activity. Plasma magnesium is usually <0.4 mg/dl; CSF levels are similarly low; and there is an absence of measurable magnesium in the urine. Plasma calcium is also moderately decreased. Treatment is an IV magnesium/calcium preparation. Postparturient hypocalcemia (milk fever) is discussed in Chapter 15. Myopathy and myositis are described in Chapters 11 and 14.

DIFFUSE CENTRAL NERVOUS SYSTEM DISORDERS

Tetanus

Etiology

Tetanospasmin, a powerful exotoxin of *Clostridium tetani*, is the cause of tetanus in humans and animals. Although not a strict anaerobe, *C. tetani* is a spore-forming gram-positive rod that is commonly found in soil and the intestinal tract of some animals. Both soil contamination and gastrointestinal flora containing *C. tetani* may be more prevalent in some geographic regions than others. Soil containing livestock feces is more likely to harbor *C. tetani*. The vegetative growth of *C. tetani* eventually will result in spore formation. Spores are viable in soil for years and are not easily destroyed. In addition to tetanospasmin, *C. tetani* produces two other exotoxins: tetanolysin and a peripherally active nonspasmogenic toxin. Of these, tetanolysin seems to contribute to pathogenicity of *C. tetani* in vivo by contributing to local tissue necrosis at sites of vegetative growth, thereby lowering oxygen tension in tissue.

Once placed into tissue, *C. tetani* spores convert to vegetative forms when tissue necrosis, relative or absolute anaerobic environments, and other microbial growth requirements contribute to the proper growth factors. Washed spores of *C. tetani* placed in healthy oxygenated tissue may never vegetate. Therefore puncture wounds, deep wounds with much necrotic tissue, heavy purulence in a wound, and mixed infections that produce many exotoxins and endotoxin that damage adjacent tissue are high risks for *C. tetani* growth.

In cattle, the most common infection sites associated with tetanus are umbilical infections in neonatal calves, dehorning wounds, castration wounds, castration by elastrator bands, nose rings, tail docking with elastrator bands, sole abscesses, ear-tag wounds, chronic sinus infections, deep necrotic wounds of any body region, necrotic lesions in the vulva or vagina secondary to dystocia, and severe metritis in recently calved cattle. Other sites of infection certainly have been observed, and in some cases, the location of the infection cannot be found. Fox suggests considering infection at the site of deciduous teeth about to be lost in younger cattle as a possibility in this instance (Fox FH, personal communication, 1970, Cornell University). However, it appears that overgrowth of massive numbers of *C. tetani* in the forestomach may occasionally result in tetanus, thereby explaining sporadic cases without obvious wounds or infection sites. This is an attractive theory, albeit difficult to prove.

Once established at the site of infection, *C. tetani* produces tetanospasmin, which seeks local vasculature and nerve endings. The toxin is thought to bind with the axons of alpha motor neurons at the neuromuscular junction and pass retrograde through the axon until reaching the neuronal cell body in the ventral horn of the spinal cord. Here, the toxin passes into the presynaptic inhibitory neurons (Renshaw cells) within the ventral gray column, and inhibits function of these neurons. The toxin inhibits glycine release from the Renshaw cells, which normally limits the duration and intensity of motor neuron discharge. In the brainstem, the release of gamma-aminobutyric acid from inhibitory interneurons is prevented; therefore tetanospasmin "inhibits the inhibition" of alpha motor

nerves resulting in a continuous contraction producing the rigidity defined as tetanus. By definition, tetanus is the clinical sign of continuous contraction of antigravity-extensor muscles that is not intermittent. Tetany is the continuous contraction of these muscles, which is intermittent. Most clinicians use the term tetanus for the disease caused by the toxin of *C. tetani*.

Signs

Clinical signs may be mild or severe, with rapid progression indicating a guarded prognosis. A stiff gait is classic for tetanus in cattle, but many confined animals are never observed walking. The stiffness may initially appear as lameness in just one limb—especially if that limb contains the source of infection (i.e., sole abscess), but this is rare. A sawhorse stance is typical because of extensor muscle rigidity and tetany in the major limb muscles. Bloat and an anxious expression characterized by ears held back, eyelids held open widely, head extended, and nostrils flared are typical in cattle (Figures 12-56 and 12-57) (see video clip 55). Bloat probably results from failure of eructation because the complex act of eructation requires interaction of striated muscles in the larynx, pharynx, and proximal esophagus—all muscles that could be affected by the toxin. The tail head is raised away from the perineum, and this response is often apparent when the animal's temperature is taken. Rather than having the tail snap back down over the anus, the tail remains elevated and should raise the clinician's index of suspicion for the disease tetanus. The muscles of mastication are involved and give rise to the layperson's term "lockjaw." Attempts to open the mouth are met with extreme rigidity of the jaws and only serve to upset the patient.

Affected cattle usually lose the ability to eat because efforts to chew result in tetany. They frequently, at least transiently, lose the ability to drink and thus may become progressively dehydrated. Prolapse of the nictitans is apparent in most, but not all, cattle. Passive prolapse of the nictitans results from the disinhibited retractor oculi muscles. Prolapse of the nictitans and other clinical signs can be accentuated by provoking muscular activity through visual, auditory, or touch stimuli applied to the patient.

Clinical signs are unmistakable in cattle with advanced tetanus but may be more subtle in milder cases. On many occasions, veterinarians have been embarrassed by misdiagnosing tetanus; the usual mistake is to concentrate on bloat as a sign of gastrointestinal disease with resulting erroneous diagnoses such as traumatic reticuloperitonitis or indigestion. Because not all patients show all of the classical signs described above, there are two physical examination techniques that will help the physician avoid overlooking tetanus in mild cases:

1. If the animal is confined (i.e., stanchion, tie stall), release her and make her move so the gait can be observed

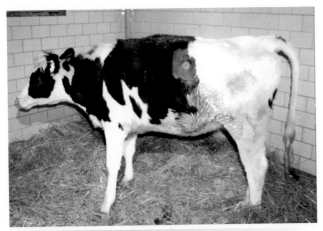

Figure 12-56

Tetanus patient showing anxious expression with ears held caudally, raised tail head, and sawhorse stance. A temporary indwelling ruminal trocar has been placed because of chronic bloat. A rumen fistula is a more useful technique than trocarization for treatment of bovine tetanus.

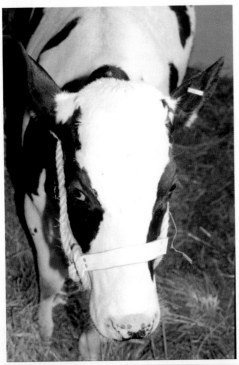

Figure 12-57

Passive protrusion of the nictitans and anxious expression with ears retracted caudally in a tetanus patient.

2. Look at the animal's face, and if necessary attempt to open the mouth

These two procedures may sound simple, but they are frequently not performed, especially on stanchioned cattle.

Depending on the severity of clinical signs and potential treatment for the site of infection, affected cattle

may have a highly variable prognosis. Severely affected animals or cattle with rapidly progressive signs may be unable to rise, continue to struggle to rise, and eventually die from respiratory failure as the muscles of respiration suffer from tetany during exertion. Regarding recumbency in tetanus patients, cattle are more fortunate than horses because they tend to lie in sternal recumbency, whereas horses prefer to lie in lateral recumbency. Once an animal with tetanus lies in lateral recumbency, it may "self-destruct" because the initial attempt to raise the neck and flex the extended limbs provokes tetany, and a vicious cycle of lateral recumbency, extensor rigidity, pain, panic, and exertion ensues.

Most cattle that die from tetanus do so because of exertion and respiratory failure. Bloat also can result in death as can aspiration pneumonia. Musculoskeletal injuries such as fractures of the femur and hip luxations are another common cause of demise of tetanus patients. Affected cattle housed on slippery floors are at much greater risk of musculoskeletal injury or difficulty in rising with resultant respiratory failure.

Diagnosis

Diagnosis is usually based on the clinical signs shown by the patient. These signs disappear after death in tetanus patients, so confirmation of premortem tetanus is based on ruling out other diseases, hoping to find the site of growth of *C. tetani*, and demonstrating the organism through Gram stain or cultures. Similarly if the site of infection is found in a patient showing signs of tetanus, pus or necrotic tissue from the site may be examined microscopically or cultured to confirm *C. tetani*. However, failure to find *C. tetani* organisms should never rule out tetanus in a patient with obvious clinical signs.

Treatment

Tetanus is one of the most frustrating diseases to diagnose in any species because no method exists for the clinician to offer an accurate prognosis for tetanus patients. Myriad complications are possible. Empathy for the patient is essential because the disease causes exquisite pain, and clinical therapeutic exuberance in neophyte clinicians often results in patient suffering rather than cure.

First, the infection that has resulted in tetanus must be addressed. If the wound or site of infection can be identified readily, it should be cleaned, débrided, and drained following sedation and analgesia of the patient. The wound should be aerated as well as possible to minimize further vegetative growth and toxin production in an anaerobic environment. Tetanus antitoxin should be administered at least once and may be repeated at 12-hour intervals for three or four total treatments in cases where the site of infection is not apparent. Tetanus antitoxin obviously cannot counteract toxin already bound to receptors but may bind any circulating toxin or toxin not yet fixed. Treatment with antitoxin is empiric, and dosages suggested vary from 1500 to 300,000 U. We usually administer 15,000 U once or twice as initial therapy.

Penicillin should be used to kill vegetative *C. tetani* at the wound site. Usually procaine penicillin at 22,000 to 33,000 U/kg body weight twice daily is used for this purpose. In calves or extremely valuable cows, crystalline penicillin administered through a jugular catheter at the same dose but four times daily will provide less discomfort for the patient.

Tetanic episodes, excitement, and the pain associated with tetanic episodes should be minimized. Therefore cotton should be packed into the patient's external ear canals to muffle sound stimuli; the animal should be kept by itself in a darkened box stall in as quiet a location as possible. All treatments should be performed by a single concerned caretaker, and footing and bedding in the stall should minimize any slippery floor conditions. Tranquilization is very helpful in most cases. Acepromazine is used for this purpose, and the dosage should be adjusted to the individual patient. Most adult patients receive 20 to 40 mg of acepromazine two to four times daily. This can be given IV through an indwelling catheter or IM. Sedation helps the animal remain calm, and most cows continue to be able to rise from sternal recumbency at this dosage. Milking machines should be brought to the cow, or she should be hand milked. Judicious use of analgesics may be indicated at the veterinarian's discretion.

A ruminal fistula (rumenotomy) should be performed in tetanus patients that have sufficient free-gas bloat to require stomach tubing. Because stomach tubing and other therapeutic measures about the head cause tremendous patient anxiety, it is best to sedate the patient, use analgesics, and following standard surgical preparation of the left paralumbar fossa and with the use of local anesthesia surgically create a ruminal fistula of 2.5 to 5.0 cm in diameter. The fistula allows free gas to escape until the patient regains the ability to eructate and allows a portal for water and alfalfa pellets to be placed in the rumen of patients unable to eat or drink. The fistula thus avoids stressful procedures that otherwise may be required two or more times daily.

Tetanus patients should be considered in critical condition for 14 days following diagnosis in most cases. Mild cases may respond within 1 week, but this is unusual. Patients that continue to deteriorate despite therapy and become recumbent or cannot rise or develop other complications usually die. Patients that stabilize within 24 to 48 hours of the onset of therapy have a chance for recovery. Many patients stabilize only to develop unforeseen complications resulting in death or necessitating euthanasia up to 5 to 10 days following initial diagnosis. Regaining the ability to drink is one of the most encouraging signs of improvement and tends to occur 3 to 5 days following the onset of treatment in cattle that initially could not drink. All possible complications must be anticipated and avoided. Cattle that assume lateral recumbency usually self-destruct. In our experience, mechanical support aids such as slings are worthless in this situation because they tend to further excite cattle that already are in severe tetanus. Patients that survive 14 days generally make full recoveries.

Prevention

Although cattle are thought to be less susceptible to tetanus than horses and other farm animals, there is no reason to tolerate blatant risks such as filthy surgery, neglected wounds, and elastrator bands. Cattle at risk or in certain geographic areas with a high incidence of tetanus can be vaccinated easily and inexpensively with tetanus toxoid twice the first year and once yearly thereafter. As with botulism, the amount of toxin associated with clinical signs of tetanus may or may not be adequate to create humoral antibodies in the patient. Therefore cattle affected with tetanus should be vaccinated twice at 2- to 4-week intervals to ensure future protection against the disease.

Congenital Tetany

An inherited congenital tetany occurs in newborn polled Hereford calves. This has been described as congenital myoclonus and hereditary neuraxial edema. Neither of these terms is correct. The clinical sign exhibited is tetany, a continuous contraction of antigravity muscles that is mildly intermittent. Myoclonus is a sudden contraction of muscles followed by immediate relaxation. When myoclonus is continuous, a tremor results. There are no microscopic lesions in the CNS, and therefore neuraxial edema is not present in this disorder. These calves have an abnormality in the gene responsible for the normal development of the glycine receptors on neuronal cell membranes (see video clip 56). Therefore the glycine released from inhibitory interneurons, the Renshaw cells, cannot bind to alpha motor neurons of extensor muscles, resulting in their lack of inhibition. Cranial motor neurons are not affected. Calves are born recumbent and unable to get up. Tetany is exacerbated by stimulation of the calf, such as just tapping it on the muzzle. The intermittent periods of mild relaxation never are enough to allow the calf to stand. This disorder is similar to an inherited glycine receptor deficiency in humans that causes episodic tetany referred to as startle syndrome or hyperekplexia.

SUGGESTED READINGS

Bratton GR, Zmudzki J, Bell MC, et al: Thiamin (vitamin B₁) effects of lead intoxication and deposition of lead in tissue: therapeutic potential, *Toxicol Appl Pharmacol* 59:164-172, 1981.

Braun U, Feige K, Schweizer G, et al: Clinical findings and treatment of 30 cattle with botulism, *Vet Rec* 156:438-441, 2005.

Cascio KE, Belknap EB, Schultheiss PC, et al: Encephalitis induced by bovine herpesvirus 5 and protection by prior vaccination or infection with bovine herpesvirus 1, *J Vet Diagn Invest* 11:134-139, 1999.

Constable PD: Ruminant neurologic diseases, *Vet Clin N Am Food Anim Pract* 20:185-434, 2004.

Coppock RW, Wagner WC, Reynolds JD, et al: Evaluation of edetate and thiamine treatment of experimentally induced environmental lead poisoning in cattle, *Am J Vet Res* 52:1860-1865, 1991.

Cox VS: Understanding the downer cow syndrome, *Compend Contin Educ Pract Vet* 3:S472-S478, 1981.

Cox VS, Breazile JE: Experimental bovine obdurator paralysis, *Vet Rec* 93:109-110, 1973.

Cox VS, Breazile JE, Hoover TR: Surgical and anatomic study of calving paralysis, *Am J Vet Res* 36:427-430, 1975.

Davis TE, Krook L, Warner RG: Bone resorption in hypovitaminosis A, *Cornell Vet* 60:90-119, 1970.

de Lahunta A: *Veterinary neuroanatomy and clinical neurology*, ed 2, Philadelphia, 1983, WB Saunders.

DeMeerschman F, Focant C, Detry J, et al: Clinical, pathological and diagnostic aspects of congenital neosporosis in a series of naturally infected calves, *Vet Rec* 157:115-118, 2005.

Divers TJ, Bartholomew RC, Messick JB, et al: Clostridium botulinum type B toxicosis in a herd of cattle and a group of mules, *J Am Vet Med Assoc* 188:382-386, 1986.

Divers TJ, Blackmon DM, Martin CL, et al: Blindness and convulsions associated with vitamin A deficiency in feedlot steers, *J Am Vet Med Assoc* 189:1579-1582, 1986.

Divers T, Sweeney R, Rebhun WC, et al: Cerebrospinal fluid evaluation in cattle: a retrospective study. In *Proceedings: Societé Francaise de Buiatrie*, 1992, pp. 207-214.

Figueiredo MD, Perkins GA, Opsina PA: Case report: discospondylitis in two first calf heifers, *Bovine Pract* 38(1):31-35, 2004.

Hemboldt CF, Jungherr EL, Eaton HD: The pathology of experimental hypovitaminosis A in young dairy animals, *Am J Vet Res* 14:343-354, 1953.

Johns JT, LaBore D, Evans JK: Ammoniated forages and bovine hysteria, *J Am Vet Med Assoc* 185:215, 1984.

Kaneps AJ, Blythe LL: Diagnosis and treatment of brachial plexus trauma resulting from dystocia in a calf, *Compend Contin Educ Pract Vet* 8:S4–S6, 1986.

Kelch WJ, Kerr LA, Pringle JK, et al: Fatal Clostridium botulinum toxicosis in eleven Holstein cattle fed round bale barley haylage, *J Vet Diagn Invest* 12:453-455, 2000.

Konold T, Gone B, Ryder S, et al: Clinical findings in 78 suspected cases of bovine spongiform encephalopathy in Great Britain, *Vet Rec* 155:659-666, 2004.

Leipold HW, Blaugh B, Huston K, et al: Weaver syndrome in Brown Swiss cattle: clinical signs and pathology, *Vet Med Small Anim Clin* 68:645-647, 1973.

McDuffee LA, Ducharme NG, Ward JL: Repair of sacral fracture in two dairy cattle, *J Am Vet Med Assoc* 202:1126-1128, 1993.

Morgan JH: Infectious keratoconjunctivitis in cattle associated with Listeria monocytogenes, *Vet Rec* 100:113-114, 1977.

Oyster R, Leipold HW, Troyer D, et al: Clinical studies of bovine progressive degenerative myeloencephalopathy of Brown Swiss cattle, *Prog Vet Neurol* 2:159-164, 1991.

Parish SM, Maag-Miller L, Besser TE, et al: Myelitis associated with protozoal infection in newborn calves, *J Am Vet Med Assoc* 191:1599-1600, 1987.

Paulsen DB, Noordsy JL, Leipold HW: Femoral nerve paralysis in cattle, *Bov Pract* 2:14-26, 1981.

Pearson EG, Kallfelz FA: A case of presumptive salt poisoning (water deprivation) in veal calves, *Cornell Vet* 72:142-149, 1982.

Perdrizet JA, Cummings JF, deLahunta A: Presumptive organophosphate-induced delayed neurotoxicity in a paralyzed bull, *Cornell Vet* 75:401-410, 1985.

Perdrizet JA, Dinsmore P: Pituitary abscess syndrome, *Compend Contin Educ Pract Vet* 8:S311-S318, 1986.

Pringle JK, Berthiaume LMM: Hypernatremia in calves, *J Vet Intern Med* 2:66-70, 1988.

Raisbeck MF: Is polioencephalomalacia associated with high sulfate diets? *J Am Vet Med Assoc* 180:1303-1305, 1982.

Rebhun WC, deLahunta A: Diagnosis and treatment of bovine listeriosis, *J Am Vet Med Assoc* 180:395-398, 1982.

Rebhun WC, et al: Compressive neoplasms affecting the bovine spinal cord, *Compend Contin Educ Pract Vet* 6:S396-S400, 1984.

Reimer JM, Donawick WJ, Reef VB, et al: Diagnosis and surgical correction of patent ductus venosus in a calf, *J Am Vet Med Assoc* 193:1539-1541, 1988.

Saunders LZ, Sweet JD, Martin SM, et al: Hereditary congenital ataxia in Jersey calves, *Cornell Vet* 42:559-611, 1952.

Schuijt G: Iatrogenic fractures of ribs and vertebrae during delivery in perinatally dying calves: 235 cases (1978-1988), *J Am Vet Med Assoc* 197:1196-1202, 1990.

Schweizer G, Ehrensperger F, Torgerson PR, et al: Clinical findings and treatment of 94 cattle presumptively diagnosed with listeriosis, *Vet Rec* 158(17):588-592, 2006.

Sherman DM, Ames TR: Vertebral body abscesses in cattle: a review of five cases, *J Am Vet Med Assoc* 188:608, 1986.

Smith JS, Mayhew IG: Horner's syndrome in large animals, *Cornell Vet* 67:529-542, 1977.

Stuart LD, Leipold HW: Pathologic findings in bovine progressive degenerative myeloencephalopathy ("weaver") of Brown Swiss cattle, *Vet Pathol* 22:13-23, 1985.

Tryphonas L, Hamilton GF, Rhodes CS: Perinatal femoral nerve degeneration and neurogenic atrophy of quadriceps femoris muscle in calves, *J Am Vet Med Assoc* 164:801-807, 1974.

Van Biervliet J, Perkins GA, Woodie B, et al: Clinical signs, computed tomographic imaging, and management of chronic otitis media/interna in dairy calves, *J Vet Intern Med* 18:907-910, 2004.

Vaughan LC: Peripheral nerve injuries: an experimental study in cattle, *Vet Rec* 76:1293-1301, 1964.

Wallis AS: Some observations on the epidemiology of tetanus in cattle, *Vet Rec* 75:188-191, 1963.

White ME, Whitlock RH, deLahunta A: A cerebellar abiotrophy of calves, *Cornell Vet* 65:476-491, 1975.

Wiedmann M, Bruce JL, Knorr R, et al: Ribotype diversity of Listeria monocytogenes strains associated with outbreaks of listeriosis in ruminants, *J Clin Microbiol* 34:1086-1990, 1996.

CHAPTER 13

Ocular Diseases

Ronald Riis

DISEASES OF THE ORBIT

Inflammatory Orbital Diseases

Orbital Cellulitis

Etiology. Puncture wounds and lacerations of the eyelids or conjunctiva that allow opportunistic bacteria to invade orbital soft tissue are the most common cause of orbital cellulitis. Hooking the eyelid on a sharp object or stanchion lock can result in a puncture wound of the palpebral conjunctiva or eyelid. Migration of plant origin fibrous foreign bodies from the oral cavity also may result in orbital cellulitis. Severe ocular infections that progress from endophthalmitis to panophthalmitis may then infect orbital soft tissue. Chronic inflammation in the orbit from cellulitis or foreign bodies may allow orbital or retrobulbar abscess formation.

Signs. Acute orbital cellulitis patients have rapid onset of a warm, painful swelling of the orbital region, lids, and nictitans, chemosis of the conjunctiva, and a degree of exophthalmos. Fever is usually present, and the exophthalmos may allow exposure keratitis to occur as the globe is pushed outward to such an extent that the lids no longer protect the central cornea (Figure 13-1).

Chronic orbital cellulitis or orbital abscess results in a more insidious but painful exophthalmos with soft-tissue swelling that may be more localized. Fever is inconsistent.

Diagnosis. Acute ophthalmic signs coupled with fever suggest acute orbital cellulitis. Definitive diagnosis is aided by the physical finding of an entry wound in the eyelid or conjunctiva. Orbital ultrasound evaluation helps rule out neoplasia or presence of a foreign body, and tissue aspirates may reveal large numbers of neutrophils. A complete blood count (CBC) is worthwhile but may be normal or show a mild neutrophilia.

Chronic orbital cellulitis or abscessation must be differentiated from orbital neoplasia and chronic frontal sinusitis (see following discussion). A complete physical examination, percussion of sinuses, orbital ultrasound, and radiographs may be required in confusing cases. Serum globulin levels may be elevated to greater than 5.7 g/dl in cases that last longer than 2 weeks, suggesting chronic inflammation or abscessation.

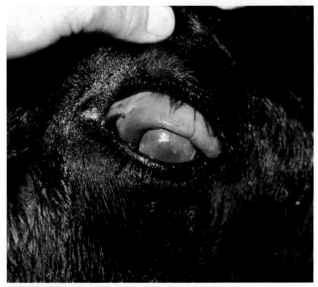

Figure 13-1

Orbital cellulitis secondary to a laceration of the palpebral conjunctiva. Swelling of the orbit and lids, and conjunctival chemosis and exposure keratitis are present.

Treatment. Acute orbital cellulitis is managed with systemic broad-spectrum antibiotics. Although penicillin may be effective because *Arcanobacterium pyogenes* is a likely causative organism, ampicillin may be a better choice. Nonsteroidal antiinflammatory agents (NSAIDs) such as aspirin (240 to 480 grains orally, twice daily) provide analgesia and mild antiinflammatory action. Warm compresses of the orbit are very helpful in reducing orbital and lid swelling, thereby lessening the degree of exophthalmos. Compresses may be applied two or three times daily for 5 minutes if labor is available. Topical antibiotic ointment or lubricant should be applied liberally to the cornea to prevent exposure keratitis. If no ulceration of the cornea has occurred, sterile ocular lubricating ointments or mastitis ointments may be used prophylactically. If exposure ulceration has occurred, the eye should be treated topically several times daily with a broad-spectrum antibiotic ointment to control infection and 1% atropine ointment to provide cycloplegia.

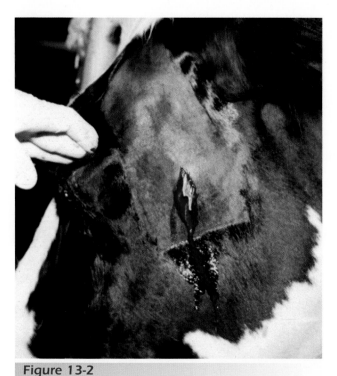

Figure 13-2

Drainage of a chronic orbital abscess in the retrobulbar region.

The prognosis for acute orbital cellulitis is good if medical and nursing care can be provided. Most cases resolve within 5 to 7 days with the aforementioned therapy.

Chronic orbital cellulitis or abscessation requires localization of the lesion to allow surgical drainage. Needle aspirates or ultrasound-guided needle aspirates confirm the location of the infection before drainage. Knowledge of the skull and orbit anatomy is helpful in avoiding injury to important structures when attempting to lance an orbital abscess (Figure 13-2). Most abscesses harbor *A. pyogenes*. Therefore systemic penicillin (22,000 U/kg once daily) should be used for 1 to 2 weeks following surgical drainage of the lesion. Gentle flushing of the abscess cavity should be performed once or twice daily, and warm compresses should be used if exophthalmos is severe enough to raise concern of exposure keratitis. Recurrent orbital abscesses or chronic cellulitis will dictate more intensive diagnostic work, including ultrasonography, radiographs, and culture-sensitivity testing to rule out foreign bodies and resistant organisms.

Inflammation of the Tissues Adjacent to the Orbit

Etiology. Chronic frontal sinusitis in dairy cattle leads to inflammatory bony expansion of the frontal sinus with ipsilateral exophthalmos that may be mild to moderate. Chronic sinusitis most commonly results from previous (months to years) dehorning or ascending respiratory infections of the sinus. *A. pyogenes* or mixed infections usually are found after dehorning, whereas *Pasteurella* spp. are most common in ascending respiratory tract infections.

Sporadic infections of the maxilla and other bones of the skull caused by *Actinomyces bovis* may occasionally cause bony expansion into the orbit, resulting in an exophthalmos.

Maxillary sinusitis also may be so severe as to expand into the ventral orbit, causing apparent ocular disease and exophthalmos. Infected tooth roots are the most common cause of maxillary sinusitis in adult dairy cattle.

Neoplasia of the frontal sinus, maxillary sinuses, or respiratory pharynx may expand the affected structures such that the orbit is compromised and ipsilateral exophthalmos with orbital swelling results. Carcinomas, fibrosarcomas, and adenocarcinomas have been diagnosed.

Signs. Mild to marked unilateral exophthalmos associated with bony expansion of the ipsilateral frontal or maxillary sinus, depression, mild ocular discharge, and fever constitute the major signs in chronic sinusitis (see Chapter 4). Fever may be transient or intermittent, depending on patency of the frontomaxillary-nasal drainage. When purulent material cannot escape, bony expansion of the sinus and fever are more constant. Purulent material can escape through sinus openings into the nasal cavity and cause unilateral purulent nasal discharge. Chronic infection causes extreme softening of the bones surrounding the sinuses and allows for variation in the appearance of the skull. The caretaker may report that the animal's skull appears swollen on some days but normal on others.

When orbital swelling is obvious, exophthalmos, lid swelling, and chemosis usually are present. Serous ocular discharge is present initially but may become mucopurulent with time. Affected cattle show signs of "headache," holding the head extended, with eyelids partially closed. Affected sinuses sound duller than normal on percussion.

A. bovis lesions that impinge or extend into the orbit are obvious bony swellings that eventually ulcerate and form draining tracts.

Sinus or skull tumors that compromise the orbital space lead to exophthalmos, ocular discharge, ipsilateral nasal discharge, and fetid breath. Inspiratory dyspnea is more common with neoplasia than infection, although fever is less common with neoplasia. Postorbital lymphosarcoma is especially common in dairy cattle.

Diagnosis. Diagnosis may be obvious following physical examination or may require radiographs, ultrasonography, aspirates for cytology, cultures, or biopsy to confirm specific diseases.

Radiographs are useful to confirm sinusitis, and aspirates for cytology and culture allow appropriate antibiotic selection. Biopsies are essential when presence of neoplasia is suspected. Radiographs are very useful to detect cheek/tooth root abnormalities in chronic maxillary sinusitis patients.

Treatment

Frontal Sinusitis Trephining of the skull in at least two areas is necessary to provide adequate drainage and lavage of chronic frontal sinusitis in adult cattle. Trephine holes should be 1.75 to 2.5 cm in diameter and drilled at the cornual area (former area of horn) and 3.75 to 4.50 cm off the skull midline along a transverse line drawn through the caudal bony orbit (see Figures 4-10 and 4-11, *A* and *B*). Some references suggest a third opening dorsocaudal to the orbit, but in Dr. Rebhun's experience, this was associated with complications such as entering the orbit. Calves and heifers *do not* have an extensive frontal sinus except at the cornual area, and trephining the sinus of heifers less than 15 to 18 months of age may lead to invasion of the calvarium.

Purulent material in the sinus should be cultured such that an appropriate antibiotic may be selected for systemic use. The most common isolates from adult cattle and bulls are *A. pyogenes* and *Pasteurella* sp. In extremely chronic cases, fluid pus may be replaced by a pyogranulomatous mass of tissue that fills the sinus. When the sinuses cannot be flushed, these patients have an extremely poor prognosis because they often develop fatal meningitis. Lavage of the sinus should be performed daily to flush away discharges and maintain patent trephine holes. Saline, dilute iodine solutions, and other nonirritating lavage solutions may be used. Analgesics such as aspirin (240 to 480 grains orally twice daily for an adult cow) are indicated to alleviate the pain associated with headache.

Successful treatment usually requires 2 weeks of local therapy, systemic antibiotics, and analgesics.

Maxillary Sinusitis Treatment of maxillary sinusitis requires differentiation of primary sinusitis, tooth root infections in the cheek, sinus cysts, and neoplasia. In dairy cattle, bad teeth that result in sinusitis usually are grossly abnormal, fractured, loose, or missing. Diseased teeth should be removed, and a trephine hole should be drilled into the sinus to allow lavage into the nasal or oral cavity (depending on cause). Because the maxillary sinus has less of a labyrinth-like anatomy than does the frontal sinus, one hole may be drilled using a 1.0- to 2.0-cm trephine or with a large Steinmann pin to allow placement of polyethylene or plastic tubing in the sinus to facilitate daily flushing. Culture of the purulent material in the sinus is essential for selection of appropriate systemic antibiotic therapy. Analgesics may relieve some of the pain associated with eating and thus improve appetite.

No treatment is practical or possible for most sinus tumors in cattle.

Actinomycosis (lumpy jaw) is best treated with sodium iodide and very long-term antibiotic therapy with penicillin (20,000 U/kg twice daily). Organic iodides, although commonly used in practice, are of unproven efficacy.

Neoplastic Disease

The most common orbital tumor in dairy cattle is lymphosarcoma. Tumors may be unilateral or bilateral and cause progressive acquired exophthalmos with exposure keratitis or proptosis (Figure 13-3). Because some Jersey, Ayrshire, and Holsteins cows have relative bilateral exophthalmos (i.e., are "bug-eyed" as a normal appearance), early detection of acquired exophthalmos may be difficult for the average caretaker. Therefore severe exophthalmos and exposure damage to the globe secondary to orbital lymphosarcoma may be reported to be acute by the caretaker. This history implies a higher likelihood of orbital cellulitis than neoplasia. However, thorough physical examination to detect other neoplastic target areas and absence of fever usually allows a proper diagnosis. In fact, even though the retrobulbar lymphoid masses obviously have been present and enlarging for some time before pathologic exophthalmos, the pathology may appear very acute once the degree of exophthalmos prevents the eyelids from completely protecting the central cornea. At this point, exposure damage and desiccation of the central cornea coupled with severe blepharospasm, chemosis, and lid swelling dramatically worsen the appearance of the eye (Figure 13-4). A visual eye with moderate exophthalmos but without exposure keratopathy may change to a blind, proptosed eye with complete corneal desiccation in less than 48 hours.

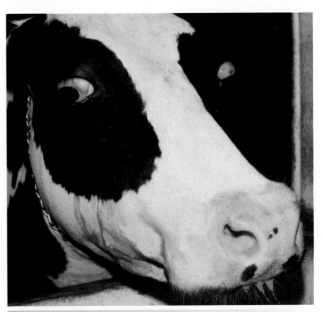

Figure 13-3

Bilateral pathologic exophthalmos and chemosis caused by retrobulbar neoplasia in a cow with widespread lymphosarcoma.

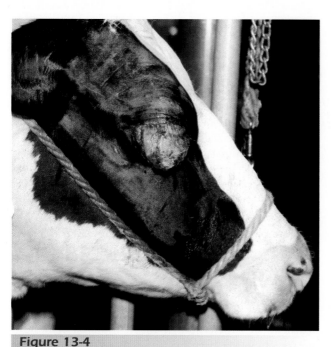

Figure 13-4

Retrobulbar lymphosarcoma causing exophthalmos, chemosis, and severe exposure keratopathy.

Diagnosis depends on finding other evidence of lymphosarcoma in the patient. Enlarged lymph nodes, melena, cardiac abnormalities, uterine masses, or neurologic signs also may be present. In some patients, the retrobulbar masses are the signal lesions, and other lesions may be undetectable. In this instance, blood for a CBC and bovine leukemia virus (BLV) agar gel immunodiffusion or enzyme-linked immunosorbent assay test is indicated to add supportive data. Most cattle with clinical lymphosarcoma test positive for BLV. This test is supportive but not conclusive because most BLV-positive cattle never develop tumors. Unlike cases with an orbital abscess, serum globulins and inflammatory markers are often normal in cattle with lymphosarcoma. Aspirates from the retrobulbar region may be helpful in some affected cattle. In questionable cases, the proptosed globe should be enucleated to alleviate the cow's pain and allow collection of tumor material from the orbit for cytology or histopathology. The lymphoid tumors can be palpated along the periorbita and in the orbital cone in most affected cattle. Although the globe usually is free of tumor, rare cases have had conjunctival, corneal, lid, or scleral involvement.

In confirmed cases, the only indication for treatment would be in extremely valuable cattle that are in the last trimester of pregnancy or candidates for embryo transfer in the near future. Enucleation is palliative to relieve the cow's pain and reduce the possibility of panophthalmitis and orbital cellulitis. Cattle with confirmed orbital lymphosarcoma usually die within 3 to 6 months as a result of diffuse lymphosarcoma. Therefore further treatment is

not warranted. Pregnant cattle with confirmed lymphosarcoma masses seldom live through more than 2 to 3 months of gestation. Those that do live to term tend to deliver small, nonviable calves. Embryo transfer attempts in cows with confirmed lymphosarcoma frequently are unsuccessful because of the cow's catabolic state.

Squamous cell carcinoma may occur in an orbital location but usually is preceded by lid, conjunctival, or corneal squamous cell carcinoma. Orbital squamous cell carcinomas are locally invasive, tend to metastasize, and have a grave prognosis. Carcinomas of respiratory epithelial origin also have been observed in older dairy cattle (more than 8 years of age). These tumors are slow growing over months to years; cause progressive unilateral exophthalmos, inspiratory stridor, and reduced airflow in the ipsilateral nasal airway; and may cause ipsilateral Horner's syndrome (see Figures 4-5 and 4-6). Although prognosis is poor, affected cattle may be productive for 1 to 3 years with these slow-growing tumors.

Cattle sent to slaughter with severe ocular or orbital neoplasia are condemned when the eye is destroyed, has draining pus, is obscured by neoplasia, has bony involvement, or is associated with lymph node enlargement or emaciation.

Neurologic Diseases

Horner's syndrome is the most common neurologic disease of the orbit observed in dairy cattle. The features of ptosis, mild miosis, and ipsilateral facial warmth coupled with dryness of the muzzle and nares are well described. Horner's syndrome in cattle is most commonly caused by injury to the cervical vagosympathetic trunk by carotid artery hematomas, cellulitis of the neck, or direct injury by traumatic venipuncture of the jugular vein (Figure 13-5). Other causes are rare, but the syndrome has been observed with skull tumors (e.g., squamous cell carcinoma, carcinoma, and adenocarcinoma) that invade the orbit causing upper respiratory dyspnea and decreased air flow from one or both nostrils, as well as Horner's syndrome.

Treatment for cervical lesions is symptomatic with topical and systemic antiinflammatory drugs. Prognosis is good for return to function. Tumors have a hopeless prognosis.

DISEASES OF THE GLOBE

Developmental Diseases of the Globe
Etiology and Signs
Developmental malformations of the globe result in megaglobus or microphthalmos (Figure 13-6). Anophthalmos, absence of all ocular tissue, is seldom an appropriate term because histologic section of orbital tissue in suspected anophthalmos cases almost always

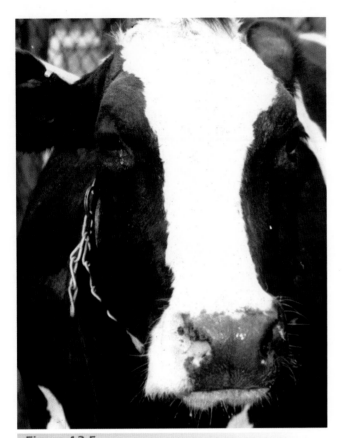

Figure 13-5

Right-sided Horner's syndrome in a cow secondary to a perivascular reaction in the right jugular vein region. Ipsilateral ptosis and dryness of the muzzle are present.

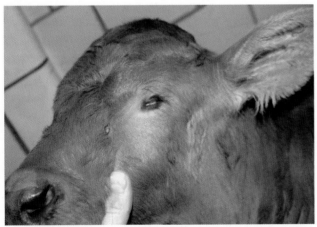

Figure 13-6

Microphthalmia in a Guernsey calf. The calf also had congenital absence of the tail and a ventricular septal defect.

produces some evidence of ocular tissue, thus making microphthalmos the proper term. Congenital microphthalmia may be unilateral or bilateral in calves. Physical, toxic, and infectious causes have been suggested but seldom are confirmed to explain all sporadic microphthalmia. In utero infection with bovine virus diarrhea virus (BVDV) during the middle trimester occasionally has resulted in microphthalmia.

Genetic causes of microphthalmia appear common in dairy cattle. In Guernsey and Holstein calves, the defect has been linked with cardiac and tail anomalies. Most commonly these calves have a ventricular septal defect and wry tail, as well as unilateral or bilateral microphthalmia. Tail defects other than wry tail have been observed in some Guernsey and Holstein calves with microphthalmia and/or ventricular septal defect. These include absence of a tail, short tail, absence of some sacral vertebrae in addition to coccygeal vertebrae, and atresia ani coupled with absence of vertebrae (see Figure 13-6). In Guernseys, these malformations are thought to be caused by a recessive trait, but in Holsteins, the exact mode of inheritance is unknown.

Congenital megaglobus results from anterior cleavage abnormalities or multiple congenital anomalies producing glaucoma in utero. Dr. Rebhun observed several calves with anterior cleavage anomalies. The lens placode had not separated from the surface ectoderm during the development of those eyes. Subsequent influx of mesodermal tissue forming the corneal stroma, endothelium, Descemet's membrane, and iris surrounds the lens. The resulting absence of an anterior chamber causes congenital glaucoma and buphthalmos. All cases to date have been unilateral, and the affected eye is noticeably buphthalmic at birth, with corneal edema, central dense opacity (lens in cornea), and no discernable anterior chamber (Figures 13-7 and 13-8).

Convergent strabismus with or without associated relative exophthalmos has been described as an inherited trait in Jersey and Shorthorn cattle. It also has been observed occasionally in Ayrshires, Holstein, and Brown Swiss cattle (Figure 13-9). Bilateral relative exophthalmos ("bug-eyed cows") is a condition that has been observed in several dairy breeds and probably is a genetic trait. Exophthalmos in these cows does not progress to a pathologic state or exposure keratitis because the eyelids still cover the cornea adequately. However, pigment migration occurs over the bulbar conjunctiva and peripheral cornea as a result of exposure of the globe to dust, air, or debris in some affected cattle.

Congenital nystagmus has been observed in several breeds and is common in Holsteins. The nystagmus is a rapid pendular nystagmus that is horizontal and constant. It persists throughout the animal's life and does not seem to interfere significantly with vision. The heritability or mode of inheritance is unknown. The trait also has been observed commonly in a herd of purebred Guernseys.

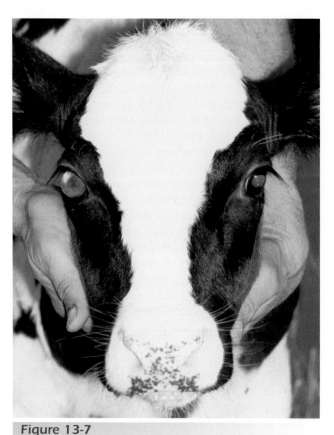

Figure 13-7

Congenital buphthalmos and glaucoma in the right eye of a calf with an anterior cleavage defect.

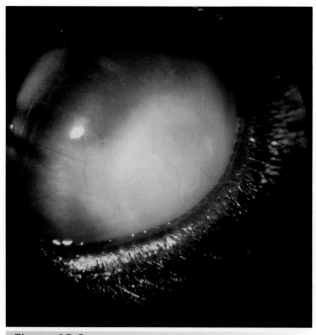

Figure 13-8

The lens can be observed as a dense circular opacity within the cornea of a calf with an anterior cleavage anomaly. Corneal edema radiates from the lens opacity.

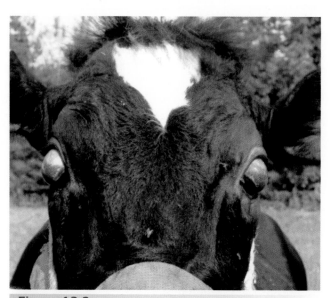

Figure 13-9

Severe convergent strabismus and congenital exophthalmos in a Holstein. The temporal bulbar conjunctiva has become pigmented as a result of chronic exposure. *(Photo courtesy Dr. Kit Blackmore.)*

Treatment

Enucleation is indicated for calves with unilateral congenital megaglobus because the affected eyes become grotesque and soon suffer exposure damage. Enucleation has been successful in these cases, and the relatively rare incidence rules against inheritance. Microphthalmic globes usually are not treated, but if no other anomalies exist, the owner may elect to raise a calf with unilateral microphthalmos. Chronic conjunctivitis occurs in some microphthalmic patients and, if persistent and severe, may dictate enucleation to stop chronic discharge and fly irritation, thereby aiding patient comfort.

Acquired Diseases

Acquired megaglobus may follow severe intraocular inflammation of exogenous or endogenous cause. Infectious bovine keratoconjunctivitis (IBK), trauma, and uveitis are the usual causes of anterior synechiae, lens luxation, and adhesions that disturb aqueous outflow, thereby creating glaucoma. Endophthalmitis and panophthalmitis secondary to septic uveitis or ocular perforation may also cause megaglobus. If megaglobus is severe enough to cause exposure keratitis, the affected globe should be enucleated to prevent eventual perforation or panophthalmitis. Adult dairy cattle with severe megaglobus treated by enucleation become comfortable and return to anticipated production within several days (Figure 13-10). Therefore it is important that acquired megaglobus is not diagnosed erroneously as a retrobulbar neoplasia.

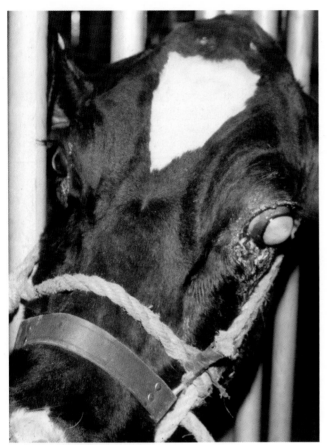

Figure 13-10

Acquired megaglobus following severe pinkeye in a Holstein cow. Enucleation of this eye resulted in rapid improvement in appetite and production as a result of resolution of pain and irritation caused by the enlarged globe.

Less frequently, megaglobus follows intraocular neoplasia or granulomatous infections of the uveal tract. Squamous cell carcinoma is the most frequent tumor to invade the globe, and tuberculosis must be considered when a granulomatous infection of the globe is diagnosed.

Phthisis bulbi (shrinking of the globe) follows ocular perforations, chronic uveal inflammation, and severe pinkeye complications such as corneal perforation and iris prolapse. If a phthisical globe is sterile and nonpainful, it may be ignored. However, if chronic conjunctivitis, facial dermatitis from discharges, and fly irritation affect the cow's production, enucleation should be performed.

DISEASES OF THE EYELIDS

Congenital Diseases

Ancillary or supernumerary nasolacrimal duct openings have been reported in 13 Brown Swiss calves and 1 Holstein calf. These calves had a depigmented, hairless puncta located a few centimeters from the medial canthus in addition to the normal puncta in the upper and lower lid margins. The lesion is likely to be inherited, but this has not been proven.

Neurologic Diseases

Unilateral facial nerve palsy causing ptosis and exposure keratitis is common in calves affected with otitis media/interna and adults affected with listeriosis. Trauma may cause facial nerve injuries resulting in neuroparalytic keratitis in bovine patients of any age. The most common cause of bilateral eyelid paralysis in cattle is "stanchion trauma" wherein a cow pulls back against a stanchion until her head is trapped along the temporal ridge between the ears and orbit. The result is a bilateral traumatic palpebral nerve paralysis.

Signs of neuroparalytic keratitis include lacrimation, ptosis, absence of palpebral response, and progressive corneal exposure damage. Treatment requires therapy for primary diseases and protection of the cornea with frequent application of antibiotic ointments or tarsorrhaphy. Cattle with facial nerve paralysis appear to be much less likely to develop corneal ulcers than in many other species. Treatment of stanchion paralysis requires warm compresses, systemic antiinflammatories, and protection of the cornea with ocular lubricants or broad-spectrum antibiotic ointment if indicated.

Flashing or protrusion of the nictitans in tetanus patients is a passive rather than active movement of the nictitans. Tetany of the retractor oculi muscles pulls the globe caudally in the orbit, allowing passive prolapse of the nictitans.

Inflammatory Diseases

Etiology and Signs

In dairy cattle, trauma to the eyelids occurs from blows to the head by other cattle or handlers, or from the cow crashing into feed troughs, stanchions, and chutes. Infection of the eyelids can result from neglected lacerations or puncture wounds from similar causes. The eyelids can be severely swollen as a result of hemorrhage or inflammation because cattle have abundant eyelid skin with a great amount of tissue elasticity. This elasticity affords the surgeon a great deal of tissue to work with if surgical or plastic repair is necessary.

Signs of trauma or laceration are obvious. Cellulitis of the eyelids and secondary orbital cellulitis are possible in neglected or dirty wounds. Lid swelling and ocular discharge accompany most traumatic injuries.

Less common causes of lid inflammation include actinobacillosis granulomas appearing at the site of previous eyelid injury and demodectic mite infestation.

Allergic reactions commonly result in eyelid swelling and conjunctival edema (chemosis). These signs usually but not always are accompanied by other systemic signs such as urticaria, skin wheals, facial swelling, and other mucocutaneous junctional swellings. Allergic reactions may occur secondary to iatrogenic administration of antibiotics, intravenous (IV) fluid, blood transfusions, and biologics. Similar reactions accompany individual animal sensitivities to various feedstuffs, plants, and milk allergy (see Chapter 7).

Treatment

Conservative measures such as cold or hot compresses, cleaning and débridement of damaged tissue, local and systemic antibiotic therapy, drainage of abscesses, and protection of the cornea with topical antibiotic ointments suffice in most cases. NSAIDs and corticosteroids are avoided unless soft tissue swelling is severe; corticosteroids are contraindicated in pregnant cattle. Lacerations of the eyelid may be closed using a two-layer technique with absorbable sutures (2-0) in the lid stroma and nonabsorbable sutures (2-0 or 3-0) in the skin. It is not necessary to suture the conjunctiva. Topical and systemic antibiotics for 5 to 7 days are indicated postoperatively to help prevent infection and subsequent wound dehiscence.

Actinobacillosis granulomas should be debulked, and the cow should be treated with 20% sodium iodide (30 g/1000 lb body weight IV) followed by 30 g of oral organic iodide powder once daily for 14 days.

Allergic reactions require treatment with avoidance or correction of the primary cause, antihistamines, antiinflammatories, or epinephrine (see Chapter 7).

Neoplastic Diseases

Etiology and Signs

Fibropapillomas or "warts" are the most common tumor to involve the eyelid of calves and young cattle. In most instances, the tumors are raised, firm masses with a gray crusty covering (see Figure 7-1).

Lymphosarcoma rarely infiltrates the eyelids as a diffuse lid swelling with conjunctival chemosis.

Squamous cell carcinomas are the most common tumor to affect the eyelids and nictitans (or third eyelid) of adult cattle. White-faced beef cattle and Holsteins that are mostly white or have nonpigmented lid margins or nictitans are at risk. In predominantly dairy practice, most bovine patients with squamous cell carcinoma ("cancer eye") are Holsteins. The tumors are pink, raised or ulcerated, cobblestone in appearance, and most commonly appear in middle-aged (5 to 10 years) cows. True squamous cell carcinoma of the eyelid usually is preceded by precursor lesions that are epitheliomas or a wartlike growth on the eyelid or eyelid margin.

Treatment

Fibropapillomas normally are self-limiting within 4 to 6 months and do not require treatment. Persistent or large fibropapillomas (Figure 13-11) may interfere with

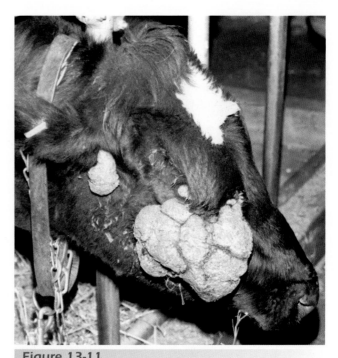

Figure 13-11

Atypical large fibropapilloma growing from the upper eyelid of a Holstein heifer.

eyelid function or cause corneal injury and require surgical treatment via cryosurgery or sharp dissection.

Squamous cell carcinomas tend to be locally invasive and may metastasize in some neglected cases. This tumor requires aggressive early therapy to prevent progression, or the cow will be lost. Many therapeutic options exist for early, small squamous cell carcinoma of the eyelids, whereas enucleation, radical exenteration, or culling may be required for large lid lesions. Recognition of early tumor formation when the mass is less than 2.0 cm in diameter allows consideration of cryosurgery, radiofrequency hyperthermia, radiation (if available), sharp surgery, and immunotherapy. Large lid masses (greater than 5.0 cm in diameter) are less likely to be treated successfully because destruction or removal of this much lid tissue may lead to ocular exposure damage (Figure 13-12). These large tumors also are more likely to invade adjacent adnexal tissue, orbital ligaments, periorbita, and bone of the skull. Tumors at the medial canthus are extremely dangerous because they need to advance only 2.0 cm along the medial orbital ligament before entering the bony orbit.

Treatment options include:
1. *Sharp surgery*: This is best performed on lesions smaller than 1.0 to 2.0 cm in diameter for which en bloc removal or wedge removal of the tumor allows complete repair of the lid margin, and it is easy to distinguish tumor margins from normal tissue. This method also is indicated for squamous cell carcinomas of the third eyelid or nictitans for which the best treatment is surgical removal of the entire

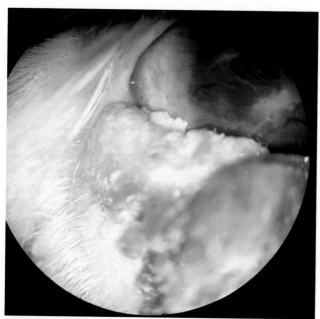

Figure 13-12

Squamous cell carcinoma of the lower eyelid. The tumor is pink, raised, ulcerative, and has a white necrotic surface discharge. Chronic superficial keratitis is present as a result of tumor irritation of the cornea.

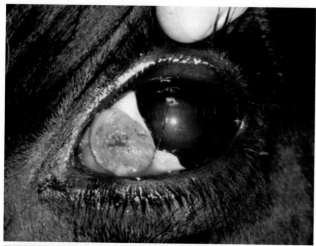

Figure 13-13

Squamous cell carcinoma of the nictitans in a Holstein cow.

third eyelid (Figure 13-13). Following sedation of the patient with xylazine, the auriculopalpebral nerve is blocked; liberal topical anesthesia (0.5% proparacaine) is applied to the eye and conjunctiva; and the nictitans then is grasped with forceps. Between 10 and 15 ml of 2% lidocaine is injected into the base of the nictitans, and the entire nictitans is removed with heavy serrated scissors. It is important to remove all of the cartilage with the nictitans, lest a sharp cartilaginous stump remains in the medial canthal region to incite further squamous

cell carcinoma through chronic irritation and tissue metaplasia. Topical antibiotics are applied to the eye for 7 days, and systemic penicillin 22,000 U/kg body weight is given intramuscularly (IM), once daily for 3 days postoperatively.

2. *Cryosurgery:* This is perhaps the best therapy for small to moderate lesions because the "freeze" can be adjusted to the size of the tumor and cosmetic results at the lid margin tend to be good, thereby preventing subsequent exposure keratitis from loss of lid margin. The cow is sedated, restrained, and the tumor site blocked by regional anesthesia. Tissue peripheral to the lesion is shielded with petroleum jelly, and a Styrofoam wedge can be applied to the cornea to act as a protective "contact lens" if the lid margin area must be frozen. The tumor is frozen by free spray or by use of any of a number of probes or cups until the periphery of the tumor adjacent to normal skin reaches −40.0° C. The tissue is allowed to thaw and then is refrozen. Cryodestruction is maximum with a quick freeze, slow thaw, and quick freeze routine. Frozen tissue sloughs over the next 7 to 14 days and gradually is replaced by granulation tissue followed by epithelialization of the wound. Frozen tissue often may remain depigmented, and returning hair will be white in most instances. Topical protective ointments should be applied to the eye. The only complication Dr. Rebhun observed with this technique was corneal ulceration caused by a large scab that was not cleared away from the lid margin in one cow.

3. *Radiofrequency hyperthermia:* This is another excellent treatment for small tumors or tumors with a small base that can be debulked before application of the device. Hyperthermia only penetrates 0.5 to 1.0 cm of tissue, so large lesions are not the best candidates for this technique. Multiple applications are possible for moderate size lesions, and an impressive cure rate for beef cattle has been quoted. Instructions are available with the kit (ThermoProbe, Hach Co., Loveland, CO, or MegaTherm, Western Instrument Co., Denver, CO).

4. *Radiation:* Squamous cell carcinoma is a radiosensitive tumor. Very small lesions less than 2 mm in depth could be treated with 7500 to 10,000 rad (1 rad = 1 centigy) of beta-radiation using a strontium[90] applicator, but the device does not penetrate deep lesions (Amersham Health, General Electric Health Care, Buckinghamshire, England NP7 9N UK). More radical radiation (e.g., radon seeds) has been used successfully on squamous cell carcinoma, but radiation safety laws limit the practicality of these options.

5. *Immunotherapy:* Many attempts at immunotherapy, including autogenous vaccines made from tumor tissue and infections of Bacillus Calmette Guérin (BCG) have been used to treat ocular squamous cell

carcinoma. Although fair results have been reported, many questions remain regarding these techniques. The major disadvantage for dairy cattle is that injections of BCG (a mycobacterium cell wall product) may render the cow positive to tuberculin testing in the future. Recently, peritumoral injections of interleukin-2 (1 million units) for 10 days resulted in tumor regression in 69% of the cases. Tumors of the third eyelid and limbus were most responsive.

6. *Enucleation*: Enucleation in the calf or cow uses the transpalpebral approach. The cow is restrained in a chute or stanchion and sedated with xylazine (20 to 40 mg IV) before routine preparation of the orbit. The face is clipped and prepared for surgery. A circumferential infiltration of 2% lidocaine is performed approximately 3.75 to 5.00 cm from the eyelid margins, and 35 ml of 2% lidocaine is deposited in the retrobulbar cone via a 8.75-cm (3.5 in), 18-gauge needle. The orbital area is surgically prepped again and draped with a fenestrated drape that can be clamped to the halter with sharp towel clamps. (It is helpful to tape the ipsilateral ear back before draping.) A circumferential incision 1.5 cm from the eyelid margins is made through the skin but not through the palpebral conjunctiva. The incision is completed to the level of the conjunctiva with scissors, and the lid margins are clamped or sewn together. The lateral ligament of the orbit is severed, and dissection continues around the globe superficial to the conjunctiva. All muscles, the optic nerve, and retrobulbar fat are cut as traction is exerted on the globe nasally. The entire nictitans and lacrimal gland are removed. Meticulous attempts at hemostasis only serve to prolong the procedure. A subcutaneous continuous suture of 2-0 catgut closes the orbit, and nonabsorbable interrupted sutures close the skin. Preoperative and postoperative systemic antibiotics are administered for 5 days in routine cases but may be necessary for a longer period in infected globes. Drains are not used unless the orbital tissues appear infected or contaminated.

7. *Exenteration*: Surgical removal of all orbital tissue is recommended if any abnormal tissue is found retrobulbarly. Closure is similar to enucleation.

DISEASES OF THE CONJUNCTIVA

Developmental Diseases

Dermoids of the conjunctiva cause irritation to the cornea because of hair growth on the dermoid and require surgical removal. A full-thickness wedge resection of the involved conjunctiva and lid followed by a two-layer repair has given excellent results.

Inflammatory Diseases

Etiology and Signs

Moraxella bovis, the cause of IBK (i.e., pinkeye), is the most important bacterial disease of the conjunctiva and cornea in cattle. The organisms and IBK will be discussed in the section on the cornea.

Pasteurella and other bacteria may also cause mucopurulent conjunctivitis in cattle occasionally. *Pasteurella* conjunctivitis occurs in conjunction with severe *Pasteurella* pneumonia or septicemia in calves. The organisms are normal inhabitants of the upper respiratory tract in cattle and therefore accessible to the conjunctiva. *Neisseria* spp. have been isolated from cattle with conjunctivitis and infectious keratitis. Atypical (winter) outbreaks of IBK-like endemics have been blamed on these other bacteria, but overwhelming evidence supports *M. bovis* as the most likely causative organism. Calves with respiratory infections caused by *Histophilus somni* may have conjunctivitis, rhinitis, laryngitis, and pneumonia. Cattle affected with bacterial conjunctivitis have a serous or mucopurulent ocular discharge, conjunctival injection, and do not appear to have ocular pain.

Mycoplasma and ureaplasma have been isolated from the eyes of cattle during herd epidemics of conjunctivitis. Affected cattle do not appear ill, but 10% to 50% of the animals have a unilateral or bilateral ocular discharge and conjunctival hyperemia. The ocular discharge is serous initially but becomes mucopurulent after 1 to 4 days. No keratitis is associated with this problem.

Infectious bovine rhinotracheitis (IBR) virus, the herpes virus 1 of cattle, may cause a severe endemic conjunctivitis in nonvaccinated cattle. The conjunctivitis may be the only lesion observed in sick cattle or may occur in conjunction with the typical respiratory form of IBR. The disease has been observed in heifers and adult cattle. Typical lesions include severe conjunctival hyperemia, heavy ocular discharge that converts from serous to mucopurulent over 48 to 72 hours, and the presence of multifocal white plaques in the palpebral conjunctiva (Figure 13-14). The lesions may be unilateral or bilateral and affect 10% to 70% of the herd. The plaque lesions are pathognomonic for IBR. Affected adult cattle have high fever (105.0 to 108.0° F/40.56 to 42.22° C), depression, and decreased milk production. Milking cattle with the conjunctival form of IBR appear ill regardless of whether the respiratory form coexists. Heifers with the conjunctival form of IBR may have fever and mild systemic illness but seldom appear as sick as adult milking cattle. The reason for this difference is not known but may be related to the stress of lactation.

Five to 9 days after the onset of disease, the white conjunctival plaques begin to coalesce and slough, and the conjunctiva becomes very chemotic. During this same time, peripheral corneal edema develops

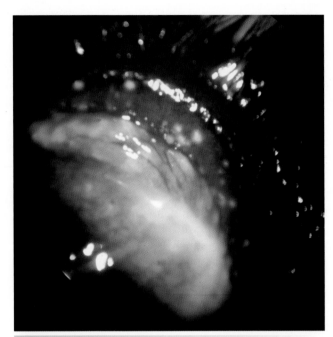

Figure 13-14

Multifocal white plaques on the palpebral conjunctiva as a result of acute infectious bovine rhinotracheitis virus conjunctivitis.

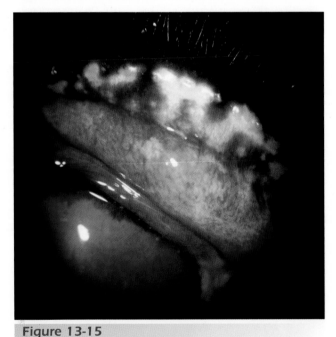

Figure 13-15

Infectious bovine rhinotracheitis conjunctivitis in a cow that has been affected 7 to 10 days. The white plaques have coalesced into nonpigmented areas of necrosis; chemosis is severe; and corneal edema is present.

in some of the more severely affected cattle (Figure 13-15). The corneal edema is circumferential edema that leaves the central cornea clear. Occasionally extremely severe cases develop complete corneal opacity with severe edema and peripheral vascularization.

These corneal opacities cause confusion with pinkeye (IBK), but no corneal ulceration occurs in IBR conjunctivitis. The early pathognomonic lesions persist for only a few days, and the virus usually cannot be recovered from the eyes for longer than 7 to 9 days following onset of disease. Cytology of the plaques yields mononuclear cells (see Table 13-2).

Although other viral diseases of cattle may cause conjunctivitis experimentally, none are important clinically.

Foreign bodies may result in persistent conjunctivitis in one or both eyes. Animals that are shipped in open trailers, kept in areas where wind is likely to raise foreign bodies, or those in lateral recumbency are at risk for foreign body conjunctivitis. Generally causative material is of plant origin. Signs include persistent epiphora, blepharospasm, conjunctival hyperemia, and chemosis. Corneal ulceration may occur in neglected cases. Conjunctival foreign bodies may be trapped in edematous folds of palpebral conjunctiva, fornix, or be positioned behind the nictitans. Parasitic conjunctivitis caused by the eye worms *Thelazia skrjabini* and *Thelazia gulosa* has been found to be prevalent in some regions of the United States.

Diagnosis

With the exception of IBR conjunctivitis, the clinical appearance seldom identifies the cause of conjunctivitis in cattle. Culture of the conjunctival discharge and cytologic examination of conjunctival scraping are the most useful diagnostic procedures when faced with a herd epidemic of conjunctivitis in calves or adult cattle. These samples should be submitted to established diagnostic laboratories familiar with bovine infectious diseases. Cytology and culture will identify bacterial causes, as well as mycoplasma and ureaplasma.

IBR can be diagnosed by fluorescent antibody tests applied to heavy conjunctival smears in acute cases, isolation of the virus in acute cases, or serology utilizing acute and convalescent (14 days) sera.

Treatment

Viral conjunctivitis, including IBR conjunctivitis, resolves without therapy. Nursing procedures such as cleansing the discharge from the patient's eyes and face certainly would aid healing but seldom is practical because of the labor involved in handling large numbers of cattle. The conjunctival form of IBR resolves after a clinical course of 14 to 20 days. Severe cases benefit from nursing care and topical treatment with broad-spectrum antibiotics to deter secondary bacterial infection. Corticosteroids of any type are contraindicated.

Bacterial conjunctivitis should be treated with appropriate broad-spectrum ophthalmic ointments approved for use in cattle. Mastitis ointments containing cephalosporin, erythromycin, or ampicillin are excellent choices and do not irritate the eye. Although dairy farmers tend to have difficulty using ⅛-oz ophthalmic ointment tubes without wasting a great deal of the ointment, it sometimes is necessary when a specific ophthalmic antibiotic is indicated. Partially used tubes should not be left uncapped in the barn because fungal agents may contaminate the ointment. The presence of foreign bodies should be ruled out by a thorough ophthalmic examination when an individual cow has persistent bacterial conjunctivitis unresponsive to antibiotic therapy.

Mycoplasma or ureaplasma may cause an insidious herd epidemic of conjunctivitis with an initial few cows having mucopurulent ocular discharge followed by several new cases during the ensuing 7 to 10 days. Caretakers report a slow spread of conjunctivitis through 10% to 50% of the cows in a typical outbreak. Most cases resolve without therapy, but cleansing of the ocular discharge coupled with topical tetracycline ophthalmic ointments speeds recovery.

Neoplastic Diseases

The most common tumor of the conjunctiva is squamous cell carcinoma. This tumor may arise from either bulbar conjunctiva, palpebral conjunctiva, or conjunctiva covering the nictitans. Treatment has been discussed in the section on lid neoplasia.

Lymphosarcoma rarely involves conjunctiva but may appear as diffuse, firm swelling of the conjunctiva in one or both eyes.

Fatty infiltration of the bulbar conjunctiva has been confused with neoplasia. Subconjunctival fat covered by bulbar conjunctiva may enlarge and appear as a soft mass between the eyelid and cornea (Figure 13-16). Treatment is not required, and affected cattle show no signs of ocular irritation.

Conjunctiva and the Systemic State

The normal palpebral conjunctiva and conjunctiva overlying the nictitans are pink and free of inflammation. The bulbar conjunctiva is thin and appears white because of the underlying sclera. Various systemic states may be reflected by the conjunctiva as one of the mucous membranes available for inspection during the physical examination. Chemosis, or edema of the conjunctiva, is observed most commonly in allergic reactions, urticaria, or hypoproteinemia. Anemia is suggested by extreme pallor of the conjunctiva, and anemia coupled with hypoalbuminemia results in extreme pallor plus chemosis. Jaundice or icterus is suggested by a yellow tint to the conjunctiva and sclera underlying the bulbar conjunctiva. Conjunctival hemorrhages are most common in newborn calves following dystocia. In newborn calves, either direct trauma to the globes or severe passive congestion resulting from a prolonged stay of the head in the vagina or protruding from the vagina may lead to subconjunctival hemorrhage. Many healthy newborn calves also have noticeable conjunctival hemorrhage. Septicemia is the most common serious cause of conjunctival hemorrhage in neonatal calves and has been associated with thrombocytopenia or other coagulopathies (Figure 13-17). In older cattle, trauma, septicemia, thrombocytopenia (e.g., BVDV, bracken fern intoxication), disseminated intravascular coagulation, and other coagulopathies may result in conjunctival hemorrhages.

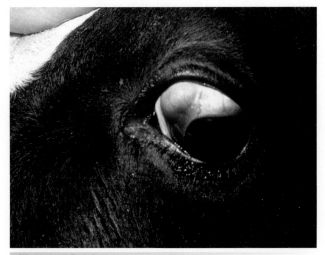

Figure 13-16

Subconjunctival fat in a Holstein that was affected bilaterally.

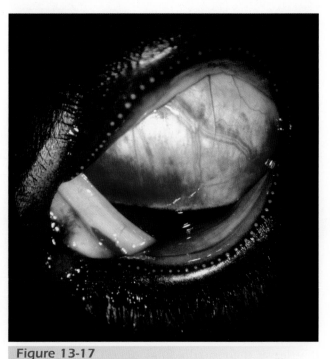

Figure 13-17

Conjunctival hemorrhage caused by thrombocytopenia in a Holstein cow.

DISEASES OF THE CORNEA

Developmental Diseases

Corneal dermoids occur infrequently in cattle. When observed, corneal dermoids usually are unilateral, originate at the limbal region, and extend a variable distance across the cornea (Figure 13-18). Removal using keratectomy is necessary to prevent persistent corneal and conjunctival irritation from the hairs growing from the dermoid. Corneal scarring is anticipated subsequent to keratectomy in some patients because rather deep keratectomies are necessary for complete removal in calves.

Congenital bilateral corneal opacities have been described in Holsteins as a recessive condition. The basic lesion is an endothelial dystrophy with subsequent corneal edema that leads to a nonpainful milky-white corneal opacity (Figure 13-19). Although blind because of rather severe corneal edema, these cattle appear otherwise normal, and some have been raised for production purposes. Obviously, affected animals should not be bred. No treatment exists.

Anterior cleavage anomalies create a severe corneal opacity that prevents intraocular ophthalmic examination. However, the ensuing glaucoma and megaglobus aid in identification of the basic lesion. This condition is further discussed in the section on the globe.

Toxic Injury

Toxic injury to the cornea most commonly results from accidental exposure of the cornea to exogenous chemicals. Chlorhexidine is extremely toxic to the corneal epithelium and stroma—both in cattle and people. Chlorhexidine disinfectants, soaps, and teat dips must be handled with great care to ovoid ocular injury to the cornea, which could lead to permanent corneal opacities. Insecticide and other chemicals, including organophosphate fly repellents, are toxic to the corneal epithelium and should not be sprayed on the periocular region of cattle. Most chemical toxicities will cause acute widespread epithelial loss.

Anhydrous ammonia, a commonly used fertilizer and silage additive, is especially dangerous to the eyes and respiratory tract of humans and animals. Leaks from broken hoses or tanks may expose cattle to this chemical. Peracute respiratory distress and corneal opacity occur in exposed cattle because the anhydrous chemical seeks water and desiccates tissues from which it has extracted the water. Severe and sometimes permanent corneal opacity develops as a result of epithelial necrosis and stromal injury.

Phenothiazine toxicity represents the classic example of endogenous corneal toxicity in cattle. Although less common today because of reduced use of phenothiazine, this toxicity still is encountered, and diagnosis is

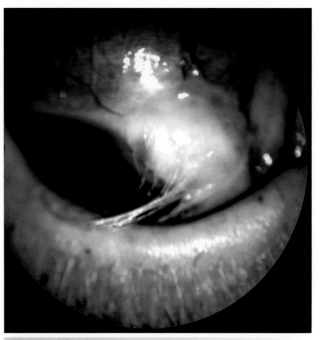

Figure 13-18

Corneoscleral dermoid in a calf. Dermoids may be pigmented or, as in this case, depigmented but usually produce hair that irritates the eye.

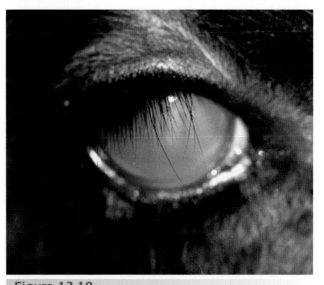

Figure 13-19

Congenital endothelial dystrophy in a Holstein calf. The lesion was bilateral.

made most easily by observing the ophthalmic manifestations. Excessive levels of phenothiazine metabolites such as phenothiazine sulfoxide circulate in the bloodstream and aqueous humor. Normally these metabolites are detoxified in the liver. Presence of phenothiazine metabolites in the aqueous coupled with exposure to sunlight (ultraviolet radiation) results in a photochemical reaction in the aqueous that releases energy

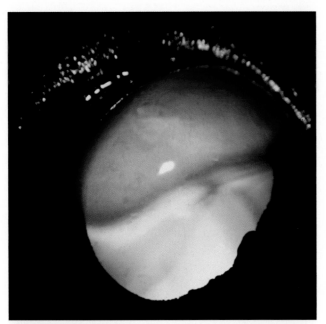

Figure 13-20

Phenothiazine toxicity. The ventral half of the cornea is edematous, secondary to photochemical damage to the corneal endothelium in this area.

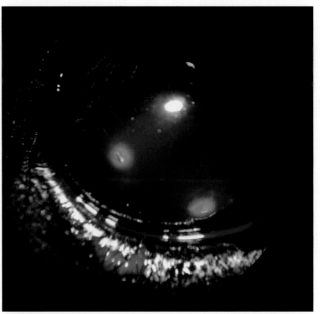

Figure 13-21

Plant material foreign body in the cornea of a Holstein. Fluorescein dye has been applied to the eye to highlight the lesion.

and heat, thereby injuring the corneal endothelium. Damage to the corneal endothelium promotes water uptake and edema of the corneal stroma because the Na^+K^+-ATPase pump of the endothelium has been damaged. Usually clinical signs include bilateral corneal edema in the ventral two thirds of the cornea. The dorsal cornea usually is unaffected because the upper eyelid protects it (Figure 13-20).

Inflammatory and Traumatic Disorders

Diseases Other Than Infectious Bovine Keratoconjunctivitis

Etiology. Traumatic injuries that cause abrasions, lacerations, or ulceration of the cornea may be caused by feedstuffs, conjunctival foreign bodies, restraint devices such as stanchions or chutes, and tail switching. Infection of corneal wounds occurs commonly because most are neglected unless they appear severely diseased. Opportunistic bacterial organisms from the conjunctival flora or inoculants carried by the offending object that caused the trauma can foster infection of any corneal wound.

Corneal foreign bodies (Figure 13-21) consisting of plant material may be embedded to variable depths in the cornea following strong winds, blowers or fans forcing feed and bedding into the eyes, or accidental trauma with plant material.

Exposure keratitis secondary to diseases of the orbit, globe, or neurologic diseases of the eyelids results in corneal desiccation and subsequent ulceration. Once

the corneal tear film no longer protects the epithelium, rapid desiccation followed by necrosis occurs in the central epithelium and underlying stroma. The result is a deep, slow-healing ulceration of the cornea that may progress to perforation if unattended.

Intrastromal abscesses in the cornea of cattle affected with the neurologic form of listeriosis have been described. However, in Dr. Rebhun's experience, the most common ocular lesion in cattle with listeriosis is exposure keratitis secondary to unilateral facial nerve paralysis.

Deep interstitial keratitis characterized by diffuse corneal edema and circumferential vascular influx from the limbus occasionally is observed in cattle with uveitis associated with septicemic conditions, endotoxemia, malignant catarrhal fever (MCF), and other systemic diseases. The conjunctival form of IBR also may result in a nonulcerative stromal keratitis.

Signs and Diagnosis. Lacrimation, blepharospasm, and photophobia are present whenever ulcerative corneal disease or corneal foreign bodies exist. Severe blepharospasm in cattle quickly leads to lid swelling from mechanical overwork of the eyelids and will be associated with conjunctival injection and ocular pain. Corneal ulcers or the opacities associated with ulceration may be apparent on inspection of the cornea, but the best means of diagnosis is via staining of epithelial defects with fluorescein dye (Fluor-I-Strip, Ayerst Laboratories, Inc., New York, NY). The epithelial defects will stain green and may be further highlighted with an ultraviolet light source that is helpful in detecting small lesions. Miosis is present in eyes with corneal ulcers as a result of reflex pain and ciliary spasm. Blocking the auriculopalpebral nerve with 2% lidocaine greatly facilitates examination of the painful bovine eye because the motor supply of cranial nerve (CN)-VII to the powerful orbicularis oculi muscle is blocked. Therefore blepharospasm no longer interferes with examination of the eye. In addition, rotation of the animal's head in a downward direction will facilitate examination of the cornea.

Corneal ulcers associated with facial nerve paralysis tend to be located in the central or lower central cornea. Absence of the palpebral response keys the diagnosis of exposure keratitis in such cases (see Chapter 12).

Infected corneal ulcers have necrotic or melting edges, more dramatic corneal edema and peripheral vascularization, a mucopurulent ocular discharge, severe miosis, and may create hypopyon or fibrin in the anterior chamber as toxins produced by bacterial organisms are absorbed through the water-soluble corneal stroma and act on the iris to cause a secondary uveitis. In general, signs of pain such as lacrimation, photophobia, and blepharospasm are more pronounced when infection complicates traumatic corneal injuries.

Most corneal foreign bodies can be identified by inspection with focal light. Magnification may occasionally be necessary to locate very small foreign bodies. Signs of ocular pain, conjunctival hyperemia, and lid swelling are present when a foreign body is present in the cornea. Initial serous ocular discharge will change to one with a mucopurulent character with chronicity or secondary infection associated with the foreign body. If a foreign body is suspected, the third eyelid should be lifted so that the conjunctiva under the lid is thoroughly examined.

Interstitial keratitis is a nonulcerative condition in which corneal edema and circumferential vascular influx from the limbus exist. Depending on severity, the vascular influx may be superficial (branching vessels) or deep (straight "paintbrush" vessels), and edema may similarly vary in severity. Rather than a specific diagnosis, interstitial keratitis usually represents a component of uveitis in cattle. Therefore it is accompanied by blepharospasm, lacrimation, photophobia, ciliary and conjunctival hyperemia, miosis, and cellular-protein accumulation in the anterior chamber. A primary systemic disease should be sought to explain the uveitis. Mycoplasma or chlamydia have not been identified as a cause of stromal keratitis in dairy cattle despite the frequency of keratoconjunctivitis caused by these organisms in sheep and goats.

Treatment. Corneal abrasions, ulcers, or nonperforating lacerations that are acute and not infected are best treated by topical broad-spectrum antibiotic ointments as prophylaxis against bacterial infection. Corticosteroids *always* are contraindicated because they reduce the eye's inherent ability to resist infection.

Subconjunctival antibiotics may be administered under the bulbar conjunctiva as an adjunct to topical antibiotics or as sole antibiotic therapy when it is impossible to catch the cow routinely for topical treatment. Veterinarians should be aware, however, that subconjunctival antibiotics are not deposit-type residual medications and are absorbed into the eye within 12 hours of administration. It is also important to utilize the bulbar conjunctiva and not a "lid injection" because absorption of drug from the lid does nothing for the eye. The only possible benefit from eyelid injections is leakage of drug from the lid puncture site onto the cornea.

Topical antibiotics should be applied as frequently as practicality and labor allow. Topical 1% atropine ophthalmic ointment is indicated (one to four times daily) to relieve ciliary spasm and dilate the pupil in extremely painful eyes. This will make the animal more comfortable and less likely to resist treatment.

Infected corneal ulcers or wounds require more aggressive antibiotic therapy. Very painful eyes with obvious deep ulcers or ulcers with necrotic edges should be assumed to be infected. Ideally scrapings should be obtained from the ulcer edges for Gram staining and culture to identify the causative organism. In practice, this is seldom done with cattle. However, for valuable animals, this diagnostic step is essential for selection of appropriate therapy just as in other species. Similarly, therapy often is compromised because of restraint difficulties with cattle. This fact should not discourage frequent treatment of the eyes of valuable calves or cows, which easily tolerate treatment, because the frequency of treatment with appropriate antibiotics is directly proportional to the speed of resolution of infection. Topical and subconjunctival antibiotics compose the major therapeutic weapons. Subconjunctival injections of penicillin (150,000 to 300,000 U) administered under the bulbar conjunctiva establish high but short-lived antibiotic levels in the cornea and anterior segment of the eye. These injections can be repeated daily if necessary. Topical antibiotics (optimally based on Gram stain of smears from the ulcer) should be applied topically as frequently as possible. Systemic antibiotics usually are not helpful. In milking cattle, antibiotic residues need to be considered and withdrawal times observed.

Topical 1% atropine again is helpful to block ciliary spasm. Atropine can be administered topically (1.25 cm length of ointment) one to four times daily or given subconjunctivally (0.05 to 0.2 mg) once daily. Discharge should be cleared away from the lids and face to prevent secondary dermatitis and to remove debris from the eye.

Corneal foreign bodies need to be removed as gently as possible to prevent further penetration of the object into or through the cornea. The easiest means to remove most foreign bodies is saline lavage. After blocking the auriculopalpebral nerve and applying topical anesthetic (0.5% proparacaine or lidocaine) to the eye, a stream of saline is directed at the corneal foreign body through a 20-ml syringe and 20-gauge needle. Most foreign material, even that which is embedded in stroma, will flush free with this technique. If flushing fails to resolve the problem, sedation of the animal, further anesthesia of the eye, and surgical manipulation of the lesion may be necessary. Once the foreign body is removed, topical or subconjunctival antibiotics are applied to the eye as prophylaxis against infection until the lesions epithelialize.

Stromal keratitis usually indicates underlying uveitis, and therapy of uveitis will be discussed below. One exception is stromal keratitis secondary to IBR conjunctivitis. This keratitis resolves spontaneously 2 to 4 weeks after onset of the viral conjunctivitis.

Exposure keratitis secondary to facial nerve lesions should be treated with topical ocular lubricants and prophylactic antibiotics if little or no ulceration exists. If central exposure damage and ulceration are present, the dried central cornea should be flushed gently with saline to remove dried crusts, hairs, necrotic corneal tissue, and other foreign material. Topical antibiotics should be applied as frequently as possible, and 1% atropine should be applied one to four times daily to improve the animal's comfort.

A temporary partial tarsorrhaphy may be fashioned by suturing the temporal third of the upper and lower eyelids together with mattress sutures that split the lid thickness. Sutures must not penetrate the lid to the level of palpebral conjunctiva, or corneal irritation may occur. Depending on the anticipated healing time for the neurologic deficit, a tarsorrhaphy may or may not be necessary. For example, acute otitis interna/media in a calf may cause facial nerve paralysis, but prompt treatment could improve facial nerve function within a few days. Therefore a tarsorrhaphy would be less necessary than in a listeriosis patient with severe facial paralysis requiring prolonged healing time. Although cattle may be less susceptible to corneal ulceration following facial paralysis than horses, exposure keratitis lesions are slow to heal compared with traumatic or infected ulcerations. Several weeks may be necessary for healing of exposure lesions, and compromised therapy predisposes to corneal perforation.

Infectious Bovine Keratoconjunctivitis (Pinkeye)

Etiology. IBK, or "pinkeye," is the most common and costly ocular disease of cattle. Management factors make the disease economically devastating to the beef industry, as well as costly and time consuming for the dairy industry. *M. bovis,* a gram-negative bacterium, is the cause of IBK. The organism exists as a virulent, hemolytic, rough colony form when pathogenic and as a nonhemolytic, smooth colony nonvirulent form in the conjunctiva of recovered cattle or calves.

The pathogenicity of the virulent form of *M. bovis* is enhanced by several characteristics. Pathogenic strains of *M. bovis* have pili that aid attachment to the corneal epithelium. The pili are made up of protein subunits known as pilin, and *M. bovis* may produce type a or type b pilin. Type b appears to be associated with pathogenicity.

In addition to pili, hemolysin is produced by virulent *M. bovis* and may contribute to the organism's cytotoxicity against bovine neutrophils. Other toxins produced by *M. bovis* appear to be proteases, but most authorities agree that these proteases do not include a collagenase. Despite the activity of *M. bovis* in corneal infection, the exact chemical mediators of stromal destruction are unknown. A dermonecrotic exotoxin has been described that may contribute to corneal "melting." Evidence also exists that chemotactic factors that recruit neutrophils and other inflammatory defenses may contribute to stromal destruction. Neutrophils are capable of collagenase release, and the "overrecruitment" of neutrophils by the *M. bovis* may encourage stromal destruction.

Infection with virulent strains confers both local and humoral immunity, but the level of protection and duration of immunity is unknown. Generally, recovered calves do not relapse or have recurrences of infection unless immunosuppressed, affected with bovine leukocyte adhesion deficit, or persistently infected with BVDV. The disease may occur in calves and cows of any age but is most common in calves and heifers (6 to 24 months of age) that are housed outside during summer months. Outbreaks in Europe have been reported when calves were on snow-covered fields. Ultraviolet light (sunlight) facilitates infection either by damaging corneal epithelial cells or activating nonhemolytic *M. bovis* in the conjunctival flora of recovered cattle. *Musca autumnalis* face flies are the major mechanical vectors for *M. bovis.* These flies carry virulent strains from the ocular or nasal secretions of infected calves to the eyes of noninfected calves. Tall grasses may also allow transmission of the infectious agent. Following recovery, most calves remain free of IBK infections in the future, suggesting a fairly lasting immunity despite difficulty reproducing this experimentally.

Pinkeye outbreaks sometimes appear during the winter months despite a paucity of sunlight and face flies. The pathogenesis in this setting is more difficult to explain, and frequently older animals or adults are involved in winter outbreaks. Although *Neisseria* spp. have been implicated in some of these "winter pinkeye epidemics," *M. bovis* remains the most likely cause, and the lesions are identical to those routinely observed in summer outbreaks of *M. bovis*-proven infections. Concurrent viral conjunctivitis or viral upper respiratory infections may trigger pinkeye outbreaks by allowing conversion of avirulent to virulent strains of *M. bovis.* Dr. Rebhun observed severe, nonresponsive pinkeye in some calves persistently infected with BVDV and during acute BVDV infection in heifers concurrently infected with *M. bovis.* In acute infections with BVDV, the deficient immune response to IBK is transient and merely awaits humoral antibody against BVDV and return of cellular immune functions. In animals persistently infected with BVDV, however, severe pinkeye lesions persist or advance. Dual infections with *M. bovis* and IBR virus can cause devastating ocular disease.

Signs and Diagnosis. Initial signs of conjunctivitis include redness and serous to mucopurulent ocular discharge. Multiple animals are affected. The lesions may be unilateral or bilateral. Within 1 to 3 days of initial infection, a circular corneal ulcer develops in the central or lower central cornea (Figure 13-22). Signs are more obvious to owners at this time because ocular pain leads to blepharospasm, lacrimation, and photophobia. Tears stain the facial region, and severe blepharospasm causes lid swelling; the animal holds the eyelids partially closed in the affected eye. Focal light examination highlights the central ulcer; initially this is circular and crater-like in appearance. Corneal edema, deep peripheral vascularization at the limbus, and miosis are present.

Following these classic early signs, the eye may deteriorate to variable endpoints, depending on management and treatment. Most patients show progression of the circular central ulcer to a less circular deep crater ulcer with melting edges that appear necrotic (Figure 13-23). The center of the ulcer may appear clear or dark in color as Descemet's membrane is approached (Figure 13-24).

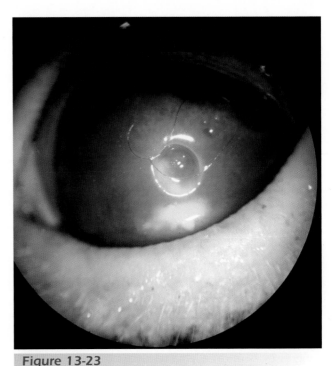

Figure 13-23

Deeper crater-like corneal ulcer in a heifer with IBK of 1 week's duration. Corneal edema surrounds the ulcer, and peripheral corneal vessels are present. Hypopyon is present in the anterior chamber as a result of secondary uveitis.

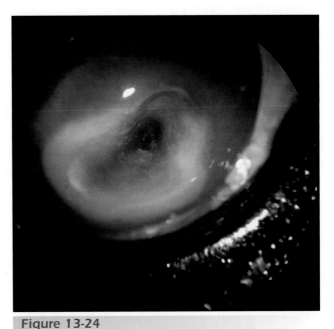

Figure 13-24

Extremely deep melting ulcer with central descemetocele (dark central area) in a heifer with IBK of 1 week's duration.

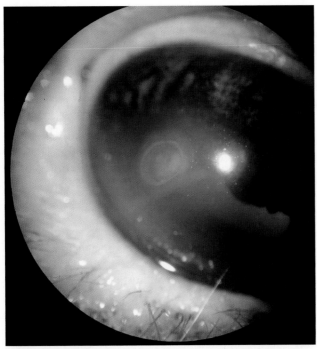

Figure 13-22

Early central corneal ulcer in a calf affected with IBK.

Corneal edema intensifies through the cornea peripheral to the ulcer, and deep corneal vascularization moves in from the limbus toward the edge of the ulcer. These vessels are necessary to provide metabolic and cellular components for completion of the healing process. At this stage, the animal suffers severe pain, and appetite and production suffer. Eyes with deep ulcers that begin to heal with or without therapy will fill in the deep crater with granulation tissue as the corneal vascularization reaches the ulcer bed. The vessels provide capillaries, and the corneal stroma contributes fibroblasts for granulation tissue. Much clinical variation exists in the appearance of infected eyes. Blue (edema), red (vessels, granulation tissue), and yellow (necrosis, stromal abscesses) are the predominant colors observed from a distance.

Superficial ulcers simply epithelialize, whereas deep ulcers fill with granulation tissue and then epithelialize during the healing process. Once epithelialization is complete, ocular pain resolves. Central corneal granulation tissue changes color from red to pink and finally to white as the corneal stroma reorganizes and healing progresses. Corneal edema resolves from the periphery first and clears progressively toward the central lesion. Corneal deep straight vessels recede, leaving only superficial branching vessels. Complete corneal remodeling requires weeks to months. Most recovered cattle have central nebulas, maculas, or leukomas but little visual loss, which is a testament to the amazing healing ability of the bovine cornea.

Eyes that are unattended or that are infected with extremely virulent strains may progress to descemetoceles, corneal perforation, or panophthalmitis. During an outbreak in a herd, all degrees of severity will be observed in affected eyes. Secondary uveitis in severe pinkeye cases may cause residual posterior synechiae and cataract formation.

The clinical signs and morbidity allow accurate diagnosis of IBK in most instances. Culture of *M. bovis* from infected corneas provides the definitive diagnosis.

Treatment. Ideal therapy would include frequent applications of topical antibiotics, daily subconjunctival antibiotic injections, and topical atropine to maintain cycloplegia. Unfortunately restraint difficulties and limited labor forces compromise therapy for IBK. Unless affected cattle are confined to tie stalls or stanchions, treatment is unlikely to be attempted more than once daily. Manageable cattle or easily confined cattle should be treated as frequently as possible to speed resolution of the *M. bovis* infection. As in other species, the rate of recovery and success of therapy will be directly correlated with the frequency of treatment.

Ideal therapy may include the following regimen (may be repeated daily for 3 days):

1. 25 mg of subconjunctival Ceftiofur (Pfizer, New York, NY) or 300,000 U of penicillin G
2. Topical application of gentamicin, erythromycin, or tobramycin ointments several times daily to affected eyes. Ophthalmic ointments or mastitis tubes may be used for this purpose. Appropriate milk and meat withdrawals should be considered before using.
3. Topical 1% atropine ointment twice daily
4. Confining the animal so as to avoid sunlight, cleansing discharges from the eye, and using fly control to discourage fly irritation on the animal's face

Less intensive therapy would include:

1. Initial subconjunctival injection of ampicillin or penicillin. Ampicillin administration requires 6 days of withdrawal time for slaughter and 48 hours for milk harvest.
2. One application of topical antibiotic and atropine
3. Repeat daily with topicals
4. 20 mg/kg long-acting oxytetracycline IM injection—repeated in 72 hours. Note: use of Liquamycin (Pfizer, New York, NY) requires a withdrawal time of 28 days for slaughter and 96 hours for milk (secretion of antibiotic in tears and selectively into conjunctival epithelium maintains effective levels against *M. bovis*).

Or

1. Tulathromycin (Draxxin; Pfizer, New York, NY) is a very good one-dose therapy at label dose for calves.
2. Pinkeye patch, tarsorrhaphy with catgut, or third eyelid flap fashioned with catgut. If the ulcer cannot be monitored and/or daily treatment is not possible, then one-dose antibiotic therapy (Naxcel subconjunctivally and either tetracycline or tulathromycin parenterally) and tarsorrhaphy is likely the best plan.

Fox (Dr. Francis Fox, personal communication, 1977, Ithaca, NY) has suggested 5% silver nitrate topically as a "last ditch" treatment for severely infected corneas that appear likely to perforate. Many other treatments have been suggested and used but cannot be recommended. Topical or subconjunctival corticosteroids are contraindicated. These drugs weaken the defense mechanisms of the infected cornea, thereby predisposing to perforation. Many practitioners advocate the use of corticosteroids, but eyes that survive treatment with these drugs do so only because the effects of topical or subconjunctival corticosteroids are short-lived (hours), and the tremendous healing power of the bovine cornea overcomes the temporary setback induced by the drug.

Although antibacterial sprays designed for ophthalmic use also are advocated, practitioners should evaluate the contents before recommending their use. Furazolidone sprays have been used in the treatment of pinkeye and appear effective but now are illegal to use. Irritating sprays containing various dyes are contraindicated, and "pinkeye powders" are inhumane when applied to an already painful eye. Empiric use of intranasal IBR vaccine applied to eyes (as advocated by some veterinarians) is contraindicated because concurrent IBR and *M. bovis* infection has been shown to worsen corneal lesions and invite perforation.

Neglected eyes that perforate or develop severe keratoconus with endophthalmitis or panophthalmitis require enucleation to prevent continual pain, irritation from flies and discharges, worsening infection, and failure of the animal to grow or produce.

Prevention. Several bacterins or other novel vaccines against *M. bovis* are currently available and used in herds where pinkeye appears annually. Although the vaccines do not prevent all new cases of pinkeye, they appear to reduce the incidence, which is advantageous because less labor, drugs, and veterinary charges are required during the pinkeye season. The beef industry, by necessity, has used more *M. bovis* bacterins than the dairy industry in most geographic regions, but results should be similar in problem dairy heifer programs. As expected, with most biologics, occasional anaphylactic reactions have been observed following administration of pinkeye bacterins, and epinephrine should be available when administering the vaccine. Some reactions may be caused by endotoxin in the vaccine rather than true anaphylaxis.

Fly control to reduce the vectors of disease is always indicated but difficult to do. Insecticide ear tags, sprays, insecticide dust bags, oral chemicals that pass in the feces and control fly larvae, and other fly control measures have been used to minimize the face fly vector. The veterinarian and producer should discuss the potential efficacy, costs, and labor involved to implement these fly control measures when considering their use. Routine clipping of the pasture may also help decrease spread.

Future technologic advances in the form of more effective vaccines and fly control offer the greatest hope for prevention of this costly disease.

Corneal Neoplasms

Squamous cell carcinoma and its precursors (e.g., epitheliomas, keratomas) are the most frequent tumors of the bovine cornea. The tumors usually originate at the temporal limbal area and extend into adjacent corneal tissue and bulbar conjunctiva (Figure 13-25). Early recognition of the lesion allows effective therapy using cryosurgery, radiofrequency hyperthermia, radiation, or keratectomy. Holsteins appear to have the highest incidence among dairy breeds. Large or neglected tumors may require enucleation to prevent metastases or further local invasion into the globe. Metastasis to regional lymph nodes—especially the parotid nodes—and lungs is possible in neglected cases.

Lymphosarcoma has been observed in the bovine cornea and globe infrequently (Figure 13-26). In these cases, the cornea was merely one of many organs involved in diffuse lymphosarcoma rather than a single tumor. Ocular lymphangiosarcoma has been confirmed as a cause of corneoscleral neoplasia in a Holstein cow.

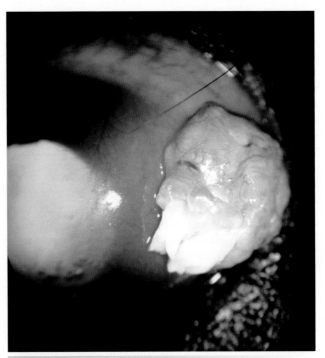
Figure 13-25
Corneal squamous cell carcinoma originating from the temporal limbus in an 8-year-old Holstein cow.

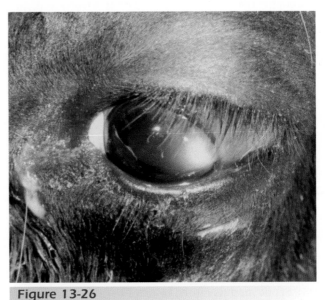
Figure 13-26
Corneal lymphosarcoma that appears as a white mass in the temporal cornea of a cow with multifocal lymphosarcoma.

Corneal Lacerations

Partial-thickness (nonperforating) corneal lacerations are treated as noninfected corneal injuries (see the earlier discussion). Perforating corneal lacerations with iris prolapse require specialized ophthalmic instrumentation, ophthalmic suture material, and general anesthesia for effective cosmetic repair. In valuable cows, referral should be suggested. If the cow's value does not warrant referral or when the initiating trauma has caused massive intraocular injury (i.e., lens or vitreous prolapse), the affected eye should be enucleated.

DISEASES OF THE UVEAL TRACT

Inflammatory Diseases of the Uveal Tract

Etiology and Signs

The iris, ciliary body, and choroid constitute the uveal tract, which is the vascular layer of the eye. The vascular nature of the uveal tract predisposes to proteinaceous and cellular exudates when these tissues are inflamed. Immune-mediated diseases also involve the uveal tract in most species. The iris is the most easily examined portion of the uveal tract, making iritis more obvious than inflammation of the ciliary body and choroid even though these tissues also may be involved.

Signs of uveitis include miosis, conjunctival and ciliary injection, hypotony, peripheral corneal edema and vascularization, edema of the iris, and cellular and fibrinous exudates accumulating in the anterior chamber. Inflammation of the iris results in vasodilation with fibrin, white blood cells, and red blood cells oozing from the inflamed iris vasculature. When white blood cells and fibrin predominate, the accumulated exudate is termed a "hypopyon," whereas if red blood cells and fibrin predominate, the exudate is termed a "hyphema." Exudates from the choroid may accumulate between the retina and choroid, resulting in either chorioretinal inflammation or serous detachment of the retina.

Uveitis is common in neonatal calves suffering from septicemia. The uveitis in these calves may be caused by direct endogenous bacterial spread to the uveal tract or endotoxemia from gram-negative organisms acting on the uveal vasculature. Hypopyon, iris swelling, and miosis appear as predominant signs in these calves (Figure 13-27). Signs of uveitis are an extremely important diagnostic clue in a comatose neonatal calf because they indicate septicemia, possible meningitis, and a poor prognosis.

Adult cattle with septicemia associated with septic mastitis, septic metritis, endocarditis, and other causes occasionally develop unilateral or bilateral uveitis (Figure 13-28). Septic mastitis caused by gram-negative organisms is the most common cause. Once again, either true septicemia or endotoxemia may trigger this inflammation.

Idiopathic unilateral or bilateral uveitis occasionally occurs in otherwise healthy cattle. Affected cattle may lose vision temporarily or permanently. Various causes have been theorized but none proven. *Leptospira* sp., *H. somni*, toxoplasmosis, *Borrelia burgdorferi*, and other organisms have been suspected. Immune-mediated uveitis also may exist in adult cattle, and the European description of *specific ophthalmia* in cattle bears resemblance to recurrent uveitis in horses and is thought to have a viral cause.

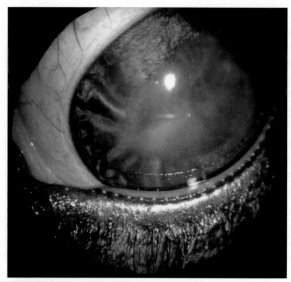

Figure 13-27

Uveitis in a neonatal calf with septicemia. The iris is edematous, and a fibrin clot obscures the miotic, occluded pupil.

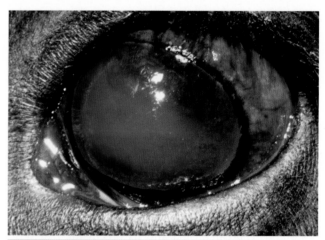

Figure 13-28

Uveitis in an adult cow with septic metritis. A large fibrin clot and hyphema fills the anterior chamber and obscures the miotic pupil.

The acute form of MCF causes a severe anterior uveitis and vasculitis that involves virtually every part of the eye except the choroid. Corneal opacity resulting from edema and peripheral vascularization may be so severe as to obscure deeper lesions, but anterior uveitis and hypopyon are usually present. The uveitis associated with MCF is bilateral and is characterized by massive influx of mononuclear cells into the anterior uveal tract (Figure 13-29). Chronic MCF or a mild form of MCF may result in more subtle signs of bilateral uveitis such as mild corneal edema, mild iritis, fibrin or hypopyon in the anterior chamber, and peripheral corneal vascularization (Figure 13-30).

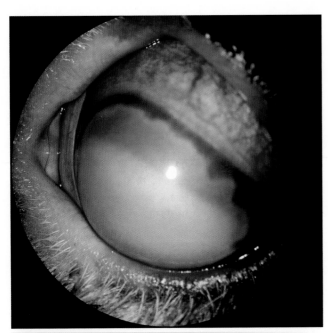

Figure 13-29

Severe uveitis in a cow with acute malignant catarrhal fever. The lesion was bilateral and consisted of severe ocular injection, corneal edema, and peripheral corneal vascularization. A dense hypopyon composed of mononuclear cells fills the ventral two thirds of the anterior chamber.

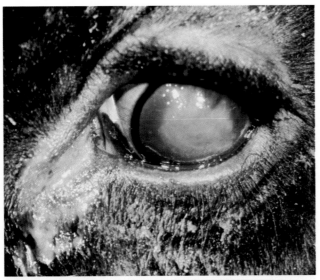

Figure 13-30

The appearance of the eye in a Holstein calf affected with chronic malignant catarrhal fever. Both eyes have suffered chronic uveitis, chronic keratitis with edema, vascularization, and edema of the cornea.

Granulomatous uveitis resulting from tuberculosis was observed occasionally before control of this disease in dairy cattle; tuberculosis should remain in the differential diagnosis when a suspicion of granulomatous uveitis coexists with weight loss and chronic respiratory

disease because of the public health implications of the disease.

Nonspecific bilateral miosis is observed commonly in "toxemia" in cattle. These cattle usually have overwhelming infections, and miosis may reflect low-grade uveitis associated with a systemic inflammatory response.

Traumatic uveitis caused by trauma to the globe occurs from head butts, stanchion and chute trauma, and rough handling of cattle by humans. Signs of traumatic uveitis are similar to those found in other types of uveitis except that hyphema tends to be a prominent finding.

Secondary uveitis is common to many serious corneal inflammatory diseases, especially pinkeye, and can cause sequelae that limit vision.

Diagnosis

Primary uveitis is diagnosed by observations of the ophthalmic lesions coupled with absence of corneal injury or fluorescein dye uptake. Primary causes of uveitis may be apparent when facial trauma is observed or septic foci such as septic mastitis are identified during the physical examination. Septicemia should be obvious in neonatal calves having depression, fever, diarrhea, a swollen navel, or other signs consistent with bacterial septicemia.

Primary sites of infection should be sought in adult cattle with uveitis. When no primary sites of infection exist and fever is absent, idiopathic uveitis should be considered. Although causes of idiopathic uveitis currently are nebulous, future efforts should be directed toward serologic investigations that might uncover etiologies. When more than one cow in a herd experiences uveitis of unknown cause, acute and convalescent serology for *Leptospira* sp., *H. somni*, toxoplasmosis, *B. burgdorferi*, and other diseases may be considered. Mucosal lesions, nasal discharge, high fever, nervous system signs, lymphadenopathy, hematuria, and other physical abnormalities are present in addition to uveitis in MCF patients.

Secondary uveitis may be obscured by severe primary corneal inflammation such as pinkeye, but miosis and hypopyon usually are apparent.

Treatment

If uveitis appears to be secondary to a septic condition (i.e., calf septicemia, septic mastitis, or endocarditis), treatment should address the possibility that bacterial pathogens have entered the uveal tract. Therefore treatment requires antibiotics topically and subconjunctivally. Whenever possible, these antibiotics should be the same antibiotics as those best suited for systemic treatment of the primary disease. For example, when a coliform mastitis is present and suspected to be the primary infection, ceftiofur may be used locally in the quarter and perhaps systemically as well if the cow appears severely ill. If this cow also develops uveitis, neomycinpolymyxin B/bacitracin topical ophthalmic ointment several times daily and subconjunctival ceftiofur (25 mg) once daily would be indicated. Similarly a neonatal calf with probable gram-negative septicemia that has uveitis may be treated with similar drugs but a lesser dose of ceftiofur subconjunctivally. Penicillin and ampicillin might be better choices for subconjunctival and topical use when a gram-positive organism was suspected as the cause of uveitis—as in a cow with endocarditis for which gram-positive organisms are likely to be causative.

Cycloplegia to control pain and establish pupillary dilation to prevent synechiae or pupil occlusion because of fibrin and cells in the anterior chamber are important adjuncts to therapy. Atropine sulfate ophthalmic ointment (1%) applied several times daily to the affected eye accomplishes these goals.

When cattle appear to have idiopathic uveitis in one or both eyes but otherwise appear normal, topical therapy includes 1% atropine several times daily to establish cycloplegia and pupil dilatation, as well as topical antibiotic-steroid preparations to counteract nonseptic uveal inflammation. Similar therapy is indicated for traumatic uveitis unless corneal abrasions or ulcers have occurred during the ocular trauma. If no corneal injury exists, traumatic uveitis is treated with 1% atropine ointment and an antibiotic-corticosteroid ophthalmic ointment each applied several times daily. NSAIDs may be helpful in the treatment of idiopathic (nonseptic, probable immune-mediated) and traumatic uveitis. Oral aspirin, flunixin meglumine, or topical flurbiprofen in standard dosages may be given to help control prostaglandin-mediated inflammation in the uveal tract and aid patient comfort.

Hemorrhage into the anterior chamber (hyphema) may occur from trauma or the many causes of thrombocytopenia (e.g., BVDV, bracken fern, idiopathic) or other clotting abnormalities. Cycloplegics and antiinflammatory topical ocular treatment can be used, but therapeutic focus is usually on the primary disease and other organ systems.

DISEASES OF THE LENS

Developmental Diseases

Etiology and Signs
Many examples of hereditary cataracts including nuclear cataracts in Holsteins and a recessive microphakia with cataract, ectopia lentis, as well as aniridia in Jerseys have been described. As in other species, a newborn calf with cataracts may represent either an inherited condition or simply a congenital accident during development of the eye. Definitive differentiation is often impossible based solely on clinical signs. If similar cataracts are found in other age-matched calves from different genetic lines, a

gestational accident such as toxicity, BVDV infection during the mid-trimester of pregnancy, or other common exposure should be investigated. When only calves from a common genetic line are involved, heredity should be suspected. Lesions in a single calf usually are impossible to differentiate unless other signs of BVDV (e.g., cerebellar hypoplasia or brachygnathism) are present. Unless inheritance can be disproven definitely, bull calves should be rejected from a bull stud if congenital cataracts are present. When BVDV is suspected as the cause of cortical cataracts in newborn calves, precolostral titers should be assessed for evidence of prenatal BVDV infection, and viral isolation from whole blood may be attempted to rule out persistent infection with BVDV.

Signs of congenital cataracts may be subtle enough to require biomicroscopy for observation of slight nuclear or cortical opacities (Figure 13-31). Other cases are obvious with the lens being completely opaque (Figure 13-32) as a result of a mature cataract. Congenital cataracts that involve only parts of the lens may progress very slowly if at all. However, when offering a prognosis, the veterinarian always should caution the owner that any cataract may progress and eventually cause blindness.

Acquired Diseases

Etiology and Signs
Acquired cataracts in cattle usually occur from either intraocular inflammation or previous trauma to the eye. Ocular inflammation associated with uveitis or severe IBK promotes posterior synechiae formation and fibrin

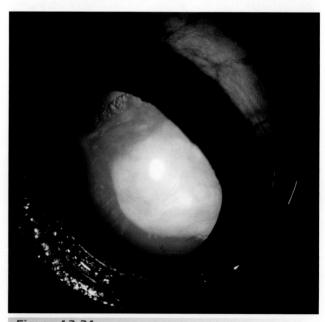

Figure 13-31

Holstein calf with a dense nuclear cataract and surrounding cortical opacities.

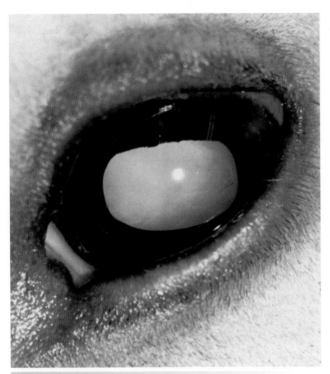

Figure 13-32

Diffuse cortical cataract in a Jersey calf.

coating the anterior lens capsule. Damage to the anterior lens capsule alters normal lens metabolism, resulting in capsular and cortical cataract formation. Cataracts formed by these mechanisms develop slowly following the initiating inflammation. Therefore the eye may appear "quiet" or free of inflammation at the time cataracts first are observed. Tell-tale markers of the previous inflammation are present, however. These markers include posterior synechiae, iris pigment rests that appear as brown or black spots on the anterior lens capsule from previous iris adhesions, and corneal scarring from previous IBK.

Similarly, traumatic uveitis may allow fibrin, hemorrhage, and iris adhesions to damage the lens capsule. Trauma may initiate lens luxation or a lens rupture in addition to uveitis and thereby further predispose to cataract formation.

Treatment

In general, bovine cataracts are not removed surgically. Few indications exist for treatment of cataracts in cattle, primarily because of economic concerns. In the rare instance that treatment is sought, referral to a veterinary ophthalmologist would be indicated.

Perhaps the greatest prevention for acquired cataracts in cattle would be increased usage of topical atropine sulfate in ophthalmic injuries, IBK infections, and uveitis of various causes. By dilating the pupil, iris adhesions (posterior synechiae) are much less likely to occur.

DISEASES OF THE VITREOUS

Developmental Diseases

Persistent hyaloid arteries are visible during ophthalmoscopy in almost all newborn calves, and the remnants of this artery are detectable in 25% to 50% of yearling cattle. In adult cattle, the fibrosed proximal end of the vessel (Bergmeister's papilla) often is visible ophthalmoscopically, floating in the vitreous but attached at the center of the optic disc.

Inflammatory Diseases

Vitreal abscesses may occur rarely in septicemic calves, and this condition progresses to endophthalmitis. Vitreitis also may be associated with MCF or embolic septic uveitis in cattle. Treatment is similar to that discussed for septic uveitis.

Congenital Inherited Diseases

Although many congenital retinopathies, retinal dysplasias, and retinal detachments may represent inherited defects, the paucity of reported cases in dairy cattle reflects a low incidence or a failure of recognition of these disorders. Retinal detachments have been observed in association with multiple congenital anomalies in four related Irish Friesian cattle.

Because dairy cattle are seldom surveyed for funduscopic lesions unless they appear blind, subtle retinal lesions may go undetected.

Nutritional Causes

Hypovitaminosis A

Etiology and Signs. Increased cerebrospinal fluid (CSF) pressure has been confirmed in experimental studies of vitamin A deficiency and is thought to be responsible for the neurologic signs observed. Increased CSF pressure results from failure of proper resorption of CSF through the abnormal arachnoid villi and thickened dura mater. The pathophysiology of visual loss is more complex. Although papilledema is a classical finding in both adult and growing vitamin A–deficient cattle, the mechanism by which papilledema occurs differs in these two age groups. In adult cattle, papilledema is thought to be secondary to chronic elevation of CSF pressure. Papilledema by itself does not lead to blindness unless it becomes chronic enough to result in vascular ischemia, interference with axonal transport, and secondary optic nerve degeneration. Increased CSF pressure probably also contributes to the papilledema observed in growing cattle. However, dural fibrodysplasia and altered bone metabolism resulting in decreased bone resorption in the optic canals causes direct optic nerve damage and may lead to papilledema. This decreased bone resorption leads to dorsoventral compression of the canals. Resultant vascular compromise, ischemic necrosis of the nerve, and direct interference with axonal transport through the optic nerve lead to more severe papilledema, edema in the nerve fiber layer of the retina, and retinal or vitreal hemorrhages as congested vessels rupture. The pathophysiology within the optic canals is irreversible in growing animals, and, when present, blindness is usually permanent.

Nyctalopia, or night blindness, has been reported as the earliest sign of visual disturbance in experimental hypovitaminosis A but seldom is observed in field outbreaks. Vitamin A is required for regeneration of the rhodopsin necessary for photoreceptor activity during dark adaptation. Rod dysfunction and subsequent loss have been shown to be greater than cone dysfunction and loss in chronic vitamin A deficiency in rats. Photoreceptor dysfunction, especially of rods, probably contributes to nyctalopia and visual loss in both adult and growing cattle. Therefore visual alterations in adult cattle are caused by photoreceptor abnormalities and papilledema. In growing calves, the same physiologic and biochemical problems occur, but additive insult occurs as a result of anatomic optic nerve compression and vascular ischemia.

Physical disruption and ischemic necrosis of the optic nerves in the stenotic optic canals are followed by their replacement with mature dense sheets of collagen as a chronic change. Destruction of the optic nerve axons at this site leads to orthograde (Wallerian) degeneration in the optic tracts and secondary astrogliosis.

Apparently male animals have a lesser tolerance of hypovitaminosis A than females. Rations persistently low in vitamin A are rare but have been found when growing cattle or feeder beef rations were formulated using either feedstuffs that had been stored for an excessive time or were composed primarily of feedstuffs (cereal grains) inherently low in vitamin A. Deficient rations must be fed for months before clinical signs of hypovitaminosis A occur. Clinical signs include blindness with dilated, nonresponsive pupils.

Ophthalmic examination confirms papilledema, retinal edema, and, in some cases, retinal hemorrhage as congested retinal vessels leak blood into the retina or vitreous (Figures 13-33 and 13-34). Although variations in the degree of visual loss and funduscopic lesions occur, papilledema is present in most animals showing neurologic or ophthalmic signs.

Diagnosis. Although clinical signs strongly support hypovitaminosis A (e.g., neurologic, ophthalmic, failure to grow), evaluation of serum or plasma vitamin A must be done to confirm the diagnosis. Serum levels less than 20 μg/100 ml support this diagnosis, and visual lesions are inversely proportional to levels less than 20 μg/100 ml. Normal values range from 25 to 60 μg/100 ml (see Table 13-1).

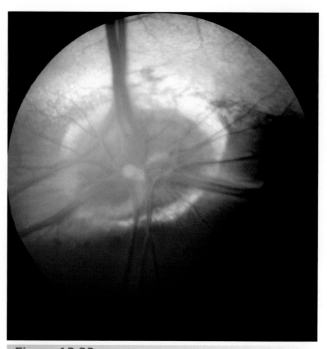

Figure 13-33

Normal bovine fundus in a Holstein cow.

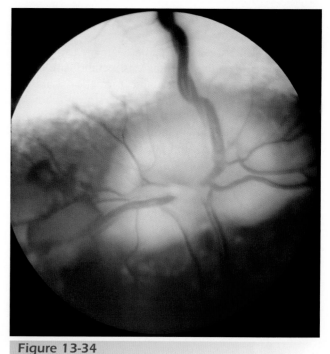

Figure 13-34

Severe papilledema, retinal edema, and preretinal hemorrhages in a Holstein steer with vitamin A deficiency.

Treatment. Correcting the deficient diet so that it provides a minimum of 40 IU of vitamin A/kg body weight is essential. Further, treatment with up to 440 IU/kg body weight for several days is indicated as initial therapy. Prognosis is poor for growing animals that are blind because permanent damage to the optic nerves as they traverse the optic canals is likely.

Male Fern Poisoning *(Dryopteris filix-mas)*

European workers have reported optic neuropathy in cattle secondary to ingestion of male fern. Variable degrees of retrobulbar optic neuritis, indigestion, and constipation are the observed signs. Papillitis, papilledema, and peripapillary hemorrhage may appear. Blindness may be temporary or permanent, depending on the amount of fern ingested.

The only treatment is removal from contaminated pasture and symptomatic laxatives.

Inflammatory Lesions

Etiology and Signs

BVDV infection of the fetus during days 75 to 150 of gestation may cause inflammatory damage to the retina and optic nerve of the fetus. Resultant visual loss may be partial or complete, depending on the degree of optic nerve damage. Retinal atrophy appearing as hyperreflective areas in the tapetal area or depigmented lesions in the nontapetum, retinal hemorrhages, and optic nerve degeneration have been observed ophthalmoscopically in affected calves at birth (Figure 13-35). If cataracts coexist (see the section on the lens), the fundus lesions may be hidden from ophthalmoscopic view. Other congenital aberrations such as brachygnathism or cerebellar hypoplasia may or may not be observed in affected calves and in other calves born about the same time in the herd.

Septicemia probably causes multifocal chorioretinal inflammation more commonly than we realize because many adult cattle have evidence of multifocal chorioretinal scarring. Ophthalmoscopic examination in acute cases shows round fluffy lesions ("cotton wool spots") of active chorioretinitis, best recognized in the nontapetal area. These lesions later appear as scars with depigmented peripheral zones and central hyperpigmented zones and have been called "bullet hole" lesions (Figure 13-36). Calf septicemia or adult septicemia caused by mastitis, metritis, and endocarditis may cause these lesions. It also is possible that the cow is asymptomatic or shows only vague illness when these lesions develop. Unless the cow loses all vision, retinal lesions are not suspected. Therefore subclinical infections with *H. somni* or other pathogens may be involved, but this has not been proven.

Treatment and Prevention

Therapy and prevention of these lesions are possible only when a direct cause and effect can be determined. For example, in utero BVDV infection may be confirmed by precolostral antibody determination coupled with attempts at viral isolation from buffy coat samples of whole blood. Control of BVDV would then be indicated as discussed in Chapter 6.

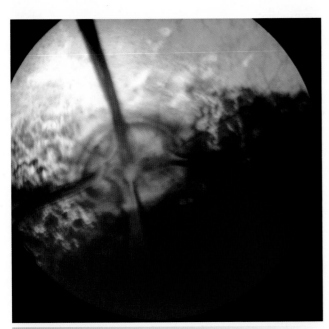

Figure 13-35

Optic nerve degeneration, peripapillary chorioretinal scarring, and tapetal hyperreflectivity in a calf that was born blind as a result of in utero BVDV infection.

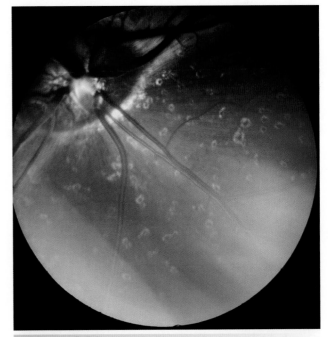

Figure 13-36

Multifocal chorioretinal scars in the nontapetum of a Holstein cow that had reduced vision in this eye. The lesions are depigmented peripherally and have a hyperpigmented center typical of "bullet hole" scars.

Vascular Lesions of the Fundus

Severe compression of the jugular veins through prolonged neck entrapment in a tight chute or accidental choking occasionally results in papilledema, retinal edema, and peripapillary retinal hemorrhages secondary to greatly increased venous pressure. Blindness with bilateral dilated and nonresponsive pupils is present. Treatment consists of freeing the trapped animal and administering dexamethasone—for nonpregnant animals—at 20 to 50 mg IV once or twice at 12-hour intervals. Most animals so affected that Dr. Rebhun diagnosed remained blind; however, none were treated during the acute phase. The ophthalmoscopic lesions are identical to those observed in vitamin A deficiency but can be differentiated easily by history of entrapment and the fact that only one animal is affected.

Polycythemia, as observed in some congenital cardiac anomalies such as tetralogy of Fallot, may cause the retinal vasculature to appear grossly enlarged (Figure 13-37). Primary and secondary causes of polycythemia should be considered. Primary polycythemia has been reported as a recessive trait in Jersey cattle.

Retinal Degeneration

Sporadic retinal degeneration with clinical features and ophthalmoscopic findings similar to progressive retinal degeneration in other species has been observed occasionally. Several unrelated cows in a Friesian herd in England developed clinical signs of retinal degeneration. The signs, ophthalmoscopic findings, and histopathology of these animals formed the basis for two reports. There appeared to be no exposure to known toxins or any evidence of genetic relationship in this herd.

Dr. Rebhun observed several sporadic instances of retinal degeneration in adult Holstein dairy cattle and one herd that had two cases of unrelated cattle at the same time. Invariably the affected cows were reported to appear clumsy, dumb, and finally were recognized as blind by the caretakers. The animals may be reluctant to move from their stalls or may behave in an unruly and anxious manner—running into people, doors, or through fences. These signs only appear when the retinal degeneration is well advanced. The pupils are dilated and either not responsive or poorly responsive to direct light stimulation. Funduscopic examination confirms generalized hyperreflectivity of the tapetal fundus, vascular attenuation, and optic atrophy (Figure 13-38).

Evidence of a possible inherited retinal degeneration was found in another herd in which the condition was diagnosed in a cow and her daughter. The animals acquired the retinal degeneration during the first 2 years of life. Histopathology showed photoreceptor degeneration, retinal thinning, and an absence of inflammatory lesions.

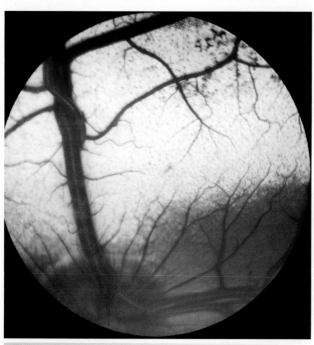

Figure 13-37

Engorged retinal vasculature in a calf with polycythemia secondary to a tetralogy of Fallot.

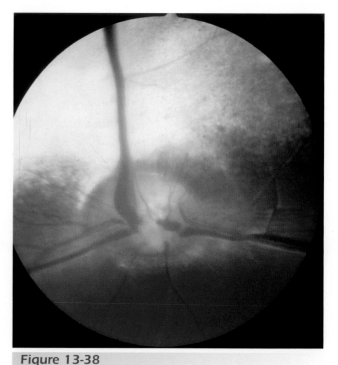

Figure 13-38

Diffuse tapetal hyperreflectivity, vascular attenuation, and peripheral demyelination of the optic disc in a Holstein with retinal degeneration.

Cortical Blindness

Cortical blindness is defined as visual loss with intact pupillary light responses and complete absence of retinal or optic nerve lesions to explain blindness. Diffuse lesions of the cerebral cortex should be suspected. Polioencephalomalacia in calves and adult cattle, lead poisoning, salt poisoning, and severe cerebral trauma should be considered in the differential diagnosis. Other less common causes include severe meningitis in calves and brain abscesses in the cerebral cortex. This latter cause may result in hemianopsia (visual from only one half of the visual field) if the abscess resides in the cerebral cortex contralateral to the blind eye.

One unusual cause of cortical blindness in adult cattle is severe ketosis. Fox and other experienced clinicians have occasionally observed severely ketotic cattle that appeared suddenly blind and remained so despite therapy that corrected acetonemia and reestablished normal appetites. Severe hypoglycemia or other metabolic factors may trigger cerebral cortical dysfunction in the visual cortex in these cows. Fortunately the syndrome is rare. Although treatment usually is futile, low-percentage IV dextrose infusions and corticosteroids can be tried. Table 13-1 lists the rule outs for CNS dysfunction and blindness in cattle, and Table 13-2 lists common ocular disorders in cattle.

TABLE 13-1	Rule Outs for CNS Dysfunction and Blindness in Cattle*		
Disease	**Signs**	**Disease**	**Signs**
Hypomagnesemia	Lactating animals affected first	Plant toxicity (e.g., locoweed, male fern, rape)	Optic neuritis, papillitis
	Low serum Mg—respond to therapy		Retinal degeneration, dry eyes
	Tetany symptoms	Polioencephalomalacia and salt poisoning	Autopsy findings, possibly papilledema
	Hyperesthesia		
	Incoordination		Often normal but variable light reflexes
Hypovitaminosis A	(Calves)		
	Exophthalmos		May progress to seizures
	Papilledema	Prussic acid toxicity	Bright red mucosa, dyspnea
	Gait abnormalities		Plant exposure, numerous animals affected
	Seizure		
Ketosis	(Nervous form)	Rabies	Blindness rare
	Ketonuria		Bellowing, ascending paralysis
	Usually in high-producing cows		Salivation, anesthesia
	Bizarre behavior but convulsions and tetany rare	Sporadic bovine encephalomyelitis	Pyrexia, respiratory signs
Lead toxicity	Muscle tremors of head and neck		Lameness, sporadic occurrence
	Mydriasis	Thromboembolic meningoencephalitis	Retinal hemorrhages, retinitis
	Mania		
	History of exposure		Cold-climate occurrence, somnolence, early death
	High lead levels in blood, kidney, liver, and feces		
Listeriosis	Dummy syndrome and convulsions	Hepatoencephalopathy (e.g., portosystemic shunts in calves, severe hepatopathy in calves or adults)	Dilated pupils
	Head deviation		Tenesmus common sign
	Facial paralysis		Photosensitization may occur with hepatopathy
	Endophthalmitis		
	Sporadic circling	Urea poisoning	
Malignant catarrhal fever	Nasal, oral and ocular lesions	Ruminal acidosis	Fluid-filled rumen, dehydration, acidosis
	Endophthalmitis		
	Deep peripheral keratitis		
	Pyrexia		

Cattle with these diseases may show blindness, nystagmus, strabismus, or nictitans proptosis—especially during convulsions.

Table extrapolated and revised from Slatter D: Fundamentals of veterinary ophthalmology, ed 3, St. Louis, 2001, Saunders.

TABLE 13-2 Common Ocular Disorders in Cattle

Disorder	Signs
Infectious bovine keratoconjunctivitis	Central corneal lesion Unilateral or bilateral Most common in young Resolves in 4-6 wk
Infectious bovine rhinotracheitis	Bilateral conjunctivitis (chemosis with plaques) Nasal discharge Pyrexia Occurs as outbreak Most recover High morbidity
Malignant catarrhal fever	Bilateral Peripheral keratitis Hypopyon Endophthalmitis Pyrexia Low morbidity High mortality
Squamous cell carcinoma	Unilateral or bilateral Affected animals >3 yr of age Painless until advanced Lesions on limbus 80%, lids 15%, nictitans 5%

SUGGESTED READINGS

Allen LJ, George LW, Willits NH: Effect of penicillin or penicillin and dexamethasone in cattle with infectious bovine keratoconjunctivitis, *J Am Vet Med Assoc* 206:1200-1203, 1995.

Anderson WI, Rebhun WC, deLahunta A, et al: The ophthalmic and neuroophthalmic effects of a vitamin A deficiency in young steers, *Vet Med* 86:1143-1148, 1991.

Angelos JA, Dueger EL, George LW, et al: Efficacy of florfenicol for treatment of naturally occurring infectious bovine keratoconjunctivitis, *J Am Vet Med Assoc* 216:62-64, 2000.

Ashton N, Barnett KC, Clay CE, et al: Congenital nuclear cataracts in cattle, *Vet Rec* 100:505-508, 1977.

Barnett KC, Palmer AC, Abrams JT: Ocular changes associated with hypovitaminosis A in cattle, *Br Vet J* 126:561-577, 1970.

Bistner SI, Robin L, Aguirre G: Development of the bovine eye, *Am J Vet Res* 34:7-12, 1973.

Bistner SI, Shaw D, Sartori R: Ocular manifestation of low level phenothiazine administration to cattle. In *Transactions: 11th Annual Scientific Program of College of Veterinary Ophthalmologists*, pp. 85-94, 1980.

Blood DC, Radostits OM, Henderson JA: *Veterinary medicine, a textbook of the diseases of cattle, sheep, pigs, goats and horses*, ed 10, London, 2007, Saunders.

Booth A, Reid M, Clark T: Hypovitaminosis A in feedlot cattle, *J Am Vet Med Assoc* 190:1305-1308, 1987.

Bradley R, Terlecki S, Clegg FG: The pathology of a retinal degeneration in Friesian cows, *J Comp Pathol* 92:69-83, 1982.

Brown MH, Brightman AH, Fenwick BW, et al: Identification of lactoferrin in bovine tears and its in vitro effect on Moraxella bovis, *Am J Vet Res* 35:437-439, 1996.

Carter-Dawson L, Kuwabara T, O'Brien PJ, et al: Structural and biochemical changes in vitamin A-deficient rat retinas, *Invest Ophthalmol Vis Sci* 18:437-446, 1979.

Clare NT: The metabolism of phenothiazine in ruminants, *Aust Vet J* 23:340-344, 1947.

Clare NT, Whitten LK, Filmer D: Identification of the photosensitizing agent in photosensitized keratitis in young cattle following use of phenothiazine as an anthelmintic, *Aust Vet J* 23:344-348, 1947.

Clegg FG, Terlecki S, Bradley R: Blindness in dairy cows, *Vet Rec* 109:101-103, 1981.

Collor JS: Safety and efficacy of Gram-negative bacterial vaccines, *Bov Pract* 29:13-17, 1994.

Cook N: Combined outbreak of the genital and conjunctival forms of bovine herpesvirus 1 infection in a UK dairy herd, *Vet Rec* 143:561-562, 1998.

Davis TE, Krook L, Warner RG: Bone resorption in hypovitaminosis A, *Cornell Vet* 60:90-119, 1970.

Deas DW: A note on hereditary opacity of the cornea in British Friesian cattle, *Vet Rec* 71:619-620, 1959.

Den Otter W, Hill FW, Klein WR, et al: Therapy of bovine ocular squamous cell carcinoma with local doses of interleukin-2, *Cancer Immunol Immunother* 41:10-14, 1995.

Divers TJ, Blackmon DM, Martin CL, et al: Blindness and convulsions associated with vitamin A deficiency in feedlot steers, *J Am Vet Med Assoc* 189:1579-1582, 1986.

Dueger EL, George LW, Angelos JA, et al: Efficacy of a long-acting formulation of ceftiofur crystalline-free acid for the treatment of naturally occurring infectious bovine keratoconjunctivitis, *Am J Vet Res* 65:1185-1188, 2004.

Eastman TG, George LW, Hird DW, et al: Combined parenteral and oral administration of oxytetracycline for control of infectious bovine keratoconjunctivitis, *J Am Vet Med Assoc* 212:560-563, 1998; comment 212:1365, 1998.

Eaton HD: Chronic bovine hypo- and hypervitaminosis A and cerebrospinal fluid pressure, *Am J Clin Nutr* 22:1070-1080, 1969.

Erb C, Nau-Staudt K, Flammer J, et al: Ascorbic acid as a free radical scavenger in porcine and bovine aqueous humour, *Ophthalmic Res* 36:38-42, 2004.

Evans K, Smith M, McDonough P, et al: Eye infections due to Listeria monocytogenes in three cows and one horse, *J Vet Diagn Invest* 16:464-469, 2004.

Fox FH: The eyes. In Fincher MG, Gibbons WJ, Mayer K, et al., editors: *Diseases of cattle*, Evanston, IL, 1956, American Veterinary Publications, pp. 385-398.

Frank SK, Gerber JD: Hydrolytic enzymes of Moraxella bovis, *J Clin Microbiol* 13:269-271, 1981.

Gearhart MS, Crissman JW, Georgi ME: Bilateral lower palpebral demodicosis in a dairy cow, *Cornell Vet* 71:305-310, 1981.

George LW: Clinical infectious bovine keratoconjunctivitis, *Compend Contin Educ Pract Vet* 6:S712-S724, 1984.

George LW, Ardans A, Mihalyi J, et al: Enhancement of infectious bovine keratoconjunctivitis by modified-live infectious bovine rhinotracheitis virus vaccine, *Am J Vet Res* 49:1800-1806, 1988.

George LW, Kagonyera G: Pathogenesis and clinical management of infectious bovine keratoconjunctivitis, *Bov Proc* 20:26-32, 1988.

George L, Mihalyi J, Edmondson A, et al: Topically applied furazolidone or parenterally administered oxytetracycline for the treatment of infectious bovine keratoconjunctivitis, *J Am Vet Med Assoc* 192:1415-1422, 1988.

George LW, Borrowman AJ, Angelos JA: Effectiveness of a cytolysin-enriched vaccine for protection of cattle against infectious bovine keratoconjunctivitis, *Am J Vet Res* 66:136-142, 2005.

Gillespie JH, Timoney JH: *Hagan and Bruner's infectious diseases of domestic animals*, ed 7, Ithaca and London, 1981, Comstock Publishing Associates.

Grahn B, Wolfer J: Diagnostic ophthalmology (orbital emphysema in a calf), *Can Vet J* 36:388-399, 1995.

Grier RL, Brewer WG Jr, Paul SR, et al: Treatment of bovine and equine ocular squamous cell carcinoma by radio-frequency hyperthermia, *J Am Vet Med Assoc* 177:55-61, 1980.

Grimes TD: Retinal detachment with associated intra-ocular abnormality in related Irish Friesian cattle. In *Transactions: 17th Annual Meeting of the American College of Veterinary Ophthahnology and Scientific Program of the International Society of Veterinary Ophthalmologists*, 1986.

Guard CL, Rebhun WC, Perdrizet JA: Cranial tumors in aged cattle causing Horner's syndrome and exophthalmos, *Cornell Vet* 74:361-365, 1984.

Hayes KC, Nielsen SW, Eaton HD: Pathogenesis of the optic nerve lesion in vitamin A deficient calves, *Arch Ophthalmol* 80:777-787, 1968.

Heider L, Wyman M, Burt J, et al: Nasolacrimal duct anomaly in calves, *J Am Vet Med Assoc* 167:145-147, 1975.

Hoffmann D, Jennings PA, Spradbrow PB: Immunotherapy of bovine ocular squamous cell carcinomas with phenol-saline extracts of allogeneic carcinomas, *Aust Vet J* 57:159-163, 1981.

Jeffrey M, Duff JP, Higgins RJ, et al: Polioencephalomalacia associated with the ingestion of ammonium sulphate by sheep and cattle, *Vet Rec* 134:343-348, 1994.

Kagonyera GM, George LW, Munn R: Light and electron microscopic changes in corneas of healthy and immunomodulated calves infected with Moraxella bovis, *Am J Vet Res* 49:386-395, 1988.

Kleinschuster SJ, Rapp HJ: Immunotherapy of bovine ocular carcinoma with BCG cell wall vaccine. In *Proceedings: 68th Annual Meeting American Association of Cancer Researchers*, 1977, p. 85.

Kopecky KE, Pugh GW Jr, McDonald TJ: Influence of outdoor winter environment on the course of infectious bovine keratoconjunctivitis, *Am J Vet Res* 42:1990-1992, 1981.

Ladouceur CA, Kazacos KR: Eye worms in cattle in Indiana, *J Am Vet Med Assoc* 178:385-387, 1981.

Lane VM, George LW, Cleaver DM: Efficacy of tulathromycin for treatment of cattle with acute ocular *Moraxella bovis* infections, *J Am Vet Med Assoc* 229(4):557-561, 2006.

Levisohn S, Garazi S, Gerchman I, et al: Diagnosis of a mixed mycoplasma infection associated with a severe outbreak of bovine pinkeye in young calves, *J Vet Diagn Invest* 16:579-581, 2004.

Marolt J, Burdnjak Z, Vekelic E, et al: Specific ophthalmia of cattle, *Zentralbl Veterinärmed* 10A:286-294, 1963.

Mason CS, Buxton D, Gartside JF: Congenital ocular abnormalities in calves associated with maternal hypovitaminosis A, *Vet Rec* 153:213-214, 2003.

McConnel CS, House JK: Infectious bovine keratoconjunctivitis vaccine development, *Aust Vet J* 83:506-510, 2005.

McConnon JM, White ME, Smith MC, et al: Pendular nystagmus in dairy cattle, *J Am Vet Med Assoc* 182:812-813, 1983.

Momke S, Distl O: Bilateral convergent strabismus with exophthalmus (BCSE) in cattle: an overview of clinical signs and genetic traits, *Vet J* 173:272-277, 2007.

Moore LA: Some ocular changes and deficiency manifest in mature cows fed a ration deficient in vitamin A, *J Dairy Sci* 24:893-902, 1941.

Moore LA, Sykes JF: Terminal CSF pressure values in vitamin A deficiency, *Am J Physiol* 134:436-439, 1941.

Moritomo Y, Koga O, Miyamoto H, et al: Congenital anophthalmia with caudal vertebral anomalies in Japanese Brown Cattle, *J Vet Med Sci* 57:693-696, 1995.

Neilsen SW, Mills JHL, Woelfel CG, et al: The pathology of marginal vitamin A deficiency in calves, *Res Vet Sci* 7:143-150, 1966.

O'Toole D, Raisbeck M, Case JC, et al: Selenium induced "blind staggers" and related myths: a commentary on the extent of historical livestock losses attributed to selenosis on Western U.S. rangelands, *Vet Pathol* 33:104-116, 1996.

Paulsen ME, Johnson LaR, Young S, et al: Blindness and sexual dimorphism associated with vitamin A deficiency in feedlot cattle, *J Am Vet Med Assoc* 194:933-937, 1989.

Pugh GW Jr, Hughes DE: Bovine infectious keratoconjunctivitis: Moraxella bovis as the sole etiologic agent in a winter epizootic, *J Am Vet Med Assoc* 161:481-486, 1972.

Raisbeck MF, Dahl ER, Sanchez DA, et al: Naturally occurring selenosis in Wyoming, *J Vet Diagn Invest* 5:84-87, 1993.

Rebhun WC, King JM, Hillman RB: Atypical actinobacillosis granulomas in cattle, *Cornell Vet* 78:125-130, 1988.

Rosen ES, Edgar JT, Smith JLS: Male fern retrobulbar neuropathy in cattle, *Trans Ophthalmol Soc UK* 89:285-299, 1969.

Rosenbusch RF, Kinyon JM, Apley M, et al: In vitro antimicrobial inhibition profiles of Mycoplasma bovis isolates recovered from various regions of the United States from 2002 to 2003, *J Vet Diagn Invest* 17:436-441, 2005.

Ruggles AJ, Irby NL, Saik JE, et al: Ocular lymphangiosarcoma in a cow, *J Am Vet Med Assoc* 200:1987-1988, 1992.

Saunders LZ, Fincher MG: Hereditary multiple eye defects in grade Jersey calves, *Cornell Vet* 41:351-366, 1951.

Saunders LZ, Rubin LF: *Ophthalmic pathology of animals*, Basel, Switzerland, 1975, S. Karger.

Shryock TR, White DW, Werner CS: Antimicrobial susceptibility of Moraxella bovis, *Vet Microbiol* 61:305-309, 1998.

Slatter D: *Fundamentals of veterinary ophthalmology*, ed 3, St. Louis, 2001, WB Saunders.

Smith JS, Mayhew IG: Horner's syndrome in large animals, *Cornell Vet* 67:529-542, 1977.

Stehman SM, Rebhun WC, Riis RC: Progressive retinal atrophy in related cattle, *Bov Pract* November:195-197, 1987.

Stewart RJ, Masztalerz A, Jacobs JJ, et al: Local interleukin-2 and interleukin-12 therapy of bovine ocular squamous cell carcinomas, *Vet Immunol Immunopathol* 106:277-284, 2005.

Stewart RJ, Masztalerz A, Jacobs JJ, et. al: Treatment of ocular squamous cell carcinomas in cattle with interleukin-2, *Vet Rec* 159(20):668-672, 2006.

Tennant B, Harrold D, Reina-Guerra M, et al: Arterial pH, PO_2 and PCO_2 of calves with familial bovine polycythemia, *Cornell Vet* 59:594-604, 1969.

Van der Woerdt A, Wilkie DA, Gilger BC: Congenital epiphora in a calf associated with dysplastic lacrimal puncta, *Agric Pract* 17:7-11, 1996.

Whittaker CSG, Gelatt KN, Wilkie DA: Food animal ophthalmology. In Gelatt KN, editor: *Veterinary ophthalmology*, ed 4, Philadelphia, 2007, Williams & Wilkins.

Whitten LK, Filmer DB: A photosensitized keratitis in young cattle following the use of phenothiazine as an anthelmintic. *Aust Vet J* 23:336-340, 1974.

Willoughby RA: Congenital eye defects in cattle, *Mod Vet Pract* 49:36, 1968.

Metabolic Diseases

Simon F. Peek and Thomas J. Divers

The common metabolic problems of early lactation, milk fever and ketosis, are really management diseases. At the herd level, disease does or does not occur as a function of how cows are fed and handled during the late dry period and during transition to the nutrient-dense rations needed to support high milk production in early lactation. Because infectious diseases are more effectively controlled by sound immunization, the economic importance of these common metabolic disorders and their prevention by sound nutritional and herd management has assumed ever greater relevance on the modern dairy. Feeding management includes sources, storage, preparation, ration formulation, delivery, and access. Good feeding management must be coupled with providing an environment as comfortable as possible to facilitate maximal feed consumption. In investigating herd problems of excessive metabolic diseases, all these factors must be considered. Individual cows may be predisposed to metabolic problems as a result of improper body conditioning, concurrent illness, genetics, and any other events that may decrease dry matter intake. In addition to calcium, the other macrominerals of relevance in dairy cattle are potassium, magnesium, and phosphorous, and although disorders involving these elements are of far lesser importance than hypocalcemia, they will also be considered within this chapter.

KETOSIS: CAUSES, CLASSIFICATION, AND PATHOPHYSIOLOGY

Ketosis occurs when cows are in negative energy balance. This most commonly happens in the last 2 weeks of pregnancy or in early lactation. In the last weeks of gestation hormonal factors and decreased rumen capacity may cause a decrease in nutrient intake and/or an increase in lipolysis. At parturition the major demand is that of milk production such that negative energy balance continues. Although the volume of milk production and lactose formation is the predominant demand for energy, there is also a secondary (or possibly primary in some cows) lipid demand for milk fat synthesis. It appears obvious to us that our ability to feed cows in

the 2 weeks before freshening to 4 weeks after calving has not kept up with our advancements in genetics for milk production. There are many categories of ketosis in cattle but most involve a similar pathophysiology of lipolysis, excessive release of nonesterified free fatty acids (NEFAs), inadequate hepatic metabolism of increased amounts of NEFAs (incomplete oxidation results in production of ketone bodies), increased fatty acid storage as triacylglycerols in the liver (kidney and muscle to a lesser extent), and, in some cows, decreased hepatic secretion of very low-density lipids (VLDLs). Certain cows with primary ketosis may be genetically predisposed to hepatic lipidosis because of their inability to properly remove triglycerides from the liver.

Pregnancy toxemia is mostly related to an inability to meet energy requirements for fetal development. It is equally common in heifers as multiparous cows and may be predisposed to by twin fetuses. Transient secondary ketosis can be defined as a transient increase in plasma beta-hydroxybutyrate (BHB) caused by a decline in feed intake directly related to another disorder (e.g., left displacement of the abomasum [LDA]).

Subclinical ketosis refers to "clinically normal" cows in the first weeks of lactation that have BHB values greater than 1400 μmol/L or 14.4 mg/dl. Clinical effects can be seen as excessive weight loss, decreased appetite and production, and diminished reproductive performance. Subclinical ketosis may be present in 30% to 50% of early lactation cows in some herds.

Primary clinical ketosis will refer to ketosis in early lactation cows (usually between 1 and 3 weeks in milk, and most commonly in cows in their second to fourth lactation) that are seemingly well fed, in proper body condition before calving, and have no other medical illness. These cows often have BHB levels greater than 3000 μmol/L or 26 mg/dl. Fat cow/fatty liver syndrome refers to the overly conditioned cow that becomes ill just before or at parturition and suffers from marked anorexia, relapsing milk fever, retained placenta, myopathy, and sepsis.

Hepatic lipidosis may take at least three forms: (1) clinically silent in subclinical ketosis, (2) chronic fat mobilization following early-onset periparturient ketosis with an individual susceptibility as a result of either genetics and/or periparturient overconditioning, and (3) periparturient ketosis in the obese cow with massive lipid accumulation in the liver within the first days of lactation.

Clinical Signs and Diagnosis of Ketosis

Primary or spontaneous ketosis is most common in the first month of lactation, with the majority of cases occurring between 2 and 4 weeks of lactation. Cows with either ketosis early (first week) in lactation or cows with persistent ketosis beyond 4 weeks of lactation are most likely to have more marked hepatic lipidosis. Cows with primary ketosis have reduced feed intake of total mixed rations (TMRs) and may prefer forages over concentrates if ingredient fed. Temperature, pulse, and respiration are normal or occasionally subnormal. The rumen in TMR-fed cows will be reduced in volume, have a lower contraction frequency, and also typically have a small fiber mat. In ingredient-fed cows, the rumen may be normal in size but with a large, doughy fiber mat. It is common to hear the heartbeat while listening to the rumen of affected cows. Ketones may be detected in the breath, urine, or milk. Some sensitive individuals can easily recognize this odor. A urine test for acetoacetate is widely available and is the most sensitive test, although specificity is not as high as with milk ketone tests. A color change to purple indicates the presence of acetoacetate (Figure 14-1). The rate and intensity of change are indicative of acetoacetate concentration, but the urine acetoacetate test may be affected by the hydration status of the cow and the concentration of the urine. Many cows with primary ketosis give a strong purple color on the urine test, although the urine of individuals with hepatic lipidosis may only cause a lighter purple coloration. The manure is drier in consistency than herdmates

at the same stage of lactation. Affected cows appear dull with a dry hair coat and piloerection. Neurological signs such as persistent licking at herself or objects, aggressive behavior, and unusual head carriage may be seen with nervous ketosis. The pathogenesis of nervous ketosis is unknown. Inability to rise or ataxia resulting from weakness may be seen in some cows with primary ketosis, and these signs are directly related to hypoglycemia. Metabolic acidosis may occur in some cows and, although unpredictable, can be severe (bicarbonate of as low as 12 mEq/L) in a few cows.

Cows with secondary ketosis have clinical signs related to the primary disease (most often displaced abomasum). Except for metritis, ketosis is rare in cows with systemic disorders such as peritonitis, septic mastitis, and salmonellosis. The urine ketostrips will often be a light purple color with secondary ketosis but may be dark purple if the cow is dehydrated and the urine concentrated. Therapy should correct the primary problem, and the ketosis should then resolve. If the ketosis persists, primary ketosis may be present. A proportion of cows with abomasal displacements will have primary ketosis, which is not surprising because there is a proven association between the two disorders. If BHB is measured and gives a concentration of greater than 1400 μmol/L, this may indicate primary ketosis.

Cows with persistent ketosis for 1 to 7 weeks usually have hepatic lipidosis. Ultrasound examination or biopsy of the liver (Figure 14-2) can be used to confirm hepatic lipidosis, but this is seldom required because the diagnosis is easy but treatment more difficult. Cows with chronic ketosis/fat mobilization and hepatic lipidosis lose considerable amounts of weight, have a poor appetite, but continue to produce moderate amounts of milk considering their poor feed intake (Figure 14-3).

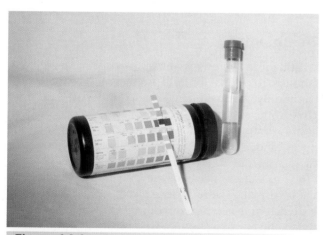

Figure 14-1

Urine ketostrip with urine-positive reaction to acetoacetate from a cow with primary ketosis.

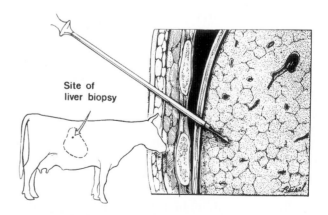

Site of liver biopsy

Figure 14-2

Drawing depicting site and method of liver biopsy in a cow. Neither liver biopsy nor ultrasound is required for diagnosis of hepatic lipidosis in most cows. The diagnosis is based mostly on history, clinical examination, and laboratory findings.

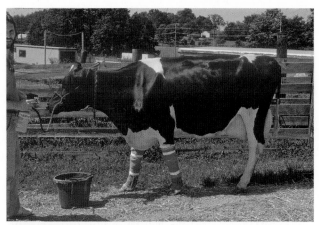

Figure 14-3

A 4-year-old Holstein cow with chronic ketosis, chronic fat mobilization, weight loss, and hepatic lipidosis. The cow recovered after 3 weeks of medical treatments.

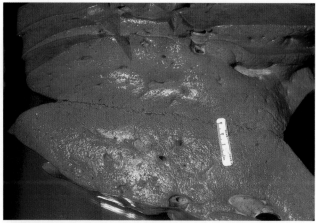

Figure 14-4

Severe hepatic lipidosis observed at necropsy. The liver was from a recently fresh and obese cow.

Affected cows may appear weak, which could be caused by hypoglycemia, muscle weakness from fatty accumulation in muscle, and/or hypokalemia. Some cows may die, be sold, or have complications caused by frequent treatment (e.g., phlebitis from glucose administration, oral trauma from forced feeding). Serum concentrations of hepatic-derived enzymes (aspartate aminotransferase [AST], gamma glutamyl transferase [GGT], and sorbitol dehydrogenase [SDH]) are often elevated, and serum cholesterol is frequently low in cows with hepatic lipidosis. However, these values are not consistently abnormal. Serum cholesterol generally returns toward normal value as the cow begins to eat better.

Cows that are overconditioned before parturition and have periparturient ketosis (although a urine ketone test may be only weakly positive) rapidly develop hepatic lipidosis and have life-threatening illness (Figure 14-4). These cows have recurrent hypocalcemia and recumbency and, because of their heavy weight, often develop fatal myopathy (Figure 14-5). Most of these obese/periparturient ketosis/hepatic lipidosis cows have retained placenta and may die of septic metritis even without a fetid smelling discharge (Figure 14-6). Their predisposition to sepsis with mild to moderate metritis may be caused by excessive fat deposition in the liver and diminished hepatic macrophage (Kupffer cells) function. Affected cows may also develop septic mastitis with repeated episodes of recumbency.

Cows in late pregnancy may become ketotic. This usually occurs with multiple fetuses and is triggered by some other illness or external event that restricts access to feed. Early signs are identical to lactational ketosis. Without prompt treatment, the signs progress to extreme constipation followed by recumbency, renal failure, and death. Cows do not become blind as do sheep with pregnancy toxemia.

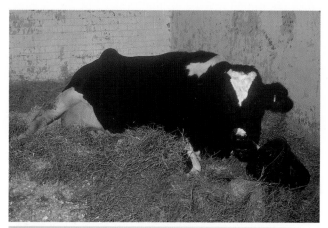

Figure 14-5

A large, overconditioned cow with ketosis and recurrent milk fever that resulted in a severe myopathy. The cow survived but required considerable therapy including flotation.

Treatment

Treatment for ketosis is aimed at restoring energy metabolism to normal for milk production. The three most commonly used treatments are 500 ml of 50% dextrose given intravenously (IV) once or twice, glucocorticoid administration (e.g., 10 to 20 mg of dexamethasone once), and 300 ml of propylene glycol orally once or twice a day for 5 days. These treatments may be combined to suit the needs of the case and the abilities of the herdsman. The propylene glycol should be given as a drench and not mixed in the feed. Full recovery requires the return to normal feed intake, and supportive therapy may need to be continued for several days to allow time for the cow to maintain normoglycemia. Offering a choice of feedstuffs (i.e., brewer's yeast) may

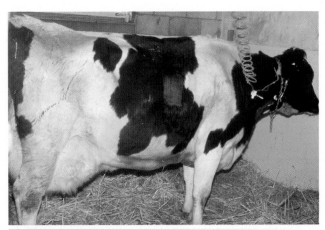

Figure 14-6

An overconditioned, fresh cow with ketosis that died of septic metritis. There was no obvious smell from the rear of the cow, and the metritis did not appear to be severe enough to make most cows systemically ill. The severe hepatic lipidosis most likely predisposed the cow to the fatal toxemia from a relatively moderate metritis.

help in restoring the cow's appetite. Cows with nervous ketosis can be treated with chloral hydrate (40 g orally daily), which serves as both a sedative and as a substrate for glucogenic-producing bacteria.

Cows with ketosis of pregnancy require more rapid intervention to prevent irreversible hepatic lipidosis and multiorgan failure. Induction of parturition or surgical delivery of the calves may be required. Intensive support of the cow with dextrose and force feeding is necessary. If therapy is discontinued in the first few days after parturition, these cows often have serious, sometimes fatal, relapses of ketosis within 48 hours.

Cows with ketosis and hepatic lipidosis or "fatty liver disease" are challenging cases to treat. Cows with chronic fat mobilization and ketosis/hepatic lipidosis are often the "best cow in the herd" and produce a high milk volume. These cows do not get better overnight with any treatment and in fact may have already been treated with the above listed traditional therapy for ketosis for 1 to 3 weeks before veterinary attention is sought. Treatment should include continual 5% glucose administration in balanced electrolyte solutions with 40 mEq of KCl added per liter of fluid. Insulin (200 IU of zinc protamine, which can be purchased from compounding pharmacies) should be given subcutaneously (SQ) every 24 to 36 hours if a continuous glucose infusion is used. Insulin will promote glucose uptake in peripheral sites, which should inhibit lipolysis. Interestingly the mammary gland and brain of the dairy cow do not require insulin for glucose uptake. Another method of increasing insulin concentration is to give 250-ml boluses of glucose IV twice daily. An attempt should be made to prevent persistent hyperglycemia because this will cause

excessive fluid loss in the urine and the hyperglycemia/hyperinsulinemia may predispose to abomasal displacements. Niacin (12 g orally daily) will also inhibit lipolysis and is frequently administered daily to cows with chronic ketosis. Multi-B vitamins are commonly administered (slowly IV) on a daily basis. The most important treatment of cows with chronic fat mobilization and hepatic lipidosis is twice-daily forced feeding. Alfalfa meal, 4 oz of KCl, and rumen transfaunation from a healthy donor cow is our traditional gruel. If these treatments do not appear to be effective after 3 to 5 days, then it may be necessary to reduce the cows' milk production by milking for 1 minute twice daily until the negative energy balance cycle is broken. Cows should test negative on the California mastitis test to qualify for the controlled milking. Usually the limited milking is required for 4 to 7 days before the ketosis is permanently resolved. We have performed this on many cows with chronic fat mobilization, and it, along with previously mentioned treatments, has been successful in all but one case. Additionally, owners have reported the milk production for the remainder of the lactation was very good. Although cows with chronic fat mobilization have delayed time of estrus and their production is diminished during the first 6 weeks of lactation, their prognosis for complete recovery is excellent. Time to recovery is variable, but most cows are well by 6 to 8 weeks into lactation. The most frequent complication associated with treatment of these cows is thrombophlebitis caused by multiple IV administrations of dextrose.

Treatment of periparturient overweight cows with ketosis and hepatic lipidosis is intensive. Affected cows are administered IV fluids to combat hypotension and lactic acidosis. Glucose and calcium are often added to the fluids, although baseline blood glucose levels may be high in some of the cows. The cows should be force fed as described above and have only limited milk removed (if there is mastitis in a quarter, it should be stripped and intramammary antibiotics administered). Insulin therapy can be used as described previously for cows with chronic fat mobilization. Reduced neutrophil and hepatic macrophage function in these cows may allow septic conditions such as even mild metritis or mastitis to overwhelm the patient. Fresh feed, clean water, and salt should be available, and the cow should be housed in either a large well-bedded box stall with excellent footing or in a grass paddock. Along with sepsis, musculoskeletal injury is the most common reason for euthanasia of overweight cows with periparturient hepatic lipidosis. Every effort should be made to maintain calcium levels within normal limits by either slow continuous infusion or SQ administration; ideally ionized calcium should be closely monitored and the cow housed in an area that will provide the best comfort for standing up and lying down. If there has been any difficulty in rising, the cow should be administered flunixin meglumine (500 mg once or even twice daily if needed). The knees should be wrapped with soft cotton bandages to provide protection to the carpus area, which is often the first anatomical site to be adversely affected in cows that have difficulty rising. Although lipotropic medications such as choline and methionine are used by some clinicians for cattle with hepatic lipidosis, their value in the treatment probably is not significant. If lipotropic medications are used, rumen-protected choline is preferred. Electrolyte imbalances also should be addressed should laboratory facilities exist that allows easy assessment of these values.

Ketosis as a Herd Problem

Ketosis can be considered a herd problem when more than an acceptable incidence occurs in the cows at greatest risk—that is, cows less than 6 weeks into lactation. The average incidence in early postpartum cows in a New York study of 35 herds was 15%. Most herd owners would agree that 20% of fresh cows with ketosis represent a herd problem. Dr. Gary Oetzel and colleagues at the University of Wisconsin use an alarm level of 10% for clinical ketosis in well-managed dairies. The underlying circumstances leading to herd level problems with ketosis are not fully understood in all situations, but some specific examples of predisposing causes are known. Ketosis and hepatic lipidosis are closely interrelated. Probably all cows with clinical ketosis have greater than physiological accumulation of lipid in hepatocytes. Some are more severely affected than others. Feeding strategies to prevent ketosis really are no more than generally recommended practices of nutrition and feed bunk management. In many herds with a high incidence of ketosis, the problems originate with nutritional mistakes during the dry period and especially in the "close up" cows, 1 to 2 weeks before calving.

Normal cows undergo a shift in their energy metabolism and its regulation as parturition approaches. There is a decrease in lipogenesis and esterification and a simultaneous increase in hormone-sensitive lipase activity. The process is initiated by prolactin and precedes the onset of lactation. Insulin secretion declines in preparation for lactation. The mammary gland of the dairy cow does not require insulin for glucose uptake, and low insulin would result in greater amounts of glucose being used by the udder for milk/lactose production and less being used via peripheral sites. There is an increase in NEFAs. The normal cow in energy equilibrium will reesterify the serum NEFAs in the liver and resecrete them as VLDLs. When energy deficits occur and NEFAs are produced in excess of liver capacity for esterification, they are oxidized to ketone bodies. This pattern of regulation of energy metabolism may persist until about 8 weeks into lactation, when lipid synthesis is again promoted. The system is also sensi-

tive to "stress," which through sympathomimetic pathways may lead to excessive lipid mobilization and hepatic fat accumulation.

The dry matter intake (DMI) of a cow frequently declines by up to 20% in late gestation to the day before calving. This decline (often from 15 kg/day DMI to 12 kg/day or less for the adult Holstein) in intake is accompanied by an increasing rate of lipid mobilization from body fat stores. The serum concentration of NEFAs correspondingly increases. NEFA levels in cows destined to develop pathologic hepatic lipidosis, when measured in the prepartum period, are above those of normal cows at their peak in early lactation. When NEFAs are measured within 7 days of calving, they can be useful in predicting the incidence of ketosis and, to some extent, displaced abomasum and retained placenta. Ideally NEFA values would remain 0.5 mmol/L or less during this period. The week before calving is the proper time to be measuring NEFAs because their measurement in random cows can be used to determine whether energy balance in the late dry period may be responsible for a high incidence of ketosis in a herd. BHB should be used postcalving to determine level of ketosis, including subclinical, in a herd. Values greater than 1400 mmol/L suggest ketosis, and many of these cows, if monitored and traced back, were only ingesting 12 kg or less DMI the week before calving and had elevated NEFAs. Milk component testing has also been used to monitor energy consumption in lactating cows. A milk fat/milk protein ratio more than 1.5 is considered a risk factor for ketosis. This could imply the importance of the demand for NEFAs for milk fat production. Attempts to decrease milk fat production in early lactation could have beneficial effects in preventing ketosis as long as milk production were not further increased.

Because all cows undergo physiological accumulation of lipid in the liver during the periparturient period, conditions that lead to excessive lipid mobilization are most likely to result in severe hepatic lipidosis and ketosis. Obesity or other diseases that restrict feed intake are both potential causes. Conversely, the force feeding via rumen fistula of the difference between intake at 3 weeks prepartum and voluntary intake until calving reduced the increase in liver triglyceride accumulation from 23% to 16%. Most data suggest that an attempt should be made to gradually increase nonfiber carbohydrates (NFCs) in the last 2 weeks of gestation in an attempt to increase dry matter intake and maintain a positive energy balance in the cow. An additional benefit is an increase in plasma insulin, which inhibits lipolysis. This increase in NFC (to between 34% and 36%) should be a gradual increase such that the cow will be continually increasing caloric intake into the first few days of lactation. Further restriction of intake in the late dry period when a decline normally occurs can be a herd problem. A separate feeding group has been recommended for the springing cows with a diet formulated to greater nutrient density than for early dry cows. Mismanagement of this group has occurred, leading to outbreaks of postpartum ketosis. Dr. Guard describes a herd with a ketosis problem that offered its close up cows an appropriate ration. There were 3 in of bunk space for 15 to 25 cows. The area in front of the bunk was a deep mudhole. In addition, there was an electric fence surrounding the bunk and strung across the top to prevent cows from stepping into the feed. Creating a new 20-m feed bunk away from mud and electricity appeared to solve the ketosis problem. Although unlikely under modern management practices, Dr. Guard also describes simple starvation resulting in death from hepatic failure of about half of the periparturient cows during a 4-week period in a 300-cow herd. The manager was so concerned about fat dry cows that intake was limited to 5 kg of poor quality grass hay. The dying cows were thin with body condition scores of 2 to 2.5, but had severe hepatic lipidosis. The late dry period is not a time to try to get cows to lose weight! Cows that lose condition during the dry period have higher rates of not only ketosis but also of abomasal displacements, milk fever, and metritis.

Ketosis and hepatic lipidosis have been produced experimentally in lactating cows by restricting intake to 80% of recommended nutrients and infusing butanediol, a precursor of BHB. In this model, hepatic lipidosis preceded clinical ketosis. This is not surprising because fatty infiltration of the liver impairs gluconeogenic capacity of rumen-derived propionate and amino acids, which are the two major substrates (55% and 25%, respectively) for hepatic gluconeogenesis. Clinical signs were not apparent in the experimental cows until hypoglycemia developed.

Long dry periods per se appear to put cows at increased risk for clinical ketosis whether obesity develops or not. Many individual cows with severe ketosis that may be refractory to routine treatments have been discovered to have preceding dry periods of 3 or more months. I have particularly noticed this to be common in cows used for embryo transfer. The pathophysiology of this phenomenon has not been described, but many practitioners have made the same observation. Body condition scores greater than 4.0 are known to increase the incidence of ketosis (see Appendix 1).

Undersupply of protein during the dry period and, in particular during the last 3 weeks before calving, has been shown experimentally to predispose cows to ketosis. The treatment group in this study was supplemented with animal source protein to increase the bypass fraction and total crude protein intake. General discussion of this work with nutritionists has suggested that simply increasing the crude protein in the diet of close up dry cows probably has the same benefit as using the more expensive animal source ingredients. If diets higher in NFC are fed to the close up cows this would provide the opportunity to increase microbial protein yield. The minimum requirement for metabolizable protein for close up cows and heifers is 900 g/day. For lactation, this increases to at least 1100 g/day. Lysine and methionine should be adequate and balanced in the diet. Excess dietary protein in any form, but particularly nonprotein nitrogen or readily soluble protein, may lead to herd problems with ketosis. Several outbreaks of ketosis affecting animals in many stages of lactation have occurred following the on-farm experimental addition of urea to the diet. Urea has been added for reasons varying from incomplete digestion of the corn grain in corn silage to just trying something because cows were not milking as expected. In all known cases of urea feeding ketosis outbreaks, recovery was spontaneous when the urea was removed from the diet. Dr. Guard worked with a 200-cow herd that developed about a 50% prevalence of ketosis during grazing of alfalfa pastures. Corrective action included confining the cows to the barn 12 hours/day, during which corn silage was offered with 120 ml of propylene glycol added per cow.

Niacin supplementation has undergone experimental evaluation as a possible means of ketosis prevention and has become popular in the management of individually valuable, overconditioned embryo transfer donor cows that have experienced protracted dry periods. In one study niacin was supplemented at 6 g/day to cows beginning 2 weeks prepartum and continued at 12 g/day postpartum for 12 weeks. Cows receiving extra niacin had higher blood glucose and lower blood BHB than controls. In a second experiment evaluating dose response, niacin was fed at 0, 3, 6, or 12 g/day for 10 weeks postpartum. There was no observable effect of feeding at the 3-g level. Cows receiving 6 or 12 g/day had slightly higher milk production and blood glucose than those receiving 0 or 3 g/day. Despite these observations, the feeding of niacin to prevent ketosis has not been widely used. Cost and the inconvenience of providing a feed ingredient only to early lactation cows have both contributed to the lack of adoption. The most effective periparturient use of niacin may be in herds with a high incidence of ketosis (clinical or subclinical) or in overconditioned periparturient cows.

The use of ionophores in close up and lactating cow diets now provides a strong management tool for the prevention of ketosis. The action of these antibiotics is to reduce acetate production and enhance propionate production by rumen bacteria. Because propionate is converted to glucose by the liver, an increase in its supply would diminish the likelihood of hypoglycemia and excessive lipid mobilization from fat stores. Administration of monensin by rumen-controlled release during the periparturient period decreased the incidence of ketosis by 50% and decreased both BHB and NEFA concentrations during this period. Intraruminal controlled release capsules are more effective than when the monensin is added to the feed. In situations where monensin is fed within a ration if dry matter intake decreases, the concentration of monensin may be too low to have the needed effect on the rumen microorganisms.

No discussion on prevention of ketosis would be complete without considering cow comfort. Adequate space for both feeding and some exercise is critically important for the periparturient cow. Additionally, proper space and environment for resting are critical if cows are expected to ruminate properly. During hot weather, misting and fans should be used to improve cow comfort and feed intake. Frequent pen moves during the late dry period should also be avoided because this has a negative impact on dry matter intake because cows repeatedly establish and reestablish their social hierarchy and familiarity with new surroundings.

HYPOCALCEMIA

Pathophysiology

The normal blood calcium concentration in adult cows is between 8.5 and 10 mg/dl, which translates into a total plasma pool of only about 3 g in a 600-kg individual. It is evident that to meet the calcium needs of colostrum production, fetal maturation, and incipient lactation at the end of gestation (collectively these requirements may reach 30 g/day), adult cows will need to mobilize substantial amounts of calcium from bone and increase the efficiency of gastrointestinal tract absorption. Intestinal absorption of calcium is heavily dependent on the production of 1,25-dihydroxyvitamin D_3 by the kidney in response to parathormone (PTH) secretion. The third component of calcium homeostasis, namely, enhanced renal absorption of calcium, is quantitatively very small in terms of its contribution to increased calcium availability in the transitioning adult cow. Regulation of calcium homeostasis within plasma levels that maintain critical muscular, nervous, and other cellular functions is achieved through the action of PTH. The normal physiologic response to decreasing calcium levels is to produce PTH, which acts to increase osteoclastic bone resorption (direct PTH effect), increase intestinal absorption (via 1,25-dihydroxyvitamin D_3), and enhance renal tubular resorption of calcium. PTH secretion is exquisitely sensitive to small decreases in plasma calcium, but the response can be blunted by hypomagnesemia, partly explaining the well-documented link between clinical hypomagnesemic tetany and hypocalcemia, even in nonlactating cattle. There are several other important factors that interfere with PTH activity at a tissue level that can serve to blunt the individual's ability to respond efficiently to the increased demands of lactation, despite appropriate PTH secretion. Perhaps the most important factor, and one that has been the subject of a great deal of interest and research in recent years, is the role that acid-base status plays. Metabolic alkalosis predis-

poses to both milk fever and subclinical hypocalcemia principally because it interferes with skeletal calcium resorption and intestinal absorption by conformationally altering the PTH-receptor interaction at the tissue level. By altering this interaction, downstream signaling events that should result in increased plasma calcium do not occur despite PTH secretion. The first observations that dietary acidification could reduce the incidence of hypocalcemia by Ender and Dishington in 1971, and the subsequent exploitation of this paradigm by many researchers such as Oetzel and Goff, have led to the widespread practice of anionic salt supplementation to the diets of dry cows as a means by which milk fever and subclinical hypocalcemia rates can be reduced because of relative acidification of cattle in late gestation. It is worth noting that strong univalent cations, such as potassium and sodium, probably influence the development of milk fever via their alkalinizing effects and subsequent diminished tissue responsiveness to PTH, far more than does calcium in the diet during the late dry and early lactational period. Low calcium diets can theoretically be fed as a means of reducing milk fever incidence because prolonged exposure to high PTH levels can overcome the negative effects of alkalinization on tissue responsiveness; however, these prolonged and low calcium diets are impractical to formulate and deliver. A more detailed discussion on cation-anion diets and the manipulation of pH in the transition cow can be found in a later section in this chapter.

There are other factors that contribute to the development of hypocalcemia in dairy cattle, specifically age, breed, and endocrinologic factors such estrogen levels. With increasing age there is a reduced pool of calcium available for absorption from bone as a result of diminishing numbers of bone cells, and this is a reason why heifers, in whom osteoblastic activity is high, do not suffer from clinical milk fever. A further age-related change is the reduction in PTH receptors in peripheral tissues of older cattle. It has long been observed by practitioners that the incidence of milk fever is higher in Jersey cattle than in Holsteins, and although the absolute explanation for this is uncertain, two factors that likely contribute to this breed predilection are the higher calcium concentration in colostrum and milk from Jerseys and the lower number of intestinal receptors for 1,25-dihydroxyvitamin D_3 within the breed compared with Holsteins. Although estrogens increase predictably in the last few days of gestation and this hormone has a negative effect on calcium mobilization from bone, it does not appear to be a significant contributor to the incidence of milk fever nor the severity of hypocalcemia.

Clinical Signs

Parturient hypocalcemia or milk fever may occur from about 24 hours before to 72 hours after parturition. The initial signs are restlessness, excitability, and anorexia.

Many cows at this stage will protrude their tongue when stimulated around the head. This activity otherwise only occurs in cows as a displacement activity when they would rather kill you or run away but cannot. The ability to regulate core temperature is gradually lost. Therefore rectal temperature will be either high or low depending on ambient temperature. Cutaneous circulation is depressed, leading to cool extremities when the ambient temperature is less than 68.0° F/20.0° C. Rumen contractions will progress from weak to absent. Skeletal muscle weakness develops over several hours. Cows may stagger or fall but more commonly are found down and unable to rise. Heart rate increases during the development of hypocalcemia, yet cardiac output decreases as a result of reduced venous return and weaker cardiac muscle. Bloat occurs because of failure to eructate. Death may occur within 12 hours of the onset of signs caused by suffocation secondary to bloat or cardiovascular collapse. Historically texts have divided hypocalcemia into three stages, with stage 1 characterized by the cow still being able to stand, stage 2 by recumbency, and stage 3 by coma and unresponsiveness.

Treatment

Parenteral administration of calcium borogluconate has been the most common treatment of hypocalcemia for many years worldwide. Concentrations of calcium, calcium salt formulations, and other elemental and carbohydrate components within the infusion solution vary widely according to personal preference and the perceived needs of the cow. There is no doubt that treatment with calcium borogluconate solutions IV or SQ leads to rapid recovery of skeletal muscle tone and smooth muscle function in the gastrointestinal tract. Cows often will eructate, defecate, or urinate during the IV administration of calcium, and many truly uncomplicated cases of stage 2 hypocalcemia are capable of standing before or shortly after the infusion is finished. Individuals with stage 3 hypocalcemia may take longer to generate the ability to stand unassisted but are still frequently able to stand within minutes of receiving IV calcium. Cattle that are recumbent on slippery surfaces such as concrete free stall alleys should be moved or slid to good footing. This procedure may help prevent exertional myopathy and other musculoskeletal injuries that are common to hypocalcemic cows that struggle to rise on slippery surfaces.

Serum calcium concentration is normally between 8.5 and 10 mg/dl. The degree of hypocalcemia that develops at parturition is not perfectly correlated with the clinical signs. At a level of 7 mg/dl, most cows will be able to stand but have moderate bloat and anorexia. At a level of 5 mg/dl, most cows will be down. At levels less than 4 mg/dl, most cows will be comatose. A standard 500-ml bottle of 23% calcium borogluconate contains 10 g of calcium. A mature Holstein in good condition weighing

700 kg will have about 210 L of extracellular fluid. If her calcium level is 5 mg/dl, her calcium deficit is 10.5 g. Thus one standard bottle of calcium will increase serum calcium to 10 mg/dl. Most practitioners will give all or part of a second bottle of calcium, perhaps giving it SQ, to provide extra calcium for anticipated ongoing losses. The heart rate normally decreases to some degree during infusion of IV calcium solutions to hypocalcemic cows. A sudden increase in heart rate or arrhythmia that develops during infusion may require slowing or stopping the infusion. Calcium solutions to be administered IV should be warmed to body temperature before administration. SQ treatment alone is inadequate for down cows because of the slow rate of absorption with impaired circulation.

Oral gels and liquids have become increasingly available and utilized by producers for treatment and/or prevention of hypocalcemia. Among the simple calcium salts, only calcium chloride has proven to be adequately bioavailable for therapy of clinical milk fever. Liquid forms of calcium chloride, when given as a drench to down cows, tend to be highly caustic and have caused aspiration pneumonia and death. The use of oral calcium supplements requires functional swallowing reflexes to prevent these caustic materials from entering the trachea such that the severity of hypocalcemia and muscle weakness should be assessed in an individual before their use. Increasingly, calcium propionate has been incorporated into drench mixtures given to early lactation cows that are off feed. A total of 1.5 lb of calcium propionate administered orally provides approximately 140 g of calcium, whereas 1 lb provides approximately 90 g of calcium and calcium propionate has the advantage of also providing an energy source (propionate) and not being caustic. Evidence-based research suggests that the relapse rates and clinical response of true milk fever cases to oral calcium administration compare favorably with those seen with conventional IV therapy. However, personal clinician and farm experience often dictates that IV calcium administration is elected for the treatment of recumbent milk fever cases, but on many dairies, calcium administration to anorectic cows that may only be mildly hypocalcemic has moved completely to the oral route.

In the majority of uncomplicated cases of milk fever, a single treatment is all that is required. Should relapse occur, consideration should be given to supplementing magnesium in addition to calcium. A convenient method for supplementing magnesium for an individual is to use magnesium hydroxide rumen laxative boluses or magnesium oxide for a few days after parturition. Excessive use may cause systemic alkalosis and decrease ionized calcium.

Practitioners vary in their advice of complete milkout of mature cows at risk of milk fever. Partial milk removal may lessen the development of hypocalcemia. However, cows not fully milked out may leak milk and be predisposed to environmental mastitis.

MILK FEVER AS A HERD PROBLEM

The 1996 and 2002 National Animal Health Monitoring System surveys document that the incidence of milk fever in dairy cows in the United States was 5.9% and 5.2%, respectively, for the 12-month periods preceding publication. When the incidence of milk fever exceeds 20% in mature cows, most veterinarians would agree that this is excessive and represents a herd problem. On well-managed dairies, the incidence of milk fever should not exceed 8% in mature cows, and I use this cutoff point as a herd alarm level at the University of Wisconsin. With the changing distribution of ages within modern dairying, such that the proportion of first-calf heifers is much higher on many dairies than was once customary, the relative parity distribution on a farm needs to be carefully considered when judging whether there is a problem with milk fever incidence on any given dairy. The most common age distribution of clinical cases of milk fever is twice the rate in third and greater lactations compared with second calvings and none in first calvings. The occurrence of milk fever is dependent on the nutritional management of cows during the dry period and, in particular, during the last 3 weeks before calving. If practitioners wish to investigate parturient hypocalcemia as a subclinical entity, I suggest sampling cattle of all ages about 12 to 24 hours after calving and using a cutoff of 30% as an alarm level for parturient hypocalcemia using adult cow reference values from the laboratory in question.

Historically, maintaining calcium intake at less than 60 g/day and keeping the dietary calcium/phosphorus ratio at around 1.5:1 was thought to be adequate for prevention of milk fever, but we now know that simplistic approach to be flawed. The 2001 National Research Council (NRC) publication on nutrient requirements states that a 680-kg mature body weight dry cow at 270 days of gestation should receive 21.5 g of absorbable calcium (because absorption coefficients for most calcium-containing feed components are between 70% and 90%, the total calcium amount in the diet on an absolute weight basis is higher than the absorbable value given here), 20 g of phosphorus, 15 g of magnesium, and 52 g of potassium per day (these NRC guidelines are for a standard diet without anionic salt supplementation). These translate into concentrations of 0.45% Ca, 0.23% P, 0.12% Mg, and 0.52% K, respectively. Many diets formulated for dry cows with conventional forages and grains will exceed all minimum requirements except for magnesium. More recent experiences have illustrated that prevention of milk fever by following traditional nutritional guidelines is sometimes impossible to achieve because of high calcium forages and high cationic (particularly potassium containing), and therefore alkalinizing, transition diets. *The maintenance of the late gestation dry cow in a state of mild metabolic acidosis by manipulation of the inorganic cation-anion difference has empirically solved some herd problems with excessive cases of milk fever.* This can best be achieved by feeding HCl containing Soy-Chlor (West Central, Ralston, IA) to the close up dry cows. The amount of the product fed (usually 2 to 3 lbs/cow/day) and its effectiveness can be easily monitored by checking urine pH. After 5 days of feeding this high-chloride supplement, the urine pH should be between 6.0 and 7.0 and it should be maintained at this level until parturition. Other nutritional advisors have approached herd problems by concentrating on the potassium/magnesium ratio in the dry cow diet to achieve similar results.

The two common problems in formulating dry cow diets to achieve a low incidence of milk fever are the farm-specific necessity to feed legume forages, which are relatively high in calcium, and the increasingly higher concentrations of potassium in forages grown on soils either fertilized with potash or those with heavy applications of manure. The latter has become more significant as liquid manure systems have become the norm. Liquid manure storage and handling is considered environmentally sound because it prevents many soluble nutrients from escaping into surface water around the barnyard and is preferred as convenient and economical on large dairies. However, as dairies have expanded and become the sole business of many farmers, the animal units per crop acre have increased with subsequently more manure to dispose of per acre. This manure in liquid form provides more soluble nutrients for plant uptake and recycling to the cows.

Oetzel reviewed the literature on diet and milk fever and found that the incidence was very low at daily calcium intakes of less than 50 g, increased with calcium intake up to about 120 g/day, and then declined at higher calcium intakes. This paradoxical relationship with calcium intake helped refute some of the earlier thinking about calcium-intake restriction being of primary importance. In evaluating these experimental diets, the cation minus anion difference was calculated. Measured cations included sodium and potassium (calcium and magnesium); anions included chloride, sulfate, and phosphate. The incidence of milk fever increased as the sum of cations minus anions increased. The equation most predictive for the incidence of milk fever was $(Na + K) - (Cl + S)$ expressed as milliequivalent per kilogram dry matter. Typical dry cow diets are +100 to +250. Further experiments to test this hypothesis of strong ion balance on calcium mobilization and activity have shown that, when the difference is manipulated around parturition, serum calcium homeostasis is altered. When cations minus anions was negative (around −100) in prepartum diets, serum calcium was increased after calving relative to controls.

Salts used to manipulate the diet of dry cows to achieve greater anionic content include ammonium chloride, ammonium sulfate, calcium sulfate (gypsum), and magnesium sulfate (Epsom salts). These salts are relatively expensive and unpalatable. Their successful use requires that they be fed in a blended diet such as a total mixed ration. Current costs for such diets are U.S. $0.30 to 0.40 per cow per day. Typically they are included in the diet of close up cows due to calve within 3 weeks. In herds without separate feeding facilities for this group, they may be fed throughout the dry period. Anionic salt feeding is discontinued at calving with the effect on serum calcium concentration persisting for a few days. There is a delayed rebound hypocalcemia following the discontinuation of anionic salt feeding. In most circumstances, this rebound occurs several days after calving when the dry matter intake of the cow is adequate to provide the calcium necessary to support the current milk production, and no clinical effects are seen. These salts have been mostly replaced by the feeding of SoyChlor (see the previous discussion on this product).

Some herds have had disappointing to disastrous results with the now nearly outdated anionic salt supplementation. When such disasters occur, there are some commonplace explanations to consider. First, there is the possibility that supplementation has negatively affected palatability to the point where dry matter intakes have decreased significantly. Unfortunately it is not uncommon for overzealous anionic salt supplementation to be instituted in the face of a milk fever outbreak, with the undesirable effect that feed intake decreases dramatically and the metabolic problems on the dairy become confounded by negative energy balance peripartum and clinical ketosis. In addition, there is concurrence that anionic salt supplementation necessitates an increase in the amount of calcium in the diet of close up cows. For example, NRC guidelines specify that under conditions of anionic salt supplementation, the amount of absorbable calcium in the diet should be increased to at least 95 g/day (0.98%). Calcium intakes of up to 150 g/day or higher may be necessary in some cases of anionic salt supplementation to prevent milk fever. Occasionally high chloride content forages will overacidify the diet of transition cows and cause ruminal acidosis.

Because the degree of dietary acidification will be ultimately related to urinary pH, measurement and monitoring of the latter are attractive tools for herd monitoring. Therefore the urine pH of dry cows has been suggested as a parameter to monitor or judge the effectiveness of any anionic salt program. Cows on unsupplemented diets typically have urine pH of 8 to 8.5. The pH may be as low as 5.5 with excessively heavy anionic salt or HCl acid supplementation. There are studies that suggest that dietary cation-anion difference (DCAD) and milk fever prevention is best served by a target urinary pH of between 6.0 and 7.0, although further research on this is warranted. Occasionally practitioners will encounter high urinary pH values (7.0 or higher) in a herd that is supposedly feeding anionic salts. In many

instances, this situation will relate to high potassium content forages, and the solution will be either higher anionic salt supplementation or less high DCAD forages being fed. The role of high potassium intake (greater than 150 g/day) during the dry period has been linked to a high incidence of milk fever regardless of dietary calcium level. It is common to find no supplemental magnesium when investigating such herds. The interaction of potassium, magnesium, and calcium is not fully understood and may be separate from the strong ion effect discussed earlier. Potassium is the major cation in forages and cereal grains. The concentration of potassium in the rumen dictates the transruminal electrical potential. As the amount of ingested potassium increases, ruminal fluid potassium concentration also increases. This reciprocally decreases rumen sodium concentration. The observed transruminal electrical potential increases from about 5 to 60 mV as sodium is isotonically replaced by potassium. The primary site of magnesium absorption in ruminants is across the rumen epithelium via passive carrier-mediated transport. The rate of absorption is inversely related to the transmural potential. The presence of sodium in rumen fluid is not observed to be important to magnesium absorption because replacement of sodium with lithium has no effect on magnesium uptake. Thus high potassium intake also directly leads to decreased bioavailability of magnesium. Supplementing the diet of the dry cow with magnesium in the form of magnesium oxide to provide 1 g of magnesium for every 4 g of potassium up to a maximum of 65 g of magnesium per day has been successful in managing many herd milk fever problems. Alternatively, magnesium sulfate could be fed to address both the K/Mg ratio and the dietary cation-anion difference. Magnesium oxide and magnesium sulfate are relatively unpalatable and must be mixed with other feeds or salt to achieve the desired intake.

Long-term success in feeding cows to minimize the incidence of milk fever and related magnesium deficiencies will be aided by better understanding of the potassium uptake by forage species. Most grasses and alfalfa respond with greater yields when soil potassium is plentiful. Manure storage systems to control environmental degradation return more potassium to the soil. As purchased grains and concentrates are brought to the farm, there is a net accumulation of potassium. As we inadvertently feed more and more potassium to our dry cows, the occurrence of fresh cow problems may be increasing. Anionic salt feeding should be viewed as a temporary solution to a milk fever problem. Other options in devising diets with a healthy balance of minerals are being developed. Land intentionally underfertilized with potash and not manured may be set aside for production of dry cow forages. Some dairy managers are purchasing feed from farms with historically low potassium supplementation and no manuring.

HYPOPHOSPHATEMIA

The clinical relevance of hypophosphatemia in high producing dairy cattle has long been a matter of conjecture and debate among practitioners and academics. Undoubtedly many veterinarians include phosphorus supplementation in either oral or IV form in their therapy of repeat milk fevers and persistently recumbent cattle, but convincing scientific evidence for hypophosphatemia as a contributor or absolute cause of recumbency is lacking. The normal reference range for plasma phosphorus is 5.6 to 6.5 mg/dl, and it is common for anorectic cattle to demonstrate blood levels below this reference range. Measurement of phosphorous levels in blood taken from the jugular vein routinely underestimates phosphorus obtained from the coccygeal vein by up to 0.8 mg/dl (Oetzel, Madison, WI, 2006, personal communication). Mild hypophosphatemia (between 2 and 4 mg/dl) is not associated with discernible clinical signs in the absence of other significant macroelement or electrolyte disturbances. Cattle with severe hypophosphatemia (plasma phosphorus <1 mg/dl) may be recumbent, but the absolute relevance of their hypophosphatemia is clouded by the fact that such individuals are usually hypocalcemic, hypoglycemic, and hypomagnesemic. It should always be remembered that most cows with milk fever will also be hypophosphatemic (cows with plasma calcium <5 mg/dl will typically have phosphorus values of <2 mg/dl) and that IV treatment with calcium alone will be followed by normalization of blood phosphorus within a few hours.

Treatment

Increasingly oral phosphorus supplementation has become an integral part of oral drenching solutions administered to nonrecumbent, but anorectic dairy cattle. The biologically active form of phosphorus is in the form of inorganic phosphate, and any attempts to therapeutically address real or perceived hypophosphatemia should reflect this. Sodium monophosphate is the preferred form of phosphorus supplementation either for oral or IV use. Sterile Fleet solutions are a good source of phosphorus and can be given subcutaneously or intravenously when diluted. Calcium or magnesium phosphate should not be given IV for fear of precipitation. Oral phosphorous supplementation can be given in the form of 200 to 250 g of sodium monophosphate (providing approximately 50 g of phosphate), usually combined with other drench components such as calcium, energy sources, and magnesium.

HYPOMAGNESEMIA

Hypomagnesemia in dairy cattle very rarely assumes the severe clinical presentation with which veterinarians who work with pastured, spring-calving beef herds will be all too familiar. Normal plasma magnesium concentration is in the range of 1.8 to 2.3 mg/dl, but it should be remembered that measured blood values are a poor indicator of whole body magnesium status for this predominantly intracellular cation. Initial muscle fasciculations, followed by hyperexcitability will be seen in cattle whose magnesium values decrease rapidly to 1.0 mg/dl or less, and untreated this will progress to convulsions, tetany, and death as levels decrease still lower. Unfortunately blood levels, particularly in advanced cases in which convulsions and tetany have led to significant muscle damage and subsequent leakage of magnesium out of cells, are an unreliable means of definitive diagnosis. Ocular fluids, urine and cerebrospinal fluid will more reliably determine the antemortem magnesium status of an animal found moribund, or if sampled within 12 hours of death. Magnesium absorption is reduced when the concentration of ammonia or ammonium is high in rumen fluid. The combined effect of a low magnesium and high nitrogen content in rapidly growing grass causes clinical signs of hypocalcemia and hypomagnesemia. The mechanism of high ammonia concentration leading to inhibition of magnesium absorption is not known. Dry cow diets based on ammoniated corn silage or the use of urea as the primary protein supplement may inadvertently lead to secondary magnesium deficiency. The clinical signs of affected cows are similar to milk fever rather than the classic grass tetany of hypomagnesemia. On rare occasions downer cows in early lactation may result if excess nonprotein nitrogen or soluble protein is fed without adequate magnesium supplementation.

It is much more common to encounter milder hypomagnesemia (plasma levels of 1.3 to 1.8 mg/dl) in anorectic dairy cattle in early lactation, and such mild hypomagnesemia is frequently accompanied by mild hypophosphatemia and mild hypocalcemia. Severely hypomagnesemic cattle are also typically mildly to moderately hypocalcemic. The clinical relevance of low grade hypomagnesemia in lactating dairy cattle is hard to characterize; however, chronic, low magnesium levels are thought to limit productivity and predispose to hypocalcemia. Sampling of individual, anorectic cows for a herd issue with hypomagnesemia is of dubious value, but the demonstration of plasma magnesium levels of less than 2.0 mg/dl in the majority of cows sampled within 12 to 24 hours of freshening on a farm should be taken as a problem with magnesium availability or absorption in the transition diet. Similar testing can be performed on groups of cows in early lactation. Because dietary magnesium absorbed in excess of requirements for maintenance and lactation is excreted in urine, a useful measure of herd magnesium status is to evaluate urinary magnesium-creatinine ratios for about 10 cows per group. This ratio corrects for the degree of water conservation by the kidney and better reflects magnesium status than does magnesium concentration alone. Guidelines for target values of this ratio have not been developed by North American laboratories as they have been in New Zealand.

There, average values for a group of cows of less than 1.0 suggest that the cows are magnesium deficient (or would respond with less disease or more milk if magnesium were supplemented).

Hypermagnesemia is rarely encountered, but when it is it usually suggests either compromised renal function or is an iatrogenic phenomenon resulting from the zealous administration of oral magnesium salts to off-feed cattle or both.

Treatment

Treatment of cattle with hypomagnesemic grass tetany represents an emergency to save the animal's life. Maniacal or convulsing cattle will occasionally first need to be sedated before parenteral administration of magnesium. Xylazine or barbiturates, depending on the severity of neurologic signs, can be used. IV magnesium administration is appropriate in such cases, but caution needs to be taken with regard to the speed of infusion because of its potential cardiotoxicity. Elevating serum magnesium from less than 1.0 mg/dl to within the normal reference range in a severely hypomagnesemic grass staggers case will require approximately 2 to 3 g of magnesium. If commercial solutions containing multiple macroelements such as calcium and phosphorus are used, the magnesium content of these should be checked before infusion to verify that there is adequate magnesium present. The infusion should be performed over at least 5 to 10 minutes. To prevent relapses over the next 12 to 24 hours, a further 250 ml of 20% magnesium sulfate solution can be administered SQ over at least four sites. It is appropriate to select infusion solutions that also contain calcium because many individuals will be concurrently hypocalcemic, and the relapse rate appears to be lower and the initial response rate greater in cattle that receive parenteral calcium also. Many practitioners will administer oral magnesium salts as further insurance against recurrence, but this requires that the animal has regained good protective upper airway reflexes and also runs the risk of overstimulation and a return to tetany if used prematurely in severe cases. Undoubtedly, however, oral magnesium supplementation is a safe and effective way to address less severe hypomagnesemia in cattle. Many drenches, commercial or home made, that are used as nonspecific supportive enteral fluid therapy in lactating cows now contain 200 to 250 g of magnesium sulfate. Repeated use of magnesium salts will result in catharsis and elevation of serum magnesium above the normal reference range; however, only IV magnesium administration represents a potentially acute cardiotoxic risk.

HYPOKALEMIA

Potassium homeostasis is a complicated issue in the periparturient cow and one that is impacted by numerous factors including dry matter intake, concurrent metabolic disease, drug treatments, acid-base balance, and inability to accurately measure the intracellular K concentration, which is 98% of the total body potassium. Moderate, clinically occult hypokalemia is an anticipated electrolyte disturbance in cattle that are off-feed for any reason. Normal plasma potassium is between 3.8 and 5.6 mEq/L, and many cattle with common postparturient diseases such as metritis, LDA, or ketosis will have measured potassium values slightly below this range. Severely hypokalemic cows in which the plasma potassium has decreased to less than 2.5 mEq/L may demonstrate progressive weakness and become recumbent. Recumbency may be anticipated when the potassium level decreases to less than 2.0 mEq/L. Typical premonitory signs of obvious muscle fasciculations and increased time lying down will have been noticed by the astute producer, but the progression to being recumbent and unable to stand can be measured in just a few hours. It should be emphasized, however, that severe hypokalemia is a rare cause of recumbency in dairy cattle compared with hypocalcemia or musculoskeletal and dystocia-related trauma. Previously there has been an observed link between the repeated use of the mixed glucocorticoid/mineralocorticoid isoflupredone acetate and the occurrence of the severe hypokalemia syndrome. Retrospective clinical observations have been validated by experimental reproduction of severe hypokalemia and weakness following multiple administrations of the drug. However, it has become evident in recent years that the condition can be seen in the absence of isoflupredone acetate administration. Consistent management and nutritional or other factors in herds experiencing this problem are uncertain; however, many affected cattle have a history of chronic refractory ketosis, or at least repeated treatments for presumed ketosis with a variety of agents that may induce hyperglycemia. Theoretically the repeated administration of hyperglycemia-inducing agents, such as 50% dextrose, propylene glycol, and glucocorticoids, will act to increase urinary loss and drive potassium intracellularly. This intracellular shifting may be exacerbated by the inevitable metabolic alkalosis that accompanies prolonged inappetence in cattle. Cattle with prolonged anorexia may also have whole body potassium depletion caused by inadequate intake in feed, coupled with continued obligate losses in urine and feces. Administration of any drugs with mineralocorticoid action will further exacerbate urinary losses. The clinical manifestation of severe hypokalemia is a flaccid paralysis (Figure 14-7, *A* and *B*) that resembles the profound weakness and flaccidity seen with botulism. Many affected animals are unable to even support the weight of their heads and hence are mistaken for more conventional milk fever cases, but fail to respond to usual calcium treatments and become downers. Aggressive oral treatment with potassium chloride appears to be as, if not more, effective than high volume potassium-supplemented IV fluid administration in correcting the severe hypokalemia. Recommendations include oral administration of up to 0.5 lb of potassium chloride orally

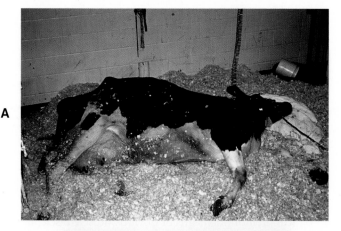

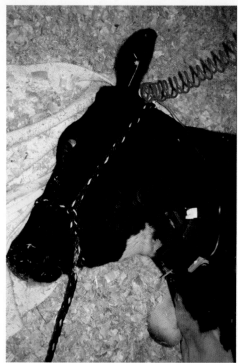

Because of the observed risk of worsening hypokalemia in cattle repeatedly treated for ketosis, it is prudent to consider lower level potassium supplementation to such individuals. Indeed, the inevitably of mild hypokalemia in association with anorexia in the postpartum cow has led to the inclusion of potassium supplementation by many practitioners to cows that receive oral fluids for whatever reason. Low level supplementation in the order of 60 to 125 g is well tolerated and safe when large volume orogastric fluids are administered.

Figure 14-7

A and **B,** Cow with severe hypokalemia and recumbency. The cow exhibited flaccid paralysis manifested as an inability to support the weight of the head or maintain herself in sternal recumbency.

twice daily to cattle with confirmed severe hypokalemia (<2.5 mEq/L) and weakness. Administration of such large amounts of potassium to cattle is inappropriate in all but the most severe hypokalemic states and will inevitably lead to catharsis in the following days. However, clinical experience suggests that recumbent individuals with severe hypokalemia do very poorly unless they regain the ability to stand within 24 to 48 hours of the onset of treatment. The use of devices such as slings, hip lifters, and flotation tanks should be considered, but severely hypokalemic cattle are potentially difficult to manage in flotation tanks as a result of their marked flaccidity.

SUGGESTED READINGS

Bertics SJ, Grummer RR, Cadorniga-Valino C, et al: Effect of prepartum dry matter intake on liver triglyceride concentration and early lactation, *J Dairy Sci* 75:1914-1922, 1992.

Bobe G, Young JW, Beitz DC: Invited review: pathology, etiology, prevention, and treatment of fatty liver in dairy cows, *J Dairy Sci* 87:3105-3124, 2004.

Carrier J, Stewart S, Godden S, et al: Evaluation and use of three cowside tests for detection of subclinical ketosis in early postpartum cows, *J Dairy Sci* 87:3725-3735, 2004.

Coffer NJ, Frank N, Elliott SB, et al: Effects of dexamethasone and isoflupredone acetate on plasma potassium concentrations and other biochemical measurements in dairy cows in early lactation, *Am J Vet Res* 67:1244-1251, 2006.

Curtis CR, Erb HN, Sniffen CJ, et al: Path analysis of dry period nutrition, postpartum metabolic and reproductive disorders, and mastitis in Holstein cows, *J Dairy Sci* 68:2347-2360, 1985.

Dann HM, Morin DE, Bollero GA, et al: Prepartum intake, postpartum induction of ketosis, and periparturient disorders affect the metabolic status of dairy cows, *J Dairy Sci* 88:3249-3264, 2005.

Drackley JK, Veenhuizen JJ, Richard MJ, et al: Metabolic changes in blood and liver of dairy cows during either feed restriction or administration of 1,3-butanediol, *J Dairy Sci* 74:4254-4264, 1991.

Duffield TF: Monitoring strategies for metabolic disease in transition dairy cows. In *Proceedings, World Buiatrics Congress, Quebec, Canada,* pp. 34-35, 2004.

Duffield TF, LeBlanc S, Bagg R, et al: Effect of a monensin controlled release capsule on metabolic parameters in transition dairy cows, *J Dairy Sci* 86:1171-1176, 2003.

Dufva GS, Bartley EE, Dayton AD, et al: Effect of niacin supplementation on milk production and ketosis of dairy cattle, *J Dairy Sci* 66:2329-2336, 1983.

Elcher R: Evaluation of the metabolic and nutritional situation in dairy herds: diagnostic use of milk components. In *Proceedings, World Buiatrics Congress, Quebec, Canada,* pp. 36-38, 2004.

Ender F, Dishington IW, Helgebostad A: Calcium balance studies in dairy cows under experimental induction and prevention of hypocalcemic paresis puerperalis, *Z Tierphysiol Tierernahr Futtermittelkd* 28:233-256, 1971.

Geishauser T, Leslie K, Kelton D, et al: Monitoring for subclinical ketosis in dairy herds, *Comp Cont Educ* 23:S65-S71, 2001.

Gerloff BJ: Feeding the dry cow to avoid metabolic disease, *Vet Clin North Am (Food Anim Pract)* 4:379-390, 1988.

Goff JP: Macromineral disorders of the transition cow, *Vet Clin North Am Food Anim Pract* 20:471-495, 2004.

Goff JP: Major advances in our understanding of nutritional influences on bovine health, *J Dairy Sci* 89:1292-1301, 2006.

Goff JP: Treatment of calcium, phosphorous and magnesium balance disorders, *Vet Clin North Am Food Anim Pract* 15:619-640, 1999.

Hayirli A: The role of exogenous insulin in the complex of hepatic lipidosis and ketosis associated with resistance phenomenon in postpartum dairy cattle, *Vet Res Commun* 30:479-774, 2006.

Head MJ, Rook JAF: Some effects of spring grass on rumen digestion and metabolism of the dairy cow, *Proc Nutr Sec (Lond)* 16:25-34, 1957.

Holtenius P, Hjort P: Studies on the pathogenesis of fatty liver in cows, *Bov Pract* 25:91-94, 1990.

Jenkins TC, Palmquist DL: Effects of fatty acids or calcium soaps on rumen and total nutrient digestibility of dairy rations (Holstein cows), *J Dairy Sci* 67:978-986, 1984.

Kim IH, Suh GH: Effect of the amount of body conditions loss from the dry to near calving periods on the subsequent body condition change, occurrence of postpartum diseases, metabolic parameters and reproductive performance in Holstein dairy cows, *Theriogenology* 60:1445-1446, 2003.

LeBlanc SJ, Lissemore KD, Kelton DF, et al: Major advances in disease prevention in dairy cattle, *J Dairy Sci* 89:1267-1279, 2006.

Martens H, Blume I: Effect of intraruminal sodium and potassium concentrations and of the transmural potential difference on magnesium absorption from the temporarily isolated rumen of sheep, *Q J Exp Physiol* 71:409-415, 1986.

Melendez P, Goff JP, Risco CA, et al: Incidence of subclinical ketosis in cows supplemented with a monensin controlled-release capsule in Holstein cattle, Florida, USA, *Prev Vet Med* 73:33-43, 2006.

Moore SJ, VandeHaar MJ, Sharma BK, et al: Effects of altering dietary cation-anion difference on calcium and energy metabolism in peripartum cows, *J Dairy Sci* 83:2095-2104, 2000.

Morrow DA, Hillman D, Dade AW, et al: Clinical investigation of a dairy herd with the fat cow syndrome, *J Am Vet Med Assoc* 174:161-167, 1979.

Oetzel GR: Meta-analysis of nutritional risk factors for milk fever in dairy cattle, *J Dairy Sci* 74:3900-3912, 1991.

Oetzel GR: Monitoring and testing dairy herds for metabolic disease, *Vet Clin North Am Food Anim Pract* 20:651-674, 2004.

Oetzel GR, Fetmian MJ, Hamar DW, et al: Screening of anionic salts for palatability, effects on acid-base status, and urinary calcium excretion in dairy cows, *J Dairy Sci* 74:965-971, 1991.

Overton TR, Waldron MR, Smith KL: Transition cow management systems in the context of varied dry period length, Cornell Dairy Nutrition Conference, 2005.

Peek SF, Divers TJ, Guard C, et al: Hypokalemia, muscle weakness and recumbency in dairy cattle, *Vet Ther Res Appl Vet Med* 1:235-244, 2000.

Pinotti L, Baldi A, Politis I, et al: Rumen-protected choline administration to transition cows: effects on milk production and vitamin E status, *J Vet Med A Physiol Pathol Clin Med* 50:18-21, 2003.

Pravettoni D, Doll K, Hummel M, et al: Insulin resistance and abomasal motility disorders in cows detected by use of abomasoduodenal electromyography after surgical correction of left displaced abomasum, *Am J Vet Res* 65:1319-1324, 2004.

Rukkwamsuk T, Kruip TA, Wensing T: Relationship between overfeeding and overconditioning in the dry period and the problems of high producing dairy cows during the postparturient period, *Vet Q* 21:71-77, 1999.

Sutherland RJ, Bell KC, McSporran KD, et al: A comparative study of diagnostic tests for the assessment of herd magnesium status in cattle, *N Z Vet J* 34:133-135, 1986.

Vernon RG: Lipid metabolism during lactation: a review of adipose tissue-liver interactions and the development of fatty liver, *J Dairy Res* 72:460-469, 2005.

West HJ: Liver function of dairy cows in late pregnancy and early lactation, *Res Vet Sci* 46:231-237, 1989.

Body Condition Scoring*

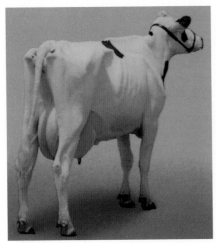

BCS=1

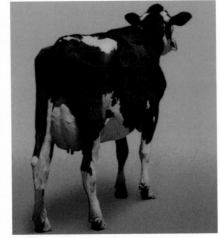

BCS=2

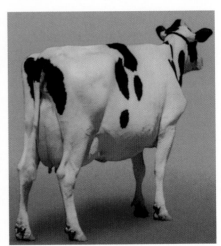

BCS=3

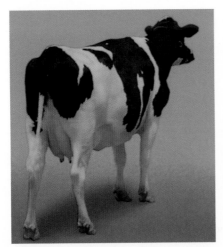

BCS=4

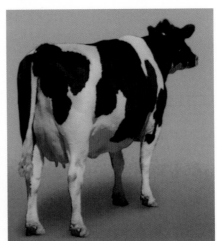

BCS=5

*Courtesy of Elanco Products Company, A Division of Eli Lilly and Company, Lilly Corporate Center, Indianapolis, Indiana 46285, U.S.A.

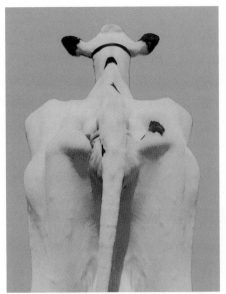

BCS=1

Deep cavity around tailhead. Bones of pelvis and short ribs sharp and easily felt. No fatty tissue in pelvic or loin area. Deep depression in loin.

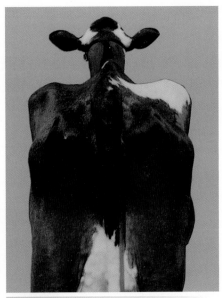

BCS=2

Shallow cavity around tailhead with some fatty tissue lining it and covering pin bones. Pelvis easily felt. Ends of short ribs feel rounded and upper surfaces can be felt with slight pressure. Depression visible in loin area.

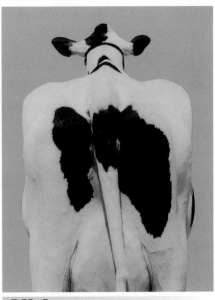

BCS=3

No cavity around tailhead and fatty tissue easily felt over whole area. Pelvis can be felt with slight pressure. Thick layer of tissue covering top of short ribs, which can still be felt with pressure. Slight depression in loin area.

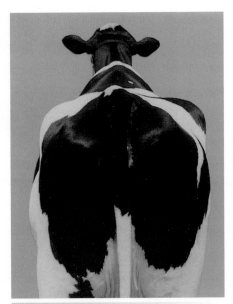

BCS=4

Folds of fatty tissue are seen around tailhead with patches of fat covering pin bones. Pelvis can be felt with firm pressure. Short ribs can no longer be felt. No depression in loin area.

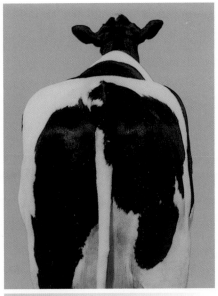

BCS=5

Tailhead is buried in thick layer of fatty tissue. Pelvic bones cannot be felt even with firm pressure. Short ribs covered with thick layer of fatty tissue.

CHAPTER 15

Miscellaneous Infectious Diseases

Franklyn Garry

CLOSTRIDIAL MYOSITIS

Etiology

Clostridial myositis is a highly fatal disease of cattle caused by the anaerobic spore-forming bacteria *Clostridium septicum*, *Clostridium chauvoei*, *Clostridium novyi*, *Clostridium sordelli*, *Clostridium perfringens*, and occasionally other opportunistic *Clostridial* spp. For clostridial myositis to develop, both the organism and a suitable anaerobic environment for its vegetative growth must be present. Therefore muscle that has been damaged by trauma, penetrating or puncture wounds, lacerations, surgical incisions, or intramuscular (IM) injections of irritating drugs or chemicals is susceptible.

C. septicum and *C. perfringens* are normal inhabitants of the gastrointestinal tract of most warm-blooded animals. Therefore contamination or inoculation of muscle with these organisms is by exogenous routes (Figure 15-1). Soil and feces may contain *C. septicum* or *C. perfringens*. *C. septicum* has been identified specifically as the cause of malignant edema, whereas *C. chauvoei* infections are referred to as "blackleg." It probably is easier to refer to all clostridial infections as clostridial myositis because clinical differentiation of the species involved is sometimes difficult, and laboratory assistance is usually required. Malignant edema—implying any clostridial myositis rather than specific *C. septicum* infections—also has been used as a general term for clostridial myositis.

C. chauvoei has the most confusing pathogenesis. The organism survives in soil, but it is not known whether it survives in both the vegetative and spore forms or only the spore form. Ingestion of *C. chauvoei* by cattle apparently allows the vegetative form to proliferate in the gut and then gain entrance to the lymphatics, bloodstream, and finally seed muscle and liver. Having reached the muscle and liver, the organism remains innocuously in the spore form unless the surrounding tissue is injured in some way that creates an anaerobic environment suitable for vegetative growth of *C. chauvoei*. Exogenous infections of muscle also are possible with *C. chauvoei* if soil contamination or inoculation of damaged tissue occurs. Farms and soils that harbor *C. chauvoei* create endemic risk of clostridial myositis for cattle grazing this ground or

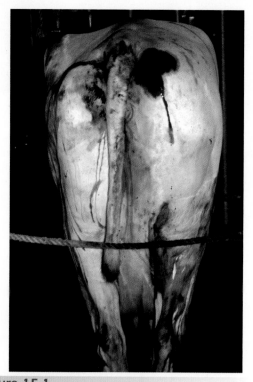

Figure 15-1

Clostridium perfringens myositis in the right hind limb of a Holstein cow subsequent to an intramuscular injection of prostaglandin.

ingesting crops harvested from such soil. Young cattle appear to be at greatest risk for *C. chauvoei* muscular infections, and most cases occur in well cared for animals 6 to 24 months of age. However, we investigated a herd epidemic of *C. chauvoei* myositis that involved several first-lactation cows that ranged between 2 and 3 years of age. The cows in this outbreak had grazed pastures the previous summer, but the epidemic occurred during the winter months and was triggered by muscle bruising and trauma as a result of crowding through a narrow passage created by a frozen doorway (Figure 15-2). *C. sordelli* may have a similar pathogenesis because it has been associated with muscle bruising in rapidly growing beef cattle.

Regardless of the species of *Clostridium* causing infection, toxemia and severe myositis ensue. Clostridial

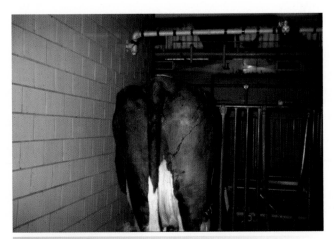

Figure 15-2

Clostridium chauvoei myositis in the right hind limb of a 2-year-old Holstein heifer secondary to repeated bruising of the hind limbs by being forced through a narrow passageway.

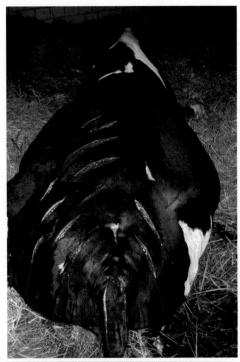

Figure 15-3

Holstein cow with *Clostridium perfringens* infection subsequent to tail docking. Note the extensive surgical fenestrations along the dorsum.

exotoxins promote spread of the infection, are detrimental to host defense mechanisms, and propagate the anaerobic environment essential for vegetative growth. *C. chauvoei*, *C. septicum*, and *C. perfringens* produce alphatoxin, which is a hemolytic and necrotizing lecithinase that is leukocidal and increases capillary permeability. In addition, *C. chauvoei* produces other toxins such as hyaluronidase; *C. septicum* produces beta-toxin (deoxyribonuclease and leukocidal), gamma-toxin (hyaluronidase), and delta-toxin (hemolysin); *C. perfringens* also may produce toxins other than the alpha-toxin, depending on the serotype involved. As a general statement, *C. chauvoei* and *C. sordelli* are linked with highest mortality, *C. perfringens* the least, and *C. septicum* in between. Occasional cases or specific geographic areas may encounter clostridial myositis as a result of *C. novyi*, *C. sordelli*, *Clostridium fallax*, or other species. *C. novyi* may cause exogenous infection or endogenous infections ("black disease") as a result of fluke-induced hepatic activation of spores to vegetative forms.

Regardless of the causative species, most clostridial myositis in dairy cattle occurs by exogenous routes. Any procedure that allows feces or dirt to gain entrance to subcutaneous locations constitutes a risk. Minor surgical procedures, tail docking, IM injections, and neglected wounds predispose to clostridial infections. Tail docking is a relatively new management practice in the northeastern United States, and farmers heretofore unfamiliar with the procedure have been performing it. Clostridial myositis, tetanus, and ascending wound infections caused by other organisms have resulted from dirty tail docking techniques. An epidemic of *C. perfringens* myositis occurred following tail docking of an entire adult herd (Figure 15-3).

Currently the most common cause of clostridial myositis in dairy cattle is IM injections. Frequent use of prostaglandin makes this drug the most common offender. However, it may not be so much the drug itself but the fact that some people injecting a drug do not clean, nor discriminate among, injection sites. Nor do some always use sterile needles and syringes. Therefore while injecting a drug, they also inoculate the IM site with clostridial organisms that are present on the hair coat or skin of the cow, present in their multiuse syringe and needle, or present in a contaminated multidose vial.

Clinical Signs

The signs of clostridial myositis include fever, depression, inappetence, toxemia, and a progressively enlarging region of swollen muscle. Lameness is severe if the myopathy involves limb musculature. Initially the skin over the affected muscle is warm, soft, and may have pitting edema. However, the primary muscle site eventually becomes firm, and the overlying skin is dark, taut, cool, and necrotic. Crepitus caused by gas formation may be palpable in the infected muscle. Soft tissue swelling progresses along fascial planes and ascends or descends, depending on anatomic location. Systemic signs are referable to toxemia induced by the potent clostridial exotoxins. Fever usually is present initially, but some patients may become so ill as a result of toxemia that normal or subnormal temperatures are recorded. Heart and respiratory rates are elevated progressively as the pathology worsens. Signs progress rapidly over a 24- to 48-hour course, and few cows survive after 3 days unless therapy is instituted. The clinical course may be so rapid as to be thought a sudden death. Usually, however, progressive swelling, toxemia, and lameness are observed before death.

Dehydration, severe lameness or recumbency, apparent neurologic signs, and shock eventually appear in advanced cases. Terminally, some cattle develop disseminated intravascular coagulation (DIC) or multiple organ failure.

Recent tail docking, recent dystocia with vulvar or vaginal lacerations, or other wounds may provide diagnostic clues. Recent injections may be suspected by "needle tracks" or be reported in the history.

Diagnosis

Clostridial myositis must be differentiated from soft tissue cellulitis, phlegmon, abscessation, seroma, or hematoma. In general, the progression of signs is too rapid for consideration of abscessation, and seroma is ruled out by fever and toxemia. Hematoma is ruled out by fever, toxemia, and absence of anemia.

Direct means to ascertain the cause of the infection and differentiate the condition from other causes of cellulitis are indicated immediately. The skin overlying the point of maximal muscular swelling should be clipped and prepared for aseptic aspiration. An aspirate usually reveals serosanguineous or brownish fluid and some gas. Gram staining and culturing the aspirate are indicated. Gram staining can allow a rapid diagnosis because large gram-positive rods are easily found. Muscle biopsies also provide excellent diagnostic samples for cytology, fluorescent antibody identification of clostridial species, and culture. Aspirate or biopsy sites do not bleed as healthy tissue would. In fact, incisions into obviously involved muscle ooze serum and serosanguineous fluid, but the blood supply to the most severely affected muscle is greatly reduced or absent. Gram stains and fluorescent antibody preparations provide the most rapid means of definitive diagnosis. Culture is helpful to identify the causative species but usually is completed too late to help an individual patient.

Although generally *C. chauvoei* produces more gas and *C. septicum* more edema (malignant edema organism), much overlap exists in the pathology. It is not possible to speciate clostridial organisms accurately based on the clinical signs they produce in affected cattle.

Blood work is not helpful to the diagnosis because neither a complete blood count (CBC) nor serum chemistry panel offers significant data. The leukogram result is extremely variable in clostridial myositis patients and most often is normal, despite the patient's overwhelming infection and toxemia. Perhaps even more surprising is

the fact that serum creatine kinase and aspartate aminotransferase values are sometimes only mildly elevated. In fact, muscle enzymes released from the region of profound myositis cannot gain access to the peripheral blood because of the self-serving vascular thrombosis and destruction created by clostridial exotoxins. Therefore absorption of enzymes and potassium from affected muscle is prevented by diminished blood supply to the lesion. Necropsy confirms the presence of black, deep red, or greenish red necrotic muscle with gas and fluid in *C. chauvoei* infections (Figure 15-4). Gas also may be present in other types of clostridial myositis, but edema and discolored muscles are the major lesions in *C. septicum* and *C. perfringens*. Serosal hemorrhages also can be observed in many tissues. Dr. John King, veterinary pathologist at Cornell University, likens the odor of affected tissue to the sickeningly sweet odor of rancid butter.

Treatment

Treatment seldom is successful unless the disease is diagnosed early in its course. Penicillin is the antibiotic of choice to kill vegetative *Clostridium* spp., and the drug should be used at very high levels (44,000 U/kg IM or subcutaneously [SQ], twice daily). Intravenous (IV) sodium or potassium penicillin given four to six times daily at the same dose is an excellent choice but may be too expensive for use in cattle. Some clinicians believe it is important to inject some of the penicillin into the region of the infection or proximal to the lesion in an affected limb. Sulfa drugs or tetracyclines also have been used successfully against clostridial myositis infections and were responsible for some of the earliest successful treatment in grade cattle. Systemic antibiotic therapy kills only those organisms that can be reached by viable

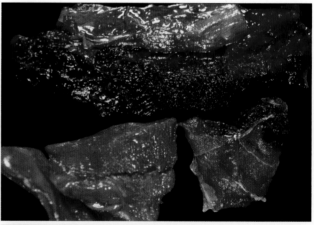

Figure 15-4

Classic blackleg *(Clostridium chauvoei)* lesion in the muscle of a 7-month-old heifer presented for fever and lameness. Two other heifers in this herd had become lame and died the day before.

circulation. Therefore it tends to counteract spread into new tissue but may not be able to attain inhibitory concentrations in the most severely affected muscle because of loss of blood supply in this tissue.

Fenestration of affected muscle with skin and fascial incisions allows direct oxygenation of the tissue and subsequent interference with the anaerobic environment required for continued replication of the organism. Acute cases should be fenestrated surgically and the wounds lavaged with saline or hydrogen peroxide. Extensive debridement is not necessary or indicated in acute cases but may become necessary if the patient survives the acute infection and progresses to a sloughing wound.

Analgesics such as nonsteroidal antiinflammatory drugs (NSAIDs) may be used to aid patient comfort, and judicious dosages are necessary if such drugs are used as maintenance therapy, lest toxic gastrointestinal or renal side effects occur.

Patients that are extremely toxemic or in shock may benefit from IV fluids and a one-time dose of soluble corticosteroids; corticosteroids should not be used repeatedly.

Improvement is signaled by stabilization of the progressive swelling, resolution of fever, reduced depression, and increased appetite. Antibiotic therapy is required for 1 to 4 weeks and can be reduced according to clinical response. Infected muscle frequently sloughs and may necessitate long-term wound care. Lameness may persist in animals that have prolonged wound healing or that suffer fibrosis and contraction of major muscle groups.

Prevention and Control

Client education may help prevent the disease when faulty injection techniques, multiple-dose vials, or dirty syringes and needles are suspected as causes. Similarly instruction in tail docking may be helpful. When *C. chauvoei* is identified as the cause, all young animals should be vaccinated against this organism. Vaccination is highly effective against blackleg and the other causes of clostridial myositis when *C. chauvoei* has been identified or whenever ongoing management conditions may predispose to clostridial myositis caused by any species. Many effective toxoids incorporating new adjuvants are available commercially and should be used according to manufacturer's recommendations because some vaccines now claim effective immunization with just one dose. In the past, with the exception of *C. chauvoei*, most bacterin-toxoids required two initial doses at a 2- to 4-week interval to protect against most species of *Clostridium* capable of causing myositis. Bacterin-toxoids are best administered after passive maternal antibodies have dwindled. If administered at less than 4 months of age, these vaccines should be repeated at 4 months or older. Herd vaccination programs should include an initial primary course and boosters such that animals have adequate protection before tail docking if performed. The preventative value of annual boosters in protecting adult dairy cattle against clostridial myositis is uncertain but makes empiric sense for both endemic farms and those with no recent history of the disease.

BACILLARY HEMOGLOBINURIA (REDWATER)

Etiology

Clostridium hemolytica, an anaerobic organism now renamed *C. novyi* type D, is the cause of bacillary hemoglobinuria in cattle. This fulminant disease results from peracute proliferation of *C. novyi* in the liver, resulting in a large necrotic infarct. The infarct and systemic signs of hemolysis and toxemia are caused by a potent beta-toxin, phospholipase C, produced by the organism.

C. novyi is endemic in some geographic areas, especially moist or swampy areas that maintain a high soil pH (approximately 8.0). The spores of *C. novyi* are extremely hardy and remain in contaminated soil for long periods. Ingested spores apparently are transported to liver and other tissue by lymphatics and blood as happens with *C. chauvoei*. Cattle harboring the organism can shed it in feces and urine but may remain healthy because *C. novyi* is a normal part of the gastrointestinal flora and can be found in the liver of healthy cattle.

Livers harboring *C. novyi* are at risk for converting spores to vegetative organisms if hepatocellular damage occurs. Unvaccinated cattle harboring *C. novyi* can have the organism activated to the virulent form by liver lesions associated with flukes, liver abscesses secondary to rumenitis, septicemia, and metabolic anoxia of the liver, hepatotoxins, and biopsy. Similar to other clostridia, the organism simply seeks a damaged area of liver with reduced oxygen tension such that anaerobic vegetative growth can occur. Vegetative growth is associated with production of potent exotoxins, including phospholipase C, which then induce hepatic necrosis, hemolysis, and profound toxemia. Liver flukes are the major biologic contributor to disease; therefore bacillary hemoglobinuria is more common in some geographic areas than others and is more common during pasturing of cattle.

Clinical Signs

The disease usually occurs in adult cattle. Peracute illness with high fever (104.0 to 106.0° F/40.0 to 41.11° C), elevated heart rate, gastrointestinal stasis, cessation of milk production, loss of appetite, an arched stance, and evidence of abdominal pain ensue. Intravascular hemolysis causes progressive anemia, eventual dyspnea, and hemoglobinuria that appears after a significant loss of red blood cells has already occurred. Icterus also may be apparent. The course of the disease is rapid, with most patients dying in 12 to 48 hours.

Diagnosis

The disease must be differentiated from acute leptospirosis (usually in calves), postparturient hemoglobinuria (fresh cows in phosphorus-deficient areas), acute pyelonephritis (hematuria, pyuria), hemorrhagic cystitis associated with malignant catarrhal fever, and bracken fern toxicity (enzootic hematuria). In certain geographic areas hemoglobinuria and/or anemia associated with parasitemic diseases such as babesiosis and anaplasmosis should be considered, but these diseases do not tend to be so peracutely fatal and anaplasmosis does not cause hemoglobinuria.

Gross necropsy findings are somewhat pathognomonic in that a large anemic liver infarct and "blackened" kidney are present (Figure 15-5, A and B) and

A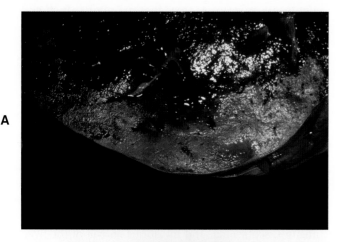

B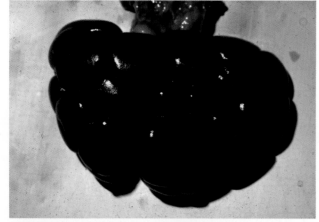

Figure 15-5

A, Liver infarct caused by *Clostridium novyi* from an adult cow found dead at pasture. **B,** Discolored kidney from the same cow with *C. novyi* infection; the discoloration is caused by hemoglobinemia/hemaglobinuria.

C. novyi can be cultured from the lesion. Despite the fact that *C. hemolytica* can be cultured from normal livers, the presence of the characteristic infarct associated with the organism usually is sufficient for diagnosis. Clostridial fluorescent antibody (FA) tests also can be helpful but may cross-react with *C. novyi* types B and C. Toxin identification is conclusive but may not be available.

Treatment

Treatment is seldom successful but should include high levels of IV sodium or potassium penicillin (44,000 U/kg four times daily), administration of whole blood, and IV fluids.

Prevention and Control

When flukes are involved in the pathogenesis of bacillary hemoglobinuria, infected pastures should be kept off limits to cattle, and the animals should be treated with appropriate and approved drugs to kill flukes. Feeding practices that predispose to rumenitis should be corrected.

Vaccination of calves with commercial bacterin-toxoids including *C. novyi* type D are protective if administered twice 3 to 4 weeks apart after maternal antibodies have worn off. Subsequent vaccination boosters should be administered twice yearly to cattle at risk.

LEPTOSPIROSIS

Etiology

Leptospirosis in cattle may be caused by non–host-specific serotypes such as *Leptospira pomona, Leptospira icterohaemorrhagiae,* and *Leptospira canicola* or host-specific types such as *Leptospira hardjo.* Pathogenic leptospira are now divided into 13 named species and four genomospecies based on DNA-DNA reassociation studies, with *Leptospira interrogans* being the most common. The species are further divided into serovars/serogroups and then into strains. The two genospecies *L. interrogans* and *Leptospira borgpetersenii* are most important in cattle. Six serovars have been identified in cattle in the United States: *pomona, canicola, icterohaemorrhagiae, hardjo, grippotyphosa,* and *szwajizak. L. borgpetersenii hardjo-bovis* appears to be the most common serovar of cattle in the United States. *Leptospira australis* and *Leptospira hebdomadis* also have been identified in cattle in Japan.

Leptospira spp. are spirochetes that are considered saprophytic aquatic organisms, and those pathogenic for humans and animals do not appear to multiply outside the host. Infection occurs by penetration of the organism through the mucous membranes of conjunctiva, digestive tract, reproductive tract, skin wounds, or moisture-damaged skin. Hematogenous spread of the organism can result in seeding of multiple organs, including the uterus, and establishment of renal infection. Most *Leptospira* spp. colonize the renal tubules and are shed in urine for variable periods of time following infection.

Many natural domestic and wild reservoirs of *L. interrogans* exist that can shed the organism into the environment of cattle. It is difficult to blame any single species in all instances because most of the serotypes are not host adapted. Dogs, swine, rats, mice, horses, deer, and other wild animals may contaminate the environment of susceptible cattle. Cattle are the maintenance host of *L. hardjo* and appear to be the only reservoir.

Following infection and bacteremia, immunoglobulin (Ig) M antibodies that are agglutinins appear within a few days, whereas IgG antibodies with neutralizing activity appear later. Although agglutinating antibodies help clear the bacteremia, they do not result in resolution of residual renal infection. Non–host-adapted *Leptospira* spp. may persist in cattle for 10 days to 4 months.

The clinical consequences of leptospira infection in cattle include both septicemic and reproductive disorders, but many leptospiral infections are subclinical and detected by serologic evidence or by presence of lesions of interstitial nephritis at slaughter. The exact prevalence of leptospirosis is not known, but serovar *hardjo* infection seems to be increasing, whereas serovar *pomona* infection rates seem to be decreasing. Some estimates suggest herd infection prevalence in U.S. dairies between 35% and 50%, mostly attributable to serovar *hardjo*.

Clinical Signs

Both experimental and natural infections with *L. pomona* have an incubation period of 3 to 9 days. Acute leptospirosis with *L. pomona* is most common in calves but can be seen in adult dairy cattle. Calves have an acute onset of fever (104.0 to 107.0° F/41.11 to 41.67° C), septicemia, hemolytic anemia, hemoglobinuria, inappetence, increased heart and respiratory rates, and depression. Petechial hemorrhages and jaundice also are possible. Mortality is high in calves less than 2 months of age. Adult cattle with acute *L. pomona* infections are septicemic, have high fever and a complete cessation of milk flow, accompanied by a slack udder with a characteristic thick mastitis secretion that is red, orange, or dark yellow in all quarters. Adult cattle may show hemoglobinuria and may abort during the septicemic phase.

Subacute or chronic infections are most common in adult dairy cattle and, unless fever, hemoglobinuria, jaundice, or mastitis appears, may go undiagnosed unless epidemic abortions occur. Abortion usually happens several weeks—on average 3 weeks—following septicemic infection of the fetus, and a cluster of animals may abort within a few days or few weeks. Aborted fetuses characteristically are in the last trimester of pregnancy but can be anywhere from 4 months gestation to term. Calves infected in utero during the terminal stages of gestation

may be born weak or dead. Because abortion follows infection by such a long time, aborted fetuses are dead and may be somewhat autolyzed. It follows that serum collected from the aborting cow usually will show seroconversion and, in effect, be a convalescent titer because the cow was infected several weeks earlier. Certain geographic areas that support *L. interrogans* serovar *pomona* or other serovars pathogenic to cattle have a high incidence of leptospira abortion unless intensive vaccination is practiced. Heifers allowed access to pasture typically abort in late summer or early fall in the northeastern United States. Failure to establish adequate primary immunity in bred heifers that are pastured is the leading management problem predisposing to abortion in this area. A different situation occurs in free stalls, where infection can occur at any time of the year in susceptible cattle exposed to the organism.

Recently *L. borgpetersenii* serovar *hardjo* has been reported to cause epidemic or endemic reproductive problems in cattle in the United States. Definitive proof of a causative relationship between *L. hardjo* infection and abortion in cattle is lacking! This host-associated serovar (*hardjo*) may have a pathogenesis slightly different from other serovars in cattle in that *L. hardjo* primarily infects the uterus and mammary gland following septicemia. The subacute to chronic form of infection is most commonly associated with reproductive problems. Studies have demonstrated that cattle naturally infected with *L. borgpetersenii* serovar *hardjo* can shed the organism in their urine for indefinite periods, with the maximal shed occurring early in infection. Acute systemic signs are possible when the disease is introduced into a herd and include fever, depression, inappetence, and a flaccid udder that secretes thick yellow to orange milk from all quarters. Abortion is believed to occur most commonly 4 to 12 weeks following initial infection of pregnant cows.

Subclinical infection and possibly abortion are most likely in herds having endemic infection caused by *L. borgpetersenii* serovar *hardjo*. Such endemic herds may have resistant adult cows but persistent reproductive problems in first-calf heifers joining the herd. Infertility and early embryonic death are seen with increased services per conception, prolonged calving intervals, and delayed return to heat. The organism is shed from the reproductive tract for several days following abortion and persists in the oviducts and uterus of infected cows for prolonged periods of weeks to months. In addition, the organism can be cultured from the oviducts up to 3 weeks following abortion or calving. Venereal spread also is possible in bull-bred herds.

Diagnosis

For acute infections in young calves showing hemoglobinuria, water intoxication is the major differential. Adult cattle showing acute septicemic disease and hemoglobinuria require differentiation from many diseases, including postparturient hemoglobinuria, bacillary hemoglobinuria, babesiosis, hemorrhagic cystitis associated with malignant catarrhal fever (MCF), enzootic hematuria, pyelonephritis, and other diseases causing "red urine." Seroconversion assessed by comparative acute and convalescent titers is the best diagnostic proof of infection. Although several antibody tests are available, the microscopic agglutination test and enzyme-linked immunosorbent assay (ELISA) are used most commonly. FA techniques or dark field examination also can be used to detect leptospira in urine during acute infections with *L. interrogans* serovar *pomona*. A fourfold increase in convalescent titer over acute titer is considered significant and is even expected with most serovars. Vaccination of cattle generally causes a relatively low agglutination titer (400 or usually less).

Leptospira borgpetersenii serovar *hardjo* does not play by the same rules, however, and titers are more difficult to interpret and quite variable. Titers of antibody against serovar *hardjo* may be low or negative at the time of abortion.

Because aborted fetuses are long dead and autolyzed, they generally are not helpful to the diagnosis. Therefore serology is indicated for abortion epidemics suspected to be *L. interrogans* serovar *pomona* or other non-*hardjo* serovars and serology coupled with detection of the organism in uterine tissue, fluids, or urine in *L. borgpetersenii* serovar *hardjo* abortions. Leptospires or their DNA can be detected by culture, immunofluorescence, special stains of tissue, or polymerase chain reaction (PCR) assay.

Treatment

Acute cases caused by *L. interrogans* serovar *pomona* can be treated with tetracycline or tilmicosin. Because streptomycin has been withdrawn from the market and causes prolonged meat residues, this highly successful treatment in cattle no longer can be recommended. Whole blood transfusions and IV fluids may be necessary supportive measures in the treatment of acute septicemic calves or cattle.

L. hardjo has been treated successfully with a single dose of long-acting oxytetracycline at 20 mg/kg IM, tilmicosin at 10 mg/kg SQ, or multiple injections of ceftiofur sodium (2.2 or 5 mg/kg IM, once daily for 5 days, or 20 mg/kg IM, once daily for 3 days). All have some efficacy in eliminating urinary shedding of *L. borgpetersenii hardjo*. Amoxicillin administered IM at 15 mg/kg, in two doses 48 hours apart, has likewise been shown to eliminate shedding of *L. borgpetersenii hardjo* in urine. Following treatment of shedding heifers with a single dose of amoxicillin at 15 mg/kg, no leptospires were isolated from the kidneys at slaughter.

Prevention

Because treatment of leptospirosis often is unsuccessful, prevention using vaccination is imperative. Whole cell bacterins must be serovar specific for protection to occur. Five-way leptospirosis bacterins (*pomona, canicola, icterohaemorrhagiae, grippotyphosa,* and *hardjo*) are most commonly used. Effective prevention against these serovars— with the exception of *hardjo*—is possible when primary vaccination of calves is followed by twice-yearly boosters. Calves should be vaccinated after maternal antibodies have diminished at 4 to 6 months of age, and two doses of vaccine are essential to establish primary immunity. Boosters are administered at 4- to 6-month intervals thereafter. The most common mistake that prevents effective vaccination is administering a single dose of bacterin to heifers and then not giving them booster shots until 6 to 12 months later, thereby never effecting primary immunization. Effective immunization against *L. borgpetersenii* serovar *hardjo* is more difficult, and only a few vaccines have demonstrated efficacy against *L. hardjo* infections. Monovalent serovar *hardjo* vaccines have been shown to protect cattle from infection, whereas pentavalent vaccines have not. Currently available monovalent vaccines formulated with *L. borgpetersenii* serovar *hardjo* (Spirovac, Pfizer Animal Health, New York, NY, and Leptavoid, Schering Plough, Coopers Animal Health, Wellington, New Zealand) have been demonstrated to induce both humoral IgG responses and cellular immune responses that confer protection against *L. hardjo* infection. Although proven disease due to *L. hardjo* is controversial, vaccination is recommended because other control measures are not available. Isolation of aborting or acutely ill cattle and prompt removal of aborted fetuses may decrease spread of the organism but is seldom a practical means of control. Antibiotic treatment to eliminate the organism in infected cattle should be part of the control strategy because vaccination will not eliminate infection.

TUBERCULOSIS

Etiology

Few diseases of cattle (other than perhaps brucellosis) generate the emotional, economic, and public health concerns that tuberculosis does. The consequences of a positive tuberculosis reactor cow or cows may entail depopulation of the herd and economic ruin—despite salvage and indemnity or compensation available through regulatory efforts. Few veterinarians in this generation have experience with the disease in dairy cattle and therefore have assumed the disease to be nearly eradicated and of little concern. However, eradication efforts directed toward tuberculosis have been hampered by confirmation of the disease in captive *Cervidae*, exotic imports and zoo animals, and cattle from Mexico. Additionally, since 1994 Michigan has recognized bovine tuberculosis caused by *Mycobacterium bovis* in wild white-tailed deer, with the discovery of tuberculosis in cattle populations since 1998. It is highly unusual to have self-sustaining bovine tuberculosis in a wild, free-ranging cervid population in North America, and it appears that high deer densities and the focal concentration caused by baiting (the practice of hunting deer over feed) and feeding may be responsible for this problem. A resurgence of surveillance efforts currently is underway to safeguard dairy cattle in the United States under the cooperative auspices of state and federal regulatory veterinary services. Surveillance programs have been diminished overall because of fiscal cutbacks at both the federal and state levels, but high-risk herds in areas where the disease has been confirmed or where cattle have had contact with infected *Cervidae* or Mexican cattle are still supported. Some states and some milkshed regions still mandate periodic tuberculin testing of all herds producing milk or supplying milk to the milkshed. Coupled with this concern of increased risk for certain cattle populations, the resurgence of tuberculosis in people has raised great concern.

M. bovis is the usual cause of tuberculosis in cattle, and the organism is capable of infecting many other species, including humans. *Mycobacterium tuberculosis* is the causative organism in people and may infect pigs, monkeys, and more rarely cattle, dogs, and parrots. *M. bovis* is very similar to *M. tuberculosis* and can infect cattle, pigs, horses, people, and rarely cats and sheep. *Mycobacterium avium* is a distinct species that rarely infects cattle, pigs, sheep, or humans. All three organisms are acid-fast, alcohol-fast, and gram-positive rods. Growth requirements are stringent, and specific media and laboratory techniques are necessary for culturing. Virulence factors include surface lipids such as 6,6′-dimycolyltrehalose or "cord factor" and other factors. The organism can survive in macrophages, in part as a result of interfering with cellular fusion of lysozymes to phagosomes and therefore are intracellular bacteria. *M. bovis* also produces proteins (stress or heat-shock proteins) that protect the organisms within phagosomes. Metabolic products of *M. bovis* are toxic for neutrophils, and immune responses to the organism eventually recruit cytotoxic T lymphocytes that kill macrophages harboring *M. bovis*.

Infection may occur following inhalation or ingestion by susceptible cattle. Inhalation is thought to be the major route of infection for adult cattle, whereas younger animals can be infected by ingestion—especially of infected milk. Following infection, primary lesions form in the infected organ or lymph nodes draining this area. Therefore inhalation of the organism usually results in small primary lesions in the lung. Because of the small size of early primary lesions, however, these lesions may be overlooked grossly, whereas larger lymph node lesions draining the organ may be more apparent. Lymph nodes may confine or "arrest" the infection for a variable length of time before spread to other lymph nodes and viscera, or generalized spread, which can occur in the most severe cases, immunosuppressed patients, or with extremely virulent types. In resistant host species or in highly resistant individuals, the tuberculosis organisms may be confined for extended periods to lymph nodes. Genetic resistance, mediated through macrophage killing of intracellular bacteria, may play a role in relative resistance to *M. bovis* in many species. Tubercles are the classic pathologic lesions that evolve in primary lesions and subsequent lymph nodes that drain the region. Tubercles result from a frustrated cellular response by the host and microscopically consist of necrotic centers with a halo of macrophages and other mononuclear cells. Calcification is common, and older lesions are calcareous and caseated. In adult cattle, the lesions are most common in the thorax because inhalation is the major source of infection. Advanced or generalized cases can have diffuse lesions. In calves, for which ingestion of the organism appears to be the major route of infection, mesenteric and other visceral lymph nodes usually are affected, and the pharyngeal lymph nodes may also develop lesions. Lesions in the gut itself are uncommon in calves.

Infected cattle shed the organism in sputum, aerosol tracheal exudates, feces (ingestion or swallowing of respiratory discharges), and other secretions, depending on the site and extent of their lesions. *M. bovis* may remain infective for weeks in feces and also persists for days in moist environments or stagnant water. Reproductive spread, although rare, is possible.

Clinical Signs

Infected cattle that have clinically detectable lesions represent the minority of infected cattle. When present, clinical signs are extremely variable and often nonspecific. Loss of body condition and failure to thrive with progressive emaciation may occur in patients with more advanced disease. Classic respiratory signs of a chronic moist cough and thoracic abnormalities on auscultation may be the most suspicious signs but do not occur with great frequency. Lymph node enlargement coupled with chronic respiratory disease may result in a higher index of suspicion. Retropharyngeal lymph node involvement may cause either respiratory signs or difficulty in swallowing or eructation. Apparent forestomach or intestinal obstruction may accompany visceral lymph node enlargement. This is usually painless and may be associated with drainage in advanced cases. Udder infections occur in the minority of cases but, when present, have drastic public health ramifications if infected unpasteurized milk is consumed by humans or animals. Fortunately pasteurization destroys *M. bovis* in milk. Reproductive tract lesions also are rare. Both reproductive and mammary tissue infections usually are accompanied by associated lymph node enlargement.

The majority of positive tuberculin reactors have minimal, if any, detectable lung lesions but are more likely to have detectable lymph node lesions. More frustrating is the fact that some severely infected cattle with generalized lesions may occasionally fail to react at all to tuberculin.

Diagnosis

Routine surveillance through intradermal tuberculin tests of herds for milk market regulations and individual cattle for sale (interstate or foreign) and slaughterhouse inspection of carcasses comprise the major means of detection of infected cattle in the United States. Accredited veterinarians perform intradermal skin testing utilizing 0.1 ml of purified protein derivative (PPD) tuberculin into either of the caudal tail folds. The test is read at 72 hours and interpreted as negative, suspicious, or positive. Any suspicious or positive reactor cattle are retested by regulatory veterinary personnel by means of a comparative (avian and bovine PPD) cervical skin test. Historically, many other tests have been used, but few other than the intradermal tests are used currently. Slaughterhouse surveillance and subsequent traceback has been the primary large-scale diagnostic test. Slaughterhouse inspection, however, suffers from a lack of sensitivity because of the small size of lesions in many cattle. Currently a gamma-interferon test coupled with tail fold intradermal testing is being used in the El Paso milkshed area, where endemic tuberculosis exists in several large dairy operations. The gamma-interferon test detects specific lymphokines produced by lymphocytes in response to tuberculosis organisms.

Because eradication of tuberculosis in cattle remains the goal in the United States, positive tuberculin reactors usually are quarantined, identified, and sent to approved slaughter plants. Owners may collect indemnity for these animals and salvage value. When infection is confirmed in positive reactors, depopulation of the herd is recommended, and traceback measures are instituted to test herds that have sold cows to or purchased cows from the infected herd. Large herds, as in the El Paso study, may undergo a quarantine procedure with removal of positive reactors, at least two negative herd tests at 60-day intervals, and finally another test 6 months later. Unfortunately this procedure does not always rid the herd of infection. The U.S. Department of Agriculture, Animal and Plant Health Inspection Service, Veterinary Services has found that, in large infected herds, up to 40% of infected herds remain infected despite testing and quarantine procedures. Therefore depopulation of infected herds is the

most helpful procedure when eradication is desired. Inherent errors in skin testing constitute the major reasons for failure of compromise programs. False-positive reaction (no gross lesions) may occur in cattle sensitized to other mycobacteria, including human or avian tuberculosis, Johne's disease, and "skin tuberculosis." False-negative reactions may occur in advanced cases, recently infected cattle, desensitized cattle, or old cattle. The current PPD tuberculin test is considered to have approximately 85% sensitivity and 98% specificity. The gamma-interferon test has similar sensitivity and specificity. However, on a herd basis—because of the current low level of tuberculosis—skin tests may have a low predictive value. In infected herds, the predictive value increases. In addition, attention to detail and technique by the testing veterinarian also can influence results.

Many states, including New York, no longer support regular tuberculin testing of all cattle but do require testing of cattle in a "high risk" category. Animals considered at high risk may include herds associated with captive *Cervidae* or those near exotic animal farms or zoos. High-risk herds obviously also include those found by traceback epidemiology from infected herds.

Accredited free states have had no known tuberculosis herds for 5 years. Such states will have this classification suspended or revoked when one or more cattle or bison herds are identified within a 48-month period. Vaccination using Bacillus Calmette Guérin (BCG) as practiced in some areas is not recommended in the United States. Similarly treatment of infected cattle is not allowed.

ULCERATIVE LYMPHANGITIS

Etiology

Lymphangitis of the lower limbs occurs sporadically in cattle. The lesion has occasionally caused a false-positive tuberculin test. Although usually present in tuberculosis-free cattle, the lesion also has been found in infected cattle. The major concern raised by the lesion is the frequency with which affected cattle react as suspicious or positive to tuberculin testing. In the past, such cattle have been labeled as "skin reactors."

Organisms that probably are saprophytic and acid-fast have been observed within the lesions, but classification of these organisms and isolation on selected media have not been accomplished. Intradermal transmission of infection through ground tissue samples has been successful in only one report. The lesions are theorized to develop secondary to front or lower limb injuries that allow seeding of the lymphatics. Affected cattle usually are healthy otherwise.

Similar lesions have been identified in cattle associated with infection by *Corynebacterium pseudotuberculosis*. In these cases, the lesions are restricted to the lower limbs with or without lymph node enlargement. The ulcerative lesions may discharge a clear, gelatinous exudate. Infection of cattle with *C. pseudotuberculosis* can also cause granulomatous cutaneous abscesses, typically located on the exposed lateral face, neck, thorax and abdomen, or less commonly mastitis and visceral infections. Because the clinical signs are markedly different than ulcerative lymphangitis, these will be discussed below.

Clinical Signs

Multiple subcutaneous nodules in the metacarpal or metatarsal region are the primary lesions. One or more limbs may be affected. The nodules ulcerate periodically and discharge pus that varies from serous to caseated. Mild lameness may be apparent before ulceration and discharge as the nodules swell and become inflamed. Lameness resolves as drainage occurs. Over time, the nodules may coalesce or form knotted cords of tissue that mainly is subcutaneous but may have a dermal component as well (Figure 15-6). Other than periodic mild lameness and ulceration, systemic signs are absent.

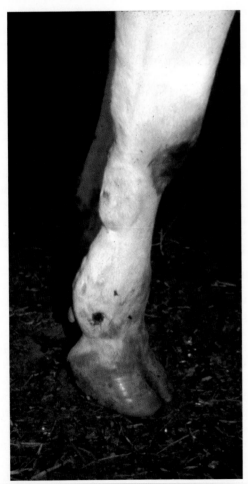

Figure 15-6

Typical lesions of ulcerative lymphangitis involving the right metacarpal area of a Holstein cow.

Diagnosis

Smears of pus or biopsy may allow identification of acid-fast organisms. Culture may be unrewarding, and saprophytic acid-fast bacilli are suspected to be the cause, but in other cases *C. pseudotuberculosis* may be identified. Suspicious tuberculin reactions in such cattle in noninfected herds usually are considered "skin reactors," but a positive reaction may require notification of regulatory veterinarians who may elect a comparative cervical test. Parenteral administration of penicillin or tetracycline may be useful in treatment.

CORYNEBACTERIUM PSEUDOTUBERCULOSIS INFECTION

C. pseudotuberculosis is commonly known as the cause of caseous lymphadenitis in sheep and goats and pigeon fever in horses but seldom is mentioned as a cause of disease in cattle. However, in California and occasionally other areas of the United States, it is identified as the cause of ulcerative necrotic skin lesions in cattle. As in small ruminants, the organism tends to become endemic in certain herds, and clinical manifestations occur as sporadic instances.

The organism survives in soil, the environment, and within infected tissues for long periods. It is generally believed to require an entry site such as mucosal or skin injury, abrasion, or laceration to infect a host. Once through the skin or mucosal barrier, the organism travels through lymphatics to lymph nodes or other tissues. In the horse, *C. pseudotuberculosis* becomes a facultative intracellular organism that survives in phagocytes and also possesses many potential weapons to maintain itself in the host such as an exotoxin (phospholipase D) that attacks sphingomyelin in erythrocytes and capillary endothelial cells. The organism also possesses a pyogenic factor and surface lipids, which may be toxic to phagocytic cells. All of these factors contribute to chronicity and maintenance of host infection by the organism and are well recognized in small ruminants.

In cattle, the cutaneous ulcerative lesions exude pus and are typically located on the exposed lateral face, neck, thorax, and abdomen. Affected cattle do not usually show other signs of disease, and the lesions may heal spontaneously in 2 to 4 weeks, although healing may be enhanced by drainage or surgical debridement. The infection often occurs as a herd problem, and up to 10% of cattle in a herd may be affected. The disease occurs more frequently in adult cattle than primiparous or nulliparous heifers. Spread of infection is apparently enhanced where housing and handling facilities cause abrasion to the lateral body surfaces. It has been assumed that skin trauma and contamination of minor skin abrasions by the organism are causative features of the disease. Affected animals are often culled. The disease has most commonly been seen in dairy cows in the arid western United States and Israel and occurs more frequently in the summer months.

Clinical Signs

Signs in cattle consist of large ulcerative lesions on the sides of the face, neck, or trunk. Necrotic material accumulates in the lesions, and granulation tissue is present deep to the necrotic material. Affected cattle do not otherwise appear ill, although decreased milk production by 4% to 6% may be noted. Sporadic cases may be recognized in endemic herds.

Diagnosis

The lesions must be differentiated from actinobacillosis granulomas, other granulomatous masses, and tumors. Culture confirms the diagnosis, and biopsies differentiate the lesion from tumors and granulomas.

Treatment

Spontaneous cure is common, but some cases benefit from debridement followed by 7 or more days of penicillin or tetracycline therapy.

BABESIOSIS

Etiology

Babesiosis is a protozoan disease of cattle that has been eradicated from the United States thanks to control of the causative ixodid ticks. The disease is also called Texas fever, redwater, piroplasmosis, or tick fever in cattle. Babesiosis may be caused by six or more species of *Babesia* that are divided morphologically into large or small types. The major large species is *Babesia bigemina*, and the major small species is *Babesia bovis*. The disease is seen primarily in tropical and subtropical climates but remains a threat to the United States from Central America and Mexico.

B. bigemina appears as paired pear-shaped bodies within erythrocytes and is transmitted by *Boophilus* spp., usually *Boophilus annulatus*. Ticks are infected by feeding on infected animals and subsequently infect their larvae through transovarian passage. *B. bigemina* continues to develop in the larvae, nymph, and eventually adult ticks, which then transmit the disease to susceptible cattle through bites. Other insects and blood-contaminated instruments also may transmit infection, but ticks are the major vector. Infection is most likely to cause clinical disease in cattle older than 6 months of age because calves are thought to have colostral passive protection or unique erythrocyte protective factors (or both) that protect against infection before 6 to 9 months of age.

B. bovis appears as a single, multiple, or paired complex within erythrocytes. The single and multiple organisms are rounded, whereas pairs may be pear shaped but joined at a more obtuse angle than *B. bigemina*. Erythrocytes infected with *B. bovis* are less numerous and more difficult to identify than with *B. bigemina* infection, and the propensity of *B. bovis* infection to localize in the capillaries of the brain has made microscopic examination of the brain a successful diagnostic test. Multiple *Boophilus* spp., including *B. annulatus* and *Boophilus microplus*, can transmit *B. bovis*, and the larval stage is the major source of infection.

Clinical Signs

Fever, anemia, hemoglobinuria, icterus, weakness, anorexia, depression, and gastrointestinal stasis are frequent signs of *B. bigemina* infections. Tachycardia, dyspnea, and pallor progress as erythrocyte destruction increases. Abortion sometimes is observed. A hemolytic anemia is responsible for intravascular hemolysis and the subsequent hemoglobinuria and jaundice. Mortality may exceed 50%. Ticks are present on affected cattle or herdmates.

B. bovis infections in cattle may be indistinguishable from those caused by *B. bigemina*, but the degree of anemia and hemoglobinuria frequently are less severe than that observed in *B. bigemina*. Relative host resistance and the organism can have an impact on the severity of disease. Neurologic signs, including opisthotonos, seizures, excitability, depression, or coma, are common in *B. bovis* infections and may explain mortality in cattle that are judged to not have life-threatening anemia. Neurologic signs are related to the propensity of infected erythrocytes to accumulate within capillaries in the brain.

Cattle that survive after the acute signs of babesiosis may have chronic disease, remain carriers, suffer recurrent infections, or die from secondary infections. Recovering cattle experience prolonged production compromise.

Diagnosis

Babesiosis must be differentiated from other causes of hemoglobinuria, hemolysis, fever, and jaundice. Therefore bacillary hemoglobinuria, leptospirosis, postparturient hemoglobinuria, toxic hepatopathies, and chronic copper poisoning may be considered in the differential diagnosis. When neurologic signs appear in *B. bovis* infections, differentiation from other diseases of the central nervous system is required. Few other neurologic diseases cause hemolysis and hemoglobinuria, however. Anaplasmosis can lead to similar signs, but hemoglobinuria is absent in anaplasmosis.

Confirmation of babesiosis requires ancillary tests in addition to the suggestive clinical signs. *B. bigemina* is more likely to be observed on Giemsa-stained blood smears than *B. bovis*, but both organisms are more likely to be found in acute infections than in chronic cases. Antibodies against *Babesia* sp. may appear in the blood of infected cattle within 1 to 3 weeks and are sought by complement fixation (CF) or indirect FA tests. The FA test may be more sensitive and can detect antibodies for a longer period following infection than the CF. Brain biopsies also have been used in the diagnosis of *B. bovis* infections but are obviously of no value antemortem. Other serologic tests are being evaluated, but all suffer from a lack of availability.

Treatment and Control

Successful treatment is possible with a number of chemotherapeutic agents. A dilemma exists in that early effective therapeutic intervention that kills all parasites may deter effective immune responses and leave the patient subject to rapid reinfection.

Trypan blue, an early effective treatment for *B. bigemina,* is not effective against *B. bovis* and other small *Babesia* spp. Imidocarb (1 to 3 mg/kg) successfully treats both infections, as do several other diamidine derivatives such as diminazene diaceturate (3 to 5 mg/kg) and aminocarbalide disethionate (5 to 10 mg/kg). Other successful treatments include quinoline and acridine derivatives.

Tick control is essential and certainly, based on the U.S. experience, necessary for eradication of babesiosis. Many effective acaricides currently are available (see Chapter 7). In some countries, tick control rather than complete eradication is practiced in the hopes of maintaining a low level of vectors to effectively immunize cattle but not enough to result in severe or widespread disease.

Vaccines for both *B. bigemina* and *B. bovis* have been used in some areas (e.g., Australia) but are not available commercially and may require judicious use of chemotherapy when live organisms are used. With recent progress toward completion of the *B. bovis* genome project, more effective vaccination strategies combining genomic and proteonomic approaches may be forthcoming.

Tick control or eradication is the ideal control method when possible.

ANAPLASMOSIS

Etiology

A rickettsial organism, *Anaplasma marginale,* is the cause of anaplasmosis in cattle. The organism parasitizes red blood cells following infection of susceptible cattle and is transmitted by ticks, biting insects, and introduced mechanically by blood-contaminated instruments that penetrate skin.

Dermacentor andersoni, other *Dermacentor* species, and *B. annulatus* are biologic vectors that pass *A. marginale* through their eggs into the next generation of ticks. Other ticks, tabanids, and mosquitoes may be mechanical vectors of the disease as they inject blood from infected cattle to susceptible cattle while feeding. Needles and veterinary instruments that become contaminated with blood during herd-wide procedures can transmit the infection. Similarly, blood-contaminated instruments used for reproductive work such as infusion cannulas, embryo transfer instruments, and insemination equipment occasionally can spread the infection.

Chronically infected cattle that usually are asymptomatic act as reservoirs of anaplasmosis, and spread of the disease tends to occur during peak vector seasons or following common surgical procedures that result in iatrogenic spread.

Cattle less than 1 year of age tend to either be resistant to infection or have very mild signs of illness. The opposite is true for adult cattle because susceptible animals more than 2 years of age often have severe illness and possible high mortality. The resistance of young animals to infection may be explained partially by passive antibodies obtained from colostrum. However, other factors appear to be important because infection in susceptible cattle up to 1 to 2 years typically results in mild signs, if any, whereas infection of susceptible cattle older than 2 years frequently causes acute, severe disease. In addition, sources of stress such as shipment, starvation, weather extremes, and experimental splenectomy apparently can overcome the natural resistance of young cattle to anaplasmosis, thereby resulting in acute disease.

Natural infection of young cattle results in a carrier state that may persist for the life of the animal. A biologic balance appears necessary to maintain immunity because clearing of infection eventually may allow susceptibility to reinfection. Seroconversion may occur despite the chronic carrier state, although it does not occur in all infected carrier cattle. Protective immunity requires both humoral and cellular immune components, including antibody against the outer cell membrane plus macrophage activation. The immune response can clear the acute rickettsemia but fail to completely clear the infection because of development of antigenic variants of the agent. Seropositive cattle are assumed to be carriers. Seronegative cattle in endemic areas are more difficult to categorize and the subject of much research. Further confusion is added by studies that demonstrate acquired immunity to clinical disease persisting following clearance of infection by chemotherapy. This immunity following chemotherapy with imidocarb or tetracycline persisted regardless of seropositive or seronegative status of the treated cattle. However, in endemic regions harboring anaplasmosis, seronegative cattle within *A. marginale*-infected herds appear susceptible to infection and illness. Therefore seronegative cows in positive herds have not necessarily developed effective immunity even if they had been seropositive previously and naturally cleared the infection later. Relative exposure rate, concurrent stresses, vector loads, and length of time between clearance of infection and subsequent reinfection all may influence the susceptibility of seronegative cattle that once had been seropositive.

Clinical Signs

As previously stated, the likelihood of clinical illness associated with *A. marginale* infection is typically proportional to the age of the susceptible animal. Exceptions do occur, especially when extraordinary stress, heavy infective doses, heavy vector parasitism, or concurrent diseases overwhelm the apparent resistance in younger cattle. Many, if not most, animals less than 1 year of age have inapparent infection or very mild signs. Incubation in natural infection ranges from 20 to 40 days and is followed by acute disease characterized by dramatic signs of fever (104.0 to 107.0° F/40.0 to 41.7° C), depression, anorexia, gastrointestinal stasis, anemia, dehydration, and cessation of milk flow. The severity of clinical signs is proportional to the degree of anemia. Icterus is present in many acute cases but may not appear unless the affected animal survives 2 or more days. Hemoglobinuria *does not* occur. Hemolysis results from erythrocyte destruction by the reticuloendothelial system and therefore is primarily extravascular. Mortality varies but may reach 50% in acute cases. Infected cattle that survive acute signs may remain weak, anemic, jaundiced, and lose significant condition. Susceptible adult cattle introduced into endemic herds may suffer peracute signs and die within 1 to 2 days after onset of signs. Infected animals are assumed to remain carriers of the organism regardless of the degree of subsequent seropositive status. Recovery from acute disease may require weeks. Abortion may occur during the acute or convalescent period.

Diagnosis

The CF and rapid card agglutination tests are the most common means of confirmation of infection but may not become positive until 1 week following acute infection. These same serologic tests are very useful to detect chronic carrier cattle that may be free of clinical signs. Diagnosis in acute cases is aided by ancillary tests that verify the severe anemia (low packed cell volume and regenerative) and also rule out liver disease as a cause of jaundice. Microscopic examination of whole blood smears stained by Wright's, new methylene blue, or Giemsa stains may allow identification of *A. marginale* in erythrocytes (Figure 15-7). The organisms appear as one or more spherical bodies in the periphery of erythrocytes and must be differentiated from basophilic stippling and Howell-Jolly bodies. PCR and competitive ELISA are newer and more sensitive tests and should be used to help determine infection and clearance of infection following treatment.

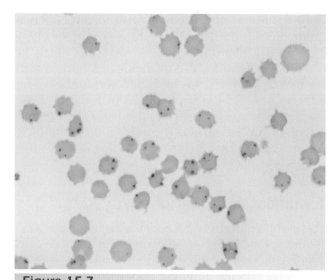

Figure 15-7

Wright's stain of blood from a heifer with *Anaplasmosis marginale*. The organism can be seen at the margin of several erythrocytes.

Treatment

Treatment with several chemotherapeutic agents is possible but inconsistently effective in clearing the organism. The most current recommendations in North America indicate oxytetracycline to be the treatment of choice. In Europe the fluoroquinolones could be used. A variety of tetracyclines can be used, and intensity of treatment may dictate whether the organism is eliminated or simply reduced in number within the host. Imidocarb dipropionate (5.0 mg/kg IM in two doses at 14-day intervals) will sterilize infected cattle, but this drug is not used in cattle in North America. Long-acting tetracycline (20 mg/kg IM—four times at 3-day intervals; Liquamycin LA 200, Pfizer, Inc., Animal Health Division) also eliminates the infection in some calves. Lesser numbers of injections of this same long-acting tetracycline may control acute infections but not eliminate the organism completely. Cattle cleared of infection may eventually be susceptible to infection again. Whole blood transfusions also may be necessary when anemia is judged to be life-threatening in acutely infected cattle.

Acaricides and fly control measures always are indicated to reduce the vector population as much as possible. These chemicals must be applied or utilized in approved manners as regards dairy cattle.

Prevention

When the incidence of infection is low, elimination of infection in acute and asymptomatic carrier cattle (as evidenced by seropositivity) coupled with insect control may allow effective control. Endemic herds or geographic regions present a more difficult challenge for control measures. In addition to vector control and treatment measures, husbandry practices must be modified. Stress should be minimized; animals from nonendemic areas should not be introduced to the herd; and common use of instruments for veterinary procedures, blood collection, and ear tagging should be avoided unless disinfected between animals. Vaccinations have been used but require care because currently none are completely free of problems. In the United States, a killed product has been utilized, and this product is formulated from infected erythrocytes. Therefore anti–red blood cell antibodies may develop in vaccinated cattle and predispose to neonatal isoerythrolysis in calves born to vaccinated cows receiving the recommended yearly boosters. Administration of boosters should not be performed during late gestation. Live vaccines are commonly used in many countries including Australia and countries in Central and South America but are not licensed in the United States because of concerns about pathogen transmission from blood-based vaccines. A product approved in California consists of modified live irradiated *A. marginale* organisms and is administered to calves less than 1 year of age to cause immunity associated with persistent infection. This vaccine may cause disease if administered to older animals. Recently another purified vaccine has been introduced and is available in the United States. This vaccine is reported to minimize the potential for neonatal isoerythrolysis in calves suckling colostrum from vaccinated dams (Am-Vax, Schering-Plough Animal Health, Kenilworth, NJ).

Continued advances in vaccine technology hold the best hope for future control of anaplasmosis in cattle.

EPERYTHROZOONOSIS (MYCOPLASMOSIS)

Etiology

Disease is caused by *Eperythrozoon wenyonii*, rickettsial organisms, which are obligate parasites of erythrocytes. The hemotrophic rickettsial species of the genus *Eperythrozoon* have recently been reclassified to the genus *Mycoplasma* based on 16S ribosomal RNA gene sequence analysis, but the former name is also used here for recognition. It appears that infection of cattle with the parasite is common because cattle splenectomized for experimental purposes commonly show parasitemia after the splenectomy. However, naturally occurring disease is uncommon, and experimental attempts to reproduce the problem by transfusion of whole blood from infected to apparently uninfected cattle have failed. Clinical disease occurs primarily in dairy heifers in early to mid-lactation and typically in the summer months, suggesting that there are susceptibility features of particular animals, but these have not been identified.

Clinical Signs

The syndrome in dairy heifers occurs with swollen teats and distal hind limbs, fever, prefemoral lymph node enlargement, decreased milk production, and mild weight loss. The disease is transient, and acute clinical signs resolve in 7 to 10 days. Most commonly the disease occurs in individual animals in a herd, but as small outbreaks with multiple cattle affected over time. A similar problem has been seen in young bulls, characterized by scrotal and hind limb edema and infertility. These signs are associated with large numbers of *Mycoplasma wenyonii* seen in blood smears, and the signs resolve as parasitemia declines. The severe anemia and hemolytic problems identified in swine and sheep with *Mycoplasma (Eperythrozoon)* infection have not been identified in the naturally occurring syndrome seen in cattle.

Diagnosis

Diagnosis is achieved by identifying typical clinical signs in dairy heifers in early to mid-lactation, followed by identification of the parasite in dried blood smears (Figure 15-8).

Treatment

Many animals that have remission of signs will also experience a decline in parasitemia to undetectable levels over 7 to 14 days. Alternatively, a good response with

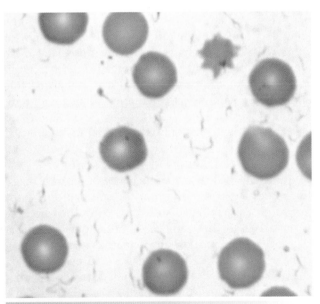

Figure 15-8

Eperythrozoon organisms in a blood smear of a heifer from a herd with multiple heifers having swollen legs. The organisms are harder to see and more centrally located than with *Anaplasma*.

rapid clearance of the organism and resolution of signs will follow a single dose of parenteral oxytetracycline.

TICKBORNE FEVER

Anaplasma phagocytophilum is the causative agent of tickborne fever. Although the organism is present in *Ixodes* spp. ticks in several areas of the United States, to our knowledge clinical disease in cattle has not been reported in North America. Fever, leukopenia, thrombocytopenia, abortions, ataxia, decreased production, and increased susceptibility to other infections have been reported in cattle in other parts of the world. Observation of the morula within white blood cells or detection of DNA in the blood by PCR is the preferred diagnostic test. Although the infection is generally self-limiting, oxytetracycline therapy would be expected to shorten the clinical course.

ANTHRAX

Etiology

Bacillus anthracis, a large gram-positive rod, causes anthrax in humans and animals. Vegetative growth in culture media is characterized by chain formation of tightly packed rods ("Medusa-head" colonies), whereas in vivo growth differs by having short chains, rounded ends to the rods, and well-formed capsules that may surround several cells. The organism is a spore-former but usually only develops spores when growing aerobically at 15.0 to 40.0° C rather than in vivo. The spores are extremely hardy and may survive in dry alkaline soils that contain high nitrogen levels for decades or more. Therefore discharges or tissue from fatal cases contaminate soils and allow the organism to remain in certain geographic pockets where the disease occurs sporadically. Rain or wet conditions coupled with temperatures greater than 15.5° C foster germination and vegetative growth that subsequently result in sporulation as dryness returns to contaminated soil. Most clinical cases occur during the grazing season.

Cattle exposed to contaminated ground may ingest the spores either directly from the soil or from plants grown on contaminated soil. The spores then become vegetative in the host. Abrasions of the oral mucosa or digestive tract may allow an edematous localized infection, which then seeds lymphatics and eventually results in bacteremia. Localized infections may occur subsequent to skin wounds and have been called "malignant carbuncle" in people. Inhalation of spores is a less common means of infection but can occur in people ("woolsorter's disease") or animals and often is fatal. Animal byproducts such as hides, slaughterhouse material, and bone meals from endemic areas may harbor the organism or spores and represent dangers to people and animals exposed to these tissues. Insects that feed on blood also may transmit the infection.

Virulence of *B. anthracis* is caused by a polyglutamic acid capsule that deters phagocytosis and lysis and a potent toxin consisting of an edema factor, a protective antigen, and a lethal factor. These three factors working together frequently form a lethal combination because they kill phagocytic cells, damage capillaries, and interfere with clotting of blood. A vicious cycle of capillary permeability, thrombosis, and tissue edema evolves.

Clinical Signs

Peracute *B. anthracis* infection in cattle may result in death so rapid as to be thought to be sudden and thus confused with other causes of sudden death such as lightning, fatal internal hemorrhage, clostridial myositis, bloat, or metabolic conditions. Blood-tinged or dark reddish-black sanguineous discharges from body orifices are common in cattle dying from acute anthrax and may lead to confusion with death resulting from caudal vena caval thrombosis, bleeding abomasal ulcers, jejunal hemorrhage syndrome, arsenic poisoning, or peracute salmonellosis.

Acute anthrax causes fever, complete loss of appetite and production, depression, and evidence of blood in most body secretions, including feces, urine, milk, and nasal discharge. Tachycardia, dyspnea, and possible neurologic signs also are present. Unless treated with intense therapy very early in the course of the disease, affected cattle become recumbent within 1 to 2 days and die. Whenever anthrax is suspected based on signs (or lack thereof) and sanguineous discharges from body orifices, necropsy *should not* be performed until other tests have been performed to rule out the disease.

Localized wound infections with *B. anthracis* are possible in cattle but uncommon and difficult to diagnose. A history of anthrax on the farm or within the locale may add a heightened index of suspicion for peracute or acute fatal cases.

Diagnosis

Blood collected from the jugular vein, mammary vein, or ear vein may provide material for cytologic examination and culture when the carcass is fresh. It is no longer necessary to send an ear from the carcass, and in fact such procedures may merely increase the risk of human exposure. Carcasses that are rotten or more than 12 hours old may be overgrown by clostridial organisms that confuse attempts at cytologic diagnosis.

Blood samples or smears should be examined at a qualified laboratory to ensure correct interpretation. Other blood tests, including an FA technique and ELISA, are available at some laboratories. Inoculation of collected material into guinea pigs has been used to diagnose anthrax in the past, but collected material may contain other opportunistic pathogens, thereby confusing the diagnosis. Although necropsy of possible anthrax cases is not recommended, it frequently is performed because other diseases may need to be ruled out. Prosectors should wear gloves, gowns, and masks whenever anthrax has been considered in the differential diagnosis of a dead cow. Splenic enlargement, widespread serosal hemorrhages, sanguineous or serosanguineous body cavity fluids, and dark red or black body orifice discharges are the major necropsy findings. A diagnosis of anthrax requires notification of regulatory veterinarians to aid in quarantine management and carcass disposal.

Treatment

Treatment seldom is possible because of the acute or peracute course of illness. Penicillin and tetracycline in high levels should be effective in early cases or the less common localized infections.

Prevention and Control

Prevention and control can be accomplished by the following:
1. Avoid infected pastures. This is seldom possible on a practical basis.
2. Spore vaccines—the Sterne strain of rough, nonencapsulated *B. anthracis* was derived through growth of virulent *B. anthracis* on 50% serum agar in 10% to 30% CO_2. The resulting avirulent organism is used in the spore form as a live vaccine for cattle, sheep, and goats. The vaccine is recommended once yearly before pasture season. Use of any vaccine in dairy cattle may require regulatory approval, although there is no evidence that milk contains spores following vaccination of lactating cows.
3. Complete disposal of infected carcasses is done by burning or burial at least 6 feet into the ground and covering the carcass with quicklime. Regulatory veterinarians should be consulted regarding appropriate disinfection techniques.

Younger veterinarians may benefit from consultation with neighboring older colleagues to learn whether and where anthrax has been diagnosed previously in their service territory.

Recently awareness of the zoonotic potential of this infection has been highlighted by discussion of the "weaponization" of the agent as a terrorist threat. Human cases of anthrax in many parts of the world have become uncommon because of the success of control measures and lack of human exposure to infected livestock. Genetically modified organisms and alternative exposure methods besides livestock have created new concerns for human and animal health. One offshoot is

the increase in research to find alternative vaccination strategies, such as DNA vaccines, which may prove useful for animal disease control in the future.

COXIELLA BURNETII INFECTION (Q FEVER)

Etiology

Coxiella burnetii, a rickettsia, causes Q fever in humans. The organism is an obligate intracellular rickettsia but, unlike many other rickettsiae, completes its life cycle in the phagosomes of nucleated host cells. The organism exists in two phases: phase I tends to be the form isolated in farm animals or ticks and reacts to antibodies in late convalescent serum, whereas phase II reacts with antibodies in early convalescent serum and can be found after repeated passage in embryonated chicken eggs.

Domestic animals, including cattle, sheep, and goats, are the reservoirs of *C. burnetii*. Infection in cattle is common based on serologic surveys. Ticks may spread the infection from one animal to another, but the major source of organisms is amniotic fluids, placenta and fetal membranes of parturient ewes, goats, and cows, as well as milk, urine, and feces of infected animals. Infected ruminants do not show clinical disease in most instances. High abortion rates are rarely observed, except in some caprine herds. Apparently the organism concentrates in the placenta and udder of pregnant animals, which then release large numbers of *C. burnetii* at parturition. Aborting animals, but also females with normal parturition, as well as cows suffering from metritis, can shed *C. burnetii* for several months. Milk shedding is more frequent and lasts longer in cows and goats than in ewes. Milk shedding in cows is not rare, and there has been some recent concern about infection increasing California mastitis test scores.. Aerosols resulting from highly contaminated secretions and tissues allow infection of people and other animals in the vicinity. Contaminated environments, hides, wool, and bedding also may allow subsequent aerosol infection of humans. Once present in the environment or on inanimate objects, the organism is extremely resistant and persistent. Dust storms may predispose to infection by inhalation in endemic areas. A solution of 1% to 2% chlorine bleach may effect disinfection, however.

In people, Q fever is an occupational disease in agricultural workers or animal researchers. The major reason for concern in dairy cattle is that infection of dairy cattle and subsequent production of milk containing *C. burnetii*, especially in recently fresh cows, is widespread. In the United States, the disease formerly was thought to be limited to western states, but now Q fever is known to exist in most states. The frequency of *C. burnetii*–contaminated milk is another reason to avoid unpasteurized milk. Pasteurization temperatures of 62.8° C (145.0° F) for 30 minutes or 71.7° C (161.0° F) for 15 seconds kill the organism; thus routine pasteurization of milk for retail sale prevents spread of disease to humans through this route. Even though oral ingestion is an infrequent route of infection, it may cause seroconversion, and raw milk may contain enough *C. burnetii* to allow aerosol infection in dairy workers.

Clinical Signs

Infected cattle usually are asymptomatic or subclinical with nonspecific signs. The disease in humans follows an incubation of 10 to 28 days and is characterized by chills, fever, headache, malaise, and muscle aches. Septicemia is probable based on a high incidence of pneumonitis and hepatitis, as well as lesser incidences of severe endocarditis.

Diagnosis

Serologic testing using CF tests is the most common means of diagnosis, but other tests, including a radioisotope precipitation test, exist. A capillary-tube agglutination test may be used to detect infected milk. Infection rates in cattle vary based on geographic location, herd size, and stage of gestation. In people, the CF test and PCR detection of the organism are used most commonly to detect infection, but serologic testing frequently may not become positive to phase II antigen until 4 weeks following the onset of clinical signs.

Treatment

Treatment is not practiced in cattle, but tetracycline is the primary chemotherapeutic agent for Q fever in people.

Prevention and Control

Awareness of the zoonotic potential of *C. burnetii* and possible bad press for dairy cattle associated with Q fever mandate concern and respect for *C. burnetii*. Drinking unpasteurized milk should be avoided and could be a problem with organic herds that are not tested! Veterinarians should be aware of the potential for disease so as to protect themselves and farm workers. Considering the potential exposure of veterinarians through obstetrical procedures among others, it would seem that bovine practitioners would be at high risk. Perhaps most have developed immunity, although documentation of this effect is lacking.

Humans deemed at high risk in laboratory or abattoir settings have been vaccinated experimentally with apparent success. Vaccination with experimental vaccines in cattle results in seroconversion but does not eliminate shedding.

BRUCELLOSIS

Etiology

Brucellosis (Bang's disease) is an infectious cause of reproductive failure in cattle and a disease having profound public health significance. As with tuberculosis, brucellosis induces fervent and emotional responses when control and eradication efforts are discussed. Much of the United States is free of brucellosis thanks to testing and control methods fostered by cooperative state and federal efforts. However, the disease persists in cattle in certain states, and bison and wild ruminants (e.g., elk and moose) may carry the disease and could represent a risk to range cattle in certain areas of the western United States.

In cattle, *Brucella abortus* is the usual cause of brucellosis, but other *Brucella* spp. such as *B. melitensis* and *B. suis* can rarely infect cattle. *Brucella* spp. tend to have favorite primary hosts but seldom limit infection to only one host species. This discussion will be limited to *B. abortus*.

B. abortus is a short gram-negative rod that is fastidious and grows best in a CO_2-enriched aerobic environment. The organism has many other complex requirements for in vitro growth, and speciation of *Brucella* spp. or identification of biotypes is difficult. Some techniques used for speciation and biotyping include CO_2 requirements, production of H_2S, growth on various dyes, bacteriophage lysis, substrate oxidation, and agglutination tests. Multiple biotypes of *B. abortus* have been identified, but in the United States, biotype 1 is the major type with biotypes 2 and 4 playing smaller roles. Despite the complex growth requirements in vitro, the organism can persist in certain animal products and the environment for prolonged periods under favorable circumstances. In general, the organism likes moisture and cool temperatures but fares poorly in sunlight, dryness, and heat. For example, *B. abortus* may survive in manure at 12° C for 250 days but is killed quickly in manure that is heated. Similarly, infected placenta and fetal tissues, refrigerated infected milk and other dairy products, and cool water may support prolonged infectivity. Fortunately pasteurization kills *B. abortus* in milk.

Infection occurs primarily by ingestion of the organism, but venereal, intramammary, and congenital spread has been documented occasionally. Ingestion of the organism by susceptible cattle is fostered through contamination of feedstuffs, pasture, or fomites by infective placental fluids, tissues, fetuses, or milk. In dairy cattle, large herd size and intensive dairy management conditions predispose to epidemic infections and continuation of endemic infections.

Once infection has occurred, the organism exists in the host as a facultative intracellular organism capable of survival in host phagocytic cells. Polysaccharides and lipopolysaccharide protein components of the cell wall compose the surface antigens that result in the production of agglutinating antibodies by the host. Detection of these antibodies forms the basis for many of the serologic tests utilized on brucellosis control programs. Cell-mediated immunity, as expected based on the facultative intracellular designation of *B. abortus,* is important but poorly understood.

B. abortus gains entrance to cattle through mucous membranes of the oral cavity, nasal cavity, conjunctiva, or broken skin. Because ingestion is the major route of infection, the pharynx is thought to be the primary site of entrance. Calves can be infected by ingesting infected milk, and venereal spread can occur in both cows and bulls. Once penetration of the mucous membranes occurs, the organism seeks out and proliferates in regional lymph nodes before causing bacteremia. Similar to *Salmonella* spp., *Listeria* spp., and other facultative intracellular organisms, *B. abortus'* septicemic spread is aided by macrophage circulation. *B. abortus* septicemia results in infection that localizes in the udder, uterus, and associated lymph nodes of these organs. Infection of the pregnant uterus, especially during the second half of gestation in the cow, results in a progressive placentitis involving the chorion followed by an endometritis and fetal placental infection. Interference with fetal blood supply, endotoxemic effects on the fetus, and infection all contribute to subsequent loss of fetal viability and abortion. Most abortions occur from 5 months' gestation to near term. Aborted fetuses have been dead for days but frequently harbor viable *B. abortus* in the lung and abomasum.

Infected cattle usually remain carriers for life, and subsequent maximal shedding of *B. abortus* in milk and reproductive tract discharges occurs in association with each parturition. Although *B. abortus* abortion is infrequent during subsequent pregnancies in infected cows, the placenta may be infected during pregnancy, and carrier cows may contaminate the environment during calving and through their discharges for variable times following calving.

Young animals are thought to possess resistance to infection. This resistance is not completely understood but probably is aided by passive colostral origin antibodies. Cattle appear more susceptible to infection after they reach puberty or become pregnant. This generality regarding age resistance in young cattle is complicated somewhat by the occasional development of so-called latent infections in calves. Latent infections in calves can occur following in utero infection by infected dams or ingestion of infected milk.

Latent infections do not result in seroconversion or clinical signs until later in life when these animals are late in gestation, calve, or abort. The exact incidence or prevalence of latency is difficult to determine but appears infrequent based on recent two generation studies.

Clinical Signs

The clinical signs in cattle are limited to abortion of fetuses—usually during the last half of gestation. Abortion storms may occur when the disease has recently been introduced in a herd, whereas abortion in first-calf heifers or new additions typifies endemic infection. Severe illness in people is possible and can be difficult to diagnose unless physicians have an index of suspicion based on historical patient data that indicates occupational risk. In people, the disease is called undulant fever and is a well-known zoonotic infection. Farm workers, veterinarians, and slaughterhouse workers are at high risk if they handle infected cattle, placentas, fetuses, or milk. Drinking unpasteurized milk or eating unpasteurized cheeses from infected cattle is extremely dangerous for humans. Brucellosis in people can masquerade as many other more common diseases and may cause fever, myalgia, or joint or eye infection. *Brucella* spp. can infect people through the mucous membranes or breaks in the skin.

Diagnosis

Although culture of *B. abortus* remains the gold standard for positive diagnosis, economics and the need for specialized bacteriologic capabilities limit the use of culture for widespread surveillance and regulatory control programs. Recent development of PCR tests for detection of the agent in aborted fetuses is replacing the need for culture and the difficulties that culturing entails. Serologic testing remains the most common means of diagnosis of infected carrier animals. Many serologic tests are available and are better understood when interpreted in light of normal bovine immune responses to *B. abortus.* Shortly after infection of susceptible cattle, IgM agglutinins appear and peak within 2 weeks. Subsequent IgG antibodies peak by 1 to 2 months and become the major detectable antibodies in chronic infections. IgG_1 antibodies are nonagglutinating, have no opsonizing activity, block IgM and IgG_2 antibodies, and may aid the persistence of *B. abortus* in the host. This also may explain why serologic evidence of high humoral antibodies does not correlate with immunity or perhaps effective immunity in clinically infected cattle. Further, protective Strain 19 vaccines primarily induce IgM antibodies and lesser IgG_1 responses, suggesting that IgG_1 nonagglutinating antibodies may be harmful host responses.

The serum tube agglutination test, the plate (or rapid) agglutination test, and the card test are the tests used commonly. The serum tube agglutination test and card test tend to detect IgM antibodies, thus aiding detection of Strain 19 antibodies or recent infection.

The rivanol and mercaptoethanol tests may be helpful in differentiating antibodies elicited by chronic infection (mainly IgG_1) from antibodies subsequent to

Strain 19 vaccination (mostly IgM). These chemicals remove most IgM from the serum, so a reduction in titer following addition of the chemical to serum suggests that the titer resulted from Strain 19 vaccine rather than true infection.

The milk ring test is used widely for surveillance of *B. abortus* infection in dairy cattle. Bulk tank milk samples from each producer are tested at regular intervals by milk plants. A hematoxylin-stained suspension of killed *B. abortus* is added to fresh milk and incubated in a water bath at 37.0° C. Agglutinating antibodies in the milk will be detected by a color change in the cream layer because fat globules cause clumps of agglutinated organisms to rise in the tube, leaving decolorized milk below. A negative test result is confirmed when the milk in the tube remains colored.

None of these tests is completely accurate or foolproof. Statistical probabilities of a positive test meaning actual infection are much less in areas having little if any brucellosis versus areas with endemic infection. Therefore epidemiologic, surveillance, and control methods are limited by available diagnostic tools—similar to the situation with tuberculosis.

The CF test is accurate when testing adults that have never been vaccinated or that were vaccinated as calves. This test only detects IgM and IgG_1, and it is thought that complement fixing antibody levels decrease more rapidly than agglutinating antibodies in calves. Therefore fewer false-positive findings may result from calfhood vaccination when the CF test is used. Accuracy, specificity, and sensitivity of serologic tests may be enhanced in the future by ELISA and other techniques.

The development of new vaccines that do not result in confusing antibody levels in currently available tests has been an exciting recent development. Strain 19 vaccine has been an extremely helpful tool to control *B. abortus* in cattle but suffers because it produces antibodies in vaccinated cattle, may cause abortion in cattle vaccinated as adults, and can cause illness in people. In calfhood vaccinates, Strain 19 origin antibodies present only an occasional problem that leads to frustration for owners when sale, show, or shipment requirements result in a positive serologic test. However, for adult vaccinates, the resulting antibody levels seriously complicate all current serologic tests and make it extremely difficult to differentiate clinically infected cattle from vaccinates. Therefore vaccines utilizing rough strains of *B. abortus* have been tested. These rough strains lack the outer membrane lipopolysaccharides that are used as the antigenic component in most available tests. Cattle vaccinated with rough forms of *B. abortus* do not react as positive on testing with current serologic tests. Consequently, for states still requiring female calfhood vaccination, the RB51 strain has now been adopted as the official calfhood vaccination strain in the United States.

Treatment

Treatment currently is not approved for brucellosis in dairy cattle. Similar to therapy in people, however, experimental treatment of infected cattle supports the use of tetracycline and streptomycin in combination.

Control

Control measures should adhere to current state and federal guidelines. In most areas where brucellosis has been eliminated or minimized, surveillance methods include regular milk ring tests, serologic tests performed randomly at slaughterhouses for traceback of positive cattle, and serologic tests performed for interstate, international, or private sales. Whenever a positive milk ring test or individual has been identified, blood testing of the entire herd, removal of reactors, and quarantine usually are carried out. Calfhood vaccination in accordance with regulatory recommendations provides added insurance against epidemic loss. Some states still require calfhood vaccination using Strain RB51 vaccine for heifer calves aged 4 to 8 months. Bull calves should not be vaccinated for fear of causing chronic infection in the reproductive organs.

In endemic large dairy herds located in the southern United States and in range beef cattle, control of infection by test and slaughter may not be possible. Calfhood vaccination and increased efforts in sanitation may minimize or eliminate brucellosis in such herds over a period of years as chronically infected cows are eliminated by attrition. Vaccination of adult cattle has been performed in some areas where heavy infection exists, but usually it is discouraged and could only be considered when regulatory veterinary personnel approve the procedure.

BOVINE LEUKEMIA VIRUS INFECTION (LEUKOSIS) (BOVINE LYMPHOSARCOMA)

Etiology

Bovine leukemia virus (BLV), a retrovirus, is the cause of most cases of bovine lymphosarcoma. Infection with BLV is referred to as enzootic bovine leukosis (EBL) or simply leukosis of adult cattle. This retrovirus is further classified into the subfamily *Oncovirinae* and, similar to other retroviruses, possesses the enzyme reverse transcriptase. Reverse transcriptase enables retroviruses to convert RNA to DNA and then integrate this viral DNA into the chromosomal DNA of the host cell. This mechanism results in lifetime infection of the host and allows the viral protein to be replicated as the host cells replicate. Host antibody production against the virus is continual and lifelong as a result of repetitive viral protein replication. The host cell for BLV is the B lymphocyte. During initial infection, the encoded viral DNA (provirus) is believed to produce true virions, escape host cells, and infect other cells. After host antibody production against the virus, however, the virus lives somewhat in limbo in the lymphocyte because host antibodies (probably against glycoprotein 51 [gp 51]) outside the cell in the bloodstream may neutralize escaping virions. Infectious virus can escape in lymphocytes, however, if infected lymphocytes are separated from the checking presence of serum antibodies by removal of infected lymphocytes from the host or dilution of antibody. Therefore horizontal spread of BLV usually requires the transfer of blood containing infected lymphocytes from an infected to a susceptible cow. Infected cells require mechanical aids or compromised surface barriers to bypass intact epithelium or mucosa and be free of neutralizing antibody in a susceptible host. Milk, colostrum, and other body secretions containing infected lymphocytes can also result in horizontal spread of BLV.

Vertical transmission of BLV from infected dams to their fetuses by transfer of virus across the placenta is also possible but probably occurs in fewer than 10% of the pregnancies in infected cattle. Higher incidences of in utero infection rates have been observed in herds with an exceedingly high prevalence of persistent lymphocytosis (PL) cows or in herds with a high incidence of lymphosarcoma. Therefore these cattle represent a higher risk factor for vertical transmission. Calves infected in utero appear to be infected after establishing immunocompetence because they have both virus and antibody against the virus in their blood at birth, before colostrum ingestion.

Specific references and research data regarding transmission of BLV from infected to susceptible cattle would require an exhaustive and lengthy text and reference list. Some review articles on these subjects are included in the bibliography.

Studies of horizontal transmission have used susceptible cattle in natural settings, susceptible cattle in experimental settings, or susceptible sheep—which are very easily infected with BLV. Infective doses of lymphocytes from BLV-infected cattle may be as low as 1000 lymphocytes, although reported dosages vary greatly from several thousand lymphocytes up to 5 or more ml of blood. This variation can likely be explained by the number of infected lymphocytes of the donor; many cows have <5% lymphocyte infection, whereas other cows have >50% lymphocyte infection, most commonly PL cows. These findings imply higher risks of horizontal transmission of BLV in herds having BLV-positive PL cows. Intradermal, SQ, IM, and IV parenteral administration of BLV-infected lymphocytes or whole blood has resulted in infection of susceptible hosts.

Horizontal transmission of blood is frequently iatrogenic by herdspeople and veterinarians through the use or reuse of common needles and syringes, dehorners, ear tattoo instruments, castrating equipment, blood collection needles, IV needles, blood transfusions, and nose leads. Intradermal tuberculin testing also is a possible, although less likely, cause of horizontal spread.

Rectal palpation using a common sleeve for examination of BLV-positive cattle followed by palpation of BLV-negative cattle also may spread BLV horizontally, but conflicting results have evolved in studies designed to assess this possibility. One epidemiologic study in a large dairy failed to detect increased risk of infection for BLV-negative cattle when a common sleeve was used by a single examiner to perform rectal examinations randomly on both BLV-positive and BLV-negative cattle. However, other studies show increased risk of transmission to BLV-negative cows palpated with a common sleeve immediately after BLV-positive cows. This discrepancy may be explained by difference in the number of PL cows in the herds. Rectal transmission by unnatural volumes of infective blood and unnatural means of rectal irritation has caused experimental infection of susceptible calves and sheep.

Infection through the use of dehorners and other surgical instruments on several animals is much less likely if the instruments are rinsed and disinfected with either chlorine bleach or chlorhexidine between animals. Blood sampling with a common needle is very dangerous, especially for susceptible cattle sampled immediately after BLV-positive cattle. Therefore individual needles are essential for this procedure and for parenteral injections.

The role of insects in horizontal spread of BLV is controversial, and most studies have used completely unrealistic materials and methods, such as injecting mouth parts of various insects that have fed on BLV-positive blood, or creating controlled populations of insects that feed on BLV-positive cattle and then are applied to BLV-negative cattle. Tabanids, mosquitoes, and ticks have, in some studies, transmitted infection, whereas stable flies and horn flies seem less likely to do so. At this time, the role of insects in the spread of BLV is unknown. It is interesting that no studies have assessed the potential for BLV transmission for lice because these parasites constitute a serious parasitic burden to many cattle during the winter months. Higher incidence of BLV infection in beef cattle in the southern states compared with northern states would support the possibility of insects playing a role in BLV transmission.

Epidemiologic studies emphasize that close contact of infected and susceptible cattle enhance the horizontal transmission of BLV. Prevalence within infected herds tends to peak during confinement, increased cattle density, or when BLV-negative cattle are suddenly grouped with BLV-positive cattle. Management procedures that result in increased density or that entail common treatment procedures as heifers come of breeding age or join milking herds seem to facilitate infection. Similarly calves and heifers housed with adult cattle probably have a greater risk of infection. Infected cattle having antibodies to the viral core protein and those that have PL represent greater risk to susceptible cattle than BLV-positive cattle having only antibodies against the gp 51 surface glycoprotein.

Because infection spreads when BLV-positive cattle are closely confined with BLV-negative cattle, many studies assessing infectivity of various secretions have been performed. Nasal secretions, saliva, bronchoalveolar washes, urine, feces, uterine flush fluid, and semen have been examined. Secretions that are highly cellular are more likely to be infective than those that are relatively acellular. Soluble fractions of secretions are seldom infective because the virus is cell associated, but in one study of urine from BLV-positive cows, BLV p25 antigen was found in the soluble portion in a majority of cattle tested. Respiratory secretions may harbor infected cells, but the natural risk of these secretions spreading infection seems low. Similarly, uterine fluid obtained during embryo transfer from BLV-positive donors is most dangerous when cell contamination occurs. Semen presents little risk when artificial insemination is used because highly cellular ejaculates are usually discarded by bull stud services, and bull studs rarely, if ever, keep BLV-positive bulls. However, BLV-positive bulls used for natural service that had reproductive tract infections causing increased numbers of infective cells in the ejaculate could spread infection to susceptible cattle. The relatively low infectivity of secretions fails to explain completely the increased risk of infection observed epidemiologically in closely confined or dense cattle populations. Physical cow interactions and management procedures (e.g., restraint equipment) may play a role. Lymphocytes in milk represent a potential source of virus and certainly represent a significant secretory source of virus. The role of milk and colostrum fed to susceptible calves will be discussed later.

In utero transmission of BLV, embryo transfer, and the feeding of infected milk or colostrum require consideration. As discussed earlier, in utero spread of BLV from infected dams to susceptible fetuses occurs in a low percentage—probably less than 10% in most infected herds. Herds with an extremely high incidence of infected cattle or herds containing many cows with PL or clinical tumors may experience higher in utero infection rates. In utero infection appears to represent a direct viral infection through the placenta. Fetuses are assumed to be infected after attaining immunocompetence because both BLV and antibodies against BLV are detectable in the blood of these animals at birth. Cows that are BLV-positive that produce an in utero–infected calf may or may not produce infected calves on subsequent pregnancies.

Embryo transfer is *not* a major source of BLV vertical transmission. Embryos from BLV-positive donors neither infect BLV-negative recipients nor result in infected fetuses. Embryos from either BLV-positive or BLV-negative cows, however, would be at risk for in utero infection if implanted into BLV-positive recipients. Therefore the key to successful management of BLV in embryo transfer is the maintenance of BLV-negative recipient stock.

Perhaps the area of greatest controversy in transmission of BLV involves feeding infected milk or colostrum. As previously stated, the colostrum and milk of BLV-positive cows may contain BLV because lymphocytes constitute a normal cellular component of milk and colostrum. The frequency with which BLV is found in the milk of BLV-positive cows is unknown. However, it must be assumed that milk or colostrum from BLV-positive cows is likely to harbor infected lymphocytes. In addition to infected lymphocytes, however, the colostrum of BLV-positive cattle contains antibody against the virus, and this antibody is thought to provide some immediate protection against infection. Infected lymphocytes given orally to susceptible newborn calves can cause infection experimentally if administered before colostral feeding. It appears that calves are most susceptible to infection by BLV in colostrum or milk from birth to 3 days of age and thereafter may not be as commonly infected by this route. Relatively few calves have been studied experimentally, however, and much remains to be learned regarding colostral transmission of the virus to neonatal calves. Colostrum containing virus and antibodies against the virus seems to be associated with limited, immediate infection. Passive antibodies against BLV can be detected in calves consuming colostrum from BLV-positive cows, and these antibodies persist for as long as 6 months.

Calves fed milk from infected cows up to weaning can become infected with BLV, but the frequency of this occurrence is difficult to determine based on conflicting experimental results. Calves having ingested colostrum with BLV antibodies, as well as those that ingested colostrum without antibodies, may be at some risk. Probably fewer than 10% of calves ingesting infected milk would become infected with BLV in most field settings. Milk containing higher numbers of infected lymphocytes, as might be found in cows with PL or lymphosarcoma, should be considered the most dangerous. Soured milk that reaches a pH of less than 4.4 and is held at 65.0° F (18.33° C) for 24 hours will kill BLV. In addition, freezing followed by thawing or pasteurizing colostrum and milk might destroy BLV in these fluids. The best recommendation regarding colostrum and milk feeding for calves is to feed colostrum from BLV-negative cows to all calves and then use a milk replacer or pasteurized milk up to weaning.

Numerous older studies have evaluated the prevalence of BLV infection in dairy and beef cattle. Results vary greatly based on geographic area and types of management. In the northeastern United States, it is assumed that 35% or more of all dairy cattle are infected, but rarely herds may have no incidence, whereas others have greater than 80% positive cattle. Estimates in some southern states reach 50% or greater positive dairy cattle. Well fewer than 5% of all infected (BLV-positive) cattle subsequently develop lymphosarcoma. This is an important statistic because veterinarians sometimes diagnose lymphosarcoma erroneously when faced with vague illness in seropositive cattle. The risk for lymphosarcoma in a BLV-infected cow is genetically related. Genetic factors allow the monoclonal proliferation of B lymphocytes in tumor-bearing cows.

A small percentage of BLV-positive cattle also may have PL in their peripheral blood. Persistent lymphocytosis has been defined as an absolute lymphocyte count at least three standard derivations above the normal mean count that persists at least 3 consecutive months. Persistent lymphocytosis is the result of benign polyclonal B-lymphocyte proliferation. More than 98% of cattle with PL test positive for BLV, and the tendency for PL may be a separately inherited trait in response to BLV infection. Clinically, genetic influences exist on both the occurrence of PL or lymphosarcoma within certain lines of purebred cattle. Further genetic relationships regarding susceptibility or resistance to BLV infection and PL have evolved from studies of bovine lymphocyte antigens (BoLAs) in cattle. The risk of lymphosarcoma in PL cattle versus non-PL, BLV-positive cattle is unproven. One study found no increased risk of lymphosarcoma in PL cows, but further studies are needed.

Clinical Signs

Two facts must be emphasized preceding a discussion of signs observed in BLV-infected adult cattle having clinical tumors or lymphosarcoma. The first is that fewer than 5% of all BLV-positive cattle develop tumors or illness associated with lymphosarcoma. Most BLV-infected cattle are asymptomatic, immune-competent, and can be as productive as their seronegative herdmates. Recent data suggest BLV-positive cattle do not remain in the herd as long as BLV-negative cattle and therefore reflect a financial loss for the farmer. The reason for this was not clear. Although several classic clinical presentations occur in lymphosarcoma cattle as a result of specific target organ involvement, the majority require careful differentiation from a multitude of other diseases. Lymphosarcoma can masquerade as a myriad of other inflammatory or debilitating diseases of cattle.

Clinical signs of lymphosarcoma seldom develop before 2 years of age and are most common in cattle between 3 and 6 years of age. Lymphosarcoma occurring in cattle less than 2 years of age is *rarely* caused by BLV infection. For example, thymic, calf-B cell, juvenile T-cell, and most skin lymphosarcoma patients are less than 2 years of age. These non-BLV (sporadic) associated forms of lymphosarcoma will be discussed later.

Lymphosarcoma may occur in peripheral lymph nodes, internal lymph nodes, and specific target organs such as the abomasum, heart, uterus, retrobulbar space, and epidural region of the central nervous system (see figures of lymphosarcoma in other chapters). Any or all of the aforementioned tissues may become neoplastic. In addition, atypical targets such as the upper and lower respiratory tract, udder, forestomach, kidney, ureter, liver, spleen, and bone marrow may be affected. Chance mix and matching of lesions in one or more locations is the rule and results in the tremendous variation in clinical signs observed in an individual patient.

Most lymphosarcoma patients have nonspecific signs of weight loss, decreased appetite, and decreased production. However, lymphosarcoma cattle with one predominant lesion, such as epidural spinal cord compression, may suffer a rapid onset of paralysis despite a normal appetite and body condition. The greater the number of tumors and the more visceral organs involved, the greater is the likelihood of weight loss, inappetence, and reduced production. If cattle with lymphosarcoma lived long enough, they might have neoplasms in many target areas. However, usually a tumor affecting one anatomic region predominates. Fever also may be present in a low percentage of lymphosarcoma patients, thereby confusing the differential diagnosis with inflammatory and infectious diseases. Fever, when present, is a result of tumor necrosis, secondary bacterial infections, or pyrogens associated with various cellular and soluble mediators of inflammation stimulated by neoplastic cells.

Peripheral lymph node enlargement of one or more external lymph nodes is common and found in approximately 25% of tumorous cows. Superficial cervical (prescapular), superficial inguinal (prefemoral), supramammary, submandibular, or retropharyngeal lymph nodes may be enlarged. Internal lymph nodes such as the sublumbars, mesenteric or others may be found to be enlarged on rectal examination or laparotomy. Lymph node enlargements sometimes result in clinical consequences such as dyspnea (retropharyngeal) (see Figure 4-4) or bloat (retropharyngeal, mediastinal). Bloat occurs as a result of failure of, or interference with, eructation associated with pharyngeal or mediastinal lymph node neoplasia. Similarly, compressive neoplastic lymph nodes may interfere with effective air movement that usually occurs in the pharyngeal or laryngeal region, causing inspiratory dyspnea.

The intestinal tract is a common site for lymphosarcoma tumors. Although the abomasum is the most commonly affected area of the gastrointestinal tract, the forestomach and intestine can also have lesions. Abomasal lymphosarcoma can result in melena, signs of vagus indigestion, or simply inappetence and weight loss. Diffuse or focal neoplasms can be found in the abomasum (see Figures 5-62 and 5-63). When a major lymphosarcoma tumor involves the pylorus, abdominal distention typical of vagus indigestion results from interference with abomasal outflow. Bleeding from ulcerative neoplasms or mucosal ulcers resulting from lymphosarcoma infiltrates in the abomasal wall can cause occult bleeding or obvious melena. Affected cattle also may grind their teeth because of nonspecific abdominal or abomasal pain. Abomasal lymphosarcoma resulting in melena must be differentiated from simple abomasal ulceration.

Lymphosarcoma tumors in the rumen, reticulum, and omasum cause varying degrees of forestomach dysfunction, weight loss, reduced appetite and production, bloat, or signs of vagus indigestion. Such tumors are difficult to diagnose unless either abdominal fluid cytology or exploratory laparotomy is performed. Focal or diffuse lymphosarcoma masses or infiltrates may rarely involve the small or large intestine.

The uterus and reproductive tract constitute another common "target" location for lymphosarcoma. Neoplasms may be focal, multifocal, or diffuse. Classical uterine lymphosarcoma lesions consist of multifocal firm nodules or masses within the uterine wall (see Figure 9-4). Palpation of such masses can be compared with palpation of caruncles and feel nodular or like raised umbilicated lesions with a central depression. Such lesions may be present in one or both uterine horns. Ovaries and oviducts occasionally are neoplastic as well. Large focal or diffuse tumors may completely involve the uterus or the entire caudal reproductive tract. Reproductive tract neoplasms are much easier to identify in nongravid tracts than in heavily pregnant cows, in which placentomes and the fetus frequently obscure the masses. Routine rectal palpations often uncover reproductive tract lymphosarcoma before development of overt systemic signs, but palpable uterine masses discovered per rectum must first be differentiated from other uterine tumors, as well as uterine and periuterine abscesses and hematomas.

Cardiac abnormalities, including arrhythmias, murmurs, pericardial effusions, muffling of heart sounds, venous distention, and signs of congestive heart failure, are possible consequences of lymphosarcoma affecting the heart or pericardium. The right atrium is reported to be the most common site of lymphosarcoma tumors in the heart of cattle, but the tumor may affect any region of the heart or pericardium (see Figure 3-10). Focal, multifocal, or diffuse neoplasia is possible, thereby explaining the plethora of potential clinical consequences. Cardiac lymphosarcoma may require differentiation from arrhythmias caused by primary electrolyte or gastrointestinal disturbances or nonneoplastic myocardial lesions, septic pericarditis, cardiomyopathy, endocarditis, and myocarditis.

Respiratory signs associated with lymphosarcoma masses include inspiratory stridor resulting from nasal or upper airway infiltrates, lymph node enlargements, or tumor masses in the upper airway. Dyspnea of lower airway origin may reflect pleural effusions, pulmonary involvement, mediastinal masses, or congestive heart failure.

Ocular signs most commonly reflect involvement of the retrobulbar area as a common target location. Therefore progressive unilateral or bilateral exophthalmos progressing to pathologic exophthalmos and exposure damage to the globe represents the most common ophthalmic manifestation of lymphosarcoma in BLV-positive cattle that develop tumors (see Figures 13-3 and 13-4). Although the retrobulbar masses or infiltrate usually progresses over several weeks, the subsequent appearance of the eye associated with pathologic exophthalmus can appear to be acute as the eyelids lose the ability to completely protect the protruding globe (Figure 15-9). Corneal exposure damage, desiccation, and profound chemosis generally develop quickly. Although the rate of progression may vary in retrobulbar areas, cattle usually are affected bilaterally if they survive long enough.

Tumors of lymphosarcoma in the epidural region of the spinal cord cause progressive paresis and eventual paralysis consistent with the anatomic location of the tumor. Posterior paresis and paralysis are most common because of the frequency of tumors in the thoracolumbar, lumbar, or sacral areas. However, cervical and cranial thoracic lesions are possible such that tetraparesis may be observed. Tumors in the extradural space may again be focal, multifocal, or diffuse. Lymphosarcoma of the brain also has been observed but is much less common than spinal cord compressive neoplasms and is rarely BLV associated. Although not a firm rule, compressive lymphosarcoma neoplasms affecting the spinal cord frequently cause neurologic signs before the patient's

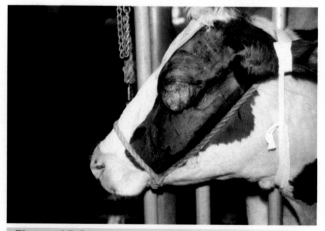

Figure 15-9

Lymphosarcoma in the left retrobulbar region causing pathologic exophthalmos and exposure damage to the globe.

physical status (e.g., appetite, condition) has deteriorated to such a degree that a neoplastic process would be considered likely. Therefore compressive lymphosarcoma lesions commonly are confused with metabolic conditions or spinal injuries (see Chapter 12). Cattle with lymphosarcoma masses compressing the spinal cord usually progress from paresis to paralysis within 2 to 7 days. During this time, they may be noticed to have difficulty rising, require manual assistance (lifting them by the tail) to rise, or make repeated attempts before being able to rise (see Figures 12-35 to 12-37). Loss of tail and anal tone and perineal desensitization may also be seen with caudal lymphosarcoma lesions involving the lumbosacral spinal cord and cauda equina. Symptomatic treatment with corticosteroids may result in temporary clinical improvement.

Neoplasms affecting the urinary system can do so by direct or indirect mechanisms. Perirenal lymph node enlargement may result in reduced renal perfusion, renal infarcts, or prerenal azotemia when both kidneys have vascular compromise. Diffuse lymphosarcoma in one or both ureters may cause hydronephrosis, hematuria, colic, or postrenal azotemia (bilateral). Neoplasms in the bladder or urethra may cause hydronephrosis, hydroureter, hematuria, tenesmus, dribbling of urine, or colic. Extradural spinal cord compressive neoplasms affecting sacral segments also may cause bladder dysfunction. Renal tumors may result in no outward signs, renal colic, renal azotemia (bilateral), hematuria, or other signs. Tumors affecting the urinary system frequently are palpable on rectal or vaginal examinations. Enlargement of the left kidney may be appreciated on routine rectal examination, and this should prompt ultrasonographic evaluation of both kidneys transrectally and/or transabdominally. Significant differentials for renal lymphosarcoma include other nonpainful, firm masses such as those encountered with renal carcinomas and renal amyloidosis. Normal shape of the kidney is often lost with renal lymphosarcoma. Definitive diagnosis may be reached by biopsy.

Lymphosarcoma tumors associated with the mammary gland or mammary lymph nodes may be occult or overt. The mammary lymph nodes are more likely to be clinically affected than the mammary glands, and neoplastic enlargement of the supramammary lymph nodes—unilateral or bilateral—is common (see Figure 8-8, A). Diffuse infiltration or focal lymphosarcoma tumors are possible in one or more mammary glands and are best detected by palpation of the glands.

Rarely skin tumors appear in adult lymphosarcoma patients. Such tumors are firm and either nodular or plaquelike. Skin tumors are usually 5 to 20 cm in diameter. The skin of the trunk or udder is generally involved (see Figure 7-10). Enlargement of hemal lymph nodes, most apparent in the region of the paralumbar fossa, is rarely associated with lymphosarcoma in dairy cattle.

Diffuse splenic neoplasia caused by BLV-positive lymphosarcoma is a form of lymphosarcoma in adult cattle and, although usually accompanied by gross or microscopic neoplasms in other visceral locations, may be the only identifiable lesion. Diffuse splenic lymphosarcoma may result in splenic capsular rupture, subsequent fatal intraabdominal hemorrhage, and acute death. This lesion is observed as the cause of fatal exsanguination approximately once yearly by the Necropsy Service at the Cornell University Veterinary College. Abdominal hemorrhage causing acute death is not rare in adult dairy cattle; most have no proven etiology; and only a few are caused by lymphosarcoma.

Lymphosarcoma masses are possible in virtually any tissue, and cattle with lymphosarcoma tumors in one or more organs may be presented without classical target organ involvement. Visceral or body cavity masses with or without lymphadenopathy can occur. Adult BLV-positive cattle with lymphosarcoma or lymphomatosis tumors seldom survive more than a few weeks to a few months, and almost all succumb within 6 months. There may be temporary response to corticosteroids, but treatment is seldom used. Occasionally cattle with lymphosarcoma that are in the last trimester of pregnancy can be successfully treated palliatively in terms of reaching parturition. However, the prognosis beyond palliative treatment for more than a few weeks is hopeless. It is possible to see some success with the use of nonabortifacient corticosteroids in late pregnancy, typically prednisone (1 mg/kg daily) or isoflupredone acetate in the treatment of cattle with retrobulbar, thoracic, or abdominal visceral tumors. It should be remembered that dexamethasone is highly unlikely to cause abortion in the first 150 days of gestation, so this may be an option for open cows with lymphosarcoma, for which the only goal is to retrieve embryos for preservation of genetic merit. Occasionally severely catabolic cows with lymphosarcoma that are "limped" through to parturition will give birth to very dysmature calves, even if they are term at delivery. These calves are also commonly infected in utero and bull calves would therefore be of little value. Such calves have high perinatal mortality rates and can be challenging to save. Clinicians at the University of Wisconsin have on occasion used specific chemotherapeutic protocols involving agents such as vincristine, L-asparaginase, and cyclophosphamide in the treatment of individual cows with lymphosarcoma that have extreme genetic and financial merit, but the use of these drugs is obviously prohibited in animals whose milk or meat is intended for human consumption, and the use of such large doses of highly toxic drugs would require hospitalization and careful removal of wastes. Palliative treatment of a late pregnant cow with pericardial lymphosarcoma by pericardectomy was performed at Cornell.

Sporadic bovine leukosis (SBL) includes the juvenile mostly T-cell, thymic, which some consider part of the juvenile form, calf mostly B-cell, and the "skin form" (T-cell) of lymphosarcoma. All are rare and mostly occur in cattle less than 2 years of age. In the sporadic form the tumors are not caused by BLV infection, and most, but not all, cattle with SBL are BLV seronegative. Tumor cells of sporadic lymphomas represent immature lineages of T and less commonly B cells. The protooncogene c-Myb is expressed in most sporadic lymphomas but not enzootic lymphomas.

Juvenile and calf form of lymphosarcoma can affect calves from birth to up to 18 months of age. Younger cattle are generally affected by the B-cell calf form. The most obvious clinical sign with either form is diffuse lymphadenopathy that results in obvious and palpable enlargement of peripheral lymph nodes (see Figure 4-3). Such calves commonly are presented for evaluation because of recurrent or persistent bloat or because of dyspnea. Rare cases of congenital lymphosarcoma are possible (Figure 15-10). Visceral tumors are possible in calves with juvenile/calf lymphosarcoma, and bone marrow lesions and peripheral leukemia are common in the 4- to 7-month-old calves. Occasionally, single tumors are found (e.g., in the cerebral cortex). The Milking Shorthorn breed seems to have a higher incidence of juvenile/calf lymphosarcoma than the other dairy breeds.

Thymic lymphosarcoma usually is observed in 6- to 24-month-old cattle. Progressive enlargement of the thymus occurs in all cases but is most apparent clinically when cervical enlargement develops. In some thymic lymphosarcoma patients, the majority of thymic enlargement remains in the thorax. Most patients, however, develop a caudal cervical swelling, which may progress in a cranial

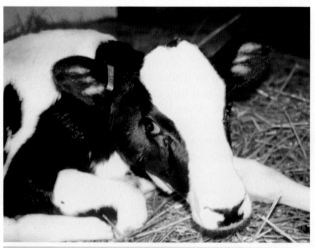

Figure 15-10

Newborn heifer calf with juvenile multicentric lymphosarcoma. Note the huge retropharyngeal lymph node enlargement. The heifer was one of a pair of twins both of whom were born with sporadic lymphosarcoma.

direction to the mid or cranial ventral cervical region. As with juvenile lymphosarcoma patients, the chief complaint for thymic lymphosarcoma heifers usually is either bloat or dyspnea (see Figure 4-50). External compression of the esophagus interferes with effective eructation, and tracheal compression, pulmonary displacement or compression, pleural effusion, and pulmonary edema contribute to signs of dyspnea. Exceptionally large thymic masses within the thorax or thoracic inlet also may cause jugular vein distention as a result of reduced venous return and thus interfere with cardiac and pulmonary function to such a degree that heart failure may be suspected. A thoracic mass may be suspected based on muffled heart sounds or reduced air sounds in the ventral hemithorax unilaterally or bilaterally. Fever is a common sign, but the exact mechanism of fever is poorly understood. The presence of fever causes clinical confusion with abscesses, cellulitis, esophageal lacerations, and other inflammatory diseases. Fever may result from tumor necrosis, tumor-induced pyrogens or mediators, or secondary respiratory infections. Palpation of cervical masses resulting from thymic lymphosarcoma can be misleading because the masses may feel soft, fluctuant, or edematous in some patients. In others, the lesions palpate as firm or hard, thus appearing more consistent with neoplasia. Cervical enlargements may be so soft, edematous, or fluctuant as to suggest fluid distention. However, attempts at aspiration reveal little, if any, fluid, whereas fine needle aspirates or biopsies will confirm the lesions as lymphosarcoma. Tumors may be present in other locations in some patients having thymic lymphosarcoma. One interesting epidemic of thymic lymphosarcoma in BLV-free herds has been described in calves 4 to 10 months of age in France during 1987 and 1988. Of the 73 calves affected, 67 were sired by the same bull. Genetic implications have not been described in the United States, possibly because of a lack of cases.

The "skin form" of lymphosarcoma is rare, sporadic, occurs in cattle less than 30 months of age, and usually affects cattle that are seronegative for BLV. Multiple skin nodules appear on the neck, trunk, and rear quarters (see Figure 7-9). The lesions become more numerous and enlarge over a period of months. Lymphadenopathy may accompany the skin lesions or appear later in the course of the disease. Lesions may become so numerous that they appear confluent (see Figure 7-9). Although cattle with skin lymphosarcoma appear otherwise healthy during the early phase of the disease, their body condition and health deteriorate over 6 to 12 months, and eventually those cattle succumb to diffuse neoplasia. Insects severely irritate cattle having skin lymphosarcoma. Insect bites may cause superficial dermatitis or bleeding from the skin nodules, and some lymph nodes may become abscessed. Scores of skin nodules are present in this form of the disease and allow clinical differentiation from adult lymphosarcoma, in which occasionally an individual or a few skin lesions accompany visceral lesions.

Diagnosis

The diagnosis of BLV infection in cattle is done using serologic techniques such as the agar gel immunodiffusion (AGID) test, ELISA, or radioimmunoassay (RIA). Recently PCR tests for identification of the agent in blood have been developed and successfully applied. Following infection with BLV virus, most cattle remain persistently infected despite the production of serum antibodies against the virus. Serologic tests use one or both of the major antigens of the BLV-p24, which is a major core protein that was the first recognized internal protein of BLV, or gp 51, which is the major external envelope glycoprotein and probably assists viral binding to host cells. The envelope gp 51 antigen may also induce neutralizing activity against BLV, inhibit activity of released virus, and deter extracellular BLV activity.

The AGID test used by most laboratories incorporates gp 51 antigen. A commercial AGID test also is available and uses gp 51 (Leukassay-B, Piunan-Moore, Washington Crossing, NJ). Some laboratories incorporate both p24 and gp 51 antigens into the AGID. All AGID tests detect specific antibodies against BLV in serum. Following infection of a susceptible cow with BLV, antibodies may be detected by the AGID in 3 to 12 weeks. Although this "lag time" between infection and AGID-detectable levels of antibody has been used to criticize AGID testing, the AGID currently is the most popular test because of high specificity, high sensitivity, simplicity, and proven ability to provide effective screening to eliminate BLV infection in cattle populations. The AGID also is required as the current test of choice for export testing of cattle.

A positive AGID or ELISA, which is commonly used now by many diagnostic laboratories, would be expected in calves that received colostral antibodies from BLV-positive dams and infection in those young animals could only be confirmed by PCR. As previously mentioned, such passively acquired antibodies usually decrease to undetectable levels by 6 to 7 months of age, but biologic variation will affect the exact length of time required for passive decay. Therefore a positive AGID in a calf less than 6 months of age may either reflect an infection or be caused by passive antibodies acquired in colostrum. False-negative findings usually result from failure to detect antibodies during early infection, usually thought to range from 3 to 12 weeks when the AGID test is used. Some false-negative findings, however, may reflect a decrease in circulating antibody levels in a BLV-infected animal. This most commonly occurs around the time of parturition as maternal antibodies, in effect, "drain" into the udder. The period from 2 weeks before parturition to 6 weeks postpartum may be associated with an overall decrease in antibody levels. If this decrease causes antibody levels to decrease below detectable AGID levels, a false-negative result may occur. Rarely a false-negative AGID results from failure of host antibody response.

RIA and ELISA tests are considered more sensitive than the AGID. RIA may detect infection by 2 weeks and also may be used to detect BLV antibodies in milk and the blood of periparturient cows. These benefits may be helpful in selected testing situations. The major disadvantage to RIA involves the greater technical and equipment requirements. The ELISA is extremely sensitive and probably equals the specificity of the AGID and is now used in many commercial laboratories. It seems likely that blood PCR tests will ultimately equal or exceed sensitivity of the serologic tests. Pooled serum samples from groups or herds may be surveyed by the ELISA test to detect low levels of infection that may prompt individual testing. Milk from the bulk tank may be tested for antibodies with the ELISA test.

Diagnostic efforts may incorporate ELISA herd screening, milk screening of bulk samples utilizing new ELISA or PCR technology, or other tests and detection of tumor-associated antigens. Tumor-associated antigens are detectable by monoclonal antibodies specific for polypeptides on lymphosarcoma cells. Seropositive BLV cattle commonly do not ($\leq 10\%$) have detectable tumor-associated antigens. However, lymphosarcoma patients and PL cattle appear almost always to have such antigens.

Lymphosarcoma patients may have "double-line positive" AGID results. The significance of this result is unknown but may reflect tumor-associated antigens or strong antibody levels against both gp 51 and p24 (when both antigens are included in the AGID media).

Diagnosis of lymphosarcoma may require only a physical examination when lymphadenopathy and obvious (or palpable) target organ neoplasia is present. However, most patients with lymphosarcoma require some diagnostic aids. The best aids are cytology or biopsy collected from effusions or target organs. A positive ELISA or other serum-antibody test adds an index of suspicion but cannot be considered definitive because fewer than 5% of all BLV-positive cattle develop tumors. Peripheral lymphocytosis adds a stronger index of suspicion but again does not equate with lymphosarcoma in all cases.

Taking samples of abdominal and thoracic fluid may be helpful when large tumors are suspected in these body cavities. Cytology of such fluid may sometimes reveal abnormal lymphocytes that confirm a suspected diagnosis. This is most helpful when thoracic effusion, pericardial effusion, or large abdominal (abomasal) tumors are present. Lymph node aspirates or biopsies confirm a diagnosis of lymphosarcoma in some patients that have obviously enlarged lymph nodes. However, it is not uncommon to have such lymph node samples interpreted as reactive or hyperplastic rather than neoplastic. Pelvic or reproductive tract masses may be aspirated or biopsied through the vagina in some cattle to confirm a diagnosis of lymphosarcoma. Ultrasound may be helpful in conjunction with aspirates or biopsies for visceral masses within body cavities, the retrobulbar space, or the heart.

Forestomach neoplasia, abomasal neoplasia, and other visceral involvement may require laparotomy to confirm diagnosis when other ancillary tests have failed to define lymphosarcoma.

Perhaps the two most difficult clinical situations in which to confirm suspected lymphosarcoma occur when compressive spinal neoplasms or abomasal infiltration occurs. Unless other target organ lesions or lymph node enlargements are apparent, diagnosis in these anatomic areas can be difficult. When the abomasum is suspected to have lymphosarcoma based on occult or gross melena, weight loss, inappetence, and bruxism, an abdominal paracentesis is indicated. If cytology of this fluid is not helpful, a laparotomy may be necessary. Compressive lymphosarcoma neoplasms causing paresis or paralysis in cattle with no other detectable evidence of lymphosarcoma require a cerebrospinal fluid (CSF) analysis—usually from the lumbosacral region when spinal cord signs predominate. The CSF from such patients often is normal but may have increased protein levels in some instances. In addition, a lesser percentage of these patients will have neoplastic lymphocytes present in the CSF. When no fluid is obtained from the lumbosacral space but the clinician is confident that the space has been entered with the spinal needle, aspirates may be obtained because the space occasionally is obliterated by a neoplastic mass (see Figure 12-37). Although uncommon (fewer than 10% of lymphosarcoma patients), true leukemia may be detected by CBCs in some lymphosarcoma patients. Serum lactic acid dehydrogenase values also may be elevated in some cattle with lymphosarcoma, but this finding is not specific for the disease.

The diagnosis of atypical (sporadic) lymphosarcoma in the juvenile, thymic, calf, and skin forms is relatively easy. Lymph node aspirates or biopsies suffice for the juvenile form, and skin biopsies confirm the skin form. The thymic form may be diagnosed by aspirates, biopsies, thoracocentesis, or ultrasound-guided biopsy.

For treatments, see page 629.

Control

Control measures for BLV infection in dairy herds may be easy when the prevalence of BLV-positive cattle is low. Serologic testing of all cattle and calves is performed. Positive cattle and calves older than 6 months could be culled. Seropositive calves less than 6 months of age can be either segregated and retested at 9 months of age or

tested by PCR. Extremely valuable BLV-positive cattle may be superovulated and their embryos placed in seronegative heifers or cows. However, the continued existence of BLV-positive cows is a detriment to eradication of BLV in the herd; this is especially true for PL cows! If serologic tests are used in this control program, limitations of the test must be recognized. Early infections may yield false-negative results as may some periparturient cows. Therefore repeat testing of the entire herd is required in 3 to 6 months. Several programs have been suggested to eliminate BLV infection from herds, and guidelines were devised by the U.S. Animal Health Association in 1980 to establish BLV-free herds. New York and some other states have also sponsored programs to achieve BLV-free status, but outcome of such programs has frequently been disappointing.

Stringent culling programs do entail economic losses and are most applicable when a low prevalence of infection exists in the herd. In addition, control measures to deter horizontal spread should be used. These measures include both veterinary and management techniques such as single needle and syringe use, electric dehorning, disinfection of all common instruments between uses (chlorhexidine or chlorine bleach), individual rectal sleeves, stringent insect control, and avoidance of purchasing new animals. Vertical and much of the horizontal transmission can be avoided by culling all PL cattle. Feeding calves colostrum or milk only from BLV-negative cows (although the precise importance of this is not known), pasteurizing or freezing BLV-positive colostrum or milk before feeding (if this is necessary), feeding milk replacer to calves after they ingest preferably BLV-negative colostrum, and using only seronegative embryo recipients are other routine recommendations.

If economics disallow test and slaughter, various other plans can be devised such as testing and segregating seropositive cattle away from seronegative cattle. Segregation must be enforced, and facilities such as milking areas must be separate. In addition, management techniques to prevent horizontal or in utero spread must be used as outlined above. Segregation does allow positive cattle to be productive and culled by attrition over time. When segregation is enforced, the seronegative herd may remain seronegative. Elimination of PL cattle and lymphosarcoma patients should be performed as quickly as possible!

When neither test-and-slaughter nor test-and-segregate is feasible because of economic or management factors, control through testing and corrective management procedures may be the only alternative. Corrective practices to reduce horizontal or vertical spread, as outlined above, may reduce the prevalence of BLV infection. Separation of young stock and adult cows may decrease prevalence when combined with corrective management techniques. Most programs devised to institute corrective measures can reduce but not eliminate BLV infection. Unfortunately the best technique for eradication remains test-and-slaughter, a program which seldom will be selected by owners of herds with a high prevalence or herds containing seropositive cows deemed of high genetic and productive value.

Experimental vaccines have been used against BLV. Inactivated virus, virus components, and lymphoblastoid cell lines from calves with lymphosarcoma have been used to instigate resistance to BLV challenge. Results have been variable and reflect experimental design, antigenic dose of vaccine, and challenge variables. Successful vaccines would require that vaccinates produce specific antibodies that could be differentiated from those antibodies produced by BLV-seropositive infected cattle. Therefore, for example, if vaccine incorporated only gp 51, diagnostic tests to detect infection would need to detect p24 or other antigens to differentiate seropositive vaccinates from infected cows. Alternatively, diagnostic tests would require identification of virus DNA from infected cattle by PCR. Infected cattle to be used as embryo donors should have embryos collected without cell contamination and implanted only in noninfected recipients, and recipients should ideally be maintained in a seronegative herd.

BOVINE IMMUNODEFICIENCY VIRUS

Etiology

Bovine immunodeficiency virus (BIV) is a lentivirus infection of cattle with a worldwide distribution. Serologic and molecular evidence of BIV infection exists in several regions including the United States, Canada, and Europe. There appears to be great variation regionally and even within herds with respect to the prevalence of infection, but with the advent of more sensitive diagnostic PCR techniques for the identification of proviral BIV sequences, it is evident that some herds may have infection rates of greater than 50%. Previous serologic surveys have only identified seroprevalence rates of between 1% and 6% in Europe and North America. It appears that infection rates are higher in dairy herds compared with beef cattle. The exact mode of transmission for BIV is uncertain, but it is probable that horizontal transmission in body fluids such as blood, milk, semen, and colostrum represents the major means of spread and that very similar risk factors would apply for the transmission of BIV as exist for the transmission of BLV. Natural transplacental infection is possible, and proviral DNA of BIV has been found in frozen-thawed semen.

Clinical Signs

The clinical relevance of BIV infection is uncertain. Although the virus was first discovered approximately 30 years ago, there have been no compelling experimental studies or reports of naturally occurring disease describing consistent signs in infected cattle. Lymphocytosis and lymphadenopathy have been documented following experimental infection, but the health consequences of BIV infection are not clear. Furthermore, the economic implications of BIV infection are similarly debatable, although trends toward lower milk production and higher incidences of other common diseases are reported in high seroprevalence herds.

Diagnosis

Diagnosis of BIV infection requires either serologic confirmation of an antibody response to the virus by either an immunofluorescent antibody (IFA) or Western blot assay or PCR amplification of proviral DNA sequences. The latter is much more sensitive but not commonly available commercially.

Treatment

Because of its questionable relevance clinically, there are no specific treatment or control measures commonly used for the prevention and/or eradication of BIV infection. In herds where diagnostic testing has demonstrated a high prevalence of infection, similar control measures as adopted for BLV may be instituted.

LYME DISEASE

Etiology

Lyme disease or Lyme borreliosis is an infectious disease of humans and animals caused by *Borrelia burgdorferi*, a spirochete. The disease is common in humans and dogs in Connecticut and other eastern areas of the United States, the Midwest, Texas, and California. Lyme disease is spread by ticks, especially deer ticks *Ixodes dammini* in the east and *Ixodes pacificus* in the west. These ticks have a complicated 2-year life cycle that involves three hosts. Adult ticks feed on vertebrate hosts during warm weather and overwinter in the ground. Adult females lay eggs in the spring, and larvae hatch from these eggs 1 month later. Larvae usually feed once and then become dormant through fall and winter before emerging the following spring as nymphs. Larvae and nymphs commonly feed on white-footed mice from which they obtain *B. burgdorferi*. Nymphs mature to adults and attach to hosts during the warm months. Although deer are the usual hosts for adult ticks, people and domestic animals may provide suitable alternatives and can therefore be infected with *B. burgdorferi* carried from the white-footed mouse to the new host by nymph or adult ticks. Nymphs of these ticks are extremely small (1 to 2 mm) and may be difficult to observe on hosts; bites may go undetected. At least one study has demonstrated significant numbers of adult ticks in pastures with heifers and dry cows, suggesting fairly high risk for exposure, whereas farmhouse yards and forage croplands appear to represent negligible risk.

Once infection occurs, several possible consequences may develop. Subclinical infections with seroconversion are common, and it is likely that only a small percentage of infected animals develop detectable clinical signs. The mechanisms that determine whether infection will produce clinical consequences are poorly understood. In most species, fever, skin rashes (early signs), lameness, neurologic signs, and visceral infections indicate a septicemic spread of the organism following an initial skin infection. A delayed inflammatory response may occur at the site of the original tick bite, and *B. burgdorferi* apparently causes delayed hypersensitivity reactions, immune complexing, and other immunologic factors involved in manifestations of disease in several anatomic areas. Therefore acute local and septicemic consequences can evolve into delayed immunologically triggered pathology. The acute infection may be mild, inapparent, or misdiagnosed, unless a characteristic skin rash is present. Because many infections apparently do not result in clinical disease, diagnostic tests that determine antibody levels are of limited value. In cattle, the organism has been found in blood and urine. Urine may provide a means of transmission because it appears some infected cattle shed *B. burgdorferi* in urine for prolonged times.

Clinical Signs

The clinical consequences of *B. burgdorferi* infection in cattle have not been well described, and there is no proof that Lyme disease exists in cattle! Clinical signs that have been observed in association with *Borrelia* seroconversion include fever, lameness, stiffness, joint distention in one or more joints, swollen lower limbs, and abortions. Cows in a district of Switzerland known to harbor ixodid ticks had *B. burgdorferi* detected in synovial fluid and milk, and signs in these animals included erythematous lesions on the hairless skin of the udder, poor general condition with a poor appetite and decreased milk production, and a stiff gait and swollen joints.

Lower limb swelling, distended joints with mononuclear cell inflammation, and other musculoskeletal consequences result in lameness, reluctance to rise or move, and secondary injuries, decubital sores, and joint distention. Therefore especially when first-calf heifers are affected with these signs, laminitis, "concrete disease" resulting from poor heifer adaptation to confinement, infection with *E. wenyonii*, and vitamin E/selenium deficiency should be ruled out before any consideration is given to Lyme disease! A study from Minnesota and Wisconsin associated high antibodies against *B. burgdorferi* with lameness in dairy cattle. Abortion appears to be either a sporadic or endemic consequence of *B. burgdorferi* infection in cattle. In one group of cattle being studied

because of persistent urinary shedding of *B. burgdorferi*, 3 of 12 subsequently aborted.

The organism may be found in milk from some infected cattle but is killed by pasteurization.

Diagnosis

Absolute diagnosis of *B. burgdorferi* infection requires a combination of clinical signs, serologic testing or identification of the agent, and judgment. Because serum antibodies do not necessarily indicate disease and may persist for long periods or even for life, diagnosis based only on serology should be avoided. At present, Western blot tests that apply suspect serum to an electrophoresis of *B. burgdorferi* proteins appear to be the most specific diagnostic tests performed in serum from clinical suspects.

When *B. burgdorferi* is considered as the cause of illness in cattle, a specialized diagnostic laboratory capable of isolation techniques and Western blot analysis of serum should be contacted for help. The incidence and prevalence of disease caused by *B. burgdorferi* in cattle are unknown. Some reports demonstrate fairly high exposure levels based on serology, but the occurrence of clinical disease is much less frequent.

Treatment

Because the disease is poorly defined, treatment is impossible to evaluate. In most species, tetracycline and penicillin are used to treat Lyme disease. Whereas antibiotics may or may not successfully clear infection, their role in counteracting immunologically mediated consequences of infection is less apparent. Tick control may be valuable for cattle in endemic regions of Lyme disease.

SARCOCYSTOSIS

Etiology

Infection of ruminant skeletal or cardiac muscle tissue by *Sarcocystis* spp. is extremely common, and although lesions may be present to some degree in up to 75% of cattle, most infections only can be detected histologically rather than grossly. However, sarcocystosis is very much a "dose-related" disease, with lower infective doses causing inapparent infection and massive doses causing acute fulminant disease characterized by anemia, anorexia, fever, neurologic signs, lameness, loss of tail switch (rat tail), or abortion.

Cattle are the secondary host for three major species: *Sarcocystis cruzi, Sarcocystis hominis,* and *Sarcocystis hirsuta,* whose definitive hosts are the dog, primates, and the cat, respectively. Definitive hosts are infected by eating contaminated tissue of cattle harboring the sporozoan. Ingested encysted sporozoites become bradyzoites, undergo sexual reproduction, form oocysts in the gut lamina propria, and oocysts evolve to sporocysts containing sporozoites. Sporulated oocysts are shed for weeks to months by the definitive host, and infection does not preclude reinfection. Cattle are infected by ingestion of feed contaminated by feces containing oocysts from a definitive host. Sporozoites are released in the abomasum and invade capillaries. Merozoites and schizonts remain in blood vessels (usually endothelial cells); more merozoites are produced and spread through the bloodstream to muscle and other organs. This life cycle is extremely complex, and further reproductive cycles may be involved. In any event, eventually *Sarcocystis* cysts are formed in muscle.

Cattle of all ages are susceptible, but infection tends to be more severe in calves or previously naive adult cattle suddenly exposed to great numbers of infective oocysts. Severely infected cattle suffer vasculitis and extravascular hemolysis leading to anemia. The hemolysis is likely immune mediated, and disseminated intravascular coagulation has been observed experimentally. Neurologic and reproductive consequences have been described but may require reevaluation and differentiation from *Neospora* spp. since the discovery of *Neospora caninum* (see Chapter 9) as a cause of abortion. Experimental infections with *Sarcocystis* spp. can cause abortion during the second trimester.

Clinical Signs

Clinical signs in cattle may appear approximately 1 to 3 months after ingestion of infective sporocysts. Experimental doses have consisted of 100,000 or more sporocysts. How frequently this level of infection occurs naturally is unknown. However, when clinical signs are observed, fever, anorexia, anemia, weight loss, lameness, lymphadenopathy, salivation, weakness, neurologic signs, and gastrointestinal abnormalities may be observed. Hair loss around the eyelids, neck, and tail switch (rat tail) has been observed. Anemia characterized as a hemolytic extravascular immune-mediated phenomenon may be life-threatening or fatal and associated with DIC and elevated indirect bilirubin levels. Abortion may occur, especially during the second trimester, and may reflect fetal infection or maternal stress.

Neurologic signs are associated with inflammatory lesions in the central nervous system, whereas weakness may reflect combined effects of myopathy and anemia.

Diagnosis

Although indirect hemagglutination, ELISA, and AGID tests are available for serologic testing of antibody levels against the parasite, these tests are largely limited to specialized laboratories. Early IgM antibody responses appear by 1 month following infection and peak at 3 to 4 months, whereas IgG increases by 6 weeks and peaks by 3 months.

Clinical signs may be very helpful in severe cases but obviously limited in subclinical or low-grade infections. Postmortem lesions in overwhelming acute infections consist of anemia, multifocal hemorrhages, lymphadenopathy, flaccid edematous striated muscle with alternating light and dark striations, myocardial hemorrhages and myopathy, and a pale liver. Histologically, inflammatory granulomatous encephalomyelitis, intravascular schizonts, or IM schizonts may be observed. Chronic infection may be detected by *Sarcocystis* cysts within striated or cardiac muscle. Frequently *Sarcocystis* cysts are found in striated muscle or cardiac muscle as incidental findings in cattle dying of other causes.

Treatment

Most references to treatment have resulted from experimental infections, and the efficacy or practicality of therapeutic intervention in field situations is unknown. Amprolium, monensin, and other ionophores may be somewhat effective for prophylaxis, but the effect of these drugs for treatment of infected cattle has not been determined.

Control

Breaking the life cycle of *Sarcocystis* spp. by prompt and complete removal of cattle carcasses and preventing definitive host feces from contaminating cattle feed appear to be the best means of control.

HEAT STROKE, HEAT STRESS

Although certainly not an infectious disease, heat stroke must be differentiated from infectious diseases because hyperthermia must be differentiated from true fever.

Etiology

High ambient temperatures and humidity predispose to heat stress and, in the most severe instances, heatstroke. The predominant dairy breeds in the United States originate from northern Europe, the British Isles, and western Europe and are well adapted to temperate climate. In the United States these animals tend to fare well in the northern states with cold winters and moderate summer temperatures. The effects of heat stress are profound on these animals that are well adapted to cold conditions. High relative humidity exacerbates the impact of ambient temperature, and therefore the potential for heat stress is more closely related to a temperature-humidity index than to environmental temperature alone. Heat stress may be a significant animal welfare challenge facing some dairy herds. The greatest heat stress problems occur in the humid southern and central states. Affected cows show increased core body temperature, altered respiration, abnormal gastrointestinal function, increased water loss, reduced feed intake, reduced and altered milk production, delivery of low birth weight calves, reduced reproductive performance, and other negative effects. The problem can also occur in northern areas of the country but generally is less common and less profound. The means to reduce the impact of heat on the cattle include modified shelters, fans that move large volumes of air around the cattle, water-spraying misters, and alterations in diet.

Cattle stressed by handling, shipment, recumbency, or confinement in poorly ventilated areas are prone to heat stroke. Cattle with preexisting respiratory diseases or pyrexia caused by other diseases also are at greater risk. Hypocalcemic cows and/or cows with hepatic lipidosis that lose thermoregulatory ability can suffer heat stroke if recumbent in poorly ventilated areas or in direct sunshine during periods of high ambient temperature and humidity. Dairy cattle that are not ventilated adequately or cooled during times of heat stress frequently have body temperatures of 103.5° F (39.72° C) or more, and minimal additional stress is necessary to increase body temperatures to 106.0° F (41.11° C) or more. Earlier than anticipated heat and humidity extremes during late spring or early summer may predispose to heat stroke in cattle and heifers that have not fully shed out winter coats and therefore have less efficient heat loss. Most heat loss in cattle occurs from the respiratory tract, and such heat loss may create a vicious cycle of progressive tachypnea, dyspnea, and ultimately pulmonary edema, which interferes with (rather than aiding) heat loss. Heat stroke is relatively common in adult dairy cattle and occasionally occurs in young stock or calves. Fatal DIC has been reported in a calf with exertional heat stress.

Clinical Signs and Diagnosis

Tachypnea (>60 breaths/min) coupled with a rectal temperature greater than 105.0° F (40.56° C) signals heat stroke. Most cows will begin to breathe with an open mouth, show salivation, and have an anxious expression. Tachycardia of 100 beats/min or more is common. Obvious pulmonary edema is apparent as frothy discharge at the mouth or nose in severe cases. Body temperature continues to increase, and prostration, weakness, and recumbency may develop at temperatures greater than 106.0° F (41.11° C). Neurologic damage is possible when temperatures reach or exceed 108.0° F (42.22° C).

Clinical signs of tachypnea, tachycardia, hyperthermia, and exertional dyspnea, pulmonary edema, and open-mouth breathing suffice for diagnosis, but associated or concurrent diseases also must be suspected, diagnosed, and treated. For example, cattle with septic mastitis, metritis, or pneumonia are already febrile and therefore are more prone to heat stroke. Hypocalcemic cattle that are recumbent in poorly ventilated areas or in direct sunshine require calcium therapy in addition to treatment of heat stroke. Handling or movement of cattle suffering from heat stroke can worsen the condition. Differential causes of extreme pyrexia should be ruled out as much as possible by a complete physical examination.

Treatment

All stress that involves treatment or movement should cease once heat stroke has been diagnosed. The animal should be cooled by hosing the entire body with cold water and placing the animal in front of a large fan whenever possible. Concurrent use of a fan facing the animal's head and cold water hosing is the best treatment. Alcohol soaks are not as efficient as cold water because it is impossible to find enough alcohol to adequately cool an adult cow. Cool water administered into the rumen via stomach tube and/or room temperature crystalloids administered IV may be helpful.

If pulmonary edema is suspected, 0.5 to 1.0 mg/kg furosemide should be administered systemically. Hypocalcemia should be treated, but great care is required when administering IV calcium because of preexisting tachycardia (often ≥120 beats/min) and the need for restraint of the patient. Excessive restraint must be avoided. NSAIDs and one dose of prednisolone sodium succinate may be helpful in advanced prostrate patients (those that are not pregnant). Concurrent inflammatory or metabolic diseases should be treated as soon as the patient is stable. Hypocalcemia is an exception to this rule because treatment of hypocalcemia is usually necessary before the animal is moved to an area where cold water is available.

Rectal temperature should be monitored until the temperature decreases below 104.0° F (40.0° C) and tachycardia and tachypnea resolve or become less severe. A strong fan should remain in place facing the animal's head. The more air that can be directed at the animal, the better.

Dr. Francis H. Fox of Cornell University has had repeated experience with heat stroke in show cattle confined to poorly ventilated stalls during periods of high temperature and humidity at state and county fairs held during the summer months. He recommends that blocks of ice be placed in feed pans in front of the cow's face and then a strong fan directed at the ice to blow cold air waves at the cow's face. Patients that have not shed out should have the hair coat completely clipped with cow clippers. The prognosis is good unless the cow is recumbent, is prostrate, develops disseminated intravascular coagulation, or cannot be moved to an area where water and fans are available. The prognosis may be poor in patients having a rectal temperature greater than 108.0° F (42.22° C).

SUGGESTED READINGS

Abt DA, Marshak RR, Kulp HW, et al: Studies on the relationship between lymphocytosis and bovine leukosis, *Bibl Haemat* 36: 527-536, 1970.

Aleman MR, Spier SJ: Corynebacterium pseudotuberculosis infection. In Smith BP, editor: *Large animal internal medicine*, St. Louis, 2002, Mosby.

Alt DP, Zuerner RL, Bolin CA: Evaluation of antibiotics for treatment of cattle infected with *Leptospira borgpetersenii* serovar hardjo, *J Am Vet Med Assoc* 219:636-639, 2001.

Animal and Plant Health Inspection Service: *Bovine tuberculosis eradication*, Washington, DC, 1989, United States Department of Agriculture.

Asahina M, Ishiguro N, Wu D, et al: The proto-oncogene c-myb is expressed in sporadic bovine lymphoma, but not in enzootic bovine leucosis, *J Vet Med Sci* 58:1169-1174, 1996.

Behymer DE, Biberstein EL, Riemann HP, et al: Q fever (*Coxiella burnetii*) investigations in dairy cattle: challenge of immunity after vaccination, *Am J Vet Res* 37:631-634, 1976.

Behymer D, Riemann HP: *Coxiella burnetii* infection (Q fever), *J Am Vet Med Assoc* 194:764-767, 1989.

Bielanski A, Simard C, Maxwell P, et al: Bovine immunodeficiency virus in relation to embryos fertilized in vitro, *Vet Res Commun* 25:663-673, 2001.

Bolin CA, Thiermann AB, Handsaker AL, et al: Effect of vaccination with a pentavalent leptospiral vaccine on *Leptospira interrogans* serovar hardjo type hardjo-bovis infection of pregnant cattle, *Am J Vet Res* 50:161-165, 1989.

Bolin CA, Alt DP: Use of a monovalent leptospiral vaccine to prevent renal colonization and urinary shedding in cattle exposed to *Leptospira borgpetersenii* serovar hardjo, *Am J Vet Res* 62:995-1000, 2001.

Brown RA, Blumerman S, Gay C, et al: Comparison of three different leptospiral vaccines for induction of a type 1 immune response to *Leptospira borgpetersenii* serovar Hardjo, *Vaccine* 21:4448-4458, 2003.

Burgess EC, Gendron-Fitzpatrick A, Wright WO: Arthritis and systemic disease caused by *Borrelia burgdorferi* infection in a cow, *J Am Vet Med Assoc* 191:1468-1469, 1987.

Burgess EC, Wachal MD, Cleven TD: *Borrelia burgdorferi* infection in dairy cows, rodents, and birds from four Wisconsin dairy farms, *Vet Microbiol* 35:61-77, 1993.

Burgess FC: *Borellia burgorferi* infection in Wisconsin USA horses and cows, *Ann N Y Acad Sci* 539:235-243, 1988, Benach JL, Bosler EM, editors [special issue published in conjunction with Lyme Disease and Related Disorders, International Conference held in New York, NY, September 14-16, 1987].

Burridge MJ, Thurmond MC, Miller JM, et al: Fall in antibody titer to bovine leukemia virus in the periparturient period, *Can J Comp Med* 46:270-271, 1982.

Burridge MJ, Thurmond MC: An overview of modes of transmission of bovine leukemia virus, *Proc US Anim Health Assoc* 85:165-169, 1981.

Catlin J, Sheehan E: Transmission of bovine brucellosis from dam to offspring, *J Am Vet Med Assoc* 188:867-869, 1986.

Cheville NF: Development, testing and commercialization of a new brucellosis vaccine for cattle, *Ann N Y Acad Sci* 916:147-153, 2000.

Cheville NF, Stevens MG, Jensen AE, et al: Immune responses and protection against infection and abortion in cattle experimentally vaccinated with mutant strains of *Brucella abortus*, *Am J Vet Res* 54:1591-1597, 1993.

Crawford RP, Huber JD, Sanders RB: Brucellosis in heifers weaned from seropositive dams, *J Am Vet Med Assoc* 189:547-549, 1986.

Daugschies A, Hintz J, Henning M, et al: Growth performance, meat quality and activities of glycolytic enzymes in the blood and muscle tissue of calves infected with Sarcocystis cruzi, *Vet Parasitol* 88:7-16, 2000.

Daugschies A, Rupp U, Rommel M: Blood clotting disorders during experimental sarcocystiosis in calves, *Int J Parasitol* 28:1187-1194, 1998.

DiGiacomo RF: Horizontal transmission of the bovine leukemia virus, *Vet Med* 87:263-271, 1992.

DiGiacomo RF: The epidemiology and control of bovine leukemia virus infection, *Vet Med* 87:248-257, 1992.

DiGiacomo RF: Vertical transmission of the bovine leukemia virus. *Vet Med* 87:258–262. 1992.

DiGiacomo RF, Hopkins SG, Darlington RI, et al: Control of bovine leukosis virus in a dairy herd by a change in dehorning, *Can J Vet Res* 51:542-544, 1987.

DiGiacomo RF, McGinnis LK, Studer E, et al: Failure of embryo transfer to transmit BLV in a dairy herd, *Vet Rec* 127:456, 1990.

Divers TJ: Transmission of bovine leukemia virus by rectal palpation—control and epidemiologic studies. In *Proceedings: American Association of Bovine Practitioners Conference*, 84-89, 1992.

Dubey JP, Fayer R: Sarcocystosis, toxoplasmosis, and cryptosporidiosis in cattle, *Vet Clin North Am (Food Anim Pract)* 2:293-298, 1986.

Dubey JP, Lindsay DS, Anderson ML, et al: Induced transplacental transmission of *Neospora caninum* in cattle, *J Am Vet Med Assoc* 201:709-713, 1992.

Ellis WA, O'Brien JJ, Cassells JA, et al: Excretion of *Leptospira interrogans* serovar hardjo following calving or abortion, *Res Vet Sci* 39:296-298, 1985.

Ellis WA, O'Brien JJ, Neill SD, et al: Bovine leptospirosis: serological findings in aborting cows, *Vet Rec* 110:178-180, 1982.

Enright JB, Sadler WW, Thomas RC: Thermal inactivation of *Coxiella burnetii* in milk pasteurization, *Public Health Monogr* 47:1-30, 1957.

Erwin BG: Experimental induction of bacillary hemoglobinuria in cattle, *Am J Vet Res* 38:1625-1627, 1977.

Essey MA: The TB challenges—how can we prevent a disastrous comeback? *Large Anim Vet* January/February:10-14, 1994.

Fayer R, Johnson AJ: Effect of amprolium on acute sarcocystosis in experimentally infected calves, *J Parasitol* 61:932-936, 1975.

Fayer R, Johnson AJ, Lunde M: Abortion and other signs of disease in cows experimentally infected with *Sarcocystis fusiformis* from dogs, *J Infect Dis* 134:624-628, 1976.

Ferrer JF, Marshak R, Abt DA, et al: Relationship between lymphosarcoma and persistent lymphocytosis in cattle: a review, *J Am Vet Med Assoc* 175:705-708, 1979.

Ferrer JF, Piper CE: Role of colostrum and milk in the natural transmission of the bovine leukemia virus, *Cancer Res* 41:4906-4909, 1981.

Fox FH, Roberts SJ: Recent experiences in the ambulatory clinic, *Cornell Vet* 39:249-260, 1949.

Frelier PF, Lewis RM: Hematologic and coagulation abnormalities in acute bovine sarcocystosis, *Am J Vet Res* 45:40-48, 1984.

Galloway DR, Baillie L: DNA vaccines against anthrax, *Expert Opin Biol Ther* 4:1661-1667, 2004.

Gasbarre LC, Suter P, Fayer R: Humoral and cellular immune responses in cattle and sheep inoculated with sarcocystis, *Am J Vet Res* 45:1592-1596, 1984.

Gerritsen MJ, Koopsman MJ, Dekker TC, et al: Effective treatment with dihydrostreptomycin of naturally infected cows shedding *Leptospira interrogans* serovar hardjo subtype hardjobovis, *Am J Vet Res* 55:339-343, 1994.

Goren MB: Phagocyte lysosomes: interactions with infectious agents, phagosomes, and experimental perturbations in function, *Annu Rev Microbiol* 31:507-533, 1977.

Grooms DL, Bolin CA: Diagnosis of fetal loss caused by bovine viral diarrhea virus and *Leptospira* spp, *Vet Clin North Am Food Anim Pract* 21:463-472, 2005.

Gunning RF, Jones JR, Jeffrey M, et al: Sarcocystis encephalomyelitis in cattle, *Vet Rec* 146:328, 2000.

Gupta P, Ferrer JF: Detection of bovine leukemia virus antigen in urine from naturally infected cattle, *Int J Cancer* 25:663-666, 1980.

Halling SM: Paradigm shifts in vaccine development: lessons learned about antigenicity, pathogenicity and virulence of Brucellae, *Vet Microbiol* 90:545-552, 2002.

Hatfield CE, Rebhun WC, Dill SG: Thymic lymphosarcoma in three heifers, *J Am Vet Med Assoc* 189:1598-1599, 1986.

Henry ET, Levine JF: Rectal transmission of bovine leukemia virus in cattle and sheep, *Am J Vet Res* 48:634-636, 1987.

Hirsh DC, MacLachlan NJ, Walker RL: *Veterinary microbiology*, ed 2, Oxford, 2004, Blackwell Publishing Ltd.

Hopkins SG, Evermann JF, DiGiacomo RF, et al: Experimental transmission of bovine leukosis virus by simulated rectal palpation, *Vet Rec* 122:389-391, 1988.

Huber NL, DiGiacomo RF, Evermann JF, et al: Bovine leukemia virus infection in a large Holstein herd: prospective comparison of production and reproductive performance in antibody-negative and antibody-positive cows, *Am J Vet Res* 42:1477-1481, 1981.

Ji B, Collins MT: Seroepidemiologic survey of Borrelia burgdorferi exposure of dairy cattle in Wisconsin, *Am J Vet Res* 55:1228-1231, 1994.

Johnson R, Kaneene JB: Bovine leukemia virus. Part I. Descriptive epidemiology, clinical manifestations, and diagnostic tests, *Compend Contin Educ Pract Vet* 13:315-327, 1991.

Johnson R, Kaneene JB: Bovine leukemia virus. Part II. Risk factors of transmission, *Compend Contin Educ Pract Vet* 13:681-691, 1991.

Johnson R, Kaneene JB: Bovine leukemia virus. Part III. Zoonotic potential, molecular epidemiology, and an animal model, *Compend Contin Educ Pract Vet* 13:1631-1640, 1991.

Johnson R, Kaneene JB: Bovine leukemia virus. Part IV. Economic impact and control measures, *Compend Contin Educ Pract Vet* 13:1727-1737, 1991.

Kabeya H, Ohashi K, Onuma M: Host immune responses in the course of bovine leukemia virus infection, *J Vet Med Sci* 63:703-708, 2001.

Kaja RW, Olson C: Non-infectivity of semen from bulls infected with bovine leukosis virus, *Theriogenology* 18:107-112, 1982.

Kim SG, Kim EH, Lafferty CJ, et al: Coxiella burnetii in bulk milk tank samples, United States, *Emerg Infect Dis* 11:619-621, 2005.

King JM: Clinical exposures: bovine splenic lymphosarcoma, *Vet Med* June:533, 1992.

Kuckleburg CJ, Chase CC, Nelson EA, et al: Detection of bovine leukemia virus in blood and milk by nested and real-time polymerase chain reactions, *J Vet Diagn Invest* 15:72-76, 2003.

Kuttler KL: Babesiosis. In Committee on Foreign Animal Diseases, editor: *Foreign animal diseases*, Richmond, VA, 1998, United States Animal Health Association.

Langston A, Ferdinand GA, Ruppanner R, et al: Comparison of production variables of bovine leukemia virus antibody-negative and antibody-positive cows in two California dairy herds, *Am J Vet Res* 39:1093-1099, 1978.

Lassauzet MLG, Thurmond MC, Walton RW: Lack of evidence of transmission of bovine leukemia virus by rectal palpation of dairy cows, *J Am Vet Med Assoc* 195:1732-1733, 1989.

Leonard FC, Quinn PJ, Ellis WA, et al: Duration of urinary excretion of leptospires by cattle naturally or experimentally infected with *Leptospira interrogans* serovar *hardjo*, *Vet Rec* 121:435-439, 1992.

Levy MG, Clabaugh G, Ristic M: Age resistance in bovine babesiosis: role of blood factors in resistant to *Babesia bovis*, *Infect Immun* 37:1127-1131, 1982.

Lewin HA, Bernoco D: Evidence for bovine lymphocyte antigen-linked resistance and susceptibility to subclinical progression of bovine leukaemia virus infection, *Anim Genet* 17:197-207, 1986.

Lincoln SD, Zaugg JL, Maas J: Bovine anaplasmosis: susceptibility of seronegative cows from an infected herd to experimental infection with *Anaplasma marginale*, *J Am Vet Med Assoc* 190:171-173, 1987.

Lischer CJ, Leutenegger CM, Braun U, et al: Diagnosis of Lyme disease in two cows by the detection of Borrelia burgdorferi DNA, *Vet Rec* 146:497-499, 2000.

Lopes CW, de Sa WF, Botelho GG: Lesions in cross-breed pregnant cows, experimentally infected with *Sarcocystis cruzi* (Hasselmann, 1923) Wenyon, 1926 (Apicomplexa: Sarcocytidae), *Rev Bras Parasitol Vet* 14:79-83, 2005.

Magnarelli LA, Bushmich SL, Sherman BA, et al: A comparison of serologic tests for the detection of serum antibodies to whole-cell and recombinant Borrelia burgdorferi antigens in cattle, *Can Vet J* 45:667-673, 2004.

Magonigle RA, Newby TJ: Response of cattle upon reexposure to *Anaplasma marginale* after elimination of chronic carrier infections, *Am J Vet Res* 45:695-697, 1984.

Magonigle RA, Simpson JE, Frank FW: Efficacy of a new oxytetracycline formulation against clinical anaplasmosis, *Am J Vet Res* 39:1407-1420, 1978.

Maurin M, Raoult DQ: Q fever, *Clin Microbiol Rev* 12:518-553, 1999.

McNab WB, Jacobs RM, Smith HE: A serological survey for bovine immunodeficiency-like virus in Ontario dairy cattle and associations between test results, production records and management practices, *Can J Vet Res* 58:36-41, 1994.

McQuiston JH, Childs JE: Q fever in humans and animals in the United States, *Vector Borne Zoonotic Dis* 2:179-191, 2002.

Meas S, Usui T, Ohashi K, et al: Vertical transmission of bovine leukemia virus and bovine immunodeficiency virus in dairy cattle herds, *Vet Microbiol* 84:275-282, 2002.

Monke DR: Noninfectivity of semen from bulls infected with bovine leukosis virus, *J Am Vet Med Assoc* 188:823-826, 1986.

Monke DR, Rohde RF, Hueston WD, et al: Estimation of the sensitivity and specificity of the agar gel immunodiffusion test for bovine leukemia virus 1296 cases 1982–1989, *J Am Vet Med Assoc* 200:2001-2004, 1992.

Moosawi M, Ardehaii M, Farzan A, et al: Isolation and identification of Clostridium strains from cattle malignant edema cases, *Arch Razi Institute* 50:65-70, 1999.

National Research Council: *Livestock disease eradication*, Washington, DC, 1994, National Research Council.

Newby TJ, Magonigle RA: Long-acting oxytetracycline injectable for the elimination of chronic bovine anaplasmosis under field conditions, *Agri-Practice* 4:5-7, 1983.

Nicoletti P: A short history of brucellosis, *Vet Microbiol* 90:5-9, 2002.

Nicoletti P: The epidemiology of bovine brucellosis, *Adv Vet Sci Comp Med* 24:69-98, 1980.

Nicoletti P, Milward FW, Hoffmann E, et al: Efficacy of long-acting oxytetracycline alone or combined with streptomycin in the treatment of bovine brucellosis, *J Am Vet Med Assoc* 187:493-495, 1985.

O'Brien DJ, Schmitt SM, Fitzgerald SD, et al: Managing the wildlife reservoir of *Mycobacterium bovis*: the Michigan, USA, experience, *Vet Microbiol* 112:313-323, 2006.

Onuma M, Hodatsu T, Yamamoto S, et al: Protection by vaccination against bovine leukemia virus infection in sheep, *Am J Vet Res* 45:1212-1215, 1984.

Onuma M, Aida Y, Okada K, et al: Usefulness of monoclonal antibodies for detection of enzootic bovine leukemia cells, *Jpn J Cancer Res* 76:959-966, 1985.

Orr KA, O'Reilly KL, Scholl DT: Estimation of sensitivity and specificity of two diagnostics tests for bovine immunodeficiency virus using Bayesian techniques, *Prev Vet Med* 61:79-89, 2003.

Ott SL, Johnson R, Wells SJ: Association between bovine-leukosis virus seroprevalence and herd-level productivity on US dairy farms, *Prev Vet Med* 61:249-262, 2003.

Palmer GH, Lincoln SD: Diseases associated with increased erythrocyte destruction—anaplasmosis. In Smith BP, editor: *Large animal internal medicine*, St. Louis, 2002, Mosby.

Palmer MV, Waters WR: Advances in bovine tuberculosis diagnosis and pathogenesis: what policy makers need to know, *Vet Microbiol* 112:181-190, 2006.

Parker JL, White KK: Lyme borreliosis in cattle and horses: a review of the literature, *Cornell Vet* 82:253-274, 1992.

Parma AE, Santisteban G, Margin RA: Analysis in in vivo assay of *Brucella abortus* agglutinating and non-agglutinating antibodies, *Vet Microbiol* 9:391-398, 1984.

Parodi AL, DaCosta B, Djilali S, et al: Preliminary report of familial thymic lymphosarcoma in Holstein calves, *Vet Rec* 125:350-352, 1989.

Pelzer KD, Sprecher DJ: Controlling BLV infection on dairy operations, *Vet Med* 88:275-281, 1993.

Piper CE, Ferrer JF, Abt DA, et al: Postnatal and prenatal transmission of the bovine leukemia virus under natural conditions, *J Natl Cancer Inst* 62:165-168, 1979.

Pollock JM, Rodgers JD, Welsh MD, et al: Pathogenesis of bovine tuberculosis: the role of experimental models of infection, *Vet Microbiol* 112:141-150, 2006.

Potgieter FT: Eperythrozoonosis, *Infect Dis Livestock* 1:573-580, 2004.

Quinn PJ, Markey BK, Carter ME, et al: *Veterinary microbiology and microbial disease*, Oxford, 2002, Blackwell Science Ltd.

Radostits OM, Gay CC, Blood DC, et al: *Veterinary medicine. A textbook of the diseases of cattle, sheep, pigs, goats and horses*, ed 10, London, 2007, WB Saunders Co Ltd.

Ragan VE: The Animal and Plant Health Inspection Service (APHIS) brucellosis eradication program in the United States, *Vet Microbiol* 90:11-18, 2002.

Ray WC, Brown RR, Stringfellow DA, et al: Bovine brucellosis: an investigation of latency in progeny of culture-positive cows, *J Am Vet Med Assoc* 192:182-186, 1988.

Rhodes JK, Pelzer KD, Johnson YJ: Economic implications of bovine leukemia virus infection in mid-Atlantic dairy herds, *J Am Vet Med Assoc* 223:346-352, 2003.

Rhodes JK, Pelzer KD, Johnson YJ, et al: Comparison of culling rates among dairy cows grouped on the basis of serologic status for bovine leukemia virus, *J Am Vet Med Assoc* 223:229-231, 2003.

Richtzenhain LJ, Cortez A, Heinemann MB, et al: A multiplex PCR for the detection of Brucella spp. and Leptospira spp. DNA from aborted bovine fetuses, *Vet Microbiol* 87:139-147, 2002.

Roberts DM, Carlyon JA, Theisen M, et al: The bdr gene families of the Lyme disease and relapsing fever spirochetes: potential influence on biology, pathogenesis, and evolution, *Emerg Infect Dis* 6:110-122, 2000.

Roby TO, Amerault TE, Mazzola V, et al: Immunity to bovine anaplasmosis after elimination of *Anaplasma marginale* infections with imidocarb, *Am J Vet Res* 35:993-995, 1974.

Roby TO, Mazzola V: Elimination of the carrier state of bovine anaplasmosis with imidocarb, *Am J Vet Res* 33:1931-1933, 1972.

Ruppanner R, Jessup DA, Ohishi I, et al: A strategy for control of bovine leukemia virus infection: test and corrective management, *Can Vet J* 24:192-195, 1983.

Schmidtmann ET, Schlater JL, Maupin GO, et al: Vegetational association of host-seeking adult blacklegged ticks, Ixodes scapularis Say (Acari: Ixodidae), on dairy farms in northwestern Wisconsin, *J Dairy Sci* 81:718-721, 1998.

Schmitt SM, O'Brien DJ, Bruning-Fann CS, et al: Bovine tuberculosis in Michigan wildlife and livestock, *Ann N Y Acad Sci* 969:262-268, 2002.

Schurig GG, Roop RM 2nd, Bagchi T, et al: Biological properties of RB51: a stable rough strain of *Brucella abortus*, *Vet Microbiol* 28:171-188, 1991.

Schurig GG, Sriranganathan N, Corbel MJ: Brucellosis vaccines: past, present and future, *Vet Microbiol* 90:479-496, 2002.

Schurr E, Malo D, Radzioch D, et al: Genetic control of innate resistance to mycobacterial infections, *Immunol Today* 12:A42-A45, 1991.

Shettigara PT, Samagh BS, Lobinowich EM: Control of bovine leukemia virus infection in dairy herds by agar gel immunodiffusion test and segregation of reactors, *Can J Vet Res* 53:108-110, 1989.

Smith CR, Corney BG, McGowan MR, et al: Amoxycillin as an alternative to dihydrostreptomycin sulphate for treating cattle infected with *Leptospira borgpetersenii* serovar hardjo, *Aust Vet J* 75:818-821, 1997.

Smith JA, Thrall MA, Smith JL, et al: *Eperythrozoon wenyonii* infection in dairy cattle, *J Am Vet Med Assoc* 196:1244-1250, 1990.

Snyder JH, Snyder SP: Bacillary hemoglobinuria. In Smith BP, editor: *Large animal internal medicine*, St. Louis, 2002, Mosby.

Stalheim HV, Fayer R, Hubbert WT: Update on bovine toxoplasmosis and sarcocystosis, with emphasis on their role in bovine abortions, *J Am Vet Med Assoc* 176:299-302, 1980.

Staples CR, Thatcher WW: Heat stress in dairy cattle. In Roginski H, Fuquay JW, Fox PF, editors: *Encyclopedia of dairy sciences*, Boston, 2003, Academic Press.

Surujballi O, Mallory M: An indirect enzyme linked immunosorbent assay for the detection of bovine antibodies to multiple Leptospira serovars, *Can J Vet Res* 68:1-6, 2004.

Sweeney R, Divers TJ, Ziemer E, et al: Intracranial lymphosarcoma in a Holstein bull, *J Am Vet Med Assoc* 189:555-556, 1986.

Tanner WB, Potter ME, Teclaw RF, et al: Public health aspects of anthrax vaccination of dairy cattle, *J Am Vet Med Assoc* 173:1465-1466, 1978.

Thurmond MC, Carter RL, Puhr DM, et al: An epidemiological study of natural in utero infection with bovine leukemia virus, *Can J Comp Med* 47:316-319, 1983.

Tripathy DN, Hanson LE, Mansfield ME, et al: Experimental infection of lactating goats with *Leptospira interrogans* serovars *pomona* and *hardjo*, *Am J Vet Res* 46:2512-2514, 1985.

Udall DH: *The practice of veterinary medicine*, ed 6, Ithaca, NY, 1954, Published by the author.

Uilenberg G, Thiaucourt F, Jongejan F: On molecular taxonomy: what is in a name? *Exp Appl Acarol* 32:301-312, 2004.

VanDerMaaten MJ, Miller JB, Schmerr MJ: Effect of colostral antibody on bovine leukemia virus infection of neonatal calves, *Am J Vet Res* 42:1498-5000, 1981.

Wagenaar J, Zuerner RL, Alt D, et al: Comparison of polymerase chain reaction assays with bacteriologic culture, immunofluorescence, and nucleic acid hybridization for detection of *Leptospira borgpetersenii* serovar hardjo in urine of cattle, *Am J Vet Res* 61:316-320, 2000.

Wells SJ, Trent AM, Robinson RA, et al: Association between clinical lameness and *Borrelia-burgdorferi* antibody in dairy cows, *Am J Vet Res* 54:398-405, 1993.

Williams BM: Clostridial myositis in cattle: bacteriology and gross pathology, *Vet Rec* 100:90-91, 1977.

Wojnarowicz C, Ngeleka M, Sawtell SS, et al: Saskatchewan: unusual winter outbreak of anthrax, *Can Vet J* 45:516-517, 2004.

Yaeger M, Holler LD: Bacterial causes of infertility and abortion. In Youngquist RS, editor: *Current therapy in large animal theriogenology*, Philadelphia, 1997, WB Saunders.

Yeruham I, Elad D, Friedman S, et al: *Corynebacterium pseudotuberculosis* infection in Israeli dairy cattle, *Epidemiol Infect* 131:947-955, 2003.

Yeruham I, Friedman S, Perl S, et al: A herd level analysis of a *Corynebacterium pseudotuberculosis* outbreak in a dairy cattle herd, *Vet Dermatol* 15:315-320, 2004.

Young DB, Mehlert A, Bal V, et al: Stress proteins and the immune response to mycobacteria antigens as virulence factors, *Antonie van Leeuwenhoek* 54:431-439, 1988.

Zaugg JL: Babesiosis. In Smith BP, editor: *Large animal internal medicine*, ed 3, St. Louis, 2002, Mosby.

16

Miscellaneous Toxicities and Deficiencies

Franklyn Garry

TABLE 16-1	Miscellaneous Toxicities and Deficiencies			
Agent	Usual Source	Signs	Diagnosis	Treatment
Blue-green algae (*Cyanobacteria*)	Farm ponds, midsummer to early autumn when warm sunny weather and wind combine to propel toxic algae to shore	Hepatotoxicosis Neurotoxicosis Bloody diarrhea Signs dependent on toxins produced by different species	Identification and culture of various toxic species	Activated charcoal, support, add $CuSO_4$ to pond water to attain a concentration of 0.2-0.4 ppm
Gossypol	Cottonseed, cottonseed meal	Cardiac failure caused by alterations in potassium levels (acute) or cardiomyopathy (chronic) Hemoglobinuria Reproductive failure Liver necrosis	History of feeding cottonseed or meal to young cattle, 100 ppm in diet support toxicity or adult cattle 1000-2000 ppm free gossypol in diet	Change diet, decrease amount fed in hot weather
Ammoniated forage toxicosis ("bovine bonkers")	Ammoniated feeds	Hyperexcitability, blinking, pupillary dilatation, altered vision, twitching, trembling, frothing, bellowing, charging	History of feeding ammoniated feeds Blood and rumen *ammonia levels normal;* toxic effects caused by pyrazines and imidazoles are implicated	Change diet Proper mixing Gradual adaptation to NPN sources Do not feed to cows that are nursing calves
Citrus pulp	Citrus pulp in total mixed ration has been associated with multiple deaths in dairy cattle. It is unknown why this occurs	Skin lesions, hemorrhage, heart failure, and systemic granulomatous disease that is similar to vetch poisoning (*Vicia*). Suggested type IV sensitivity.	Clinical signs and history of citrus pulp feeding	Citrus pulp is often fed with no problems, so there may be a specific toxin that occurs with specific but unknown conditions
*Other byproducts fed to cattle	Food oils, pretzels, and so on may sporadically cause acute or subacute toxicosis in cattle	Variable but may include ruminal atony, diarrhea, neurological signs, in addition to renal or hepatic failure in some cases	A specific toxin is usually not identified, and in many outbreaks similar byproducts have been fed without problems	Symptomatic

*www.wisc.edu/dysci/uwex/nutritn/Pubs/ByProducts/ByproductFeedStuffs.html

TABLE 16-1 Miscellaneous Toxicities and Deficiencies—cont'd

Agent	Usual Source	Signs	Diagnosis	Treatment
Nonprotein nitrogen (NPN)–induced ammonia toxicosis (urea toxicosis)	Urea, ammoniated feed, ammonium salts	Rapid onset (maybe sudden death) Colic, bloat, excitement, bellowing, neurologic signs, collapse, salivation	History of consumption Determine NPN in ration Rumen pH >8.0 (in live patients or very fresh postmortem) Blood or vitreous ammonia >1.0 mg/dl	Remove source Administer 2-6 L vinegar and 20-30 L cold water through stomach tube Do not feed more than one third of nitrogen in diet as NPN Do not feed more than 1% of total ration as urea unless animals' diet is gradually increased to higher levels
Monensin/lasalocid toxicity	Ionophores fed in excess or improperly mixed, especially in young calves! Simultaneous feeding of macrolide antibiotic increases risk of monensin toxicity	*Acute:* anorexia, pica, diarrhea, depression, dyspnea, central nervous system (CNS) signs (lasalocid), and acute death *Subacute/chronic:* heart failure, dyspnea, weakness, diarrhea	Hemorrhage and necrosis in cardiac and skeletal muscle Hydrothorax, ascites, edema, enlarged firm, bluish liver (may occur days to months after ingestion) Feed analysis	Supportive, parenteral selenium/vitamin E
Boron	Boron fertilizer	Neurologic: weak, depressed, fasciculations, seizures Diarrhea	Colorimetric assay on ashed tissue Minimum lethal dose 200-600 mg/kg	Supportive
Iron toxicosis	Hep/Hematinic preparations	Icterus, nervous signs	History of administration, increased liver enzymes	Supportive, blood removal
Iron deficiency	Total milk diet, chronic blood loss	Weakness, tachycardia, pallor	History, clinical signs, microcytic, microchromic nonregenerative anemia with HCT often <12%, serum iron extremely low, iron-binding capacity normal or high	Blood transfusion Parenteral iron
Zinc toxicosis	Milk replacer (veal calves) Contaminated water (adult cattle)	Pneumonia, exophthalmos, chemosis, diarrhea, anorexia, bloat, cardiac arrhythmia, convulsions, polyuria/polydipsia Constipation Reduced milk yield	Preruminant diets containing more than 100 μg/g Zn	Removal of source or add roughage to diet
Lead toxicosis	Old paints, batteries, drained motor oil, lead shot in feed	Cortical blindness, hyperesthesia, ataxia, tremors, seizures, grinding teeth, rumen atony, and occasionally diarrhea	Signs, possible exposure, look for oil in rumen sample, blood lead concentration >0.35 ppm Liver/kidney >10 ppm	Thiamine 1 g IV daily; CaEDTA 35 mg/kg IV every 12 hr for at least 3-5 days Rumenotomy Na or Mg sulphate orally

Continued

TABLE 16-1 Miscellaneous Toxicities and Deficiencies—cont'd

Agent	Usual Source	Signs	Diagnosis	Treatment
Fluoride poisoning (fluorosis)	Acute weed treatment and wood preservative Plants and soils downwind from manufacturing plants that process fluoride-containing substances	Acute—gastroenteritis, renal failure, and neurologic Chronic (typical)—lameness caused by exostoses and other bone lesions Dental abnormalities—excessive wear and discoloration	Acute—urine, tissue, and rumen contents >5500 ppm fluoride in compact bone >7000 ppm fluoride in cancellous bone	None
Nitrate and nitrite poisoning	Nitrate-accumulating plants—sorghum, Sudan grass, pigweed stems, cereal grains Fertilizer-contaminated water Nitrate converted to nitrite by rumen. Nitrite is usually toxic ion	Methemoglobinemia (brown blood) Dyspnea, weakness Abortion/infertility caused by fetal anoxia	Acute poisoning may be caused by forage nitrate levels >10,000 ppm or water nitrate levels >1500 ppm National Academy of Science cautions that drinking water should not have more than 440 mg nitrates/L or 33 mg nitrites/L Aqueous humor of eye levels >40 μg/ml nitrate confirms diagnosis (40 ppm) Field tests using 1% diphenylamine for plant or aqueous nitrate levels	1% Methylene blue solution 4-15 mg/kg IV; not approved in food animals. Tissue staining may occur for months postadministration Feeds should contain <0.6% nitrate
Petroleum hydrocarbons and crude oil	Contamination of water sources or accidental exposure	Enteric—bloat, regurgitation caused by vaporization and expansion of volatile hydrocarbons Pneumonia caused by aspiration of volatile products into the lungs or aspiration during eructation Neurologic signs possible	Confirmation of volatile hydrocarbons in gut contents, feces, or lungs Mix rumen contents with water and look for oil Submit rumen contents for confirmation	Rumenotomy and supportive therapy
Organophosphate toxicosis	Access or accidental exposure to organophosphate insecticides	Ingestion—signs within hours Dermal—signs may be delayed 1 to 7 days or more Signs vary depending on specific toxin and variable muscarinic or nicotinic effects Usually salivation, miosis, tremors, weakness, dyspnea, dehydration Diarrhea typical, but chlorpyrifos in bulls also causes profound rumen stasis	Reduced cholinesterase activity in blood, blood clots, brain, retina, and other tissues Samples should be delivered to lab chilled in less than 24 hr. Frozen samples may be acceptable for several days. Cholinesterase levels decreased over 50% from controls	Atropine: 0.25-0.50 mg/kg body weight. Repeat only if necessary Oral dose of 1-2 lb activated charcoal 2-PAM*: 20-50 mg/kg IM. Best given during first 24-48 hr For dermal exposure, gently wash with water and detergent

*Protopam chloride, Ayerst Labs, New York, NY.

TABLE 16-1   Miscellaneous Toxicities and Deficiencies—cont'd

Agent	Usual Source	Signs	Diagnosis	Treatment
Carbamate toxicosis	Access or accidental exposure to carbamates	Same as organophosphates	Same as organophosphates	Similar to organophosphates but 2-PAM not used for carbamate toxicosis
Organochlorine toxicosis or exposure	Residual or improperly discarded restricted products such as aldrin, methoxychlor, among others, most of which are currently illegal	Acute—seizures and other neurologic signs Residues—none or minimal signs but milk fat and meat contamination	History, signs, blood, or tissue residues Collect samples in glass or metal containers Toxic concentrations in adipose tissue (brain, liver, blood) vary with each product, but all lead to contaminated tissues or milk for months or years	Acute—supportive Residues—prolonged excretion; may try to enhance metabolic loss of drugs through various manipulations of pharmacokinetics Cull affected cattle
Anhydrous ammonia	Agricultural liquid fertilizer (often stolen for methamphetamine labs that can result in accidental spills near livestock facilities)	Sudden deaths, corneal ulceration, necrosis of the upper respiratory and bronchial mucosa	Detection of ammonia or history of anhydrous ammonia spill	Supportive
Mycotoxins				
Zearalenone (F-2)	Usually stored corn contaminated with *Fusarium* as a result of warm moist conditions followed by cold weather	Hyperestrogenism—premature udder development, swollen vulvas, prolapses, abortion, infertility	Feed analysis for zearalenone Usually ≥5 ppm to cause signs	Removal of contaminated feed
Trichothecenes (T-2) (DON, vomitoxin) (DAS)	Forages harvested late because of wet weather Corn, wheat, barley, and other grains	Feed refusal—most common! Necrotic oral mucosal lesions Coagulopathies possible Immunosuppression Reproductive failure	T-2 and DAS >10 ppm = toxic	Removal of contaminated feed
Slaframine (slobber factor)	Legumes (often red clover) contaminated with *Rhizoctonia leguminicola*	Salivation that increases over 24 hr followed by anorexia, frequent urination, diarrhea	Clinical signs and identification of specific fungus in forage	Removal of contaminated feed Atropine in severe cases (0.25 mg/kg)
Ergot	Grains contaminated with sclerotia of *Claviceps purpurea*	Dry gangrene of extremities, lameness	Diets containing 0.3-1.0% ergot	Removal of contaminated feed
Aflatoxins (B_1 most toxic)	Seed grains (especially corn) having too great a moisture content	Reduced productivity Hepatotoxicity (central lobular) Immunosuppression	Dietary concentrations ≥20 ppb Milk concentrations should be less than 0.5 ppb	Removal of contaminated feed

Continued

TABLE 16-1   Miscellaneous Toxicities and Deficiencies—cont'd

Agent	Usual Source	Signs	Diagnosis	Treatment
Fescue toxicosis ("summer syndrome")	Fescue grass contaminated with *Acremonium coenophialum*	Poor growth, salivation, dyspnea, nervousness, poor heat tolerance Reduced pregnancy rates	Endophyte identification in fescue Measure ergopeptide levels in fescue grass	Symptomatic Overseed with legumes and supplement with grain Use low endophyte seed varieties
Fescue foot (usually fall or winter)	Fescue grass contaminated with *A. coenophialum*	Lameness, sloughing of extremities Reduced weight gain	Endophyte identification in fescue Measure ergopeptide levels in fescue grass	Overseed with legumes and supplement with grain Use low endophyte seed varieties
Fescue fat necrosis	Fescue grass contaminated with *A. coenophialum*	Abdominal fat necrosis (often in Channel Island breeds)	Endophyte identification in fescue Measure ergopeptide levels in fescue grass	Overseed with non-fertilized legumes and supplement with grain Use low endophyte seed varieties
Tremorogenic toxins	Dallis grass infected with *Claviceps paspali* Bermuda grass (fall) tremors *Phalaris* spp. staggers Perennial ryegrass staggers— contaminated with *Acremonium loliae* Annual ryegrass (corynetoxins) Tremorogenic mycotoxins caused by various *Penicillium* and *Aspergillus* spp. Penitrem is one such toxin White snake root, rayless goldenrod, Jimmy fern, mountain laurel	Tremors accentuated by exercise, hyperexcitability, ataxia, hypermetria, tetany, collapse followed by relaxation White snake root excreted in milk, toxic to calves or people drinking milk from exposed cows	Identify plant and appropriate time of year	Remove from exposure
Iodine toxicosis	Excessive supplementation or therapeutic administration in diet	Respiratory tract disease Naso-ocular discharge Dry scaly coats Immune suppression Decreased production, growth, and fertility	Iodine intake far exceeding 12 mg/head/day Serum iodide or milk iodide ≥20 μg/dl	Maximum of 0.60 ppm in diet for adults Maximum of 0.25 ppm in diet for young stock

TABLE 16-1 Miscellaneous Toxicities and Deficiencies—cont'd

Agent	Usual Source	Signs	Diagnosis	Treatment
Arsenic toxico-sis	Wood preservatives Burn piles Outdated insecticides Rodenticides Herbicides Slag from previous mining Poultry and swine feed additives	Gastroenteritis and diarrhea (sometimes hemorrhagic) Some nervous signs Tooth grinding Possible renal lesions Skin necrosis if topical	>3 ppm arsenic (wet weight) in liver and kidney	Thioctic acid 20% solution 50 mg/kg IM thrice daily or sodium thiosulfate 30 g orally once daily for 4 days
Halogenated cyclic hydro-carbons (PCB, PBB) poison-ing	Residual environ-mental contamina-tion by com-pounds no longer produced or trans-former accidents	Wasting, skin lesions, hy-perkeratosis, immuno-suppression, reproduc-tive problems, liver and kidney lesions *Prolonged residues*	Tissue levels, milk levels as-sessed by qualified labora-tories. Fat deposition	None Culling may be required
Dicoumarol or coumarin toxicities	Rodenticides such as warfarin or second-generation antico-agulants such as brodifacoum Also moldy sweet clover hay or silage Sweet vernal hay (*Anthoxanthum*)	Bleeding caused by vita-min K antagonism lead-ing to decreased pro-duction of clotting factors in the liver. Re-sultant hypoprothrom-binemia and inability to convert prothrombin to thrombin occurs Hematomas, hemarthro-sis, gastrointestinal bleeding, epistaxis, bleeding from insect bites, ecchymoses, anemia, abortions, and so on	Signs Prolonged clotting time Prolonged prothrombin time—always Prolonged activated partial thromboplastin time—sometimes Platelets and FDP values normal	Vitamin K_1 0.5-2.5 mg/kg body weight IM or SQ several times (second-generation rodenti-cides may require therapy for weeks) Fresh whole blood transfusion, especially if life-threatening anemia is present
Bracken fern	Pasture or hay consumption of bracken	May be delayed after long-term ingestion (1-3 mo) Bleeding and aplastic anemia Enzootic hematuria and bladder neoplasms	Thrombocytopenia Leukopenia Anemia (nonregenerative) Hematuria and bladder masses	None practical other than avoid-ance and whole blood transfu-sions
Oak or acorn poisoning	Oak leaves or acorns Oak buds in spring and acorns in the fall	Anorexia, rumen stasis, hemorrhagic enteritis, subcutaneous edema, renal disease	Characteristic signs Laboratory confirmation of renal disease by testing se-rum and urine Necropsy findings of en-larged kidneys, perirenal edema and hemorrhage, gastrointestinal lesions, oak or acorns in rumen	Fluid therapy Rumenotomy
Oxalate poison-ing	*Rumex* sp. plants (sorrels and docks)	Renal failure, hypocalce-mia, often with hyperphosphatemia, hyperkalemia, and hypernatremia	Confirm renal disease with oxalate crystals Find plant in rumen	Fluid therapy Rumenotomy

Continued

TABLE 16-1   Miscellaneous Toxicities and Deficiencies—cont'd

Agent	Usual Source	Signs	Diagnosis	Treatment
Redroot pigweed poisoning	*Amaranthus retroflexus*—leafy portions of plants especially during drought conditions; A common source of nitrates and oxalates	Subcutaneous edema, hypoproteinemia, renal failure	Confirmation of renal failure and ingestion of plant	Fluid therapy; Rumenotomy
Cyanogenic plants	Sorghum, Sudan grass (usually fresh cut rather than stored forage), *Prunus* sp. trees, Johnson grass	Polypnea, anxiety, progressive weakness and dyspnea followed by death; Bright red color to venous blood	Confirmed exposure to cyanogenic plants and signs	0.5 g/kg body weight sodium thiosulfate as a 30-40% solution IV. Also administer orally
Yews (*Taxus*)	Discarded trimmings from shrubs or overgrown shrubs	Sudden death common or cardiac dysrhythmias and death several days later	History and finding plant in rumen	None
Pyrrolizidine alkaloid poisoning	*Senecio* sp., *Crotalaria* sp., *Heliotropium* sp., *Amsinckia* sp., *Cynoglossum officinale*	Hepatic failure, icterus, tenesmus, rectal prolapses, hepatic encephalopathy, gastrointestinal signs, photosensitization possible	History, signs, hepatic failure based on serum chemistry, typical histopathology findings in liver	Avoidance
Kochia scoparia poisoning	Pasture exposure	Photosensitization secondary to toxic hepatic damage; Polioencephalomalacia	History, signs, confirmation of hepatic disease by serum chemistry, biopsy, or necropsy	Avoidance
Cassia sp. (e.g., sicklepod, coffee senna)	Chopped forage containing high levels of plants or pasture exposure	Myopathy, weakness, recumbency, myoglobinuria	Elevated CK and AST; Myoglobinuria; Rule out selenium deficiency and exertional myopathy	Avoidance or removal of contaminating feed
Eupatorium rugosum, White snake root	Pasture plant in the northeastern states	Muscle tremors, weakness, ataxia caused by the effects of tremetone	Detection of the plant, signs of muscle tremors, myopathy	Remove source of tremetone
Cocklebur (*Xanthium* spp.)	Pastures containing two leafed seedlings toxic	Weakness, depression, dyspnea, neurologic signs including convulsions	History, typical gastrointestinal, hepatic, and renal lesions	Pasture management to control plant
Perilla mint (*Perilla frutescens*)	Cattle grazing forest land	Acute respiratory distress with expiratory grunt	History, clinical signs, ruling out infectious causes. Pulmonary edema and emphysema of lungs on autopsy	Remove from pasture, supportive (diuretics, antiinflammatories).
High tryptophan grasses	Introduced to new lush pasture 4-14 days before signs			Ionophores in feed may be preventive before exposure
4-Ipomeanol (moldy sweet potato)	Sweet potato infected with *Fusarium solani*			
Brassica spp. (turnips, rape, kale)	Pasturing on turnips or other *Brassica* spp.	Several possible syndromes, including: Polioencephalomalacia, acute bovine pulmonary emphysema and edema, bloat, hemolytic anemia	History, signs	Avoidance or limitation of access; Feed roughage

TABLE 16-1	Miscellaneous Toxicities and Deficiencies—cont'd			
Agent	**Usual Source**	**Signs**	**Diagnosis**	**Treatment**
Pentachloro-phenol (PCP or Penta)	Wood preservative	Local irritation (salivation, inflamed oral mucosa, skin lesions) Systemic absorption through skin and lungs may cause acute (neurologic) or chronic (wasting) signs Prolonged residues	Whole blood analysis for PCP	Do not use treated wood indoors
Larkspurs (*Delphinium* spp.)	Pastures	Curare-like neuromuscular blockade Dose-dependent signs of anxiety, excitability, stiffness, base-wide stance, collapse, bloat, vomiting, constipation Sudden death	History, signs	Physostigmine 0.08 mg/kg body weight IV *or* Neostigmine 0.01 to 0.02 mg/kg body weight IM
Oleander	Pasture, hay, or trimmings	Cardiotoxic glycosides Sudden death Cardiac arrhythmia	History, signs	Atropine for arrhythmias
Onion (*Allium* sp.)	Wild onions in spring pasture	Onion odor, hemoglobinuria	Exposure and Heinz bodies in red blood cells	Supportive, antioxidants; treatment often not required
Rye grass	Annual ryegrass pasture/hay	Hemoglobinuria or Staggers (Lolitrem toxicity)	Measure Lolitrem in hay	
Selenium poisoning	Selenium converter plants in selenium-rich soils (*Astragalus* spp.) and so on, causing dietary intake of 5-40 ppm Se Overdosage of selenium products	*Acute*—respiratory distress, heart failure, diarrhea, death *Chronic*—dullness, weight loss, lameness, poor hair coat, rat tail, deformed hooves "blind staggers"	Hair Se levels >5 ppm Blood Se levels >1.5 ppm	Remove from source Selenium deficiency is a bigger problem—see section on white muscle disease
Copper poisoning	Accidental ingestion—cattle may be poisoned by 200 or more mg/kg $CuSO_4$ Normal Cu + low Mb in diet Hepatotoxic plants (pyrrolizidine alkaloids) that cause excessive Cu retention in liver	*Acute*—severe gastrointestinal signs and death *Chronic*—methemoglobinemia, brown mucous membranes, anemia, dyspnea, hemoglobinuria Copper deficiency (see p. 649)	Elevated blood, liver, and kidney copper levels Normal blood Cu = 0.7 to 1.3 ppm—blood may not reflect body tissue levels!! Normal liver Cu = 30.0 to 140.0 ppm (wet weight) Normal kidney Cu ≤15.0 ppm (wet weight) Postmortem: blue-black kidneys, hemoglobinuria, icterus, enlarged liver	Remove source Reduce copper or add molybdenum to diet to reduce Cu/Mb ratio 3 g sodium molybdate and 5 g sodium thiosulfate can be added to diet/head/day for 2 weeks and then tapered

Continued

TABLE 16-1   Miscellaneous Toxicities and Deficiencies—cont'd

Agent	Usual Source	Signs	Diagnosis	Treatment
Sulfate poisoning	High sulphate-containing plants and/or water	Blindness, recumbency, seizures, death Subacute: visual impairment, ataxia, twitching of ears and facial muscles	Polioencephalomalacia High hydrogen sulfide levels in rumen gas. Rations exceeding 0.4% total sulfur on a dry matter basis. Note: Not all animals consuming greater than 0.4% sulfur are affected by clinical disease. Note: Considerable sulfur intake may occur from water and must be considered as part of sulfur calculated in ration.	Supportive Thiamine treatment Glucocorticoid therapy Removal of affected animals from high-sulfur sources and provision of low-sulfur rations
Molybdenum poisoning	Cu/Mb dietary ration <2:1 or dietary Mb >10 ppm	Chronic severe diarrhea, poor condition, anemia, lameness, and faded coat with depigmentation around the eyes—same as Cu deficiency Acute—kidney and liver necrosis	Cu = Mo dietary ratios Blood Mo >0.10 mg/kg	Reduce Mo or add Cu as 1-2% $CuSO_4$ to diet
Zinc deficiency	Forage from low zinc soils, especially if soil is alkaline and is fertilized heavily with nitrogen and phosphorus	Parakeratosis and alopecia of head, neck, tail head, and limb flexion sites Poor condition and growth Lameness	Serum zinc levels much lower than normal (80-120 μg/dl)	Add zinc to ration. Minimum daily requirement is 40 ppm (dry matter basis)
Magnesium poisoning Magnesium deficiency less common in dairy cattle than beef cattle—see metabolic diseases	Overzealous administration of Mg products, especially to dehydrated cattle	Weakness, recumbency, hypotension	History, clinical signs, azotemia, blood Mg usually >5 mg/dl	Calcium borogluconate slowly IV in crystalloids
Manganese deficiency	Forages from low Mn soils or alkaline soils with marginal Mn levels	Infertility, calves with congenital limb deformities and knuckling at fetlocks Poor growth and poor hair coats	Blood and tissue levels variable	40 ppm Mn in diet

TABLE 16-1   Miscellaneous Toxicities and Deficiencies—cont'd

Agent	Usual Source	Signs	Diagnosis	Treatment
Sodium chloride deficiency	Lack of supplementation or availability	Polyuria, polydipsia, pica, drinking urine, salt hunger, and loss of appetite, weight, and production	Salivary sodium normal = 140-150 mEq/L Deficient = 70-100 mEq/L	Salt fed at 0.5% of diet
Salt toxicity— (see chapter 12)	Most commonly from iatrogenic oral administration of abnormally concentrated electrolyte supplements to calves as treatment for diarrhea. Also may occur if calves are fed high salt milk replacers without free water access	Blind, seizure, coma	Plasma sodium > 160 mEq/L	Slowly correct the hypernatremia with sodium-containing fluids and administer thiamine
Iodine deficiency	Iodine-deficient soils High intake of calcium Diets high in *Brassica* spp.	Enlarged thyroid and weakness in newborn calves Stillbirths	Assess blood and forage for iodine	Lactating and dry cows 0.6-0.8 mg/kg dry weight feed Calves 0.1-0.3 mg/kg dry weight feed
Vitamin D_3 toxicosis and/or Overzealous and prolonged parenteral calcium administration	Large parenteral doses to cattle; most commonly young calves or periparturient cows. Jerseys seem more susceptible	Tachycardia, weakness, signs of heart failure	Hypercalcemia, calcification of heart, and greater vessels	Steroids, magnesium, diuresis, and supportive care
Copper deficiency	Primary—forage grown on deficient soils and diet not supplemented adequately Secondary—high molybdenum or low Cu/Mb ratio High zinc, iron, lead, or calcium carbonate Also inorganic sulfates potentiate effect of Mb on copper	*Calves*—Poor growth, rough hair coat, faded or bleached hair coat, diarrhea, musculoskeletal abnormalities *Adult*—Loss of condition and production, anemia, bleached rough hair coat, chronic diarrhea (usually in secondary Cu deficiency), falling disease (myocardial degeneration)	Pasture having <3 mg Cu/kg dry matter Blood and liver copper levels vary greatly and overlap occurs between deficient, marginal and normal values—therefore response to copper supplementation may provide clinical confirmation of suspected deficiencies Plasma copper: 19-57 µg/dl = marginal <19 µg/dl = low Supplementing mineral and salt content of diet to 3-5% copper sulfate Liver copper: >100 mg/dl dry weight = normal <30 mg/kg dry weight = low Clinical signs Dietary levels of Cu, Mb, sulfates, and so on	Oral $CuSO_4$: Calves = 4 g/day for 3-5 wk Cows = 8-10 g/day for 3-5 wk Diet should contain 10 mg copper/kg dry matter for prevention

Continued

TABLE 16-1 Miscellaneous Toxicities and Deficiencies—cont'd

Agent	Usual Source	Signs	Diagnosis	Treatment
Cobalt deficiency	Pastures or diets deficient in cobalt Cobalt deficiency impairs B_{12} production and prevents propionic acid metabolism	Progressive loss of appetite, weight, and production Anemia, weakness, pica	Liver B_{12} levels: normal >0.3 mg/kg liver Codeficient <0.1 mg/kg liver	To prevent: 0.11 mg cobalt/kg (dry matter basis) To treat: B_{12} injection IM, 1 mg cobalt orally, once daily

TABLE 16-2 Diagnostic Sample Submission for Suspected Toxicities

Alive	Dead
CBC	Aqueous humor, 2 ml
Chemistry	1 kg rumen contents:
Coagulation profile (blue tube)	frozen, check pH
Save EDTA and heparin samples separated from cells	100 g feces: frozen
Serum sample	Liver and kidney:
Special tubes for mineral analysis	100 g frozen and
Urine	another sample in
Feed: 1 refrigerated and 1 frozen in airtight container	formalin
Water sample: same as feed storage	Brain: frozen and formalin
Rumen contents and feces: 100 g leak-proof container and refrigerated	Fat (omental or abdominal): 100 g frozen
Suspect materials, e.g., pasture, chemicals	

SUGGESTED READINGS

Burrows GE, editor: Clinical toxicology, *Vet Clin North Am (Food Anim Pract)*, vol 5, Philadelphia, 1989, WB Saunders.

Committee on Minerals and Toxic Substances in Diets and Water for Animals, Board on Agriculture and Natural Resources, Division on Earth and Life Studies, National Research Council of the National Academies: *Mineral tolerance of animals*, Washington, DC, 2005, National Academy Press.

Gabor LJ, Downing GM: Monensin toxicity in preruminant dairy heifers, *Aust Vet J* 81:476-478, 2003.

Gonzalez M, Barkema HW, Keefe GP: Monensin toxicosis in a diary herd, *Can Vet J* 46:910-912, 2005.

Iizuka A, Haritani M, Shiono M, et al: An outbreak of systemic granulomatous disease in cows with high milk yields, *J Vet Med Sci* 67:693-699, 2005.

Kaur R, Sharma S, Rampal S: Effect of sub-chronic selenium toxicosis on lipid peroxidation, glutathione redox cycle and antioxidant enzymes in calves, *Vet Hum Toxicol* 45:190-192, 2003.

Knight AP: *A guide to plant poisoning of animals in North America*, Jackson, WY, 2001, Teton New Media.

Lopez-Alonso M, Crespo A, Miranda M, et al: Assessment of some blood parameters as potential markers of hepatic copper accumulation in cattle, *J Vet Diagn Invest* 18:71-75, 2006.

Osweiler GD: Physical and chemical diseases. In Howard JL, Smith RA, editors: *Current veterinary therapy 4: food animal practice*, ed 4, Philadelphia, 1999, WB Saunders.

Osweiler GD, Galey FD, editors: Toxicology, *Vet Clin North Am (Food Anim Pract)*, vol 16, Philadelphia, 2000, WB Saunders.

Radostits OM, Gay CC, Blood DC, et al: Veterinary medicine. *A textbook of the diseases of cattle, sheep, pigs, goats and horses*, eds 9 and 10, Philadelphia, 2000 and 2006, WB Saunders Co Ltd.

Santos JE, Villasenor M, Robinson PH, et al: Type of cottonseed and level of gossypol in diets of lactating dairy cows: plasma gossypol, health, and reproductive performance, *J Dairy Sci* 86:892-905, 2003.

Saunders GK, Blodgett DJ, Hutchins TA, et al: Suspected citrus pulp toxicosis in dairy cattle, *J Vet Diagn Invest* 12:269-271, 2000.

Subcommittee on Dairy Cattle Nutrition, Committee on Animal Nutrition, Board on Agriculture and Natural Resources, National Research Council of the National Academies: *Nutrient requirements of dairy cattle*, ed 7, Washington, DC, 2001, National Academy Press.

Velasquez-Pereira J, Risco CA, McDowell LR, et al: Long-term effects of feeding gossypol and vitamin E to dairy calves, *J Dairy Sci* 82:1240-1251, 1999.

Important Web Links and Phone Numbers for Dairy Practitioners

Food Animal Residue Avoidance Databank
FARAD expert-mediated assistance
Call 1-888-USFARAD
OR
E-mail farad@ncsu.edu
http://www.farad.org/
Activities have been suspended.

Milk and Dairy Beef Quality Assurance Center
http://www.dqacenter.org/

Center for Veterinary Medicine
7519 Standish Place
Rockville, MD 20855-0001
240-276-9300 or 1-888-INFO-FDA
http://www.fda.gov/cvm/default.html

CVM Counterterrorism Coordinator
Center for Veterinary Medicine
Office of Surveillance and Compliance—HFV-200
7519 Standish Place
Rockville, MD 20855-0001
240-453-6830
http://www.fda.gov/cvm/counterterror.htm

CDC List of Biological Agents and Diseases Posing Threats to Public Health
http://www.bt.cdc.gov/agent/agentlist.asp

USDA High Consequence Pathogen List
http://www.aphis.usda.gov/programs/ag_selectagent/
ag_bioterr_toxinslist.html

Selection of Disinfectants
http://www.cfsph.iastate.edu/BRM/disinfectants.htm

USDA Animal Health—Import/Export Health Requirements
http://www.aphis.usda.gov/animal_health/lab_info_
services/
Link for import and export requirements is:
http://www.aphis.usda.gov/import_export/index.shtml

USDA Office of Emergency Response
http://www.aphis.usda.gov/emergency_response/index.
shtml

USDA Center for Veterinary Biologics
http://www.aphis.usda.gov/animal_health/vet_biologics/
or http://www.aphis.usda.gov/vs/cvb/

APHIS-USDA Center for Veterinary Biologics—Adverse Event Reporting
http://www.aphis.usda.gov/vs/cvb/html/
adverseeventreport.html

National Center for Foreign Animal and Zoonotic Disease Defense
http://fazd.tamu.edu/

Foreign Animal Diseases
http://www.vet.uga.edu/vpp/gray_book02/index.php#

National Animal Health Laboratory Network
http://www.aphis.usda.gov/vs/nahln/html/
Laboratories.html

ASPCA Animal Poison Control Center
College of Veterinary Medicine
University of Illinois
888-426-4435 800-548-2423
http://www.aspca.org

Poisonous Plants
http://www.ansci.cornell.edu/plants/anispecies.html
http://cal.vet.upenn.edu/poison/index.html
http://texnat.tamu.edu/cmplants/toxic/livestock/cattle.
html

By-Products Fed to Dairy Cattle
www.ag.ndsu.edu/pubs/ansci/dairy/as1180w.htm
www.wisc.edu/dysci/uwex/nutritn/pubs/ByProducts/
ByproductFeedstuffs.html

Necropsy Findings
http://w3.vet.cornell.edu/nst/nst.asp?Fun=Asrch

Consultant
http://www.vet.cornell.edu/consultant/consult.asp

Other Suggested Web Pages:

World Organization for Animal Health (OIE)—General
http://www.oie.int

World Animal Health Information Database WAHID (OIE)
http://www.oie.int/wahid-prod/public.php?page=home

Food and Agriculture Organization (FAO)—Emergency Prevention System for Transboundary Animal and Plant Pests and Diseases (EMPRES)
http://www.fao.org/ag/againfo/programmes/en/empres/home.asp

USDA Foreign Agriculture Service, Dairy, Livestock and Poultry Division Bovine Spongiform Encephalopathy Information
http://www.fas.usda.gov/dlp/BSE/bse.html

Legends for Video Clips

Amy E. Yeager, Alexander de Lahunta, Simon F. Peek,
Norm Ducharme, and Thomas J. Divers

Video clip 1: A 5-year-old Holstein cow with cardiac lymphosarcoma demonstrating true jugular pulsation associated with right sided heart failure.

Note rapid "hosepipe" like filling of jugular from thoracic inlet to mandible with head held in neutral position. Persistent jugular distention is also evident, as is the arrhythmic nature of the pulse waves.

Video clip 2: A 10-year-old red and white Holstein with 1-week history of fever and decreased appetite.

Sonogram of the heart (first segment) of a 10-year-old female Holstein with pleuritis and pericarditis. A vector 4 to 1 MHz scan head is located at right 5th intercostal space. Caudoventral is to the left. The pericardium is thick (0.8 cm) and the pericardial sac contains fluid and fibrin (1.9 cm thick). Right ventricular wall and chamber are normal.

Diagnosis: Idiopathic pericarditis; inflammatory but not septic. The cow was treated with antibiotics systemically and dexamethasone in the pericardial space and recovered.

Video clip 3: A 9-month-old Holstein heifer was examined because of stertorous breathing since birth. The difficulty in breathing was accentuated by increased environmental temperature. The heifer was otherwise healthy.

Endoscopy findings: The initial part of the video shows the normally large nasopharyngeal septum, but in the distance a normal size opening to the nasopharynx cannot be seen. The larynx appears normal, but as the scope is withdrawn from the larynx or advanced toward the larynx, a collapse of the pharyngeal wall is noted. A diagnosis of functional pharyngeal collapse was made. The heifer's respiratory signs have remained unchanged, but she calved normally 1 year later. The owners report she is smaller than other 2 year olds on the farm and she moves slower than the other cows in the summer months.

Video clip 4: A 9-year-old Brown Swiss cow with a 2-week history of fever and coughing with sudden progression to respiratory distress with stridor.

Endoscopy findings: Evidence of arytenoid chondritis that nearly obstructs the airways. A tracheostomy was performed and, with local anesthetic, the necrotic arytenoid was grasped and removed. The cow was treated with ceftiofur, penicillin, and flunixin and was doing well at 6-month follow-up.

Diagnosis: Necrotic arytenoid chondritis

Video clip 5: A 2-year-old Holstein had been making an audible upper respiratory noise since shortly after birth. The noise had become louder over time and was beginning to cause some respiratory distress.

Endoscopy findings: A mass is observed on the right ventricle of the larynx. This mass was incised (last segment of the video) and thick mucus material was drained. A biopsy and histopathology of the wall of the mass suggested this was a branchial cyst. Following general anesthesia, the lining of the cyst was removed by laser surgery. The cow recovered and has remained normal without any respiratory noise.

Video clip 6: A 2-month-old Holstein bull calf with a 3-week history of progressive dyspnea and upper respiratory stridor.

Endoscopy findings: Swelling of arytenoid cartilages and exudates draining from the left arytenoid area. A tracheostomy was performed followed by surgical exploration under general anesthesia. The dorsal portion of the left arytenoid cartilage was necrotic and draining pus. The necrotic area was curetted (not shown in video) and the calf treated with penicillin. The diagnosis was necrotic laryngitis and the calf recovered.

Video clip 7: An adult Holstein cow with a 5-day history of upper respiratory stridor. There had been some transient improvement in the clinical signs following a combination of corticosteroid and antimicrobial therapy.

Endoscopy: (7a) An inflamed larynx with little movement of the arytenoid cartilages can be noted. A mass can be seen caudal and dorsal to the cartilages. Following a tracheostomy, the abscess and the diseased arytenoid cartilage were surgically removed. Three days later on recheck, endoscopy (7b) revealed significant improvement in laryngeal function. The cow was treated with penicillin for 2 weeks and received a single dose of dexamethasone immediately following surgery. The cow recovered and was healthy at a 6-month follow-up.

Diagnosis: Arcanobacterium pyogenes arytenoid abscess

Video clip 8: A 2-month-old Holstein heifer was examined because of a 1-month history of progressive respiratory distress with stridor. Tilmicosin, dexamethasone, and flunixin meglumine had been used as treatment, but had not been effective.

Endoscopy: There is evidence of laryngitis, severe edema of the trachea and larynx, and deformity of the right arytenoid cartilage. A tracheostomy was performed as an emergency procedure and surgery was recommended. The owners declined and the calf was euthanized.

Diagnosis (necropsy): Chronic necrosuppurative laryngitis, tracheitis, and pneumonia

Video clip 9: An 8-year-old Holstein with fevers and cough following calving 1 week earlier.

Sonogram video of the right side of the thorax of an 8-year-old female Holstein with pleuropneumonia. A vector 4 to 1 MHz scan head is used. Ventral is to the left side of the image. The pleural space contains large abscesses. These are the two compartments of fluid with waving tags of fibrin, 5 cm and 18 cm, with distinct 1 cm thick capsules. The lung is poorly visualized as the dorsal (right side of the image), triangular, hyperechoic structure at 5-10 cm depth. Lung is adhered to the pleural abscesses.

Diagnosis: Pleuropneumonia, pleural abscess. *A. pyogenes* and *Clostridium perfringens* cultured

Video clip 10: A 4-year-old Holstein with weight loss, decreased appetite, and abdominal distention.

Sonogram video (first segment) of the cranioventral abdomen of a 4-year-old female Holstein with lymphoma. A convex 5 to 2 MHz scan head is used and cranial is to the left side of the image. Viscera are viewed in the following order: first abomasum, then rumen, reticulum, liver, and again reticulum. The lymphoma is the peritoneal mass, 6.5 x 8 cm, hypoechoic, irregularly interdigitating with abnormally hyperechoic fat and blending with the wall of the reticulum and, to a lesser extent, the wall of the abomasum. The sonographic appearance of lymphoma may resemble abomasitis, reticulitis, and peritonitis. In this case, the diagnosis of lymphoma was confirmed by fine needle aspirate cytology.

Static sonogram demonstrates first the lymphoma and then the right side of the liver made with vector 4 to 1 MHz scan head. Ventral is to the left side of the image. In the liver is a 4 x 7 cm hypoechoic mass, most likely lymphoma.

Sonogram video (second segment) of normal left craniodorsal abdomen of a 4-year-old female Holstein. A vector 4 to 1 MHz scan head is placed dorsally in a caudal intercostal space and travels ventrally. Ventral is to the left side of the image. Seen first is a very hyperechoic interface oriented parallel to the body wall and casting reverberation artifact—the normal air-filled lung. Ventral to this is a triangular hyperechoic homogenous soft tissue structure, height about 13 cm, containing a vein in cross-section—the normal spleen. Ventral to the spleen is a curved very hyperechoic structure casting hypoechoic shadow—the lumen contents of the normal rumen. Note that the wall of the rumen is thin (about 1-2 mm) and difficult to detect. This sequence repeats twice.

Sonogram video (third segment) of normal small intestines of a 4-year-old female Holstein. A vector 4 to 1 MHz scan head is placed caudal to the costal arch on the right side. Ventral is to the left side of the image. The small intestines are the circular structures with normal motility. Intestine diameter is normal (2.2 to 4.0 cm), intestinal walls are normal (thin) and the lumen contains normal granular hyperechoic ingesta.

Diagnosis: Lymphoma

Video clip 11: A 6-year-old Holstein with fever, inappetence, decreased production, decreased rumination, and hunched posture since freshening 1 month earlier.

Sonogram video of right cranial dorsal abdomen showing normal viscera of a 6-year-old female Holstein with fever and hunched stance.

A vector 4 to 1 MHz scan head is used. The sonogram begins dorsally in the 11th intercostal space and travels ventrally. Ventral is to the left side of the image.

At the beginning of the study (first segment), air-filled right caudal lung lobe, anechoic pleural fluid (abnormal), and normal liver are shown. At times, in the lower left region of the image are aorta and caudal vena cava (1.5 cm diameter).

The scan head travels further ventrally (second segment) and is centered on the right kidney. In the center of the kidney are a few 1-2 cm, intensely hyperechoic foci that cast faint acoustic shadow. These are calculi. Otherwise, the kidney is normal with normal size (height and width are about 9 cm), lobulated contour, hypoechoic medulla clearly distinguished from cortex, and cortex about 1 cm thick.

The normal right adrenal gland (4.5 x 1.5 cm) is visible between the right kidney and caudal vena cava and aorta (third segment). Rumen is the deepest viscera in the image (16 cm deep). Ventral to right kidney is more liver (fourth segment). Ventrally between liver and rumen are portal vein, pancreas (3 cm thick), and lymph nodes (2 cm thick). The lymph nodes might be slightly large. When the probe is tipped cranially, the portal vein is larger (2.5 cm diameter). In many adult bovines, right adrenal gland, pancreas, and periportal lymph nodes are not visible. In this case, conditions were favorable for detecting smaller deeper viscera because the cow was thin, the bowel was small due to anorexia, and the cow was not pregnant.

Sonogram video (fifth segment) of right cranioventral abdomen showing focal peritonitis. A convex 5 to 3 MHz scan head is used. Medial is to the left side of the image. The abomasum is between the body wall and rumen. It is small (6 cm height) because the lumen is nearly empty. Its wall is normal with layer echogenicity, rugal folds, and about 0.5 cm thick between folds. In the peritoneal cavity lateral to the abomasum is focal peritonitis, a large (12 cm) irregularly margined region of compartmentalized peritoneal fluid.

Sonogram video (sixth segment) of left cranioventral abdomen showing a peritoneal abscess. A convex 5 to 3 MHz scan head is used. Cranial is to the left side of the image. The sonogram starts at a 12 cm abscess with hypoechoic fluid surrounded by a distinct capsule and a dorsal gas cap. Next, the scan head travels cranially to the normal reticulum (note the characteristic convex shape of the reticulum), returns to the abscess, and then travels caudally to abnormal hyperechoic fat near the abomasum and then more caudally to show the rumen and peritoneal (or omental) fluid and fibrin.

Diagnosis: Focal peritonitis from a perforated abomasal ulcer

Video clip 12: A 3-year-old Holstein with acute onset of anorexia and decreased production.

Sonogram video of a 3-year-old female Holstein with omental bursitis. The convex 5 to 3 MHz scan head is oriented in the transverse plane at the midabdomen. The video begins at ventral mid-line and progresses dorsally through the right side of the midabdomen.

The distended (8 cm) omental bursa is seen as a distinct fluid compartment located between the body wall and the peritoneal cavity. Deep to the omental bursa, the peritoneal cavity is seen to contain a triangle of anechoic fluid between the rumen ventrally and the small intestine dorsally.

The fluid within the omental bursa contains irregular webs of fibrin, in this case indicating inflammation.

Diagnosis: Peritonitis (omental bursitis)

Video clip 13: A 4-year-old Holstein fresh 5 weeks with intermittently poor appetite and decreased production for 10 days.

Sonogram video (first segment) and static image of the liver demonstrating 5 choleliths in a hepatic duct. The convex 5 to 2 MHz scan head is located at a right intercostal space. Ventral is to the left side of the image. The choleliths are the five < 1 cm, well margined, oval, very hyperechoic structures that cast acoustic shadow. These are located in a hepatic duct as evidenced by their linear distribution and location immediately adjacent and parallel to a portal vein. Normal rumen is deep to the liver.

Sonogram video of the liver at a right intercostal space using a vector 4 to 1 MHz scan head demonstrating that deeper portions of the liver contain multifocal choleliths (second segment). These are in hepatic ducts, which are the many hyperechoic branching linear structures parallel to portal veins.

Additionally, liver has abnormal increased attenuation of sound resulting in poor penetration and therefore poor visualization of the deepest portions of the liver. This is a typical but not exclusive finding of lipidosis.

Diagnosis: Hepatic lipidosis, cholelithiasis

Video clip 14: A 6-year-old Holstein with anorexia, lethargy, decreased production, and jaundice for 3 days.

Sonogram of the liver and gallbladder of a 6-year-old female Holstein with depression, anorexia, and jaundice. A convex 4 to 2 MHz scan head is used. Dorsal is to the left side of the image (first segment). Liver contains too many anechoic, branching, tubular structures, some of which are enlarged hepatic ducts. Normally, hepatic ducts are too small to easily detect. Gallbladder is also enlarged (13 cm diameter) (second segment). Extrahepatic bile duct obstruction was suspected.

Enlarged hepatic ducts (third segment) can be distinguished from enlarged hepatic veins because hepatic ducts are largest (in this case 4.5 cm) at the porta hepatis and enlarged hepatic ducts frequently have tortuous shape. Congested hepatic veins are largest near the caudal vena cava (not demonstrated in this study) and are typically not tortuous. Liver biopsy showed chronic cholangiohepatitis and liver sample was submitted.

Diagnosis: Cholangiohepatitis. *Fusobacterium necrophorum* and *Streptococcus* sp. group D were cultured from the liver biopsy.

Video clip 15: Normal udder ultrasound

Longitudinal sonogram of the normal left caudal quarter of the udder at the gland and teat sinus. These are patent and filled with hypoechoic milk. The gland cistern has normal full diameter (2.7 cm) and the lactiferous ducts are also full.

Video clip 16: Normal teat ultrasound

Transverse sonogram of normal left caudal teat beginning at the udder and moving distally to the teat sphincter. Distal is to the left side of the image. A linear 12 to 5 MHz probe is used. The teat sinus is patent and filled with hypoechoic milk. Note the ring of blood vessels around the teat sinus. The teat sphincter appears as a centrally located hyperechoic dot, 1 mm.

Video clip 17: A 2-year-old Holstein cow, recently fresh and minimal production from the right rear quarter

Transverse sonogram of right caudal teat beginning at the udder and moving to the teat sphincter (distal is to the left of the image). A linear 12 to 5 MHz probe is used. The proximal portion of the *teat cistern is obstructed by many soft tissue webs.* Distally, the teat sinus is patent, having normal diameter lumen (8 mm) containing hypoechoic fluid (milk). At the tip of the teat the sphincter is normal, appearing as a centrally located hyperechoic dot, 1 mm.

Video clip 18: A 2-year-old Holstein cow—difficult to milk out the right rear quarter

Longitudinal sonogram of the obstructed right caudal teat beginning at the teat sphincter and moving toward the udder. Distal is to the left of the image. A linear 12 to 5 MHz probe is used. The length of the teat is 3.6 cm. The teat sphincter is normal and appears as a 9 mm length x 1.5 mm thick hyperechoic stripe at the tip of the teat. The distal $1/3$ of the teat sinus has normal 9 mm wide lumen filled with hypoechoic fluid (milk). The proximal $2/3$ of *teat sinus is obstructed by many soft tissue webs.* These extend into the gland sinus.

Video clip 19: A 2-year-old Holstein, recently fresh but milk cannot be obtained from one quarter

Longitudinal sonogram of abnormal right caudal quarter at the gland cistern. (Distal is to the left of the image.) A convex 8 to 5 MHz probe is used.

The *teat and gland cistern are obstructed because the lumen contains many soft tissue webs.* The gland cistern is also small diameter (1.9 cm). Udder parenchyma is normal (hyperechoic background tissue) and lactiferous ducts are normal hypoechoic branching structures full of milk (1 cm lumen diameter).

Video clip 20: A 2½-month-old Holstein with poor growth and dribbling urine since birth.

Sonogram video of a 2½-month-old male Holstein with unilateral pyelonephritis. This is a transverse image of the right kidney made with a convex 5 to 3 MHz scan head. The kidney is large (10 cm diameter) because all of the calyces and the pelvis are enlarged (2-4 cm). These contain anechoic fluid and round hypoechoic material that could be caseated pus, necrotic debris, or blood clot. Renal cortex is very thin (< 5 mm). Right nephrectomy was performed.

Diagnosis: Pyelonephritis—suspect ectopic ureter

Video clip 21: A 5-year-old Holstein with decreased appetite and milk production and appearance of white crystals in the urine.

Sonogram (first segment) of the right kidney of a 5-year-old female Holstein with renal failure and calculi. A vector 4 to 1 MHz scan head is used. The center of the kidney contains many oval discrete hyperechoic structures that cast strong (dark) acoustic shadow. These are calculi with variable diameter as large as 2.7 cm. Also in the center of the kidney are five to ten, 2 cm anechoic fluid cavities. There are enlarged calyces and pelvis. The calculi are located dependently in these. Kidney shape (lobulated contour), size, and corticomedullary definition are normal.

Kidney size is normal (11 x 17 cm). Calyces and pelvis are enlarged probably because of obstruction of right ureter by calculi. Right ureter cannot be seen in the sonograms because it is obscured by the acoustic shadow from the renal calculi.

At necropsy, right renal parenchyma was atrophied and right ureter and pelvis were enlarged (8 cm wide) and contained hundreds of calculi (0.1 to 2 cm). The wall of the pelvis was thick and fibrotic.

Sonogram (second segment) of the left kidney of the same 5-year-old female Holstein with renal failure and calculi. A 4 to 1 MHz vector scan head is used. The left kidney is difficult to visualize, partly because it is so large (approximately 20 x 30 cm) that its margin extends beyond the equipment's maximum field of view (26.3 cm deep). The left kidney is also difficult to visualize because portions of the renal capsule are poorly defined and portions of the kidney have poor corticomedullary definition. Several 2 cm renal calculi and multiple fluid cavities, some as large as 2 cm diameter, are detected. Some of these are centrally located and are enlarged calyces or pelvis. Other fluid cavities are peripheral and it is uncertain whether these are parenchymal or capsular. These may be necrosis, abscess, or hematoma.

At necropsy, the renal capsule contained a large hematoma. Renal parenchyma had two infarcts (4 cm and 9 cm). Kidney was enlarged. Pelvis and ureter contained hundreds of calculi (0.1 to 2 cm).

Diagnosis: Chronic pyelonephritis—renal calculi

Video clip 22: A 2-year-old Holstein cow with a 1-week history of hematuria and progressive inappetence. The urinalysis had degenerative neutrophils and large numbers of bacteria.

Endoscopy: Endoscopy revealed an edematous and inflamed-appearing bladder with exudate and blood clots on the floor of the bladder. There is also an ulcerative lesion on the ventral bladder mucosa. A biopsy of this confirmed necrotic cystitis. The cow was treated with penicillin and improved, but long-term follow-up was not available.

Diagnosis: Necrotic cystitis caused by *Corynebacterium renale*

Video clip 23: An 11-year-old Holstein cow with a 6-month history of hematuria and stranguria. The cow was in good body condition and all other examination findings were normal.

Endoscopy: Endoscopy reveals a large proliferative mass on the ventral floor of the bladder. In the middle of the video, the apex of the bladder can be seen when the scope is retroflexed (causing the image to be upside down). The ureters can be seen traversing through the dorsal bladder wall and opening, with urine flow at the trigone.

Diagnosis: A biopsy confirmed a transitional cell carcinoma

Video clip 24: A 2½-month-old Holstein with poor growth

Static sonograms of a 2½-month-old female Holstein with an umbilical mass. The umbilical mass is displayed in longitudinal (first segment) and is cranial to the left side of the image and transverse (second segment) planes. The sector 5 to 3 MHz scan head is placed on the ventral aspect of the umbilical mass. The umbilical mass has findings typical of an abscess. It is a large (15 cm) single compartment containing echoic fluid and surrounded by a distinct capsule. Real-time, it has no motility. The abscess extends caudally in the peritoneal cavity and has a tubular shape, indicating involvement of urachus or umbilical artery. The peritoneal cavity is deep in the image, beginning at the calipers.

Sonogram video (third segment) of the umbilical abscess and the normal peritoneal cavity cranial to the abscess demonstrating that the abscess does not involve the abomasum. The convex 8 to 5 MHz scan head is oriented in the transverse plane and begins on the ventral aspect of the umbilical mass and proceeds cranially. The umbilical mass is an abscess with a thick capsule containing echoic fluid. When the scan head reaches the peritoneal cavity, the abscess is no longer detected and the image changes to show normal abomasum, which has a thin wall (1.2 mm) with layers, thin rugal folds, and normal ingesta that is of much greater echogenicity than the abscess fluid.

Sonogram video (fourth segment) of urachus or umbilical artery abscess demonstrating that the abscess contains gas. The convex 8 to 5 MHz scan head is oriented in the transverse plane in the caudoventral abdomen. The video begins at the apex of the urinary bladder, which contains anechoic urine and has a mildly thick wall (9 mm). The video proceeds caudally to show an 8 cm diameter abscess in the peritoneal cavity immediately cranial to the urinary bladder. In addition to the distinct thick capsule and echoic fluid, the abscess has a dorsal gas cap forming a straight, smooth, very echoic, linear interface that casts acoustic shadow at the deep edge of the fluid.

Sonogram of the urachus or umbilical artery abscess and urinary bladder in the longitudinal plane (cranial is to the left side of the image) using a convex 8 to 5 MHz scan head (static image—fifth segment). The capsule of the abscess is continuous with and distorts the cranial aspect of the urinary bladder.

Diagnosis: Urachal abscess (abscess umbilical artery)

Bovine Neurology Videos: Signalment and history (**H**) are given first followed by:
AD = Anatomic Diagnosis (neuroanatomical location of dysfunction)
CD = Clinical (or Pathologic) Diagnosis

Video clip 25: A 3-week-old Holstein calf
H: Abnormal gait since birth with no change in the signs.
AD: Cerebellum
CD: Necropsy diagnosis of cerebellar hypoplasia and atrophy. Presumptive in utero BVD viral infection.

Video clip 26: Three Holstein calves born from different cows on one farm in a 10-day period
H: All unable to stand since birth.
AD: Cerebellum
CD: Necropsy diagnosis of cerebellar hypoplasia and atrophy. Presumptive in utero BVD viral infection.

Video clip 27: Two Holstein calves—1 and 2 weeks old
H: Both unable to stand since birth.
AD: Cerebellum
CD: The first calf had no lesions at necropsy and is an example of a presumptive congenital functional cerebellar disorder. The second calf had lesions of a presumptive in utero BVD viral infection. There are no obvious clinical differences.

Video clip 28: A 4-day-old Holstein calf
H: Born unable to get up with diffuse tremors associated with any muscle activity. When recumbent and totally relaxed, the tremors disappear.
AD: Diffuse central nervous system (CNS)
CD: Necropsy diagnosis of hypomyelinogenesis. Presumptive in utero BVD viral infection.

Video clip 29: A 5-day-old Holstein calf
H: Since birth, action-related tremors have been present primarily in the pelvic limb and trunk muscles. When recumbent and totally relaxed, the tremors disappear.
AD: Diffuse CNS
Whole body tremors require a diffuse disturbance of CNS neurons or their myelin.
CD: Necropsy diagnosis of diffuse axonopathy most pronounced in the spinal cord. Presumptive inherited disorder.

Video clip 30: Two 2-day-old polled Hereford calves
H: Unable to stand since birth. Diffuse tremors are associated with any muscle activity. When recumbent and totally relaxed, the tremors disappear.
AD: Diffuse CNS
CD: Necropsy diagnosis of diffuse CNS edema ("cerebral edema"), a form of spongiform degeneration, which is an inherited autosomal recessive metabolic disorder of polled Herefords.

Video clip 31: A 4-week-old Angus calf
H: Two weeks of progressive depression and ataxia. Recumbent for three days.
AD: Cerebellum-pons-midbrain
Opisthotonus occurs with disorders of these anatomic sites.
CD: CSF contained elevated levels of protein and degenerate neutrophils. Necropsy diagnosis of suppurative meningitis.

Video clip 32: A 6-month-old Holstein calf
H: One week of depression, excessive recumbency, sialosis, and tongue protrusion.
AD: Cranial nerves II through XII, caudal brain stem for the mild ataxia/paresis (upper motor neuron/general proprioception [UMN/GP] systems)—more likely parenchymal lesion.
CD: Necropsy diagnosis of probable pituitary abscess that ruptured and extended caudally along the ventral surface of the brain stem.

Video clip 33: An 18-month-old Holstein
H: Depression progressing over 48 hours to obtundation and reluctance to move.
AD: Diencephalon

Based on the severe obtundation from interference with the ascending reticular activating system in an animal that is still able to walk.
CD: Necropsy diagnosis of a large focal pituitary abscess.

Video clip 34: A 3-year-old Holstein
H: Six days of intermittent circling to the right and inability to eat normally.
AD: Cranial nerves III through XII—left pons, medulla.
This cow had vision but could not close the eyelids due to the bilateral facial paralysis. The extensive cranial nerve dysfunction with the mild gait disorder suggested an extramedullary lesion, which turned out to be incorrect in this cow.
CD: Lumbosacral CSF contained 26 WBC/µl with 60% macrophages. Necropsy diagnosis of listeriosis with extensive involvement of cranial nerve nuclei.

Video clip 35: A 2-year-old Hereford
H: Ten days of progressive depression and dysphagia.
AD: Pons, medulla
CD: Necropsy diagnosis of listeriosis.

Video clip 36: A 5-year-old Holstein
H: Five days of progressive difficulty using the pelvic limbs associated with overflexed tarsi and buckled fetlocks. She was recumbent at hospitalization, unable to urinate, and on rectal exam had a large bladder. Loss of tail movement and anal reflex developed within the first 6 hours after hospital admission. She became quite agitated and acted in discomfort.
AD: Lumbosacrocaudal spinal cord segments or spinal nerves.
Unusual "stringhalt-like" flexor reflex action in the paretic pelvic limbs, which probably reflected disturbed inhibition in the lumbosacral grey matter.
Lumbosacral CSF contained 9 WBC/µl (lymphocytes and macrophages) and 97 mg protein/dl.
CD: Necropsy diagnosis of rabies viral myelitis.

Video clip 37: A 6-month-old Holstein calf
H: Acute onset of lethargy, loss of vision, and ataxia. Progressed to recumbency in 24 hours. Improved following therapy.
AD: Prosencephalon. Note depression and loss of vision but the ability to walk. The pupils were small and still reactive to light. The initial signs reflected a diffuse brain lesion that had recovered to just the prosencephalic signs seen on the videotape.
CD: Presumptive vitamin B–deficient polioencephalomalacia.

Video clip 38: A 6-month-old Holstein calf
H: Acute onset of lethargy, loss of vision, and ataxia. Became recumbent in 24 hours.
AD: Diffuse brain
CD: Necropsy diagnosis of a polioencephalomalacia. Presumptive thiamin deficiency, but beware of sulfur and lead toxicity that cause the same lesions.

Video clip 39a: A 2-month-old Holstein calf
H: One week of "swaying" gait and progressive depression with loss of vision.
AD: Cortical disorder

CD: Blood ammonia was > 600 μmol/L (normal <40). At necropsy, a portocaval shunt was found and a diffuse hepatic form of encephalomyelopathy. On rare occasion spinal cord signs without obvious cerebral signs have been observed in other calves with portosystemic shunts (see 39b).

Video clip 39b: A 2-month-old Holstein calf
H: One week of abnormal gait.
AD: C1 to C5 spinal cord segments—focal or diffuse.
CD: A discospondylitis or abscess was suspected. Radiographs were normal. At necropsy, a portocaval shunt was found and a diffuse hepatic form of encephalomyelopathy. No cerebral signs were reported or observed. Similar spinal cord signs have been observed in other calves with portosystemic shunts.

Video clip 40a: A 3-year-old Jersey
H: Two weeks postpartum, acute depression, decreased milk production, and abnormal behavior. Videotape shows the maniacal chewing, neck extension, and closed palpebral fissures all observed on hospital admission.
AD: Prosencephalon (limbic system)
CD: Strong elevation of urine ketones, decreased bicarbonate, and increased anion gap diagnosed as ketoacidosis. The clinical signs of nervous ketosis resolved with dextrose therapy.

Video clip 40b: An 18-month-old Holstein heifer
H: Escaped from barn 2 days earlier, now demonstrating blindness, hyperesthesia, and ataxia.
AD: Prosencephalon (limbic system) and diffuse brain
CD: Elevated blood lead concentrations (from licking old battery), and clinical signs are diagnostic for lead poisoning.

Video clip 41: A 2-week-old Holstein calf
H: Since birth, unable to stand and walk with the pelvic limbs.
AD: T3 to L3 spinal cord segments—focal or diffuse. The simultaneous use of the pelvic limbs, referred to as bunny hopping, is a very reliable sign of some form of myelodysplasia. This simultaneous activity is also observed on testing the flexor reflex. Spinal cord malformations are often accompanied by vertebral column malformations. The latter was palpated at L2 and L3 in this calf.
CD: Radiographs and CT images (see the video clip) diagnosed an L2, L3 malformation. The CT shows segmental spinal cord hypoplasia at this level. Necropsy diagnosis of thoracolumbar myelodysplasia with segmental hypoplasia of the L2 and L3 segments and sacral segment diplomyelia.

Video clip 42: A 2-day-old Simmental cross calf
H: Recumbent since birth.
AD: T10-T11 focal transverse lesion.
This was based on the paraplegia and the T13 line of analgesia. The simultaneous pelvic limb movements were all uninhibited reflex actions similar to spinal walking. There were no vertebrae palpated from T13 to L2.
CD: Myelodysplasia and vertebral malformation were confirmed at necropsy. There were no vertebral arches between T13 and L2 and there were no spinal cord segments from T13 through L3. There was myelodysplasia in the caudal thoracic segments and from L4 through the caudal segments. The extreme pelvic limb

hyperreflexia seen here was due to the complete absence of any brain stem inhibition of the lumbosacral grey matter.

Video clip 43: A 1-week-old Holstein calf
H: Abnormal use of the pelvic limbs since birth.
AD: T3 to L3 spinal cord segments—focal or diffuse.
The scoliosis indicates a vertebral malformation and the congenital simultaneous pelvic limb action indicates a myelodysplasia.
CD: Necropsy diagnosis of multiple thoracolumbar spinal cord segment myelodysplasia.

Video clip 44: A 1-month-old Holstein calf
H: Rapid progression of inability to stand and walk with the pelvic limbs.
AD: T3 to L3 spinal cord segments—focal or diffuse.
This is based on the spastic paresis (UMN dysfunction) and pelvic limb ataxia (GP dysfunction) with retained spinal reflexes and nociception.
CD: Radiographic diagnosis of discospondylitis at the T13-L1 articulation with a compression fracture of T13.

Video clip 45: A 1-year-old Holstein heifer
H: Found at pasture with an abnormal gait.
AD: Cranial thoracic spinal cord segments.
Spastic paraparesis and pelvic limb ataxia with LMN signs of short strides in the thoracic limbs suggest a C5-T2 spinal cord segment anatomic diagnosis, but note the strength shown by this heifer in her thoracic limbs when she stumbles and is able to get back up. This suggests that the UMN/GP lesion is in the cranial thoracic spinal cord segments and there is loss of thoracolumbar axial muscle function.
CD: Necropsy diagnosis of a fracture of T4 with displacement into the vertebral foramen. The cause of the fracture is unknown. There were no lesions of any vertebral body infection.

Video clip 46: A 5-month-old Holstein calf
H: One month of progressive abnormal gait in the left pelvic limb.
AD: Sciatic-tibial nerve / S1, S2 spinal cord segment—gamma efferent dysfunction.
CD: These signs of extreme hyperextension of the tarsus when attempts are made to protract the limb are typical of the functional disorder referred to as spastic paresis or "Elso heel." There are no microscopic lesions. The hyperactive gastrocnemius muscle activity is due to uninhibited gamma efferents in the sacral spinal cord segments. This is an inherited disorder in many breeds of cattle.

Video clip 47: A 3-month-old Hereford calf
H: Abnormal use of the right pelvic limb since birth with no change in the clinical signs.
AD: Right femoral nerve—L4-L5 spinal cord segments or spinal roots—nerves.
Note the inability to support weight when the right pelvic limb is protracted.
CD: Presumptive dystocia with overextension of the hip during calving and injury to the femoral nerve as it emerges from the iliopsoas muscle or avulsion of its nerve roots. At necropsy, the latter was found in this calf.

Video clip 48: A 3-day-old Holstein calf
H: Abnormal use of the pelvic limbs since birth.
AD: Bilateral femoral nerve—L4-L5 spinal cord segments or spinal roots—nerves.
The lack of pelvic limb support is most severe in the left pelvic limb. Note the intact nociception on the medial side of the left crus, which is innervated by the saphenous nerve, a branch of the femoral nerve. This suggests a better prognosis.
CD: Presumed femoral nerve injury secondary to a dystocia. This calf recovered in a few weeks.

Video clip 49: A 4-year-old Holstein
H: Two months of progressive gait abnormality in both pelvic limbs that began in the right pelvic limb.
AD: Bilateral tibial nerve—S1, S2 spinal cord segments—spinal nerves.
The latter is less likely with the normal tail, anus, and perineum. Note the overflexion of the tarsus typical of a tibial nerve dysfunction. The buckling dorsally of the fetlock is a unique sign of tibial nerve dysfunction seen only in cattle.
CD: On rectal exam, a bony defect was palpated on the ventral surface of the sacrum. At necropsy, there was a healed displaced fracture of S2 with fibrosis of the intervertebral foramina entrapping the S1 and S2 spinal nerves. The fracture was presumed to be due to this cow having been ridden by another cow or bull.

Video clip 50: A 2-year-old Holstein
H: Rapidly progressive abnormal gait in both pelvic limbs.
AD: Bilateral L6, sacral, and caudal nerves or spinal cord segments.
Compared to case in video clip 49, note the loss of tail tone and severe hypalgesia of the sacrocaudal dermatomes in this animal.
CD: Necropsy diagnosis of extensive L6-S1 discospondylitis, with suppurative inflammation involving multiple lumbosacral spinal nerves.

Video clip 51: Two Holstein calves—2 and 4 months old
H: Ten days of progressive ataxia, head tilt, and ear droop.
AD: Two-month-old calf—right cranial nerves VII and VIII
AD: Four-month-old calf—left cranial nerve VII, pons, and medulla.
Note the depression, the need for assistance to stand, and the neck extension.
CD: Two-month-old calf—radiographic diagnosis of otitis media-interna. This is a very common cause of facial nerve and/or vestibulocochlear nerve dysfunction in calves.
CD: Four-month-old calf—necropsy diagnosis of suppurative otitis media-interna, with meningitis and abscess formation in the left side of the pons and medulla.

Video clip 52: A 1-month-old Holstein calf
H: Bilateral ear droop developed over a few days.
AD: Bilateral facial nerve.
CD: Bilateral otitis media diagnosed on CT imaging.

Video clip 53: A 12-year-old Holstein
H: Two months prior to the videotaping, the farmer/owner of this cow treated her for "milk fever" with calcium gluconate presumably administered intravenously in the right external jugular vein. A large mass slowly developed at the injection site. The farmer noted that on cold mornings, there was less mist emerging from the cow's right naris during expiration.
AD: Right sympathetic innervation of the head. The right side of the muzzle is dry; the right ear is warmer than the left. There is a smaller right palpebral fissure. Miosis and third eyelid protrusion were minimal. Loss of vasoconstriction in the right nasal cavity would explain the decreased air flow and less mist seen on expiration on a cold morning.
CD: Presumptive dysfunction of the right cervical sympathetic trunk due to the granuloma on the right side of the neck caused by the extravascular injection of calcium gluconate.

Video clip 54: A 1-week-old Holstein calf
H: Since birth, this calf was inactive, walked with short strides, and preferred to remain recumbent.
AD: Diffuse neuromuscular
CD: The response to intravenous Tensilon suggests congenital myasthenia gravis. Over the next few weeks, this calf improved to normal. A delay in the development of normal neuromuscular receptors was presumed.

Video clip 55: A 1-month-old Holstein calf
H: This calf developed a stiff gait and became recumbent over a few days.
AD: Diffuse spinal cord ventral grey columns and brain stem nuclei. Note the typical facial expression with the ears held caudally and the tight lips.
CD: Tetanus due to infection with *Clostridium tetani*. This calf died from respiratory deficiency 2 days later.

Video clip 56: A 6-week-old polled Hereford calf
H: Since birth this calf has been recumbent, unable to stand, and exhibits extensor rigidity.
AD: Diffuse spinal cord ventral grey columns. The clinical signs observed are tetany, the prolonged extensor muscle activity when stimulated with mild relaxation between stimuli, and not attempting to move.
CD: This is hereditary tetany of polled Herefords caused by an autosomal recessive gene, which results in the abnormal formation of glycine receptors on motor neuronal cell membranes.

Index

Page numbers in italics refer to figures. Page numbers followed by "t" refer to tables.

Watch and Learn

with the Companion DVD!

You'll quickly master essential diagnostic, surgical, and treatment techniques for cattle when you watch the **Companion DVD** for *Rebhun's Diseases of Dairy Cattle, 2nd Edition*. Real-time videos guide you through key procedures and illustrate important concepts to help you effectively manage a wide range of bovine diseases and disorders.

COMPANION DVD

Rebhun's
DISEASES OF DAIRY CATTLE

SAUNDERS
ELSEVIER

WIN/MAC

Divers
Peek

Second Edition

9996026604

Copyright © 2007 by Saunders, an imprint of Elsevier Inc.
All rights reserved.
Produced in China.

The Companion DVD offers video presentations of:

- < Neurologic case studies
- < Ultrasound examinations
- < Endoscopic procedures
- < Cutting-edge imaging techniques
- < State-of-the-art equipment protocols

SEE the essential procedures and techniques presented in the book —

Start using the Companion DVD today!